Vascular Intervention
A Clinical Approach

Vascular Intervention
A Clinical Approach

Edited by

Bruce A. Perler, MD, FACS

Professor of Surgery
The Johns Hopkins University School of Medicine
Director of the Vascular Surgery Fellowship and
Vascular Noninvasive Laboratory
The Johns Hopkins Hospital
Baltimore, MD

Gary J. Becker, MD, FSCVIR, FACC, FACR

Medical Director
Interventional Radiology
Miami Cardiac and Vascular Institute
Baptist Hospital
Clinical Professor of Radiology
University of Miami School of Medicine
Miami, FL

1998

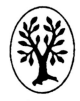

Thieme
New York * Stuttgart

Thieme Medical Publishers, Inc.
333 Seventh Avenue
New York, NY 10001

Vascular Intervention: A Clinical Approach
Bruce A. Perler, MD, FACS
Gary J. Becker, MD, FSCVIR, FACC, FACR

Library of Congress Cataloging-in-Publication Data
Vascular intervention : a clinical approach / Bruce A. Perler, Gary J. Becker, editors.
    p. cm.
    Includes bibliographical references and index.
    ISBN 0-86577-694-6 (hardcover). — ISBN 3-13-108041-8 (GTV :
hardcover)
    1. Blood-vessels—Diseases.   2. Blood-vessels—Surgery.
3. Arteries—Diseases.   4. Arteries—Surgery.   5. Cerebrovascular
disease.   I. Perler, Bruce A.   II. Becker, Gary J.
    [DNLM: 1. Vascular Diseases—therapy.   WG 500 V33185 1997]
RC691.V383   1997
616. 1′3—dc21
DNLM/DLC
for Library of Congress   97-30187
                                                  CIP

Important note: Medical knowledge is ever-changing. As new research and clinical experience broaden our knowledge, changes in treatment and drug therapy may be required. The authors and editors of the material herein have consulted sources believed to be reliable in their efforts to provide information that is complete and in accord with the standards accepted at the time of publication. However, in view of the possibility of human error by the authors, editors, or publisher of the work herein, or changes in medical knowledge, neither the authors, editors, publisher, nor any other party who has been involved in the preparation of this work, warrants that the information contained herein is in every respect accurate or complete, and they are not responsible for any errors or omissions or for the results obtained from use of such information. Readers are encouraged to confirm the information contained herein with other sources. For example, readers are advised to check the product information sheet included in the package of each drug they plan to administer to be certain that the information contained in this publication is accurate and that changes have not been made in the recommended dose or in the contraindications for administration. This recommendation is of particular importance in connection with new or infrequently used drugs.

Some of the product names, patents, and registered designs referred to in this book are in fact registered trademarks or proprietary names even though specific reference to this fact is not always made in the text. Therefore, the appearance of a name without designation as proprietary is not to be construed as a representation by the publisher that it is in the public domain.

Printed in the United States of America

5 4 3 2 1

TMP ISBN 0-86577-694-6
GTV ISBN 3-13-108041-8

To Mason and Rachel, the stars of my universe, the light of my life;
and to Patti, whose unconditional love shows me the way.

Bruce A. Perler, M.D.

To my parents, who have lovingly provided opportunity
To Allison, Aaron, and Samantha, who prove daily that I am blessed
To Pat, my loving and understanding partner in life

Gary J. Becker, M.D.

Contents

Acute Peripheral Arterial Occlusive Disease

Arterial Aneurysm Disease

Cerebrovascular Disease

Visceral Vascular Disease

Venous Disease

Contributors

EDITORS

Bruce A. Perler, MD, FACS
Professor of Surgery
The Johns Hopkins University School of
    Medicine
Director of the Vascular Surgery Fellowship and
    Vascular Noninvasive Laboratory
The Johns Hopkins Hospital
Baltimore, MD

Gary J. Becker, MD, FSCVIR, FACC, FACR
Medical Director
Interventional Radiology
Miami Cardiac and Vascular Institute
Baptist Hospital
Clinical Professor of Radiology
University of Miami School of Medicine
Miami, FL

CONTRIBUTORS

Samuel S. Ahn, MD (17)
Associate Clinical Professor of Surgery
UCLA School of Medicine
Los Angeles, CA

Cameron M. Akbari, MD (20)
Division of Vascular Surgery
Department of Surgery
Deaconess Hospital
Harvard Medical School
Boston, MA

Robert C. Allen, MD (25)
Division of Vascular Surgery
Department of Surgery
Stanford University Medical Center
Stanford, CA

John F. Angle, MD (56)
Department of Radiology
Division of Amgiography and Interventional
    Radiology
University of Virginia Health Sciences Center
Charlottesville, VA

Niren Angle, MD (65)
Senior Surgery Resident
Department of Surgery
UCSD Medical Center
San Diego, CA

Robert G. Atnip, MD (54)
Associate Professor of Surgery
Section of Vascular Surgery
The College of Medicine
The Pennsylvania State University
The Milton S. Hershey Medical Center
Hershey, PA

Curtis W. Bakal, MD, MPH, FSCVIR (16)
Chief, Vascular and Interventional Radiology
The University Hospital for the Albert Einstein
    College of Medicine
Montefiore Medical Center
Bronx, NY

Dennis F. Bandyk, MD (14)
Professor of Surgery
Director, Vascular Surgery Division
University South Florida College of Medicine
Tampa, FL

Robert W. Barnes, MD (66)
Professor and Chairman
Department of Surgery
University of Arkansas for Medical Sciences and
    the Surgical Services
Veterans Affairs Medical Center
Little Rock, AR

Stanley L. Barnwell, MD, PhD (51)
Associate Professor of Neurosurgery and
    Radiology
The Dotter Interventional Institute
Oregon Health Sciences University
Portland OR

Richard A. Baum, MD (4)
Department of Radiology
University of Pennsylvania Medical Center
Hospital of the University of Pennsylvania
Philadelphia, PA

Michael Belkin, MD (13)
Department of Surgery
Brigham and Women's Hospital
Harvard Medical School
Boston, MA

William R. Bell, MD (26)
Anne E. and Hubert E. Rogers Scholar
Edythe Harris Lucas-Clara Lucas Lynn Professor
Department of Medicine
Division of Hematology
The Johns Hopkins University School of
    Medicine
Baltimore, MD

James F. Benenati, MD (39)
Medical Director
Peripheral Vascular Laboratory
Interventional Radiologist
Miami Cardiac and Vascular Institute
Miami, FL

Marshall E. Benjamin, MD, RVT (3, 57)
Assistant Professor
Division of Vascular Surgery
University of Maryland Medical Center
Baltimore, MD

John J. Bergan, MD, FACS, FRCS(Eng) (65)
Professor of Surgery
Loma Linda University Medical Center
Loma Linda, CA
Professor of Surgery
University of California, San Diego
San Diego, CA

Henry D. Berkowitz MD (18)
Associate Professor of Surgery
University of Pennsylvania Medical School
Chief of Vascular Surgery
University of Pennsylvania Health System
Philadelphia, PA

Ramin Beygui, M.D. (25)

Joseph J. Bookstein, MD, FSCVIR (29)
Professor Emeritus
Research Professor of Radiology
University of California
San Diego, CA

David C. Brewster, MD (35)
Clinical Professor of Surgery
Massachusetts General Hospital
Harvard Medical School
Boston, MA

Richard P. Cambria, MD (46)
Associate Professor of Surgery
Harvard Medical School
Visiting Surgeon
Division of Vascular Surgery
Massachusetts General Hospital
Boston, MA

Elliot L. Chaikof, MD, PhD (8)
Assistant Professor of Surgery
Division of Vascular Surgery
Emory University School of Medicine
Atlanta, GA

Kenneth J. Cherry, MD (47)
Chairman, Division of Vascular Surgery
Professor of Surgery
Mayo Medical School
Mayo Clinic
Rochester, MN

Wayne M. Clark, MD (51)
Director of Organ Stroke Center
Associate Professor of Neurology
The Dotter Interventional Institute
Oregon Health Sciences University
Portland, OR

Michael D. Colburn, MD (45)
Vascular Surgery
UCLA School of Medicine
Los Angeles, CA

Anthony J. Comerota, MD, FACS (31)
Department of Surgery
Section of Vascular Surgery
Temple University Hospital
Philadelphia, PA

Blessie Concepcion, Bsc (17)
Section of Vascular Surgery
UCLA Center for the Health Sciences
Los Angeles, CA

P. Macke Consigny, PhD (1)
Departments of Radiology and Physiology
Thomas Jefferson University
Jefferson Medical College
Philadelphia, PA

Constantin Cope, MD, FACP, FSCVIR (4)
Department of Radiology
University of Pennsylvania Medical Center
Hospital of the University of Pennsylvania
Philadelphia, PA

Jack L. Cronenwett, MD (33)
Professor of Surgery
Dartmouth Medical School
Chief, Section of Vascular Surgery
Dartmouth-Hitchcock Medical Center
Lebanon, NH

Jacob Cynamon, MD, FSCVIR (16)
Associate Chief
Vascular and Interventional Radiology
Associate Professor of Radiology
Albert Einstein College of Medicine
Montefiore Medical Center
Bronx, NY

Michael Dake, MD (41, 42)
Assistant Professor of Radiology and Medicine
Chief, Cardiovascular and Interventional
    Radiology
Stanford University Medical Center
Stanford, CA

Richard H. Dean, MD (57)
Professor and Director of Division of Surgical
    Sciences
Department of General Surgery
The Bowman Gray School of Medicine
Winston-Salem, NC

Donald F. Denny, MD, FSCVIR (74)
Attending Physician
Department of Radiology
The Medical Center at Princeton
Princeton, NJ
Associate Clinical Professor of Radiology
Yale University School of Medicine
New Haven, CT

James A. DeWeese, MD (34)
Emeritus, Chief of Cardiothoracic and Vascular
    Surgery
University of Rochester School of Medicine and
    Dentistry
Rochester, NY

Edward B. Diethrich, MD (50)
Medical Director
Arizona Heart Institute
Chief of Cardiovascular Surgery
Arizona Heart Hospital
Phoenix, AZ

Paul DiMuzio, MD (55)
Assistant Professor of Surgery
Department of Surgery
Division of Vascular Surgery
Jefferson Medical College
Philadelphia, PA

Magruder C. Donaldson, MD (13)
Department of Surgery
Brigham and Women's Hospital
Harvard Medical School
Boston, MA

Gary S. Dorfman, MD, FSCVIR (70)
Professor of Diagnostic Imaging
Brown University School of Medicine
Department of Diagnostic Imaging
Rhode Island Hospital
Providence, RI

James M. Edwards, MD (23)
Division of Vascular Surgery
Oregon Health Sciences University
Portland, OR

Calvin B. Ernst, MD (36)
Clinical Professor of Surgery
University of Michigan Medical School
Ann Arbor, MI
Head, Division of Vascular Surgery
Henry Ford Hospital
Detroit, MI

James Farrell, MD (61)
The Johns Hopkins University School of
    Medicine
Baltimore, MD

J William R. Flinn, MD (3)
Chief and Professor
Division of Vascular Surgery
University of Maryland Medical Center
Baltimore, MD

John A. Flynn, MD (24)
Department of Medicine
The Johns Hopkins University School of
    Medicine
Baltimore, MD

Thomas J. Fogarty, MD (25)
Professor of Surgery
Department of Surgery
Stanford University Medical Center
Stanford, CA

Elizabeth A. Forsyth, MD (21)
Vascular Research Resident
VA Medical Center
Washington, DC

Bruce L. Gewertz, MD (53)
Dallas B. Phemister Professor and Chairman
Department of Surgery
University of Chicago
Chicago, IL

David L. Gillespie, MD (2)
Assistant Chief Vascular Surgery Service
Walter Reed Army Medical Center
Washington, DC
Assistant Professor of Surgery
Uniformed Services University of the Health
    Sciences
Bethesda, MD

Lazar J. Greenfield, MD (72)
Department of Surgery
University of Michigan
Ann Arbor, MI

Signe H. Haughton, BA, CCRC (71)
Medical College of Wisconsin
Milwaukee, WI

David B. Hellmann, MD (24)
Executive Vice Chairman
Mary Betty Stevens Professor of Medicine
Department of Medicine
The Johns Hopkins University School of
    Medicine
Baltimore, MD

H. Franklin Herlong, MD (61)
Associate Professor of Medicine
The Johns Hopkins University School of
    Medicine
Baltimore, MD

William R. Hiatt, MD (6)
Professor of Medicine
Section of Vascular Medicine
University of Colorado Health Sciences Center
Denver, CO

Timothy C. Hodges, MD (33)
Section of Vascular Surgery
Dartmouth-Hitchcock Medical Center
Lebanon, NH

David R. Holt, MD (62)
Surgical Director
Liver Transplantation
Inova Transplant Center
Falls Church, VA

Michael Horgan, MD (51)
Resident
Division of Neurosurgery
Oregon Health Sciences University
Portland, OR

Jeffrey M. Isner, MD (5)
Professor of Medicine and Pathology
Tufts University School of Medicine
Chief, Cardiovascular Research
St. Elizabeth's Medical Center
Boston, MA

Brad L. Johnson (14)
Assistant Professor
Vascular Surgery Division
College of Medicine
University of South Florida
Tampa, Florida

**Barry T. Katzen, MD, FACR, FACC, FSCVIR
(39)**
Medical Director
Miami Cardiac and Vascular Institute
Baptist Hospital
Clinical Professor of Radiology
University of Miami School of Medicine
Miami, FL

Richard R. Keen, MD (19)
Attending Surgeon
Department of Surgery
Division of Vascular Surgery
Cook County Hospital
Chicago, IL

Andrew S. Klein MD (62)
Associate Professor of Surgery
Director of Comprehensive Transplant Center
The Johns Hopkins University School of
    Medicine
Baltimore, MD

Robert A. Koenigsberg, DO (52)
Assistant Professor of Radiology
Director of Neuroradiology
Allegheny University - MCP
Philadelphia, PA

Katharine L. Krol, MD (48)
Vascular Radiology
Northwest Radiologists
Indianapolis, IN

Paul C. Lakin, MD (63, 73)
Associate Professor
Dotter Interventional Institute
Oregon Health Sciences University
Portland, OR

Sophie M. Lanzkron, MD (26)
Dotter Interventional Institute
Oregon Health Sciences University
Portland, OR

Timothy K. Liem, MD (27)
Department of Surgery
University of Missouri-Columbia
Columbia, MO

David A. Lipski, MD (36)
Fellow, Division of Vascular Surgery
Henry Ford Hospital
Detroit, MI

James D. Lutz, MD (15)
Clinical Assistant Professor
Department of Radiology
University of Texas Health Science Center
San Antonio, TX

Herbert I. Machleder, MD (67)
Professor of Surgery
Vascular Surgical Services
UCLA School of Medicine
Los Angeles, CA

Michael L. Marin, MD (12, 40)
Assistant Professor of Surgery
Division of Vascular Surgery
Montefiore Medical Center
New York, NY

Eric C. Martin, FRCP, FRCR, FSCVIR (9)
Professor of Radiology
College of Physicians and Surgeons of Columbia
    University
Director of Cardiovascular and Interventional
    Radiology
Columbia-Presbyterian Medical Center
New York, NY

Robert Martinez, MD (50)
Interventional Fellow
Arizona Heart Institute
Phoenix, AZ

Alan H. Matsumoto, MD (56)
Associate Professor
Director, Division of Angiography and
    Interventional Radiology
University of Virginia Health Sciences Center
Charlottesville, VA

Robert B. McLafferty, MD (23)
Division of Vascular Surgery
Oregon Health Sciences University
Portland, OR

Thomas O. McNamara, MD, FSCVIR (11)
Professor of Radiological Sciences
UCLA Medical Center
School of Medicine
Los Angeles, CA

Mark Mewissen, MD (71)
Associate Professor of Radiology
Director, Vascular and Interventional Radiology
Medical College of Wisconsin
Milwaukee, WI

Stanley L. Minken, MD (2)
Associate Professor
Division of Vascular Surgery
The Johns Hopkins University School of
    Medicine
Baltimore, MD

Sally E. Mitchell, MD, FSCVIR (30)
Associate Professor of Radiology and Surgery
Department of Radiology
The Johns Hopkins University School of
    Medicine
Baltimore, MD

Wesley S. Moore, MD (45)
Professor of Surgery/Vascular
UCLA School of Medicine
Los Angeles, CA

Timothy P. Murphy, MD, FSCVIR (10)
Director, Vascular and Interventional Radiology
Department of Radiology
Rhode Island Hospital
Brown University School of Medicine
Providence, RI

Robert R. Murray, Jr., MD (15)
Department of Radiology
Hill County Memorial Hospital
Fredericksburg, TX

Gary M. Nesbit, MD (51)
Assistant Professor of Radiology and
   Neurosurgery
The Dotter Interventional Institute
Oregon Health Sciences University
Portland, OR

M. Lee Nix, BSN, RVT (66)
Chief Technologist
Vascular Laboratory
University of Arkansas for Medical Sciences and
   the Surgical Service
Veterans Affairs Medical Center
Little Rock, AR

Thomas F. O'Donnell, Jr., MD (69)
Chief Executive Officer and President
New England Medical Center
Boston, MA

Jeffrey W. Olin, DO (7)
Chairman
Department of Vascular Medicine
Cleveland Clinic Foundation
Cleveland, OH

Stephen Oppenheimer, MD (44)
Director
Cerebrovascular Program and the Laboratories
   of Neurocardiology
The Johns Hopkins University School of
   Medicine
Baltimore, MD

Kenneth S. Ostrow, MD (41)
Clinical Instructor
Cardiovascular and Interventional Radiology
Stanford University Medical Center
Stanford, CA

Kenneth Ouriel, MD (28)
Associate Professor of Surgery
Section of Vascular Surgery
Strong Memorial Hospital
The University of Rochester
Rochester, NY

Bryan D. Petersen, MD (73)
Dotter International Institute
Oregon Health Sciences University
Portland, OR

Frank B. Pomposelli, Jr., MD (20)
Assistant Professor of Surgery
Harvard Medical School
Vascular Surgeon
Beth Israel Deaconess Medical Center
Boston, MA

John M. Porter, MD (23)
Division of Vascular Surgery
Oregon Health Sciences University
Portland, OR

Mary C. Proctor, MS (72)
Department of Surgery
The University of Michigan Hospital
Ann Arbor, MI

Peter N. Purcell, MD (46)
Division of Vascular Surgery
Massachusetts General Hospital
Boston, MA

Seshadri Raju, MD, FACS (68)
Emeritus Professor of Surgery
The University of Mississippi Medical Center
Jackson, MS

Norman M. Rich, MD, FACS (22)
Chief, Division of Vascular Surgery
Professor and Chairman/Department of Surgery
Uniformed Services University of the Health
   Sciences
Bethesda, MD

Patrick N. Riggs, MD (34)
Assistant Clinical Professor of Surgery
University of Rochester School of Medicine and
    Dentistry
Rochester, NY

Anne C. Roberts, MD, FSCVIR (43)
Associate Professor and Chief of Vascular/
    Interventional Radiology
UCSD Medical Center
Thornton Hospital
La Jolla, CA

Josef Rösch, MD, FSCVIR (73)
Professor and Director of Research
Dotter Interventional Institute
Oregon Health Sciences University
Portland, OR

Kenneth Rosenfield, MD (5)
Departments of Medicine (Cardiology) and
    Biomedical Research
St. Elizabeth's School of Medicine
Tufts University School of Medicine
Boston, MA

Gail P. Sandager, RN, RVT (3)
Division of Vascular Surgery
University of Maryland Medical Center
Baltimore, MD

Scott J. Savader, MD, FSCVIR (38)
Associate Professor of Radiology and Surgery
Russell H. Morgan Department of Radiology and
    Radiological Sciences
Division of Cardiovascular and Interventional
    Radiology
The Johns Hopkins University Medical Center
Baltimore, MD

Richard R. Saxon, MD (63)
Assistant Professor
Dotter Interventional Institute
Oregon Health Sciences University
Portland, OR

Robert Schainfeld, MD (5)
Departments of Medicine (Cardiology) and
    Biomedical Research
St. Elizabeth's School of Medicine
Tufts University School of Medicine
Boston, MA

Donald E. Schwarten, MD, FSCVIR (48)
Director, Peripheral Vascular Services
Northside Cardiology, PC
Indianapolis, IN

Lewis B. Schwartz, M.D. (53)
Department of Surgery
University of Chicago
Chicago, IL

Charles P. Semba, MD (41, 42)
Assistant Professor of Radiology
Cardiovascular and Interventional Radiology
Stanford University Medical Center
Stanford, CA

Anton N. Sidawy, MD (21)
Chief, Surgical Services
VA Medical Center
Associate Professor of Surgery
George Washington University
Washington, DC

Donald Silver, MD (27)
W. Alton Jones Professor and Chair
Department of Surgery
University of Missouri-Columbia
Columbia, MO

Robert P. Smilanich, MD (54)
Department of Surgery
The College of Medicine
The Pennsylvania State University
The Milton S. Hershey Medical Center
Hershey, PA

Robert B. Smith, III, MD (8)
Professor of Surgery and Head
General Vascular Surgery
Emory University School of Medicine
Atlanta, GA

Thomas A. Sos, MD, FSCVIR (59)
Professor of Radiology
Associate Director of Cardiovascular and
    Interventional Radiology
The New York Hospital—Cornell Medical
    Center
New York, NY

James C. Stanley, MD (58)
Professor of Surgery
Head, Section of Vascular Surgery
University of Michigan
Ann Arbor, MI

Ronald J. Stoney, MD (55)
Professor of Surgery Emeritus
Department of Surgery
Division of Vascular Surgery
University of California
San Francisco, CA

Charles J. Tegtmeyer, MD, FSCVIR (56)
Department of Radiology
Division of Angiography and Interventional
    Radiology
University of Virginia Health Sciences Center
Charlottesville, VA

Scott O. Trerotola, MD, FSCVIR (60)
Associate Professor of Radiology
Director, Vascular and Interventional Radiology
Indiana University Medical Center
Indianapolis, IN

David W. Trost, MD (59)
Assistant Professor of Radiology
Division of Cardiovascular and Interventional
    Radiology
The New York Hospital—Cornell Medical Center
New York, NY

Fong Y. Tsai, MD (52)
Professor of Radiology
Chairman, Department of Radiology
The Medical College of Pennsylvania and
    Hahnemann University
Philadelphia, PA

Frank J. Veith, MD (12, 40)
Division of Vascular Surgery
Department of Surgery
Montefiore Medical Center
The University Hospital for the Albert Einstein
    College of Medicine
New York, NY

Anthony C. Venbrux, MD (64)
Associate Professor of Radiology and Surgery
Acting Director of Cardiovascular Diagnostic
    Laboratory
The Johns Hopkins University School of
    Medicine
Baltimore, MD

John J. Vignati, MD (35)
Clinical and Research Fellow
Massachusetts General Hospital
Harvard Medical School
Boston, MA

Michael S. Webb, MD (70)
Department of Radiology
Rhode Island Hospital
Providence, RI

Harold J. Welch, MD (69)
Department of Vascular Surgery
Lahey Hitchcock Clinic
Burlington, MA
Assistant Professor of Surgery
Tufts University School of Medicine
Boston, MA

Anthony D. Whittemore, MD (13)
Department of Surgery
Brigham and Women's Hospital
Harvard Medical School
Boston, MA

Eric S. Williams, MD (66)
Vascular Research Fellow
Division of Vascular Surgery
Department of Surgery
University of Arkansas for Medical Sciences and
    the Surgical Service
Veterans Affairs Medical Center
Little Rock, AR

G. Melville Williams, MD (37)
Division of Vascular Surgery
The Johns Hopkins Medical Institutions
Baltimore, MD

James S. T. Yao, MD, PhD (19)
Magerstadt Professor of Surgery
Department of Surgery
Northwestern University Medical School
Chicago, IL

Christopher K. Zarins, MD (32)
Chidester Professor of Surgery
Chief of Vascular Surgery
Stanford University School of Medicine
Stanford, CA

Gerald Zemel, MD (39)
Director
Miami Cardiac and Vascular Institute
Baptist Hospital
Clinical Assistant Professor of Radiology
University of Miami School of Medicine
Miami, FL

Preface

As we move into the next era of vascular intervention, the economic pressures to which we allude to in the Introduction require clinicians to carefully assess the outcomes of all percutaneous and surgical interventions. It will be exceedingly important to demonstrate that outcomes match the promise of new technology. It is with this ultimate goal in mind that *Vascular Intervention: A Clinical Approach* has been created.

The multidisciplinary editorship of this book reflects our philosophy of patient care and our goal of producing a text of value both to interventionalists and to vascular surgeons, as well as to noninterventional physicians caring for patients with circulatory disease. The material provided will allow the interventionalist and surgeon to understand and compare their respective approaches to a variety of common and not so common arterial and venous disorders. It will also provide the information with which the internist, family practitioner, or cardiologist can decide whether referral for a formal vascular evaluation is indicated. As the reader will note, contributors to this book include widely recognized leaders in interventional radiology and vascular surgery, as well as specialists from the disciplines of internal medicine, vascular medicine, cardiology, neurology, and hematology. Authors were invited to contribute not only because of their significant contributions to their respective specialties and their academic reputations, but also because we know that they, like we, are busy clinicians who practice what they write.

In the ideal practice setting, all of these disciplines must be available to optimize the management of the vascular patient. This book epitomizes that philosophy. Our goal is to make it of value to clinicians in training, as well to experienced specialists in this rapidly evolving field. Ultimately, it is the clinician who must dictate the proper treatment strategy and who in the future will have an increasing number of promising options for managing the vascular patient.

When evaluating new or alternative strategies for treating old problems, it is useful to consider the words of one of the great surgical innovators of this century, Dr. Mark Ravitch, who once said: "it behooves each of us every day to justify every operation we do, to be learned enough, thoughtful enough, rigorous enough in our thinking, and compassionate enough, to do the right thing by our patients, at the same time that we strive to advance our healing art" (*Ann Surg* 1984;200:231–246).

We hope that this text will help the clinician meet Dr. Ravitch's challenge.

Foreword

It is a privilege and an honor to write a Foreword to *Vascular Intervention: A Clinical Approach.* I have known and appreciated the scientific contributions of both editors as friends and colleagues interested in the advancement of education and clinical management of vascular disease for many years. They have combined their talents as a vascular surgeon, Bruce Perler, and a vascular interventionalist, Gary Becker, to create an outstanding collection by expert contributors who are experienced clinicians in the field. The result is an exceptionally useful reference on vascular disease and its management today.

The introductory chapters define the pathology and pathophysiology of atherosclerotic disease with clinical evaluation, both through history and physical examination and through an objective measure of its extent with noninvasive technologies such as ultrasound, segmental plethysmography, and magnetic resonance imaging. A thorough discussion of the use of intravascular ultrasound is included, showing the delineation of the atherosclerotic disease and the effects of interventions. The medical management of patients with atherosclerosis is included to complete the holistic care of the patient.

There are collections of chapters that focus on aortoiliac disease, infrainguinal pathology, and visceral occlusive disease. These include surgical and percutaneous therapies and specialized clinical problems (e.g., the diabetic foot, Buerger's disease, and atheroemboli). The standard therapies of angioplasty, surgical bypass options, stents, and atherectomy are included, as are the newer materials and methods of covered stent prostheses and mechanical thromboembolectomy. Medical management of chronic and acute occlusive events is also given strong consideration.

A wide variety of venous thrombotic problems are discussed, with sensitivity to the combined use of thrombolysis, embolectomy, and angioplasty with and without stent intervention together with surgical reconstruction. Discussions of the prevention and treatment of pulmonary embolic disease include both extensive evaluation of inferior vena cava filters and pulmonary embolectomy. Therapy of portal hypertension using the TIPS procedure is included as a maturing therapy. A detailed evaluation of central venous catheter placement and the materials available to a vascular interventionalist shows the evolution of purely surgical care into less invasive therapies by interventional physicians.

The book includes potentially inflammatory topics such as the use of covered stent management of aortic aneurysmal disease and angioplasty with and without stent therapy of carotid vascular occulsive disease. These topics are well treated here, with realistic and thoughtful discussions that await large-scale evaluations. These, of course, will be carried out with some difficulty, given the continuing evolution of both the methods and the materials.

In many of the individual chapters there is careful weighing of the data for the appropriate selection of patients and the options for intervention with the various therapies available. The editors and contributors are to be congratulated on beginning what will be an evolving intense discourse on the therapeutic election for care of the patient with vascular disease. The spectrum of disease is great and the writing is clean and well organized, with useful and clear illustrations. Because of its timeliness and the combination of clinical research and experience brought by its contributors, this compendium is destined to become a standard reference in vascular disease management.

Arthur C. Waltman, M.D.
Associate Professor of Radiology
Harvard Medical School
Massachusetts General Hospital
Director, Division of Vascular Radiology
Boston, Massachusetts

Introduction

As the new millennium approaches, we continue to witness improvements in the care of patients with circulatory disease. The rate of evolution in vascular evaluation and therapy is rapidly accelerating. With unprecedented precision, safety, and success we are able to diagnose and treat arterial and venous disease. As a result, vascular physicians now face a time of great challenge and opportunity.

At a minimum, the treatment of circulatory disease represents a growth area in medical practice. The elderly, in whom vascular disease is most prevalent, represent the fastest-growing segment of the population. In the United States, the number of individuals over the age of 65 will increase by 35%, and those over the age of 85 by 600%, over the next three decades. It has been estimated that by 2030 roughly 25% of the population will be 65 or older and 7% will be 85 or older. Often a 65-year-old man in the vascular specialist's waiting room today is the son of the patient rather than the patient himself! Whereas just a few years ago performing an abdominal aortic aneurysm repair or carotid endarterectomy on an octogenarian raised eyebrows in many hospitals, today these procedures are being carried out on a routine basis.

Rapid technologic advance is providing a growing number and variety of increasingly sophisticated and accurate diagnostic modalities. Color flow Doppler studies have rendered diagnostic venography an historic relic in the workup of patients with suspected deep venous thrombosis. Instead of grading the severity of chronic venous insufficiency in the most subjective, qualitative terms, such as ulcer presence, location, and size, we now can identify the anatomic location and precisely measure the volume of venous reflux. Therefore, patients can now be objectively selected for surgical repair of their diseased valves. Duplex graft surveillance has dramatically enhanced our diagnostic sensitivity and ability to detect the failing infrainguinal bypass graft before thrombosis occurs. As a result, we have been able to markedly improve long-term graft patency. Intravascular ultrasound provides an immediate anatomic depiction of the results of percutaneous transluminal angioplasty (PTA) so that the need for stent deployment can be properly determined. The role of magnetic resonance angiography in selecting candidates for lower limb salvage by distal reconstruction continues to evolve.

Furthermore, although surgical reconstructive procedures are being performed on increasing numbers of older and sicker patients, outcomes have improved and operative morbidity has declined to very low levels. For example, the operative mortality associated with abdominal aortic aneurysm repair has declined from double digits to well under 5%, and aortic reconstructive surgery for occlusive disease has witnessed a decline in operative mortality from over 10% to approximately 2% in most busy centers today. Although as recently as 15 years ago in many institutions extensive infrageniculate occlusive disease mandated a primary below- or above-knee amputation, today bypasses are being routinely performed to vessels at the ankle and beyond, with limb salvage achieved in the vast majority of cases. In fact, over the last decade, the primary amputation rate has declined from roughly 40% to 5% or less in specialized centers. Carotid endarterectomy has become the most frequently performed peripheral vascular operation in the United States, and several randomized prospective clinical trials have firmly established its safety and superiority compared to the medical management of patients with carotid bifurcation atherosclerosis. Operations are now being performed on patients into their 90s, with operative mortality rates under 1% and comparable improvement in perioperative stroke rates. Progress in venous reconstructive surgery has matched that of arterial repair. For decades the management of patients with the postphlebitic syndrome consisted exclusively of the use of elastic support stockings, intermittent leg elevation, and prophylactic skin care. Today large numbers of patients are undergoing direct surgical repair of the diseased valve segments, with remarkable symptomatic relief and improvement in well-being.

Perhaps even more remarkable has been the rapid growth and development of the endovascular treatment of circulatory disease. Indeed, interventional radiology has evolved as a separate and vitally important subspecialty in the evaluation and management of patients with arterial and venous disorders. Based on its compelling record of safety and efficacy, PTA has assumed an accepted place in the therapeutic armamentarium for treating arterial occlusive disease in diverse anatomic sites. The safety and long-term results of iliac angioplasty, for example, support its performance as the initial intervention for patients with localized aortoiliac occlusive disease. Patients who only a decade ago would have undergone transabdoininal surgical revascularization under general anesthesia now avoid those surgical risks and relatively lengthy hospitalization by undergoing percutaneous treatment. Stents have further enhanced the clinical outcome in this patient population. The use of angioplasty in the extremities is being expanded to selected patients with renal, visceral, and, perhaps most excitingly, cerebrovascular occlusive disease. Percutaneous techniques have revolutionized the management of patients with portal hypertension, Budd-Chiari syndrome, and other central venous occlusive disorders. Over the past 15 years, thrombolytic therapy has evolved from intravenous to intra-arterial administration, with markedly improved outcomes, reduced morbidity, and shorter infusion periods. Newer approaches such as pulse spray thrombolysis and percutaneous suction thromboembolectomy are further reducing the duration of thrombolytic infusions. Early administration of thrombolytic agents can prevent the evolution of strokes in selected patients with acute intracerebral arterial occlusions. Our growing experience with thrombolytic therapy has stimulated surgeons to use these drugs selectively in the operating room as an adjust to limb salvage surgical revascularization.

The remarkable progress that has occurred to date is the prologue to even more dramatic future refinements in care. It is undeniable that some of the most important advances in the management of vascular disease during the next decade will evolve from current conventional endovascular technology. Just as large numbers of patients who formerly would have undergone aortofemoral bypass are now being treated exclusively by angioplasty, or as an adjunct to less invasive extra-anatomic surgical procedures, a significant percentage of patients who would have required surgical aortic aneurysm repair will be treated instead by endovascular stent grafts. Exclusion of the aneurysm via transfemoral stent graft insertions should further reduce the morbidity associated with abdominal and especially thoracic aortic aneurysms. In the next few years, randomized trials will allow us to critically compare carotid stents with surgical endarterectomy in the treatment of carotid atherosclerosis.

Progress in the management of circulatory disease will occur in an era of unprecedented uncertainty and external scrutiny within our health care system. What is clear is that society will not have limitless resources to support the increasingly sophisticated technology that vascular specialists bring to the clinical arena. Vascular specialists, like all health care providers, will be practicing in an environment of increasing financial constraint. Careful clinical judgment will be required to select appropriate candidates for intervention and determine the most appropriate method of treatment. The potential long-term benefit of less invasive endovascular alternatives will have to be assessed within the context of the acute risks and proven long-term track record of conventional surgical procedures. Both of these approaches will have to be weighed against the natural history of the disease without intervention. Consequently, interventionalists have become involved in the preprocedural clinical evaluation and postprocedural follow-up of their patients: *the interventionalist as clinician.* Conversely, fear of being excluded from the management of this patient population has stimulated increasing numbers of vascular surgeons to seek expertise in endovascular intervention: *the endo-vascular surgeon.* Unfortunately, in some communities this has resulted in turf battles over control of the patient. We are concerned that as the economic pressures facing health care providers increase, and as endovascular technology continues to develop and expand, this turf battle mentality may increase, with a deleterious impact on the respective specialties and, most important, on the delivery of patient care.

Acknowledging that practice models will vary from community to community depending on the distribution of specialists and a number of other factors, and that newer innovative training programs may evolve to produce multispecialty skilled prac-titioners, we believe that in the ideal situation today and in the forseeable future, inter-ventionalists and surgeons can and should work in a cooperative relationship. This is how we have always practiced at the Johns Hopkins Hospital and the Miami Vascular Institute. Despite the concerns of some in the surgical community, interventionalists will not replace vascular surgeons. The tremendous growth in the performance of PTA has been matched by a significant increase in the number of bypass operations carried out for occlusive disease. Indeed, it appears that the availablility of PTA has allowed sig-nificant numbers of patients with diffuse, severe disease who formerly would have been considered unacceptable medical risks for complex multilevel surgical reconstructive procedures to undergo revascularization, including proximal PTA and distal bypass. The aging of our population will only enhance this trend. On the other hand, it seems to us that most vascular surgeons in practice today will be unable to acquire the endo-vascular skills necessary to perform complex endovascular procedures. Collaboration will continue to be essential to the delivery of superior patient care.

It is in that spirit that this book was conceived, and has been produced.

Vascular Intervention
A Clinical Approach

Section 1

Chronic Peripheral
Arterial Occlusive Disease

1

Atherosclerotic Lesions and Their Development

P. Macke Consigny, Ph.D.

The purpose of this chapter is twofold. The first purpose is to describe the six types of atheromatous lesions as recently defined by the American Heart Association. The second purpose to provide an explanation of how these six types of lesions might develop.

TYPES OF ATHEROSCLEROTIC LESIONS

Although atherosclerosis is a progressive disease that develops over decades, atherosclerotic lesions can be divided into several types based on their morphologic appearance. In the past, atherosclerotic lesions were divided into three types—fatty streaks, fibrotic lesions, and complicated lesions.[1,2] However, over the past several years, the Committee on Vascular Lesions of the Council on Arteriosclerosis, American Heart Associa-

tion has issued a series of three papers[3-5] that have reclassified atherosclerotic lesions into six types. This new schema, which is summarized in the text below and in Table 1–1 and Figures 1–1 to 1–7, is based on an extensive macroscopic, light and electron microscopic, histochemical, and immunohistochemical examination of both normal and atherosclerotic arteries.

Normal Arterial Intima

The normal artery (Fig. 1–1) is composed of three layers: an inner intima, a media, and an outer adventitia. The intima, where atherosclerotic lesions develop, is normally composed of a monolayer of endothelial cells and an underlying subendothelial matrix. The subendothelial matrix is composed of an inner layer of pro-

Table 1–1. Characteristics of Atherosclerotic Lesion Types

Lesion Type	Lesion Characteristics
Type I (initial)	Intima contains microscopic lesions composed of monocyte/macrophages containing lipid droplets (foam cells).
Type II (fatty streak)	Macroscopically visible lesions composed of layers of macrophages, smooth muscle cells, and lipid droplet-containing foam cells of macrophage and smooth muscle origin. Some lesions are prone to progression (type IIa), while others are not (type IIb).
Type III (intermediate)	Fatty streaks with microscopically visible extracellular lipid deposits.
Type IV (atheromatous)	Lesions with a thin, fibrotic cap overlying the core of extracellular lipid. Peripheral edges of the fibrotic cap contain high concentrations of macrophages and occasional T cells.
Type V (fibrotic)	Lesions with thickened, fibrous cap containing smooth muscle cells and collagen that overlies a core of lipid (type Va), calcific (type Vb), or fibrotic (type Vc) material.
Type VI (complicated)	Type IV or V lesion that has fractured or ulcerated, resulting in luminal thrombosis or intramural hemorrhage.

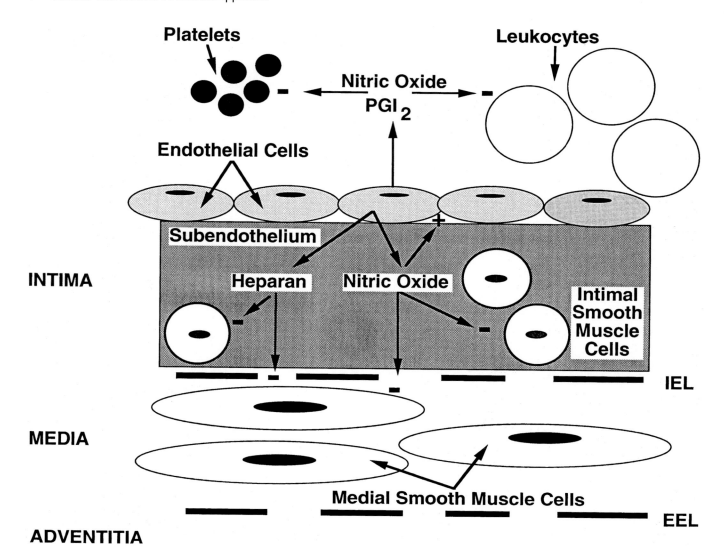

Figure 1-1. Diagram of a normal muscular artery. The normal artery is composed of three layers: an intima, a media bordered by the internal (IEL) and external (EEL) elastic laminae, and an adventitia. The normal intima is composed of a monolayer of endothelial cells attached to a subendothelial matrix. The normal endothelium releases a number of factors that inhibit processes that contribute to the development of an atherosclerotic lesion. Those processes (and the factors involved) include maintenance of limited endothelial permeability (nitric oxide), inhibition of platelet adhesion and aggregation (nitric oxide and prostacyclin or PGI_2, inhibition of leukocyte recruitment (nitric oxide), and inhibition of smooth muscle cell migration and proliferation (nitric oxide, heparan).

teoglycans (chondroitin sulfate, dermatan sulfate, heparan sulfate) containing occasional single smooth muscle cells and an outer musculoelastic layer containing numerous smooth muscle cells and elastic fibers.

The intima of the normal arteries often varies in thickness. In many regions of normal arteries, areas of increased intimal thickening are present. These thickenings, which are either focal, eccentric thickenings or diffuse, concentric thickenings, typically occur in regions where wall shear stress is reduced or where oscillatory and/or circumferential wall stress is elevated. In addition, because these lesions can be found in arteries obtained shortly after birth, it is thought that these thickenings are an adaptive response by arteries to return local shear and mechani-

cal stresses to control levels. Regions of arteries that develop intimal thickenings are also the regions that are most prone to the development of atherosclerotic lesions, suggesting that the stress factors that promote intimal thickenings may also promote atherosclerotic lesion development.[3,6]

Type I (Initial) Lesion

The earliest atherosclerotic lesions (Fig. 1–2) can only be detected using microscopic or chemical methods. The lesions are composed of small, isolated groups of macrophages and macrophages containing lipid droplets (macrophage foam cells). These macrophages are recruited to the intima in response to the accumula-

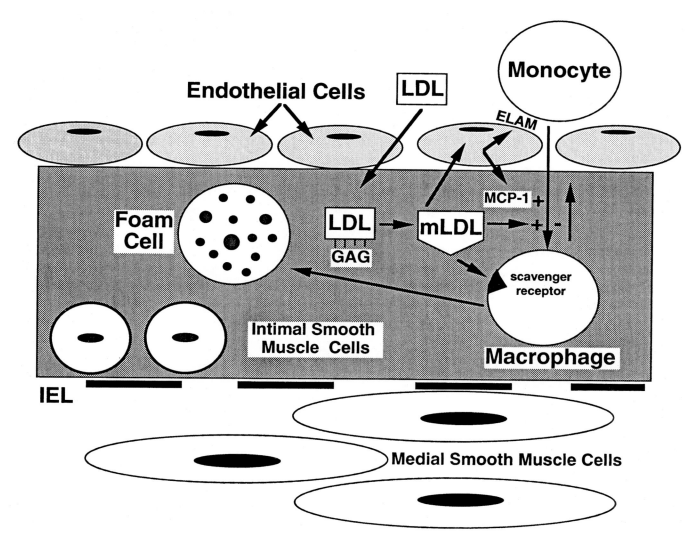

Figure 1–2. Diagram of type I (initial) lesion. Type I atherosclerotic lesions are microscopic lesions composed of individual macrophage foam cells of monocyte origin. Risk factor–mediated endothelial injury increases the permeability of the endothelium to LDL. On entry into the subendothelium, LDL binds to glycosaminoglycans (GAGs), where it undergoes oxidative modification to form modified LDL (mLDL). The mLDL stimulates endothelial cells to express binding sites including endothelial leukocyte adhesion molecule (ELAM) for the recruitment of monocytes. These endothelial cells also produce monocyte chemoattractant protein (MCP-1), which further promotes monocyte recruitment. After recruitment to the subendothelium, monocytes change to become macrophages. Using scavenger receptors expressed on their cell surfaces, these macrophages bind and internalize mLDL in an uncontrolled fashion, resulting in the formation of foam cells.

tion of lipoproteins in the intima. Initial lesions can be found in both children and adults and most frequently appear in areas of hemodynamic or mechanical stress.[4]

Type II (Fatty Streak) Lesion

Fatty streaks (Fig. 1–3) are lesions that are macroscopically visible as colored patches or streaks on the luminal surface of the artery. The lesions are composed of stratified layers of macrophages and foam cells of macrophage and smooth muscle cell origin. T lymphocytes are also present. Many of the macrophages in these lesions are activated, expressing major histocompatibility complex, CD antigen, cytokines, and growth factors,

and many are undergoing proliferation. Smooth muscle cells, presumably of intimal origin, are present in both the superficial and deep layers of the intima. These cells typically have a noncontractile, synthetic appearance characterized by the presence of a rough endoplasmic reticulum. The proteoglycan content of these lesions is typically elevated, particularly chondroitin sulfate and dermatan sulfate, which have a high affinity for plasma low density lipoprotein (LDL). The lipids in these lesions are predominantly intracellular, with some thinly dispersed extracellular droplets, presumably of foam cell or extracellular lipoprotein origin. There is some evidence of endothelial cell

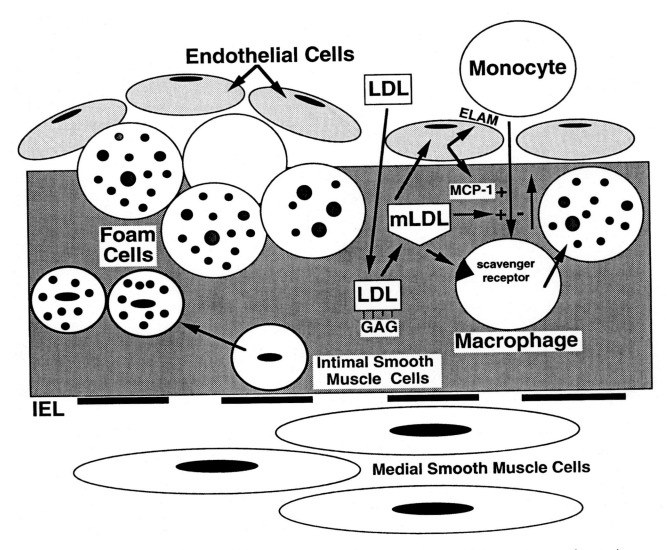

Figure 1–3. Diagram of a type II (fatty streak) lesion. The processes that produced a type I lesion continue, resulting in the formation of a macroscopic fatty streak composed of foam cells of monocyte-macrophage and intimal smooth muscle cell origin.

dysfunction in these lesions. For example, the endothelial cells overlying these lesions appear rounded and are no longer aligned in the direction of blood flow. In addition, there is increased endothelial cell turnover, but there is no evidence of cell necrosis or disruption. Type II lesions are present in the aorta of almost all children 2 years of age or older but do not appear in coronary arteries until puberty. Some type II lesions, particularly those located in areas where hemodynamic and mechanical forces promote the influx of lipid into the lesion, are prone to progression and are referred to as type IIa lesions. Other type II lesions are resistant to progression and are referred to as type IIb lesions.[4]

Type III (Intermediate) Lesion

Type III lesions (Fig. 1–4) are lesions that contain pools of microscopically visible extracellular lipid droplets. These extracellular droplets are present among layers of smooth muscle cells and foam cells of smooth muscle cell origin that lie beneath more superficial layers of macrophages and macrophage foam cells. These lipid droplets are dispersed, so no well-delineated lipid core is present. These intermediate lesions are found in progression-prone regions of arteries where type IIa lesions occur.[4]

Type IV (Atheroma) Lesion

Type IV lesions (Fig. 1–5) are advanced atherosclerotic lesions characterized by the accumulation of extracellular lipid into a lipid core that presumably results from the joining of the small extracellular lipid pools present in type III lesions. These lesions are macroscopically visible, eccentric lesions that may or may not encroach on the lumen, depending on the ability of the artery to undergo a compensatory enlargement. A thin fibrotic cap is present above the extracellular lipid pool.

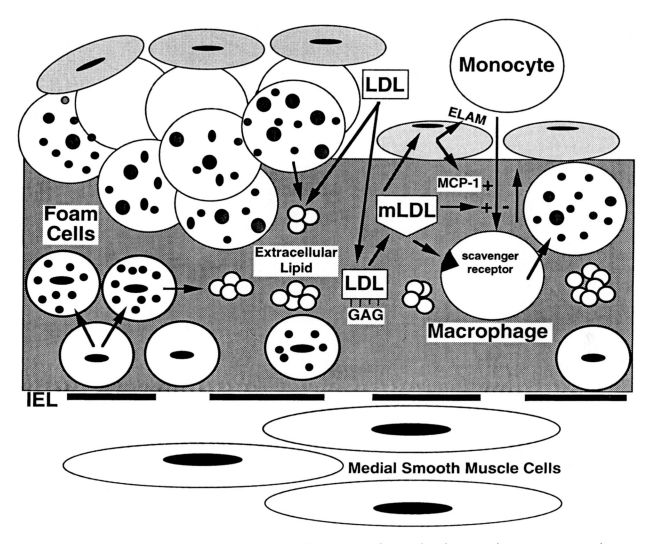

Figure 1–4. Diagram of a type III (intermediate) lesion. The processes that produced a type II lesion continue, resulting in the formation of a fatty streak that now contains microscopically visible extracellular lipid droplets. These droplets may be of foam cell origin or they may be aggregates of LDL.

This cap is composed of an endothelium covering a proteoglycan-rich subendothelium that contains macrophages and smooth muscle cells, with and without intracellular lipid droplets. The thinness and composition of this cap make these lesions particularly susceptible to fissuring and the formation of type VI lesions. At the peripheral edges of the lipid pool, concentrations of macrophages, macrophage foam cells, and T lymphocytes can be found. Within the lipid pool, calcium particles appear.[5]

Type V (Fibrotic) Lesion

Type V lesions (Fig. 1–6), like type IV lesions, have a fibrotic cap composed of a superficial monolayer of endothelial cells overlying layers of macrophages, smooth muscle cells, and foam cells of macrophage and smooth muscle cell origin. However, unlike type IV lesions, the fibrous cap in type V lesions has an abundance of fibrous connective tissue, particularly collagen. Type V fibrotic lesions can be divided into three subtypes based on the material underlying this thickened fibrotic cap. In type Va fibroatheroma lesions, lipid cores composed of one or more multiple layers lie beneath the fibrous cap. In type Vb calcific lesions, the core has undergone considerable mineralization and calcification. In type Vc fibrotic lesions, the core is composed of fibrotic material that is relatively lipid free. In type V lesions, changes are also observed in the media and adventitia of the artery, including medial thinning, the accumulation of macrophages, macrophage foam cells and T lymphocytes in the media, and the presence of lymphocytes and mast cells in the adventitia.[5]

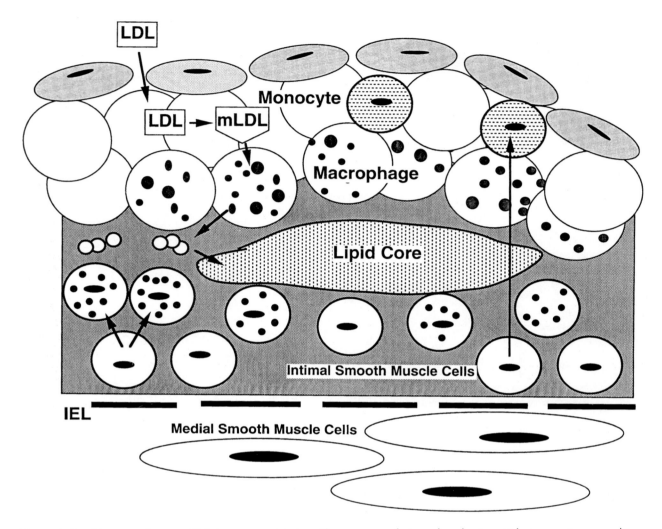

Figure 1–5. Diagram of a type IV (atheromatous) lesion. The processes that produced a type III lesion continue, resulting in the formation of an atheromatous lesion characterized by the presence an extracellular lipid pool beneath a thin, fibrous cap.

Type VI (Complicated) Lesion

Type VI lesions (Fig. 1–7) are type IV or type V lesions that have become more complex as a result of disruption of the lesion. In type VIa lesions, defects ranging from microscopic areas of focal endothelial cell loss to macroscopic ulcerations, fissures, or tears are present on the surface of the lesion. In type VIb lesions, hematomas are present as a result of plaque disruption or hemorrhage of intramural microvessels. In type VIc lesions, platelet aggregates and fibrin deposits are present on the surface of the lesion.[5]

DEVELOPMENT OF AN ATHEROSCLEROTIC LESION

The interrelation between the above six types of atherosclerotic lesions can perhaps be more completely appreciated by following the growth of a lesion from its inception to its development into a complicated (type VI) lesion. The progression described below and depicted in Figures 1–2 to 1–7 presumes that endothelial cell injury and lipid insudation are the causative factors. It should be noted, however, that several alternative explanations for the genesis of atherosclerosis have been proposed, including a monoclonal mechanism,[7] a viral mechanism,[8,9] and an immune mechanism.[10]

Endothelial Injury

Many of the risk factors associated with the development of atherosclerosis, including hyperlipidemia, diabetes, smoking, and hypertension, have one element in common—they injure the endothelium. This injury promotes the development of atherosclerosis by converting normal endothelium into a dysfunctional endothelium. In this dysfunctional state, the release of endothelium-derived factors that normally blunt the development of atherosclerosis is diminished, and the

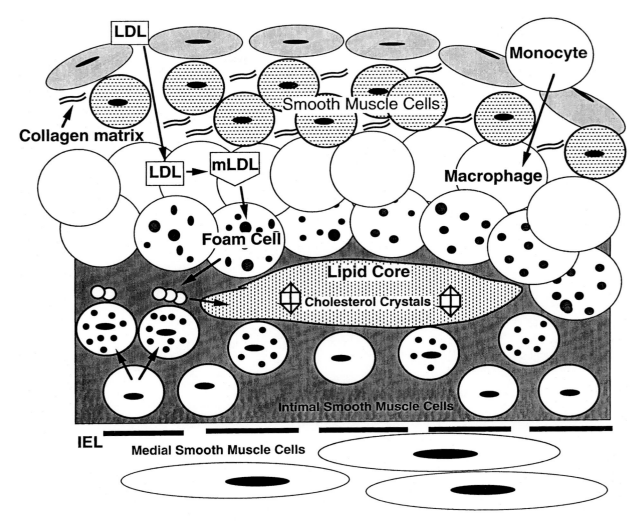

Figure 1-6. Diagram of a type V (fibrotic) lesion. The processes that produced a type IV lesion continue, resulting in the formation of a fibrotic lesion that is characterized by the presence of a thickened, fibrotic cap composed of smooth muscle cells and strengthened by the presence of collagen. The core beneath the fibrotic cap may be composed of lipid (type Va), calcific (type Vb), or fibrotic (type Vc) material.

release of endothelium-derived factors that promote atherosclerosis is increasd[11–14] (Table 1–2).

Influx of LDL and Its Binding to Glycosaminoglycans (GAG) in the Subendothelium Matrix

One of the changes associated with endothelial cell dysfunction is a change in cell shape and a concomitant increase in endothelial permeability. The increase in permeability permits LDL and other large molecules to pass from the circulation into the subendothelium (Fig. 1–2). LDL that has entered the subendothelium has a high affinity for GAGs in the subendothelial matrix. The binding of LDL to these GAGs increases the length of time that these molecules reside in the subendothelium and thereby increases the probability that they will undergo oxidative modification.[1,15–17]

Initial LDL Modification and Monocyte-Macrophage Recruitment

The LDL that has diffused into the subendothelium may undergo mild oxidation by endothelium-derived factors, resulting in the formation of a mildly modified form of LDL (Fig. 1–2). This mildly modified LDL is capable of stimulating endothelial cells and activating certain transcription factors, including a (NFkB)-like transcription factor, resulting in the expression of certain genes that produce factors that promote the recruitment of circulating monocytes. These gene products include a monocyte chemoattractant (monocyte chemoattractant protein-1, or MCP-1) and endothelial membrane receptors that bind and recruit monocytes (intercellular adhesion molecule-1, or ICAM-1, and vascular cell adhesion molecule-1, or VCAM-l). Additional factors in the subendothelium,

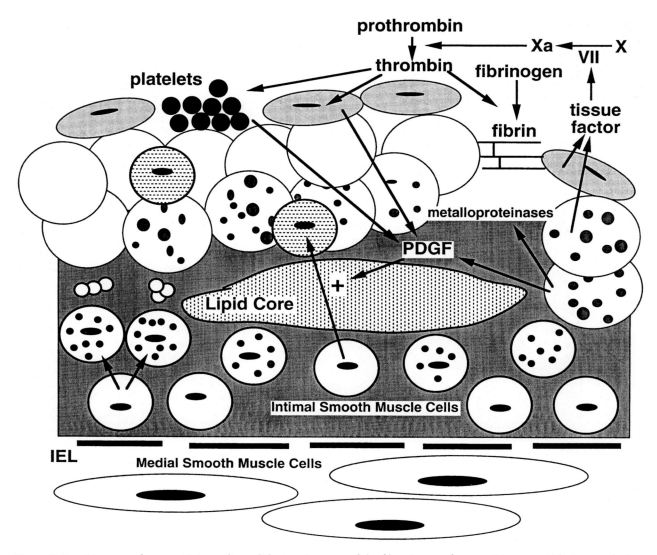

Figure 1–7.   Diagram of a type VI (complicated) lesion. Fracture of the fibrotic cap of a type IV or type V lesion results in thrombosis. The release of tissue factor stimulates the extrinsic coagulation pathway, resulting in the formation of fibrin. Thrombin, which is formed during the coagulation process, stimulates platelet aggregation. Activated platelets, endothelial cells, and macrophages release platelet-derived growth factor (PDGF), which promotes the recruitment and proliferation of smooth muscle cells.

including colony-stimulating factor, tumor necrosis factor-alpha, and oxidized LDL, may further attract these monocytes and stimulate their conversion into macrophages.[1,16–18]

Further Lipid Oxidation and Foam Cell Formation

Macrophages are capable of further modifying LDL to a more highly oxidized form that can then be internalized into macrophages by way of scavenger receptors (Fig. 1–2). Unlike normal LDL receptors that are downregulated in the presence of LDL, scavenger receptors are not regulated. Consequently, large amounts of oxidized LDL can be incorporated into the macrophages, resulting in the formation of foam cells,

so named because the lipid droplets found in their cytoplasm give the cells a foamy appearance.[15,18,19]

Accumulation of Foam Cells of Macrophage and Smooth Muscle Origin

The acumulation of foam cells beneath the endothelium results in the formation of a visible lesion referred to as a *fatty streak* (Fig. 1–3). This foam cell accumulation is due in part to continued monocyte recruitment, macrophage proliferation, and the inhibition of macrophage egress by MCP-1–induced expression of fibronectin receptors on the macrophage cell surface. Foam cell accumulation is also due to the incorporation of lipids into intimal smooth muscle cells.[1,16–18]

Table 1-2 Functions of the Vascular Endothelium in Normal and Injured States

Function	Normal Endothelium	Injured/Dysfunctional Endothelium
Permeability	Tight cell-to-cell junctions prevent passage of large molecules into subendothelium.	Loss of tight junctions increases penetration of large molecules into subendothelium.
Thrombogenicity	Platelets are repelled by negative surface charge of endothelial cells. Platelet aggregation is inhibited by prostacyclin and nitric oxide release. Thrombolysis is promoted by tissue plasminogen activator release.	Antithrombotic function is decreased by diminished release of prostacyclin, nitric oxide, and tissue plasminogen activator. Thrombosis is promoted by increased release of plasminogen activator inhibitor and tissue factor.
Vasomotor tone	Vasodilation is promoted by release of prostacyclin and nitric oxide.	Vasoconstriction is promoted by diminished release of prostacyclin and nitric oxide and by increased release of endothelin-1.
Vascular smooth muscle migration and proliferation	Smooth muscle migration and proliferation are inhibited by release of heparan sulfate and nitric oxide.	Smooth muscle proliferation is promated by diminished nitric oxide release and increased release of platelet-derived growth factor and endothelin-1.
Inflammation	Inflammatory cells are not recruited to the artery.	Leukocytes are recruited to sites of endothelial injury by expression of adhesion molecules and by release of chemotactic factors.

Source: Table modified from Reference 2.

Formation of Extracellular Lipid Pools

Type III (intermediate) lesions (Fig. 1–4) are characterized by the presence of microscopically visible extracellular lipid droplets, predominantly in the musculoelastic layer of the intima. Some of the extracellular lipid is in the form of cholesterol ester-rich oily droplets, suggesting that their formation is the result of plasma lipoprotein aggregation/fusion. Additional extracellular lipid is in the form of vesicles or crystals of free cholesterol, suggesting that their formation is the result of cell death, the extrusion of blebs of cell membrane, or the extrusion of lysosomal contents. Possible causes of cell death include the buildup of toxic lipids, apoptosis (programmed cell death), the release of free radicals, and/or ischemia due to the increased diffusion distance between the tissue and the blood. In more advanced type IV atheromatous lesions, these lipid pools have coalesced to form a macroscopic lipid pool.[1,4,20]

Plaque Fracture

Type VI (complicated) lesions (Fig. 1–7) develop when the fibrotic cap of type IV (intermediate) lesions fractures. The sites of plaque fracture are typically found near lipid pools. One factor that affects the vulnerability of these sites to fracture is the size of the lipid core; plaque fractures typically occur in areas where the lipid pool occupies 40% or more of the plaque. The fracture at these sites is due, at least in part, to an increased tensile load placed on the fibrotic cap overlying the lipid pool because the tensile strength in the area of the lipid pool is reduced. A second factor that may determine plaque fracture is the thickness of the fibrous cap; thin fibrous caps lacking smooth muscle cells and extracellular collagen matrix are more susceptible to fracture than more mature fibrotic caps containing smooth muscle cells and collagen. A third factor is the presence of inflammatory cells within the fibrotic cap; shoulder regions of fibrotic caps typically contain high numbers of macrophages that, when activated, release matrix-degrading metalloproteinases (MMPs) including interstitial collagenase (MMP-1), gelatinases (MMP-2, MMP-9), and stromelysins that degrade the matrices that provide tensile strength to the cap. Finally, cap fatigue secondary to shear, repeated bending, or compression can result in plaque fracture.[15,21–25]

Thrombus Formation

Subsequent to plaque fracture, thrombosis ensues, resulting in the formation of a complicated (type VI) lesion (Fig. 1–7). Thrombosis involves activation of the coagulation cascade by exposure of the blood to collagen within the plaque and by the release of tissue factor (tissue thromboplastin), which is found in high concentration in association with endothelial cells and macrophages within the atherosclerotic lesion. Tissue factor enables factor VII to activate factor X, which catalyzes the conversion of prothrombin to thrombin. Thrombin catalyzes the conversion of fibrinogen into monomeric fibrin, which then undergoes polymerization and stabilizes the thrombus. Thrombin may also stimulate cellular proliferation within the atherosclerotic lesion and within the thrombus by stimulating additional platelet aggregation and by inducing cells within the lesion to synthesize and release platelet-derived growth factor (PDGF). Thrombosis may be further potentiated by lipoprotein (a), which inhibits thrombolysis by competitively inhibiting the conversion of plasminogen into plasmin. Depending on the balance between thrombotic and thrombolytic processes, the thrombus may undergo dissolution, with no clinical sequelae. Alternatively, clinical sequelae may ensue if the thrombus enlarges to occlude the artery or sloughs off and occludes a more distal vessel.[5,24–27]

Fibrotic Cap Formation

In the normal artery, smooth muscle cells reside in the intima, particularly in the deeper musculoelastic layer of the subendothelium. After fracture of a type IV (atheromatous) or type V (fibrotic) lesion, platelets adhere to and aggregate at the site of fracture (Fig. 1–7). These platelets release PDGF, a potent smooth muscle chemoattractant. This PDGF, alone or in combination with additional PDGF released from activated endothelial cells and macrophages, stimulates smooth muscle cells to migrate from the deeper intima and possibly the media toward the luminal surface of the lesion, where they recellularize the thrombus. In addition, cells within the atherosclerotic plaque, including platelets, smooth muscle cells, macrophages, and endothelial cells, are capable of releasing a number of growth factors, including PDGF, insulin growth factor, and basic fibroblast growth factor, that stimulate some of these smooth muscle cells to proliferate. This proliferation is further promoted by the presence of a dysfunctional endothelium that releases less than normal amounts of nitric oxide, a factor that inhibits smooth muscle migration and proliferation. Following cell migration and proliferation, the smooth muscle cells secrete a collagenous extracellular matrix, thereby producing the thickened, fibrotic cap that is characteristic of type V (fibrotic) lesions (Fig. 1–7). Beneath the fibrotic cap, calcium hydroxyapatite deposits may be found secondary to either calcium crystallization on preexisting cholesterol crystals or secondary to the osteogenic activity of macrophages and smooth muscle cells within the lesion. Microvessels may also be found; they are the result of angiogenic processes occurring within the intima and media.[1,5,28–30]

SUMMARY

Atherosclerosis is a progressive disease that begins as a thickening of the intima in areas of hemodynamic or mechanical stress. With the development of a dysfunctional endothelium, atherosclerotic lesions slowly develop over decades of life. Eventually, a lesion may become a type V (fibrotic) lesion of sufficient size to restrict blood flow during periods of increased demand, resulting in clinical entities such as angina and intermittent claudication. Alternatively, a type IV (atheromatous) lesions may fracture, thrombose, and form a type VI (complicated) lesion that either transiently or permanently occludes blood flow, resulting in either a transient (angina at rest, transient ischemic attacks) or a permanent change (myocardial or brain infarct). The key to preventing these clinical events is to minimize the development of significant endothelial cell dysfunction by controlling the risk factors that induce the dysfunction.

REFERENCES

1. Ross R. the pathogenesis of atherosclerosis: A perspective for the 1990s. *Nature* 1993; 362:801–809.
2. Consigny PM. Pathogenesis of atherosclerosis. *AJR* 1996;164:553–558.
3. Stary HC, Blankenhorn DH, Chandler AB, et al. A definition of the intima of human arteries and of its atherosclerosis-prone regions. A report from the Committee on Vascular Lesions of the Council on Arteriosclerosis, American Heart Association. *Circulation* 1992;85:391–405.
4. Stary HC, Chandler AB, Glagov S, et al. A definition of initial, fatty streak, and intermediate lesions of atherosclerosis. A report from the Committee on Vascular Lesions of the Council on Arteriosclerosis, American Heart Association. *Arteriosclerosis Thromb* 1994;14:840–856.
5. Stary HC, Chandler, AB, Dinsmore RE, et al. A definition of advanced types of atherosclerotic lesions and a histological classification of atherosclerosis. A report from the Committee on Vascular Lesions of the Council on Arteriosclerosis, American Heart Association. *Arteriosclerosis Thromb Vasc Biol* 1995;15:1512–1531.
6. Schwartz SM, deBlois, D, O'Brien ERM. The intima. Soil for atherosclerosis and restenosis. *Circ Res* 1995;77:445–465.
7. Benditt EP, Benditt JM. Evidence for a monoclonal origin of human atherosclerotic plaques. *Proc Natl Acad Sci USA* 1973;70:1753–1756.
8. Minick CR, Fabricant CG, Fabricant J, and Litrenta MM. Atheroarteriosclerosis induced by infection with a herpes virus. *Am J Pathol* 1979;96:673–706.
9. Benditt EP, Barrett T, McDougall JK. Viruses in the etiology of atherosclerosis. *Proc Natl Acad Sci USA* 1983;80:6386–6389.
10. Hansson GK, Jonasson L, Seifert PS, and Stemme S. Immune mechanisms in atherosclerosis. *Arteriosclerosis* 1989;9:567–578.
11. Flavahan NA. Atherosclerosis or lipoprotein-induced endothelial dysfunction. Potential mechanisms underlying reduction in EDRF/nitric oxide activity. *Circulation* 1992;85:1927–1938.
12. Glasser SP, Selwyn AP, Ganz P. Atherosclerosis: risk factors and the vascular endothelium. *Am Heart J* 1996; 131:379–384.
13. Griendling KK, Alexander RW. Endothelial control of the cardiovascular system: recent advances. *FASEB J* 1996;10:283–292.
14. Shireman PK, Pearce WH. Endothelial cell function: biologic and physiologic functions in health and disease. *AJR* 1996;166:7–13.

15. Goldstein JL, Brown MS. The low-density lipoprotein pathway and its relation to atherosclerosis. *Annu Rev Biochem* 1977;46:897–930.
16. Berliner JA, Nabab M, Fogelman AM, et al. Atherosclerosis: basic mechanisms. Oxidation, inflammation, and genetics. *Circulation* 1995;91:2488–2496.
17. Navab M, Fogelman AM, Berliner JA, et al. Pathogenesis of atherosclerosis. *Am J Cardiol* 1995;76:18C–23C.
18. Raines EW, Rosenfeld ME, Ross R. The role of macrophages. In: Fuster V, Ross R, Topol EJ (eds.): *Atherosclerosis and Coronary Artery Disease.* Philadelphia: Lippincott-Raven, 1996;539–555.
19. Wu H, Moulton KS, Glass CK. Macrophage scavenger receptors and atherosclerosis. *Trends Cardiovasc Med* 1992;2:220–225.
20. Guyton JR, Klemp KF. Development of the lipid-rich core in human atherosclerosis. *Arterioscl Thromb Vasc Biol* 1996;16:4–11.
21. Richardson PD, Davies MJ, Born GVR. Influence of plaque configuration and stress distribution on fissuring of coronary atherosclerotic plaques. *Lancet* 1989;2:941–944.
22. Galis, ZS, Sukhova GK, Lark MW, Libby P. Increased expression of matrix metalloproteinases and matrix degrading activity in vulnerable regions of human atherosclerotic plaques. *J Clin Invest* 1994;94:2493–2503.
23. Loree HM, Tobias BJ, Gibson LJ, Kamm RD, Small DM, Lee RT. Mechanical properties of model atherosclerotic lesion lipid pools. *Arterioscl Thromb* 1994;14:230–234.
24. Falk E, Shah PK, Fuster V. Coronary plaque disruption. *Circulation* 1995;92:657–671.
25. Fuster V. Elucidation of the role of plaque instability and rupture in acute coronary events. *Am J Cardiol* 1995;76:24C–33C.
26. Liu AC, Lawn RM. Lipoprotein (a) and atherogenesis. *Trends Cardiovasc Med* 1994;4:40–44.
27. Falk E, Fernandez-Ortiz A. Role of thrombosis in atherosclerosis and its complications. *Am J Cardiol* 1995;75:5B–11B.
28. Demer LL, Watson KE, Bostrom K. Mechanism of calcification in atherosclerosis. *Trends Cardiovasc Med* 1994;4:45–49.
29. O'Brien ER, Garvin MR, DCev R, Stewart DK, Hinohara T, Simpson JB. Angiogenesis in human coronary atherosclerotic plaques. *Am J Pathol* 1994;145:883–894.
30. Bostrom K, Watson KE, Stanford WP, Demer LL. Atherosclerotic calcification: relation to developmental osteogenesis. *Am J Cardiol* 1995;75:88B–91B.

2

Clinical Assessment of the Patient with Peripheral Arterial Occlusive Disease: The History and Physical Examination

Stanley L. Minken, M.D., F.A.C.S.
David L. Gillespie, M.D.

At a time of increasing sophistication in diagnostic technology, it cannot be overemphasized that a careful history and a well-performed physical examination remain the most important part of the evaluation of patients with peripheral arterial occlusive disease (PAOD). The initial evaluation of the patient with suspected circulatory disease requires that the examiner characterize the problem in both physiologic and anatomic terms. In essence, this requires answering a number of dichotomous questions. At the most fundamental level, one must determine if the presenting complaint likely reflects vascular disease or some other etiology. If the problem appears to be vascular, is it arterial or venous/lymphatic? Once it has been established that arterial insufficiency is the most likely etiology, one must determine if the ischemic process is acute or chronic and if the level of ischemia is limb-threatening or non-limb-threatening. This information, which is critical in determining the necessity for diagnosis and therapy and selecting specific strategies, can be easily gathered through a relatively brief, careful history including an assessment of demographic and other arteriosclerotic risk factors. Once the ischemic process has been characterized clinically, the anatomic level of disease and the severity of ischemia should be further characterized through a careful physical examination including palpation of peripheral pulses, auscultation of bruits, and visual inspection of associated cutaneous lesions.[1]

Patients who present primarily with PAOD often are afflicted with multisystemic problems that require a thorough overall medical evaluation. In this regard, vascular specialists often find themselves serving in the role of primary care physicians, investigating diverse organ systems in order to formulate a comprehensive picture of the patient's status. This chapter will focus primarily on the vascular history and physical examination while recognizing the need for a careful assessment of the patient's overall condition.

THE HISTORY: GENERAL CONSIDERATIONS

The medical history should focus on those variables particularly relevant to the development and characterization of the patient's arterial disease. For example, the social history is extremely relevant. Long-term tobacco use is particularly noteworthy, as it is the single most important risk factor for arteriosclerotic disease. In addition, continued smoking is associated with a relatively poorer response to conservative treatment, as well as earlier and higher failure rates following revascularization procedures, both surgical and endovascular. The family history also offers insight into the genetic and developmental aspects of the patient's overall medical condition. Evidence of significant parental or sibling peripheral occlusive disease, cardiac disease, or lipid abnormalities should be sought. A family history of diabetes is also important.

The patient's past medical history allows the vascular specialist to determine the severity of associated comorbidity, which is crucial in making judgments with respect to the advisability of attempting revascularization and the method to be used. Diabetes mellitus is not only a risk factor for PAOD, but may also increase its severity and complicate its management.[2] The clear

15

association of cerebrovascular and coronary artery disease with PAOD mandates that patients presenting primarily with symptoms in one of these systems be assessed for the presence of these other associated atherosclerotic complications. Hypertension is another important risk factor for PAOD, and the presence of poorly or marginally controlled hypertension requires the examiner to investigate further the possibility of renal artery disease.

In addition, a detailed review of systems will often uncover subtle hints that may indicate the need for a more detailed investigation of parts of the vascular system other than that directly related to the presenting complaint. As an example, vague neurologic symptoms may point to previously unrecognized carotid artery disease. Intermittent abdominal discomfort with weight loss or new-onset hypertension may indicate early visceral or renal artery stenoses, respectively. The potentially diverse systemic manifestations of atherosclerotic disease must always be considered in the evaluation of this patient population.

THE PULSE EXAMINATION

The femoral pulse, which is easily palpated at or just inferior to the groin crease 2 to 3 cm lateral to the pubic tubercle, is normally approximately 1 to 2 cm in diameter. A wider or unusually prominent pulsation may indicate a femoral artery aneurysm (see Chapter 34). The pulse is felt by applying gentle pressure with the middle three fingers over the area of the entrance below the inguinal ligament. In obese patients the vessel may be obscured by a thick layer of tissue, requiring increased pressure or even Doppler identification of the artery's location. It is useful to develop a grading system of pulse strength for future comparisons. Although somewhat arbitrary, one system ranges from 0 for an absent pulse to 2+ for a normal pulse to 3+/4+ for a dilated/aneurysmal vessel. One should also auscultate the groin for a bruit, indicative of turbulent flow and suggestive of stenotic arterial disease.

The popliteal pulse is examined with the patient in the supine position. The examiner's hands are gently cupped, fingertip to fingertip, in the center of the popliteal space between the medial and lateral heads of the gastrocnemius muscle. With the patient's leg relaxed and slightly bent, gentle pressure is applied until the pulsation is felt. In obese patients, manipulation of the popliteal fat pad may be required. In a small percentage of individuals, the popliteal pulse may be detectable only by Doppler examination. Once identified, the popliteal pulse should also be graded in terms of intensity and width. The normal popliteal pulse is no more than 2 cm in width. A more dilated or unusually strong pulsation may indicate a popliteal aneurysm requiring further investigation (see Chapter 34).

Evaluation of the pedal pulses is carried out with the patient in the supine position and the ankle joint relaxed. The dorsalis pedis pulse is palpated over the central aspect of the foot, usually at midfoot level. Occasionally, the vessel may be found somewhat more medial or lateral to the midline. In a small number of normal individuals, the anterior tibial artery may arborize proximal to the foot and thus be nonpalpable at the usual dorsalis pedis level. The posterior tibial pulse is found posterior to the medial malleolus and is examined by applying gentle forehand pressure behind the malleolus with the second and third fingers. Back handing should be avoided, as it often leads to erroneously missed pulses.

The physical examination of the pedal pulses should be supplemented with a study employing a handheld, continuous-wave Doppler ultrasound scanner. Although covered more comprehensively later in this text (see Chapter 3), office or bedside measurement of the ankle/branchial index (ABI) should be an integral part of the initial evaluation of the patient with suspected PAOD. Systolic pressure of the ankle is determined by placing a standard blood pressure cuff just superior to the ankle, auscultating the dorsalis pedis artery with the Doppler probe, inflating the cuff until the signal is no longer audible, and then slowly deflating until the pulse reappears. The pressure at which the pulse returns is the systolic pressure in that vessel. The process is then repeated with the posterior tibial artery. The higher of the two ankle pressures is divided by the highest brachial systolic pressure to yield the ABI. Repeat measurement of the ABIs during serial follow-up is crucial in assessing disease stability, progression, or improvement. Table 2–1 shows the general levels of ABI and associated symptomatology, although one may anticipate significant overlap between these relatively arbitrary groups. As noted in Chapter 3, patients with diabetes often develop extensive arterial calcinosis, so that artifactually elevated ankle pressures, reflecting noncompressible vessels, may be noted. In this situation, a recording Doppler scan may show an abnormal arterial waveform in the presence of normal or suprasystemic systolic pressures (Fig. 2–1).

In addition to the peripheral pulse examination, the skin as well as the musculoskeletal system should be assessed. The presence, site, and size of skin ulcers; hair distribution; and other cutaneous observations should

Table 2–1. Relationship of ABI and Symptoms

ABI	Symptoms
1–0.8	None
0.8-0.6	Arterial claudication
0.6-0.3	Rest pain
0.3-0	Tissue loss

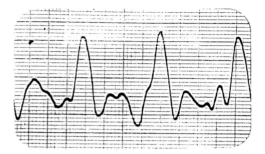 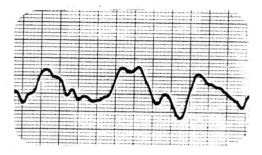

Figure 2–1. Normal triphasic arterial Doppler waveform (left) and markedly abnormal waveform due to occlusive disease (right).

be carefully documented. Care must be taken to identify small fissures and ulcers beneath calluses and between toes, as well as areas of discoloration and necrosis. Muscle mass and leg circumference should be assessed. Bony abnormalities, especially in the feet, should be identified and are particularly important in diabetic patients. Examination of the feet should include an assessment of capillary refill and venous return times. Prolongation of these parameters is indicative of more advanced arterial insufficiency. Capillary refill time is determined by compressing and rapidly releasing the pulp. Color to the nail bed should return in a few seconds. Venous return time is measured by placing the limb in the dependent position immediately after elevation. Superficial vein filling should be noted within 5 to 10 seconds in the individual with normal arterial perfusion.

ACUTE ISCHEMIA: THE HISTORY AND PHYSICAL EXAMINATION

Acute arterial insufficiency is typically manifested by a constellation of signs and symptoms known as the *five Ps* (Table 2–2). Patients can invariably recall the exact moment at which the occlusion occurred by the sudden onset of severe pain in the involved extremity. This is especially true in the patient with an embolic occlusion, whereas if the etiology is thrombosis superimposed on a preexisting chronic stenosis, the onset may be more gradual. In the patient with chronic symptoms of intermittent claudication (vida infra), the acute thrombotic process may be manifested primarily by the sudden worsening of those claudication symptoms, that is, symptoms occurring while walking for significantly shorter distances. The extremity distal to the site of occlusion typically will be pale and cool. The presence/

Table 2–2.   The Five Ps

Pain
Pallor
Pulselessness
Paresthesias
Paralysis

absence of palpable pulses is useful in determining the anatomic site of the occlusion. It is important to examine the uninvolved extremity carefully since an abnormal pulse exam in that limb, implying chronic arterial occlusive disease, may suggest a thrombotic rather than an embolic etiology in the acutely ischemic extremity. During the initial hours of the ischemic process, the patient may experience paresthesias in the affected extremity. With progressive ischemia, however, paralysis may develop. It cannot be overemphasized that profound neurologic deficits are completely consistent with a diagnosis of severe arterial insufficiency. Failure to recognize this point, and the associated signs of arterial insufficiency, has led to the incorrect diagnosis of acute neurologic injury in some patients, resulting in significant delay in attempted revascularization and a poor outcome. In addition to acute neurologic disease, the differential diagnosis of the acutely ischemic limb includes acute deep venous thrombosis and orthopedic injury.

Determining the need for, and most appropriate method of, revascularization in the patient with acute limb ischemia depends on an accurate assessment of the severity of the ischemic process as well as the suspected etiology. To allow more reliable and scientific assessment of therapeutic interventions, the Ad Hoc Committee on Reporting Standards, Society for Vascular Surgery/North American Chapter, International Society for Cardiovascular Surgery has published criteria for describing more objectively the acutely ischemic limb.[3] It is acknowledged that this categorization, while very useful in guiding therapeutic decision making, is not definitive. Ultimately, careful clinical judgment remains an important element in electing further therapy. The *viable* limb is characterized by intact capillary refill, normal motor and sensory function, and the presence of arterial and venous Doppler signals. The *threatened* limb requires urgent intervention to achieve limb salvage. Capillary refill is slow, and there may be mild motor and/or sensory abnormalities. Usually, distal arterial Doppler signals are inaudible, but venous signals remain present. *Irreversible* ischemia is characterized by absent capillary refill, marked motor abnormality or frank paralysis, significant sensory loss or anesthesia, and inaudible arterial and venous Doppler signals in the distal extremity. This diagnosis implies that amputation is inevitable, so attempts at revascularization are generally not warranted, and potentially deleterious.

In addition to determining that the limb is salvageable and grading the severity of ischemia, the clinician should try to ascertain the most likely underlying etiology, that is, embolic versus thrombotic occlusion. The necessity for diagnostic arteriography and the most appropriate method of attempting revascularization will depend in part on that differentiation. While the clinical presentation may provide important clues which allow the examiner to distinguish between thrombotic and embolic occlusions (Table 2–3), in reality establishing the correct etiology has become increasingly problematic in recent years. The incidence of rheumatic heart disease has declined, so increasingly, cardiogenic emboli originate from mural thrombi secondary to previous myocardial infarction or valve damage due to ischemic disease. In addition, in part as a consequence of the dramatic aging of the U.S. population, we are increasingly seeing acute embolic occlusions occurring in patients with preexistent chronic PAOD. In view of this situation, although in most cases of uncomplicated embolic occlusion, surgical embolectomy may be successfully performed without the necessity for preoperative arteriography, in some cases even when the most likely etiology is embolus, arteriography can provide useful information preoperatively. An angiographic study is favored by many vascular surgeons when the most likely etiology is thrombosis and when the severity of limb ischemia will allow the time necessary to perform the imaging study.

CHRONIC ISCHEMIA

Patients presenting with chronic PAOD should be characterized as experiencing either non-limb-threatening, or limb-threatening ischemia.

Non-Limb-Threatening Ischemia

Intermittent claudication, defined as pain that occurs with exercise and is relieved by rest, is the classic symptom of non-limb-threatening PAOD. Patients with intermittent claudication will, by definition, generally be asymptomatic at rest and will have no or only subtle peripheral manifestations suggestive of arterial disease. From the history, one should ascertain the walking distances at which symptoms first occur and at which the patient must first stop to rest, the time required for the pain to resolve completely with rest, the leg muscles involved, the duration of this symptomatic complaint, and any change (improvement or worsening) in recent weeks. Walking distances are remarkably stable from day to day when ambient conditions are relatively stable, so any significant worsening of symptoms will typically reflect anatomically progressive disease. In general, symptoms occur in muscles distal to the site of the occlusive process, so that from the history (and supplemented by the physical examination), one may begin to differentiate inflow (aortoiliac) from outflow (femoro-popliteal-tibial) occlusive disease. The patient's description of the discomfort may vary from a mild ache to muscle tightening to hard cramping or may be characterized as intense fatigue with numbness.[4,5]

The differential diagnosis of intermittent claudication includes a number of causes of leg discomfort. The most important and frequent differential diagnostic entity is neurogenic claudication (pseudoclaudication) due to spinal stenosis. Discomfort of neurogenic origin occurs generally in the buttock and/or thigh and descends to the calf in some patients. It may be associated with paresthesias or weakness. Often there is an antecedent history of a back disorder, and the patient may also describe positional pain with bending or stooping. Individuals with pseudoclaudication typically have a normal arterial physical examination, although on occasion one may encounter a patient with an element of arterial occlusive disease superimposed on more classic spinal stenosis symptomatology. Frequently, patients will manifest diminished ankle reflexes with reduced sensation in the first web space or lateral foot. Often the pain occurs with standing or sitting and may actually improve with ambulation, which tends to differentiate it from intermittent claudication. Venous claudication presents as an intense ache or bursting sensation, primarily in the calf, with ambulation. This discomfort is not totally relieved with a brief period of rest but rather may persist for hours. Patients with venous claudication usually have other signs of venous insufficiency such as brawny edema, lipodermatosclerosis, or ulcers, and may have a history of deep venous thrombosis. On physical examination, these patients usually have normal arterial pulsations unless there is associated arterial occlusive disease. Other differential diagnostic considerations include night cramps, muscle strain, and arthritis.

Table 2–3. Acute Arterial Occlusion: Thrombotic versus Embolic

	Thrombotic	Embolic
Onset	Progressive to sudden	Sudden
Previous symptoms	Frequent	Infrequent
Distal pulses	Absent	Absent
Countralateral extremity pulses	Frequently abnormal	Frequently normal
Cardiac disease	Common	Common

Limb-Threatening Ischemia

Limb-threatening ischemia is defined by the presence of pain at rest, nonhealing ulcers, or frank gangrene. Ischemic rest pain is an extremely debilitating symptom, characterized as an intense, continuous ache over the dorsum of the foot or toes and usually occurring after the patient assumes the supine position when going to bed. The pain is relentless and minimally responsive to oral analgesies. Patients often will attempt to augment arterial flow and relieve the pain via gravity by hanging the leg off the bed or by sleeping in a chair with the legs dependent. In these patients, severe leg edema and congestive skin changes secondary to positional stress on the extremities are not uncommon.

The patient with rest pain typically will manifest extremity hair loss, with dry, cracked skin over the toes. Pallor on elevation and dependent rubor occur commonly, and arterial pulsations are severely diminished and, in most patients, nonpalpable distally. Doppler examination shows low-amplitude monophasic or biphasic waveforms and an ABI generally less than 0.5.

The differential diagnosis of ischemic rest pain includes reflex sympathetic dystrophy (RSD) and musculoskeletal night cramps. A history of extremity trauma usually precedes the development of RSD. Typical complaints include burning or shooting pain that is exacerbated by contact with the extremity. The pain is not necessarily isolated to the dorsum of the foot, although otherwise it may closely mimic the rest pain of severe arterial insufficiency. Rubor of the involved extremity may be present, but it does not disappear when the extremity is elevated. In contrast to patients with ischemic rest pain, these patients rarely find relief by placing the extremity in the dependent position, and they usually have normal pulsations and no associated skin changes typically seen with severe arterial insufficiency.

Night cramps are a common complaint of many older individuals. This painful syndrome results in muscle spasms rather than ischemia. Historically, the cramps occur at rest, usually at night, often awakening the patient from sleep. The calf is the most common location, but the arch and toes may also be involved, thus mimicking ischemic rest pain. Although the onset of discomfort may be related to muscle stretching, the cramps are not altered by positional change. There are no characteristic physical findings associated with this condition, and the arterial examination is typically unremarkable.

The most advanced stage of arterial insufficiency is marked by tissue breakdown, that is, ischemic ulcerations or gangrenous necrosis of the extremity. Ischemic ulcers are most commonly found on the lateral aspects of the leg or foot, typically at pressure points, but may occur in other areas of the extremity. The ulcers are usually deep, with irregular borders and necrotic, poorly granulating bases. In most cases, these ulcerations are quite painful and often exhibit considerable suppuration.

Other types of leg ulcers, such as those caused by venous insufficiency, and neurotrophic changes must be distinguished from the ischemic ulcer. Venous ulcers are usually found on the medial surface of the ankle or leg. They develop serpiginous borders with shallow bases that often display interrupted islands of granulation tissue. There is usually only mild to moderate associated pain. By contrast, neurotrophic ulcers are small, with deep recesses, and are frequently associated with surrounding callus or pressure areas secondary to bony prominences. These ulcers have little associated pain.

The presence of tissue necrosis is frequently complicated by the development of a mixed flora infection. Ischemic ulcers usualy exhibit a yellow, shaggy base with a fibrinous exudate and may be covered by an eschar hiding frank pus. Gangrene may present in a dry, dessicated state, which causes minimal pain and rarely presents as a major source of infection; alternatively, wet gangrene with infection may be present. Wet gangrene frequently is associated with systemic signs of infection, including elevated temperature and leukocytosis. The necrotic area is suppurative and usually malodorous. The necrotic cavity may penetrate to a bone or joint space. Pain is severe, usually arising from inflammation at the transitional area with viable tissue, and is very difficult to control with oral analgesics. Diabetics are at increased risk of fulminant foot infections from infected ischemic ulcers or active gangrene. These infections often begin in plantar or web space lesions (see Chapter 20).

It is not widely recognized that lower extremity edema may be associated with advanced PAOD. Patients who suffer from rest pain often resort to sleeping in the sitting position, which commonly results in significant morning pedal edema, as noted above. However, the swelling typically resolves with leg elevation. This dependent edema must be distinguished from the chronic edema of venous insufficiency, in which the swelling is minimal in the morning and worsens as the day progresses. On the other hand, lymphedema tends to be constant. Finally, because many of these patients have severe cardiac disease, some element of congestive heart failure may be contributing to the edema experienced by patients with severe arterial insufficiency.

It is important to differentiate ischemic ulcers from tissue loss due to venous insufficiency. Most patients with venous ulcers have a history of prior venous thrombosis or varicose veins. Ulceration typically occurs in the perimalleolar area of the medial aspect of the leg and is often associated with dark pigment deposition, brawny edema, and lipodermatosclerosis. In addition, venous ulcers are usually larger than ischemic ulcers, and while a fibrinous exudate may be present, some granulation tissue is usually seen at the base. Palpation of arterial pulses may be difficult in these patients due to the location of the ulcers and the associated edema, although in most patients with venous ulcerations arterial perfusion is completely within normal limits.

REFERENCES

1. Bates B. The peripheral vascular system. In: Bates B, Bickley L, Hoekelman R, eds. *A Guide to Physical Examination and History Taking*, 6th ed., vol 1. Philadelphia: JB Lippincott; 1995:274–276.
2. Logerfo F, Coffman J. Vascular and microvascular disease of the foot in diabetes. *N Engl J Med* 1984;311:1615–1618.
3. Rutherford RB, Flanigan DP, Gupta SK, et al. Suggested standards for reports dealing with lower extremity ischemia. *J Vasc Surg* 1986;4:80–94.
4. Porter J, Taylor L. *Basic Data Underlying Clinical Decision Making Vascular Surgery*, vol. 1. St Louis: Quality Medical, 1994.
5. Rutherford R. The vascular consultation. In: Rutherford R, ed. *Vascular Surgery*, 4th ed., vol 1. Philadelphia: WB Saunders, 1995:2–5.

3

The Role of the Vascular Laboratory in the Evaluation of the Patient with Peripheral Arterial Occlusive Disease

Marshall E. Benjamin, M.D., R.V.T.
Gail P. Sandager, R.N., R.V.T.
William R. Flinn, M.D.

Noninvasive vascular testing has had an important impact on the evaluation of patients with known or suspected peripheral arterial disease (PAD). In the past, patients with a history or physical findings suggestive of PAD often had arteriography as their only option for further diagnostic testing. Arteriography produced anatomic confirmation of PAD but provided no hemodynamic information that would allow a quantitative assessment of the severity of the disease in an individual patient, or help determine the need for treatment. Contrast arteriography also involves potential risks, discomfort, and expense and is not essential in most cases. Today in dedicated vascular laboratories, noninvasive diagnostic testing is available for the evaluation of patients with virtually all vascular disorders. Noninvasive testing can confirm the presence of significant arterial occlusive disease, provide information about the anatomic distribution of occlusive lesions, quantitate the severity of the limb ischemia, and provide information about possible treatment options—all without subjecting the patient to any risk or discomfort. Noninvasive vascular testing can be used to identify patients who will benefit from more invasive diagnostic evaluation, such as arteriography, or possibly to select patients who may be eligible for treatments such as percutaneous transluminal angioplasty (PTA) or bypass surgery.

Preliminary noninvasive evaluation of patients with suspected PAD may be performed at the bedside or in the office setting. Indeed, a thorough physical examination is always the first noninvasive examination. However, pulse palpation and the accurate identification of aneurysms or other vascular pathology by physical examination alone can be inaccurate. The simplest noninvasive vascular testing tool is the hand-held, continuous-wave (CW) Doppler flowmeter, which is relatively inexpensive and uncomplicated. A modest understanding of this instrumentation and some of its limitations provides the practicing clinician with an accurate interpretation of the findings in a setting outside the dedicated vascular laboratory. More recently, the routine use of duplex ultrasound (including color-flow scanning) in the vascular laboratory has added a new and much more sophisticated element to noninvasive vascular testing by supplying more specific anatomic and physiologic information. Duplex scanning technology is not routinely available in the office setting, and it is important for the practicing physician to understand the specific diagnostic information that this technology can provide. A description of the standard noninvasive examination for evaluation of patients with PAD in the extremities follows. Exams with special applications will also be described, and strategies for the initial evaluation as well as the long-term follow-up of patients treated for PAD will be explained. It is hoped that this discussion will provide a series of algorithms so that the practicing physician can utilize most effectively and efficiently the diagnostic testing modalities available in the modern vascular laboratory.

PRINCIPLES OF DOPPLER ULTRASOUND APPLICATIONS

CW Doppler

The simplest and most versatile noninvasive vascular evaluations are performed using the CW Doppler ultrasound probe. In almost all applications, the Doppler probe consists of a transmission source that emits ultrasound waves at a fixed frequency (F) and a receiving crystal to collect the reflected sound waves (Fig. 3–1). Ultrasound waves are transmitted into the soft tissues and reflected off moving targets, theoretically the red blood cells that are circulating within a vessel at a given velocity (V). The Doppler equation reflects the observation that the frequency of transmitted ultrasound will be altered, or shifted, when it is reflected off the moving targets (red blood cells) and that this measured *Doppler frequency shift* (f_D) will be proportional to the

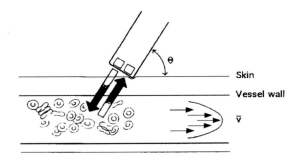

$$f_D = \frac{2FV\,(\cos \emptyset)}{c}$$

f_D = Doppler frequency shift

F = Frequency of transmitted ultrasound

V = Velocity of blood flow

$\emptyset$ = Angle of the incident ultrasound beam

c = Speed of sound

$$V = cf_D \Big/ 2F(\cos \emptyset)$$

Figure 3–1. This schematic representation illustrates the basic Doppler ultrasound assessment of blood flow. The Doppler equation demonstrates that the detected frequency shift (f_D) in the reflected ultrasound is proportional to the velocity of the moving red blood cells. The more complex duplex ultrasound instrumentation allows direct, real-time calculation of blood flow velocity throughout the cardiac cycle by "solving" the Doppler equation.

velocity of the targets (velocity of blood flow). The Doppler frequency shift (f_D) becomes the fundamental measurement of virtually all vascular Doppler systems, and this f_D can then be processed in a variety of ways for clinical use. Following is a description of some of the way the f_D is processed, but it should be recognized that this description is a vast oversimplification of the principles involved, as well as of the basic research supporting those principles.

The simplest and most universally applied technique used to process the f_D is through a preamplifier/amplifier system where an audible arterial (or venous) flow signal is produced. An audible arterial flow signal allows segmental arterial blood pressure to be measured in an extremity, similar to standard blood pressure measurement by the detection of the Korotkoff sounds with a stethoscope in the brachial artery. Blood pressure measurement in the pedal arteries is not feasible using a standard stethoscope, particularly when distal arterial perfusion is compromised due to PAD. However, with most commercially available, hand-held CW Doppler flowmeters, flow will be audible in distal arteries down to a perfusion pressure of 20 to 30 mm Hg. This allows perfusion pressures to be measured accurately at the ankle level even in the presence of relatively severe arterial occlusions. The highest Doppler-derived ankle systolic blood pressure is then compared to the brachial artery systolic pressure (using brachial pressure as a reflection of the patient's normal systemic pressure), and the resultant fractional comparison is termed the *ankle/brachial index (ABI)*,[1] sometimes referred to as the *ischemic index*. For example, if the ankle pressure measured from the dorsalis pedis or posterior tibial arteries is 60 mm Hg and the brachial systolic pressure is 120 mm Hg, the ABI is 0.5, and we can reliably predict that arterial perfusion to the foot is approximately 50% of normal. This simple examination can be done in the office or at the bedside. However, examination in the dedicated, noninvasive vascular laboratory will provide an increased degree of sophistication, as explained below.

In addition to the generation of an audible flow signal, simultaneous processing of the basic f_D through a frequency:voltage converter allows transmission through a strip-chart recorder and generation of flow waveforms. Arterial flow, and thus the Doppler waveform of a normal extremity arterial flow, is triphasic, with an initial phase of rapid forward flow during early systole (and a rapid deceleration during late systole). Then, during early diastole, the second phase is a brief reversal of flow caused by vessel wall elastic rebound during mid-diastole. Finally, there is a return to a low-velocity forward flow during late diastole as the third phase (Fig. 3–2). When a proximal occlusion is present, the acceleration and deceleration components have a lower slope, and there is loss of the negative flow com-

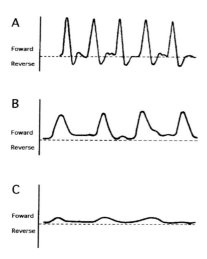

Figure 3–2. Normal and abnormal Doppler velocity waveforms. (A) The waveform of normal peripheral artery flow is triphasic but becomes biphasic (B) and then monophasic (C) with increasing proximal occlusive disease.

ponent. These changes in the flow velocity waveform progress with more severe ischemia until identifiable pulsatile flow is lost.

Pulse Volume Recordings

Pulse volume recording (PVR) is another method for noninvasive study of limb perfusion. PVR measures changes in the volume of the limb throughout the cardiac cycle; since the quantity of muscle, bone, fat, skin, and venous blood remains relatively constant over time, volume changes in the resting limb reflect changes in arterial flow. To perform this plethysmographic test, a cuff is inflated to either a known pressure or a known volume, and pulsatile waveforms are recorded from the cuffs positioned around the thighs, above and below the knee, above the ankle, and at the transmetatarsal and first toe levels.[2,3] Calibration allows for a 1-mm Hg change in cuff pressure to be reflected as a 20-mm defection on the chart recorder. The changes in volume of the respective cuffs during the cardiac cycle identify the presence of arterial occlusions by reduction in the pulsatile flow at the sites of the respective cuffs. The PVR recordings may be useful in patients with diabetes mellitus or other causes of diffuse vascular calcification in whom Doppler-derived ABIs may be unreliable. Vascular calcification will not affect the reliability of the PVR waveform. However, since PVRs, like Doppler-derived pressures, are indirect hemodynamic measurements, precise localization of the disease is compromised, and the information obtained cannot accurately distinguish between high-grade stenosis and segmental arterial occlusion.

Duplex Ultrasound Scanning

Duplex scanning currently represents the most technologically sophisticated form of noninvasive vascular testing. Duplex scan technology was initially developed for the diagnosis of extracranial carotid artery occlusive disease, but it has been adapted for noninvasive diagnosis in a wide variety of vascular disorders. The most recent application has been for the diagnosis of acute venous thrombosis, where it has virtually eliminated the need for venography in the majority of cases. Duplex ultrasound scanning has also been used for the evaluation of PAD in the extremities, but this application has been much more selective, as will be discussed below.

Duplex scanning, as the name implies, has two major components: (1) B-mode ultrasound imaging and (2) pulsed-Doppler frequency spectral analysis. The B-mode imaging component is identical to the standard ultrasound imaging that has been used to evaluate the gallbladder, pancreas, aorta, and other organs. Direct ultrasound imaging of specific vessels selected for examination allows a more accurate and specific Doppler examination. The Pulsed Doppler (in comparison to CW Doppler) allows a focused sampling of the f_D information directly from vessels using the B-mode ultrasound image as a guide. In combination, duplex scanning facilitates an image-directed Doppler exam of specific arteries or their branches. The critical importance of this combination becomes evident if one thinks about a Doppler exam of the neck. The hand-held Doppler instrument would readily allow auscultation of an arterial flow signal in the neck along the course of the carotid artery, but there would be no way to determine specifically from which artery (eg, internal carotid or external carotid) that signal originated. However, by first imaging the vessels, the duplex scan allows specific, individual Doppler examination of the common carotid, external carotid, and internal carotid arteries.

Pulsed-Doppler spectral analysis, the second component of the duplex scan, is simply a more sophisticated way of processing the basic f_D information. The microprocessor units in available instruments allow on-line analysis of the f_D changes throughout systole and diastole in the area of the vessel being examined. The Doppler equation is simultaneously solved (Fig. 3–1), allowing display of the arterial flow velocities and flow-velocity waveforms as a representation of the distribution of the spectrum of different velocities of blood flow throughout systole and diastole. It is known from experimental observations and from direct clinicial correlations that arterial occlusive lesions of progressive severity are associated with characteristic changes in systolic and diastolic flow velocities. Thus, from measurement of specific components of the flow-velocity waveforms, such as peak systolic velocity or end-diastolic velocity, it is possible to predict the severity of a focal arterial occlusive lesion. The image-directed sampling provided by the B-mode scan allows the examiner to identify the precise anatomic location of the lesion.

Further sophistication and clinical usefulness has been added to duplex ultrasound technology by the development of *color-flow* or *color-Doppler* systems, which arbitrarily assign colors to the in vivo Doppler-derived flow velocities based on the direction and the absolute velocity of flow. In a typical vascular examination, flow toward the ultrasound probe (arterial) would be assigned red, and flow away from the probe (vein) would be assigned blue. Variations in hue are produced by significant variations in flow velocities, such as the marked increase in velocity produced by the turbulent flow across a focal stenosis. Color-flow systems provide several advantages. They allow a more rapid identification of standard vascular anatomy during B-mode imaging, which facilitates a more efficient examination. They also allow more rapid identification of areas of arterial pathology by the visual identification of color changes (produced by the blood-flow velocity changes) that signal the presence of focal areas of turbulence produced by severe disease. Finally, these systems allow the visual identification of areas in the artery where flow is absent (no color is seen), which would imply that the artery is occluded in that region. This latter distinction between a severe stenosis and a complete occlusion of an arterial segment may have implications for the subsequent management of the lesion.

All or most of the technologies discussed above are employed in the modern noninvasive vascular laboratory, although different techniques are utilized in different clihnical situations. Other refinements or adjunctive studies may also be performed to increase the accuracy of the overall diagnostic evaluation of each patient. In the case of PAD of the extremities, this might include treadmill exercise testing for patients with claudication, or a cold stimulation test to evaluate patients with suspected Raynaud's phenomenon in the hands. The following discussion will emphasize the standard noninvasive vascular laboratory examinations to assess PAD in the extremities so that the practitioner may select the most useful and appropriate studies for evaluation of the individual patient and understand some of the limitations of these examinations.

PERIPHERAL ARTERIAL TESTING

Standard Noninvasive Examination: Lower Extremity Arterial Exam

The standard lower extremity arterial examination consists of a combination of Doppler-derived segmental

arterial pressures and flow waveforms using the CW Doppler. Flow waveforms are recorded at the common femoral, popliteal, posterior tibial, and dorsalis pedis arteries. Segmental pressures are measured at the popliteal and ankle levels (Fig. 3–3), and ABIs are recorded for both pedal vessels. A part of the standard examination frequently overlooked by clinicians is that the brachial systolic pressure is recorded from both arms of each patient, and the ABI is calculated from the higher brachial pressure. This is done to avoid the possibility of a falsely reduced brachial pressure that might be produce by a proximal subclavian stenosis (the most frequent atherosclerotic lesion in the upper extremity). Generally, if the gradient between the arms exceeds 20 mm Hg, this will be recorded as part of the findings. Such a finding can also have other clinical implications, such as in the assessment of blood pressure control. A clinical algorithm for vascular labora-

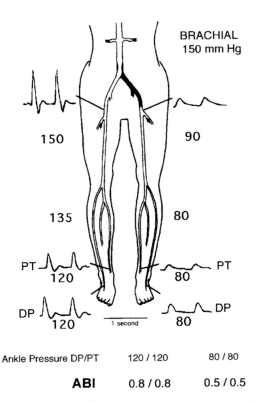

Figure 3–3. A routine lower extremity Doppler arterial examination with segmental pressure measurements and flow waveforms. Note the triphasic waveforms throughout the right limb. Velocity waveforms obtained from the left femoral and distal vessels are monophasic and have a corresponding drop in arterial pressure at the distal thigh and ankle levels. These findings are consistent with a significant occlusive lesion above the common femoral artery. Duplex scanning can then be employed to determine the presence of a left iliac artery occlusion. PT, posterior tibial artery; DP, dorsalis pedis artery.

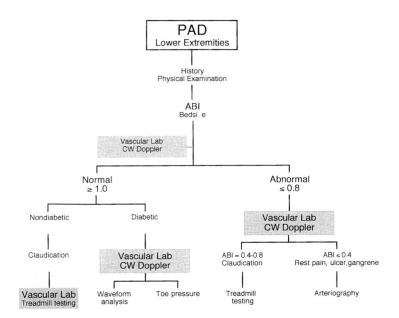

Figure 3–4. A suggested algorithm for clinical applications of the noninvasive vascular laboratory in patients with lower extremity PAD.

tory testing in patients with lower extremity PAD is provided in Figure 3–4.

Severity of Disease

The Doppler instrumentation used in the vascular laboratory is more sophisticated and reliable than portable units. The statistical variation in ABI in most laboratories is only 0.10 to 0.15, so these examinations provide reproducible, objective documentation of the presence of significant arterial occlusive lesions.[4,5] An ABI of ≤0.85 indicates the presence of some arterial occlusive disease. An ABI of 0.4 to 0.8 indicates the presence of major segmental arterial occlusions and is generally classified as moderate ischemia. Patients with typical uncomplicated vascular claudication are often found to have an ABI in this range. However, patients with cutaneous ulceration or even minor peronychial or intertriginous infection may have a significant delay or a failure to heal, with an ABI in the 0.4 to 0.6 range. Even when delayed healing occurs, it may not be permanent and recurrent skin breakdown may occur. It remains for the clinician to monitor the response to standard therapy, but when this response appears to be compromised, further, more invasive diagnostic evaluation including arteriography and a consideration of revascularization may be necessary.

Patients with an ABI at rest of ≤0.4 usually have multisegmental arterial occlusive disease. This is believed to represent more severe limb ischemia and may be associated with complaints of ischemic rest pain. Local foot infection or skin ulceration would not be expected to heal in such circumstances, and these patients are at risk for limb loss. In these cases, further diagnostic evaluation should be considered because improved arterial perfusion will be required to achieve definitive healing and, ultimately, limb salvage (Fig. 3–4).

The standard lower extremity CW Doppler examination can accurately and objectively document the presence of significant arterial occlusive disease, quantitate its severity in most cases, and help determine the anatomic location of significant occlusive lesions. As noted previously, normal Doppler waveforms are triphasic. When normal waveforms are present at the common femoral artery and those below are abnormal, we know that the patient has femoropopliteal or femorotibial occlusive disease. When normal waveforms are recorded from both the femoral and popliteal arteries and the ABI is reduced, this is indicative of infrapopliteal occlusive disease, as typically seen in diabetic patients. Monophasic waveforms throughout the lower extremity indicate the presence of proximal aortoiliac occlusions (Fig. 3–3).

One of the well-recognized shortcomings of Doppler-derived segmental pressure measurements is the presence of diffuse, severe vascular calcification. Vessel wall calcification is a natural part of the atherosclerotic process, but typically the proximal arteries are more heavily diseased and the distal arterial tree is spared. The notable exceptions to this rule include patients with long-standing diabetes mellitus and those with an associated predisposition to systemic hypercalcemia, such as that seen in chronic renal failure. Tibial vessels in these patients will be rigid and incompressible, and thus the Doppler-derived ankle pressure and the ABI will be falsely elevated, often ≥1.0. A simple ankle pressure measured in the office or at the bedside in these cases may give the managing physician the false impression that the patient has normal distal arterial perfusion. The standard examination in the vascular laboratory employs two strategies for the detection of significant foot ischemia in these patients. First, waveform analysis may demonstrate abnormal monophasic or nonpulsatile flow waveforms at the pedal vessels. This finding indicates significant arterial occlusive disease despite a normal or elevated (≥1.0) ABI. Second, forefoot or toe systolic blood pressure can be measured using specialized instrumentation and pressure cuffs. The process of vascular calcification rarely involves the digital vessels, so this technique can provide objective information about the adequacy of forefoot perfusion. However, the quantitative analysis of toe pressure measurements is not as reliable and reproducible as the standard ABI. Nevertheless, a forefoot or toe perfusion pressure ≤40 mm Hg is indicative of significant ischemia, and cutaneous lesions are unlikely to heal with this level of perfusion.[6]

Treadmill Exercise Testing

Claudication is a relatively benign symptom of PAD since population studies have indicated that few claudicants go on to develop more severe, limb-threatening ischemia or require major amputation. Nevertheless, claudication may be disabling for many patients. Overall, the functional limitations imposed by claudication are probably greatly underestimated by those whose walking is unimpaired.

Although the symptoms of lower extremity claudication are usually quite characteristic, in some cases even experienced vascular specialists may have difficulty distinguishing vascular claudication from symptoms of neurospinal compression syndromes, so-called neurogenic claudication. True vascular claudication occurs only with ambulation. Pain in the thigh or calf while sitting or recumbent is more likely due to neuropathic disorders like spinal stenosis or herniated nucleus pulposis—common clinical disorders. Similarly, the "night cramps" experienced by many elderly patients

are not related to vascular disease (see Chapter 2). It should also be remembered that patients with true vascular claudication may have a normal *resting* lower extremity vascular exam. Also, patients with known, stable PAD may have good compensatory collateral flow and normal ambulatory hemodynamics. Thus, the most accurate diagnosis of vascular claudication is provided by an ambulatory examination: the treadmill exercise test (Fig. 3–5).

The treadmill test for claudication is similar to a standard cardiac stress test, and some vascular laboratories routinely employ continuous cardiac monitoring during the period of treadmill walking. Because patients with PAD have an increased incidence of coronary artery disease, the physician must determine whether this exercise test poses any undue risk for the patient.

A standard resting lower extremity Doppler arterial examination is performed prior to treadmill exercise testing. The patient then walks on the treadmill at a speed of approximately 1 to 1.5 mi/hr and at a 10% grade. Patients are instructed to walk until significant claudication symptoms cause them to stop or for a maximum period of 5 minutes. Doppler-derived ankle systolic pressure measurements are recorded from the symptomatic limb(s) at 1-minute intervals following the cessation of exercise. An abnormal examination is indicated by a significant drop in the postexercise ankle perfusion pressure followed by a gradual return to baseline levels within 5 to 10 minutes[3,7] (Fig. 3–5). This objective demonstration of abnormal ambulatory hemodynamics is diagnostic of vascular claudication. When revascularization is elected, one can be confident that restoration of normal distal perfusion will reliably result in symptomatic relief.

Postprocedural Testing

The noninvasive vascular laboratory also provides prompt, accurate, and objective assessment of the immediate efficacy of any form of intervention, includ-

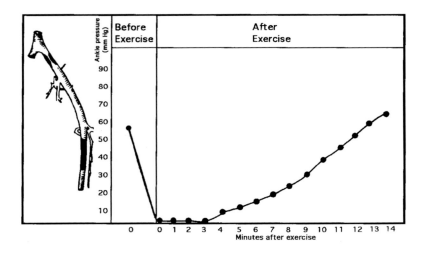

Figure 3–5. Graphic display of resting and postexercise ankle pressures in a patient with claudication. The drop in ankle pressure following treadmill exercise confirms the presence of abnormal ambulatory hemodynamics with exercise-induced ischemia.

ing medical, radiologic, and surgical therapy. These techniques also allow interval follow-up of treated patients and can serve as a baseline for evaluation of new (or recurrent) symptoms. Reliable relief of initial ischemic symptoms and/or healing of ischemic tissues depends on the provision of a measurable, hemodynamically significant improvement in distal arterial perfusion. Following endovascular (eg, PTA, vascular stent placement) treatment, a repeat Doppler arterial examination is generally performed. A postprocedural Doppler exam should demonstrate a significant improvement in the ABI (an increase ≥0.15) to be considered successful. Failure to demonstrate a measurable improvement after treatment requires further diagnostic investigation, which may include duplex ultrasound scanning (see below) or arteriography. Figure 3–6 provides a suggested plan for the noninvasive evaluation and follow-up of patients after various treatment regimens.

Upper Extremity Arterial Exam

Arterial occlusive disease occurs less frequently in the upper extremities than in the lower extremities. Atherosclerosis is the most frequent etiology of arterial occlusions in the upper extremities, but a variety of other disorders may also produce symptoms and require noninvasive evaluation. This includes patients with Raynaud's syndrome and those suspected of having thoracic outlet compression syndromes. As noted below, these clinical conditions may require more specialized testing.

The standard upper extremity Doppler arterial examination includes flow waveform recordings at the axillary, brachial, radial, and ulnar arteries. Segmental

Doppler-derived systolic pressure measurements are made at the brachial, radial, and ulnar arteries. Similar to the lower extremity examination, this allows identification of major occlusive lesions and measurement of the severity of ischemia. It also helps determine the anatomic location of the lesions.

Patients with symptoms suggestive of Raynaud's syndrome may have vasospasm, organic arterial occlusive disease of the digital vessels, or a combination of both (see Chapter 23). Examination of these patients may include digital arterial pressure measurements. A significant reduction in the resting digital arterial pressure indicates the presence of organic arterial occlusive disease, and the precise cause must then be clarified by further diagnostic evaluation. Digital ischemia may be seen with an arteritis such as Buerger's disease or a rheumatoid vasculitis; a collagen vascular disease like scleroderma; or embolization from a more proximal subclavian artery aneurysm. However, organic occlusive lesions are not produced by vasospasm alone. Patients with true Raynaud's disease (vasospasm) have normal resting digital perfusion but an intense vasospastic response to cold stimuli. This can be assessed in patients by measurement of fingertip temperature using digital thermisters. The hands are briefly immersed in ice water, and the temperature response is observed. In patients with Raynaud's disease there is a marked drop in digital temperature, as well as a prolonged time (>20 minutes) for return to the baseline temperature after immersion.

Some patients may be suspected of having arterial involvement in the thoracic outlet syndrome (TOS). This usually is due to compression of the subclavian artery by musculoskeletal abnormalities such as cervi-

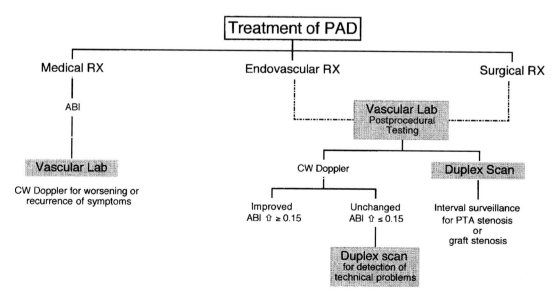

Figure 3–6. A suggested protocol for noninvasive follow-up of patients undergoing various treatments for PAD. RX, therapy.

cal ribs, the scalenus anticus muscle, or (most commonly) costo-clavicular compression between the clavicle and the first rib. These patients have normal arterial examinations at rest unless other complications (eg, embolization or arterial thrombosis) have already occurred. Specific diagnosis of these disorders requires some provocative anatomic maneuver at the time of diagnostic testing. Using a Doppler flowmeter or a photoplethysmographic pulse detector, abduction and external rotation of the shoulder are performed. These manuevers cause obliteration of the audible Doppler signal or the recorded waveform in most cases of vascular compression due to thoracic outlet compression syndrome. This very simple, noninvasive test can confirm the presence of TOS but should be specifically requested because it is not part of the routine upper extremity examination.

Special Applications: Duplex Ultrasound Scanning

Lower Extremity Testing

As noted above, duplex scanning represents a significant advance in the technological sophistication of noninvasive arterial testing. The combination of direct arterial imaging and focused, image-directed hemodynamic assessment of specific arterial occlusive lesions has led some to regard this as an "ultrasonic arteriogram." It has been suggested that duplex scanning be performed preferentially in all patients with lower extremity PAD because it provides a much more anatomically specific localization of the occlusive lesions than the standard CW Doppler examinations.[8-11] However, duplex scanning is more time-consuming and expensive than the standard lower extremity Doppler examination, and the majority of patients with PAD do not require such a detailed initial examination. Figure 3-7 is one suggested clinical algorithm for the utilization of duplex scanning in patients with lower extremity arterial occlusive disease.

Lower extremity duplex scanning may be particularly useful for evaluation of the morphology of a selected occlusive lesion. An ABI measurement alone is really a whole-limb assessment and simply identifies the presence and severity of occlusive disease. The addition of flow waveforms may help to determine the anatomic location of the lesion but does nothing to clarify the morphology of the lesion even if its anatomic location is generally known. With available endovascular treatments such as balloon angioplasty or stenting, it may be very useful to determine whether there is a stenosis or an occlusion of the involved vessel. A focal arterial stenosis is the ideal occlusive lesion for endovascular treatment, and some short-segment occlusions can also be managed using these techniques. However, long-segment occlusions or diffuse, multifocal disease generally responds less well to endovascular treatment. Duplex scanning can examine specific arterial segments and determine the presence of a stenosis or an occlusion, as well as the anatomic extent of the local disease, because it can directly image the vessel walls. The effective combination of noninvasive technologies (standard CW Doppler and duplex scanning) in selected patients can determine the presence of PAD, its severity, its anatomic location, and perhaps even

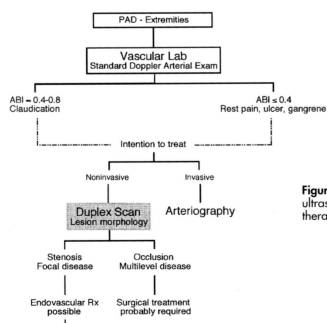

Figure 3–7. A clinical algorithm for selected used of duplex ultrasound scanning in patients with PAD requiring treatment. RX, therapy.

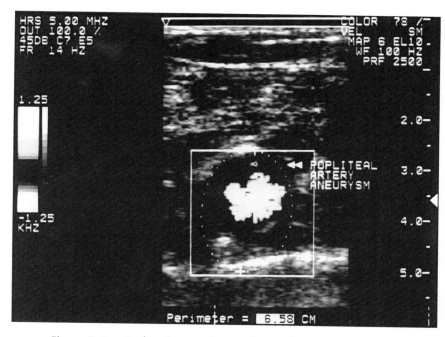

Figure 3–8. Duplex ultrasound scan of a popliteal artery aneurysm.

suggest the possible therapeutic options even before arteriography or other invasive interventions are used.[12,13]

Duplex ultrasound is also commonly used to examine the femoral and popliteal arteries for the presence of aneurysms (Fig. 3–8). Aneurysm size can be determined and mural thrombus within the lesion can be identified.

Postprocedural Testing

Lower extremity duplex scanning may also be useful in the follow-up of patients after revascularization. As noted previously, standard CW Doppler testing is an effective method for determining the initial hemodynamic improvement after lower limb PTA or bypass. However, because duplex scanning can specifically examine focal lesions, it is particularly useful for the examination of diseased arterial segments following treatment by PTA or stent placement.[14] Because there is a 10 to 40% incidence of restenosis following PTA, this noninvasive form of follow-up may be particularly useful for the early detection of recurrent lesions. Also, as noted above, duplex scanning may be employed if the post-treatment standard Doppler exam does not demonstrate a significant initial hemodynamic improvement (ie, ABI increase ≥ 0.15). Direct duplex examination of the treated lesion usually can determine the cause of failure and help determine subsequent therapeutic options.

Duplex ultrasound scanning is particularly useful in the follow-up of patients who have undergone femoropopliteal or femorotibial bypass grafting, especially using saphenous vein. (see Chapter 14). If standard

ABIs fail to demonstrate improvement immediately after bypass, duplex scanning can be used to visualize the graft directly and identify any technical problems requiring immediate revision. A duplex scan of the graft is almost routinely performed 2 to 4 weeks after discharge to serve as a baseline for further follow-up. Surveillance duplex scans of vein bypass grafts are then performed at 3-month intervals for the first 2 years in the authors' institution. Duplex scans can detect significant reductions in flow velocity within the grafts and directly identify graft stenoses (Fig. 3–9). It has been observed that up to 30% of vein grafts develop stenotic lesions,[15–18] which if not identified and repaired are likely to lead to graft thrombosis. Once vein graft thrombosis has occurred, secondary patency is poor, and far inferior to that seen after revision of the stenotic but patent vein graft. Neither clinical symptoms nor the standard ABI measurements are as sensitive as duplex scanning for detection of these lesions.[17] Duplex scan surveillance of infrainguinal vein bypass grafts is clearly useful to help extend the patency of these grafts and to prolong limb salvage.

SUMMARY

The focus of this discussion has been on atherosclerotic disease of the extremities, particularly the lower extremities, because this is the most frequent application of noninvasive testing for peripheral arterial disease. Numerous other applications of noninvasive testing, such as carotid, venous, renal, and mesenteric duplex scanning, are covered elsewhere in this text. While diagnosis still begins with a compulsory history

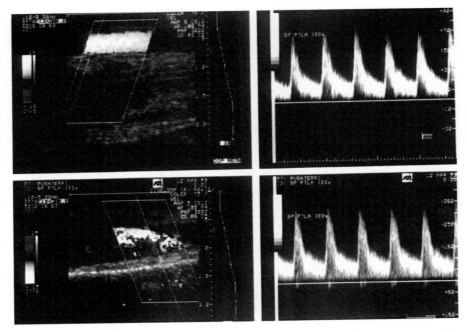

Figure 3–9. Duplex ultrasound scan of an in situ vein bypass graft revealing a graft stenosis that was detected on routine postoperative surveillance.

and physical examination, the subsequent diagnostic algorithm for patients with known or suspected vascular disorders almost always includes noninvasive vascular testing in the dedicated vascular laboratory.

REFERENCES

1. Yao JST. Haemodynamic studies in peripheral arterial disease. *Br J Surg* 1970;57:761.
2. Raines JK. Vascular laboratory criteria for the management of peripheral vascular disease of the lower extremities. *Surgery* 1976;79:21.
3. Raines JK. The pulse volume recorder in peripheral arterial disease. In: Bernstein EF ed. *Vascular Diagnosis*, 4th ed. St Louis: Mosby Year Book; 1993:534–543.
4. Esses GE, Bandyk DF. Noninvasive studies of vascular disease. In: Dean RH, Yao JST, Brewster DC, eds. *Current Diagnosis and Treatment in Vascular Surgery*. Norwalk, CT: Appleton & Lange; 1995:5–12.
5. Strandness DE Jr. Indirect noninvasive testing. In: Strandness DE, Van Breda A, eds. *Vascular Disease: Surgical and Interventional Therapy*. New York: Churchhill Livingstone; 1994:139–156.
6. Yao JST. Pressure measurement in the extremity. In Bernstein EF ed. *Vascular Diagnosis*, 4th ed. St Louis: CV Mosby; 1993:169–175.
7. Strandness DE, Zierler: Exercise ankle pressure measurements in arterial disease. In: Bernstein EF, ed. *Vascular Diagnosis*, 4th ed. St Louis: Mosby Year Book; 1993:547–553.
8. Strandness DE Jr. Noninvasive vascular laboratory and vascular imaging. In: Graor RA, Olin JW, et al, eds. *Peripheral Vascular Diseases*. St Louis: Mosby Year Book; 1991: 39–69.
9. Moneta GL, Yeager RA, Lee RW, et al. Noninvasive localization of arterial occlusive disease: a comparison of segmental Doppler pressures and arterial duplex mapping. *J Vasc Surg* 1993;17:578–582.
10. Hatsukami TS, Primozich JF, Zierler RE, et al. Color Doppler imaging of infrainguinal arterial occlusive disease. *J Vasc Surg* 1992;527–533.
11. Kohler TR, Nance DR, et al. Duplex scanning for the diagnosis of aortoiliac and femoropopliteal disease: a prospective study. *Circulation* 1978;76:1074.
12. van der Heijden FH, Legemate DA, van Leeuwen MS, et al. Value of duplex scanning in the selection of patients for percutaneous transluminal angioplasty. *Eur J Vasc Surg* 1993;7:71–76.
13. Edwards JM, Coldwell DM, Goldman ML, et al. The role of duplex scanning in the selection of patients for transluminal angioplasty. *J Vasc Surg* 1991;13:69–74.
14. Mewissen MW, Kinney EV, Bandyk DF, et al. The role of duplex scanning versus angiography in predicting outcome after balloon angioplasty in the femoropopliteal artery. *J Vasc Surg* 1992;15:860–866.
15. Bandyk DF, Cato RF, Towne JB. A low flow velocity predicts failure of femoropopliteal and femorotibial bypass grafts. *Surgery* 1985;98:799–809.
16. Bandyk DF, Schmitt DD, Seabrook GR, et al. Monitoring functional patency of in situ saphenous vein bypasses: the impact of a surveillance protocol and elective revision. *J Vasc Surg* 1989;9:286–296.
17. Idu MM, Blankenstein JD, de Gier P, et al. Impact of a color-flow duplex surveillance program on infrainguinal vein graft patency: a five-year experience. *J Vasc Surg* 1993;17:42–53.
18. Mattos MA, van Bemmelen PS, Hodgson KJ, et al. Does correction of stenoses identified with color duplex scanning improve infrainguinal graft patency? *J Vasc Surg* 1993;17:54–66.

4

The Role of MRA in the Evaluation of Peripheral Arterial Occlusive Disease (PVD)

Constantin Cope, M.D., F.A.C.P.
Richard A. Baum, M.D.

There has been rapid progress in the development of magnetic resonance imaging in the past two decades. Magnetic resonance angiography (MRA) has also been intensively investigated as a noninvasive technique for imaging the extra- and intracranial cerebral circulation, the heart, the thoracic and abdominal aorta, and the main abdominal visceral arteries, as well as the superior and inferior vena cava and their major inflow veins. Little attention was initially paid to MR study of the peripheral circulation because, firstly, PVD workup with Doppler ultrasound and arteriographic examinations was considered perfectly satisfactory and, secondly, because it was thought that the lively triphasic blood flow of the iliofemoral arterial circulation would give rise to too many artifacts.

Following an interpretive error that led to surgical exploration of the wrong leg compartment, we became interested 6 years ago in MRA of the leg with the hope that it could be used to better identify trifurcation vessel segments in patients with severe PVD. To our surprise, we found that MRA provided excellent depiction of infrainguinal arteries in patients with severe PVD due to the slow monophasic blood flow, with no reversal of direction during diastole. Sheline et al[1] showed that MRA axial cuts obtained by two-dimensional time of flight (2D TOF) were accurate in identifying named arteries or arterial segments below the knee (Fig. 4–1).

Despite subsequent prospective studies supporting the accuracy [2–4] and potential cost effectiveness[5] of peripheral MRA, many still feel that this technique does not yet have a role in the workup for PVD because it cannot match the combined precision of standardized, noninvasive studies and arteriography[6] and is not cost efficient. We would like to point out some of the limitations of these accepted studies to provide a back-ground for presenting the potential usefulness of MRA for complementing and at times replacing arteriography.

STANDARD PVD WORKUP

Although a good history and physical examination are invaluable for patients with possible PVD to make the diagnosis and assess the degree of impairment, the error rate for this initial evaluation can be significant.[7] Intermittent leg claudication must be clearly differentiated from the symptomatology of such diseases as osteoarthritis and neurologic entrapment syndromes. The noninvasive vascular laboratory can provide important physiologic data that can document the diagnosis and correlate it with the patient's symptoms. In the final analysis, it can provide objective, repeatable values that allow the clinician to estimate the severity and general location of PVD and is therefore most valuable as a guide for initial assessment and follow-up during conservative treatment, for timing interventions, and for evaluating postintervention benefits and long-term results. Although duplex ultrasound scanners can be used to image lesions and estimate local velocity changes by pulsed Doppler, their resolution is generally insufficient to gauge the degree of vascular stenosis except in very superficial vessels and subcutaneous bypass grafts.[8] Although these noninvasive tests correlate well with the severity of ischemic symptoms, they do not differentiate focal lesions from long segmental occlusions and can be inaccurate for evaluating suprainguinal lesions and calcified vessels.

Once the decision has been made to intervene, it is important to have a complete vascular map extending from the aorta to the toes in order to study the loca-

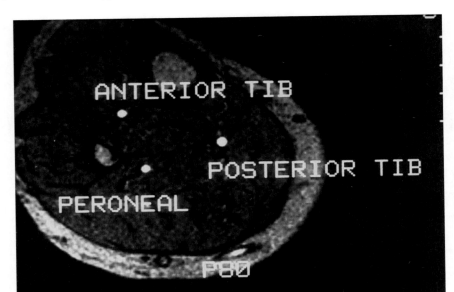

Figure 4–1. 2D TOF axial section of the midcalf shows the known relationship of named vessels to bone and muscle.

tion and extent of significant stenoses, as well as the adequacy of the peripheral runoff. For the past 50 years, contrast arteriography has been considered the gold standard for presurgical examination of the diseased iliofemoral vascular tree. Although in earlier years angiographers often had difficulty clearly demonstrating vessels below the midcalf due to the use of primitive serial screen film techniques and underpowered X-ray generators, these inferior studies were usually adequate in an age when the femoropopliteal graft was the mainstay of the vascular surgeon and amputation was often the rule when there was severe infrapopliteal vascular disease. However, when it became technically possible and safe to perform percutaneous balloon angioplasty of trifurcation vessels and/or to insert in situ or reversed long vein grafts surgically in the lower leg and foot, it then became essential for the angiographer to demonstrate distal target vessels accurately.[9] It has also become important to assess the quality of the pedal runoff in order to predict the likelihood of limb salvage. The equipment necessary to clearly opacify the lower leg vessels was developed in the past 10 to 15 years because of technological advances in X-ray generators, increased sensitivity of films and screens, and, most importantly, the introduction of sophisticated electronic digital subtraction angiography (DSA). Although the cut film technique provides excellent resolution, it requires the injection of a large volume of contrast medium into the lower aorta or iliac arteries,[10] which may have to be repeated because of bolus mistiming in the lower leg or the need to identify a poorly defined vessel segment in another projection if DSA is not available. In general, focused questions about vessels that remain after aorto-

peripheral angiography are easily answered by selective low-volume injections and digital subtraction acquisition. Because of greater sensitivity in the DSA mode, the femoral tree can be opacified equally well with smaller volumes of more dilute contrast medium. Because the flow of contrast is followed under real-time fluoroscopy and the bone is subtracted, there is less need for repeat injections unless the patient moves. In many centers, DSA is used to study the aorta, iliacs, femoral bifurcations, and lower legs, while cut films are reserved for the simultaneous vascular opacification of both legs. In a prospective study, cut film and DSA techniques were equally accurate in demonstrating significant peripheral vascular disease.[11] High-quality peripheral arteriograms can be obtained in most patients with moderate to fairly advanced atherosclerotic disease. We still find, however, a certain number of patients with severe pain at rest with significant inflow and diffuse arterial disease in whom it is difficult to opacify distal named vessels despite the use of large contrast volumes, vasodilators, or reactive hyperemia. In cases where only fine collaterals are visualized at the ankle, it is not possible to rule out occult vessels suitable for bypass except by intraoperative arteriography. There has been ample documentation in the surgical literature indicating that widely patent named arterial segments may often be demonstrated by intraoperative arteriography or ultrasound that previously either could not be opacified or appeared to be of such poor quality that they were of no use for planning bypass surgery. In clinical laboratories with state-of-the-art DSA, this problem should occur only rarely and only in instances of severe combined inflow and outflow occlusions. Patel et al make the additional point that even at intra-operative arteriography, the reconstituted pedal arch may be missed if vessel cannulation is not performed close enough to the ankle.[12] It is also interesting to note that, in a series of 94 diabetics who were carefully studied with DSA for possible pedal artery bypass, patent dorsalis pedis arteries were missed in 11.5% of 104 limbs.[13]

Because patients with limb-threatening ischemia have fixed resistance to blood flow from stenoses and occlusions of named vessels, perfusion of the distal limb is mostly dependent on the adequacy of the collateral supply, which itself can vary greatly from one patient to another even when they may have the same pattern of occlusive disease. The extent of collateral flow in a diseased limb depends on many factors, such as rapidity of arterial occlusion, atherosclerotic occlusion of collateral feeders, and the potential for developing enosculating anastomoses, as well as the actions of various vascular growth factors. It has been shown that the resistance of collaterals increases with the severity of the disease. Vasodilating techniques can reduce resistance by 30% in patients with claudications but only by 5% in those with pain at rest.[14] We find, perhaps related to this pathophysiological difference, that despite the best arteriographic techniques, it is still possible in a small percentage of cases to miss patent distal tibial-pedal arteries in advanced PVD. Some of the reasons are as follows:

1. Slow blood flow prevents good distal limb opacification because of poor mixing due to stasis and layering of the heavier-than-blood contrast medium in the proximal limb, dilution of contrast medium, and loss of contrast medium in the proximal pelvic and thigh arteries and collateral beds due to sumping.
2. Certain patterns of arterial occlusion can lead to balanced or retrograde blood flow.
3. Contrast medium can be shunted away from the feet by natural arteriovenous shunts, which are commonly seen in advanced PVD.

Although diagnostic arteriography is considered a benign procedure,[15] it is associated in older patients with severe PVD[16] with a low but significant morbidity rate of 2.9%, which is mainly related to puncture site vascular damage such as thrombosis, major hematomas, pseudoaneurysms, arteriovenous fistulae, dissections, and contrast-induced renal failure.

THE STATUS OF MRA IN PVD

One of the most interesting phenomena associated with MR is its ability to image flowing blood without the need for contrast medium. Of the many sequences available for imaging blood flow, 2D TOF has been found to be the most useful for studying the lower extremity.[17] Imaging the lower extremity is ideally suited for 2D TOF because, in addition to the slow monophasic blood flow that reduces pulsatility artifacts, the vessels are straight and run perpendicularly through the axial imaging slice, a relationship that provides maximum signal intensity for flow-related enhancement.

Basic Technique

The parameters that we currently use for lower extremity MRA are as follows[18]: repetition time (TR) 33 to 36 msec, echo time (TE) 6.2 to 7.7 msec, field of view (FOV) 14 to 16 cm, and flip angle (FA) 60 degrees. A saturation band is placed inferior to the imaging section to eliminate the venous signal. To obtain high resolution of small vessels, it is important to use extremity coils (Fig. 4–2) from the midthigh down to the foot, as well as to image very thin cross sections (2 mm or less). This MRA technique is very effective in suppressing static spins (soft tissues) and enhancing moving spins (blood flow). Thus, each axial image section provides a ghostly but easily recognizable representation of muscle groups, on which is superimposed a bright cross-sectional image of flowing arterial blood (Fig. 4–1). Pedal vessels must be realigned along the long axis by plantar-flexing the foot to maintain optimal flow-related enhancement. In comparison to studies of the legs, 2D TOF studies of inflow vessels that are performed with a body coil can be of poor quality, especially when the lower aorta and the iliac vessels are markedly diseased, dilated, and tortuous. Imaging artifacts are caused by turbulence, retrograde flow, and misalignment of blood flow from the cephalocaudad axis. If the 2D TOF study is unsatisfactory, we have found that excellent images of the aortoiliac vessels can be obtained by intravenously injecting a bolus of 40 to 60 mL of gadolinium during a 20-sec breath hold, using an ultrafast three-dimensional (3D) spoiled-gradient MR technique. This eliminates most artifacts because the signal intensity of the resultant images is related only to the gadolinium T1 effects rather than to flow-related enhancement[19] (Fig. 4–3A,B). Demonstration of iliac stenosis alone may be misleading, however. The measurement of pressure gradients with and without a vasodilator challenge may be required for assessment of significance.

MRA is displayed to resemble a conventional angiogram by stacking axial images to create a 3D data set from which a maximum-intensity projection image of flowing arterial blood is derived. Although these images are essentially a quick way of reviewing the study in any projection desired, they can occasionally be misleading because small vessels and filling defects may be obscured if they are surrounded by high signal intensity from flowing blood. One should always refer back to the axial images to evaluate problem areas.

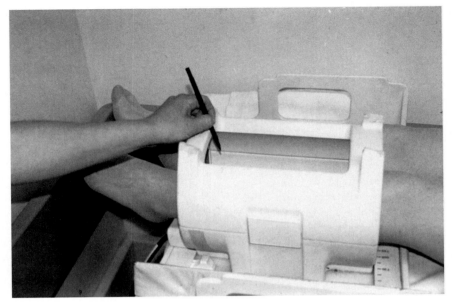

Figure 4–2.   Extremity coil used for 2D TOF MRA.

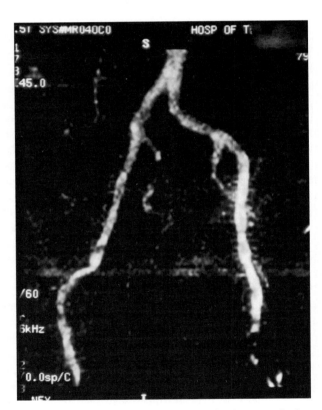

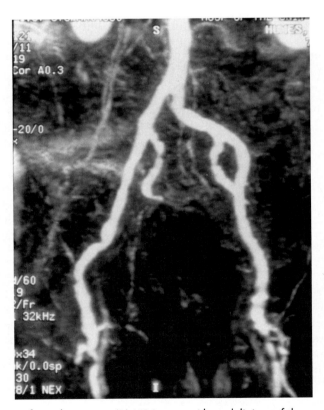

Figure 4–3.   (A) 2D TOF MRA scan of pelvic vessels shows many artifactual stenoses. (B) MRA scan with gadolinium of the same patient shows a true representation of iliofemoral disease.

MRA ARTIFACTS IN THE PERIPHERAL CIRCULATION

As with any imaging modality, it is important for the clinician to understand the pitfalls of MRA techniques and interpretation. Although artifacts can mimic vascular stenoses or occlusions, they fortunately have specific patterns that can usually be recognized, discounted, or corrected.[18] It is most important to appreciate that because maximum flow intensity occurs at a right angle to the imaging plane, it follows that any significant deviation of blood flow from the long axis will result in decreased flow enhancement and the appearance of artifacts due to in-plane flow. These can appear as pseudostenoses or staircase effects, which are typically seen in the projected images of tortuous iliacs, proximal anterior tibials, and dorsiflexed feet. Similarly, the saturation band that is used to bar the appearance of veins will also affect arterial segments that demonstrate balanced or retrograde blood flow due to significant proximal occlusive lesions. As a result, these vessels may appear to be partially or completely occluded due to spin saturation. Other commonly seen artifacts are caused by limb motion or isolated muscle contractions (focal misalignment of vessel projections), pulsatility (image ghosts or bands), metallic clips, or implants (signal void). Potential artifacts that appear on the reconstructed image projections of the vascular tree are usually easily differentiated from significant lesions by referring back to the axial source images and by having an intimate knowledge of vascular patterns of disease states.

The introduction of gadolinium-enhanced 3D TOF imaging of the lower aorta, iliacs, and proximal femoral arteries in combination with 2D TOF imaging of the symptomatic leg has markedly decreased scanning time in the magnet to an hour or less. This can now allow busy MR centers to accommodate more vascular cases on their schedule. Peripheral MRA is best accomplished in a center in which there is close collaboration between the MR radiologist, the interventional radiologist, and the vascular surgeon. Because imaging quality greatly depends on the type of equipment available and the MR programming used, it is imperative to have institutional validation of the accuracy of MRA against state-of-the-art contrast angiography before using this technique to guide percutaneous or surgical interventions.

PATIENT POSITIONING IN THE MAGNET

Following a careful history and physical examination of the patient to rule out hazardous ferromagnetic devices such as pacemakers, metal clips, prostheses, or dentures, the patient is positioned supine on the magnet table with the foot in the extremity coil (Fig. 4–2). Appropriate sedation or pain medication is administered if needed to calm the patient. For patients who are known to be claustrophobic, our MR nurse has found that premedication with Ativan (Wyeth-Ayerst Labs) followed by occasional small intravenous doses of Versed (Roche Labs) almost always allows the study to be completed. The patient's vital signs and oxygen saturation are monitored with MR-compatible equipment. Imaging of one lower extremity from the lower aorta to the foot requires six MRA stations, which take about 10 minutes each to image. It is always better to start imaging the foot and the lower leg, so that if the patient is not able to tolerate the complete examination, vital information concerning the patency of the infrapopliteal vessels will still be available for review by the clinicians. Moreover, once intravenous MR contrast is given to image the inflow vessels, one can no longer perform 2D TOF of the legs.

MRA VALIDATION

MRA has been evaluated firstly to assess its ability to image vessels that cannot be visualized or definitely identified by angiography, secondly to assess its accuracy with regard to the degree of stenosis, and finally to assess the long-term success of bypass leg grafts performed solely on the basis of MRA findings.

Identification of Vessel and Vessel Patency

MRA is more sensitive to slow blood flow (less than 2 cm/s) than arteriography because its imaging is a function of flowing protons in blood and is not limited by the delivery of viscous, hyperosmotic contrast medium through high-resistance vessels.[20] We have found that in comparative studies of patients with severe PVD, MRA was more accurate than conventional contrast DSA in identifying the presence of patent infrapopliteal and pedal arteries. Carpenter et al.[21] reported in one series that bypass surgery was successful in 18% of 51 patients with limb-threatening ischemia when a target vessel could not be identified by contrast angiography, based solely on the demonstration of occult vessels by MRA and subsequently verified by intraoperative arteriography. In assessing the outcomes and conclusions of such studies, however, the reader must make an effort to assess whether or not both the MRA and the angiography described were state-of-the-art. If not, then differences can contribute meaningfully to the ultimate conclusions. Not only could these occult vessels or vessel segments be clearly depicted in varying image projections, but their exact identity could always be recognized on the axial images by examining their well-known relationship to the muscle groups and bones. By providing the vascular surgeon with the exact location of a potential bypass target vessel, MRA may considerably shorten exploratory operative time, which may

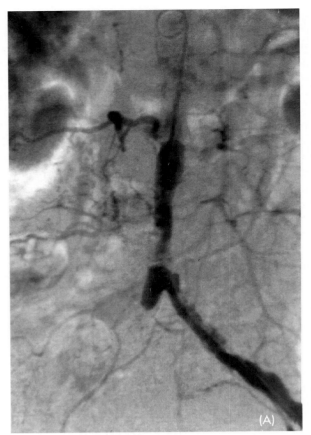

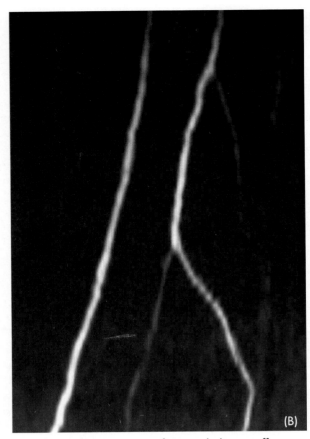

Figure 4–4. (A) Aortogram in a diabetic patient with severe iliofemoral occlusive disease; no significant right leg runoff demonstrated by DSA. (B) 2D TOF MRA, however, demonstrated excellent anterior tibial and peroneal artery runoff at the ankle.

result in lower morbidity due to decreased tissue trauma and possibly greater cost effectiveness.

Accuracy of MRA Arterial Stenoses

Due to the relatively large pixel size of the MRA digital system, the degree of stenosis in small vessels is commonly underestimated by 5 to 15% when reading the individual axial images and to an even larger extent on the reconstructed projections. For example, flow through a 0.3-mm focal narrowing in a 3-mm vessel can be overestimated as a 0.63 × 1.25 mm stenosis because this is the size of the pixel. On occasion, this vessel may even appear to be double in size if there is sufficient flow-related enhancement to straddle two voxels[18]!

Several early clinical comparative studies done in our institution to evaluate the accuracy of MRA with regard to patency, significant stenosis, and complete occlusion against standard arteriography and/or intraoperative arteriography[21,22] were very promising. In 48% of 55 limbs studied, MRA showed arterial segments which were not evident on the contrast arteriogram (Fig. 4–4A,B). Although 20 focal stenoses were identified with both techniques, it was possible to identify 7 additional stenoses by MRA that had been graded as normal or occluded by arteriography. In addition, it was possible to

identify correctly five patent arterial segments by MRA that had been misread on the arteriogram (Fig. 4–5A,B). These studies were criticized because DSA had not been used in all patients. A prospective multicenter trial using intraoperative arteriography as the gold standard was recently completed.[4] In interpreting the results of this study, the same caveat mentioned above must be applied. Multiple segments from the lower thigh to the foot were graded as "no disease," "minimally diseased with less than 50% focal stenosis," "focal stenosis greater than 50%," "diffuse significant disease," and "complete occlusion." Compared with intraoperative angiography, the sensitivity and specificity of MRA were 85% and 81%, respectively, whereas those of standard arteriography were 83% and 81%, respectively. Again, because MRA demonstrated more patent segments than percutaneous arteriography, surgical plans were changed in 15% of patients due to the MR study.

There were concerns that the angiographically occult vessels imaged solely by MRA might have too poor a pedal runoff to support long-term graft patency. Over a 4-year period, 14 such patients were compared with 138 patients who received grafts on the basis of a standard contrast arteriogram. There was no significant difference in patency rate between the two groups based

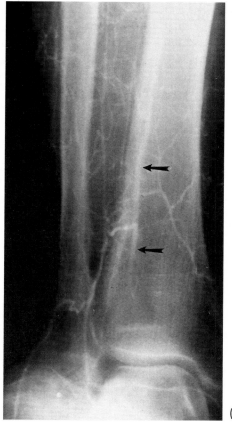

(A)

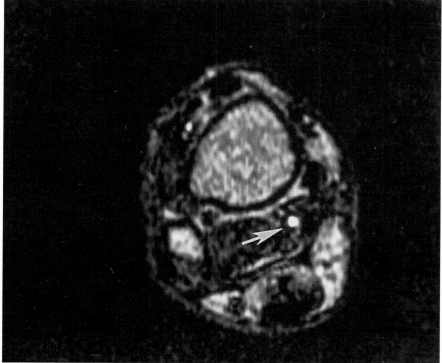

(B)

Figure 4–5.   (A) In this patient with limb-threatening ischemia, it was difficult to identify the distal crural artery (arrows). (B) On cross-sectional MRA imaging, the vessel is easily identifiable as a posterior tibial artery (arrow).

on a life-table analysis[23] with regard to either graft patency (Table 4–1) or limb salvage (Table 4–2).

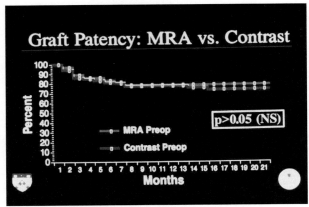

Table 4–1. Graft Patency

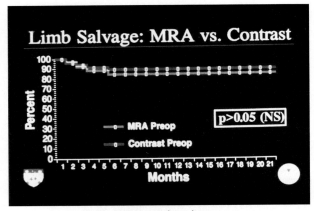

Table 4–2. Limb Salvage

SUGGESTED CLINICAL APPLICATIONS OF MRA IN PVD

At present, the most common procedure for performing MRA in our institution is to make an initial evaluation of patients with limb-threatening ischemia and/or renal failure, from which revascularization plans can be formulated by the surgeon and/or the interventional radiologist (Fig. 4–6). If, in cases of severe atherosclerotic disease, the peripheral MRA scan is of adequate quality for planning bypass surgery, this will be performed without the need for standard contrast arteriography[24] (Fig. 4–7). When appropriate, patients with less advanced disease may be scheduled for percutaneous transluminal angioplasty (PTA) (Fig. 4–8A,B), either as the sole treatment or serially in combination with bypass surgery. If the MRA scan is not considered satisfactory due to flow or metal artifacts, a "directed" arteriogram is performed to reassess solely the vascular segments that were not adequately visualized. By performing only a limited study rather than a complete aortogram and runoff examination, it is possible to greatly decrease the contrast load and the associated potential toxicity to the kidneys commonly seen in elderly and diabetic patients.

MRA can replace angiography in providing a road map for reconstructive surgery, especially involving the head, neck, and extremities. At our institution, it was possible to accurately identify suitable donor and recipient vessels in all of 38 patients, except for 1 patient with Raynaud syndrome who had severe peripheral vasospasm.[25]

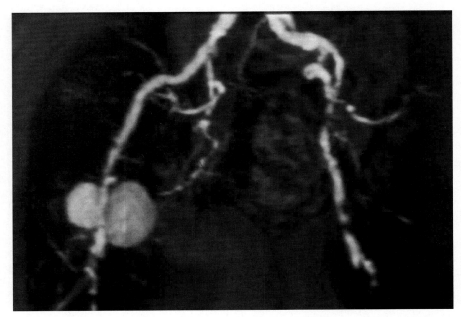

Figure 4–6. Pulsatile groin mass following cardiac catheterization. The creatinine level is elevated. MRA scan with gadolinium shows a large pseudoaneurysm of the common femoral artery.

We have found that MRA can be used to replace arteriography for the follow-up reevaluation of protocol patients who have had atherectomy and percutaneous transluminal angioplasty (PTA). In addition to providing an accurate demonstration of restenosis and occlusion, this technique makes it possible to observe healing of subintimal dissections and focal imaging abnormalities in the arterial wall.[26]

FUTURE DEVELOPMENTS

The wide acceptance of MRA at present is limited by the lack of standardization of equipment and techniques and the lack of validation of its accuracy in many centers. It cannot be considered cost effective until it can provide shorter examination times, allow simultaneous study of both legs, and effectively replace preinterventional angiography.

With further progress in the field of MRA, it is anticipated that this noninvasive technique will eventually supplant most diagnostic angiography by providing accurate and speedy vascular mapping in multiple planes as well as blood flow measurements.[27] If and when this occurs, standard contrasts arteriography will evolve into a more directed, focused procedure, in which a specific surgical question is answered or a percutaneous transcatheter therapy pursued.

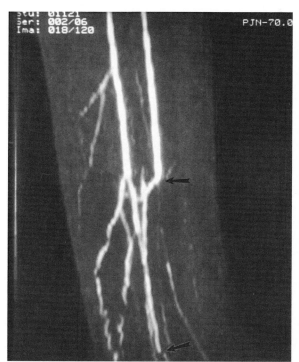

Figure 4–7. Leg MRA on a patient who suddenly developed foot ischemia shows abrupt termination of tibial vessels (arrows). A surgical embolectomy was performed without the need for a formal arteriogram.

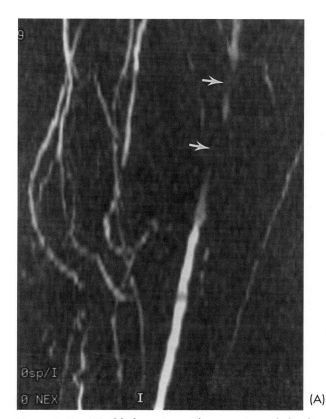 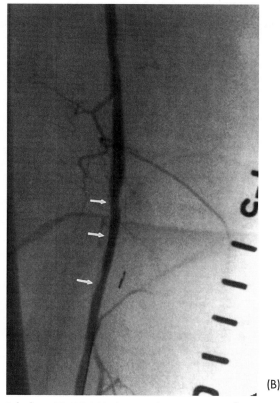

Figure 4–8. (A) Elderly patient with azotemia and claudication of the right leg. 2D TOF MRA scan shows segmental occlusion of the (SFA) (arrows) and diffuse distal arterial disease. (B) SFA recanalized by PTA-assisted atherectomy with minimal intra-arterial contrast requirements. At the 6-month follow-up, MRA showed reocclusion of the SFA.

REFERENCES

1. Sheline ME, Shlansky-Goldberg RD, Owen R. Three dimensional relationship of vessels at the ankle. *JVIR* 1991;2:20.
2. Owen RS, Carpenter JP, Baum RA, et al. Magnetic resonance imaging of angiographically occult run-off vessels in peripheral arterial occlusive disease. *N Engl J Med* 1992;326:1577–1580.
3. McCauley TR, Monib A, Dickey KW, et al. Peripheral occlusive disease: accuracy and reliability of time-of-flight MR angiography. *Radiology* 1994;192:351–357.
4. Baum RA, Rutter CM, Sunshine JH, et al. Multicenter trial to evaluate vascular magnetic resonance angiography of the lower extremity. *JAMA* 1995;274:875–880.
5. Yin D, Baum RA, Carpenter JP, et al. Cost-effectiveness of MR angiography in cases of limb-threatening peripheral vascular disease. *Radiology* 1995;194:757–764.
6. Picus D, Hicks ME, Darcy MD, Vesely TM. Magnetic resonance imaging of angiographically occult run-off vessels in peripheral arterial occlusive disease. Critical review and authors' response. *Invest Radiol* 1993;7:656–658.
7. Kepczinski RF. The role of noninvasive testing in the evaluation of lower extremity arterial insufficiency. In: Kempczinski RF ed: *The Ischemic Leg*. Chicago: Year Book Medical Publishers, 1994.
8. Moneta GL, Yeager RA, Antonovic R, et al. Accuracy of lower extremity arterial duplex scanning. *J Vasc Surg* 1992;15:275–284.
9. Ascer E, Veith FJ, Gupta SK, et al. Bypasses to plantar arteries and other tibial branches: an extended approach to limb salvage. *J Vasc Surg* 1988;8:434–441.
10. Darcy MD. Lower extremity arteriography: current approach and techniques. *Radiology* 1991;178:615–621.
11. Smith TP, Cragg AH, Berbaum KS, Nakagawa N. Comparison of the efficacy of digital subtraction and film-screen angiography of the lower limb: prospective study in 50 patients. *AJR* 1992;158:431–436.
12. Patel KR, Semel L, Clauss RH. Extended reconstruction rate for limb salvage with intraoperative prereconstruction angiography. *J Vasc Surg* 1988;2:531–537.
13. Pomposelli FB, Jepsen SJ, Gibbons GW, et al. Efficacy of the dorsal pedal bypass for limb salvage in diabetic patients: short term observations. *J Vasc Surg* 1990;11:745–752.
14. Lubbrook J. Collateral artery resistances in the human lower limb. *J Surg Res* 1966;6:427–434.
15. Hessel SJ, Adams DF, Abrams HL. Complications of angiography. *Radiology* 1981;138:273–281.
16. Egglin TKP, O'Moore PV, Feinstein AR, et al. Complications of peripheral arteriography: a new system to identify patients at increased risk. *J Vasc Surg* 1995;22:787–794.
17. Owen SO, Baum RA, Carpenter JP, et al. Symptomatic peripheral vascular disease: selection of imaging parameters and clinical evaluation with MR angiography. *Radiology* 1993;187:1–3.
18. Schnall MD, Holland GA, Baum RA, et al. MR angiography of the peripheral vasculature. *Radiographics* 1993;13:920–930.
19. Holland GA, Carpenter JP, Baum RA, et al. Breath-hold ultrafast 3D MR angiography of the abdominal aorta, renal vessels and the visceral vessels performed with gadolinium: preliminary experience. *JVIR* 1996;7:106–107.
20. Scheibler ML, Listerud J, Baum RA, et al. Magnetic resonance angiography of the pelvis and lower extremities *Magn Reson Q* 1993;9:755–764.
21. Carpenter JP, Owen RS, Baum RA, et al. Magnetic resonance angiography of peripheral runoff vessels. *J Vasc Surg* 1992; 16:807–815.
22. Hertz SM, Baum RA, Owen RS, et al. Comparison of magnetic resonance angiography and contrast arteriography in peripheral arterial stenosis. *Am J Surg* 1993;166:112–116.
23. Baum RA, Holland GA, Carpenter JP. Results of bypasses performed to angiographically occult runoff vessels detected with use of MR angiography (abstract). *JVIR* 1996;7:107–108.
24. Carpenter JP, Baum RA, Holland GA, et al. Peripheral vascular surgery with magnetic resonance angiography as the sole preoperative modality. *J Vasc Surg* 1994;20:861–869.
25. Baum RA, Holland GA, Partington M, et al. Microvascular surgery guided with MR angiography. *Radiology* 1993; 189(P):251.
26. Hertz SM, Baum RA, Holland GA, et al. Magnetic resonance angiographic imaging of angioplasty and atherectomy sites. *J Cardiovasc Surg* 1994;35:1–6.
27. Mostbeck GH, Caputo GR, Higgins CB. MR measurements of blood flow in the cardiovascular system. *AJR* 1992;159:453–461.

5

The Role of Intravascular Ultrasound in the Evaluation of Peripheral Arterial Occlusive Disease

Jeffrey M. Isner, M.D.
Kenneth Rosenfield, M.D.
Robert Schainfeld, M.D.

Advances in interventional technology have intensified the need for improved vascular imaging capabilities. Conventional contrast angiography has been the time-honored approach for lesion characterization and assessment. Angiography, however, remains limited by several factors that have been well described.[1–10] These limitations relate principally to the fact that contrast angiography depicts the vessel lumen only; plaque and vessel wall are viewed as a "negative imprint" on the contrast-filled lumen. While this allows for characterization of lumen topography, irregularities in the plaque/wall topography may only be inferred from the negative imprint. Thus angiography does not allow visualization or characterization of tissue elements below the intimal surface. This becomes particularly problematic in a vessel with diffuse disease, in which case the vessel may appear angiographically normal due to the ubiquitous distribution of atherosclerotic plaque. Furthermore, contrast angiography is limited to a single planar view per injection; therefore, information regarding the circumferential nature of the vessel–lumen interface cannot be directly recorded. Visualization of the vessel from alternative angles is possible, but only at the expense of additional injections of contrast material. As a consequence of uniplanar viewing, direct measurement of luminal cross-sectional area is not feasible; instead, estimates of cross-sectional area must be derived from algorithms based on diameter measurements obtained from a single, potentially nonrepresentative plane.

Intravascular ultrasound (IVUS) imaging offers a potential solution to many of these limitations inherent in conventional contrast angiography. IVUS is unequivically superior to contrast angiography in its ability to demonstrate detailed characteristics at the lumen–vessel wall interface, as well as to depict structures within the plaque and vessel wall. Several investigators[11–15] have demonstrated that IVUS is exquisitely sensitive in detecting plaque and other details that are angiographically "silent." IVUS now provides the opportunity for the first time to accurately assess qualitative and quantitative effects of interventional therapy in vivo.[16–29] As a result, the mechanisms by which balloon angioplasty increases luminal patency, as well as the device-specific effects of directional and rotational atherectomy, laser angioplasty, and stent deployment, may be more clearly elucidated.

Technological developments, as well as an expanding library of clinical experience with image interpretation, have facilitated the clinical applications of IVUS. In this chapter, we review some of the early studies that laid the foundation for the current and potential future applications of IVUS, describe clinical experience with IVUS, and review the result of both combination (imaging/therapeutic) devices and three-dimensional reconstruction of serial IVUS images.

IN VITRO VALIDATION OF IVUS

Images of vessels derived from IVUS typically demonstrate a layered appearance surrounding the probe, as

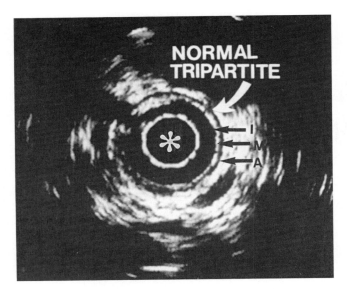

Figure 5–1. Architecture of the normal arterial wall as seen by IVUS. Asterisk indicates tranducer, positioned within arterial lumen. Three-layered appearance of a normal arterial wall includes echogenic intima (I), echolucent media (M), and surrounding adventitia (A), again echogenic.

illustrated by the appearance of the normal arterial wall in Figure 5–1. The presentation of distinct layers is a consequence of the differing acoustic reflectivity of different tissues. Dense, hyperreflective tissues are represented by bright echoes, and less dense tissues produce hypoechoic signals. While the acoustic property of each tissue is critical in determining the brightness of the signal produced, it appears that "acoustic discrepancy" or "mismatch" (e.g., a change in sono-reflectivity between adjacent structures) is the most important factor in defining the border between structures.[30] Accordingly, even a minor difference between tissue echogenicity can enable delineation of a border.

IVUS enables high-resolution imaging of the vessel wall and lumen. Because of the intraluminal location of the probe and the ability of ultrasound energy to penetrate tissues, IVUS provides information regarding the arterial wall previously unavailable by in vivo examinations. Indeed, experimental and clinical experience to date indicates that IVUS images correlate remarkably well with the results of the histologic examination, qualitatively as well as quantitatively. Numerous in vitro comparison studies have established the relationship between echos seen on IVUS images and structures seen histologically.[27,30–36] Each layer of the arterial wall can be recognized by a typical ultrasound "signature": in normal, muscular arteries, intima yields a hyperechoic signal, media a hypoechoic one, and adventitia a hyperechoic one. Siegel et al further confirmed the pathoanatomic correlates of the three layers by peeling away sequential layers of the vessel using microdissection techniques.[37,38] IVUS images were obtained at each stage of dissection and, despite the limitation that

vessels were formalin-fixed, the results supported previous assignments of the three layers to intima, media, and adventitia. Pathologic or abnormal elements also have their own characteristic ultrasound appearance: calcium, for example, consistently produces bright echo reflections with acoustic shadowing or dropout of the subjacent ultrasound signal.

In addition to the qualitative similarity between IVUS and histology, quantitative measurements of the thickness of the arterial wall correlate remarkably well; Mallery et al found correlation coefficients for total wall thickness and media alone of 0.85 and 0.83, respectively;[39] Potkin et al found a similar correlation of 0.92 for linear wall thickness, including plaque and media combined.[33] Despite these results, because the correlation between IVUS and histologic measurements for intima alone is less optimal than when intima and media are combined, there remains some controversy regarding the accuracy of IVUS in determining the thickness of the intimal layer. Several investigators have demonstrated that the inner echogenic layer by IVUS is often thicker than the intimal layer measured histologically.[40,41] The presumed cause is radial spreading or "blooming" of the ultrasound reflections; that is, the signal created by the interface between blood and intima is sufficiently bright relative to the subjacent echolucent media that it "overlaps" into the medial area.

Normal elastic arteries, in contrast to muscular arteries, do not demonstrate a distinct border between intima and media.[16,31,34,42] Consequently, the vessel wall is more homogeneous and lacks the three-layered appearance. This is likely to be due to the presence of highly sono-reflective elastic and fibrous tissue in the medial layer. It is the absence of this tissue in muscular arteries that renders the media more sonolucent and therefore creates the three-layered appearance.

Nishimura et al observed in vitro that even muscular arteries may not exhibit the typical tripartite appearance if the intima is truly normal (eg, only a few cell layers thick).[34] This finding was confirmed in vivo by Yeung et al.[43] Although this phenomenon was originally presumed to be due to the relative lack of resolution of the 20-MHz device employed in their study, work by Fitzgerald et al confirmed the absence of an intimal signal in histologically normal vessels, even using a higher-resolution 30-MHz instrument.[30] Explanted muscular coronary arteries from young patients (mean age = 27 years) had a homogeneous, nonlayered IVUS appearance; in contrast, older (mean age 42 = years) vessels demonstrated the typical tripartite layering. Histologic analysis demonstrated that an intimal thickness ≥178 μm was required to generate sufficient sono-reflectivity to be apparent on a IVUS examination; in young, normal patients, intimal thickness was typically <178 μm and was therefore sonographically silent. The implication of these findings is that intimal thickening increases with advancing age. Previous descriptions[27] of the three-layered appearance as the norm were based on studies from relatively normal vessels in patients with high-grade stenoses elsewhere; not unexpectedly, even so-called normal sites in these patients had evident intimal thickening. A second factor that may account for the increased echogenicity of the intima with advancing age is a gradual change in the composition of the intima, with an increase in echogenic material; such an age-related change would be consistent with gradual loss of compliance and elasticity. Whether due to subtle intimal thickening or to age-related changes in the composition of the intimal layer, differences demonstrated by IVUS between "young" and "old" intima underscore the ability of IVUS to identify subtle abnormalities of the vasular wall.

IVUS DETECTION OF "SILENT" PLAQUE

Studies in our own laboratory,[27] as well as those by Tobis et al,[44] Nissen et al.[45] and Davidson et al,[11] have shown that IVUS frequently demonstrates plaque not detected angiographically. Davidson et al observed that among 46% of patients in whom plaque was identified by IVUS, the sites examined were normal by angiography. In reports[14,46] comparing IVUS examinations to angiographic studies in cardiac transplant recipients, St. Goar et al demonstrated that among patients studied 1 year after cardiac transplantation, all exhibited intimal thickening by IVUS.[46] Despite this, corresponding angiograms were normal in 42 of the 60 patients studied; in 21 of the 42, the thickening was severe or moderate. Angiography was likewise found to be less sensitive than IVUS for assessment of progressive intimal thickening in transplant recipients.[47] The fact that diffuse, uniform intimal thickening is not detected angiographically has been documented in multiple previous angiographic–histologic correlative studies.[6,9] Interestingly, of the 20 patients studied by St. Goar et al within 1 month after transplantation, the intima was visualized in only 7 (35%); this is consistent with the findings described above regarding the "invisible"[48] nature of the intima on the IVUS exam in young, normal, muscular arteries and suggests that the thickness of the intimal layer was <178 µm in these vessels (ie, below the resolution of the IVUS instrument).

In our own experience in imaging patients during interventional procedures, the finding of angiographically "silent" plaque has been the rule rather than the exception. Angiographically normal sites that are adjacent to lesions and that would typically be identified as "normal reference vessels" are almost always significantly diseased by IVUS. Again, this highlights one of the major liabilities of angiography: the degree of disease at one site is typically (and for lack of any other valuable standard) evaluated in relation to a *normal-appearing* adjacent site.[5,27]

TISSUE/PLAQUE CHARACTERIZATION

Previous studies have attempted to use IVUS to determine the composition of plaque.[22,31,33,34,39] Fibrous plaque appears as bright, homogeneous echos. Calcific deposits clearly and consistently generate intensely echogenic bright signals, which create an "acoustic shadow" that shields subjacent structures. In our experience, reproducible characterization of plaque as fibrous versus "fatty" is not as consistently possible by IVUS; this is almost certainly due in part to the fact that few plaques are ever purely fatty, and the lipid component of most plaques is, in fact, minor. In occasional cases, identification of thrombus by IVUS has been well documented.[20] Although some investigators have suggested that thrombus may be regularly distinguished from low-density plaque,[49] we have not found any reliable characteristics to differentiate these two entities. Indeed, the appearance of thrombus may be variable even in the same patient. Seigel et al likewise found IVUS to be insensitive for the identification of thrombus.[35] Detection of thrombus and associated unstable plaque appears to be one area in which angioscopy is superior to both IVUS and angiography.[50,51]

In occasional cases, IVUS may be uniquely informative with regard to details of plaque/wall pathology. The images shown in Figure 5–4, for example, were recorded from a patient with onset of disabling claudication; hypoechoic foci that suggested plaque rupture and hemorrhage were responsible for the patient's accelerated symptoms[52] (Fig. 5–2). Tissue obtained by directional atherectomy documented findings of plaque fissure and hemorrhage (Fig. 5–3), confirming plaque rupture as the mechanism for the patient's acute onset of symptoms.

Preliminary investigation using so-called back-scatter analysis and ice-pick imaging may better define the acoustic properties of given tissues and allow more reproducible and accurate tissue characterization in vivo.[53]

UTILITY OF IVUS FOR QUANTIFICATION OF VESSEL DIMENSIONS

The most critical advantage of IVUS for clinical work derives from its unequivocally superior ability to define luminal dimensions, particularly cross-sectional area. Early in vitro studies by Nishimura et al demonstrated the accuracy (correlation coefficient = 0.98) of IVUS lumen measurements compared to histology.[34] Nissen et al, using live animals, found a correlation for diameter between quantitative angiography and IVUS of 0.98 for normal sites and 0.89 for experimentally induced concentric stenoses.[45] Subsequent studies in

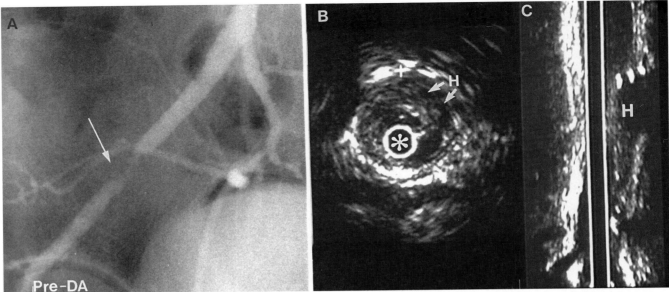

Figure 5–2. Angiographic and intravascular ultrasound findings in a patient with crescendo claudication. (*A*) Diagnostic arteriogram showing irregular, high-grade stenosis (*arrow*) in right external iliac artery. (*B*) Two-dimensional intravascular ultrasound image (asterisk indicates the ultrasound transducer) obtained before atherectomy shows heterogeneous plaque with hypoechoic foci that are consistent with plaque hemorrhage (H, *arrows*), suggesting plaque rupture as a possible mechanism for patient's recent onset of symptoms. (*C*) Three-dimensional reconstruction of serial intravascular ultrasound images showing right external iliac artery narrowed by segmental stenosis that abuts ultrasound catheter, encroaching on lumen (hypoechoic foci of plaque hemorrhage, H).

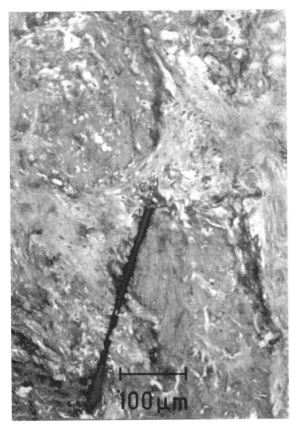

Figure 5–3. Histopathologic findings implicating plaque rupture as the cause of crescendo claudication in the patientin Figure 5–2. Atherectomy specimen from the right iliac artery shows foci of plaque hemorrhage within a fibrous, hypocellular plaque.

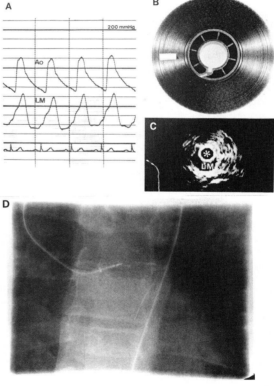

Figure 5–4. IVUS obviates the need for multiple orthogonal views. (*A*) In this patient, recurrent damping of coronary arterial pressure was observed upon engaging left main (LM) coronary artery. (*B*) Ambiguous angiographic appearance of LM required multiple angulated projections, resulting in protracted cine recording. (*C*) IVUS inspection of LM promptly excluded significant LM stenosis. (*D*) Cine frame of IVUS catheter in LM coronary artery. (Ao, aorta; *, IVUS catheter).

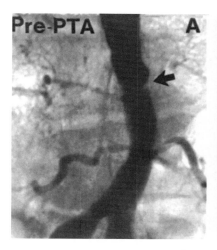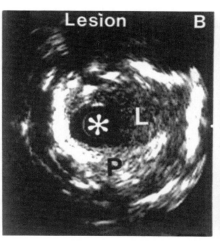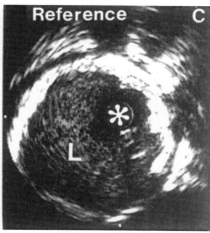

Figure 5–5. Superior imaging of an eccentric aortic lesion by IVUS compared to angiography. This 63-year-old woman presented with accelerated bilateral buttocks claudication, occurring at one or two blocks. (A) Conventional anteroposterior angiography failed to disclose any significant stenosis; mild irregularity (arrow) was seen within the distal aorta. After a large pressure gradient was discovered, IVUS exam was performed: (B) IVUS image depicting focal, eccentric plaque (P) narrowing the lumen (L) in distal aorta. (C) IVUS from a reference site distal to stenosis depicts normal lumen dimensions. Postangioplasty/stent, gradient and symptoms resolved. *, IVUS catheter.

humans found similarly close correlations (0.80 to 0.95) between cross-sectional area in normal or near-normal vessels measured by IVUS versus quantitative angiography.[11,15,54] Diseased, nondilated vessels demonstrated a smaller but still respectable correlation (r = 0.86).[15] While these data demonstrate a good *correlation* between cross-sectional area measured by IVUS and measurements derived from quantitative angiographic algorithms, the *absolute* values for area may differ substantially. Furthermore, because algorithms developed for quantitative angiography fail to address the problems posed by diffusely diseased vessels,[7] the *relative* degree of compromise of a given site may be better determined by IVUS.

To the extent that IVUS may directly demonstrate luminal cross-sectional area in cases in which angiography is complicated by certain anatomic factors, IVUS may be useful as a *diagnostic* tool. Angiographic assessment of the left main coronary artery, for example, has been a well-documented[5] source of ambiguity. IVUS imaging has been useful in such cases for elucidating the extent of luminal compromise[55] (Fig. 5–4). IVUS may also clarify lesion severity in instances in which the presence of bends, vessel overlap, or branch points obscures the border of contrast during angiography (Fig. 5–5). IVUS can also be particularly helpful when it is necessary to define components of the arterial wall. While difficulty in assessing pathology in the tortuous coronary tree is not uncommon, IVUS may be specifically useful for defining the severity of aorto-ostial lesions in renal and mesenteric vessels[56] (Figs. 5–6, 5–7); stenoses at these sites are often difficult to visualize angiographically due to their proximity to the aorta,

the brisk flow of contrast, and the abundance of calcium.

Postintervention, there is significantly more discrepancy between vessel dimensions determined by IVUS and angiography.[57] This was graphically demonstrated in the assessment of 13 consecutive patients, in whom the results of balloon (10) or laser (3) angioplasty were quantified by both quantitative angiographic analysis and intravascular ultrasound.[23] Minimal luminal diameter and cross-sectional area were calculated for interventional sites and nearby reference sites. Corresponding ultrasound frames from both interventional and reference sites were digitized, and the minimal luminal diameter was measured directly; cross-sectional area was obtained by tracing the perimeter of the lumen. Luminal diameter for reference sites measured 3.9 mm by IVUS versus 3.3 mm by quantitative angiography ($p < 0.05$). Regression analysis disclosed a correlation coefficient of 0.87. For cross-sectional area of *reference sites*, the absolute difference between ultrasound and angiography—12.6 versus 9.6 mm^2—was also statistically significant ($p < 0.05$). Regression analysis disclosed a correlation coefficient of 0.92, similar to that calculated for analysis of the luminal diameter. Luminal diameter for *interventional sites* measured 2.8 mm by IVUS versus 1.8 mm by angiography ($p < 0.01$). Regression analysis disclosed a poorer correlation—0.62—than that calculated for reference sites. Similarly, for cross-sectional area of interventional sites, there was a highly statistically significant difference between absolute measurements made by ultrasound (6.9) versus quantitative angiography (2.8; $p < 0.01$).

There is good reason to believe that cross-sectional area measurements are more accurate by IVUS than by

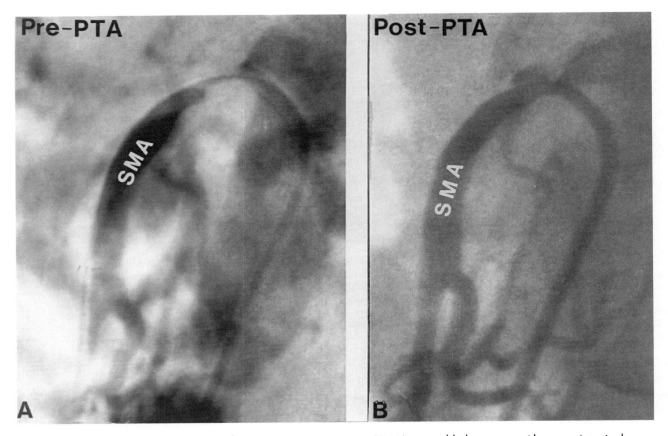

Figure 5–6.   Balloon angioplasty (PTA) of a superior mesentic artery (SMA) in an elderly woman with severe intestinal angina. (*A*) Selective angiography before PTA demonstrates critical ostial stenosis. The angiogram depicted was obtained only after test injections in many other, less optimal angles. (*B*) Post-PTA plaque fracture is evident. Presence and distribution of calcium are difficult to discern by angiography and fluoroscopy.

quantitative angiography, especially postintervention. Figure 5–8 illustrates certain of the advantages inherent in IVUS imaging. First, IVUS provides accurate delineation of luminal borders and obviates the need for multiple orthogonal angiographic views. Second, IVUS provides the ability to directly planimeter cross-sectional area, eliminating the dependence on algorithms that derive area from diameter measurements, making potentially incorrect assumptions about luminal geometry. Third, in contrast to quantitative angiography, where the catheter used for calibration may be located at a distance from the segment being measured, with IVUS the calibration instrument is, by definition, within the plane of measurement. Fourth, with IVUS, the area being measured occupies nearly the entire field of view on the screen; in contrast, for angiographic analysis, the vascular region of interest involves only a small fraction of the cine frame from which it is measured.

UTILITY OF IVUS TO DEFINE THE MECHANISM OF BALLOON ANGIOPLASTY

The most extensive clinical experience with IVUS to date, and the application in which IVUS appears to

offer the greatest practical clinical utility, is in the assessment of the intravascular effects of percutaneous therapy in coronary and peripheral vessels. Contrast angiography, while routinely performed pre- and postinstrumentation, provides only a profile of luminal diameter rather than depiction of cross-sectional area; this fact, along with other methodological limitations described previously,[1,2,4–6] has compromised its usefulness for the study of angioplasty mechanisms. In vitro studies have demonstrated that IVUS consistently provides exquisite detail regarding morphologic alterations in the arterial wall and subjacent plaque resulting from the barotrauma of balloon inflation.[33,36,58–60]

Experience with in vivo imaging postdilation has confirmed the in vitro data. In the few patients studied at necropsy after (PTA) in whom IVUS had also been performed, IVUS images displayed the identical morphologic abnormalities seen by light microscopy[60,61] (Fig. 5–9). The fact that IVUS routinely depicts tomographic full-thickness images of the arterial wall allows one to gain—in vivo—a perspective similar to that achieved by histologic examination. Furthermore, the ability to perform serial examinations in vivo enables documentation of pathologic alterations attributable to specific

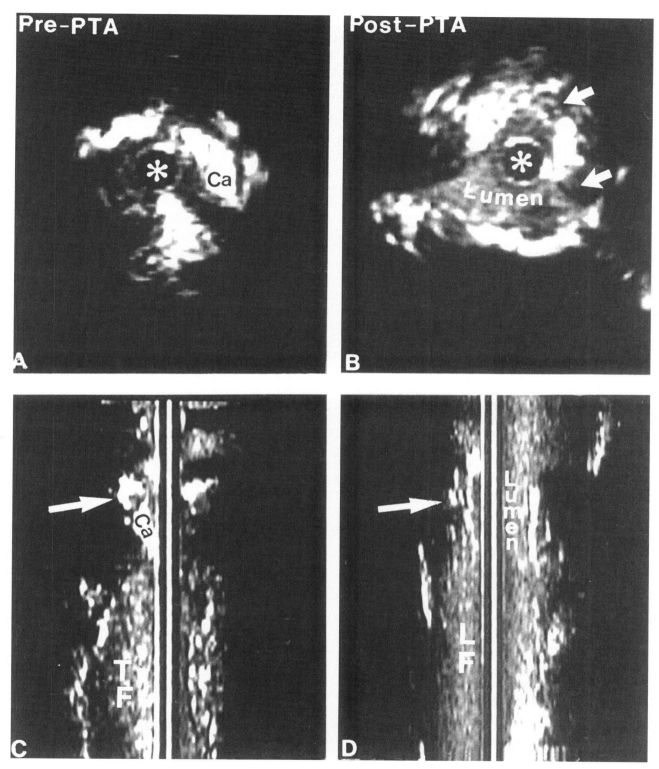

Figure 5–7.   IVUS and sagittal three-dimensional reconstruction during ballon angioplasty (PTA) of SMA from Figure 5–2. (A) IVUS before PTA demonstrates heavily calcified (ca) plaque surrounding probe (asterisk), not appreciated by angiography (Fig. 5–2). (B) IVUS after PTA shows enlargement of lumen due to increased separation/fracture (arrows) between calcific deposits. (C) Sagittal image from serial IVUS frames reconstructs vessel longitudinally, similar in orientation to the angiogram, and shows calcific plaque (arrow) encroaching on lumen, which has normal dimensions more distally. Coarse echoes in distal lumen indicate turbulent flow (TF) through stenosis. (D) Sagittal view following PTA. Proximal lumen is partially enlarged at lesion site (arrow), and echo signals corresponding to blood flow are now more uniform, indicating more laminar flow (LF).

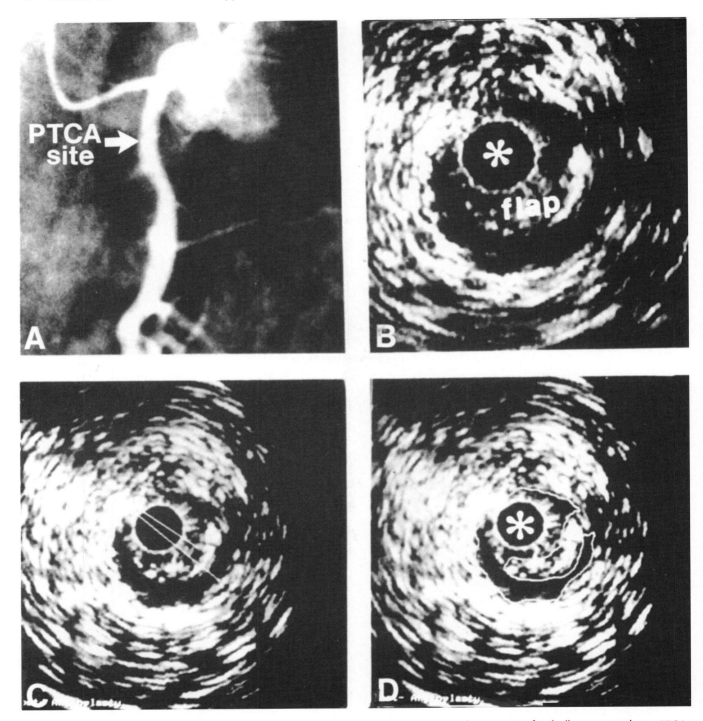

Figure 5–8.   Angiographic versus IVUS assessment of postinterventional cross-sectional area. (*A*) After balloon angioplasty, PTCA site in proximal right coronary artery appears widely patent. (*B*) IVUS image of PTCA site discloses tissue flap resulting from crescentic fracture. (*C*) Determination of post-PTCA luminal diameter, angiographically or even by IVUS using a cross-sectional view, is problematic: peninsular "flap" creates ambiguity regarding minimum versus maximum diameter. (*D*) Determination of luminal cross-sectional area of even the nongeometric, complicated lumen resulting from PTCA is straightforward using plianmetered area from IVUS cross-sectional image.

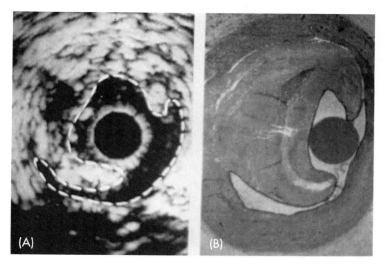

instrumentation employed. These unique features of IVUS have been used to good advantage to study the mechanisms by which balloon angioplasty improves luminal patency (Figs. 5–10 to 5–12). Observations from IVUS at our own institution[27] and others[62] suggest that plaque fracture and/or dissection is associated with balloon dilation in the overwhelming majority of angiographically and hemodynamically successful procedures. Indeed, data [63,64] suggest that at least some degree of plaque fracture must be seen by IVUS to achieve a successful long-term result; vessels that display no tearing may be much more prone to recoil or restenosis.

Figure 5–9. Correlation between IVUS and histology. (A) IVUS image obtained from angioplasty (PTA) site in iliac artery demonstrating extensive plaque fracture. Patient died 24 hours later from unrelated cause. (B) Histologic section corresponding to PTA site (A) depicting morphologic features nearly identical to those seen on IVUS.

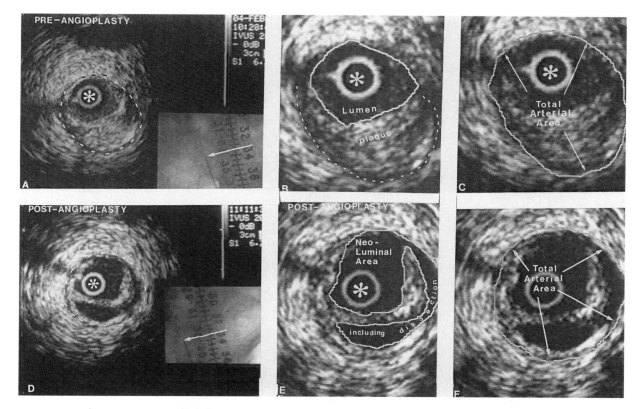

Figure 5–10. Panel A: IVUS image of left iliac artery at site of stenosis before angioplasty. Asterisk denotes IVUS catheter. Echolucent band (dashed line) represents media of arterial wall. Split screen shows simultaneous floroscopic recording of catheter position during IVUS imaging; arrow marks position of IVUS transducer at time of image acquisition. Panel B: digitized IVUS image of stenosis site before angioplasty. Luminal area, confirmed by injection of agitated saline, is traced. Large, eccentric plaque occupies area between lumen and media (dashed line) of vessel wall. Panel C: digitized IVUS image of stenosis site showing computerized tracing of medial border of assessment of total arterial area before angioplasty. Panel D: IVUS image of same site in iliac artery after angioplasty. Dashed line traces medial border. Arrow confirms transducer location identical to preangioplasty site. Panel E: digitized postangioplasty image with computerized measurement of neoluminal area. Large, crescent-shaped dissection contributes significant portion of the neoluminal area. Injection of agitated saline confirmed that this dissection was functional part of postangioplasty lumen. Panel F: digitized IVUS image of postangioplasty artery with computerized measurement of total arterial area.

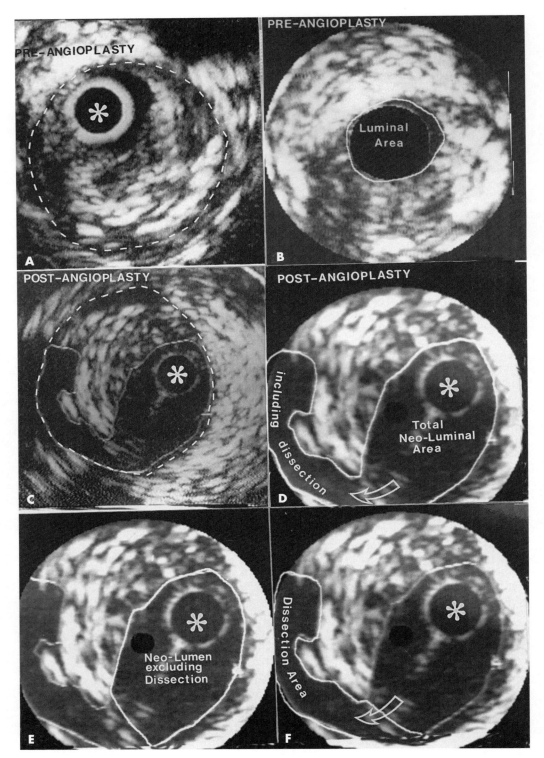

Figure 5–11. Panel A: IVUS image of iliac artery at site of stenosis before angioplasty. Asterisk denotes IVUS catheter. Lumen of vessel, black and crescent-shaped, surrounds IVUS catheter. Dashed line marks outer border of media of vessel wall. Area between lumen and media is filled with heterogeneous-appearing plaque. Panel B: digitized IVUS image at site of stenosis before angioplasty. Central black area represents computerized removal of IVUS catheter during digitizing process. Measurement of lumen area is demonstrated. Panel C: IVUS image of same stenotic site after angioplasty. Dotted line along outer medial border denotes outer wall of the artery. Line tracing denotes neolumen, confirmed by injection of agitated saline during IVUS imaging. Panel D: digitized image of postangioplasty treatment site. Neoluminal area has now been measured and includes a large dissection. Panel E; tracing of the neolumen excluding the area contributed by the dissection. Panel F: tracing of area contributed to neolumen by dissection area.

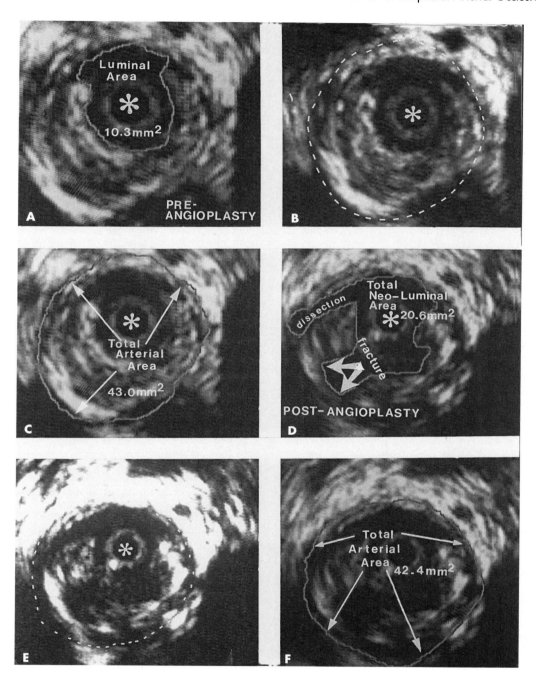

Figure 5–12.   Panel A: digitized IVUS image of iliac artery before angioplasty demonstrating measurement of luminal area. Asterisk marks IVUS catheter. Panel B: primary, unprocessed IVUS image from which digitized images were obtained. Dashed line traces media of vessel wall. Panel C: digitized image demonstrating measurement of total arterial area. Panel D: Postangioplasty measurement of neoluminal area. Comparison with preangioplasty image (immediately to left) reveals that a significant part of the increase in luminal area is supplied by accessory lumen resulting from plaque fracture. Panel E: primary unprocessed IVUS image after angioplasty from which digitized images for quantification were obtained. Dashed line traces outer border of media of arterial wall. Panel F: measurement of total arterial area after angioplasty from digitized IVUS image.

The relative contribution of plaque fractures, as opposed to other factors, to the overall increase in luminal area seen following balloon angioplasty has been elucidated by IVUS (Figs. 5–13 and 5–14). Tobis et al[36] demonstrated in vitro that diseased vessels sub-jected to balloon dilation tended to tear longitudinally at the thinnest region of the plaque; they suggested that these tears account for the enlargement of luminal cross-sectional area. Losordo et al[65] evaluated IVUS images obtained before and after PTA performed in 40

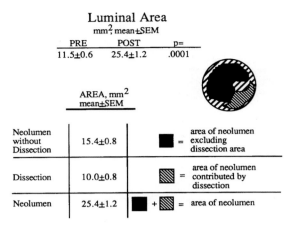

Luminal Area
mm², mean±SEM

PRE	POST	p=
11.5±0.6	25.4±1.2	.0001

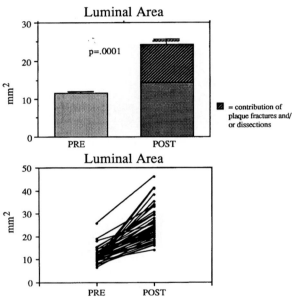

	AREA, mm² mean±SEM	
Neolumen without Dissection	15.4±0.8	■ = area of neolumen excluding dissection area
Dissection	10.0±0.8	▨ = area of neolumen contributed by dissection
Neolumen	25.4±1.2	■ + ▨ = area of neolumen

Plaque Area
mm², mean±SEM

PRE	POST	p=
33.8±1.8	22.5±1.5	.0001

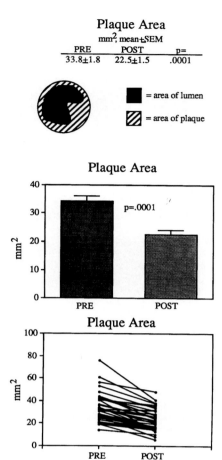

■ = area of lumen

▨ = area of plaque

Figure 5–13. Luminal cross-sectional area measured by IVUS before and after angioplasty. Top panel: diagram: luminal area excluding the contribution of plaque fractures and dissections is represented in black; area contributed by fractures and dissections is represented by narrow diagonal stripes. Wide diagonal stripes denote atherosclerotic plaque. Middle panel: bar graph showing luminal area (mean ± SEM) measured by IVUS before and after angioplasty for entire cohort. Area contributed by IVUS-defined fractures and dissections is denoted by narrow diagonal stripes. Bottom panel: graph showing luminal area before and after angioplasty measured by IVUS for 40 individual arteries.

Figure 5–14. Plaque area before and after angioplasty. Top panel: diagram: lumen is indicated schematically in black; plaque is indicated by wide diagonal stripes. Middle panel: bar graph showing plaque area (mean ± SEM) before and after angioplasty for entire cohort. Bottom panel: graph showing plaque area before and after angioplasty measured by IVUS for 40 individual arteries.

patients, and quantified the relative contributions of plaque fracture, plaque compression, and arterial stretch to the enhanced overall luminal area. Luminal cross-sectional area more than doubled, from 11.5 mm² pre-PTA to 25.4 mm² post-PTA. The neolumen created by plaque fractures accounted for the majority (72%) of the total increase in luminal area. Compression of plaque was seen in all treated vessels and made an important, but quantitatively less significant, contribution to the postangioplasty increase in luminal area.

Arterial stretching was demonstrated in only 25% of patients, and even in this group, its contribution to the increased area was minimal. These data confirm previous observations suggesting that plaque fracture constitutes the principal mechanism responsible for increased luminal patency after balloon angioplasty. These results consequently contradict conclusions based on prior in vitro studies[66,67] and a smaller in vivo study[68] that implicated stretching of the vessel wall as a major factor contributing to increased lumen size.

In an attempt to categorize the degree of plaque fracture observed by IVUS following balloon angioplasty. Honye et al[64] have identified six characteristic morphologic patterns of vessel disruption (Table 5–1). In their proposed scheme (Fig. 5–15), patterns A through D represent increasing degrees of plaque tearing and separation from subjacent structures, while pattern E represents stretching without obvious tearing. In 66 coronary lesions subjected to balloon dilation,

PTA MORPHOLOGY by IVUS

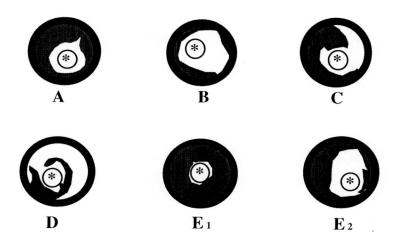

Figure 5–15.   Classification of morphologic patterns of vessel disruption postangioplasty (after reference 69).

Honye et al observed fairly equal distribution of the different morphologic subtypes, with a slight predominance in types B, C, and especially E. Interestingly, in their preliminary analysis, Type E1 lesions displayed a greater tendency toward restenosis at 6-month follow-up.

Calcified plaque (Fig. 5–16) is detected by IVUS in most vessels undergoing angioplasty, a feature that is underappreciated by angiography and that may be important in understanding the mechanism of PTA. Honye et al, for example, identified calcific deposits in 14 versus 83% of patients studied by angiography and ultrasound, respectively.[69] Our experience has been similar.[22,27] Waller et al previously suggested that tears and fractures typically occur along the border between calcific plaque and softer tissue[70]; assuming that such is

the case, then the increased sensitivity of IVUS in detecting calcific deposits may be clinically relevant. Indeed, observations[71,72] lend further support to the notion that the presence of calcium may predict the location and extent of plaque fracture. Fitzgerald et al, for example, imaged 41 patients following angioplasty; they found that in 87% of patients with focal deposits of calcium who also demonstrated dissections, the fracture site was located adjacent to the calcified plaque. Furthermore, the extent of dissection was greater in the patients with calcified vessels than in those with noncalcified vessels.[71] To the extent that large dissections may portend a poor angioplasty outcome, including specifically a higher risk of abrupt closure, the detection and localization of calcium may become an important practical application of IVUS. Further studies are necessary, however, to determine the characteristic features or patterns of calcific deposition that might be a harbinger of a poor result with percutaneous transluminal coronary angioplasty (PTCA).

Preliminary evidence from in vivo IVUS studies has also provided insight regarding the mechanisms by which directional atherectomy, stent deployment, and laser angioplasty enhance the luminal area. In contrast to vessels undergoing balloon angioplasty, vessels in which directional atherectomy is performed demonstrate less prominent plaque-arterial wall disruption; instead, the perimeter of the neolumen is typically smooth and uninterrupted. In our initial series of patients,[27] no plaque cracks were observed on post-atherectomy IVUS examination. Instead, discrete "bites" corresponding to individual passes of the cutting blade were often observed, consistent with tissue

Table 5–1.   Morphologc Patterns of Vessel Disruption Following PTCA

Type A:	partial-thickness tear in plaque not extending to subjacent tissue
Type B:	full-thickness tear in plaque extending to media, with separation of the two edges of torn plaque
Type C:	full-thickness tear, with separation (dissection) of plaque from underlying media for an arc of up to 180 degrees
Type D:	full-thickness tear, with separation of plaque extending circumferentially >180 degrees; plaque largely or entirely pulled away from subjacent tissues
Type E:	stretching of concentric (E1) or eccentric (E2) plaque, without obvious separation of plaque fracture

Source: Adapted from Reference 64.

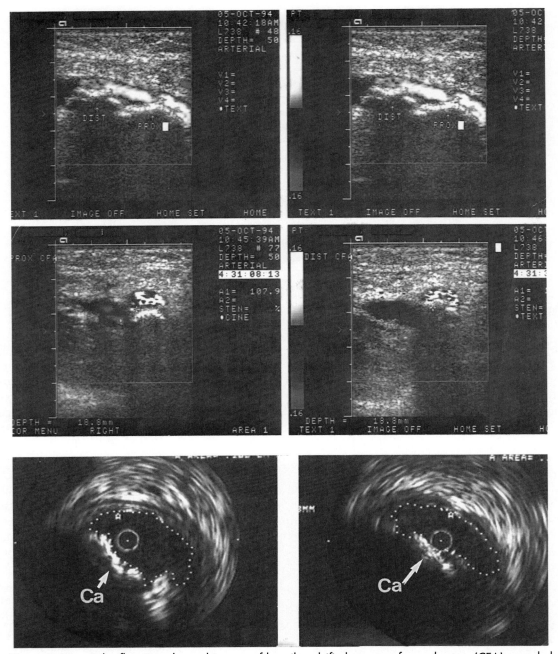

Figure 5–16.   Color-flow Doppler and images of heavily calcified common femoral artery (CFA) recorded 1 day post-IVUS for CFA angioplasty. Top: two longitudinal views of CFA (red) show eccentric calcific spur at site of minimum luminal diameter. Common femoral vein (CFV) is indicated in blue. Middle: two cross-sectional views of CFA (color mosaic indicates turbulent flow at site of heavy calcific deposit.) CFV appears blue. Bottom: two cross-sectional views of CFA recorded immediately postangioplasty. Heavy calcific deposit attenuates image of subjacent arterial wall. Note correspondence of lumen geometry between IVUS and color-flow images (luminal boundaries in IVUS images have been plianmetered to measure cross-sectional area. Patient remains asymptomatic at 1 year follow-up.

removal. Similar findings have been reported by Yock et al,[73] Smucker et al,[74] and Tenaglia et al,[17] all of whom reported a relatively low incidence of plaque fracture. Controversy persists regarding the extent to which inflation of the eccentric balloon of the Simpson Atherocath contributes to an increased luminal area; indeed, angiographic studies have suggested that the amount of tissue retrieved is not enough to account for the resultant increase in luminal diameter,[75,76] and in certain cases, the Dotter effect of the catheter and the effects of balloon inflation have been documented to produce the majority of luminal patency.

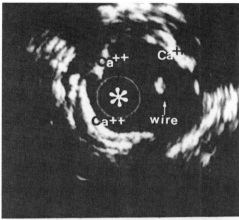

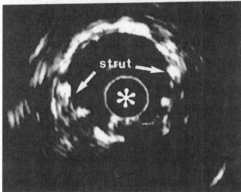

Figure 5–17. Top: Heavily calcified (Ca^{2+}) lesion with multiple plaque fractures postangioplasty. Bottom: arterial wall trauma is effaced by deployed endovascular stent.

Signs of arterial wall trauma are most completely effaced on IVUS images recorded following delivery of an endovascular stent (Fig. 5–17); the fact that extensive trauma is observed at these same sites after balloon insertion (before stenting) suggests that stent implantation acutely ameliorates arterial wall pathology.[27,77,78]

VASCULAR REMODELING

The term *vascular remodeling*[79] has been clinically regarded as a naturally occurring adaptation to atherosclerosis,[80] but more recently it has been used to define a response of the vascular wall to percutaneous revascularization.[81] The former implies segmental arterial enlargement, while the latter involves segmental arterial constriction. The application of IVUS to both aspects of remodeling illustrates the utility of this imaging modality for studying pathogenetic mechanisms involving the intact arterial circulation of live patients. Glagov et al[80] described the enlargement of atherosclerotic left main coronary arteries in a population of human hearts obtained at post mortem. The conclusion that arterial enlargement occurred in response to the accumulation of atherosclerotic plaque was based on a regression analysis correlating the size of the left

main coronary arteries with the degree of atherosclerotic plaque accumulation. Subsequent similarly performed pathologic studies[82] reproduced these findings. Epicardial echocardiography[83] was also used to compare coronary arterial dimensions in normal and atherosclerotic arteries, yielding similar results.

In vivo analysis of human arteries using IVUS of paired, adjacent normal and atherosclerotic arterial segments disclosed progressive focal dilatation of the outer arterial wall in response to the incremental accumulation of atherosclerotic plaque[84] (Fig. 5–18). Quantitative analysis of arterial morphometry showed that as the cross-sectional area of plaque within a diseased vessel segment increased, the outer wall of the artery expanded in an attempt to compensate for this accumulation of plaque. Two points regarding the enlargement of arteries in response to plaque accumulation are worth emphasizing. First, the increase in total arterial area was proportional to the amount of plaque at the diseased site, as demonstrated by the positive correlation between these variables. Second, the enlargement of the artery was a focal response that did not affect the adjacent normal segments of the artery.

Two important benefits of IVUS provided a unique opportunity to demonstrate that arterial enlargement occurs as a local response of the artery wall to the development of atherosclerotic plaque. First, morphologic data were collected without the perturbation of tissue architecture, a prerequisite for the standard pathologic examination.[85,86] Second, because adjacent normal or near-normal and diseased arterial segments within the same artery were examined, patients could serve as their own internal controls, avoiding the potential hazards of comparisons made between normal and abnormal individuals.

More recently, Post et al[81] used the term *remodeling* to describe arterial constriction that develops postangioplasty and appears to constitute the pathogenetic mechanism explaining those cases of restenosis that lack a significant proliferative component. This concept was investigated in vivo by Mintz and coworkers,[87–89] who used IVUS to evaluate serially the acute and chronic response to percutaneous revascularization in human patients. Because their approach permitted direct area measurements of both wall and lumen, the authors' findings support the contention that late lumen loss is not limited to encroachment by atherosclerotic plaque but rather is related in part to a demonstrable reduction in total arterial cross-sectional area. These in vivo studies were extended to the lower extremity vasculature by Post et al. Using serial IVUS analyses of human patients undergoing percutaneous lower extremity revascularization,[90] they confirmed the interpretation that they had initially developed on the basis of live animal studies. Shown in Figure 5–19 is an extreme form of constrictive vascular remodeling due

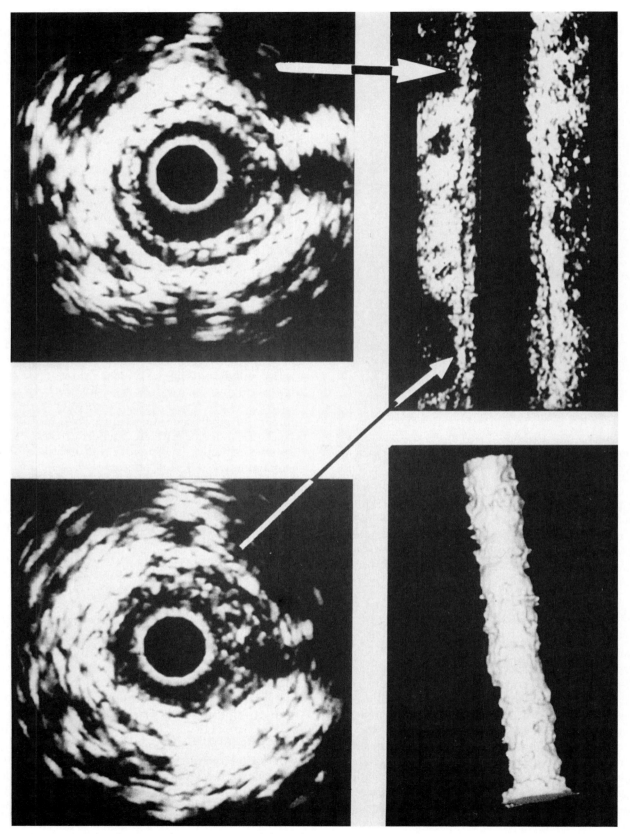

Figure 5–18. Two-dimensional (2D) images and three-dimensional (3D) reconstructions of IVUS recording illustrating compensatory dilation. Top: 2D image shows minimal plaque. Bottom: 2D image shows moderate luminal narrowing. Corresponding sites on 3D sagittal image, indicated by arrows, shows increased arterial diameter (media stripe to media stripe) at site of moderate antherosclerotic narrowing. As 3D cast image of bottom right shows, such focal dilation preserves similar luminal dimensions over entire length of diseased as well as normal artery.

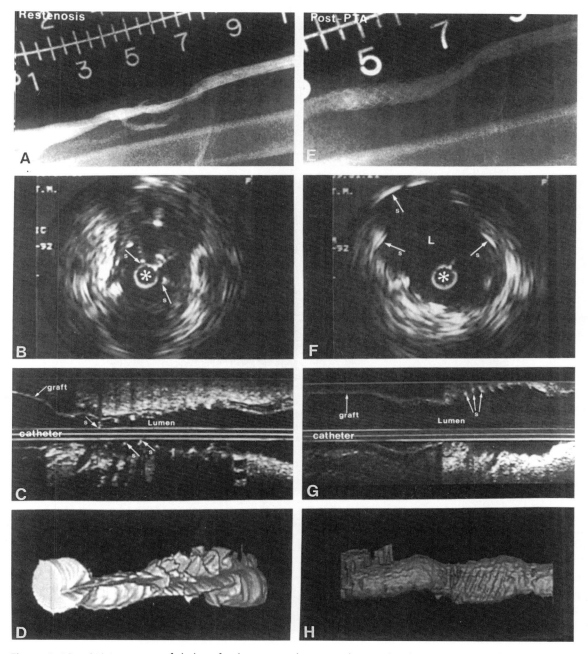

Figure 5-19. (A) Restenosis of dialysis fistula appears by angioplasty to be due to neointimal thickening (left); in fact, IVUS (B) shows stent struts (s, arrows) abutting IVUS catheter. Sagittal 3D reconstruction shows same finding in longitudinal format (C). Consequent luminal narrowing is illustrated by cast 3D reconstruction (D). Postangioplasty, angiographic luminal diameter is restored (E). IVUS (2D in B, 3D sagittal in C) shows stent struts no longer abutting IVUS; catheter luminal cast (D) shows augmented luminal patency.

to stent collapse. IVUS clarified the basis for restenosis in this case and altered the proposed treatment strategy: whereas directional atherectomy had been planned, based on angiographic findings, recognition of stent collapse by IVUS dictated that balloon inflation alone be usd to reexpand the collapsed stent.

UTILITY OF IVUS TO GUIDE INTERVENTIONS

Although the ultimate role of IVUS vis-à-vis contrast angiography remains to be determined, we have used IVUS as the primary (sole) imaging modality to guide

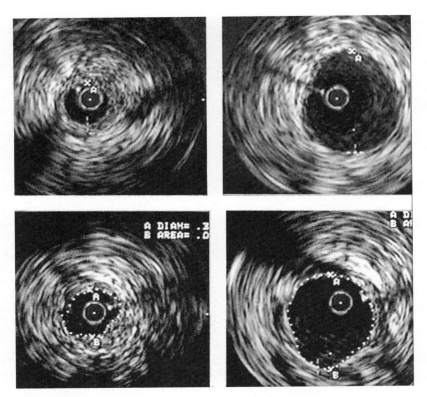

Figure 5–20. Use of IVUS to size interventional device. Top left: minimum luminal diameter of dialysis fistula measures 2.64 mm. A burr measuring 3.0 mm in diameter is therefore selected to perform rotational atherectomy. Bottom left: rotational atherectomy results in minimum lumen diameter of 3.0 mm. Top right: reference diameter of upstream segment of fistula measures 6.4 cm in minimum lumen diameter. An angioplasty (PTA) balloon (Blue Max, Boston Scientific) measuring 6 mm in diameter is selected for dilation. Bottom right: final cross-sectional area post-PTA measures 6.0 mm in diameter.

interventional procedures.[91] In a series of 46 patients undergoing iliac or femoro-popliteal revascularization, serial IVUS imging was performed to assess the results of balloon dilation, directional atherectomy, and/or physiologic low-stress angioplasty. Decisions regarding whether the procedure's result was satisfactory and whether to treat further were made on the basis of IVUS exams alone, without any angiographic informtion. Repeat intervention was deemed necessary by IVUS in approximately one-third of patients; the specific adjunctive treatment modality, including repeat balloon inflation, adjunctive atherectomy, or stent deployment, was determined based on interpretation of the quantitative and qualitative findings on IVUS exam. Angiograms were performed after completion of the recanalization procedure, both to confirm the adequacy of the result by the traditional standard and to determine if IVUS had failed to define a significant residual narrowing. In only 2 of 46 patients did information obtained on completion angiography indicate the need for repeat intervention.

A number of reports support the notion that IVUS enhances definition of residual luminal narrowing and morphometry postintervention and that this information may influence subsequent therapeutic management.[26,92–95] Several of these studies have explored the lesion- and device-specific use of IVUS[96–98] and, in addition to supporting its use to determine the procedural outcome, implicate a potential role for IVUS in identifying the optimal interventional therapy. Examples of this include determination of appropriate device/balloon size based on accurate measurement of vessel dimensions (Fig. 5–20); selection of a directional, rather than a concentric, atherectomy device based on the finding of eccentric plaque; and choosing a device that is better suited for debulking of calcium in the case of a heavily calcified lesion.

IVUS is uniquely suited for guidance in the deployment of endovascular stents[27,77,99–103] (Fig. 5–21). Whereas evaluation of the interface between stent struts and endoluminal surface is difficult by fluoroscopy (where one sees the stent but not the vessel wall) and by angiography (where one sees the vessel but the contrast column may obscure the stent), such evaluation is straightforward by IVUS. IVUS is specifically useful during stent deployment in several respects. First, IVUS

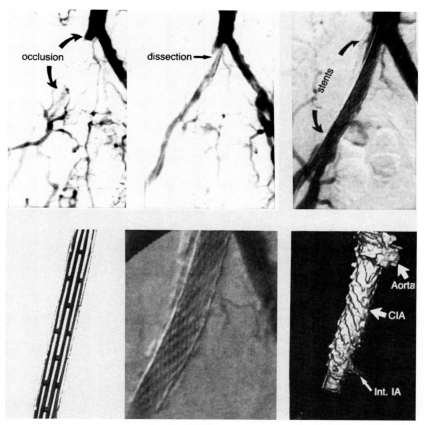

Figure 5–21. Amelioration of post-PTA dissection of iliac artery using stents. Top left: baseline angiogram of occluded iliac artery. Top middle: postangioplasty. Top right: following deployment of two Palmaz stents, an excellent angiographic result is obtained. Bottom left: Unexpanded Palmaz stent. Bottom middle: digital radiographic image of deployed stents. Bottom right: (3D) reconstruction of serial IVUS images creates a "cast" of the vascular lumen, of stented common iliac artery (CIA). (Int. IA, internal iliac artery)

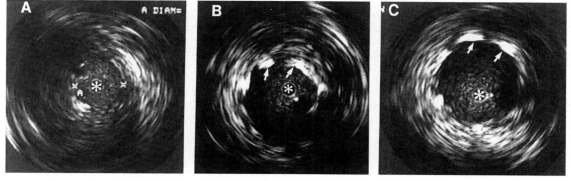

Figure 5–22. IVUS during subclavian PTA/stenting. (A) IVUS after 7-mm balloon dilation. Maximum diameter is 4.8 mm, indicating significant recoil. (B) Following stent deployment with 8-mm balloon, struts (*arrows*) still protrude slightly into lumen. (C) Post-PTA 9 mm, struts (*arrows*) now well apposed to arterial wall. *, IVUS catheter.

may assist in determining the need to stent a vessel post-PTA by identifying an inadequate luminal area (Fig. 5–22), severe plaque disruption, or the presence of a flow-limiting flap or dissection not apparent by angiography. Second, the target vessel may be measured by IVUS to ensure appropriate stent sizing (Fig. 5–23). Because balloon/stent undersizing may predispose to abrupt closure and because oversizing is associated with a hyperproliferative response leading to increased restenosis, exact sizing may directly affect the clinical outcome. Third, IVUS permits identification of the origin as well as the end sites of a dissection, and

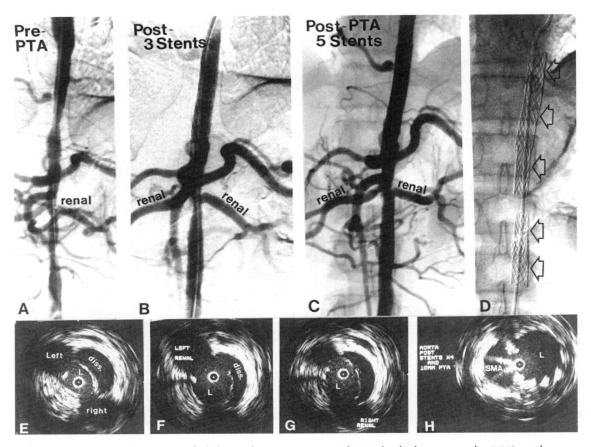

Figure 2–23. Revascularization of abdominal aortic stenosis with PTA/multiple stents under IVUS guidance. This 30-year-old woman presented with malignant hypertension and nonpalpable femoral pulses due to abdominal aortic coarctation, thought to be secondary to Takayasu's disease, now apparently quiescent. (A) Angiogram pre-PTA demonstrates extensive disease in the aorta, both above and below the renal arteries. (B) Following PTA above and below the renal arteries and placement of three stents, result appears reasonable by angiography, although moderate stenosis remains below/at level of renal arteries. IVUS image (E) at take-off of renals ("left" and "right") demonstrates large dissection (diss.) extending from proximal PTA site, encroaching on renal artery ostia and narrowing aortic lumen (L). (C) Redilated aorta, with two additional stents, shows no encroachment at level of renal arteries; IVUS frames (F) and (G) confirm persistence of dissection (diss.), but concurrent enlargement of aortic lumen (L) and elimination of obstruction leading into renal arteries ("left renal," "right renal"). (D) Stents (arrows) in aorta. (H), IVUS of stent in midaorta depicts struts overlying origin of superior mesenteric artery (SMA); struts cast "shadows" into SMA but do not compromise blood flow (C). Patient is asymptomatic and normotensive at 1-year follow-up.

thus easily identifies the longitudinal extent of a vessel that requires stenting. Fourth, IVUS may identify sites of inadequate stent expansion (Figs. 5–24, 5–25), nonapposition of struts to the underlying arterial wall. This has been specifically implicated as a basis for stent thrombosis, and optimal stent expansion guided by IVUS has led some investigators to reduce the need for associated anticoagulation.[101,102] Fifth, for complex deployment, as in the case of stenting the bifurcation of the distal aorta (Fig. 5–26), IVUS may facilitate stent positioning and subsequently confirm the adequacy of the reconstructed bifurcation. Finally, IVUS is invaluable in, and perhaps uniquely capable of, clarifying the basis for restenosis after stent deployment (Figs. 5–27, 5–28).

INSTRUMENTS FOR COMBINED ULTRASOUND IMAGING AND PERCUTANEOUS REVASCULARIZATION

Initial attempts by Mallery et al to combine intravascular ultrasound imaging with balloon angioplasty and/or mechanical atherectomy employed a 4.5F balloon dilatation catheter fitted with an array of eight 20-MHz transducers mounted radially around the catheter.[104] The transducers were positioned within and midway between the two ends of a 3-cm polyethylene balloon; images were recorded perpendicular to the long axis of the catheter through the balloon.

Hodgson et al[105] performed in vivo imaging in normal canine coronary arteries using an alternative design with a ring of modified phased-array transducers

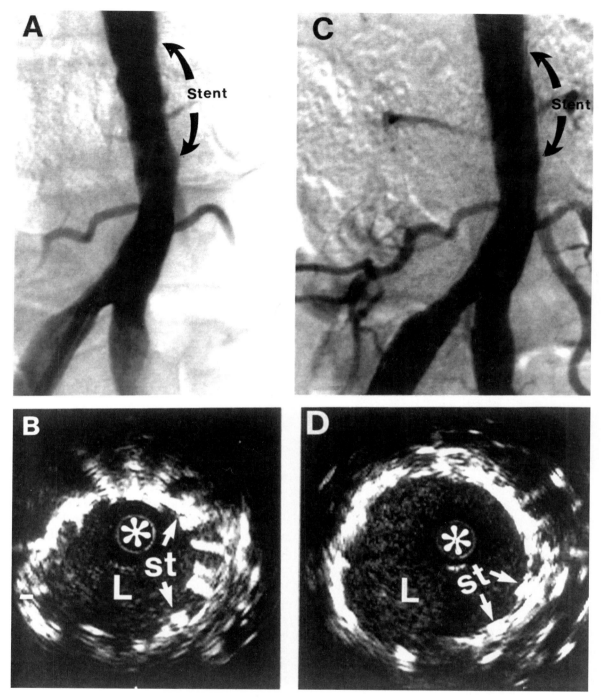

Figure 5–24.   Stent underexpansion detected by IVUS. PTA and stent deployment in eccentric aorta lesion from Figure 5–13. (*A*) Angiogram after deployment of Palmaz stent with 9-mm balloon depicts ostensibly good result, without obvious compromise in lumen or stent. (*B*) Although lumen (L) is now enlarged compared to pre-PTA (Fig. 5–13), IVUS after placement of 9-mm PTA/stent demonstrates stent underexpansion, with all struts (st) between 2 and 5 o'clock not in apposition to arterial wall. (*C*) Angiogram following 12-mm PTA shows slight decrease in luminal irregularity where stent has been redilated (*arrows*). (*D*) IVUS after 12-mm PTA demonstrates complete expansion of stent, with all struts (st) now completely apposed to arterial wall and overall lumen (L) area further increased.

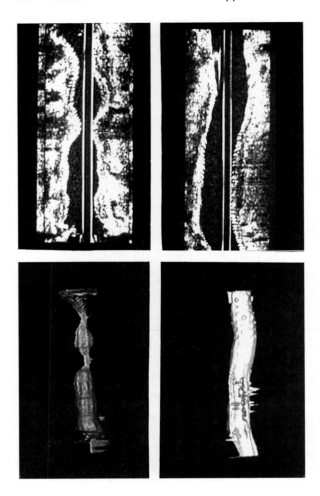

Figure 5–25.   Suboptimal expansion of Wallstent (Schneider) deployed in iliac artery is illustrated in sagittal (top left) and lumen cast (bottom left) 3-D reconstructions of IVUS recordings. Following supplementary balloon dilation, sagittal (top right) and cast (bottom right) images show satisfactory luminal dimensions.

trailing the balloon. The design of this device was intended to permit pre- and postdilation imaging without the requirement for multiple catheter exchanges. In vivo studies using this so-called Oracle in humans during PTCA[92,106] suggest that images obtained immediately before and after balloon dilation using this device may influence procedural strategy.

Clinical investigation in our laboratory has confirmed that it is feasible to perform on-line IVUS imaging during percutaneous revascularization, monitoring the effects of angioplasty on the arterial wall *during* balloon inflation as opposed to the post hoc evaluation described above. The so-called balloon ultrasound imaging catheter (BUIC; Boston Scientific), which we have employed, is a hybrid device that incorporates both diagnostic and therapeutic functions, imaging through polyethylene balloon material, the thickness of which is standard for peripheral angioplasty balloons.[63] In 8 of 10 patients pre-PTA and in 9 of 10 patients post-PTA, images recorded from the BUIC permitted rapid quantitative analysis of minimum luminal diameter and luminal cross-sectional area. The measurements obtained were nearly indistinguishable from those recorded using a nonballoon ultrasound catheter.

Quantitative findings provided by the BUIC were specifically useful for defining the contribution of elastic recoil, long inferred to constitute a mechanical reason for loss of gain achieved during balloon inflation.[61,107,108] Previous investigators employed quantitative angiographic techniques to analyze the extent to which recoil complicates standard PTCA. Nobuyoshi et al,[108] for example, observed that "restenosis" (>50% loss of gain in absolute diameter assessed by cinevideodensitometry) was already present in 27 (14.6%) of 185 patients or in 27 (11.4%) of 237 lesions 1 day post-PTCA, and was therefore interpreted to represent evidence of elastic recoil.

Measurements recorded using the BUIC confirm the observations made using angiographic techniques, and establish that the phenomenon of recoil is common to peripheral as well as coronary angioplasty and that such recoil is instantaneous. Interestingly, the single patient in our series in whom clinical evidence of restenosis has thus far been observed was the one in whom recoil was most severe.

Finally, on-line ultrasound monitoring of balloon inflation also facilitates identification of the initiation of plaque fracture. Images recorded from the BUIC dis-

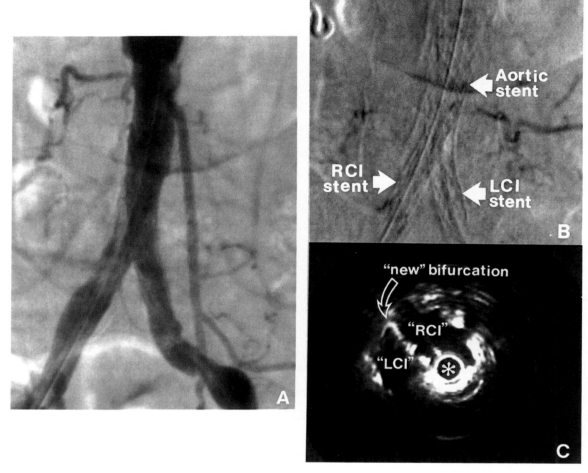

Figure 5–26. Percutaneous reconstruction of aortic bifurcation using balloon angioplasty and stent deployment. (A) Final angiogram. (B) Digital radiographic image of deployed aortic stent and common iliac stents; the latter were deployed using "kissing balloon" technique. (C) Cross-sectional IVUS image (catheter in right common iliac (RCI) demonstrates interface of RCI and left common iliac (LCI) stents, that is, the "new bifurcation."

closed that plaque fractures were initiated by dilation at low (<2 atmospheres) inflation pressures. This is consistent with previous clinical observations. Hjemdahl-Monsen et al, for example, found that most improvement in luminal size occurred at inflation pressures <2 atmospheres.[109] As suggested by Kleiman et al,[110] any technique that permits immediate on-line recognition of plaque fracture might theoretically be employed to modify the remainder of the dilatation procedure in an attempt to prevent the development of a flow-limiting dissection.

Yock et al investigated a prototype catheter that combined a 30-MHz transducer with a modified version of the Simpson directional atherectomy catheter.[111] Preliminary experiments performed in vitro and in vivo demonstrated that this device could be used to monitor the depth to which plaque was mechanically excised. Furthermore, the availability of on-line imaging from within the cutting window of the device permits the operator to assign directionality to the

subsequent cut(s). The ability to debulk plaque selectively has obvious positive implications; by facilitating more complete and selective plaque removal and avoidance of normal elements in the arterial wall, the potential beneficial therapeutic effect of the Simpson device may be maximized.

The theoretical advantages of a combined laser/IVUS device are similar to those described above, including the enhanced ability to "aim" and thereby achieve precise tissue ablation and controlled plaque removal. Preliminary attempts to combine IVUS with laser ablation by Aretz et al[112] and Linker et al[113] suggested that the development of microcavitations during laser activation might preclude effective IVUS imaging. We used a combination laser/IVUS catheter in vivo to guide and assess the results of laser-induced ablation of plaque.[114] The catheter consists of a conventional multifiber laser catheter, the wire lumen of which has been used to accommodate a mechanical ultrasound transducer. Images recorded by IVUS simul-

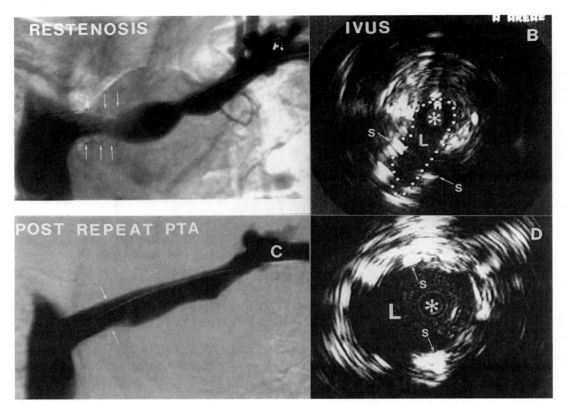

Figure 5–27. Restenosis due to eccentric stent collapse. (A) Angiogram of subclavian vein proximal to a dialysis graft 4 months postangioplasty and Palmaz stent deployment. Narrowed contrast column within stent, whose edges (*arrow*) show full expansion, suggests classic restenosis due to neointimal proliferation. (B) IVUS image from restenotic site depicts absence of neointimal growth within stent but instead confirms eccentric collapse of the stent. Approximation of opposing struts (*arrows*) gives a narrowed, slit-like configuration to the stented lumen. (C) Angiogram after repeat PTA depicts restoration of lumen. Contrast column now approaches stent borders (*arrows*) (D) IVUS demonstrates reexpansion of stent to circular configuration and enlargement of lumen (L) area.

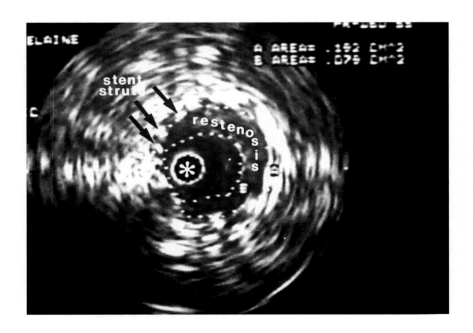

Figure 5–28. IVUS of restenosis within stent in renal artery. Stent configuration remains circular and fully expanded, but crescent of neointimal tissue growth ("restenosis") narrows the lumen's cross-sectional area by approximately 50%. *, IVUS catheter.

taneously with excimer (308-nm) laser irradiation disclosed abrupt formation of cavitations, as previously described, that transiently attenuated the ultrasound image. On cessation of laser irradiation, normal blood flow cleared the excimer-generated gas, restoring the ultrasound image and documenting the extent of reduced plaque volume.

THREE-DIMENSIONAL RECONSTRUCTION

The introduction of three-dimensional reconstruction[21,56,62,99,115–126] has eliminated certain limitations inherent in the spatial display formats of current IVUS imaging systems. Conventional two-dimensional IVUS displays tomographic sections of the lumen and arterial wall in sequential fashion as a video recording. Comparison of individual segments examined by IVUS to adjacent or more distant segments requires repeated review of serially recorded images to reconstruct, in the mind's eye, the spatial relationship of the segments of interest. For example, while one tomographic image obtained during IVUS examination may offer high-resolution definition of a plaque fracture resulting from balloon angioplasty, details regarding the longitudinal distribution of the same plaque fracture at one site relative to proximal and distal sites cannot be displayed in a single image. In contrast, conventional angiography preserves the advantage of displaying each segment in longitudinal relationship to adjacent and more distant segments; once contrast medium has opacified the artery of interest, any segment may be compared to adjacent and distant segments, limited only by the field of view.

For IVUS to provide the same capability—for example, to compre adjacent segments within the vessel—simultaneous viewing of the data from multiple sequential cross-sectional slices is necessary. The liability of IVUS that provides for only one tomographic view at a time, without a longitudina perspective, may be resolved by "stacking" (Fig. 5–29) sequential IVUS frames recorded during a catheter pullback through a given vascular segment. Computer-based reconstruction of these serially acquired IVUS frames creates a longitudinal, three-dimensional format for IVUS data. Thus, the benefits of detailed tomographic imaging are preserved while providing an efficient method to review the cumulative IVUS data.

Original attempts to perform three-dimensional reconstructions in our laboratory involved the use of software (SigmaScan, Jandel Scientific, Corte Madera, CA) that required manual morphometric tracing of each serial tomographic image followed by a computer-aided reconstruction.[119] The more detail intended, the more images were required, and consequently the more labor-intensive was the reconstruction. The principal liability of this approach, however, related to the fact that the modeling technique was based exclusively

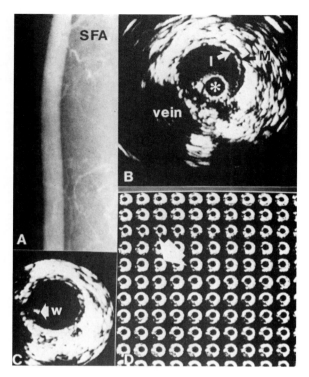

Figure 5–29. (A) Angiogram of normal superficial femoral artery (SFA). (B) Representative 2D cross-sectional IVUS image of SFA (I, intima; asterisk, IVUS catheter) and adjacent vein. (C) Digitized version of (B). (D) "Stack" of digitized 2D IVUS images used to create 3D reconstruction (arrow indicates image shown in B, C).

on boundary depiction and therefore allowed three-dimensional reconstruction of the lumen but not the arterial wall. Such an approach would clearly squander one of the chief assets of intravascular ultrasound, namely, the capability to image the vessel wall and thereby evaluate characteristics of the native wall, as well as pathologic alterations resulting from interventional therapies.

Automated three-dimensional reconstruction of intravascular ultrasound images was investigated in a preliminary fashion by Kitney et al,[127] using voxel modeling. This approach considers each voxel, or volume element, as an extension to three-dimensional space of the digital image element, or pixel (picture element). Voxel modeling is a particularly attractive option for three-dimensional reconstruction of the vasculature because it preserves detailed ultrasound data and thereby allows representation of the arterial wall, rather than simply surface features that would limit the reconstruction to the arterial lumen.

To thereby preserve information regarding the arterial wall and plaque in the reconstructed imge. Image-Comm Systems (Santa Clara, CA) developed for us a personal computer (PC)-based system using algorithms[128,129] designed specifically for analysis of images recorded during IVUS examination (Omniview, Pura

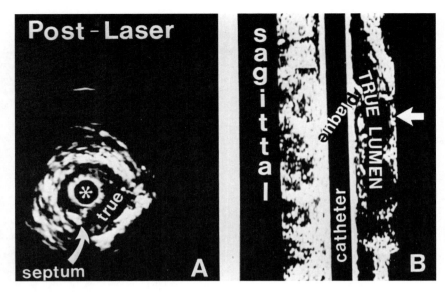

Figure 5–30.   Subintimal channel created during recanalization of 8-cm occlusion in superficial femoral artery (SFA) using guidewire (Terumo) followed by excimer laser angioplasty. (*A*) Inspection by conventional two-dimensional reconstruction (2DR) IVUS demonstrates "double-barrel" lumen. IVUS probe (asterisk) in subintimal channel separated by "septum" from second ("true") lumen. (*B*) Sagittal image rendered by on-line three-dimensional reconstruction (3DR) depicts subintimal pathway of ultrasound catheter as it enters atherosclerotic plaque, which separates catheter from true lumen at right. Arrow depicts level of ultrasound frame shown in (*A*).

Labs, Brea, CA). This software employs a surface rendering process predicated on segmented boundary formation, but includes interpolative algorithms designed to link boundary elements and thereby preserve the capability of viewing the arterial wall as well as the lumen. Three distinct display formats are currently available for reconstructed IVUS data: *sagittal, cylindrical,* and *lumen cast* modes. In the sagittal mode, a planar view of the IVUS data is displayed in longitudinal relief and can be revolved around the long axis of the IVUS catheter. Use of the sagittal format, in particular, not only facilitates comparative analysis of adjacent tomographic images, but offers the additional advantage of displaying the ultrasound data in a longitudinal profile-type format more familiar to the angiographer.

While similar in orientation to an angiogram, sagittal reconstruction substantially augments the information available from conventional angiography in two important ways. First, limitless orthogonal views can be rendered by incremental rotation of the imaging plane about the reference catheter. Given the documented importance of orthogonal views in the assessment of luminal narrowing[130] on the one hand, and the logistical factors that frequently obviate the possibility of obtaining orthogonal views on the other, this feature may ultimately prove to be the principal advantage of three-dimensional reconstruction. Second, informtion regarding pathologic alteration of the arterial wall is provided simultaneously with the conventional assess-

ment of luminal diameter narrowing. Experience with patients undergoing percutaneous revascularization indicates that certain features of arterial wall pathology are particularly well defined in such a longitudinal format. For example, three-dimensional reconstruction in the sagittal mode graphically demonstrated that recanalization of a lengthy total occlusion was achieved by tunneling a false lumen through calcified plaque (Figs. 5–30, 5–31). Such a mechanism of recanalization has been previously described in vitro[131,132] and is frequently inferred to occur in vivo.[133] While the individual tomographic ultrasound images indicated the creation of a "double-barrel" lumen, the full extent of pathologic disruption was more immediately apparent from inspection of the sagittal reconstructions. Similarly, sagittal reconstructions of balloon-dilated, nonoccluded vessels demonstrate the longitudinal distribution of barotraumatic injury, otherwise evident as only local, isolated plaque fractures on the tomographic two-dimensional IVUS images. Use of the three-dimensional formats facilitates delineation of the extent of a dissection, as well as selection and deployment of endovascular stents.

The cylindrical three-dimensional mode preserves the wall and lumen as an intact cylinder and thus provides true three-dimensional—as opposed to planar—views. Experience with the cylindrical format suggests that this mode of three-dimensional reconstruction—particularly when the reconstructed vascular segment is

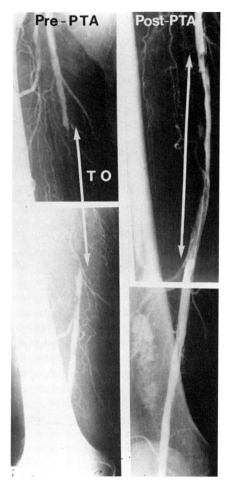

Figure 5–31. Angiograms pre- and postrevascularization from patient illustrated in Figure 5–30. "Double-barrel" lumen is less well defined by angiography than by IVUS.

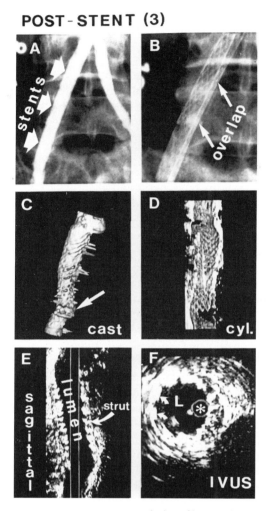

Figure 5–32. Angiogram (A) and plain film (B) show three stents in right common iliac artery. Final lumen is illustrated in 3D reconstructions of IVUS images, shown here in lumen cast (C) cylindrical (cyl.) (D), and sagittal (E). Note cobblestone appearance of luminal surface of stent in cylindrical 3D reconstruction (D). Representative 2D IVUS image of stent is shown in (F).

hemisected—is optimally suited for those cases in which direct inspection of luminal topography is of special interest, such as analysis of implanted endovascular prostheses (Fig. 5–32). Details of the "cobblestoned" neointima lining the stent cannot be appreciated angiographically or even by intravascular ultrasound when viewed in standard video format[77]; the algorithms developed to accomplish the cylindrical reconstruction serve the dual functions of joining together the series of adjacent elements representing the neointima and then rotating the reconstructed image 90 degrees to permit viewing of the endoluminal surface en face. The sagittal reconstruction supplements the cylindrical format by facilitating analysis of the arterial contour proximal and distal to the stent; such analysis is otherwise not feasible using the unassembled tomographic images.

While sagittal and cylindrical three-dimensional formats facilitate qualitative assessment of pathologic alterations involving plaque arterial wall, neither format allows quantitative analysis of residual luminal cross-sectional area narrowing. Therefore, to take advantage

of the unique ability to planimeter the cross-sectional area from tomographic IVUS images, the lumen cast format was developed,[115,116,120,123] reconstructing a cast of the lumen by isolating it from the underlying arterial wall. Each sequential, stored IVUS frame is analyzed by projecting rays radially outward from the center of the transducer. Based on a preselected threshold valve, these rays automatically detect the luminal border; the borders detected by the rays are integrated to create a disc-like cross-sectional area "map" for each IVUS frame. Maps from sequential frames are then stacked to create a three-dimensional cast of the lumen. The area of each map or disc is determined by precalibration with the known size of the IVUS probe, and the resulting series of cross-sectional area determinations is plotted linearly, allowing near-instantaneous quantitative analysis of the cross-sectional area along the entire length of the vascular segment examined. Inspection of the plot permits rapid identification of sites of residual cross-sectional narrowing.

Preliminary in vitro[134] and in vivo[120] investigations have provided evidence validating the algorithm employed for quantitative analysis in the lumen cast format. While the lumen cast display forfeits information regarding qualitative alterations in the plaque and the underlying wall, this format greatly facilitates on-line interpretation of the extent to which satisfactory luminal dimensions have been achieved. The cast graphically depicts residual sites of luminal narrowing, and as a cursor is directed to any suspicious site, the cast provides automated quantitative assessment of the luminal cross-sectional area and the percentage of narrowing at that site. Moreover, because movement of the cursor to a specific level of the luminal cast simultaneously brings up the corresponding two-dimensional tomographic image on the upper left quadrant of the ImageComm workstation screen, the operator retains the option of inspecting the two-dimensional image to confirm the quantitative readout derived from analysis of the luminal cast. Our experience in employing the lumen cast algorithm on-line during interventional precedures suggests that it is useful in accurately and rapidly identifying sites of residual narrowing, including sites that might otherwise be overlooked during routine two-dimensional IVUS exam due to their focal nature.

Certain limitations of current attempts to perform three-dimensional reconstruction must be acknowledged. First, it is apparent that the quality of the three-dimensional reconstructions can only be as good as the original two-dimensional imges. Details that are absent from the original recordings will likewise be absent from the reconstructed images. In those instances when calcific deposits, for example, are observed on the two-dimensional images to attenuate echoes from the subjacent plaque and/or wall, these portions of the plaque and/or wall will not be incorporated into the reconstructed image.

Second, *ring-down artifact*, resulting from dead space in the acoustic transmission path and manifested on the two-dimensional image as a white halo immediately peripheral to the transducer, may obscure near-field structures in smaller, particularly stenotic, vessels. In our preliminary work, this artifact was routinely masked out of the three-dimensional reconstructions; in those cases in which reconstruction is applied to two-dimensional images with little or no lumen peripheral to the transducer, such masking could overestimate three-dimensional depiction of luminal patency. Current attempts by the manufacturers of mechanical transducer systems to eliminate this artifact will hopefully resolve this issue.

Third, while major branch points, such as the aortic bifurcation, are accurately depicted in the three-dimensional reconstruction, the two-dimensional images are otherwise reassembled as a straight tube; sharp bends in the artery are not faithfully reconstructed on either the two- or three-dimensional images. While this is typically not a severe libility in evaluation of the peripheral and renal circulations, it may become more significant in the assessment of the more tortuous coronary circrulion.

Fourth, three-dimensional reconstruction shares with conventional intravascular ultrasound imaging the difficulty of matching the rotational orienttion of the ultrasound transducer to that of the imaged vessel. Furthermore, if the ultrasound probe is inadvertently twisted during the pullback recording, the three-dimensional reconstruction will reflect this rotational event.

Fifth, in most studies performed to date, the two-dimensional images hve been acquired during a slow, timed catheter pullback; this strategy is intendd to optimize the number of images acquired over a given segment length and provide equal representation for each portion of the artery in the reconstructed image. Such catheter pullback, however, is entirely operator dependent, and small variations in the rate of pullback may ultimately influence the three-dimensional representation. For example, if the catheter withdrawal rate is slowed during pullback through an abnormal segment of vessel and subsequently accelerated through a more normal segment, the abnormal segment will occupy proportionally more than its true length of the resulting reconstruction. This phenomenon is particularly likely to occur when the operator tends to slow catheter movement through abnormal segments to achieve closer inspection of morphologic disruptions. Modifications in acquisition technique include automated imge registration utilizing motorized pullback devices, rendering the technique less operator dependent.[135]

Sixth, current software does not gate imge acquisition to phases of the cardiac cycle. While this is not a significant liability in three-dimensional reconstruction of peripheral vessels, it remains a major source of artifact in reconstruction of coronary and renal vessels.

Beyond these limitations, many of which are currently being addressed, the extent to which three-dimensional reconstruction will be employed clinically is principally dependent on two factors: the time required for reconstruction and the prognostic implications of the resulting images. With regard to the former, image processing time has been reduced considerably through a combination of modifications in software and memory expansion. Whereas early reconstructions typically required 20 to 40 minutes to assemble, current sagittal reconstructions are performed and visualized in real time, concurrent with catheter pullback[117] (Fig. 5–33). Cylindrical and lumen

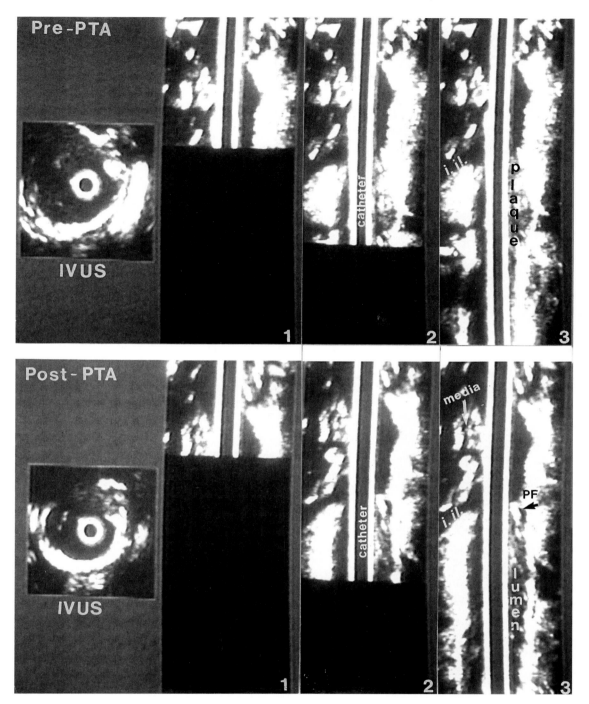

Figure 5–33.   Real-time three-dimensional reconstruction (3DR) of saggital images during intravascular ultrasound (IU) catheter pullback. Upper panel: pre-PTA, representative two-dimensional (2D) iu image stored from the beginning of the pullback is seen at left. This is one of the 220 individual images incorporated into saggital 3DR image, shown expanding in frames 1 to 3. IU catheter, located within vascular lumen, is abutted by atherescleroyic plaque (frane 3). Origin of internal iliac artery (i.il.) is demonstrated branching off to left one-third of way down reconstructed vessel. Lower panel: post-PTA, representative 2D IU image is shown at left. Frames 1 to 3 depict expanded 3D saggitel image, reconstructed concurrent with posy-PTA IU pullback (eg., real-time). In saggitel angle shown in frame 3, lumen diameter is increased from pre-PTA; plaque fracture (PF) in dilated site is demonstrated in longitudinal relief on reconstructed image. (Reconstructed view facilitates assessment of longitudinal extent of PF resulting from balloon angioplasty.)

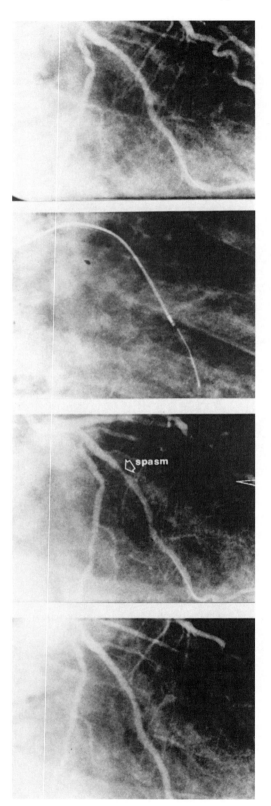

Figure 5–35.   In young childern or transplant donors with pristine coronary arteries, the absence of any intimal thickening precludes demonstration by IVUS of three-layered appearance; as intimal thickening begins to develop to a mild degree, the three-layered appearance becomes visible. Subsequently, however, as atherosclerotic narrowing begins to encroach on the lumen, the plaque appears to also encroach on the intima–media border. As a result, the three-layered appearance is gradually eroded. With the development of a high-grade lesion, frequently little remains of the three-layered appearance, making unambiguous demarcation of the internal and external elastic membranes (and, by inference, the media and the adventitia) less feasible.

COMING AND GOING OF THE 3-LAYERED APPEARANCE

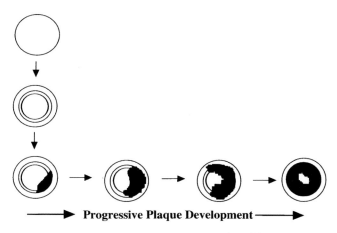

Figure 5-34. Coronary artery spasms induced by IVUS.

cast reconstructions are routinely available within 30 seconds of completing the pullback recording.[122] Thus, the time required to reconstruct and review the reconstructed images is comparable to that required to review the video playback of a contrast angiogram.

CURRENT LIMITATIONS OF IVUS FOR CLINICAL USE

Initial clinical applications of IVUS have also revealed certain limitations of this technology. Perhaps the most decisive limitation concerns the inability of currently available IVUS devices to consistently discriminate boundaries between the three layers of the arterial wall at sites of severe narrowing by atherosclerotic plaque. With advanced degrees of atherosclerosis, the characteristic ultrasound patterns become blurred. This is due principally to two factors: first, emaciation of the media typically accompanies progression of the atherosclerotic process.[136] Second, extensive calcific deposits, because they are often blanketed across the intimal–medial boundary, and because they attenuate or "shadow" the ultrasound reflections from the deeper layers of the wall, further obscure the normal ultrasound depiction of the arterial wall. Ambiguity regarding the boundary between intimal thickening and media reduces the precision with which any given measurement of wall thickness can be determined to represent atherosclerotic plaque versus normal wall.[39]

A second limitation of all currently available IVUS devices is that the design of these devices allows only for side viewing. Because forward-viewing devices[137] are not yet available for routine clinical applications, IVUS cannot be currently employed to determine the composition—for example, thrombus versus plaque—of a total occlusion prior to recanalization. Nor can

IVUS direct the advancement of a wire into an occluded segment. For this particular aspect of percutaneous interventional therapy, angioscopy may have superior utility. However, once through the occlusion, IVUS may identify whether the neolumen is intravascular or subintimal.[94]

Lastly, it should be pointed out that the application of IVUS imaging is not without risk, especially in the coronary circulation.[138] Because of the relatively large size of currently available catheters, imaging must be performed more expeditiously than is usually the case in the peripheral circulation. In addition, introduction of the IVUS catheter may occasionally precipitate spasm[139,140] (Fig. 5–34); accordingly, it is recommended that a final angiogram be recorded following IVUS examination of the coronary circulation.

REFERENCES

1. Vlodaver Z, Frech R, Van Tassel RA, et al. Correlations of the ante-mortem arteriogram and the post-mortem specimen. *Circulation* 1973;47:162.
2. Grondin CM, Dyrda I, Pasternac A, et al. Discrepancies between cineangiographic and post-mortem findings in patients with coronary artery disease and recent myocardial revascularization. *Circulation* 1974;49:703.
3. Pepine CJ, Feldman RL, Nichols WW. Coronary arteriography: potentially serious sources of error in interpretation. *Cardiovasc Med* 1977;2:747.
4. Arnett EN, Isner JM, Redwood CR, et al. Coronary artery narrowing in coronary heart disease: comparison of cineangiographic and necropsy findings. *Ann Intern Med* 1979;91:350.
5. Isner JM, Kishel J, Kent KM, et al. Accuracy of angiographic determination of left main coronary arterial narrowing: angiographic-histologic correlative analysis in 28 patients. *Circulation* 63:1056.
6. Isner JM, Donaldson RF. Coronary angiographic and morphologic correlation. *Cardiol Clin* 1984;2:571.
7. de Feyter PJ, Serruys PW, Davies MJ, et al. Quantitative coronary angiography to measure progression and regression of coronary atherosclerosis. *Circulation* 1991;84:412.
8. Marcus ML, Skorton DJ, Johnson MR, et al. Visual estimates of percent diameter coronary stenosis: "a battered gold standard." *JACC* 1988;11:882.
9. Dietz WA, Tobis JM, Isner JM. Failure of angiography to accurately depict the extent of coronary artery narrowing in three fatal cases of percutaneous transluminal coronary angioplasty. *JACC* 1992;19:1261.
10. White CW, Wright CB, Doty DB. Does visual interpretation of the coronary arteriogram predict the physiologic importance of a coronary stenosis? *N Engl J Med* 1984; 310:819.
11. Davidson CJ, Sheikh KH, Harrison JK, et al. Intravascular ultrasonography versus digital subtraction angiography: a human in vivo comparison of vessel size and morphology. *JACC* 1990;16:633.
12. Gussenhoven WJ, Essed CE, Frietman P, et al. Intravascular echographic assessment of vessel wall characteristics: a correlation with histology. *Int J Cardiol Imag* 1989;4:105.
13. Hodgson JMB, Graham SP, Savakus AD. Clinical percutaneous imaging of coronary anatomy using an over-the-wire ultrasound catheter system. *Int J Cardiac Imag* 1989;4:187.

14. St. Goar FG, Pinto FJ, Alderman EL, et al. Detection of coronary atherosclerosis in young adult heart using intravascular ultrasound. *Circulation* 1992;86:756.

15. Nissen SE, Guley JC, Grines CL, et al. Intravascular ultrasound assessment of lumen size and wall morphology in normal subjects and patients with coronary artery disease. *Circulation* 1991;84:1087.

16. Isner JM, Kaufman J, Rosenfield K, et al. Combined physiologic and anatomic assessment of percutaneous revascularization using a Doppler guidewire and ultrasound catheter. *JACC* 1993;71:70D.

17. Tenaglia AN, Buller CE, Kisslo KB, et al. Mechanisms of Balloon angioplasty and directional coronary atherectomy as assessed by intracoronary ultrasound. *Am J Cardiol* 1992;20:685.

18. Tenaglia AN, Tcheng JE, Kisslo KB, et al. Intracoronary ultrasound ealuation of excimer laser angioplasty. *Circulation* 1992;86:I-516. Abstract.

19. Yock PG, Fitzgerald PJ, Linker DT, et al. Intravascular ultrasound guidance for catheter-based coronary interventions. *JACC* 1992;17:39B.

20. Comess K, Fitzgerald PJ, Yock PG. Intracoronary ultrasound imaging of graft thrombosis. *N Engl J Med* 1992;327:1691.

21. Rosenfield K, Kaufman J, Pieczek A, et al. On-line three-dimensional reconstruction from 2D IVUS: utility for guiding interventional procedures. *JACC* 1992;19:224A. Abstract.

22. Rosenfield K, Losordo DW, Ramaswamy K, et al. Qualitative assessment of peripheral vessels by intravascular ultrasound before and after interventions. *JACC* 1990;15:107A. Abstract.

23. Rosenfield K, Voelker W, Losordo DW, et al. Assessment of coronary arterial stenoses post-intervention by quantitative angiography versus intracoronary ultrasound in 13 patients undergoing balloon and/or laser coronary angioplasty. *JACC* 1991;17:46A. Abstract.

24. The GUIDE trial investigators: lumen enlargement following angioplasty is related to plaque characteristics. A report from the GUIDE trial. *Circulation* 1992;86:I-531. Abstract.

25. Tobis JM, Mahon DJ, Lehmann KG, et al. Intracoronary ultrasound imaging after balloon angioplasty. *Circulation* 1990;82:III-676. Abstract.

26. Mintz GS, Leon MB, Satler LF, et al. Pre-intervention intravascular ultrasound imaging influences transcatheter coronary treatment strategies. *Circulation* 1992;86:I-323. Abstract.

27. Isner JM, Rosenfield K, Kelly K, et al. Percutaneous intravascular ultrasound examination as an adjunct to catheter-based interventions: preliminary experience in patients with peripheral vascular disease. *Radiology* 1990;175:61.

28. Gussenhoven eJ, The SHK, Serruys PW, et al. Intravascular ultrasound and vascular intervention. *J Int Cardiol* 1991;4:41.

29. Gurley JC, Nissen SE, Grines CL, et al. Comparison of intravascular ultrasound and angiography following percutaneous transluminal coronary angioplasty. *Circulation* 1990;82:III-72. Abstract.

30. Fitzgerald PJ, St. Goar FG, Connolly AJ, et al. Intravascular ultrasound imaging of coronary arteries. Is three layers the norm? *Circulation* 1992;86:154.

31. Gussenhoven WJ, Essed CE, Lance CT, et al. Arterial wall characteristics determined by intravascular ultrasound imaging: an in vitro study. *JACC* 1989;14:947.

32. Gussenhoven EJ, Essed CE, Frietman P, et al. Intravascular ultrasonic imaging; histologic and echographic correlation. *Eur J Vasc Surg* 1989;3:571.

33. Potkin BN, Bartorelli AL, Gessert JM, et al. Coronary artery imaging with intravascular high-frequency ultrasound. *Circulation* 1990;81:1575.

34. Nishimura RA, Edwards WD, Warness CA, et al. Intravascular ultrasound imaging: in vitro validation and pathologic correlation. *JACC* 1990;16:145.

35. Siegel RJ, Ariani M, Fishbein MC, et al. Histopathologic validation of angioscopy and intravascular ultrasound. *Circulation.* 1991;84:109.

36. Tobis JM, Mallery JA, Gessert JM, et al. Intravascular ultrasound cross-sectional arterial imaging before and after balloon angioplasty in vitro. *Circulation* 1989;80:873.

37. Coy KM, Maurer G, Siegel RJ. Intravascular ultrasound imaging: a current perspective. *JACC* 1991; 18:1811.

38. Siegel RJ, Fishbein MC, Chae JS, et al. Origin of the three-ringed appearance of human arteries by ultrasound: microdissection with ultrasonic and histologic correlation. *JACC* 1990;15:17A. Abstract.

39. Mallery JA, Tobis JM, Griffith JM, et al. Assessment of normal and atherosclerotic arterial wall thickness with an intravascular ultrasound imaging catheter. *Am Heart J* 1990;119:1392.

40. Yock PG, Linker DT. Intravascular ultrasound. Looking below the surface of vascular disease. *Circulation* 1990; 81:1715.

41. Webb JG, Yock PG, Slepian MJ. Intravascular ultrasound: significance of the three-layered appearance of normal muscular arteries. *JACC* 1990;15:17A. Abstract.

42. Lockwood GR, Ryan LK, Gotlieb AI, et al. In vitro high resolution intravascular imaging in muscular and elastic arteries. *JACC* 1992;20:153.

43. Young AC, Ryan TJ, Isner JM, et al. Correlation of intravascular ultrasound characteristics with endothelium-dependent vasodilator function in the coronary arteries of cardiac transplant patients. *Circulation* 1991;84:II-703.

44. Tobis JM, Mallery JA, Mahon DJ, et al. Intravascular ultrasound imaging of human coronary arteries in vivo. *Circulation* 1991;83:913.

45. Nissen SE, Grines CL, Gurley JC, et al. Application of a new phased-array ultrasound imaging catheter in the assessment of vascular dimensions. In vivo comparison to cineangiography. *Circulation* 1990;81:660.

46. St. Goar FG, Pinto FJ, Alderman EL, et al. Intracoronary ultrasound in cardiac transplant recipients: in vivo evidence of "angiographically silent" intimal thickening. *Circulation* 1992;85:979.

47. Pinto FJ, Chenzbraun A, Botas J, et al. Feasibility of serial intracoronary ultrasound imaging for assessment of progression of intimal proliferation in cardiac transplant recipients. *Circulation* 1994;90:2348.

48. Tuzcu EM, Hobbs RE, Rincon G, et al. Occult and frequent transmission of atherosclerotic coronary disease with cardiac transplantation. Insights from intravascular ultrasound. *Circulation* 1995;91:1706.

49. Pandian NG, Kreis A, Brockway B. Detection of intraarterial thrombus by intravascular high frequency two-dimensional ultrasound imaging: in vitro and in vivo studies. *Am J Cardiol* 1990;65:1280.

50. Siegel RJ, Chae JS, Forrester JS, et al. Angiography, angioscopy, and ultrasound imaging before and after percutaneous balloon angioplasty. *Am Heart J* 1990;120:1086.

51. Johnson C. Hansen DD, Vracko R, et al. Angioscopy: more sensitive for identifying thrombus, distal emboli, and subintimal dissection. *JACC* 1989;13:146A. Abstract.

52. Mecley M, Rosenfield K, Kaufman J, et al. Atherosclerotic plaque hemorrhage and rupture associated with crescendo claudication. *Ann Intern Med* 1992;117:663.
53. Yock PG, Linker DT. Catheter-based two-dimensional ultrasound imaging. In: Topol EJ (ed): *Textbook of Interventional Cardiology*. Philadelphia: WB Saunders, 19??;816–827.
54. Tabbara M, White RA, Cavaye D, et al. In vivo human comparison of intravascular ultrasonography and angiography. *J Vasc Surg* 1991;14:496.
55. Isner JM, Rosenfield K. Enough with the fantastic voyage: will IVUS pay in Peoria? *Cathet Cardiovasc Diagn* 1992;26:192.
56. Rosenfield K, Losordo DW, Harding M, et al. Intravascular ultrasound of renal arteries in patients undergoing percutaneous transluminal angioplasty: feasibility, safety, and initial findings, including 3-dimensional reconstruction of renal arteries. *JACC* 1992;17:204A. Abstract.
57. Nakamura S, Mahon DJ, Maheswaran B, et al. An explanation for discrepancy between angiographic and intravascular ultrasound measurements after percutaneous transluminal coronary angioplasty. *JACC* 1995;25:633.
58. Graham SP, Brands D, Savakus AD, et al. Utility of an intravascular ultrasound imaging device for arterial wall definition and atherectomy guidance. *JACC* 1989; 13:222A. Abstract.
59. Waller BF, Pinkerton CA, Slack JD. Intravascular ultrasound—a histologic study of vessels during life. The new "gold standard" for vascular imaging. *Circulation* 1992;85:2305.
60. Waller BF, Orr CM, Pinkerton CA, et al. Coronary balloon angioplasty dissections: "The Good, the Bad and the Ugly." *JACC* 1992;20:701.
61. Waller BF. Pathology of new interventions used in the treatment of coronary heart disease. *Curr Probl Cardiol* 1986;11:666.
62. Coy KM, Park JC, Fishbein MC, et al. In vitro validation of three-dimensional intravascular ultrasound for the evaluation of arterial injury after balloon angioplasty. *JACC* 1992;20:692.
63. Isner JM, Rosenfield K, Losordo DW, et al. Combination balloon-ultrasound imaging catheter for percutaneous transluminal angioplasty. *Circulation* 1991;84:739.
64. Honye J, Mahon DJ, Jain A, et al. Morphological effects of coronary balloon angioplasty in vivo assessed by intravascular ultrasound imaging. *Circulation* 1992;85:1012.
65. Losordo DW, Rosenfield K, Pieczek A, et al. How does angioplasty work? Serial analysis of human iliac arteries using intravascular ultrasound. *Circulation* 1992;86:1845.
66. Farb A, Virmani R, Atkinson JB, et al. Plaque morphology and pathologic changes in arteries from patients dying after coronary balloon angioplasty. *JACC* 1990; 16:1421.
67. Castaneda-Zuniga WR, Formanek A, Tadavarthy M. The mechanism of balloon angioplasty. *Radiology* 1980; 135:565.
68. The SHK, Gussenhoven EJ, Zhong Y, et al. Effect of balloon angioplasty on femoral artery evaluated with intravascular ultrasound imaging. *Circulation* 1992;86:483.
69. Honye J, Mahon DJ, Nakamura S, et al. Enhanced diagnostic ability of intravascular ultrasound imaging compared with angiography. *Circulation* 1992;86:I-324. Abstract.
70. Waller BF, Miller J, Morgan R, et al. Atherosclerotic plaque calcific deposits: an important factor in success or failure of transluminal coronary angioplasty. *Circulation* 1988;78:II-376. Abstract.
71. Fitzgerald PJ, Ports TA, Yock PG. Contribution of localized calcium deposits to dissecton after angioplasty. An observational study using intravascular ultrasound. *Circulation* 1992;86:64.
72. Mintz GS, Douek P, Pichard AD, et al. Target lesion calcification in coronary artery disease: an intravascular ultrasound study. *JACC* 1992;20:1149.
73. Yock PG, Fitzgerald PJ, Sykes C, et al. Morphologic features of successful coronary atherectomy determined by intravascular ultrasound imaging. *Circulation* 1990;82:III-676. Abstract.
74. Smucker ML, Scherb DE, Howard PF, et al. Intracoronary ultrasound: how much "angioplasty effect" in atherectomy. *Circulation* 1990;82:III-676. Abstract.
75. Penny WF, Schmidt DA, Safian RD, et al. Insights into the mechanism of luminal improvement after directional coronary atherectomy. *Am J Cardiol* 1991;67:435.
76. Safian RD, Gelbfish JS, Erny RE, et al. Coronary atherectomy. Clinical, angiographic, and histological findings and observations regarding potential mechanisms. *Circulation* 1990;82:69.
77. Chokshi SK, Hogan J, Desai V, et al. Intravascular ultrasound assessment of implanted stents. *JACC* 1990;15:29A. Abstract.
78. Rutherford RB, Flanigan DP, Guptka SK, et al. Sugested standards for reports dealing with lower extremity ischemia. *J Vasc Surg* 1986;4:80.
79. Isner JM. Vascular remodeling. Honey, I think I shrunk the artery. *Circulation* 1994;89:2937.
80. Glagov S, Weisenberg E, Zarins CK, et al. Compensatory enlargement of human atherosclerotic coronary arteries. *N Engl J Med* 1987;316:1371.
81. Post MJ, Borst C, Kuntz RE. The relative importance of arterial remodeling compared with intimal hyperplasia in lumen renarrowing after balloon angioplasty: a study in the normal rabbit and the hypercholesterolemic. Yucatan micropig. *Circulation* 1994;89:2816.
82. Zarins CK, Weisenberg E, Kolettis G, et al. Differential enlargement of artery segments in response to enlarging atherosclerotic plaques. *J Vasc Surg* 1988;7:386.
83. McPherson DD, Hiratzka LF, Lambert WC. Delineation of the extent of coronary atherosclerosis by high-frequency epidardial echocardiography. *N Engl J Med* 1987;316:304.
84. Losordo DW, Rosenfield K, Kaufman J, et al. Focal compensatory enlargement of human arteries in response to progressive atherosclerosis in vivo documentation using intravascular ultrasound. *Circulation* 1994;89:2570.
85. Glagov S, Grande J, Vesselinovitch D, et al. Quantitation of cells and fibers in histologic sections of arterial walls: advantages of contour tracing on a digitizing plate. In: McDonald TF, Chandler AB (eds): *Connective Tissues in Arterial and Pulmonary Disease*. New York: Springer-Verlag, 1981;57–93.
86. Siegel RJ, Swan K, Edwards G, et al. Limitations of post-mortem assessment of human coronary artery size and luminal narrowing: differential effects of tissue fixation and processing on vessels with different degrees of atherosclerosis. *JACC* 1985;5:342.
87. Mintz GS, Kovach JA, Javier SP, et al. Geometric remodeling is the predominant mechanism of late lumen loss after coronary angioplasty. *Circulation* 1983;88:I-654. Abstract.
88. Mintz GS, Kovach JA, Pichard AD, et al. Geometric remodeling is the predominant mechanism of clinical restenosis after coronary angioplasty. *JACC* 1994;23:138A. Abstract.

89. Kovach JA, Mintz GS, Kent KM, et al. Serial intravascular ultrasound studies indicate that chronic recoil is an important mechanism of restenosis following transcatheter therapy. *JACC* 1993;21:484. Abstract.

90. Pasterkamp G, Wensing PJW, Post JMJ, et al. Paradoxical arterial wall shrinkage may contribute to luminal narrowing of human atherosclerotic femoral arteries. *Circulation* 1995;91:1444.

91. Isner JM, Rosenfield K, Mosseri M, et al. How reliable are images obtained by intravascular ultrasound for making decisions during percutaneous interventions? Experience with intravascular ultrasound employed in lieu of contrast angiography to guide peripheral balloon angioplasty in 16 patients. *Circulation* 1990;82:III-440. Abstract.

92. Hodgson JMcB, Nair R. Efficacy abd usefulness of a combined intracoronary ultrasound-angioplasty balloon catheter: results of the multicenter Oracle trial. *Circulation* 1992; 86:I–321. Abstract.

93. Fitzgerald PJ, Muhlberger VA, Moes NY, et al. Calcium location within plaque as a predictor of atherectomy tissue retrieval: an intravascular ultrasound study. *Circulation* 1992;86:I–516. Abstract.

94. Rees MR, Sivananthan MU, Verma SP. The role of intravascular ultrasound and angioscopy in the placement and followup of coronary stents. *Circulation* 1992;86:I-364. Abstract.

95. Sahn S, Rothman A, Shiota T, et al. Acute and follow-up intravascular ultrasound findings after balloon dilation of coarctation of the aorta. *Circulation* 1994;90:340.

96. Kimura BJ, Fitzgerald PJ, Sudhir K, et al. Guidance of directed coronary atherectomy by intracoronary ultrasound imaging. *Am Heart J* 1992;124:1365.

97. Matar FA, Mintz GS, Pinnow E, et al. Multivariate predictors of intravascular end points after directional coronary atherectomy. *JACC* 1995;25:318.

98. Mintz GS, Potkin BN, Keren G, et al. Intravascular ultrasound evaluation of the effect of rotational atherectomy in obstructive atherosclerotic coronary artery disease. *Circulation* 1992;86:1383.

99. Rosenfield K, Losordo DW, Ramaswamy K, et al. Three-dimensional reconstruction of human coronary and peripheral arteries from images recorded during two-dimensional intravascular ultrasound examination. *Circulation* 1991;84:1938.

100. Tanaglia AN, Kisslo K, Kelly S, et al. Ultrasound guide wire-directed stent deployment. *Am Heart J* 1993; 125:1213.

101. Colombo A, Hall P, Nakamura S, et al. Intracoronary stenting without anticoagulation accomplished with intravascular ultrasound guidance. *Circulation* 1995; 91:1676.

102. Goldberg SL, Colombo A, Nakamura S, et al. Benefit of intracoronary ultrasound in the deployment of Palmaz-Schatz stents. *JACC* 1994;24:996.

103. Rosenfield K, Schainfeld RM, Khan W, et al. Restenosis of stented dialysis conduits caused by stent collapse, not neointimal proliferation. *JACC* 1995;25:262A.

104. Mallery JA, Gregory K, Morcos NC, et al. Evaluation of ultrasound balloon dilation imaging catheter. *Circulation* 1987;76:IV–371. Abstract.

105. Hodgson JMcB, Cacchione JG, Berry J, et al. Combined intracoronary ultrasound imaging and angioplasty catheter: initial in vivo studies. *Circulation* 1990;82:III–676.

106. Mudra H, Blasini R, Klauss V, et al. Diagnostic intracoronary ultrasound facility within a therapeutic balloon catheter has impact on PTCA strategy. *Circulation* 1992;86:I–324. Abstract.

107. Sanders M; Angiographic changes thirty minutes following percutaneous transluminal coronary angioplasty. *Angiology* 1985;36:419.

108. Nobuyoshi M, Kimura T, Nosaka H, et al. Restenosis after successful percutaneous transluminal coronary angioplasty: serial angiographic follow-up of 229 patients. *JACC* 1988;12–616.

109. Hjemdahl-Monsen CE, Ambrose JA, Borrico S, et al. Angiographic patterns of balloon inflation during percutaneous transluminal coronary angioplasty: role of pressure-diameter curves in studying distensibility and elasticity of the stenotic lesion and the mechanism of dilation. *JACC* 1990;16:569.

110. Kleiman NS, Raizner AE, Roberts R. Percutaneous transluminal coronary angioplasty: is what we see what we get? *JACC* 1990;16:576.

111. Yock PG, Fitzgerald PJ, Jang Y-T, et al. Initial trials of a combined ultrasound imaging/mechanical atherectomy catheter. *JACC* 1990;15:105A. Abstract.

112. Aretz HT, Martinelli MA, LeDet EF. Intraluminal ultrasound guidance of transverse laser coronary atherectomy. *Int J. Cardiac Imag* 1989;4:153.

113. Linker DR, Bylock A, Amin AB. Catheter ultrasound imaging demonstrates the extent of tissue disruption of excimer laser irradiation of human aorta. *Circulation* 1989;80(suppl II:II–581. Abstract.

114. Kasprzyk DJ, Crowley RJ, Isner JM. Excimer laser angioplasty in conjunction with intravascular ultrasonic imaging. *SPIE Proc Diagn Ther Cardiovasc Interventions II* 1992;1642:147.

115. Rosenfield K, Isner JM. Quantitative analysis by 3-dimensional intravascular ultrasound. *JIC* 1992;4:205.

116. Isner JM, Rosenfield K, Kelly S, et al. Percutaneous intravascular ultrasound for assessment of interventional techniques: initial findings in patients undergoing balloon angioplasty, atherectomy, and endovascular stent implants. *Circulation* 1989;11:579. Abstract.

117. Rosenfield K, Kaufman J, Langevin RE, et al. Real-time three-dimensional reconstruction of intravascular ultrasound images of iliac arteries. *Am J Cardiol* 1992;70:412.

118. Schryver TE, Popma JJ, Kent KM, et al. Use of the intracoronary ultrasound to identify the "true" coronary lumen in chronic coronary dissection treated with intracoronary stenting. *Am J Cardiol* 1992;69:1107.

119. DeJesus ST, Rosenfield K, Gal D, et al. 3-Dimensional reconstruction of vascular lumen from images recorded during percutaneous 2-D intravascular ultrasound. *Clin Res* 1989;37:838A. Abstract.

120. Rosenfield K, Losordo DW, Ramaswamy K, et al. Quantitative analysis of luminal cross-sectional area from 3-dimensional reconstruction of 2-dimensional intravascular ultrasound: validation of a novel technique. *Circulation* 1991;84:II–542. Abstract.

121. Rosenfield K, Harding M, Pieczek A, et al. 3-Dimensional reconstruction of balloon dilated coronary, renal, and femoropopliteal arteries from 2-D intravascular ultrasound images: analysis of longitudinal sagitttal versus cylindrical views. *JACC* 1991;17:234A. Abstract.

122. Rosenfield K, Kaufman J, Pieczek A, et al. Human coronary and peripheral arteries: on-line three-dimensional reconstruction from two-dimensioanl intravascular ultrasound scans. *Radiology* 1992;184:823.

123. Rosenfield K, Kaufman J. Pieczek A, et al. Lumen cast analysis: a quantitative format to expedite on-line analy-

sis for 3-D intravascular ultrasound images. *JACC* 1992;19:115A. Abstract.

124. Rosenfield K, Losordo DW, Harding M, et al. Three-dimensional reconstruction of coronary and peripheral vessels from 2-D IVUS images: determination of optimal image acquisition rate during timed pullback. *JACC* 1991;17:262A. Abstract.

125. Rosenfield K, Losordo DW, Palefsky P, et al. On-line 3-D reconstruction of 2-D intravascular ultrasound images during balloon angioplasty: clinical application in patients undergoing percutaneous balloon angioplasty. *JACC* 1991;17:156A. Abstract.

126. Rosenfield K, Losordo DW, Ramaswamy K, et al. 3-Dimensional reconstruction of intravascular ultrasound images recorded in 68 consecutive patients following percutaneous revascularization of totally occluded arteries: in vivo evidence that the neolumen frequently includes a subintimal component. *Circulation* 1991;84:II–686. Abstract.

127. Kitney RI, Moura L, Straughen K. 3-D visualization of arterial structures using ultrasound and Voxel modeling. *Int J Cardiac Imag* 1989;4:177.

128. Raya SQ, Udupa JK, Barrett WA. A PC-based 3-D imaging system: algorithms, software, and hardware considerations. *Comp Med Imag Graph* 1990;14:353.

129. Raya SP: SOFTVU—a software package for multidimensional medical image analysis. *Proc SPIE Med Imag IV* 1990;1232:152.

130. Spears JR, Sandor T, Baim DS, et al. The minimum error in estimating coronary luminal cross-sectional area from cineangiographic diameter measurements. *Cathet Cardiovasc Diagn* 1983;9:119.

131. Tobis JM, Smolin M, Mallery JA, et al. Laser-assisted angioplasty in human peripheral artery occlusions: mechanism of recanalization. *JACC* 1989; 13:1547.

132. Isner JM, Donaldson RF, Funai JT, et al. Factors contributing to perforations resulting from laser coronary angioplasty. Observations in an intact human post-mortem model of intra-operative laser coronary angioplasty. *Circulation* 1985;72:II–191.

133. Melchior JP, Meir B, Urban P, et al. Percutaneous transluminal coronary angioplasty for chronic total arterial occlusion. *Am J. Cardiol* 1987;59:535.

134. Zientek DM, Rodriguez ER, Liebson PR, et al. Validation of computerized three-dimensional reconstruction on intravascular ultrasound: measurements of absolute luminal diameter and cross-sectional area in ex vivo human coronary arteries. *JIC* 1992;4:179.

135. Mintz GS, Keller MB, Fay KG. Motorized IVUS transducer pullback permits accurate quantitative axial length measurements. *Circulation* 1992;86:I–323. Abstract.

136. Isner JM, Donaldson RF, Fortin AH, et al. Attenuation of the media in coronary arteries in advanced atherosclerosis. *Am J Cardiol* 1986;58:937.

137. Evans JL, Ng K-H, Vonesh MJ, et al. Arterial imaging with a new forward-viewing intravascular ultrasound cathter, I: initial studies. *Circulation* 1994;89:712.

138. Hausmann D, Erbel R, Alibelli-Chemarin M-J, et al. The safety of intracoronary ultrasound. A multicenter survey of 2207 examinations. *Circulation* 1995;91:623.

139. Isner JM, Rosenfield K, Losordo DW, et al. Clinical experience with intravascular ultrasound as an adjunct to percutaneous revascularization. In: Tobis JM, Yock P (eds): *Intravascular Ultrasound Imaging*. New York: Churchill Livingstone, Inc., 1992;171–197.

140. Alfonso F. Macaya C, Goicolea J, et al. Angiographic changes induced by intracoronary ultrasound imaging before and after coronary angioplasty. *Am Heart J* 1993;125:877.

6

Intermittent Claudication: Natural History, Medical Management, and Patient Selection for Intervention

William R. Hiatt, M.D.

Peripheral arterial occlusive disease (PAOD) affects a large segment of the adult population, with an age-adjusted prevalence of 12 to 20%.[1,2] Approximately 50% of patients with PAOD (diagnosed by noninvasive testing) are asymptomatic, 45% have intermittent claudication, and only a small minority have severe symptoms of ischemic pain at rest, ulceration, or gangrene.[3] Intermittent claudication occurs with walking when the limited arterial blood supply does not meet the metabolic demand of the muscles in the legs, resulting in muscle ischemia. This symptom causes a walking impairment that may profoundly disrupt the activities of daily life. Up to 38% of patients under the age of 55 years seeking treatment for claudication are disabled and require public assistance.[4] In addition, the yearly health care costs of patients with symptomatic PAOD were estimated to be $30.5 million in 1989 in the state of Maryland alone.[5]

Patients with PAOD have a greatly increased risk of cardiovascular mortality compared to age-matched controls. Therefore, given the prevalence of PAOD and claudication, as well as the significant risk of cardiovascular morbidity and mortality, a number of medical and interventional treatment strategies have been developed to manage the disease. This chapter will address the natural history and medical management of patients with PAOD. Although there are many medical therapies that must be considered in the management of the patient with PAOD, interventional treatment should be reserved for the most symptomatic patients.

NATURAL HISTORY OF CLAUDICATION

Patients with PAOD have a four- to sixfold increased risk of cardiovascular mortality compared to healthy, age-matched individuals.[6] The mortality risk increases with more severe vascular disease, as assessed by the ankle/brachial index (ABI),[7,8] or with more severe symptoms.[9] In a review of the literature, the mortality rate in this patient population averaged 5.7% per year, with higher mortality rates in patients who continued to smoke and in diabetic patients.[3] In contrast, patients with intermittent claudication have a fairly stable natural history.[10,11] Over 5 years, approximately 70% of patients with claudication will have stable symptoms and 30% will progress to tissue loss, with need for bypass surgery or amputation.[3] This natural history influences treatment decisions for most patients with claudication as the primary symptom; specifically, the major goals are to reduce the risk of cardiovascular mortality and to relieve intermittent claudication.

MEDICAL MANAGEMENT

Identification and Management of Vascular Disease Risk Factors

Diabetes Mellitus

Patients with diabetes have a two- to fourfold increased risk of developing intermittent claudication compared to nondiabetics.[12,13] In addition, diabetics tend to have a greater atherosclerotic disease burden, with a more distal distribution of peripheral arterial occlusions, and a worse natural history than nondiabetics with PAOD.[3,14] Complicating the management of the diabetic with claudication is the associated peripheral neuropathy and susceptibility to foot infections. Thus, a multifactorial approach must be used in treating these patients.

Although diabetes is a major risk factor for PAOD, at the time of presentation the degree of glycemic control, as assessed by blood sugar level or glycosylated hemoglobin level, is not well correlated with the presence or severity of PAOD.[15] However, in the diabetic, the associated risk factors of smoking and hyperlipidemia correlate strongly with disease severity.[15,16] Management of these patients should include excellent glycemic control, but more importantly, the clinician must also attempt to address the lipid status and smoking behavior of diabetic patients with vascular disease.[17] In diabetics, exercise training improves glycemic control and lipid profiles.[18] Although exercise programs for diabetics with PAOD have not been evaluated, exercise training in these patients may help to relieve symptoms of claudication and improve glycemic control and other cardiovascular risk factors.

Hyperlipidemia

The major lipid risk factors for PAOD are a low high density lipoprotein (HDL) cholesterol and elevated triglyceride levels.[19,20] Several trials have been conducted to evaluate the change in femoral atherosclerosis with the treatment of hyperlipidemia. In the majority of the studies, cholesterol-lowering agents were used as the primary intervention, with niacin added to increase HDL cholesterol. Recent trials support the observation that lipid modification is associated with stabilization or regression of femoral atherosclerosis.[21,22] In adition, cholesterol-lowering drug therapy decreases cardiac morbidity and mortality.[23–25] Because coronary artery disease is very prevalent in patients with PAOD, the goal of lipid therapy should be similar in both populations. The current American Heart Association recommendation is a low density lipoprotein (LDL) cholesterol level of 100 mg/dL or less.[25] In the majority of patients, this goal can be achieved only with lipid-lowering drug therapy.

Cigarette Smoking

In smokers, the risk of developing PAOD is increased two- to threefold, and smoking correlates more closely with the development of intermittent claudication than with any other cardiovascular risk factor.[3,26,27] Patients with PAOD who continue to smoke have a greater likelihood of vascular disease progression, myocardial infarction, stroke, and death than those who quit smoking.[28] In contrast, smoking cessation is associated with improvement in the symptoms of claudication and

better surgical results.[3,29] In patients with very severe PAOD, smoking can cause cutaneous vasoconstriction, which retards the healing of ischemic ulcers. Therefore, smoking cessation is critical in the management of the claudicator.

Hypertension

Hypertension is an independent risk factor for patients with claudication, raising the risk approximately twofold.[26] Hypertension needs to be treated aggressively in this patient population to reduce the risk of stroke and other adverse cardiovascular outcomes. However, when drug therapy results in a large decrease in systemic blood pressure, some patients may experience a slight worsening of their claudication symptoms.[30]

Homocysteine Level

Several reports have shown a strong association between increases in plasma homocysteine concentration and PAOD.[31–33] This is an important risk factor in patients who present with claudication at all ages, but particularly under the age of 50 years.[34] The genetic causes of disorders of homocysteine metabolism are relatively rare, but nutritional deficiencies of vitamins B_6, B_{12}, and folate may be more common causes of elevated homocysteine levels. The mechanism of homocysteine-induced atherosclerosis is multifactorial but may include impaired endothelial production of nitric oxide, proliferation of vascular smooth muscle cells, and thrombosis.[35] Screening for this disorder is generally not recommended because there are as yet no results from intervention trials. However, when selected patients are evaluated for the disorder, it is important to measure homocysteine and the oxidized products of homocysteine because these compounds may be atherogenic. Treatment involves primarily the administration of folate, in combination with vitamins B_6 and B_{12} when appropriate.[35]

Pharmacologic Management of Peripheral Arterial Disease

The primary goal of medical management in all patients with PAOD is to decrease the risk of cardiovascular morbidity and mortality. All patients with PAOD should be evaluated aggressively for the cardiovascular risk factors discussed above, with appropriate treatment provided. In particular, a high percentage of these patients will need drug therapy for management of their lipid disorders, as well as control of their hypertension and diabetes.

Other therapies have also been developed to slow the progression of peripheral atherosclerosis, as well as to decrease cardiovascular mortality. Antiplatelet therapy has been used extensively in patients with cardiovascular disease to reduce mortality. In patients with PAOD, antiplatelet therapy (primarily aspirin) has been shown to reduce the risk of myocardial infarction, stroke, and vascular death from 11.8% with placebo to 9.7% with drugs.[36] Ticlopidine has also been shown to reduce vascular morbidity and mortality in patients with PAOD, perhaps to a greater extent than aspirin.[37,38] Other antiplatelet therapies have been developed to reduce cardiovascular mortality, including clopidogrel (Lancet 1996;348:1329–39) and a new class of antiplatelet agents that block the GP llb/III receptor on platelets. Aspirin has also been shown to reduce the need for peripheral arterial surgery in the Physician's Health Study.[39] These studies demonstrate that a multifactorial approach may be necessary to alter the natural history of peripheral atherosclerosis.

Pharmacologic Management of Claudication

Vasodilators

Arteriolar vasodilators were the first class of agents used to treat claudication. However, these drugs have not been shown to have clinical efficacy in randomized, controlled trials[30,41,42] and therefore are not currently recommended for claudication.

Anticoagulant/Antiplatelet Drugs

As discussed above, the use of aspirin and other antiplatelet agents may be important in the long-term treatment of peripheral atherosclerosis. In selected patients, aspirin combined with warfarin has been used empirically following bypass surgery to prevent graft thrombosis. However, studies evaluating the effects of aspirin or coumarin on the treatment of claudication have shown no benefit.[43] Ticlopidine is a potent inhibitor of platelet aggregation that also has hemorrheologic effects. In one randomized, placebo-controlled trial, ticlopidine was shown to improve claudication symptoms and exercise performance.[44]

Hemorrheologic Agents

Pentoxifylline is currently the only approved drug for claudication. In early controlled trials, the drug produced a 22% improvement over placebo in walking distance prior to the onset of claudication and a 12% increase in maximal walking distance.[45] More recent studies suggest that patients with symptoms for longer than a year and an ankle/arm systolic blood pressure ratio below 0.80 are the subgroup most likely to respond to the drug.[46]

Metabolic Agents

Patients with PAOD not only have limited arterial blood flow, but also develop metabolic abnormalities in their skeletal muscle.[47] In patients with PAOD, carnitine is an important cofactor for skeletal muscle intermediary metabolism during exercise. Carnitine is required for the mitochondrial oxidation of long-chain fatty acids and also helps to maintain normal cellular metabolism under conditions of metabolic or hypoxic stress.[48] It has thus been hypothesized that carnitine supplementation would improve ischemic muscle metabolism. Carnitine, and an acyl form of carnitine (propionyl-L-carnitine), are experimental drugs that have been shown to increase exercise performance and improve claudication symptoms in patients with PAOD.[49,50] Several large clinical trials are in progress to establish the role of carnitine supplementation in treating patients with claudication.

Prostaglandin Drugs

Various prostaglandin analogues have been developed to treat patients with critical leg ischemia and claudication.[51] Preliminary results are encouraging, and several large clinical trials are in progress to evaluate the efficacy of these compounds.

Other Claudication Drugs

Chelation therapy has been touted as a means to treat atherosclerosis and relieve symptoms of cardiovascular disease. However, there is no scientific basis to support these claims. One randomized, double-blind multicenter trial of ethylene diamine tetraacetic acid (EDTA) has been conducted in patients with PAOD.[52] The drug was not shown to be effective in treating the symptoms of claudication or improving the ABI.

Exercise Rehabilitation

Many of the basic principles of exercise rehabilitation in diseased populations were originally developed for patients with coronary artery disease. However, the specific methods used to train patients with PAOD differ from the techniques used in cardiac rehabilitation. Supervised treadmill exercise is the most effective mode of exercise therapy for claudicators. Exercise sessions are typically held three times a week for approximately 1 hour each, and 3 to 6 months of training are customary. The beginning training workload is determined from the symptom-limited maximal treadmill test on entry; that is, the intensity of the treadmill exercise is set to the workload that initially brings on claudication pain in the patient. During the exercise sessions, rest periods (induced by claudication) are interspersed with sessions of treadmill walking. In subsequent visits, the speed or grade is increased if the patient is able to walk for 10 minutes or longer at the lower workload without experiencing moderate claudication pain. The initial training session is 35 minutes long, with subsequent increases of 5 minutes per session until a 50-minute session is possible.

A supervised exercise rehabilitation program is a highly effective treatment for patients with claudication. Walking exercise training is associated with well-established changes in treadmill exercise performance and community-based walking ability, as well as functional status in this patient population. Therefore, some form of exercise training has been recommended for nearly 50 years to help patients with PAOD improve their walking ability. Many previous trials of exercise conditioning in this patient population were not randomized or controlled. However, a recent meta-analysis of 18 nonrandomized studies involving 548 patients has shown that an exercise program will significantly improve treadmill exercise performance.[53] On average, there was a 179% improvement in pain-free walking distance from 126 ± 57 m on entry to 351 ± 189 m after therapy. Maximal walking distance increased 122%, from 326 ± 148 m on entry to 723 ± 592 m after rehabilitation. Therefore, the ability to walk for longer periods with less claudication pain is improved by training.

To date, eight randomized trials have been carried out to evaluate the efficacy of exercise rehabilitation. Seven of these trials had a nonexercising control group, and three compared exercise training to an interventional or active drug therapy. The most recent two trials also used questionnaire assessment to evaluate the change in community-based functional status.

In 1966 the first randomized, controlled trial of exercise training in patients with PAOD was published.[54] Fourteen patients with claudication were paired and then randomized into exercise and control groups. The exercise group was instructed to take a 1-hour daily walk with a pedometer and record the distance walked for 6 months, while the placebo group took a lactose tablet twice daily. Maximal walking time increased in the exercise-treated group by 183% and pain-free walking distance by 106%. In contrast, the treadmill walking distance did not change in the control group.

Two studies done in the 1970s evaluated the benefits of a program of "dynamic leg exercises" (including walking, running, dancing, and playing ball games) for improving walking ability in persons with PAOD.[55,56] In these trials, treated patients improved their maximal walking distance significantly, with increases ranging from 117% to 135%, and their pain-free walking distance from 170% to 220%.

The effect of 6 months of exercise training alone or combined with antiplatelet therapy (dipyridamole and aspirin) was evaluated in 30 patients with PAOD.[57] After 6 months of treatment, the pain-free walking time and maximal walking time improved in all three groups compared to baseline. In the group receiving drugs only, maximal walking time improved by 38% and pain-free walking time by 35%. In the group receiving exercise training only, maximal walking time improved by 86% and pain-free walking time by 90%. Finally, in the group receiving both treatments, maximal walking time improved by 105% and pain-free walking time by 120%. The differences in walking time between the group receiving drugs only and the two groups receiving exercise therapy were significant, but there were no differences between the two exercise groups.

Lundgren et al[58] conducted a randomized, controlled trial comparing the effects of peripheral bypass surgery, surgery followed by 6 months of supervised exercise training (dynamic leg exercises), or 6 months of supervised exercise training along in 75 patients with claudication. After 13 months, walking ability was improved in all three groups. In this study, the most effective treatment to improve functional status was exercise training plus surgery. The changes in maximal walking distance were 173% for the surgical group, 263% for the group that received both therapies, and 151% for the exercise-trained group. The authors found that although all surgically treated patients increased their walking distance more than patients who received only exercise training, they also had a higher rate of complications than the exercise group.

Another randomized study compared percutaneous transluminal angioplasty ($n = 20$) to a supervised program of dynamic leg exercises ($n = 16$).[59] After angioplasty, mean ABI values were significantly improved, but only at 3 months was maximum walking distance improved over baseline. In the exercise group, despite no improvement in the ABI, maximal and pain-free walking distances were progressively increased at each follow-up, with significant increases at 6, 9, and 12 months. Pain-free walking distance increased by 296% and maximum walking distance by 442% at 12 months in the exercise-trained group.

Two randomized, controlled trials of exercise conditioning for patients with PAOD have been performed using graded treadmill protocols.[60–62] In the first study,[60] 20 patients with walking impairment due to PAOD were randomized into an exercising group or a control group. The exercise program consisted of 3 months of supervised treadmill walking, with the training intensity progressively increased on a weekly basis. After 12 weeks, treated subjects increased their maximal walking time by 123%, maximal oxygen consumption by 30%, and pain-free walking time by 165%. Controls had a 20% increase in maximal walking time but no change in pain-free walking time, maximal oxygen consumption, or any other measures of treadmill exercise performance.

In a more recent trial,[61,62] 29 patients with disabling claudication were randomized to one of two exercise programs or a control group. In addition to assessing the value of a treadmill exercise training program, a secondary goal was to investigate strength training as an alternative training modality in the PAOD population. After the first 12 weeks, patients in the treadmill-trained group had a 74 ± 58% increase in maximal walking time, as well as improved maximal oxygen consumption and a prolonged pain-free walking time. Twelve additional weeks of treadmill exercise resulted in a 128% increase in maximal walking time. The treadmill training program also improved functional status in terms of walking distance, stair-climbing ability, overall physical activity, and physical functioning. After 12 weeks of strength training, patients improved their maximal walking time but no other marker of treadmill exercise performance. Minimal benefits to functional status, measured by questionnaire, resulted from strength training. Control subjects showed no change in treadmill or community-based functional variables. Thus, a supervised treadmill walking exercise program was an effective means to improve exercise performance and functional status in patients with intermittent claudication, with continued improvement over 24 weeks of training. In contrast, 12 weeks of strength training alone was much less effective than 12 weeks of supervised treadmill walking exercise.

PATIENT SELECTION FOR INTERVENTION

Asymptomatic Patients

Patients with asymptomatic atherosclerotic PAOD may be identified by a screening vascular laboratory study, or by the presence of vascular bruits or absent pulses on physical examination. If vascular disease is documented, these patients should undergo aggressive risk factor identification and modification in an attempt to reduce cardiovascular mortality and slow disease progression to the symptomatic phase. Interventional therapy is not warranted in asymptomatic patients with PAOD.

Patients with Claudication

In patients with symptomatic claudication, risk factor modification is of primary importance. Next, the physician must ascertain the severity of the claudication symptoms and the degree of disability experienced by the patient. Treadmill testing is an objective means of quantifying exercise impairment in the patient with claudication,[63] as well as documenting the amount of improvement in exercise performance after any intervention for claudication. A thorough discussion of treadmill testing methodologies in the PAOD population has been published.[63]

It is also critically important to determine the patient's assessment of his or her claudication severity in the community setting, as well as the degree of improvement from treatment. In this regard, several questionnaires have been developed and validated in the PAOD population. The PAD Walking Impairment Questionnaire (WIQ) evaluates patient-reported walking speed, distance, stair-climbing ability, and limita-

tions in walking ability due to specific symptoms. This questionnaire is sensitive to changes in community-based walking ability after exercise training and bypass surgery.[62,64] The Physical Activity Recall (PAR) provides a more global measure of impairment by assessing the energy expenditure of the patient at work, as well as during home and leisure-time activities.[65] This questionnaire can detect an increase in weekly energy expenditure after an exercise rehabilitation program.[62] Finally, the Medical Outcomes Study questionnaire has also been applied to the PAOD population. Exercise training was shown to improve the physical functioning scores.[62]

REFERENCES

1. Hiatt WR, Marshall JA, Baxter J, et al. Diagnostic methods for peripheral arterial disease in the San Luis Valley Diabetes Study. *J Clin Epidemiol* 1990;43:597–606.
2. Criqui MH, Fronek A, Barrett-Connor E, Klauber MR, Gabriel S, Goodman D. The prevalence of peripheral arterial disease in a defined population. *Circulation* 1985;71:510–515.
3. McDaniel MD, Cronenwett JL. Basic data related to the natural history of intermittent claudication. *Ann Vasc Surg* 1989;3:273–277.
4. Olsen PS, Gustafsen J, Rasmussen L, Lorentzen JE. Long-term results after arterial surgery for arteriosclerosis of the lower limbs in young adults. *Eur J Vasc Surg* 1988;2:15–18.
5. Tunis SR, Bass EB, Steinberg EP. The use of angioplasty, bypass surgery, and amputation in the management of peripheral vascular disease. *N Engl J Med* 1991;325:556–562.
6. McKenna M, Wolfson S, Kuller L. The ratio of ankle and arm arterial pressure as an independent predictor of mortality. *Atherosclerosis* 1991;87:119–128.
7. Newman AB, Siscovick DS, Manolio TA, et al. Ankle-arm index as a marker of atherosclerosis in the cardiovascular health study. *Circulation* 1993;88:837–845.
8. Vogt MT, Cauley JA, Newman AB, Kuller LH, Hulley SB. Decreased ankle/arm blood pressure index and mortality in elderly women. *JAMA* 1993;270:465–469.
9. Criqui MH, Langer RD, Fronek A, et al. Mortality over a period of 10 years in patients with peripheral arterial disease. *N Engl J Med* 1992; 326:381–386.
10. Jelnes R, Gaardsting O, Hougaard Jensen K, Baekgaard N, Tonnesen KH. Fate in intermittent claudication: outcome and risk factors. *Br Med J* 1986;293:1137–1140.
11. Singer A, Rob C. The fate of the claudicator. *Br Med J* 1960;633–636.
12. Kannel WB, McGee DL. Diabetes and cardiovascular disease. The Framingham Study. *JAMA* 1979;241:2035–2038.
13. Brand FN, Abbott RD, Kannel WB. Diabetes, intermittent claudication, and risk of cardiovascular events. *Diabetes* 1989;38:504–509.
14. Hertzer NR. The natural history of peripheral vascular disease. Implications for its management. *Circulation* 1991;83(suppl I):I-12–I-19.
15. Beach KW, Strandness DE. Arteriosclerosis obliterans and associated risk factors in insulin-dependent and non-insulin-dependent diabetes. *Diabetes* 1980;29:882–888.
16. Reunanen A, Takkunen H, Aromaa A. Prevalence of intermittent claudication and its effect on mortality. *Acta Med Scand* 1991;211:249–256.

17. Orchard TJ, Strandness DE, Cavanagh PR, et al. Assessment of peripheral vascular disease in diabetes. Report and recommendations of an international workshop. *Circulation* 1993;88:819–828.

18. Ronnemaa T, Mattila K, Lehtonen A, Kallio V. A controlled randomized study on the effect of long-term physical exercise on the metabolic control in type 2 diabetic patients. *Acta Med Scand* 1986;220:219–224.

19. Pomrehn P, Duncan B, Weissfeld L, et al. The association of dyslipoproteinemia with symptoms and signs of peripheral arterial disease. The lipids research clinics program prevalence study. *Circulation* 1986;73(suppl I):I-100–I-107.

20. Montanari G, Vaccarino V, Franeschini G, Sirtori M, Bondioli A, Sirtori CR. Metabolic approach to the diagnosis and treatment of atherosclerotic peripheral vascular disease. *Int Angiol* 1987;6:339–349.

21. Olsson AG, Ruhn G, Erikson U. The effect of serum lipid regulation on the development of femoral atherosclerosis in hyperlipidaemia: a non-randomized controlled study. *J Int Med* 1990;227:381–390.

22. Blankenhorn DH, Azen SP, Crawford DW, et al. Effects of colestipol-niacin therapy on human femoral atherosclerosis. *Circulation* 1991;83:438–447.

23. Frick MH, Elo O, Haapa K, et al. Helsinki Heart Study: primary-prevention trial with gemfibrozil in middle-aged men with dyslipidemia. Safety of treatment, changes in risk factors, and incidence of coronary heart disease. *N Engl J Med* 1987;317:1237–1245.

24. Gotto AM. Lipid lowering, regression, and coronary events. A review of the interdisciplinary council on lipids and cardiovascular risk intervention, seventh council meeting. *Circulation* 1995;92:646–656.

25. Superko HR, Krauss RM. Coronary artery disease regression. Convincing evidence for the benefit of aggressive lipoprotein management. *Circulation* 1994;90:1056–1069.

26. Kannel WB, McGee DL. Update on some epidemiologic features of intermittent claudication: the Framingham Study. *J Am Geriatr Soc* 1985;33:13–18.

27. Gofin R, Kark JD, Friedlander Y, et al. Peripheral vascular disease in a middle-aged population sample. The Jerusalem lipid research clinic prevalence study. *Isr J Med Sci* 1987;23:157–167.

28. Juergens JL, Barker NW, Hines EA. Arteriosclerosis obliterans: a review of 520 cases with special reference to pathogenic and prognostic factors. *Circulation* 1960;21:188–195.

29. Krupski WC. The peripheral vascular consequences of smoking. *Ann Vasc Surg* 1991;5:291–304.

30. Solomon SA, Ramsay LE, Yeo WW, Parnell L, Morris-Jones W. B blockade and intermittent claudication: placebo controlled trial of atenolol and nifedipine and their combination. *Br Med J* 1991;303:1100–1104.

31. Clarke R, Daly L, Robinson K, et al. Hyperhomocysteinemia: an independent risk factor for vascular disease. *N Engl J Med* 1991;324:1149–1155.

32. Molgaard J, Malinow MR, Lassvik C, Holm AC, Upson B, Olsson AG. Hyperhomocyst(e)inaemia: an independent risk factor for intermittent claudication. *J Int Med* 1992;231:273–279.

33. Taylor LM, DeFrang RD, Harris EJ, Poroter JM. The association of elevated plasma homocyst(e)ine with progression of symptomatic peripheral arterial disease. *J Vasc Surg* 1991;13:128–136.

34. Brattstrom L, Israelsson B, Norrving B, et al. Impaired homocysteine metabolism in early-onset cerebral and peripheral occlusive arterial disease. *Atherosclerosis* 1990; 81:51–60.

35. Stampfer MJ, Malinow MR. Can lowering homocysteine levels reduce cardiovascular risk? *N Engl J Med* 1995; 332:328–329.

36. Antiplatelet Trialists' Collaboration. Secondary prevention of vascular disease by prolonged antiplatelet treatment. *Br Med J* 1988;296:320–331.

37. Bokissel JP, Peyrieux JC, Destors JM. Is it possible to reduce the risk of cardiovascular events in subjects suffering from intermittent claudication of the lower limbs? *Thromb Haemost* 1996;62:681–685.

38. Janzon L, Bergqvist D, Boberg J, et al. Prevention of myocardial infarction and stroke in patients with intermittent claudication; effects of ticlopidine. Results from STIMS, the Swedish Ticlopidine Multicenter Study. *J Int Med* 1990; 227:301–308.

39. CAPRIE Steering Committee. A randomized, blinded, trial of clopidogrel versus aspirin in patients at risk of ischaemic events (CAPRIE). *Lancet* 1996;348:1329–1339.

40. Goldhaber SZ, Manson JE, Stampfer MJ, et al. Low-dose aspirin and subsequent peripheral arterial surgery in the physicians' health study. *Lancet* 1992;340:143–145.

41. Coffman JD. Vasodilator drugs in peripheral vascular disease. *N Engl J Med* 1979;300:713–717.

42. Spence JD, Arnold JMO, Munoz, CE, et al. Angiotensin-converting enzyme inhibition with cliazapril does not improve blood flow, walking time, or plasma lipids in patients with intermittent claudication. *J Vasc Med Biol* 1993;4:23–28.

43. Deutschinoff A, Grozdinsky L. Rheological and anticoagulant therapy of patients with chronic peripheral occlusive arterial disease (COAD). *Angiology* 1987;38:351–357.

44. Balsano F, Coccheri S, Libretti A, et al. Ticlopidine in the treatment of intermittent claudication: a 21-month double-blind trial. *J Lab Clin Med* 1989;114:84–91.

45. Porter JM, Cutler BS, Lee BY, et al. Pentoxifylline efficacy in the treatment of intermittent claudication: multicenter controlled double-blind trial with objective assessment of chronic occlusive arterial disease patients. *Am Heart J* 1982;104:66–72.

46. Lindgarde F, Jelnes R, Bjorkman H, et al. Conservative drug treatment in patients with moderately severe chronic occlusive peripheral arterial disease. *Circulation* 1989;80:1549–1556.

47. Hiatt WR, Wolfel EE, Regensteiner JG, Brass EP. Skeletal muscle carnitine metabolism in patients with unilateral peripheral arterial disease. *J Appl Physiol* 1992;73:346–353.

48. Bieber LL. Carnitine. *Annu Rev Biochem* 1988;57:261–283.

49. Brevetti G, Chiariello M, Ferulano G, et al. Increases in walking distance in patients with peripheral vascular disease treated with L-carnitine: a double-blind, cross-over study. *Circulation* 1988;77:767–773.

50. Brevetti G, Perna S, Sabba C, et al. Superiority of L-propionyl carnitine vs L-carnitine in improving walking capacity in patients with peripheral vascular disease: an acute, intravenous, double-blind, cross-over study. *Eur Heart J* 1992;13:251–255.

51. Scheffler P, de la Hamette D, Gross J, Mueller H, Schieffer H. Intensive vascular training in stage IIb of peripheral arterial occlusive disease. The additive effects of intravenous prostaglandin E1 or intravenous pentoxifylline during training. *Circulation* 1994;90:818–822.

52. Guldager B, Jelnes R, Jorgensen SJ, et al. EDTA treatment of intermittent claudication—a double blind, placebo-controlled study. *J Int Med* 1992;231:261–267.

53. Gardner AW, Poehlman ET. Exercise rehabilitation programs for the treatment of claudication pain. A meta-analysis. *JAMA* 1995;274:975–980.

54. Larsen OA, Lassen NA. Effect of daily muscular exercise in patients with intermittent claudication. *Lancet* 1966;2:1093–1096.

55. Dahllof A, Bjorntorp P, Holm J, Schersten T. Metabolic activity of skeletal muscle in patients with peripheral arterial insufficiency. Effect of physical training. *Eur J Clin Invest* 1974;4:9–15.

56. Holm J, Dahllof A, Bjorntorp P, Schersten T. Enzyme studies in muscles of patients with intermittent claudication. Effect of training. *Scand J Clin Lab Invest* 1973 (suppl 128);31:201–205.

57. Mannarino E, Pasqualini L, Innocente S, Scricciolo V, Rignanese A, Ciuffetti G. Physical training and antiplatelet treatment in stage II peripheral arterial occlusive disease: alone or combined? *Angiology* 1991;42:513–521.

58. Lundgren F, Dahllof A, Lundholm K, Schersten T, Volkmann R. Intermittent claudication—surgical reconstruction or physical training? A prospective randomied trial of treatment efficiency. *Ann Surg* 1989;209:346–355.

59. Creasy TS, McMillan PJ, Fletcher EWL, Collin J, Morris PJ. Is percutaneous transluminal angioplasty better than exercise for claudication? Preliminary results from a prospective randomized trial. *Eur J Vasc Surg* 1990;4:135–140.

60. Hiatt WR, Regensteiner JG, Hargarten ME, Wolfel EE, Brass EP. Benefit of exercise conditioning for patients with peripheral arterial disease. *Circulation* 1990;81:602–609.

61. Hiatt WR, Wolfel EE, Meier RH, Regensteiner JG. Superiority of treadmill walking exercise vs. strength training for patients with peripheral arterial disease. Implications for the mechanism of the training response. *Circulation* 1994;90:1866–1874.

62. Regensteiner JG, Steiner JF, Hiatt WR. Exercise training improves functional status in patients with peripheral arterial disease. *J Vasc Surg* 1996;23:104–115.

63. Hiatt WR, Hirsch AT, Regensteiner JG, Brass EP, the Vascular Clinical Trialists. Clinical trials for claudication. Assessment of exercise performance, functional status, and clinical end points. *Circulation* 1995;92:614–621.

64. Regensteiner JG, Hargarten ME, Rutherford RB, Hiatt WR. Functional benefits of peripheral vascular bypass surgery for patients with intermittent claudication. *Angiology* 1993;44:1–10.

65. Sallis JF, Haskell WL, Wood PD, et al. Physical activity assessment methodology in the five-city project. *Am J Epidemiol* 1985;121:91–106.

7

Hyperlipidemia: When and How to Treat

Jeffrey W. Olin, D.O.

There is unequivocal evidence that increased serum total cholesterol (TC), as well as increased low density lipoprotein cholesterol (LDL-C) levels and decreased high density lipoprotein cholesterol (HDL-C) levels, are strongly associated with the development of complications resulting from atherosclerotic vascular disease.[1] In the Multiple Risk Factor Intervention Trial,[2] the relationship between the TC level and death from coronary heart disease deaths was continuous and graded; the higher the cholesterol level, the greater the risk.

Since the time of these early observations, an enormous amount of data has been published regarding the role of cholesterol-lowering therapy for patients with coronary artery and peripheral vascular disease. When these data are carefully analyzed, the evidence is clear that cholesterol-lowering therapy decreases coronary heart disease events and death. In addition, recent studies have also shown a decrease in all-cause mortality as well.[3,4] Regression of atherosclerosis has been shown in virtually every study performed to assess the role of lipid-lowering therapy in the progression and regression of atherosclerosis. There is emerging evidence demonstrating that lipid-lowering therapy [specifically with hydroxy methylglutaryl coenzyme A (HMG Co-A) reductase inhibitors] may improve endothelial cell function, and the restoration of endothelial function appears to be an important factor in the mechanism by which lipid-lowering therapy decreases coronary event rates and prevents the progression of atherosclerosis.

There are still unanswered questions regarding lipid management, such as the most appropriate treatment for women or the elderly who do not have evidence of vascular disease (primary prevention) and the treatment of isolated low HDL-C. However, the central issues regarding cholesterol management in patients with clinical evidence of atherosclerosis (secondary pre-vention) or in primary prevention in men have been resolved.

EVIDENCE THAT CHOLESTEROL-LOWERING THERAPY REDUCES CARDIOVASCULAR RISK

The Coronary Drug Project[5] was a secondary prevention trial, completed in the 1960s assessing the effects of various drugs in 8341 men with a history of myocardial infarction. After 15 years of follow-up, the subjects treated with niacin had an 11% decrease in all-cause mortality compared to those treated with placebo ($p = 0.0004$). In the 1970s and early 1980s, two large-scale primary prevention trials were completed. The Lipid Research Clinics Coronary Primary Prevention Trial (LRC-CPPT)[6,7] was a randomized, placebo-controlled, double-blind, multicenter trial comparing the effectiveness of the bile acid sequestrant cholestyramine with placebo. There was a 19% reduction in primary end-points (definite non-fatal myocardial infarction and coronary heart disease death) in patients treated with cholestyramine compared to the placebo group ($p < 0.05$). The Helsinki Heart Study[8] was a randomized, double-blind, 5-year primary prevention trial comparing placebo with the fibric acid derivative gemfibrozil in 4081 middle-aged men (40 to 55 years). Gemfibrozil produced a 9% decrease in TC and an 8% decrease in LDL-C. There was a 34% reduction in the incidence of fatal and nonfatal myocardial infarction and cardiac death in the gemfibrozil-treated group compared to the placebo group. This reduction in cardiac events is greater than expected with only an 8% reduction in LDL-C. The most likely reason for this degree of reduction in cardiac event rates was the beneficial effect that gemfibrozil had on HDL-C and triglyceride levels. However, in both of these trials, there was no decrease in all-cause mortality between the placebo group and the drug-treated group. This may be explained, in part, by the relatively modest decrease in TC and LDL-C in each of these studies. In the LRC-CPPT,[6,7] the mean TC at 1 and 7 years in the placebo group was 275 mg/dL and 277 mg/dL respectively, and in the cholestyramine-treated group it was 239 mg/dL and 257 mg/dL respectively. Gould and colleagues[9] performed a meta-analysis of all randomized trials of more than 2 years' duration ($n = 35$ trials) and demonstrated that the greater the reduction in cholesterol, the greater the decrease in coronary heart disease mortality. For every 10 percentage point reduction in cholesterol, coronary heart disease mortality was reduced by 13% ($p < 0.002$) and total mortality by 10% ($p < 0.03$). There was no effect on noncoronary heart disease mortality.

However, two recently published large-scale studies [the Scandinavian Simvastatin Survival Study (4S)[3] and the West of Scotland Coronary Prevention Study[4]] demonstrated that not only coronary heart disease event and death rates can be decreased, but all-cause mortality as well[10] (Table 7–1). Both of these studies used HMG Co-A reductase inhibitors to lower TC and LDL-C; these are the most potent drugs currently available to lower LDL-C. The 4S Study[3] was a randomized, double-blind placebo-controlled secondary prevention trial involving 4444 patients. Simvastatin lowered the TC by 25%, lowered the LDL-C by 35%, and raised the HDL-C by 8%. At just over 5 years of follow-up, the relative risk of all deaths in the treated group was 0.70

(95% confidence interval 0.58 to 0.85), $p = 0.0003$). A clinical benefit became apparent in the simvastatin-treated group by 6 months, and these differences became statistically significant by 18 months. The relative risk of all coronary deaths was 0.58, and that of all cardiovascular deaths was 0.65. Women represented 18.6% of the study population and achieved a reduction in major coronary event rates similar to that of men. The overall mortality in women was low, so that no overall difference in all-cause mortality was seen in women receiving simvastatin compared to placebo. This is the first study to show that all-cause mortality and major coronary events can be significantly decreased in subjects more than 60 years of age.

The West of Scotland Coronary Prevention Study[4] addressed the role of cholesterol reduction in 6595 men between the ages of 45 and 64 who had not experienced a myocardial infarction (primary prevention). Patients were randomized to one of two groups, taking 40 mg of the HMG Co-A reductase inhibitor pravastatin every evening or placebo. The average follow-up period was 4.9 years. There was a 26% decrease in LDL-C, a 20% decrease in TC, a 12% decrease in triglycerides, and a 5% increase in HDL-C in the pravastatin-treated group. There was a 31% reduction in definite coronary events ($p < 0.001$), a 31% decrease in non-fatal myocardial infarction ($p < 0.001$), and a 32% decrease in death from all cardiovascular causes ($p = 0.033$) in the

Table 7–1.

	West of Scotland Coronary Prevention Study[4]	Scandinavian Simvastatin Survival Study (4S)[3]
Study design	Randomized, double-blind, and placebo-controlled	Randomized, double-blind, and placebo-controlled
Number of patients	6595	4444
Gender	Men (100%)	Men (81%) and women (19%)
Age (years)	45–64	35–70
Lipid-lowering agent	Pravastatin, 40 mg daily	Simvastatin, 20–40 mg daily
Mean follow-up (years)	4.9	5.4
Primary prevention	90%	—
Secondary prevention	10% had angina	100% (angina or MI)
Change in lipids		
TC	–20%	–25%
LDL-C	–26%	–35%
HDL-C	+5%	+8%
Triglycerides	–12%	–10%
Endpoints (% risk reduction)		
Nonfatal MI or death from CHD	31% ($p < 0.001$)	34% ($p < 0.00001$) 35% ($p = 0.01$) for women
PTCA or CABG	37% ($p = 0.009$)	37% ($p = 0.0001$)
CHD death (definite and suspected)	33% ($p = 0.042$)	42% (0.0001)
Death from any cause	22% ($p = 0.051$)	30% ($p = 0.0003$)

Source: Reference 10.

Abbreviations: MI, myocardial infarction; CHD, coronary heart disease; PTCA, percutaneous transluminal coronary angioplasty; CABG, coronary artery bypass graft.

pravastatin-treated group. There was no excess death from noncardiovascular causes in the actively treated group. There was a 22% (95% confidence interval 0 to 40%, $p = 0.051$) reduction in death from any cause. Reductions in LDL-C in the West of Scotland Coronary Primary Prevention Study[4] and the 4S Study[3] were much more substantial than those observed in the LRC-CPPT[6,7] and the Helsinki Heart Study,[8] possibly explaining the more marked reduction in cardiovascular events and in all-cause mortality.

Although some investigators have suggested that mortality is increased when TC values are < 160 mg/dL, an (NHLBI) Consensus Conference concluded that there was little evidence to support this adverse effect of cholesterol-lowering therapy.[11] Recently, Newman and Hulley[12] suggested that cholesterol-lowering medication caused cancer in rodents and extrapolated that the hypolipidemic medications may have the same effects on humans. In an elegant editorial, Dalen and Dalton[13] contested these conclusions. Three large meta-analyses[14–16] addressing the issue of cancer deaths and cholesterol lowering medications concluded that there is no evidence supporting such an association.

REGRESSION OF ATHEROSCLEROSIS

Numerous animal studies over the last 30 to 40 years have demonstrated that regression of atherosclerosis is possible with a low-cholesterol, low-saturated-fat diet. Over the last two decades, a large body of literature has emerged showing that regression of atherosclerosis is also possible in humans.[17–36] Most of the recently reported regression studies used quantitative angiography to measure progression and regression of coronary and peripheral atherosclerosis. The actual degree of regression measured by quantitative arteriography is small, suggesting that something other than changes in luminal diameter accounted for the marked reduction in atherosclerotic events that occurred in these trials. A detailed description of every regression study published to date is beyond the scope of this chapter. However, it should be noted that the degree of LDL reduction is substantial in virtually all of the regression trials. Most of the studies used an HMG Co-A reductase inhibitor, a bile acid resin, and/or niacin in combination with dietary therapy. Virtually every study published to date has demonstrated regression of atherosclerosis, and most of these studies have shown a decrease in cardiac event rates.

While most investigations have used lipid-lowering therapy to achieve regression of atherosclerosis, the Lifestyle Heart Trial[24] utilized intensive lifestyle modifications such as diet, exercise, and stress management to lower lipid values and decrease coronary heart disease events. In the programs on the surgical control of the hyperlipidemias (POSCH) Trial,[20] patients with a previous myocardial infarction were randomized to one of two groups, diet alone or diet and partial ileal bypass, as a means of lowering cholesterol. There was a 35% reduction in the coronary heart disease event rate in the patients undergoing partial ileal bypass compared to the control group. In addition, more regression occurred in the actively treated group. Blankenhorn and Hodis[36] performed a meta-analysis using the data from the NHLBI Type II,[17] CLAS,[18] POSCH,[20] UCSF-SCOR,[21] FATS,[22] St. Thomas' Atherosclerosis Regression Study (STARS),[23] and the Lifestyle Heart Trial[24] to evaluate the role of lipid-lowering therapy in regression of atherosclerosis and in secondary prevention of coronary heart disease. In the actively treated group of patients ($n = 688$), the odds ratio of achieving regression of atherosclerosis was 2.0 and progression of atherosclerosis was 0.4 compared to control subjects ($n = 593$) (Fig. 7–1). A total of 793 treated patients and 708 control patients were further analyzed. Cardiovascular disease events, revascularization, and deaths were significantly less in the treated group compared to the control group. The odds ratio for all-cause mortality was reduced but fell short of the 95% confidence level for significance (Fig. 7–2).

There have also been numerous studies on the use of noninvasive imaging (B-mode ultrasound) of the carotid and peripheral arteries to document the extent of atherosclerotic disease and to determine whether or not regression of atherosclerosis had occurred. A population-based ultrasonography study of eastern Finnish men demonstrated a strong association between intima-media thickness (IMT), measured by B-mode ultrasound, and the presence of cardiovascular disease.[37] The Cholesterol Lowering Atherosclerosis Study[33] reported that patients receiving placebo had an increase in IMT compared to a significant decrease in patients receiving active drug, over a 48-month period.

It is apparent that the beneficial effects of cholesterol lowering occur early, long before significant regression of atherosclerosis occurs. Benzuly and colleagues[38] have shown that functional improvement (measured as an abnormal vasoconstrictor response to serotonin) occurs before there are detectable changes in the atherosclerotic lesion. Gould and associates[39] showed that lowering cholesterol over a 90-day period decreased the size and severity of perfusion abnormalities on positron emission tomography well before structural regression of atherosclerosis could be demonstrated. Recently, data from the Cholesterol Lowering Atherosclerosis Study[40] showed that the risk of clinical coronary events (need for revascularization, non-fatal acute myocardial infarction, and coronary death) correlated with coronary lesion progression ($p < 0.05$). New lesion formation in bypass grafts ($p = 0.02$) and progression of mild/moderate lesions (<50% stenosis) were predictive of clinical coronary events ($p < 0.01$).

Regression of atherosclerosis is dependent on the composition of the plaque (such as lipid components,

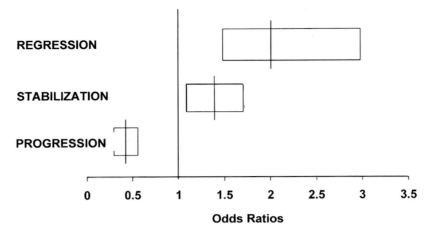

Figure 7–1. Graph showing odds ratios and 95% confidence limits for regression, stabilization, and progression comparing 688 treated subjects with 593 control subjects with entrance and exit angiograms derived from seven coronary angiographic trials. From Blankenhorn DH and Hodis HN, Arterioscler and Thromb 12:177, 1994 with permission.

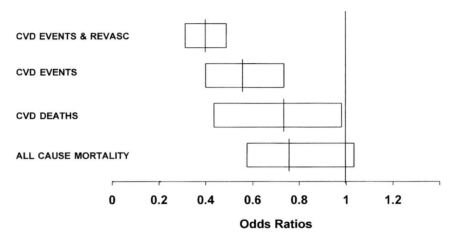

Figure 7–2. Graph showing odds ratios and 95% confidence limit for clinical coronary events and all-cause mortality, comparing 793 treated with 708 control subjects from seven coronary angiographic trials. From Blankenhorn DH and Hodis HN, Arterioscler and Thromb 12:177, 1994 with permission.

macrophages, smooth muscle cells, and connective tissue). Calcification or fibrous tissue makes regression less likely. Other mechanisms, such as lysis of occlusive thrombi or mural thrombi, healing or remodeling of an acutely disruptive plaque, physiologic remodeling independent of plaque size, relaxation of arterial vasomotor tone (vasodilator or vasoconstrictor responses), and the role of the endothelium itself, may be important.[41] Numerous factors are related to plaque instability and disruption.[42] Plaque disruption occurs most frequently when the fibrous cap is thinnest and most heavily infiltrated by foam cells. Falk and colleagues[42] have suggested that plaque rupture depends on the size and consistency of the atheromatous core, the thickness and collagen content of the fibrous cap covering the core, inflammation within the cap, and cap

"fatigue." Data from animal experiments suggest that lipid-lowering therapy depletes plaque lipid, with a reduction in cholesterol esters resulting in a stiffer, more stable atheromatous lesion.

In a randomized, double-blind, placebo-controlled trial, Treasure and colleagues[43] demonstrated that cholesterol-lowering therapy with lovastatin significantly improved endothelium-mediated responses in coronary arteries in patients with atherosclerosis. In a similar study, Anderson et al[44] randomly assigned 49 patients with coronary artery disease to receive one of three treatments: the American Heart Association Step I diet (diet group, $n = 11$), lovastatin and cholestyramine (LDL-lowering group, $n = 21$), or lovastatin and probucol (LDL-lowering–antioxidant group, $n = 17$). Endothelium-dependent coronary artery vasomotion and the response to intracoronary infusion of acetylcholine (an endothelium-dependent vasodilator) were assessed at baseline and after 1 year of therapy. Patients with coronary artery disease demonstrated vasoconstriction (an abnormal physiologic response) when acetylcholine was infused. The greatest improvement in vasoconstrictor response occurred in the LDL-lowering–antioxidant group compared to the diet group ($p < 0.01$), with a lesser response in the LDL-lowering diet group compared to the diet group ($p = 0.08$). These studies suggest that improvement in endothelial function may, at least in part, account for the decreased event rate that occurs early in patients treated with lipid-lowering therapy. In addition, improvement in endothelium-mediated relaxation may also signal the stabilization of atherosclerotic plaque. Endothelium-dependent vasomotor responses to acetylcholine and flow-mediated vasodilatation in the brachial artery closely parallel the coronary artery endothelium-dependent vasomotor responses.[45]

TREATMENT GUIDELINES

The second report of the National Cholesterol Education Program Expert Panel on the Detection, Evaluation and Treatment of High Blood Cholesterol in Adults (Adult Treatment Panel II)[46] provided specific guidelines for managing elevated blood lipid levels. Treatment decisions are based on the level of LDL-C in the presence or absence of preexisting heart or vascular disease (Table 7–2). In patients with clinical evidence of coronary heart disease or peripheral vascular disease, the goal LDL-C is <100 mg/dL. This goal should be achieved with a combination of dietary therapy, hormone replacement therapy (in the post-menopausal patient), and lipid-lowering drug therapy.

The initial steps to lower cholesterol are dietary, and useful dietary guidelines are outlined in the National Cholesterol Education Program guidelines published

Table 7–2. Treatment Decisions Based on LDL-Level

Patient Category	Initiation Level	LDL Goal
Dietary Therapy		
No CHD, <2 risk factors	≥160 mg/dL	<160 mg/dL
No CHD, ≥2 risk factors	≥130 mg/dL	<130 mg/dL
CHD, other vascular disease	>100 mg/dL	≤100 mg/dL
Drug Therapy		
No CHD, <2 risk factors	≥190 mg/dL	<160 mg/dL
No CHD, ≥2 risk factors	≥160 mg/dL	<130 mg/dL
CHD, other vascular disease	≥130 mg/dL	≤100 mg/dL

Abbreviations: CHD, coronary heart disease
Source: National Cholesterol Education Program Guidelines, Adult Treatment Panel II. *JAMA* 1993;269:3015–3023.

in 1988.[47] It is also clear that hormone replacement therapy with estrogens, cycled with progesterone, causes not only an improvement in lipoprotein values but also a decrease in coronary event rates. Adult treatment guidelines of the National Cholesterol Education Program advise consideration of estrogen replacement therapy for post-menopausal women with elevated cholesterol, particularly if they have coronary artery or peripheral vascular disease.

Pharmacologic therapy of patients with lipid abnormalities generally involves the use of drugs that reduce LDL-C concentrations. The major drug classes include the bile acid sequestrants, nicotinic acid, and the HMG Co-A reductase inhibitors. Gemfibrozil and other fibric acid derivatives are primarily triglyceride-lowering agents and tend to increase HDL-C concentrations. Nicotinic acid is the most potent HDL-C-raising agent currently available. Probucol lowers LDL-C but also lowers HDL-C, therefore, it is not widely used in clinical practice. The commonly used drugs, dosages, mechanisms of actions, and side effects are shown in Table 7–3.[48]

Combinations of drugs may be particularly effective when the drugs have different mechanisms of action, as well as major effects on different lipid and lipoprotein components. For example, nicotinic acid and the bile acid binding resins were a very effective combination in a number of clinical trials.[18,19] Another very effective drug combination for patients with marked increases in LDL-C is HMG Co-A reductase inhibitors and bile acid binders.[49] Furthermore, many lipid experts find that using low doses of more than one agent frequently reduces side effects and increases efficacy. Hence, there is a trend away from using full doses of a single medication before moving to another medication. Increasingly, it has become necessary to use a fibric acid derivative such as gemfibrozil and an HMG Co-A reductase inhibitor in combination. The risk of myositis is approximately 5 to 7% with this combination. However if the patient is educated about this possibility and followed frequently, this combination of drugs can be safely administered.

Patients who have evidence of coronary heart disease or peripheral vascular disease, or who have undergone intervention for any form of atherosclerosis, should have their lipid abnormalities treated aggressively. Often combination drug therapy using several different classes of hypolipidemic agents is necessary to adequately control the LDL-C level and optionally raise the HDL-C level. The goal of treatment is to prevent the progression of atherosclerosis, allow regression of atherosclerosis to occur, stabilize the atherosclerotic plaque, improve endothelial function, and decrease coronary heart disease events. Unfortunately, lipid-lowering therapy has not been demonstrated to decrease the incidence of restenosis after percutaneous transluminal angioplasty or stent placement.

Table 7–3. Lipid-Lowering Drugs

Type of Drug	Usual Dosage (total/day)	Times (per day)	Mechanism of Action	Comments

Bile acid sequestrants*
Cholestyramine
Colestipol
	
	4–24 g
	5–30 g
		
		2–3
		2–3
			Increases clearance of cholesterol-binding bile acids; increases LDL receptor-mediated catabolism of LDL-C	Anticipated side effects
				  Bloating
				  Midepigastric fullness or pain
				  Constipation (may be decreased by adding 3–4 g psyllium to each dose of resin)
				Tolerance increased by slow upward dose titration
				Colestipol also available in caplet form
				Possible binding of other agents including antihypertensive agents: in general, give other drugs at least 1 hour before or 4 hours after resin.
				Avoid giving with serum triglyceride levels >400 mg/dL unless gemfibrozil or niacin is also given

Nicotinic acid	1000–4000 mg	2–3	Inhibits lipoprotein and apo-lipoprotein B synthesis	Anticipated side effects
				  Flushing—especially with regular crystalline niacin preparations; usually diminished with time, administration with food, and/or addition of low-dose aspirin
				  Gastrointestinal distress/dyspepsia—probably more common with slow-release preparations and may represent early symptoms of chemical hepatitis
				May cause itching, headache, insomnia, recurrence of gout, unmasking of glucose intolerance, or diabetes mellitus; may cause toxic amblyopia, acanthosis nigricans, dry skin, or myositis (particularly when combined with an HMG CoA reductase inhibitor)

HMG CoA reductase inhibitors
  Lovastatin
  Pravastatin
 	
  Simvastatin
  Fluvastatin
	
	20–80 mg
	10–40 mg
	
	10–40 mg
	20–40 mg
		
		1–2
		1
		
		1
		1
			Inhibits the rate-limiting enzyme in cholesterol synthesis; increases LDL receptor-mediated catabolism of LDL-C	Capable of lowering LDL-C by 35–45% in high percentage of patients
				Side effects infrequent; liver enzyme elevations frequently occur but are of questionable significance; liver function testing still recommended
				Mainly lowers LDL-C level; modest elevation of HDL-C level and reduction of serum triglyceride level also occur
				Do not cause cataracts; most feared side effect is myositis, which is rare except when used with niacin, gemfibrozil, cyclosporin, or possibly erythromycin
				Most cost-effective use may be in high-risk patients; addition of low-dose resin therapy may be particularly effective

Gemfibrozil	1200 mg	2	Increases lipoprotein lipase activity	Most potent and consistently effective triglyceride-lowering agent; tends to increase HDL-C level and reduce LDL-C level by 10–20%; seems to be more effective in reducing primary CHD risk in hypertriglyceridemic patients with high LDL-C/HDL-C ratios than predicted by its LDL-C–lowering effect

*May be given as a single dose at bedtime (1 or 2 scoops or packets). Daytime doses should be given before meals.
Abbreviation: HMG CoA, hydroxy methylglutaryl coenzyme A.
From Young JR, Olin JW, Bartholomew JR (eds). *Peripheral Vascular Diseases.* C.V. Mosby Co., second edition, 1996.

REFERENCES

1. Kannel WB, Castelli WP, Gordon T, McNamara P. Serum cholesterol, lipoprotein, and the risk of coronary heart disease. The Framingham Study. *Ann Intern Med* 1971;74:1–12.
2. Multiple Risk Factor Intervention Trial Research Group. Multiple Risk Factor Intervention Trial: Risk factor changes and mortality rates. *JAMA* 1982;248:1465–1477.
3. Scandinavian Simvastatin Survival Study Group. Randomized trial of cholesterol lowering in 4,444 patients with coronary heart disease. The Scandinavian Simvastatin Survival Study (4S). *Lancet* 1994;344:1363–1389.
4. Shepherd J, Cobbe SM, Ford I, et al. Prevention of coronary heart disease with pravastatin in men with hypercholesterolemia. *N Engl J Med* 1995;333:1301–1307.
5. Canner PL, Berge KG, Wenger NK, et al. Fifteen year mortality in Coronary Drug Project patients: long-term benefit with niacin. *J Am Coll Cardiol* 1986;8:1245–1255.
6. Lipid Research Clinics Program. The Lipid Research Clinics Primary Trial Results. I. Reduction in incidence of coronary heart disease. *JAMA* 1984;351–364.
7. Lipid Research Clinics Program: The Lipid Research Clinics Coronary Primary Prevention Trial Results. II. The relationship of reduction and incidence of coronary heart disease to cholesterol lowering. *JAMA* 1984;251:365–374.
8. Frick MH, Elo O, Haapa K, et al. Helsinki Heart Study: Primary Prevention Trial with gemfibrozil in middle-aged men with dyslipidemia. Safety of treatment, changes in risk factors, and incidence of coronary heart disease. *N Engl J Med* 1987;317:237–1245.
9. Gould AL, Rossouw JE, Santanello NC, Heise JF, Furberg CD. Cholesterol reduction yields clinical benefit. A new look at old data. *Circulation* 1995;91:2274–2282.
10. Olin JW. Cholesterol lowering: perspectives on the 4S and West of Scotland studies. *Cleve Clin J Med* 1996;63:1–4.
11. Jacobs D, Blackburn H, Higgins M, et al. Report of the conference on low blood cholesterol: mortality associations. *Circulation* 1992;86:1046–1060.
12. Newman TB, Hulley SB. Carcinogenicity of lipid-lowering drugs. *JAMA* 1996;275:55–60.
13. Dalen JE, Dalton WS. Does lowering cholesterol cause cancer? *JAMA* 1996;275:67–69.
14. Davey Smith G, Pekkanen J. Should there be a moratorium on the use of cholesterol lowering drugs? *Br Med J* 1992;304:431–434.
15. Kritchevsky SB, Kritchevsky D. Serum cholesterol and cancer risk: an epidemiologic perspective. *Annu Rev Nutr* 1992;391–416.
16. Law MR, Thompson SG, Wald NJ. Assessing possible hazards of reducing serum cholesterol. *Br Med J* 1994;308:373–379.
17. Brensike JF, Levy RI, Kelsey SF, et al. Effects of therapy with cholestyramine on progression of coronary arteriosclerosis. Results of the NHLBI Type II Coronary Intervention Study. *Circulation* 1984;69:313–324.
18. Blankenhorn DH, Nessim SA, Johnson RL, et al. Beneficial effects of combined colestipol-niacin therapy on coronary atherosclerosis and coronary bypass grafts. *JAMA* 1987;257:3233–3240.
19. Cashin-Hemphill L, Mack WJ, Pogoda JM, et al. Beneficial effects of colestipol-niacin on coronary atherosclerosis: a four year follow up. *JAMA* 1990;264:3013–3017.
20. Buchwald H, Varco RL, Matts JP, et al. Effect of partial ileal bypass surgery on mortality and morbidity from coronary heart disease in patients with hypercholesterolemia. Report of the Programs on the Surgical Control of the Hyperlipidemias (POSCH). *N Engl J Med* 1990;323:946–955.
21. Kane JP, Malloy MJ, Ports TA, et al. Regression of coronary atherosclerosis during treatment of familial hypercholesterolemia with combined drug regimens. *JAMA* 1990;264:3007–3012.
22. Brown G, Albers JJ, Fisher LD, et al. Regression of coronary artery disease as a result of intensive lipid-lowering therapy in men with high levels of apolipoprotein B. *N Engl J Med* 1990;323:1289–1298.
23. Watts GF, Lewis B, Brunt JNH, et al. Effects of coronary artery disease of a lipid lowering diet, or a diet plus cholestyramine. In: St. Thomas' Atherosclerosis Regression Study (STARS). *Lancet* 1992;339:563–569.
24. Ornish D, Brown SE, Scherwitz LW, et al. Can lifestyle changes reverse coronary heart disease? The Lifestyle Heart Trial. *Lancet* 1990;336:129–133.
25. Blankenhorn DH, Azen SP, Krams CH, et al. Coronary angiographic changes with lovastatin therapy: The Monitored Atherosclerosis Regression Study (MARS). *Ann Intern Med* 1993;119:969–976.
26. Waters D, Higginson L, Gladstone P, et al. Effects of monotherapy with an HMG Co-A reductase inhibitor on the progression of coronary atherosclerosis as assessed by serial quantitative arteriography: the Canadian Coronary Atherosclerosis Intervention Trial. *Circulation* 1994;89:959–968.
27. Pitt B, Mancini GBJ, Ellis SG, et al. Pravastatin limitation of atherosclerosis in the coronary arteries (PLAC I): reduction in atherosclerosis, progression and clinical events. *J Am Coll Cardiol* 1995;26:1133–1139.
28. Alderman EL, Haskell WL, Fair JM, et al. Beneficial angiographic and clinical response to multifactor modification in the Stanford Coronary Risk Intervention Project (SCRIP). *Circulation* 1994;89:979–990.
29. Crouse JR III, Byington RP, Bond MG, et al. Pravastatin, lipids and atherosclerosis in the carotid arteries (PLAC II). *Am J Cardiol* 1995;75:455–459.
30. Jukema JW, Bruschke AVG, van Boven AJ, et al. Effects of lipid lowering by pravastatin on progression and regression of coronary artery disease in symptomatic men with normal to moderately elevated serum cholesterol levels. The Regression Growth Evaluation Statin Study (REGRESS). *Circulation* 1995;91:2528–2540.
31. Furberg CD, Adams HP Jr, Applegate WB, et al. Effects of lovastatin on early carotid atherosclerosis and cardiovascular events. *Circulation* 1994;90:1679–1687.
32. Blankenhorn DH, Azen SP, Crawford DW, et al. Effects of colestipol-niacin therapy on human femoral atherosclerosis. *Circulation* 1991;83:438–447.
33. Blankenhorn DH, Selzer RH, Crawford DW, et al. Beneficial effects of colestipol-niacin on the common carotid artery: Two- and four-year reduction in intima-media thickness measured by ultrasound. *Circulation* 1993;88:20–28.
34. Gotto AM. Lipid lowering, regression and coronary events. A review of the Interdisciplinary Council on Lipids and Cardiovascular Risk Intervention, 7th Council meeting. *Circulation* 1995;92:646–656.
35. Brown BG, Zhao X, Sacco DE, Albers JJ. Lipid lowering and plaque regression. New insights into prevention of plaque disruption and clinical events in coronary disease. *Circulation* 1993;87:1781–1791.

36. Blankenhorn DH, Hodis HN. Arterial imaging and atherosclerosis reversal. *Arterioscler Thromb* 1994;14:177–192.
37. Salonen R, Salonen JT. Determinants of carotid intima-media thickness: population based ultrasonography study in eastern Finnish men. *J Intern Med* 1991;229:225–231.
38. Benzuly KH, Padgett RC, Kaul S, et al. Functional improvement precedes structural regression of atherosclerosis. *Circulation* 1994;89:1810–1818.
39. Gould KL, Martucci JP, Goldberg DI, et al. Short-term cholesterol lowering decreases size and severity of perfusion abnormalities by positron emission tomography after dipyridamole in patients with coronary artery disease. A potential noninvasive marker of healing coronary endothelium. *Circulation* 1994;89:1530–1538.
40. Azen SP, Mack WJ, Cashin-Hemphill L, et al. Progression of coronary artery disease predicts clinical coronary events. Long-term follow-up from the Cholesterol Lowering Atherosclerosis Study. *Circulation* 1996;93:34–41.
41. Loscalzo J. Regression of coronary atherosclerosis. *N Engl J Med* 1990;323:1337–1339.
42. Falk E, Shah PK, Fuster V. Coronary plaque disruption. *Circulation* 1995;92:657–671.
43. Treasure CB, Klein JL, Weintraub WS, et al. Beneficial effects of cholesterol-lowering therapy on the coronary endothelium in patients with coronary artery disease. *N Engl J Med* 1995;332:481–487.
44. Anderson TJ, Meredith IT, Yeung AC, et al. The effect of cholesterol-lowering and antioxidant therapy on endothelium-dependent coronary vasomotion. *N Engl J Med* 1995; 332:488–495.
45. Anderson TJ, Uehata A, Gerhard MD, et al. Close relation of endothelial function in human coronary and peripheral circulations. *J Am Coll Cardiol* 1995;26:1235–1241.
46. Expert Panel on Detection, Evaluation and Treatment of High Blood Cholesterol in Adults. Summary of the Second Report of the National Cholesterol Education Program (NCEP). Expert Panel on Detection, Evaluation and Treatment of High Blood Cholesterol in Adults. *JAMA* 1993;269:3015–3023.
47. The Expert Panel. Report of the National Cholesterol Education Program Expert Panel on Detection, Evaluation and Treatment of High Blood Cholesterol in Adults. *Arch Intern Med* 1988;148:36–69.
48. Olin JW, Cressman MD, Hoogwerf B, Weinstein C. Diagnosis and treatment of lipid disturbances. In: *Peripheral Vascular Diseases.* 2nd ed. Young JR, Olin JW, Bartholomew JR (eds.) St. Louis: CV Mosby, 1996.
49. Sprecher DL, Abrams J, Allen JW, et al. Low-dose combined therapy with fluvastatin and cholestyramine in hyperlipidemic patients. *Ann Intern Med* 1994;120:537–543.

8

The Surgical Treatment of Aortoiliac Occlusive Disease: Options and Results

Elliot L. Chaikof, M.D., Ph.D.
Robert B. Smith, III, M.D.

In 10 years, performing an aortobifemoral bypass may well be an act of medical malpractice.

> Edward B. Diethrich, M.D.
> Arizona Heart Institute, April 1996

I submit that in the absence of proof of efficacy, all [endovascular] interventional procedures must be regarded as experimental.

> John M. Porter, M.D.
> *J Vasc Surg* 1995;21:995.

There remains little doubt that treatment options for occlusive disease are currently in a state of flux and a subject of divergent opinions. The development and continued refinement of a variety of minimally invasive approaches, including angioplasty, stenting, and endovascular graft placement, as described in this text, will likely alter the need for or at least the frequency of either anatomic or extra-anatomic surgical approaches for arterial occlusive disease. This chapter will review these standard surgical apaproaches to aortoiliac disease, including current indications for treatment, surgical decision making, operative strategy, and clinical outcomes. Importantly, in the evolution of new treatment strategies for aortoiliac occlusive disease, critical evaluation will require comparison with these operative procedures because the effectiveness of surgery in the treatment of symptomatic aortoiliac occlusive disease is well established and remains the benchmark for proposed new treatment strategies.

OPERATIVE INDICATIONS

In the mid-nineteenth century, the best advice a surgeon could offer to the patient with arterial occlusive disease was to moderate activity accordingly. The development of a variety of successful surgical options has improved our ability to intervene effectively in the dis-ease process. Nonetheless, we are now left with the greater challenge of interceding in a rational manner for appropriate indications. Limb-threatening ischemic symptoms, including pain at rest, a nonhealing ulcer, and gangrene, remain unequivocal indications for the treatment of aortoiliac occlusive disease. While it is recognized that pain at rest or an ischemic ulcer may not uniformly predict eventual limb loss, the natural history of the untreated patient is characterized, more often than not, by the eventual requirement of a major amputation. Thus, studies that have demonstrated ulcer healing or symptom improvement in 25 to 50% of untreated patients highlight the spectrum of ischemic disease and the uncertainty of our current predictive tests.[1-4] Fortunately, the results of aortoiliac revascularization are much more predictable and the potential for a catastrophic outcome is avoidable.

The decision to revascularize the patient with claudication symptoms alone must be individualized. In the otherwise low-risk patient, surgical intervention is deemed advisable if the symptoms significantly impair the usual acts of daily life, either related to livelihood or a desired lifestyle. These recommendations are particularly well established for occlusive disease limited to the aortoiliac segment. In such cases, reconstruction is durable and the results are uniformly good. It is noteworthy that claudication may not necessarily be associated with a benign prognosis, particularly when associated with multilevel disease. For example, Cronenwett et al[5] have demonstrated that when objective criteria are utilized to document arterial insufficiency in the claudicant, the outcome in the untreated patient may be surprisingly poor. Specifically, symptoms worsened in nearly 50% of patients, and tissue loss or surgery was required in 20% over a 30-month observation period. Similarly, Bowers et al[6] observed that one-third of patients with stable claudication and a toe pressure of less than 40 mm Hg deteriorated during a 6-month follow-up period. Gertler et al[7] have reported similar findings. While these data do not necessarily justify prophylactic intervention in the otherwise stable patient, they emphasize the importance of close patient observation when surgery is deferred.

In addition, atheromatous embolization from proximal aortoiliac disease is also an indication for revascularization. If the clinical findings are characteristic of microembolization and angiography confirm the presence of ulcerative disease, bypass grafting with exclusion of endarterectomy of the aortoiliac segment is appropriate[8,9] (see Chapter 20).

Advanced age or associated medical problems, such as coronary artery disease or pulmonary insufficiency, may influence the choice of operative procedure but are rarely considered absolute contraindications for aortoiliac revascularization. We do believe, however, that the prevalence of associated cardiac disease, which may exceed 50% in patients with aortoiliac occlusive disease, necessitates an aggressive approach with regard to preoperative screening.[10] While the motivation has been largely driven by the desire to avoid a life-threatening perioperative event, Rihal et al have demonstrated that coronary artery surgery appears to have a long-term survival benefit in patients with peripheral vascular disease.[11]

THERAPEUTIC OPTIONS

Overview

In recognizing the limits of surgical therapy, we must understand that our ability to relieve symptoms and prevent limb loss is inherently independent of a fundamental alteration in the underlying disease process. Despite the development of a variety of promising pharmaceutical agents, atherosclerosis is progressive and intervention palliative. With these issues in mind, the optimal choice of a procedure for occlusive disease is most dependent on the experience of the surgeon, the severity and distribution of occlusive disease, and the overall condition of the patient.

To date, the most durable and successful results have been achieved by anatomic bilateral aortoiliac reconstruction, characteristically using prosthetic bypass grafts.[12-15] Historically, the popularity of aortobifemoral bypass grew out of its demonstrated advantages over extensive aorto-iliofemoral endarterectomy. Bypass grafting was associated with decreased operative time, blood loss, mortality rates, and initial failures and with an improvement in late patency. In the young, otherwise healthy patient with mostly unilateral iliac artery disease, aortobifemoral bypass remains the most definitive procedure. Although bypass of the asymptomatic contralateral iliac artery does not halt the disease process, as noted above, there is a demonstrated risk of progressive occlusive disease. While the true incidence of contralateral progression is unknown, the necessity for reoperation following a unilateral procedure ranges from 10 to 30%.[16] In the patient with isolated external iliac artery involvement, an iliofemoral bypass may be an appropriate alternative. This bypass can be performed with an anticipated reduced morbidity, reduced recovery time, and an acceptable late patency.[17,18]

Despite the limitations of endarterectomy, which were well recognized during the 1950s and 1960s, this technique remains the procedure of choice in the young patient with localized disease.[19-21] Because the reconstruction is autogenous, the risk of graft-related complications, including infection and pseudoaneurysm formation, is virtually eliminated. The development of a variety of operative adjuncts, including improved fixed retractors and autotransfusion systems, has most recently helped to reduce blood loss and the technical challenges of this approach. For example, in our experience at the Emory University Hospital between 1990 and 1994, 15 patients underwent aortoiliac endarterectomy, with a median operative time and blood loss of 3.5 hours and 400 mL, respectively. Three patients received transfusions, and there was no major morbidity or postoperative death. After a median follow-up interval of 24 months, recurrent claudication symptoms were noted after 1 year in a single patient. All others remained symptom free. The advantages of an autogenous approach are coupled with superior patency rates when compared with a concurrent cohort of patients undergoing aortobifemoral bypass grafting. The caveat is that such success can be assured only if the atherosclerotic process remains limited to the aortic bifurcation and proximal iliac segments. Further, the presence of aneurysmal dilation precludes this approach. Finally, it should be recognized that the requirement for more extensive dissection may increase the risk of postoperative male sexual dysfunction if care is not taken to preserve the sympathetic plexus that crosses the left iliac artery. Given these constrains, in current practice endarterectomy often represents less than 5% of all procedures performed for aortoiliac occlusive disease.

Standard anatomic reconstruction may not be advisable in the patient with serious comorbid conditions. Additionally, a previous history of irradiation, multiple prior operations, colostomies, or ileal conduits presents the surgeon with a classic "hostile" abdomen and its attendant technical challenge. In this patient subgroup, extra-anatomic bypasses such as a femorofemoral or axillofemoral bypass may be preferable. If occlusive disease can be reliably excluded from the donor iliac artery by both biplanar arteriography and the absence of a measured gradient, a femorofemoral bypass is a useful procedure.[18,22,23] Not only does it have a role in treating isolated iliac artery disease, but it also may provide inflow for a femorodistal bypass or outflow for an axillofemoral graft. Additionally, if thrombectomy fails to reestablish blood flow in an occluded limb of an aortobifemoral bypass, a femorofemoral crossover is most often the procedure of choice. While the long-term patency of this graft is inferior to that of the aortobifemoral bypass, the incidence of other theoretical disadvantages such as "steal" from the donor limb or the pelvic circulation is exceedingly rare. In the high-risk patient with bilateral iliac disease, the axillofemoral bypass has been an important option. While early reported patency data were disappointing, significant improvement has recently been achieved through the use of externally supported prostheses of either Dacron or expanded polytetrafluoroethylene (PTFE)[24,25]

The occasional requirement of an additional outflow procedure following aortoiliac revascularization is worthy of comment. In retrospective reviews published in the 1970s, the frequency of this occurrence varied from 10 to 56%. In general, however, we believe that the necessity of simultaneous procedures is well below 10%. Unfortunately, preoperative identification of the patient who will require both aortoiliac and infrainguinal procedures is generally unreliable. Although several reports have documented acceptable operative mortality rates when simultaneous procedures were performed by two complete operative teams, others have noted a sobering 19% mortality rate, with significant blood loss and operative times approaching 9 hours.[26–29] These results likely represent the expected outcome when a single team undertakes both operations. In our opinion, staging represents the more prudent approach when faced with the need for both inflow and outflow procedures.

Aortofemoral and Iliofemoral Bypass

The explosive growth of polymer technology during the decade preceding World War II set the stage for the development of appropriate prosthetic materials for bypass procedures. While our recent preference has been for a collagen-impregnated knitted Dacron prosthesis, there are few data to substantiate the advantage of any specific textile pattern. In fact, a randomized

trial has failed to demonstrate a statistically significant difference in patency rates between PTFE and Dacron when used as aortic bifurcation grafts.[30]

In performing an aortobifemoral bypass, several technical features bear emphasis. The proximal aortic anastomosis may be constructed either in an end-to-end or end-to-side fashion. The end-to-end anastomosis offers the advantages of better hemodynamics and a reduced risk of kinking, while the end-to-side anastomosis is technically easier and faster to perform. Furthermore, if the graft occludes, complete lower extremity ischemia is less likely to occur. Randomized studies have not established a significant difference in patency. In deciding which anastomisis best suits a given anatomic picture, several factors are important to consider. While an accessory renal artery or inferior mesenteric artery can be reimplanted using a Carrell patch technique, the end-to-side anastomosis provides an expeditious alternative when preservation of prograde flow in these vessels is considered critical. Three additional scenarios also favor the end-to-side anastomosis. The first is when maintenance of hypogastric perfusion is essential for reducing the risk of colonic or spinal ischemia. If retrograde flow via the femoral arteries cannot be anticipated due to severe external iliac artery disease, an end-to-side anastomosis is mandatory. Second, an occasional female patient will present with a very small or hypoplastic aorta. The use of a bypass graft with a diameter less than 12 mm is associated with an increased possibility of thrombotic occlusion. Technically, size matching with the small aorta is easier if an end-to-side anastomosis is utilized. Finally, this anastomosis may be useful if circumferential dissection of the aorta cannot be achieved because of extensive scarring. Nevertheless, the end-to-side anastomosis is clearly contraindicated in the presence of aneurysmal disease or aortic occlusion that extends to the level of the renal arteries. Furthermore, the risk of graft limb occlusion secondary to competitive flow, inherent in the end-to-side construction, is particularly high when the iliac artery is only moderately narrowed and runoff is poor. An end-to-end connection is therefore the superior option in that circumstance.

Regardless of the choice of anastomosis, it should be positioned as far proximally as possible on the infrarenal aorta, where calcification is often less extensive and the risk of recurrent disease is minimized (Fig. 8.1). If suprarenal clamping is required because of complete aortic occlusion, control of the renal arteries prior to placement of the aortic cross clamp will lessen the risk of postoperative renal failure due to embolic debris. With an end-to-end anastomosis, thrombectomy of the aortic cuff can be performed and the cross clamp then moved to an infrarenal position.

Coverage of the graft is essential to minimize the possibility of a late aortoenteric fistula. In an end-to-end

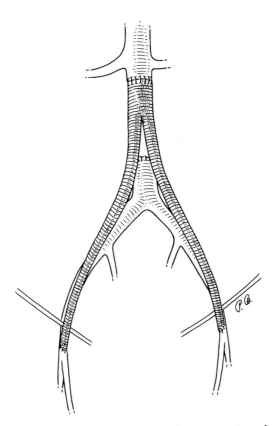

Figure 8–1. Operative principles in the construction of an aortobifemoral bypass graft with an end-to-end proximal anastomosis include (a) placing the proximal anastomosis as high as possible on the infrarenal aorta and (b) resecting a small segment of aorta so that the graft lies in the correct anatomic position.

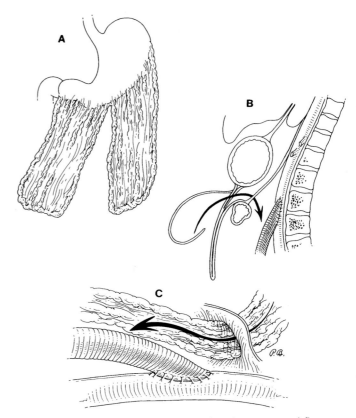

Figure 8–2. (A–C) Covering the graft with an omental flap provides a convenient solution to prevent a late aortoenteric fistula if perigraft soft tissue is inadequate.

anastomosis, this is facilitated by resecting a small segment of aorta so that the graft lies in the correct anatomic position. If perigraft soft tissue is inadequate, particularly in an end-to-side anastomosis, we have found that an omental flap provides a convenient solution (Fig. 8.2). An opening is first created adjacent to the transverse colon to provide access to the lesser sac. Then an opening in the avascular portion of the transverse mesocolon is created. After the omental flap has been created, it can be rotated around the transverse colon into the lesser sac and through the mesocolon to lie directly on top of the graft. Although bringing a portion of omentum directly onto the graft without resorting to a rotationary maneuver is simpler, the risk of inadvertently producing a small bowel trap should be recognized, and reoperation, at times, is more difficult.

In patients with aortoiliac occlusive disease, the distal anastomosis is preferentially performed at the level of the femoral artery. Exposure is simpler, and prior concerns about an increased risk of graft infection or pseudoaneurysm formation have not been confirmed. Furthermore, the profunda femoris artery is the major

outflow source and is often a critical determinant of late patency. A useful rule of thumb for determining the adequacy of this outflow vessel is its ability to accept a 4-mm dilator and a 20-cm length of uninflated catheter. If the profunda orifice is narrowed, the toe of the distal anastomosis can be extended onto the artery as a patch profundoplasty. If the external iliac arteries appear to be free of disease on the basis of biplanar angiography and the absence of a pullback pressure gradient, the distal anastomosis can be performed at the iliac level. This may be particularly advantageous when the risk of groin infection is increased, as in the obese patient with an intertriginous rash in the inguinal crease.

As previously stated, the unilateral iliofemoral bypass is a useful option in the symptomatic patient with isolated external iliac artery occlusive disease (Fig. 8.3). The proximal common iliac artery can be exposed retroperitoneally through an oblique incision 3 inches above the inguinal ligament. An 8-mm conduit, tunneled anatomically, will usually suffice.

Aortoiliac Endarterectomy

The concept of endarterectomy was first established in 1884 when the Rumanian surgeon Severeanu probed a plugged popliteal artery with a fine urethral sound dur-

pliant. The common, internal, and external iliac arteries are mobilized, and the lumbar and medial sacral arteries are identified and controlled with clips. Preservation of the sympathetic plexus across the left common iliac artery is important in the male patient to avoid postoperative impotence and retrograde ejaculation. It can often be suspended using a 0.25-inch Penrose drain. After systemic heparinization, we prefer to open the aorta and right common iliac artery using a single longitudinal incision. The left common iliac artery is then opened with a separate longitudinal incision distal to the aortic bifurcation. Endarterectomy from the aorta to the bifurcation of the right common iliac artery is completed, and the proximal left common iliac artery is endarterectomized from the aorta to the level of the distal iliac incision. Endarterectomy of the external iliac artery is difficult. Tacking sutures of 5-0 Prolene are used to secure distal intimal flaps, if present, and a Dacron patch angioplasty of the iliac arteries is performed if narrowing of the vessel lumen is a concern. The arteriotomy is closed with a running 5-0 Prolene suture (Fig. 8.4).

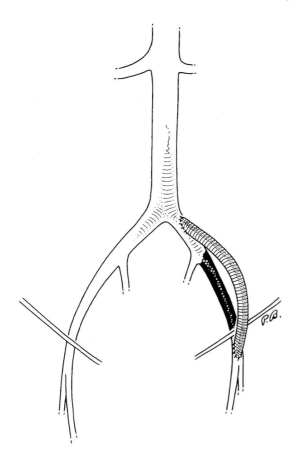

Figure 8–3. A unilateral iliofemoral bypass can be constructed by exposing the common iliac artery through an oblique incision 3 inches above the inguinal ligament.

ing an amputation.[31] The artery was unplugged and a free, pulsating flow of blood obtained. The ability to perform an endarterectomy was all the more astonishing because no pathologist had ever recognized a cleavage plane between the atherosclerotic plaque and the arterial wall. Dos Santos[32] and Reboul and Laubry[33] were the first to describe in detail the procedure and its potential in the treatment of occlusive disease. Variations in technique included the use of a single long arteriotomy or multiple short incisions. By 1950, Arnulf had reported his experience with aortoiliac endarterectomy in 40 patients.[34] Operative mortality was 20%, and the success rate in surviving patients was only 50%. Nonetheless, while these results were far from excellent, homografts provided the only alternative, and were associated with a far more dismal outcome. Norman Freeman and Richard Warren popularized this method in the United States.

Currently, the decision to perform an endarterectomy can only be made after intraoperative assessment of the external iliac arteries. If there is significant external iliac disease, aortofemoral bypass grafting is performed. Otherwise, the aorta is mobilized proximal to the inferior mesenteric artery until the wall feels com-

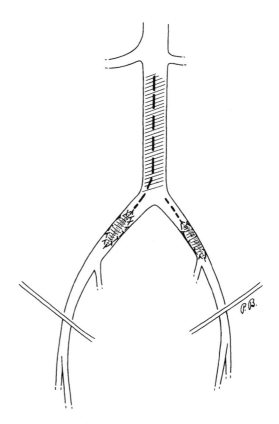

Figure 8–4. In performing an aortoiliac endarterectomy, the aorta and right common iliac artery are opened using a single longitudinal incision. The left common iliac artery is then opened with a separate longitudinal incision distal to the aortic bifurcation. Dacron patch angioplasty of the iliac arteries is performed to prevent luminal narrowing.

Extra-anatomic Reconstruction: Femorofemoral and Axillofemoral Bypass

Long-term success of the femorofemoral bypass is dependent on the adequacy of the donor iliac artery. Several authors have emphasized that in the absence of pull-out pressure measurements, 10 to 20% of patients may have a significant residual gradient despite the presence of a palpable femoral pulse and a patent iliac artery on the angiogram.[35,36] If inadequate inflow is suspected or a gradient demonstrated at operation, options include axillofemoral grafting or intraoperative angioplasty and stent placement. Otherwise, femorofemoral bypass is technically straightforward. We prefer to use an 8-mm ringed PTFE prosthesis, although the superiority of a given graft type has not been proven. Ensuring the adequacy of the profunda femoris artery as the significant outflow source is essential, as with aortofemoral or iliofemoral bypass.

If an axillobifemoral graft is chosen because of bilateral iliac disease, an 8-mm conduit will usually suffice. We have most often used a ringed PTFE prosthesis, although reported patency data are comparable to those of externally supported Dacron. The right axillary artery is the usual donor site because it is less commonly affected by occlusive disease. Nonetheless, preoperative assessment of the brachial blood pressure should be performed to ensure its suitability as a donor vessel. The axillary artery can be exposed via an oblique infraclavicular incision. The fibers of the pectoralis major muscle are separated and the underlying clavipectoral fascia incised. The anastomosis should be performed medial to the insertion of the pectoralis minor muscle to minimize potential tension on the anastomosis during arm abduction. The graft is then tunneled between the pectoralis major and minor muscles. A number of arrangements have been described for performing the crossover graft, including running a side limb to the contralateral femoral artery or creating a femorofemoral bypass either prior to or after completion of the distal axillofemoral anastomosis. We have usually connected the axillofemoral anastomosis to the ipsilateral hood of the crossover graft.

RESULTS

For the treatment of bilateral iliac occlusive disease, the aortobifemoral bypass continues to be associated with the highest level of long-term efficacy and a very low rate of procedure-related adverse events. Five-year and 10-year cumulative patency rates approach 88 and 75%, respectively.[12–15] Perioperative mortality is less than 2% and the early complication rate is in the range of 5%, predominantly due to nonfatal myocardial infarction. Other potential early complications, including bleeding, bowel or spinal ischemia, embolization, graft thrombosis, and wound infection, are infrequent events. The most frequent late complication is graft limb occlusion, most commonly related to progressive disease in the outflow tract. Thrombectomy, when combined with patch angioplasty of the distal anastomosis or an infrainguinal bypass, can increase the 5-year limb patency to 75%.[37] The incidence of other late events such as graft infection, aortoenteric fistula formation, or anastomotic pseudoaneurysm formation is in the range of 1 to 2%. Coronary artery disease remains the most common cause of the late death, with 5- and 10-year survival rates of approximately 75% and 50%, respectively. We suspect that the aggressive treatment of coronary artery disease will likely improve these statistics in the future.[11] While the iliofemoral bypass can be performed with a lower overall morbidity rate, an accompanying reduction in cumulative 5-year patency (79%) has been reported in at least one series of carefully selected patients.[17]

The advantages of the femorofemoral and axillofemoral bypass were outlined earlier. While the stress of these procedures is undeniably less and the recovery time shorter, patency rates are significantly lower than those achieved with an aortobifemoral graft. Five-year patency rates of the femorofemoral bypass in several recent series range from 55 to 75%.[38–41] Notably, if the donor iliac artery requires angioplasty or stenting prior to femorofemoral grafting, the results do not appear to be compromised.[42]

Historically, the 5-year patency rates for the axillofemoral bypass have ranged between 20% and 60%. Study trends in the past have favored the bifemoral over the unifemoral bypass, although the more recent reports of Schneider et al,[43] El-Massry et al,[25] and Mohan et al[44] have failed to demonstrate a significant difference. Recently, both El-Massry et al[25] and Taylor et al[24] have observed an improvement in patency using externally supported Dacron and PTFE, respectively. Both articles reported primary patency rates of 70% at 3 to 5 years. In general, these data are somewhat more difficult to analyze because the indications for bypass are more heterogeneous. Included are not only bypasses placed for the primary treatment of occlusive disease, but also secondary attempts at revascularization for a failing graft in which the original indication may have been aneurysmal disease.

It is worthwhile to conclude with a cautionary note regarding the treatment of advanced aortoiliac occlusive disease in the young adult. While Cronenwett et al[20] and Jensen and Egeblad[45] have both reported impressive 4-year patency data (89 to 93%) after aortobifemoral bypass grafting in the young adult, other surgeons have had much poorer outcomes in this population. In fact, many reports have documented that atherosclerotic occlusive disease is a particularly virulent multilevel process, especially in patients under 40 years of age. For example, McCready et al[46] noted that in their series 36% of women required reoperation, and Valentine and coauthors[47] observed a 51% incidence of graft limb occlusion within a mean interval of 31 months after aortic reconstruction. In the latter report, the 3-year cumulative patency rate was 65%. In these and other reviews, the rate of limb loss has ranged from 17% to 23%.[48] In a recent report, Allen et al[19] noted a revision rate of 29% in patients who underwent an initial operation when younger than 50 years of age. Although the differences were not statistically significant, fewer reoperations were required for patients who underwent endarterectomy (15%) than aortobifemoral bypass (38%). Most sobering is a report by van Goor and colleagues,[49] who reviewed their experience with 29 adults under the age of 40 years. Twenty-three of the 29 patients had an inflow procedure. At a mean follow-up interval of 12 years, there was a 76% incidence of reoperation and a 17% amputation rate, and only 25% of the surviving 20 patients were asymptomatic. Eventually, the majority of patients experienced the same walking distance limitations encountered before their initial surgery. These data highlight the need for both careful patient selection when an operation is considered and close postoperative surveillance.

REFERENCES

1. Schuler JJ, Flanigan DP, Holcroft JW, et al. Efficacy of prostaglandin E1 in the treatment of lower extremity ischemic ulcers secondary to peripheral vascular occlusive disease: results of a postoperative randomized, double-blind, multicenter clinical trial. *J Vasc Surg* 1984;1:160–170.
2. Eklund AE, Eriksson G, Olsson AG. A controlled study showing significant short term effect of prostaglandin E1 in healing ischemic ulcers in the lower limb in man. *Prostaglandins Leukotrienes Med* 1982;8:265.
3. Cronenwett JL, Zelenock GB, Whitehouse WM Jr. et al. Prostacyclin treatment of ischemic ulcers and rest pain in unreconstructable peripheral arterial occlusive disease. *Surgery* 1986;100:369–375.
4. Belch JJF, McArdle B, Pollack JG, et al. Epoprostenol (prostacyclin) and severe arterial disease: a double-blind trial. *Lancet* 1983;1:315–317.
5. Cronenwett JL, Warner KG, Zelenock GB, et al. Intermittent claudication: current results of nonoperative management. *Arch Surg* 1984;119:430–436.
6. Bowers BL, Valentine RJ, Myers SI, et al. The natural history of patients with claudication with toe pressures of 40 mm Hg or less *J Vasc Surg* 1993;18:506–511.
7. Gertler JP, Headley A, L'Italien G, et al. Claudication in the setting of plethysmographic criteria for resting ischemia: is surgery justified? *Ann Vasc Surg* 1993;7:249–253.
8. Kaufman JL, Saifi J, Chang BB, et al. The role of extraanatomic bypass exclusion bypass in the treatment of disseminated atheroembolism syndrome. *Ann Vasc Surg* 1990;4:260–263.
9. Baumann DS, McGraw D, Rubin BG, et al. An institutional experience with arterial atheroembolism. *Ann Vasc Surg* 1994;8:258–265.
10. Hertzer NR, Beven EG, Young JR, et al. Coronary artery disease in peripheral vascular patients: a classification of 1000 coronary angiograms and results of surgical management. *Ann Surg* 1984;199:223–233.
11. Rihal CS, Eagle KA, Mickel MC, et al. Surgical therapy for coronary artery disease among patients with combined coronary artery and peripheral vascular disease. *Circulation* 1995;91:46–53.
12. Perdue GD, Long WD, Smith RB III. Perspective concerning aorto-femoral arterial reconstruction. *Ann Surg* 1971;173:940–944.
13. Malone JM, Moore WS, Goldstone J. The natural history of bilateral aortofemoral bypass grafts for ischemia of the lower extremities. *Arch Surg* 1975;110:1300–1306.
14. Brewster DC, Darling RC Jr. Optimal methods of aortoiliac reconstruction. *Surgery* 1978;84:739–748.
15. Martinez BD, Hertzer NR, Beven EG. Influence of distal arterial occlusive disease on prognosis following aortobifemoral bypass. *Surgery* 1980;88:795–805.
16. Brewster DC. Clinical and anatomic considerations for surgery in aortoiliac disease and results of surgical treatment. *Circulation* 1991;83(suppl I):1–42.
17. Darling RC III, Leather RP, Chang BB, et al. Is the iliac artery a suitable inflow conduit for iliofemoral occlusive disease?: An analysis of 514 aortoiliac reconstructions. *J Vasc Surg* 1993;17:15–19.
18. Kalman PG, Hosang M, Johnston KW, et al. Unilateral iliac disease: the role of iliofemoral bypass. *J Vasc Surg* 1987;6;139–143.
19. Allen BT, Rubin BG, Reily JM, et al. Limb salvage and patency after aortic reconstruction in younger patients. *Am J Surg* 1995;170:188–192.
20. Cronenwett JL, Davis Jr JT, Gooch JB, et al. Aortoiliac occlusive disease in women. *Surgery* 1980;88:775–784.
21. van den Akker PJ, van Schilgaarde R, Brand R, et al. Long-term results of prosthetic and non-prosthetic reconstruction for obstructive aorto-iliac disease. *Eur J Vasc Surg* 1992;6:53–61.
22. Criado E, Burnham SJ, Tinsley EA Jr, et al. Femorofemoral bypass graft: analysis of patency and factors influencing long-term outcome. *J Vasc Surg* 1993;18:495–504.
23. Lorenzi G, Domanin M, Costantini A, et al. Role of bypass, endarterectomy, extra-anatomic bypass and endovascular surgery in unilateral iliac occlusive disease: a review of 1257 cases. *Cardiovasc Surg* 1994;2:370–373.
24. Taylor LJ, Moneta G, McConnell D, et al. Axillofemoral grafting with externally supported polytetrafluoroethylene. *Arch Surg* 1994;129:588–595.
25. El-Massry S, Saad E, Sauvage LR, et al. Axillofemoral bypass with externally supported, knitted Dacron grafts: a follow-up through twelve years. *J Vasc Surg* 1993;17:107–115.
26. Eidt J, Charlesworth D. Combined aortobifemoral and femorodistal bypass in the management of patients with extensive atherosclerosis. *Ann Vasc Surg* 1986;1:453–459.
27. Harris PL, Cave Bigley DJ, McSweeney L. Aortofemoral bypass and the role of concomitant femorodistal reconstruction. *Br J Surg* 1985;72:317–320.
28. Dalman RL, Taylor LM Jr, Moneta GL, et al. Simultaneous operative repair of multilevel lower extremity occlusive disease. *J Vasc Surg* 1991;13:211–221.
29. Harward TRS, Ingegno MD, Carlton L, et al. Limb-threatening ischemia due to multilevel arterial occlusive disease. *Ann Surg* 1995;221:498–506.
30. Polterauer P, Prager M, Holzenbein T, et al. Dacron versus polytetrafluoroethylene for Y-aortic bifurcation grafts:

A six-year prospective, randomized trial. *Surgery* 1992; 111:626–633.

31. Bazy L. L'endarterectomie pour artérite obliterante des membres inférieurs. *J Int Chir* 1949;9:95.

32. dos Santos CJ. Sur la désobstruction des thromboses artérielles anciennes. *Mem Acad Chir* 1947;73:409.

33. Reboul H, Laubry H. Endarterectomy in treatment of chronic endarteritis obliterans of limbs and abdominal aorta. *Proc R Soc Med* 1950;43:547.

34. Arnulf G. *Chirugie arterielle.* Paris: Masson, 1950.

35. Brenner BJ, Brief DK, Alpert J, et al. Femorofemoral bypass: A twenty-five year experience. In: Yao JST, Pearce WH (eds): *Long-term Results in Vascular Surgery.* East Norwalk, CT: Appleton & Lange, 1993;385–393.

36. Gupta SK, Veith JF, Kram HB, et al. Signficance and management of inflow gradients unexpectedly generated after femorofemoral, femoropopliteal, and femoroinfrapopliteal bypass grafting. *J Vasc Surg* 1990;12:278–283.

37. Brewster DC, Meir GH, Darling RC, et al. Reoperation for aortofemoral graft limb occlusion: optimal methods and long-term results. *J Vasc Surg* 1987;5:363–374.

38. Schneider JR, Besso SR, Walsh DB, et al. Femorofemoral versus aortobifemoral bypass: outcome and hemodynamic results. *J Vasc Surg* 1994;19:43–47.

39. Ng, RL, Gillies TE, Davies AH, et al. Iliofemoral versus femorofemoral bypass: A 6-year audit. *Br J Surg* 1992; 79:1011–1013.

40. Ricco JB. Unilateral iliac artery occlusive disease: a randomized multicenter trial examining direct revascularization versus crossover bypass. *Ann Vasc Surg* 1992;6:209–219.

41. Gupta S, Landa R, Veith F. Femorofemoral bypass for aortoiliac occlusive disease. In: Stanley JC, Ernst CB (eds): *Current Therapy in Vascular Surgery.* 3rd ed. St. Louis: Mosby-Year Book, 1995;393–396.

42. Shah RM, Peer RM, Upson JF, et al. Donor iliac angioplasty and crossover femorofemoral bypass. *Am J Surg* 1992; 164:295–298.

43. Schneider JR, McDaniel MD, Walsh DB, et al. Axillofemoral bypass: outcome and hemodynamic results in high-risk patients. *J Vasc Surg* 1992;15:952–963.

44. Mohan CR, Sharp WJ, Hoballah JJ, et al. A comparative evaluation of externally supported polytetrafluoroethylene axillobifemoral and axillounifemoral bypass grafts. *J Vasc Surg* 1995;21:801–808.

45. Jensen BV, Egeblad K. Aorto-iliac arteriosclerotic disease in young human adults. *Eur J Vasc Surg* 1990;4:583–586.

46. McCready RA, Vincet AE, Schwartz RW, et al. Atherosclerosis in the young: a virulent disease. *Surgery* 1984;96:863–869.

47. Valentine RJ, MacGillvray DC, DeNobile JW, et al. Intermittent claudication caused by atherosclerosis in patients aged forty years and younger. *Surgery* 1990;107:560–565.

48. Olsen PS, Gustafsen J, Rasmussen L, et al. Long-term results after arterial surgery for arteriosclerosis of the lower limbs in young adults. *Eur J Vasc Surg* 1988;2:15–18.

49. van Goor H, Boontje AH. Results of vascular reconstructions for atherosclerotic arterial occlusive disease of the lower limbs in young adults. *Eur J Vasc Endovasc Surg* 1995;10:323–326.

9

Aortoiliac Angioplasty: Patient Selection and Results

Eric C. Martin, F.R.C.P., F.R.C.R.

Although iliac angioplasty was first described in the 1970s,[1] it was not until the 1980s that it was established as a valuable and valid technique. Vascular stents, which were developed in the late 1980s, have yet to be proven superior, although they certainly offer a significant adjunctive role in iliac angioplasty. And the newer endovascular techniques of intravascular grafting, while very interesting, remain in their infancy and are unlikely to challenge iliac angioplasty's role in the management of aortoiliac disease for the next few years, at least in the United States.

Although angioplasty was first described by Dotter and Judkins in 1964,[2] it was unavailable for the iliac arteries until a device with a significant expansion ratio was developed. The Dotter technique, after all, creates a lumen only the size of the catheter. Balloon catheters were clearly the answer, but latex balloons did not have the correct characteristics. A caged latex balloon was developed by Porstmann in 1973 to overcome some of the problems.[1] In 1974, Gruntzig and Hopff developed the double-lumen, polyvinyl balloon catheter, which, although compliant by modern standards, did not change in diameter by more than 1 to 2 mm over its working pressure of 2 to 6 atmospheres.[3] Since then, less compliant materials, like polyethylene, have maintained fixed diameters through a wide range of pressures. Latex balloons increase in diameter with increasing pressure. Gruntzig's contribution was to conceive of a balloon that inflated to a fixed diameter despite increasing pressure.

There have also been significant advances in balloon technology, particularly in size, trackability, and profile, and there have been concomitant advances in the pharmacologic adjuncts to angioplasty. This progress, when combined with the improvement in image intensification and digital subtraction imaging, has contributed to the increasing efficacy and safety of the procedure and the slow growth in the number of procedures performed.

TECHNIQUE OF ANGIOPLASTY

The standard approach is retrograde and most iliac lesions are dilated at the time of the diagnostic study. Today, most diagnostic studies are performed with No. 4 French catheters, and an exchange is then made over a wire for an appropriate No. 5 French balloon. Lesions need to be marked so that the waist is in the center of the balloon catheter. Searching for a stenosis by multiple dilatations is poor technique, leading to too much intima damage and an increased risk of restenosis. Most patients receive heparin during angioplasty, and most patients are premedicated with nifedipine. Intraarterial nitroglycerine is useful, although spasm is not the problem that it is in the femoral system. Balloons are chosen to be about 1 mm larger than the vessel being dilated. This may be judged from the vessel on either side of the stenosis or even on the opposite side, although modern posteroanterior imaging with Puck film changers or digital subtraction angiography (DSA) is associated with 30 to 40% magnification.

Crossing stenoses is seldom a problem, but great care must be taken to stay in the lumen and not to dissect. Dilatations between the intima and the media are likely to restenose and may even rupture.

In the past, hockey stock catheters were useful in combination with soft guidewires. Now, steerable hydrophylic wires in combination with digital road mapping are preferred. Dissection must be avoided with hydrophylic wires, and they should protrude a considerable distance from the catheter tip so that they are not artificially stiffened.

On occasion, it may be useful to cross lesions by going around the bifurcation, but with the advent of bailout stenting, this has become less desirable. Seldom should common iliac lesions be managed in this man-

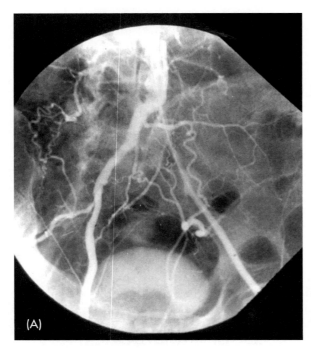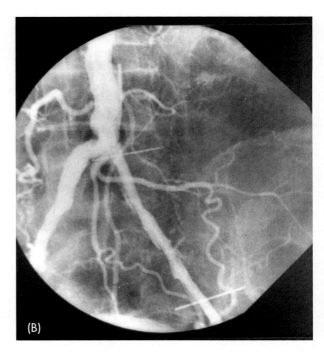

Figure 9–1.   (A) A tight left common iliac stenosis in which the catheter is occlusive. (B) After angioplasty the intimal split may be seen parallel to the vessel.

ner, but it may be desirable for low external iliac lesions. Once crossed, an exchange is made, usually over a Rosen wire or another relatively stiff-bodied exchange wire, for the appropriate balloon catheter, and dilatation performed for approximately 1 minute to remove the waist. It is ironic that as the trackability of catheters has improved, the indications for contralateral iliac catheterization for angioplasty have diminished, save for urokinase therapy distally.

Occlusions are also usually crossed from below if there is to be a primary angioplasty or stent. Again, soft hydrophylic wires are preferred and dissection must be avoided. An alternative technique, now losing favor, is a contralateral approach with urokinase therapy followed by angioplasty of the underlying lesion. Still, urokinese is indicated when the clinical story is one of acute or subacute worsening, the angiogram shows fewer than expected number of collaterals, and the occlusion is found to be soft and readily traversed with the guidewire.

As with stenoses, a good cosmetic result is the goal and the gradient should be completely removed (Fig. 9–1). In the past, an unsatisfactory result was managed by redilatation, often with a larger balloon. Today, an unsatisfactory result is an indication for stenting. Elastic recoil, frequently related to eccentric plaques, dissection, severe calcification, a residual gradient, and a poor cosmetic result are the most frequent reasons for lack of complete success. (Fig. 9–2).

Standards of care during angioplasty have been published and guidelines agreed to in a multicouncil document of the American Heart Association.[4] These should be followed. The reporting of results should follow the reporting standards of Rutherford and Becker.[5]

DISTRIBUTION OF ILIAC DISEASE

The distribution of iliac disease is relevant to the question of who should have angioplasty. A report of 440 consecutive peripheral arteriograms performed for vascular disease goes some way toward answering this question.[6,7] Only significant lesions were considered. The patient population came from six centers in the United States, two of which admitted a significant number of patients of interventional radiologists and two of which appeared to be conservative in their indications for surgery. Probably, therefore, the series is a representative sample of vascular practice around the country. The study found that femoropopliteal disease was three to five times more frequent than iliac disease. Among patients with iliac disease, stenoses were three times more frequent than occlusions, a distribution that was reversed in the femoropopliteal system.

When one plots the relative frequency against length of both iliac stenoses and occlusions, the distribution of stenoses is essentially asymptotic, with 80% of iliac stenoses being 5 cm or less in length (Fig. 9–3). The distribution of occlusions is approximately linear, with 25% being 5 cm or less in length. If one excludes occlusions from consideration for angioplasty, then, because stenoses predominate, about 60% of patients with iliac

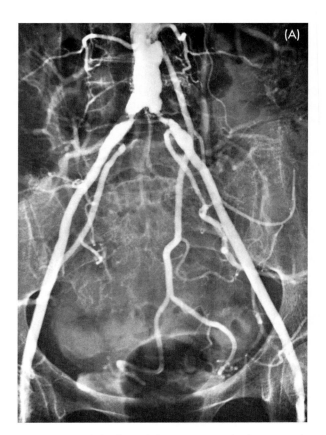 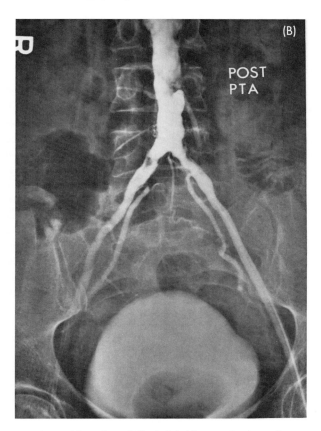

Figure 9–2. (A) Bilateral iliac stenoses. The lesion on the right is eccentric and heavily calcified. (B) After angioplasty the eccentric lesion on the right is still significantly stenotic. The patient went on to stent placement.

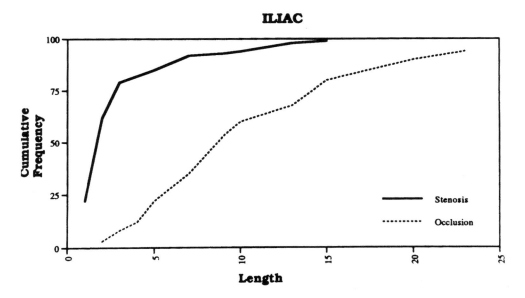

Figure 9–3. Cumulative frequency of lesions is plotted against length for iliac stenosis and occlusions. (Reprinted with permission.)

lesions will be suitable for angioplasty. In this particular series, 204 lesions underwent angioplasty, so about 40% of iliac stenoses were so treated. Because the curve for stenoses is asymptotic, the majority of lesions are short, and it is therefore reasonable to be cautious in performing angioplasty alone on the shorter lesions. Extending the attempted length adds few extra patients, and the success rate declines. If short-segment occlusions were included, then potentially 65 to 70% of patients would be suitable for angioplasty.

INDICATIONS FOR ANGIOPLASTY

Essentially for the period 1974 to 1990 but predominantly in the last decade, iliac angioplasty was the only valid endovascular technique that offered an alternative to surgery in some patients, and during that period the indications became fairly well defined. First, iliac angioplasty should be performed only in patients who are symptomatic. Although the complication rate is low, the procedure cannot be justified in asymptomatic patients except to preserve a distal bypass. The ideal candidates are patients with claudication who have a discrete stenosis. *Guidelines for Peripheral Percutaneous Transluminal Angioplasty of the Abdominal Aorta and Lower Extremity Vessels*, authored by the American Heart Association and approved by the Councils of Cardiovascular Surgery, Clinical Cardiology, Epidemiology, and Cardiovascular Radiology, categorized iliac lesions according to their degree of suitability for angioplasty.[4] Category 1 lesions are concentric, uncalcified stenoses less than 3 cm in length. Category 2 lesions are stenoses 3 to 5 cm in length and calcified or eccentric stenoses less than 3 cm in length. Category 3 lesions are stenoses 5 to 10 cm in length and occlusions less than 5 cm in length after thrombolytic therapy. Category 4 lesions are stenoses more than 10 cm in length, occlusions longer than 5 cm, extensive bilateral disease, iliac stenoses in patients with abdominal aortic aneurysms, or other lesions requiring aortoiliac surgery.

Category 4 lesions should have surgical therapy. Category 1 and 2 lesions should anticipate an 80% 5-year patency with percutaneous transluminal angioplasty (PTA), while category 3 lesions would anticipate a 65 to 75% 5-year patency. Angioplasty should therefore be performed in category 1, 2, and 3 lesions.

Not considered in this classification is the combination of iliac angioplasty with surgery. Because femorofemoral bypass grafts are frequently preferred for an iliac occlusion in higher-risk patients, angioplasty should be performed on an iliac stenosis that provides inflow. Equally, an inflow angioplasty should be performed before a femoropopliteal bypass graft in tandem diseases. This approach has been strongly advocated by Veith et al and others.[8] When both procedures were performed surgically, they were usually staged. Now iliac angioplasty may precede on infralinguinal bypass graft when it is obvious that the dominant disease is distal. It is preferable, however, to perform iliac angioplasty and then reassess the patient by noninvasive testing before proceeding. The distal operation may be unnecessary.

Because therapy is provided for patients and not for their anatomic lesions, comorbidity may influence these decisions. In high-risk patients one may extend the indications for angioplasty and be prepared to accept a lower patency rate than one would for surgery, even if it means accepting the possibility of a repeat procedure. In young patients, while one accepts surgery as more desirable, the patients may prefer angioplasty, even with the understanding that it may have to be repeated.

It is not the purpose of this chapter to consider the results of stenting in the iliac artery. Nevertheless, because the Palmaz stent has been available in the United States since 1990, it has influenced these decisions. While there are no data demonstrating that stenting allows category 4 lesions to be treated percutaneously, it seems likely that interventional radiologists are more comfortable with the availability of a bailout device and may, in high-risk patients, extend the indications for angioplasty beyond those of the earlier period.

RESULTS OF ILIAC ANGIOPLASTY

In 1989, Becker et al reviewed data from 2697 iliac artery angioplasties reported in the literature and calculated a mean 2-year patency rate of 81% and a 5-year patency of 72%.[9]

An excellent early article by Spence et al in 1981 considered 148 iliac angioplasties.[10] The 3-year patency rate, by plethysmographic criteria, was 79% (Fig. 9–4). The authors noted a difference between patients treated for claudication compared to limb salvage: 79% versus 50% at 2 years. Theirs was one of the first articles to make the observation—since substantiated repeatedly—that failures tend to occur in the first 18 months, after which time the survival (patency or cumulative clinical success) curve is relatively flat, largely altered by the progression of disease.

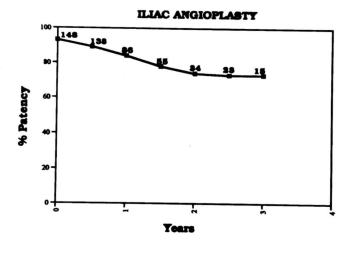

Figure 9–4. Three year patency by life table analysis. (Reprinted from Ref. 10 with permission.)

These data correlate well with an early article of Gallino et al, who in 1984 described angioplasty in 131 patients with iliac stenoses, 92% of whom had claudication. The 5 year patency rate was 83% but this appears to be a secondary patency. However, it did include all failures. There were 12 patients who underwent redilatation.[11] A more recent series is that of Tegtmeyer et al, who in 1991 reported on 340 iliac angioplasties in 200 patients followed for a mean period of 28 months.[12] Fifty-eight percent of the patients were in the Society of Vascular Surgery (SVS) grade 1, 23% were in grade 2, and 16% were in grade 3. Follow-up was clinical in 176 patients, 31 of whom had angiography. Tegtmeyer et al reported on 89% 3-year patency rate. This number excludes the 7% of primary failures and, therefore, may be corrected to 82%. Its weakness is in the follow-up, the details of which were inadequately described.

The largest series in the literature is that of Johnston et al, who reported 5-year results in 1987.[13] Their series of 984 angioplasties included 684 aortoiliac lesions, of which 80 were occlusions. Follow-up was both clinical and hemodynamic, and required improvement by one clinical grade *and* an increase in the ankle/brachial index (ABI) of 0.1. Using these criteria, the authors reported a 60% 5-year patency rate in the common iliac artery and a 48% 5-year patency rate in the external iliac artery. Common iliac stenoses with good runoff had a 65% 5-year patency rate, compared to 52% for those with poor runoff. Patients with occlusions did less well, with a 50% 5-year patency rate with good runoff and a 34% 5-year patency rate with poor runoff. These are primary patencies that include initial failures.

In 1993, Johnston reanalyzed the results he had presented in 1987. There was no change in the criteria for success.[14] For stenotic disease, patency rates were as follows: 1 year, 96%; 2 years, 77%; 3 years, 67%; and 5 years, 59%. No statistically significant variables were seen in the common iliac artery stenoses, but external iliac stenoses did worse than common iliac stenoses, with a 3-year patency of 62% versus 71%. Among patients with external iliac stenoses, females had less successful results than males: 34% versus 57%. Patients with both common and external iliac stenoses had a 60% 3-year patency rate, but those with poor runoff did significantly worse than those with good runoff: 30% versus 73% at 3 years.

The indication for angioplasty (claudication versus limb salvage), the presence or absence of diabetes, and the pretreatment ABI (greater than 0.5 or < 0.5) were also said to be significant variables.

Eighty-two patients had iliac occlusions. The 1-month patency rate was 75% (18 lesions could not be crossed). At 1 year patency was 60%, at 2 years 53%, and at 3 years 48%. The life table curve for occlusions is parallel to the curve for stenoses, and the confounding variable is obviously the inability to cross 18% of the lesions in this series dating from the early 1980s. Johnston recognized this by publishing figures with technical failures excluded and a 3-year patency of 59%.

If an iliac occlusion was dilated in association with a tandem lesion, then the 3-year patency rate was 17% versus 66% for an occlusion alone. However, a confounding variable is present here because the initial success in tandem lesions was only 45%, so the true significance of this finding is doubtful.

Johnston's conclusions are more enthusiastic after the reanalysis than before: "PTA of common iliac stenosis yields excellent results. . . . Thus iliac PTA has an important role in the management of arterial occlusive disease."

Rutherford has commented on Johnston's method of reporting as giving results that are falsely low because patients with iliac disease may develop femoropopliteal artery disease or, indeed, any other progression of disease, which will lower their ABI, and they will be regarded as having developed an iliac restenosis.[15] Rutherford reported the incidence of this over a 3-year period to be 16%, and over a 5-year period it may be as high as 25%. Rutherford has therefore suggested the use of the thigh/brachial index (TBI) which gives a 5-year patency rate of about 74%, in his experience.

Fradet et al were the first to use the TBI when they reviewed iliac angioplasties in 60 patients in 1984.[15] They reported a 95% 1-year patency rate by TBI compared with an 86% patency rate by ABI in the same patient population.

Rutherford and Durham recently reviewed iliac angioplasty and produced a composite life table curve from the available data.[16] This yielded a 70% 5-year patency rate. The authors stressed the importance of including the initial failures in the analysis because not doing so may hide trends in the data. However, the initial failure rate of iliac angioplasty is so low that it is unlikely to confound the data, except in iliac occlusions. Nevertheless, this is not a reason for not conforming to the reporting standards recently proposed by Rutherford[17,18] and modified by Rutherford and Becker.[5] These standards have since been adopted by the *Journal of Vascular and Interventional Radiology* and by *Radiology* for future publications.

In 1990, Stokes et al reported on 70 iliac angioplasties performed on patients with diabetes.[19] The overall 5-year patency rate was 35%. In patients with good runoff, the 5-year patency rate was 76%, while with poor runoff it was 20% (Fig. 9–5). For patients with claudication the 5-year patency was 70% while for those with ischemia it was 29%. The vast majority of patients with ischemia who had iliac angioplasty had subsequent femoropopliteal artery bypass grafts, and the majority of these bypasses were said to be open at the time of iliac restenosis. How this was documented is not clear from the article. The flaw in this analysis is the number

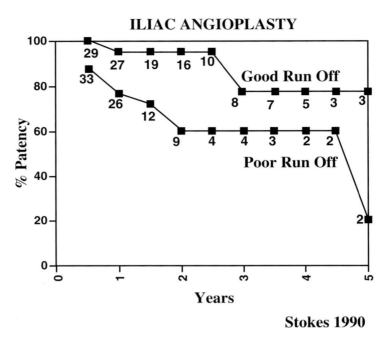

Figure 9–5.   Long term results of iliac angioplasty in diabetics with good and poor runoff. (Reprinted from Ref. 19 with permission.)

of patients involved. The 5-year patency rate was derived from five patients overall, with three and two patients, respectively, in each of the two subgroups of runoff and clinical status. The standard errors were not calculated, but they are certainly more than 10%, and the number of patients is such that only the 3-year figures have any validity. The 3-year patency rate overall for iliac angioplasty in these diabetic patients, predominantly with severe distal disease, was 65%. For patients with good runoff, the 3-year patency rate was 65%, and for those with poor runoff it was 60%. For claudication it was 70% and for gangrene 65%. These differences are not significant.

An excellent recent article is by In der Maur et al, published in 1990.[20] They followed 157 iliac angioplasties, 80% performed for claudication. All patients had short-segment lesions only. Patency was concluded over the long term when the ABI normalized at greater than 0.9 or when there was a substained increase of 0.15. The 1-year patency rate was 84% (excluding the 3% primary failure rate). Log rank tests applied to the customary variables failed to identify statistically significant differences specifically for runoff or the presence of diabetes. These results confirm the data of Stokes et al,[19] which show that for disease of similar severity, diabetes is not a significant variable.

The only randomized trial comparing angioplasty to surgery involved 263 patients reported by Wilson et al from the Veterans Administration in 1989.[21] Seventy-six patients with iliac disease were entered into the surgical arm, and 81 patients had angioplasty. At 3 years, the longest period with an adequate number of

patients, there was no significant difference between the results of surgery and angioplasty. In this series, 72% had claudication and all patients had to be suitable for both angioplasty and surgery, so they did not have extensive disease.

RESULTS IN ILIAC OCCLUSIONS

In 1982 Ring et al published an article entitled "Percutaneous Recanalization of Common Iliac Occlusions: An Unacceptable Occlusion Rate?"[22] They described angioplasty in 10 patients, of whom they were successful in crossing the lesion in 5. In two of these five patients there was contralateral embolization. Ring et al questioned whether two contralateral emboli in five patients was an unacceptably high complication rate. Since then, iliac angioplasty in complete iliac occlusions has seldom been practiced. Katzen et al advocated perfusing complete occlusions with urokinase, reducing them to an underlying stenosis, and then performing angioplasty, with good results.[23,24] Nevertheless, aortobifemoral bypass grafting or femorofemoral cross-over grafting remains the standard.

In 1986 Colapinto et al reported their attempts at angioplasty in 68 complete occlusions ranging in length from 1 to 19 cm, with an average length of 6 cm.[25] They were successful in treating 50 patients. In the lesions 5 cm or less in length, they had a 92% primary success rate. This decreased to 70% in lesions longer than 5 cm. Among those they were able to cross, the 3-year patency rate was 78%, as judged clinically and plethysmographically. When all the unsuccessful attempts (seven lesions over 15 cm in length) are included, the data can be revised downward to a 3-year patency rate of 52%.

Clearly, angioplasty in iliac occlusions has a significant primary failure rate, but if the lesion can be crossed, the results are comparable to those achieved with stenoses. However, customary practice in high-risk patients has been to use a femorofemoral crossover graft, while low-risk patients receive an aorto-bifemoral bypass graft. Angioplasty for iliac occlusion has remained an underused technique. Recent results with iliac stenting have demonstrated that iliac occlusions may be crossed with a 92% success rate; not surprisingly, primary stenting is producing results superior to those of Colapinto et al.[26]

RESULTS IN AORTIC DISEASE

Isolated aortic stenoses are uncommon, so aortic angioplasty is seldom practiced. However, one of the more common sites of iliac disease is the aortic bifurcation, and some authors have used this as a justification for the generic term *aortoiliac angioplasty*. Others regard bilateral aortoiliac bifurcation disease as a special category because it involves differences in the technique of angioplasty, but in terms of results it is no different. In 1990 Ravimandalam et al reviewed dilatation in 27 patients, 2 of whom suffered embolic complications.[27] Excellent long-term patency was reported. Odurny et al reported on 25 patients with 100% success.[28] The mean follow-up period was 38 months, with a 70% 5-year patency rate. There were no embolic complications.

The largest series is presented by Yakes et al and concerns 32 patients, all successfully treated without complications.[29] At a mean follow-up period of 25 months, 25 of 28 patients who had follow-up were asymptomatic, with maintenance of their postangioplasty TBI. It would appear, therefore, that aortic angioplasty is as successful as or more successful than iliac angioplasty.

COMPLICATIONS

There is no doubt that the complications of iliac angioplasty are significantly fewer than those of aortoiliac surgery. The largest single angiographic series is that of Belli et al, who reported on 1642 patients with a mortality rate of 0.1%.[30] Twenty-six percent of the patients had rest pain or tissue loss. Of this group, 2.8% developed complications requiring surgery but only 0.9% required a bypass. Among the patients with claudication, 0.7% required surgery and 0.5% needed a bypass. The majority of these patients had femoropopliteal disease. With modern No. 5 French catheters, groin complications are about 3%, and the complications requiring surgery include aneurysm and anteriovenous (AV) fistula repair.

The American Heart Association recently published thresholds for complications of angioplasty in a multi-Council document.[4] The complications included significant bleeding (3.4%), false aneurysm (0.5%), AV fistula (0.1%), thrombosis at the angioplasty site (3.2%), and distal embolization (2.3%). Complications occurring above these thresholds should trigger a review.

Recent experience with duplex sonography has identified many more false aneurysms, and one recent series, looking predominantly at patients who had coronary angioplasty, showed an incidence of 14%.[31] However, most of these lesions may now be treated by compression using ultrasound guidance, so the incidence of surgery should now fall.

CRITIQUE OF RESULTS OF ILIAC ANGIOPLASTY

The majority of articles concerning iliac angioplasty report on stenoses rather than occlusions: 80 to 90% in most series. Furthermore, the majority of patients have claudication, again about 80 to 90%, so a direct comparison with the results of surgery cannot be made. The article by Wilson et al is invalidated in this regard because, by virtue of the randomization, patients had to be eligible for both arm of the study.[21] As such, these patients do not compare with patients undergoing aortobifemoral bypass grafting, who tend to have more extensive aortoiliac disease.

However, the vast majority of patients with isolated iliac disease do have claudication, and it is usually only when the iliac disease is combined with severe distal disease that patients have rest pain or ischemia. Only the article of Stokes et al, among those referenced, addresses this matter, and it is not clear that there is a significant diminution in patency in this patient population.[19]

Two further articles are relevant. In 1982 Kadir et al reported on 43 patients who had angioplasty as an adjunct to surgery; in 23 patients it was performed in conjunction with planned vascular reconstruction.[32] Patency of the vascular graft was maintained in 22 of the 23 patients during a mean follow-up period of 9 months.

In 1989 Brewster et al analyzed 75 patients with tandem disease in 79 limbs who had iliac angioplasty followed by infrainguinal bypass (55 patients), femoropopliteal artery bypass (18 patients), or profundoplasty (6 patients).[33] Seventy-eight percent of the patients were operated on for limb salvage, and 22% had incapacitating claudication. The mean follow-up period was 43 months. By life table analysis, the 5-year primary patency rate of the surgery was 76% and the secondary patency rate was 88%. Because 25% of the operations involved a prosthetic conduit, these results are at least 10% better than might be expected for femoropopliteal artery bypass alone. While the results of iliac angioplasty may be worse in moderate distal disease, this is by no means proven, and Johnston's reanalysis of tandem disease is, to a large extent, invalidated by the 45% primary failure rate.[14]

If we accept these data as demonstrating about a 70 to 75% 5-year patency rate, we can certainly accept iliac angioplasty as a durable procedure. Furthermore, we know from the data of Capek et al concerning the femoral system that long-term patency from 5 to 10 years changes little and is influenced significantly only by the progression of the disease.[34] We also know from the femoral literature that if one can cross an occlusion, there is no significant difference in long-term patency between stenoses and occlusions if they are relatively short; this seems to be true in the iliac series as well.

One feature that has not emerged from the literature is the maximum length of iliac lesions suitable for angioplasty with good long-term success. Capek's article established an upper limit of 10 cm in the femoropopliteal system,[34] but there is no comparable article in the aortoiliac literature. The American Heart Association guidelines place lesions 5 to 10 cm in length in category 3 and those over 10 cm in category 4.[4] While few experienced interventional radiologists would dispute these assignments, there is little factual evidence for this choice. This is unfortunate because, as new techniques such as stenting or endovascular grafting appear, the true parameters of angioplasty have not been explored sufficiently for good comparisons to be made.

By the same token, there are very few series of iliac angioplasty in complete occlusions. In fact, the results are quite satisfactory in the reported series. But the usual practice is for iliac occlusions to be treated by aortobifemoral bypass surgery or femorofemoral bypass grafts. Vorwerk and Gunther have advocated primary iliac stenting,[35] but a randomized trial is still awaited, as it is for stenting against angioplasty alone. One reason for the diminished enthusiasm for angioplasty for occlusions was Ring's early article suggesting that the embolic risk might be too high.[22] This was further confounded by Katzen et al, who advocated urokinase therapy of iliac occlusions before proceeding to angioplasty.[23,24] Colapinto et al's report of iliac angioplasty was largely ignored.[25] Primary stenting for iliac occlusions may forever mask the true results of iliac angioplasty.

Angioplasty is probably suitable for about 60% of patients with aortoiliac disease, and about a 70 to 75% 5-year patency rate may be expected. As newer endovascular techniques are developed, it will be interesting to see if the patency rate can be improved. More interesting will be whether the indications for percutaneous therapy can be expanded and fewer patients operated on. Can aortoiliac surgery be almost completely replaced for atherosclerotic occlusive disease?

REFERENCES

1. Portsmann W. Ein neuer Korsett-Ballonkatheter zur transluminalen Rekanalisation nach Dotter unter besonderer Berucksichtigung von Obliterationen an den Beckenarterien. *Radoil Diagn (Berl)* 1993;2:239.
2. Dotter CT, Judkins MP. Transluminal treatment of arteriosclerotic obstruction: description of a new technique and a preliminary report of its application. *Circulation* 1964;30:654–670.
3. Gruntzig A, Hopff H. Percutane rekanalisation chronischer arterieller verschlusse mit einem neven dilatationskatheter. *Tsch Med Wochenschr* 1974;99:2502.
4. Pentecost MJ, Criqui MH, Dorros G, et al. Guidelines for peripheral percutaneous transluminal angioplasty of the abdominal and lower extremity vessels. *Circulation* 1994;89:511–531.
5. Rutherford RB. Becker GJ. Standards for evaluating and reporting the results of surgical and percutaneous therapy for peripheral disease. *JVIR* 1991;2:169–174.
6. Martin EC. The impact of angioplasty: a perspective., *JVIR* 1992;3:511–514.
7. Martin EC. Transcatheter therapies in peripheral amd noncoronary vascular disease. *Circulation* 1991;(suppl I):I1–I5
8. Veith FJ, Gupta SK, Wentgerter KR, et al. Changing arteriosclerotic disease patterns and management strategies in lower-limb-threatening ischemia. *Ann Rura* 1990; 212:402–412.
9. Becker GJ, Katzen BJ, Dake MD. Noncoronary angioplasty. *Radiology* 1989;170;403–412.
10. Spence RK, Freiman DB, Gatenby R, et al. Long-term results of transluminal angioplasty of the iliac and femoral arteries. *Arch Surg* 1981;116:1377–1386.
11. Gallino A, Mahler F, Probst P, et al. Percutaneous transluminal angioplasty of the arteries of the lower limbs: a 5-year follow-up. *Circulation* 1984;70:619–623.
12. Tegtmeyer Cj, Hartwell GD, Sellby JB. Results and complications of angioplasty in aortoiliac disease. *Circulation* 1991(Suppl);83:53–60.
13. Johnston KW, Rae M, Hogg-Johnston SA, et al. Five-year results of a prospective study of percutaneous transluminal angioplasty. *Ann Surg* 1987;206:403–413.
14. Johnston KW, Iliac arteries: reanalysis of results of balloon angioplasty. *Radiology* 1993;186:207–212.
15. Fradet G. Lidstone D, Herba M, et al. Percutaneous transluminal angioplasty of iliac arteries: the importance of functional studies. *Can J Surg* 1984;27:359–361.
16. Rutherford RB, Durham J. Percutaneous balloon angioplasty for arteriosclerosis obliterans: long-term results. In: Yao JST, Pearce WH, eds. *Technologies in Vascular Surgery*. Philadelphia: WB Saunders, 1993;329–345.
17. Rutherford RB, Flanigan DP, Gupta SK, et al. Suggested standards for reports dealing with lower extremity ischemia. *J Vasc Surg* 1986;4:80–94.
18. Rutherford RB. Standards for evaluating results of interventional therapy for peripheral vascular disease. *Circulation* 1991;83(suppl I):I6–1–11.
19. Stokes KR, Strunk HM, Campbell DR, et al. Five-year results of iliac and femoropopliteal angioplasty in diabetic patients. *Radiology* 1990;174:977–982.
20. In der Maur GAP, de Boot T, Boeve J, et al. Angioplasty of the iliac and femoral arteries. Initial and long-term results in short stenotic lesions. *Eur J Radiol* 1990;11:163–167.

21. Wilson SE, Wolf GL, Cross AP. Percutaneous transluminal angioplasty versus operation for peripheral arteriosclerosis. *J Vasc Surg* 1989;9:1–9.
22. Ring EJ, Freiman DB, McLean GK, et al. Percutaneous recanalization of common iliac artery occlusions: an unacceptable complication rate. *Am J Roentgenol* 1982;139:587–589.
23. Katzen BT, vanBreda A. Low dose streptokinase in the treatment of arterial occlusions. *Am J Roentgenol* 1981;136:1171–1175.
24. Katzen BT, Edwards KC, Albert AS, et al. Low dose fibrinolysis in peripheral vascular disease. *J Vasc Surg* 1984;1:718.
25. Colapinto RF, Stronell RD, Johnston KW. Transluminal angioplasty of complete iliac obstructions. *Am J Roentgenol* 1986;146:859–862.
26. Vorwerk D, Gunther RW. Chronic iliac artery occlusion. Presented at the International Congress, University of Heidelberg, Zermatt, April 1993.
27. Ravimandalam K, Rao VRK, Kumar S, et al. Obstruction of the infrarenal portion of the abdominal aorta: results of treatment with balloon angioplasty. *Am J Roentgenol* 1991;156:1257–1262.
28. Odunry A, Colapinto RF, Sniderman KW, et al. Percutaneous transluminal aortic angioplasty of abdominal aortic stenoses. *Cardiovasc Intervent Radiol* 1989;12:1–6.
29. Yakes WF, Kumpe DA, Brown SB, et al. Percutaneous transluminal aortic angioplasty: techniques and results. *Radiology* 1989:172:965–970.
30. Belli AM, Cumberland DC, Knox AM, et al. The complication rate of percutaneous peripheral balloon angioplasty. *Clin Radiol* 1990;41:380–383.
31. Katzenschlager R, Ugurluoglu A, Ahmadi A, et al. Incidence of pseudoaneurysm after diagnostic and therapeutic angiography. *Radiology* 1995;195:463–466.
32. Kadir S, Smith GW, White, RI Jr, et al. Percutaneous transluminal angioplasty as an adjunct to the surgical management of peripheral vascular disease. *Ann Surg* 1982;195:786–795.
33. Brewster DC, Cambria RP, Darling C, et al. long-term results of combined iliac balloon angioplasty and distal surgical revascularization. *Ann Surg* 1989;210:324–331.
34. Capek P, McLean GK, Berkowitz JD. Femoropopliteal angioplasty: factors influencing long-term success. *Circulation* 1991;83(suppl I):I70–I80.
35. Vorwek D, Gunther RW. Mechanical revascularization of occluded iliac arteries with use of self-expandable endoprotheses. *Radiology* 1990;175:411–415.

10

The Role of Stents in Aortoiliac Occlusive Disease

Timothy P. Murphy, M.D.

BACKGROUND

Intra-arterial stent placement to treat atherosclerotic obstruction was proposed by Dotter and Judkins in 1964[1]. Dotter subsequently placed coil-spring stents in popliteal arteries in dogs and followed the duration of their patency.[2] The first intra-arterial stent used in humans was the Maass double helix spiral prosthesis[3] (Fig. 10–1), which was used in two patients with dissecting aortic aneurysms.[3,4] This device required a 7-mm-diameter introducer and therefore had to be placed by surgical cutdown.[3,4]

Palmaz began construction of a balloon-expandable stent in 1983,[5] with a report on its experimental use appearing in 1985.[6] The first described use of percutaneously implanted stents in human arteries is the 1987 report of Sigwart et al on the use of the Wallstent (Fig. 10–2) (Schneider, Inc., Minneapolis, MN) in coronary, iliac, and femoral arteries.[7] Shortly thereafter, results achieved with the Palmaz stent (Fig. 10–3) (Johnson & Johnson Interventional Systems, Warren, NJ) in the iliac arteries appeared.[8]

The Palmaz stent received approval from the U.S. Food and Drug Administration for use in human iliac arteries in 1991, and the Wallstent was approved in 1996. The Palmaz-Schatz stent has been approved for use in the coronary arteries since 1994. The Gianturco-Roubin coronary artery stent (Cook, Inc., Bloomington, IN), a balloon-expandable stent with a continuous coil design, is undergoing trials in the United States at this time.[9] Other stents, such as the knitted, balloon-expandable Strecker stent[10] (Fig. 10–4), the Cragg nitinol stent[11,12] (Fig. 10–5), and the self-expanding Gianturco-Z stent (Cook, Inc., Bloomington, IN),[13] were developed in the 1980s. Experience with these stents in other countries has been reported, but currently they are not marketed for intra-arterial use in the United States.

CHARACTERISTICS OF STENTS

Available Stents

The Palmaz stent and the Wallstent are the most widely used stents in the aorta and iliac arteries in the United States. The Palmaz stent is made of 316L stainless steel and, prior to placement, is a hollow cylinder containing multiple longitudinal slits, which become diamond-shaped fenestrations when the stent is expanded. The stent is rigid; wall thickness is 0.13 mm for the large stent (8–12 mm in diameter) and 0.14 for the medium-sized stent (4 to 9 mm in diameter). The large version measures 3.1 mm in diameter and is up to 30 mm long prior to placement. The Palmaz stent is crimped onto an angioplasty balloon, and the large stent is placed through a No. 10 French introducer sheath.[14] The medium-sized version is suitable for most iliac lesions but is not currently approved for use in the iliac arteries. This stent can be introduced by a No. 7 French sheath.

The Wallstent is a flexible metallic tubular braid composed of Elgiloy, a stainless steel–cobalt alloy. It is woven on a mandrel from filaments 0.1 mm in diameter. The stent is mounted on a No. 7 French introducer catheter, and in its initial configuration was covered by a rolling membrane that required "priming" by contrast material injected at 3.5 atmospheres of pressure.[15,16] This priming step has been eliminated, and the current version of the stent is covered by a single membrane that is simply retracted off the stent. The stent introducer is placed through a No. 7 French sheath[15,16] and is very flexible, allowing placement around the aortic bifurcation from the contralateral femoral artery.

111

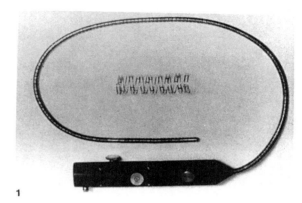

Figure 10–1. The Maass double helix. (Reprinted from Ref. 4 with permission.)

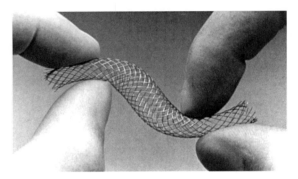

Figure 10–2. The Wallstent.

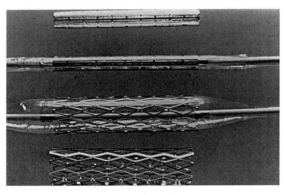

Figure 10–3. The Palmaz stent.

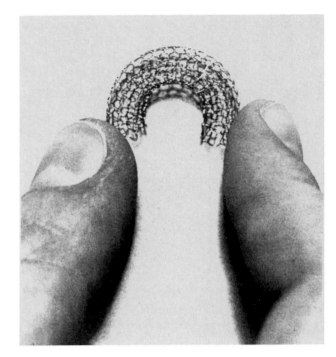

Figure 10–4. The Strecker stent. (Reprinted from Ref. 4 with permission.)

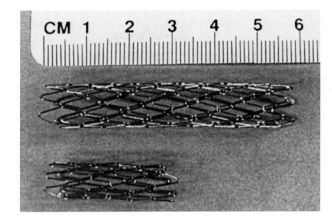

Figure 10–5. The Cragg stent. (Reprinted from Ref. 12 with permission.)

The Strecker stent is a tube that is knitted from 0.1-mm-diameter tantalum wire.[17] The tantalum filaments are loosely connected, and this stent demonstrates excellent longitudinal and radial flexibility. It is attached to an angioplasty balloon by silicone sleeves at its ends and deployed by expansion of the balloon. The surface of this stent is electronegative, and it should not contact stents that are electropositive (such as the Wallstent or Palmaz stent), as galvanic currents will result in ionic solutions.[15] This may lead to corrosion.[15] The

Cragg stent is a nitinol thermal-memory stent constructed by winding a 0.28-mm nitinol filament on a mandrel in a zigzag configuration and hled together by polypropylene sutures. This stent self-expands when deployed (Fig. 10–5). The Gianturco stent is self-expanding.[13] It is made of stainless steel wire 0.25 mm in diameter shaped in a zigzag configuration and wrapped into a tubular configuration. The stent is rigid and is placed through a No. 7 French introducer.[13]

Mechanical Properties of Stents

The ideal stent should be deployed through a small arteriotomy or puncture site but able to achieve large diameters and thus have a large expansion ratio. It should be longitudinally flexible in the undeployed and deployed states but sufficiently strong to resist elastic recoil from calcified or eccentric stenoses. It also should be biocompatible and completely covered with endothelium shortly after placement, but it should incite minimal neointima formation to preserve early gains of the procedure. Stent surface area should be minimized.

The medium-sized Palmaz stent and the Wallstent represent fundamentally different designs and demonstrate significantly different physical characteristics. Some of these characteristics have known clinical significance, others may be potentially relevant, and still others are theoretical or clinically insignificant.

The Palmaz stent is introduced through a No. 7 French sheath (4 to 9 mm diameter stent) or a No. 10 French sheath (8 to 12 mm diameter stent). It has an expansion ratio of 4:1, and the manufacturer claims a metal surface area of 10% when fully expanded. The large stent shortens to 28.9 mm (4% shortening) at 8 mm in diameter, 27.8 mm at 10 mm in diameter (7%), and 26.2 mm at 12 mm in diameter (13% shortening). It is possible to introduce the large Palmaz stent through a No. 7.5 or 8 French sheath,[18,19] but this is not recommended by the manufacturer. The 10-mm-diameter Wallstent is placed through a No. 7 French sheath; the 12-mm-diameter Wallstent requires a No. 8 French sheath. The Wallstent has an expansion ratio of 4.4:1, and the metal surface area has been measured at 20% when the stent is fully expanded at 10 mm.[20] The

68-mm-long stent shortens from 100 mm (undeployed length) to 79 mm (21% shortening) and 65 mm (35% shortening) in length at 8 and 10 mm in diameter, respectively.[21] The Palmaz stent is slightly more radiopaque than the Wallstent.

The Palmaz stent is balloon-expandable, and the Wallstent is self-expanding. The Palmaz stent is inelastic and undergoes permanent plastic deformation.[22,23] The Wallstent is almost completely elastic.[22,23] Materials that undergo plastic deformation maintain their conformation while under stress until they reach their *yield point*, at which the material collapses under the force and does not reexpand. In contrast, the Wallstent gives way evenly and proportionally to applied forces, and once the force is removed, it resumes its previous shape.[22,23]

Hoop strength is the ability of a stent to resist circular loads. This is believed to be a more relevant test of the strength of a stent than resistance to point or area loads due to the frequent use of stents in concentric stenoses. Of the two most often used stents, the Palmaz stent has hoop strength superior to that of the Wallstent. To achieve a reduction of stent circumference by 1 and 2 mm under a circular load (diameter reduction of 0.33 and 0.64 mm), approximately six times as much force is required for the PS30 Palmaz stent than for the constrained 10-mm-diameter Wallstent[23] (Fig. 10–6). The Cragg stent and the Strecker stent require approximately half as much force as the Wallstent for these minimal changes in stent diameter,[23] but with larger diameter reduction, the Wallstent[22] and the Cragg stent[11] exhibit nonlinear increases in hoop strength. With a reduction in diameter of 55%, the Cragg stent has greater hoop strength than the Wallstent.[11] Others have confirmed a significant hoop strength advantage with the Palmaz stent.[24]

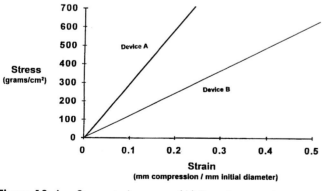

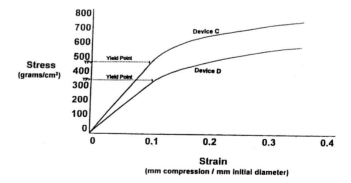

Figure 10–6. Stress-strain curves. (A) Two stress-strain curves are shown. Both materials undergo elastic deformation under the ranges of stress considered. Device A has a steeper slope, which indicates a higher modulus of elasticity (Young's modulus) than device B. Device A is more stiff than device B. (B) Two different devices, which undergo elastic deformation up to their yield point, where they undergo plastic (permanent) deformation. Device C is more stiff than device D. (Reprinted from Ref. 22 with permission.)

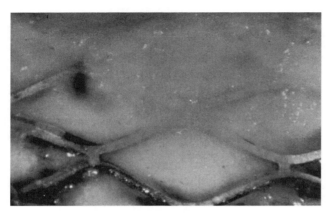

Figure 10–7. After incorporation of metallic stents, a process that takes 2 to 4 weeks, a thin neointima coats most of the stent surface. Endothelial cells are present on the surface of this neointima.

Stent Biocompatibility

Following intra-arterial stent deployment, a variable amount of thrombus and blood proteins is deposited on the stent surface; these are modified over 24 hours so that acellular proteins predominate in the neointima.[25] This neointima, which is usually less than 0.5 mm thick, is covered with endothelium within 3 or 4 weeks after stent placement[25] (Fig. 10–7). Thus, stents are incorporated into the wall of the stented artery and are considered biocompatible rather than simply biologically inert.

The amount of thrombus deposition and the thickness of subsequent neointimal hyperplasia depend on stent composition and surface properties. Surface properties such as roughness, electrical charge, and free sur-

face energy determine the thrombogenicity and biocompatibility of metals.[25]

Most metals demonstrate a positive electric charge in electrolytic solutions that results in the attraction of plasma proteins, such as fibrinogen, immediately after placement.[25] This insulates the metal surface and reduces the free surface energy, thereby decreasing the thrombogenicity of the stent.[25] Stents composed of or coated with metals that demonstrate strong electropositivity, such as gold or platinum, accumulate less thrombus immediately after placement[26] and demonstrate less neointimal hyperplasia.[27] Thrombus deposition after stent placement also can be attenuated by the use of anticoagulants and platelet inhibitors, and is maximized by the use of heparin, aspirin, dipyridamole, and dextran.[25]

Incorporation of stents into the artery wall and intimal thickness within the stent may be affected by the flexibility or rigidity of the stent. However, these effects are unclear. In one study, increased stent rigidity was associated with less intimal thickening in the common femoral artery in dogs.[28] However, other studies have shown more intimal thickening when rigid stents were placed in swine iliac arteries.[29] No clinically significant differences in biocompatibility of the Palmaz stent and the Wallstent have been convincingly demonstrated.

PROCEDURE

Indications for Stent Placement

Stents were developed for use in angioplasty failures, and this remains a frequent indication for stent use[30] (Fig. 10–8). However, stents have broadened the indi-

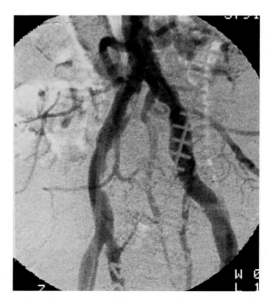

Figure 10–8. (A) Image obtained after angioplasty of an eccentric lesion in the right common iliac artery demonstrates elastic recoil and 50% residual stenosis (arrow). No improvement in the transstenotic pressure gradient was observed. (B) After placement of a Palmaz stent, the gradient was eliminated and no significant residual stenosis was seen angiographically.

cations for percutaneous revascularization in the aorta and iliac arteries. Prior to the advent of stents, only 60% of patients with aortoiliac insufficiency were believed to be suitable for angioplasty,[31] and the percentage who received angioplasty was probably considerably less. Criteria such as the length of the stenosis or the presence of chronic arterial occlusion previously were used to exclude patients from percutaneous therapy due to low technical success rates and high complication rates of angioplasty alone.[32–34] Stents have demonstrated improved long-term patency compared with balloon angioplasty in focal lesions.[35] Results using stents have been satisfactory in patients with diffuse arterial narrowing or chronic occlusion, with comparable technical success, complication, and long-term patency rates achieved with balloon angioplasty in focal stenoses. Current indications also include diffuse stenosis (>3 cm in length), chronic occlusion, flow-limiting dissection, and eccentric lesions.

Balloon angioplasty alone should be considered a viable option for focal (<3 cm), concentric, noncalcified aortoiliac stenoses (American Heart Association [AHA] category I).[36] However, the threshold for stent placement in these patients if results are unsatisfactory should be low. Balloon angioplasty without stent placement is not appropriate in patients with more severe angiographic disease (AHA category II or higher) or for those with flow-limiting dissection.[37] With the use of stents, nearly all patients with inflow to the infrarenal aorta and outflow from the common femoral arteries, except some patients with extensive diffuse aortoiliac disease who are good surgical candidates, warrant an attempt at percutaneous revascularization.

Patient Preparation

Patients should be seen by the interventional radiologist during a preadmission clinic visit.[38,39] At that time, a history should be taken and a physical examination performed. The physical examination should be directed toward determining both the severity of peripheral vascular disease and the most suitable approach for the study or intervention.

Patients with aortoiliac insufficiency often have diminished or absent femoral pulses. Although absent femoral pulses traditionally required performance of the diagnostic study by the axillary or translumbar approach,[40] elective aortoiliac interventions are optimally performed by the transfemoral approach, and current revascularization techniques permit access via the transfemoral route in most patients.

Results of noninvasive tests and other examinations should be reviewed during the preadmission visit, and any other necessary preprocedural tests can be ordered. Patients without complicating medical conditions can safely have diagnostic studies performed by a common femoral puncture without prepro-

cedure screening for coagulation disorders,[41] as abnormalities in these screening tests are rarely detected in patients without a history suspicious for bleeding difficulties.[42–45] As most patients undergoing aortography receive a significant volume of contrast (1 to 2 mL/kg), screening for baseline renal dysfunction with blood urea nitrogen and serum creatinine levels is recommended.[41] Routine cardiac screening is not indicated,[46,47] as elective coronary artery bypass surgery or angioplasty in patients found to have reversible myocardial ischemia are associated with mortality rates of 2 to 5% and 1 to 2.5%, respectively.[46] Both of these coronary revascularization procedures have higher mortality rates than aortoiliac stenting in patients who do not undergo preprocedure cardiac evaluation.[41] However, patients with a history of angina pectoris warrant a cardiac evaluation prior to invasive procedures.

Diabetic patients taking insulin should have their dose reduced by half on the day of the procedure. Patients should be instructed to discontinue taking other medications, such as warfarin compounds or metformin hydrochloride (Glucophage, Bristol-Meyers Squibb Co., Princeton, NJ) prior to their procedure. Patients are instructed to maintain a clear liquid diet for at least 8 hours prior to the procedure.

Patient preparation on the day of the procedure includes placement of a 20-gauge or larger peripheral intravenous line to allow for hydration and administration of sedatives, analgesics, heparin, or other medications as necessary. If the patient does not take aspirin, one 325-mg aspirin tablet is routinely given prior to the procedure. Both groins should be shaved prior to admission to the procedure room. A catheter should be placed in the urinary bladder routinely in patients with suspected aortoiliac insufficiency prior to diagnostic arteriography.

Diagnostic Technique

Single-plane angiography is performed, and we prefer to use dilute (30%) contrast material with digital subtraction angiography to minimize the cumulative contrast dose. Although many angiographers favor oblique images of the pelvis to evaluate the iliac arteries, it has been shown that measurement of arterial pressures is more accurate than angiography in detecting hemodynamically significant stenoses[48,49] and in determining the adequacy of interventions.[50]

Pressures should be measured simultaneously using two catheters or a single catheter through an appropriately sized vascular sheath with a side arm. The presence of an arterial occlusion is a priori evidence of hemodynamic significance, and measurement of a gradient prior to intervention is not required. Changes in systolic pressure, diastolic pressure, mean pressure, and pulse pressure have all been used to assess the significance of arterial obstruction.[51] However, for practical reasons, we favor changes in mean pressure across a stenosis, which is more static and reproducible than systolic gradients. We use a mean transstenotic gradient of 5 mm Hg as the lower limit of a hemodynamically significant lesion; this usually corresponds to a systolic gradient of 10 to 15 mm Hg.[48] Patients with intermittent claudication may have noncritical stenoses at rest and may not demonstrate a significant transstenotic gradient. In these patients, potentiation or augmentation of the gradient by intra-arterial injection of a vasodilator is desirable. In such cases, a mean gradient of 10 mm Hg is considered consistent with a significant stenosis.[52] Diastolic differences are insensitive to moderate stenoses.

Occasionally, reconstitution below an occluded external iliac artery may occur at the level of the profunda femoris artery without demonstration of the common femoral artery. However, this can be seen without significant atherosclerotic obstruction in the common femoral artery. If this pattern is observed angiographically, access to the common femoral artery is indicated. Injection of contrast material in the common femoral artery may reveal a suitable outflow artery for external iliac artery stent placement (Fig. 10–9). If the common femoral artery demonstrates hemodynamically significant stenosis, stent procedures should be done in conjunction with or in temporal proximity to femoral endarterectomy.

Stent Selection

As previously stated, the Wallstent and the Palmaz stent are the only stents currently marketed in the United States for iliac artery use. The Palmaz is the most rigid stent available and is the preferred stent for focal aortic or iliac stenoses, especially those that are calcified or eccentric, or for ostial stenoses.[23] Due to its flexibility, the Wallstent conforms to the shape of the native artery after deployment (Fig. 10–10). It is available in lengths up to 94 mm and therefore can be used to revascularize patients with diffuse iliac artery disease. The Palmaz stent is available in lengths up to 4 cm. While multiple Palmaz stents can be overlapped to treat diffuse iliac artery stenoses, their inelasticity prevents motion in the stented artery. As motion of the artery is required, stress risors can develop within the stents, which may result in stent fracture due to metal fatigue[53] (Fig. 10–11). Alternatively, if the stents are not overlapped but rather are placed contiguously, stent motion may result in shearing of the artery and pseudoaneurysm formation in the gap between the stents.

The Wallstent may be introduced through the contralateral femoral artery around the aortic bifurcation. The Palmaz stent usually does not pass through a sheath around the aortic bifurcation, but by advancing the stent and sheath in toto around the aortic bifurcation, contralateral placement of the Palmaz stent is possible.

Stent Deployment

Most patients receive full anticoagulation with heparin during the procedure in addition to antiplatelet therapy.[15] Early in the experience with stents, patients were treated with anti-vitamin K therapy for 6 months in addition to aspirin. However, in one study it was demonstrated that there was no difference in the incidence of stent thrombosis in patients undergoing this regimen compared to those treated with aspirin alone.[15]

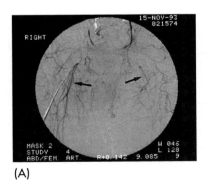
(A)

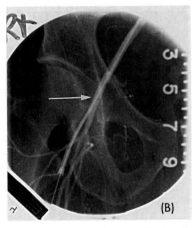
(B)

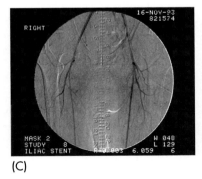
(C)

Figure 10–9. (A) Digital subtraction image of the lower pelvis and upper thighs after injection in the infrarenal aorta in this patient with chronic occlusion of the infrarenal aorta and iliac arteries. There is reconstitution of the profunda femoris arteries (arrows) without opacification of the common femoral arteries. (B) Selective injection in the external iliac artery demonstrates a right common femoral artery that is a suitable outflow artery for percutaneous aortoiliac ravascularization (arrow). Similar findings were demonstrated after access was gained in the left common femoral artery. (C) Following thrombolysis and stent placement, adequate outflow through the common femoral arteries is seen bilaterally. Nonselective contrast injections are inadequate to evaluate the status of the common femoral arteries in patients with iliac artery occlusion.

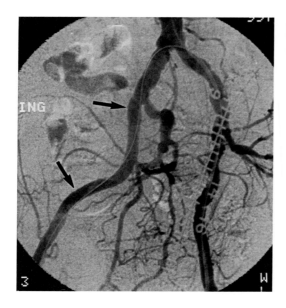

Figure 10–10. Pelvic arteriogram demonstrated occlusion of the right external iliac artery. After thrombolysis and placement of a 68-mm-long Wallstent, this oblique pelvic image demonstrates the stent (arrows) conforming to the shape of the external iliac artery.

Once the occlusion or stenosis is traversed, the stent is deployed. If stenosis involves the ostium of the common iliac artery, the properly placed stent projects into the lumen of the distal aorta for a few millimeters. A stent may need to be placed in the contralateral common iliac artery to preserve its ostium, depending on the caliber of the distal aorta and the amount of projection into the aorta that is required. Angioplasty is usually not performed prior to stent deployment if a self-expanding stent is used,[54] as this increases the likelihood of distal embolization.[10]

Stent diameters of 10 to 15 mm in the aorta, 8 to 10 mm in the common iliac artery, and 7 to 9 mm in the external iliac artery usually can be achieved. The diameter achieved after stent placement is reduced by 0.5 to 1 mm by the development of neointima within the stent,[8] and this must be considered when sizing stent dilations. Lumen diameter after stent incorporation into the artery wall of at least 6 mm is desirable, as this is the minimum iliac limb diameter that does not result in a decrease in the ankle/brachial index after aortofemoral bypass surgery.[55] However, patients who are poor surgical candidates treated for limb-salvage indications, particularly those with small body habitus underdilatation of the common iliac arteries to 7 mm, and underdilatation of the external iliac arteries to 6 mm may be satisfactory to reverse critical ischemia at rest. The diameter of self-expanding stents usually does not continue to enlarge more than the diameter of the angioplasty balloon used after deployment, but this increase in diameter has been observed in up to 12% of cases when self-expanding stents are placed in chronically occluded iliac arteries without prior thrombolysis.[56,57]

It is prudent not to stent below the inguinal ligament so that the common femoral can be used for bypass surgery should this be needed, although stenting across the hip joint can be successfully accomplished with the Wallstent in selected patients (Fig. 10–12). Stents placed over the ostium of the internal iliac artery do not occlude this artery in 83 to 89% of cases[15,56] unless stenosis of the internal iliac artery was present or, occasionally, if multiple stents are required in this area. Narrowing of the origin of the internal iliac artery may be seen in up to one-third,[15] however, and this poses the theoretical risk of decreased erectile function in males when stents are placed over the ostium of the internal iliac artery. However, impotence related to internal iliac artery insufficiency has not been reported after stent placement. Conversely, improvement in erectile function can be observed when flow through the aorta or common iliac artery to the internal iliac artery is improved with stents or angioplasty.[58]

Patients often experience discomfort during stent inflation, and this may limit the diameter that can be achieved. Pain is a sign of adventitial stretching and may herald arterial rupture.[59] Although arterial rupture can be observed with low inflation pressures, in general, stent inflation up to 6 or 8 atmospheres with mild or moderate discomfort is well tolerated. If pain is severe and excessive pressure is required to reduce a waist on an angioplasty balloon, further inflation is not advised.

If arterial rupture occurs, the patient should be stabilized by tamponading the rent with the angioplasty balloon inflated to low pressure (3 atmospheres) and then evaluated by contrast material injections to exclude continued blood loss. Blood specimens should be sent for hemoglobin, hematocrit, and type and crossmatch. Replacement fluid should be administered and vasovagal reactions treated with atropine.[59] Prolonged inflation of an angioplasty balloon has been described as therapy for arterial rupture,[15] but this is unlikely to be effective in a patent artery. After stabili-

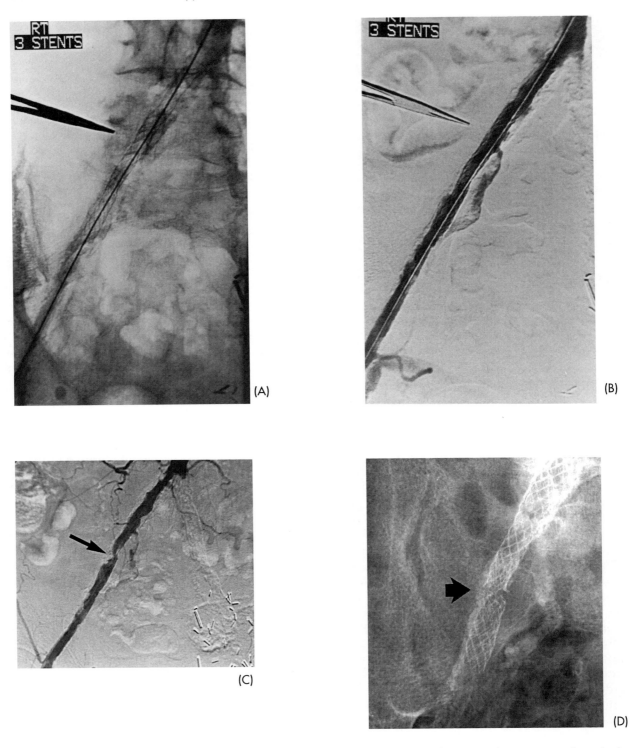

Figure 10–11.   (A) Digital radiograph of the pelvis obtained after placement of three overlapping Palmaz stents in the right iliac system. (B) Postprocedure iliac arteriogram. (C) Restenosis 13 months later (arrow) was refractory to treatment due to multiple balloon ruptures. (D) Radiograph of the pelvis shows fracture of the stents (arrow). (Reprinted from Ref. 53 with permission.)

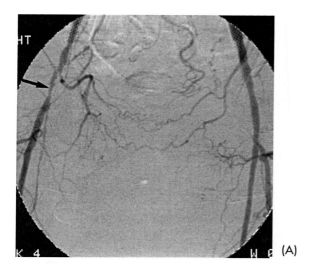 (A)

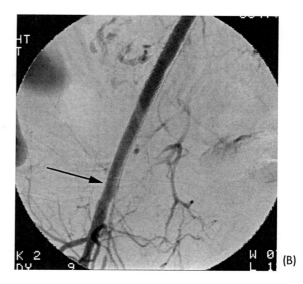 (B)

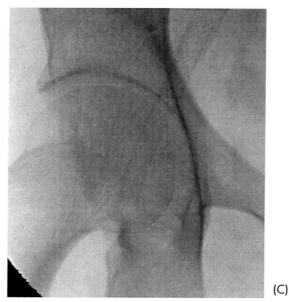 (C)

Figure 10–12. (A) A 58-year-old man with a history of multiple myocardial infarctions, ejection fraction of 20%, and a previous right infrainguinal bypass. Stents were placed in the right iliac system for chronic occlusion. One year after the procedure, mild claudication recurred and the ankle/brachial index decreased by 0.25. Duplex ultrasound showed a focal increase in velocity from 1.0 to 2.6 m/sec. Arteriography showed stenosis in the right common femoral artery distal to the stents (arrow). As this patient was not considered a surgical candidate, a stent was placed across the common femoral artery to the profunda origin. (B) Poststent arteriogram of the femoral artery showing extension of stents to the common femoral bifurcation (arrow) without residual stenosis. (C) Postprocedure digital radiograph demonstrating stents across the hip joint. Three years later, symptoms had not recurred. Most patients benefit by preserving the common femoral artery without stents to permit surgical access.

zation, attempts to manage the rupture with stent grafts should be made (Fig. 10–13). If a patient with chronic iliac artery occlusion is believed to be at high risk for arterial rupture, such as a patient taking steroids or having hypoplastic aortoiliac syndrome, alternative therapies should be considered. Predilatation (percutaneous transluminal angioplasty [PTA]) in an occluded artery without stent deployment may minimize blood loss should rupture occur.

Pressure differences should always be rechecked after intervention. Elastic recoil occasionally may compromise the lumen when the Wallstent is used and very rarely with use of the Palmaz stent. Additional placement of a rigid stent in the area of stent recoil is preferable to overdilatation; the resulting hoop strength of the two stents is additive.[22] Aortoiliac interventions should not be considered successful until pressure measurements demonstrate that transstenotic gradients

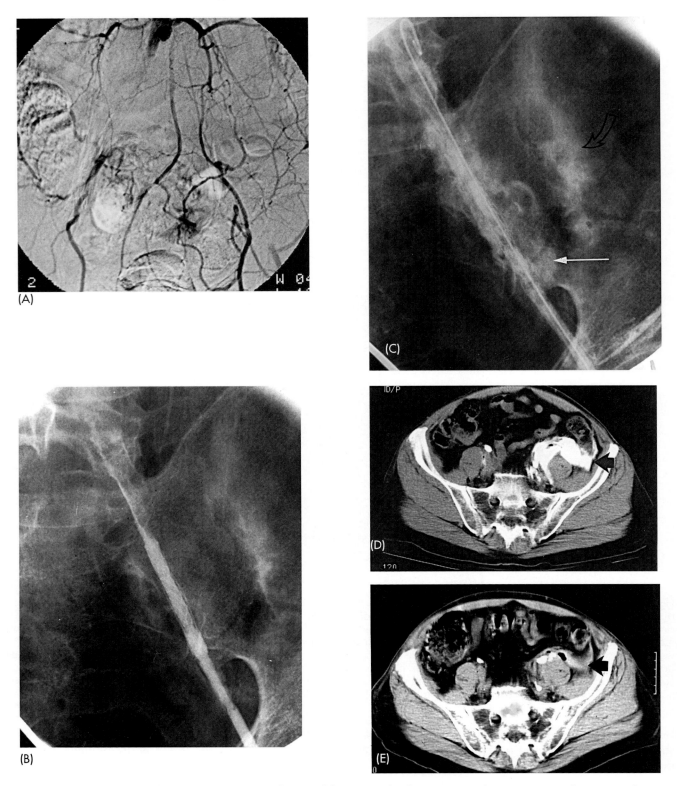

Figure 10–13. A 72-year-old man on chronic steroids treated for severe claudication. (A) Pelvic arteriogram demonstrated complete occlusion of the iliac arteries. (B) Contrast injection after angioplasty demonstrated periadventitial staining (arrow). Free extravasation in the retroperitoneum was observed fluoroscopically (curved arrow). (C) After placement of three stent grafts, no further contrast extravasation was observed. The procedure was terminated at this time. (D) Computed tomogram immediately after the procedure showed retroperitoneal hematoma containing a large amount of contrast (arrow). Hemorrhage was limited by performance of angioplasty prior to stent deployment. (E) Computed tomogram obtained the next day showed resorbtion of the hematoma (arrow). Hemoglobin and hematocrit levels remained stable.

have been reduced to below hemodynamically significant levels. Angiography is repeated after stent placement to assess the results and to check for distal embolization. If the dose of contrast material is excessive, limiting arteriography to the femoral and popliteal artery bifurcations is sufficient if the ankle/brachial index normalizes, or to just the proximal thigh if the superficial femoral artery is occluded.

Patients with multilevel disease may require adjunctive infrainguinal bypass surgery, but in our experience such operations usually should be delayed, as most patients demonstrate satisfactory results with aortoiliac revascularization alone and do not require infrainguinal bypass. The exception is patients with gangrene requiring amputation, even at the digital level, who are best served by infrainguinal bypass in addition to aortoiliac stenting to establish continuous flow to the foot and optimize healing.

Chronic Iliac Artery Occlusions

Technically successful stent placement usually is achieved in patients with stenoses unless procedure-limiting complications occur. Chronic occlusions can also be treated with technical success rates and long-term patency rates similar to those of stenoses,[60] although some have reported lower technical success rates due to the inability to traverse some chronic iliac artery occlusions.[57] Because angioplasty was infrequently performed in chronically occluded arteries prior to the availability of stents, and because chronic occlusions represent a challenging subset of patients, the percutaneous management of chronic arterial occlusions using stents deserves special consideration.

In a chronic arterial occlusion, a "true lumen" may not exist. Resistance to traversal of such chronic occlusions is often greatest at the proximal end of the obstruction, particularly when the common iliac artery is involved. Hydrophilic guidewires facilitate occlusion traversal in chronically occluded arteries.[61] Occasionally, the occluded segment can be partially traversed by antegrade and retrograde approaches, but it cannot be completely traversed by either approach. In such cases, it is often useful to snare a guidewire and pull it through the occlusion, which achieves guidewire access across the stenosis, permitting revascularization[62] (Fig. 10–14).

Successful thrombolysis of chronic arterial occlusions prior to stent placement offers the potential benefit of facilitating percutaneous revascularization by reestablishing a lumen and removing thrombus that may limit the diameter of stent inflation. Successful thrombolysis also may reduce the incidence of distal embolization. The trade-off is increased cost and prolonged hospitalization, as well as the risk of complications with thrombolysis.

Catheter-based intra-arterial infusion of low doses of streptokinase increased technical success rates to approximately 70% compared with approximately 20% for intravenous streptokinase.[63–65] Early reports on the use of intra-arterial streptokinase for peripheral arterial occlusions emphasized this treatment in acute arterial occlusions,[66–70] due in part to previous poor clinical results when thrombolysis was attempted in patients with chronic symptoms[65] and also because patients with acute occlusion often had underlying stenoses that were amenable to percutaneous or surgical therapy. Limited use of thrombolysis in patients with chronic arterial occlusions continued after the introduction of urokinase.[71–74]

To optimize the results of stent placement, we performed thrombolysis in 34 chronic iliac artery occlusions (when symptoms were stable for more than 2 weeks) in 28 patients who could tolerate the treatment.[75] Considering only those patients in whom a reliable duration of stable symptoms could be determined, a patent lumen after thrombolysis was observed in 81% of 29 limbs, with exacerbation of ischemia within 6 months, but only in one-third when stable symptoms were present for more than 6 months, and in 14% when stable symptoms were present for more than 1 year[75] (Fig. 10–15).

Distal embolization rates with stent placement in chronic iliac artery occlusions without thrombolysis vary from 0% to 14%.[15,76,77] When we used thrombolysis of chronic iliac artery occlusions prior to stent placement, a 3% rate of distal embolization was observed.[75] Distal embolization may be more likely in patients undergoing stent placement without thrombolysis if symptoms have worsened within the preceding 6 months. At present, we generally do not perform thrombolysis prior to stent placement in patients with stable symptoms for more than 6 months unless intraluminal filling defects are observed during occlusion traversal (Fig. 10–16). Contrast injections during occlusion traversal may be informative. In some patients with long occlusions, particularly those involving the aorta, the underlying stenosis is relatively short, with most of the remainder of the obstruction made up of chronic thrombus (Fig. 10–17). In such patients, revascularization without thrombolysis is impractical.

Some chronic arterial occlusions resist guidewire traversal, and most technical failures of percutaneous aortoiliac revascularization are attributed to inability to traverse an occlusion.[78–82] Although hydrophilic guidewires (Terumo, Meditech, Watertown, MA) are often useful in crossing chronic iliac artery occlusions, they achieve a subintimal course more easily than do spring-coil guidewires.[61] Prior to the advent of stents, subintimal dissection was usually considered a procedure-ending complication, as renegotiating the true lumen often proved difficult or impossible.[78,83–85] Stent placement has been avoided by many radiologists in this situation for fear of arterial rupture.[79]

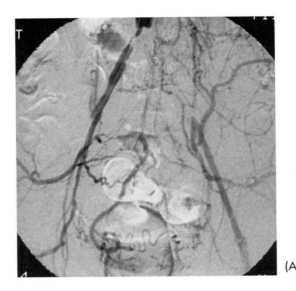

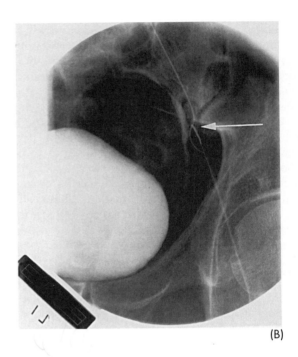

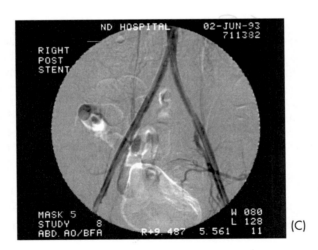

Figure 10–14. (A) Pelvic arteriogram shows occlusion of the left common iliac artery, several stenosis of the proximal right common iliac artery, and stenosis of the right external iliac artery. (B) Antegrade and retrograde accesses into the occlusion were achieved, but the occlusion could not be traversed by either approach. The antegrade guidewire was snared (arrow) and pulled through the left femoral artery. (C) This permitted completion of the procedure.

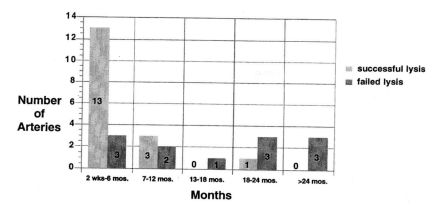

Figure 10–15. Graph of patency after thrombolysis for chronic iliac occlusion. In patients with symptoms for more than 2 weeks and less than 6 months, 81% demonstrated arterial patency after thrombolysis before angioplasty or stent placement.

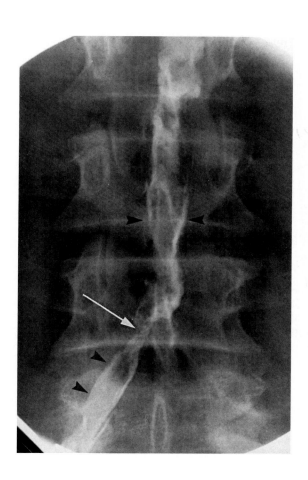

Figure 10–16. Spot film obtained during traversal of a chronic occlusion demonstrating high-grade stenosis of the proximal common iliac artery (arrow) with filling defects in the common iliac artery and aorta (arrowheads).

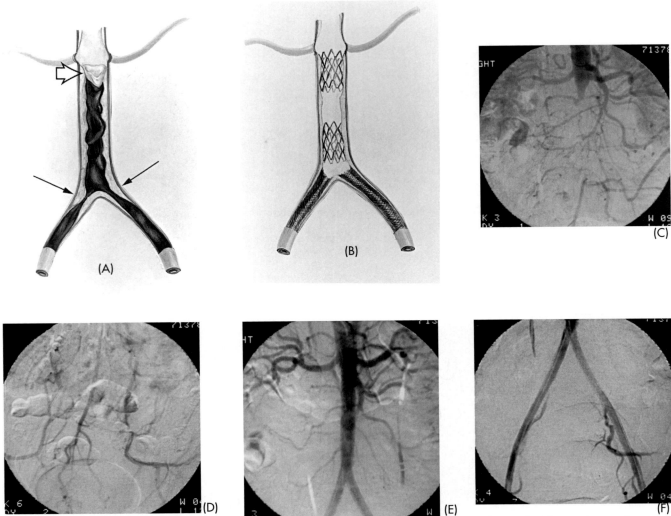

Figure 10–17. (A) Chronic arterial occlusions consist of hemodynamically significant stenosis (arrows) with superimposed thrombosis. Firm chronic thrombus (open arrow) is often present at the proximal end of chronic arterial occlusions and can be resistant to thrombolysis. (B) After thrombolysis and stent placement. (C–F) Corresponding arteriographic images. (Reprinted from Murphy TP. Nonsurgical management of aortoiliac insufficiency. *App Radiol* 1996;25(5):29–31 with permission.)

However, stents represent a suitable treatment for arterial dissections,[37] and subintimal stent placement can be used safely to revascularize chronically occluded iliac arteries.[86] The intraluminal location above and below the occluded segment must be confirmed by catheter injection, and lack of adventitial perforation must be demonstrated by pullback injection of a catheter over a guidewire throughout the entire occlusion. Contrast material must be contained throughout the subintimal course to limit pseudoaneurysm formation or hemorrhage following stent deployment and dilatation.[84,85] It is unknown whether subintimal revascularization of chronic iliac occlusions predisposes the patient to a higher risk of arterial rupture than does intraluminal revascularization, but this treatment appears to be well tolerated. However, angioplasty prior to stent deployment in a subintimal tract is advised, so that if arterial rupture occurs, the rent will not be

stented open and in contact with flowing blood. Subintimal revascularization should be accepted only after attempts at revascularization within the true lumen have failed.

Once a subintimal passage has been created, true-lumen reentry may be difficult, and advanced techniques similar to those used to fenestrate or revascularize dissection flaps in patients with spontaneous aortic dissection may be required. Puncture of intimal flaps in aortic dissections prior to fenestration has been described using the stiff end of an 0.018-inch guidewire.[87] A similar method for fenestration of a dissection flap using a Rosch-Uchida system (22-gauge needle) (Cook, Inc., Bloomington, IN) targeted at an angioplasty balloon has also been described[88] (Fig. 10–18). Although these maneuvers are traumatic and are not performed under direct visualization, they may be safely accomplished during subintimal revasculariza-

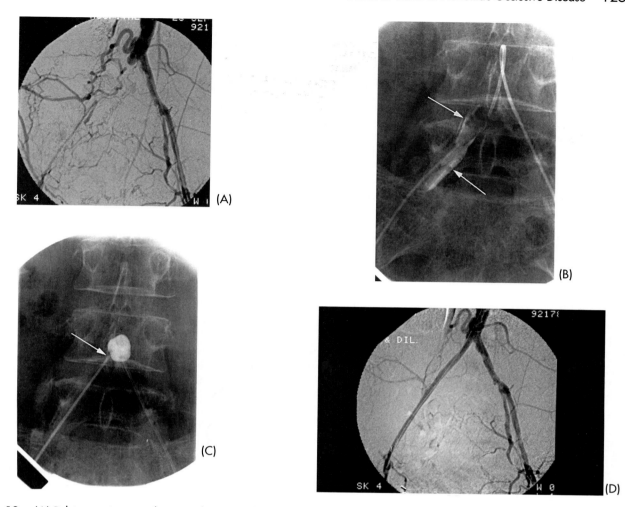

Figure 10–18. (A) Pelvic arteriogram showing chronic occlusion of the right common iliac artery and diffuse narrowing of the right external iliac artery. (B) During attempts at occlusion traversal, a subintimal passage was created (arrows), with inability to reenter the true lumen. (C) An occlusion balloon was placed in the terminal aorta to serve as a target for puncture by an 18-gauge curved needle (arrow) to reestablish access to the true lumen. (D) Completion arteriogram after placement of a Wallstent in the right iliac system and a Palmaz stent at the ostium of the right common iliac artery. No pressure gradient or angiographic stenosis was present after the procedure. (Reprinted from Murphy TP, Marks MJ, Webb MS. Use of a curved needle for true lumen re-entry during subintimal iliac artery revascularization. *JVIR*, in press. Used with permission.)

tion of chronic iliac artery occlusions if (1) the distance between the needle tip and the balloon in the true lumen is minimized; (2) an occlusion balloon is used to provide resistance against collapse of the true lumen from a needle in the false lumen; (3) the occlusion balloon is used as a target, with indentation of the balloon indicating correct needle orientation, prior to needle advance; and (4) pullback contrast injections are done after the tract is created to ensure lack of adventitial perforation.

Patient Follow-up

Catheters or sheaths are removed after sufficient time has passed to reduce the effect of anticoagulants, usually within 2 or 3 hours. Partial thromboplastin time (PTT) can be checked after 1 hour to estimate when catheters can be removed safely. Ideally, the PTT will be less than twice the control value prior to catheter removal. Alternatively, the activated coagulation time (ACT) may be tested with a Hemachron analyzer. The sheaths may be removed when the ACT is <200 seconds.

If flow through the common femoral artery is limited due to a small artery diameter or stenosis, reversal of anticoagulation with protamine after completion of the procedure may be desirable to speed catheter removal. However, protamine can cause hypotension or precipitate anaphylaxis and should be used with caution.

After hemostasis is achieved, the ankle/brachial index should be obtained to determine the results of the intervention and to establish a baseline for follow-up. The patient should remain in bed, and the access site and distal pulses should be monitored closely for 8 hours. Urine output should be monitored; if it decreases, urine samples should be sent for analysis and serum creatinine levels followed to assess for contrast-induced renal failure. After this observation period, the bladder catheter can be removed and the patient can begin to ambulate. If the patient can void, take liquids and solids orally, and ambulate, the patient may be discharged, usually the day after the procedure. Patients should be given written discharge instructions, including activity restrictions and telephone numbers to use for questions or problems. Patients should ambulate only when necessary for the first 24 hours. Stenuous activity should be avoided for the first week after the procedure.

Follow-up should be done by the physician who performed the procedure within 2 weeks, at which time the patient is interviewed and examined and ankle/brachial pressure is obtained. This should be repeated at 3 months, 1 year, and 2 years, when intimal hyperplasia is most likely to compromise the results. If symptoms worsen or noninvasive studies indicate recurrent arterial insufficiency, segmental limb pressures or color duplex ultrasound may be useful in distinguishing recurrent stenosis from new infrainguinal disease (Fig. 10–19). If restenosis is suspected, angiography is indicated so that it may be treated prior to thrombosis.

RESULTS OF AORTOILIAC STENT PLACEMENT

The vast majority of patients with aortoiliac insufficiency have predominantly or exclusively iliac artery disease. Approximately 6% of patients with iliac artery insufficiency have hemodynamically significant stenoses in the infrarenal aorta or at the aortic bifurcation in addition,[60] and a smaller percentage have disease limited to the abdominal aorta, without significant iliac artery insufficiency. While the results of aortic stenting have been described,[89–91] most published reports involve predominantly iliac artery stent placement. Often patients who undergo aortic stenting in addition to iliac artery stenting are not separated from those who undergo iliac artery intervention alone when results are reported.

Stents have demonstrated improved results compared to angioplasty alone in the iliac arteries by randomized comparison[35] and by meta-analysis of published data.[92] In a randomized trial, patients with focal stenoses received either angioplasty or stent placement.[35] Technical success was achieved in 121 of 123 stent placements compared with 113 of 124 angioplasties ($p < 0.01$). The clinical success rate at 5 years was 93% in stent patients and 70% in angioplasty patients ($p < 0.02$). Results of a second randomized trial have not yet been published.[50]

In a meta-analysis, eight studies of aortoiliac stent placement published after 1990 in the English-language literature that specifically reported patency data according to accepted reporting standards[93] were compared with six previous reports of iliac artery angioplasty.[92] Technical success was found to be higher after stent placement (96%) than after balloon angioplasty (91%).[92] Complication and mortality rates were similar, but the 4-year primary patency rate for claudication was 77% after stenting and 68% after balloon angioplasty.[92] For patients with limb-threatening ischemia, 4-year primary patency was 67% after stenting and 55% after angioplasty.[91] The relative risk of failure after stent placement was 0.61 compared with angioplasty.[92]

It was noted that in two of the eight angioplasty series, a large percentage of patients underwent stent placement without prior angioplasty.[57,60] One of these was a report of 103 chronic iliac artery occlusions[57] and the other consisted of 94 iliac limbs, of which 39 were chronically occluded, with a mean lesion length of 6.5 cm.[60] Thus, stents have demonstrated benefit in patients with focal lesions in comparison with angioplasty. They also have made percutaneous management of patients whose lesions are not suitable for angioplasty alone feasible.

Immediate Outcome

Since 1989, results of aortoiliac stent placement have been reported in at least 18 individual series with 1948 patients, excluding earlier reports from the same authors that may have included some of the same patients[10,15,16,30,54,60,77,94–104] (Table 10.1). Of these, 6 reported results using the Wallstent,[16,54,60,77,98,104] 7 with the Palmaz stent,[3,94,95,99–102] 3 with the Strecker stent,[10,97,104] 1 with mostly the Wallstent but also with some Strecker stents,[15] and one with all 3.[97] Technical success, complications, mortality, and patency rates are

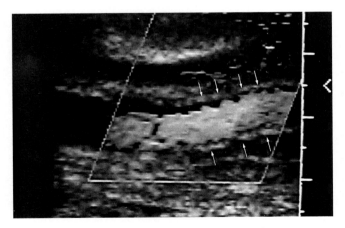

Figure 10–19. Color Doppler stent follow-up. The common iliac artery stent is well visualized as the interrupted echogenic lines (arrows). No stenosis or turbulence was visualized, and Doppler waveform analysis was normal. Murphy TP.
(Reprinted from Nonsurgical management of aortoiliac insufficiency. *App Radiol* 1996;25(5):29–31 with permission.)

Table 10–1. Results of Iliac Artery Stent Placement

First Author	Year	Stent	No. of Patients	No. of Limbs	Tech. Success	30-Day Mortality	Complications‡	Surgery Required
Rees[89]	1989	Palmaz	12	12	100%	0	17%	17%
Bonn[95]	1990	Palmaz	19	27	97%	0	16%	5%
Gunther[16]	1991	Wallstent	91	91	97%	0	3%	?
Long[15]	1991	Wallstent*	49	52	100%	2.0%	6%	0%
Vorwerk[54]	1992	Wallstent	125	137	91%	0	4%	2%
Palmaz[30]	1992	Palmaz	486	567	?	1.9%	8%	?
Liermann[96]	1992	Strecker	52	52	?	0	0%	0%
Hausegger[92]	1992	P/W/S	79	82	94%	0	9%	3%
Dyet[98]	1993	Wallstent	43	50	100%	0	2%	2%
Wolf[99]	1993	Palmaz	37	56	98%	2.7%	11%	0%
Williams[100]	1994	Palmaz	83	?	?	0	10%	1%
Cikrit[101]	1995	Palmaz	34	38	100%	5.8%	15%	12%
Henry[102]	1995	Palmaz	184	184	100%	?	2%	2%
Long[103]	1995	Strecker	64	63	98%	0	8%	0%
Murphy	1996	Wallstent	66	94	91%	1.5%	9%	5%
Martin[104]	1995	Wallstent	140	163	97%	2.9%	4%	0%
Sapoval	1996	Wallstent	95	101	99%	1.0%	9%	1%
Strecker[10]	1996	Strecker	289	289	99.6%	?	5%	1%
Total			1,948	2,058†	97%	1.4%	6%	1.2%

*Five patients received Strecker stents.
**One reference (75) includes one patient lost to follow-up within 20 days.
†One reference does not specify the number of limbs and is excluded.
‡Hematoma not considered a complication unless therapy required.

similar in most of these reports. However, due to lack of uniformity in reporting, data cannot be pooled from all of these studies for each of these parameters. The cumulative data reported below represents data that was explicitly described in the reports. If the incidence of a particular outcome was not clear from the report, whether due to incomplete reporting of the outcome or to the number of patients eligible for the outcome, the report was not included in the analysis of the parameter.

In 16 of these reports, technical success ranged from 91 to 100%, with a weighted average of 97%, in a total of 1512 iliac limbs in 1410 patients.[10,15,16,54,60,77,94,95,97–104] While many of these reports included patients who were selected for percutaneous intervention on the basis of angiographic lesion morphology or symptomatology, some included consecutive patients who were not selected using these criteria, with comparable technical success rates.[10,60] This indicates the potential for nonsurgical management of all patients with aortoiliac insufficiency with stents.

Definitions of complications vary widely, with some studies reporting complications such as inappropriate stent positioning, requiring another stent,[96] and others including groin hematomas that required no therapy,[98] or without specifying if they required any therapy or resulted in morbidity.[30] For purposes of this complication analysis, major complications are considered those that could have resulted in morbidity or mortality or required therapy (eg, surgery or blood transfusion) or prolonged hospitalization. Major complications were observed in 18 series in 6% of 1948 patients (2058 limbs).[10,15,16,30,54,60,77,94–104] The most frequent major complications were distal embolization, aortic or iliac artery rupture, and hematoma, pseudoaneurysm, or arteriovenous fistula at the puncture site.[10,15,16,30,54,60,77,94–104] Only 1.8% of the patients treated had complications that required surgical intervention.[10,15,54,60,77,94–104]

The most severe complications that have been observed include aorta or iliac artery rupture, contrast reactions, and infections. Management of arterial rupture has already been described. Local infections are uncommon when procedures are done percutaneously, but they were reported in 6 of 83 patients (7%) in one series in which 58 to 62% of procedures were done using surgical exposure of the femoral artery.[100]

Septic arteritis has been reported after stent placement but is rare[106–108] (Fig. 10–20). It results in fever and pain, and may cause pseudoaneurysm formation or aneurysmal dilatation of the treated artery.[106,108] Sepsis may ensue, and blood cultures are usually positive. This is the most serious complication of percutaneous stent placement, resulting in a high incidence of ampu-

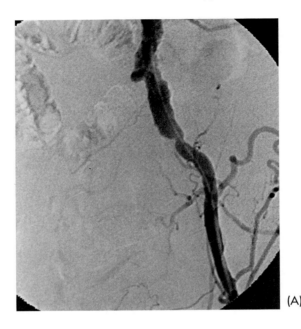

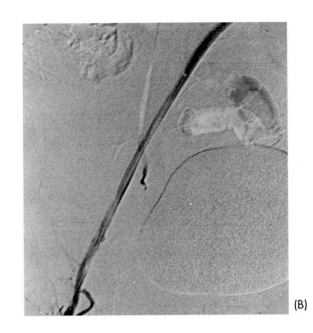

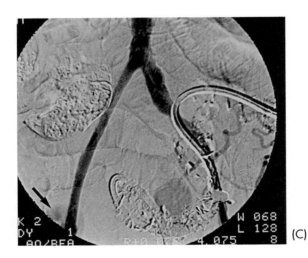

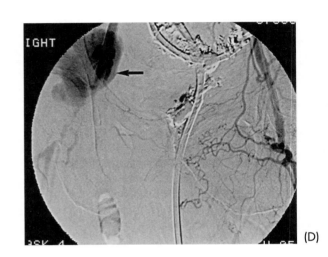

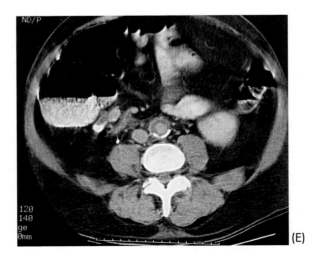

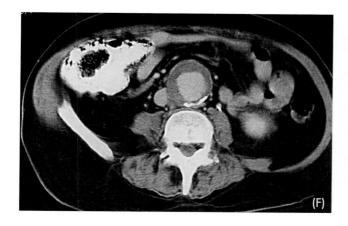
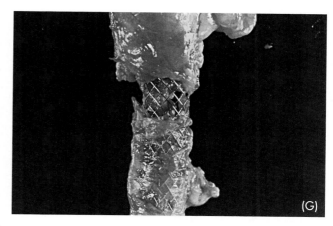

Figure 10–20. Stent infection. (A) Pelvic arteriogram shows complete occlusion of the right iliac system. (B) After stent placement, the right iliac system was patent, without stenosis or a gradient. (C, D) Two weeks later, the patient presented with right lower quadrant pain and developed acute right lower extremity ischemia. Arteriography revealed a contained rupture of the distal external artery (arrows). Surgery was done and the external iliac and common femoral arteries were litigated. Due to irreversible ischemia, a right above-the-knee amputation was performed. Stents were not removed at this time, and infection progressed to involve the abdominal aorta. (E) Baseline computed tomogram of the abdomen showed no aneurysm. (F) Two weeks later, a computed tomogram showed aneurysmal transformation of the distal aorta. (G) Specimen shows marked thinning of the wall of the artery in the region of the stent. Histology revealed lymphocyte infiltration and gram-positive cocci. Cultures grew *Staphylococcus aureus.* (Reprinted from Ref. 108 with permission.)

tation or death.[106–108] If it is suspected, removal of the stent with debridement of infected arteries and soft tissues is mandatory and should be done early. Most authors do not use prophylactic antibiotics prior to stent placement, but this practice is not universal.[102] Use of prophylactic antibiotics in immunocompromised patients seems prudent.[108]

These complications compare favorably in number and severity to those observed after aortoiliac bypass surgery. In six large surgical series of 1270 patients undergoing aortoiliac bypass for arterial insufficiency published since 1993,[109–114] the weighted complication rate is 21%. Complications include myocardial infarction, congestive heart failure, multisystem organ failure, stroke, spinal cord ischemia, intestinal infarction, aortoenteric fistula, acute renal failure, respiratory failure, and so on. However, it is likely that patients undergoing aortoiliac surgery since 1993 are not comparable in disease severity or risk factos to those undergoing aortoiliac reconstruction with stents. A randomized trial would help to determine any true difference in the frequency and severity of complications.

Mortality

Mortality data can be pooled from 15 series in which 30-day mortality was explicitly reported or in which all patients had at least 1 month of follow-up, with follow-up mortality described.[15,30,54,60,77,94–101, 103,104] This can be separated into procedure-related and -unrelated mortality in 14 of these 15 reports.[15,30,54,60,77,94–101,103] Cumulative 30-day mortality from aortoiliac stenting is 1.4% in 1384 patients, with a range of 0% to 6%.[15,30,54,60,77,94–101,103,104] Eight

of these reports described no deaths within 30 days of the procedure.[54,94–98,100,103] Procedure-related mortality was reported in 0.4% of 1289 patients.[15,30,54,60,77,94–101,103] It should be remembered that at many of the institutions reporting aortoiliac stent results, other patients with aortoiliac insufficiency were treated surgically. Presumably, high-risk patients were more likely to undergo percutaneous revascularization. Therefore, procedure-related and 30-day mortality rates are expected to be lower in unselected populations.

Although these data are not derived from direct comparison, overall mortality for aortofemoral bypass surgery reported in 13 series published since 1978[109–121] with 5249 patients treated for aortoiliac insufficiency is 4% (some series[109,110,112] include patients treated for aneurysm, but these patients are excluded from this analysis). Excluding the earlier experiences and considering only those reports that have been published since 1993 reveals six published surgical experiences with 1270 patients undergoing aortofemoral bypass for aortoiliac insufficiency.[109–114] In these reports, weighted surgical mortality is unchanged at 4%.

Patency

Seven series report patency according to accepted reporting standards, namely, including prospective trials with calculation of patency by life table analysis on an intention-to-treat basis, with life tables that state how many patients are at risk for failure at each interval.[93] Technical failures are included in such analyses. Primary patency at 1 year, 3 years, and 5 years ranges from 78 to 95%, 53 to 88%, and 58 to 82%, respectively, with weighted averages (not a life table analysis) of 86%,

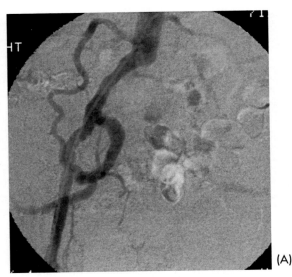 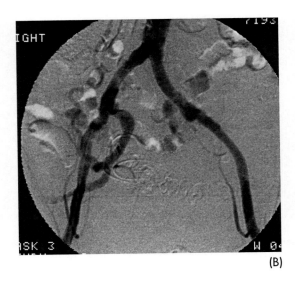

Figure 10–21.   (A) A 65-year-old diabetic male with limb-threatening ischemia on the left. Pelvic arterigram showed complete occlusion of the left iliac system. (B) Arteriogram performed 2 years after revascularization using Wallstents demonstrated continued primary patency with no significant intimal hyperplasia. (Reprinted from Ref. 60 with permission.)

74%, and 73%.[10,60,77,102–104,122] Secondary patency at 1 year, 3 years, and 5 years ranges from 86 to 98%, 81 to 94%, and 78 to 91%, respectively, with weighted averages of 92, 87, and 85%.[60,77,102–104,122]

The 5-year secondary patency rate of 78 to 91% indicates that percutaneous stent placement is an effective long-term treatment for patients with aortoiliac insufficiency (Fig. 10–21). It has been shown that secondary interventions for restenosis in aortoiliac stents are associated wiht technical success and complication rates similar to those of the original procedures, and that the durability of the secondary interventions is comparable to that of primary interventions.[60,123,124] While some patients require secondary procedures for restenosis, these are usually readily performed and often are technically easier than the original procedure, particularly if the original lesion was a chronic occlusion[60,123,124] Fig. 10–22).

Long-term patency of balloon angioplasty in the common iliac artery is superior to that in the external iliac artery.[125] However, stent placement in the common iliac artery has not demonstrated better long-term results than in the external iliac artery.[60,77] When both the common iliac and external iliac arteries are involved, long-term patency tends to be lower than if stenosis or occlusion is limited to only one of these segments.[60] Patients treated for chronic occlusion have demonstrated a nonstatistically significant trend toward lower long-term patency than patients treated for stenosis.[60] However, technical success is slightly less when chronic occlusions are treated; patients who undergo successful percutaneous treatment for chronic iliac occlusion using stents probably do not demonstrate significantly different long-term results than those successfully treated for stenosis. Patients who are treated for

limb-threatening ischemia demonstrate long-tern patency similar to that of patients treated for intermittent claudication.[60]

The effect of continued tobacco use is unclear. Patients who continued to smoke cigarettes, a known risk factor for the development of atherosclerosis,[126,127] demonstrated a poorer long-term outcome after iliac artery stent placement than those who did not smoke in one study with a mean follow-up period of 29 months.[77] However, there was no significant difference in another group of patients with a mean follow-up period of 14 months.[60] Patency of the superficial femoral artery, which has improved in those treated with angioplasty or bypass surgery,[117,128] has also shown mixed results with percutaneous stent placement. In one study, a strong relationship between long-term patency and patency of the superficial femoral artery was observed.[77] However, in another study, no statistically significant difference was observed, and the trend was actually toward lower long-term patency in patients with patent superficial femoral arteries.[60]

Better primary patency for aortofemoral surgery cannot be disputed when compared to aortoiliac stenting, although secondary patency may be similar. Patency rates of 85 to 91% at 5 years and 78 to 80% at 10 years have been reported for aortofemoral bypass surgery.[115–118] However, all surgical series from which these patency rates are derived are retrospective reviews,[109–121] except for one registry[118] and one recently published prospective trial.[114] Patency rates reported in most of these articles are secondary rates, and most use criteria for patency that fall short of currently accepted reporting standards.[93] Prospectively derived 5-year patency rates have been reported only once.[114] In this series, 5-year primary and secondary

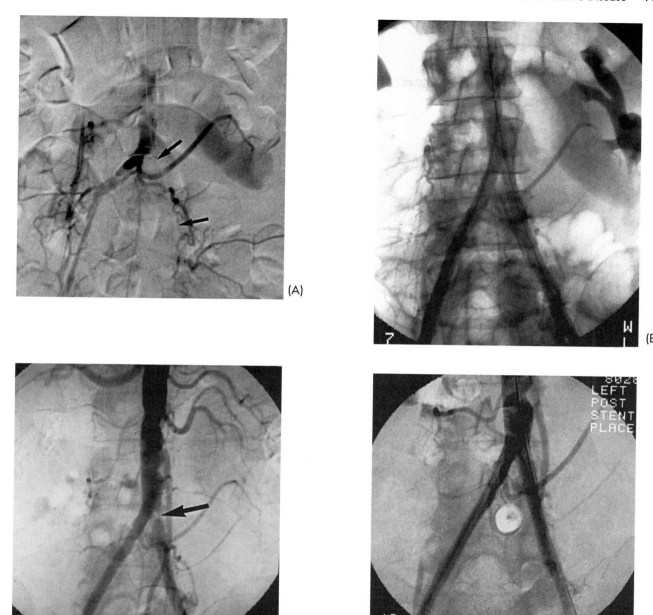

Figure 10–22. (A) Pelvic arteriogram shows occlusion of the left common and external iliac arteries. A sheath is present in the left iliac system (arrows), extending across the aortic bifurcation to the right common iliac artery. Stenosis of the right common iliac artery is present. An accessory left renal artery in the lower pole is seen arising from the right common iliac artery (arrowhead). (B) After stent placement, no residual stenosis or pressure gradient was present on either side. (C) Two years later, a decrease in the ankle/brachial index on the left was observed. Arteriography revealed focal restenosis in the origin of the left common iliac artery (arrow). (D) This was treated by placement of a Palmaz stent, with no residual gradient. Revisions often are performed more readily than the original procedure.

patency rates were 80% and 92% respectively.[114] Ten-year surgical patency rates using current reporting standards do not exist.

Patient Outcomes

Patient outcomes can be elicited using questionnaires that are administered during follow-up visits. Such medical outcomes studies elicit patient satisfaction with

the therapy received and may be more useful in determining who should receive the therapy than traditional outcome measures such as ankle pressures. These questionnaires may be nondisease-specific. One of these, the Medical Outcomes Study (MOS) SF-36 (short-form 36) assesses the patient's sense of general health, role functioning, mental health, bodily pain, social functioning, physical functioning, and vitality.[125–127] Other such surveys are disease-specific. One frequently used questionnaire for peripheral vascular disease is the Walking Impairment Questionnaire (WIQ), which assesses patient-reported community walking ability.[128]

Baseline information concerning quality of life has demonstrated physical function and health perception in patients with peripheral vascular disease (PVD) comparable to those with congestive heart failure or recent myocardial infarction, and levels of bodily pain worse in those with PVD than in those with these cardiac syndromes.[129] Patients with intermittent claudication have mean functional values, social lives, and emotional states significantly less than the ideal maximum, indicative of a reduced state of well-being.[130] Thus, disability as perceived by those with peripheral vascular disease is significant.

Improvements in quality-of-life measures in patients with peripheral vascular disease have been shown in patients undergoing invasive treatment. In one retrospective series, 187 patients who had intermittent claudication (due to inflow or outflow disease) managed invasively (surgery or balloon angioplasty) or noninvasively were evaluated using the SF-36 and the WIQ, as well as with other questions unique to the study that concerned patients' satisfaction with their care.[131] The results showed significantly better self-reported physical functioning, walking ability, and leg symptom improvement in those managed invasively.[131]

We studied 34 patients with intermittent claudication and a history of aortoiliac insufficiency who underwent aortoiliac stenting using the SF-36 and the WIQ.[132] We compared these patients to 41 patients with intermittent claudication who did not undergo arteriography, but did receive a 12-week supervised exercise program. Patients who underwent supervised exercise were not limited to those with inflow disease. Patients who underwent stent placement reported general health perceptions, mental health index, physical functioning, role-physical functioning, and vitality similar to U.S. norms for age.[132] Social function was higher, but bodily pain index and role-emotional function were slightly lower than U.S. norms (not statistically significant). Adjusted mean physical functioning was marginally better in patients managed with stents than in claudicators managed noninvasively ($p = 0.11$).[132] Multiple regression analyses identified the history of hospitalization since the intervention, a history of stroke, and advanced age as factors associated with lower physical functioning scores in stented patients.[132]

Patients with limb-threatening ischemia or intermittent claudication perceive significant disability in themselves. Invasive management (surgery or angioplasty) has demonstrated improvement in self-reported physical functioning and walking ability superior to that achieved with conservative therapy.[131] Whereas prior to the availability of stents many considered it inappropri-

ate to manage patients with intermittent claudication and inflow disease surgically, aortoiliac stent placement represents a low-morbidity option that may improve patient perceptions of physical functioning more than exercise therapy.[132]

Costs

While charge information is more readily available than cost data, charges are more variable than costs and less accurately reflect true costs to providers of providing therapy.[133] Even more elusive is information on lost wages and the cost to society of recuperation following therapy, the cost of complications, and the cost of expected secondary procedures or therapy that might be required.[133]

Of all available therapies for peripheral vascular disease, the least expensive are risk factor modification and exercise therapy. While these should be encouraged in all persons, this strategy alone is not adequate for limb-threatening ischemia and is often unsatisfactory for patients with intermittent claudication, particularly those with inflow disease.[134]

Assessment of the expense associated with invasive management of aortoiliac insufficiency has found percutaneous aortoiliac revascularization to be significantly more affordable than surgical revascularization. In one study of 83 patients, aortoiliac stenting was found to result in a 33 to 82% shorter hospital stay than bypass surgery, with most patients requiring only 1 day in the hospital.[100] Hospital charges for bilateral iliac artery stenting were approximately one-third those for aortobifemoral bypass surgery ($15,647 vs $46,253).[100] A similar difference was found when comparing the costs of these two therapies in Europe.[98] While such studies did not consider the expense associated with secondary procedures required in patients who experienced restenosis, the difference is substantial and would remain so despite this further analysis.

Conclusions

Clinical experience with aortoiliac stenting began in the late 1980s. This experience has shown that stents have better patency than balloon angioplasty alone by randomized comparison and by meta-analysis of published data. Technical success of aortoiliac stent placement has been reported in 97% of cases in 18 published series, with major complications in 6%. The most frequently observed major complications are distal embolization, arterial rupture, hematoma, and pseudoaneurysm. Rarely, arterial infections are seen, and are associated with high amputation and mortality rates. However, only 1.8% of patients experienced major complications that required surgery. More important, reported 30-day mortality is 1.4%, with procedure-related mortality in 0.4%, in patients who usually do not undergo preprocedure cardiac scanning and often are referred for percutaneous therapy because they are considered to be at high risk. Percutaneous aortoiliac revascularization results in significantly lower morbidity and mortality than does surgical revascularization.

Because of the development of intra-arterial stents, patients do not need to be selected for percutaneous therapy in the aorta or iliac arteries based on angiographic lesion morphology or symptom severity. Technical success can be achieved in most patients and has been demonstrated in consecutive patients. The costs of percutaneous therapy are significantly less than those of bypass surgery.

Patient satisfaction with aortoiliac stent placement is high. Patients with intermittent claudication, whose morbidity generally is not considered to warrant surgery, often opt for percutaneous revascularization. Such patients have shown improvements in quality-of-life measures with invasive management of intermittent claudication compared with exercise therapy, and due to the low risk of aortoiliac stent placement, this procedure is appropriate in patients with intermittent claudication due to inflow disease. The only drawback of percutaneous aortoiliac revascularization is its lower primary patency. However, stent revisions usually can be achieved more readily than initial revascularization, and secondary patency is excellent. With appropriate patient follow-up and reintervention as needed, most patients who present with aortoiliac insufficiency can be managed indefinitely without surgery.

REFERENCES

1. Dotter CT, Judkins MP. Transluminal treatment of arteriosclerotic obstruction. *Circulation* 1964;30:654–670.
2. Dotter CT. Transluminally placed coil-spring endarterial tube grafts: long term patency in canine popliteal artery. *Invest Radiol* 1969;4:329–332.
3. Maass D, Zollikofer CHL, Largiader F, Senning A. Radiological follow-up of transluminally inserted vascular endoprostheses: an experimental study using expanding spirals. *Radiology* 1984;152:659–663.
4. Zollikofer CL, Antonucci F, Stuckmann G, Mattias P, Salomonowitz EK. Historical overview on the development and characteristics of stents and future outlooks. *Cardiovasc Intervent Radiol* 1992;15:272–278.
5. Levin DC. The Palmaz stent: a possible technique for prevention of postangioplasty restenosis. *Radiology* 1988;168:873–874.
6. Palmaz JC, Sibbitt RR, Reuter SR, Tio FO, Rice WJ. Expandable intraluminal graft: a preliminary study. *Radiology* 1984;156:73–77.
7. Sigwart U, Puel J. Mirkovitch V, Jorrfe F, Kappenberger L. Intravascular stents to prevent occlusion and restenosis after transluminal angioplasty. *N Engl J Med* 1987;316:701–706.
8. Palmaz JC, Richter GM, Noeldge G, et al. Intraluminal stents in atherosclerotic iliac artery stenosis: preliminanry report of a multicenter study. *Radiology* 1988;168:727–731.
9. Roubin GS, Cannon AD, Agrawal SK, et al. Intracoronary stenting for acute or threatened closure complicating percutaneous transluminal coronary angioplasty. *Circulation* 1992;85:916–927.
10. Strecker EP, Boos IB, Hagen B. Flexible tantalum stents for the treatment of iliac artery lesions: long-term patency complications, and risk factors. *Radiology* 1996;199:641–647.
11. Cragg A, Lund G, Rysavy J, Castaneda F, Castaneda-Zuniga WR, Amplatz K. Nonsurgical palcement of arterial endoprostheses: a new technique using nitinol wire. *Radiology* 1983;147:261–263.
12. Hausegger KA, Cragg AH, Lammer J, et al. Iliac artery stent placement: clinical experience with a nitinol stent. *Radiology* 1994;190:199–202.
13. Kichikawa K, Uchida H, Yoshioka T, et al. Iliac artery stenosis and occlusion: preliminary results of treatment with Gianturco-Z expandable metallic stents. *Radiology* 1990;177:799–802.
14. Palmaz JC, Garcia OJ, Schatz RA, et al. Placement of balloon-expandable intraluminal stents in iliac arteries: first 171 procedures. *Radiology* 1990;174:969–975.
15. Long AL, Page PE, Raynaud AC, et al. Percutaneous iliac artery stent: angiographic long-term follow-up. *Radiology* 1991;180:771–778.
16. Gunther RW, Vorwerk D, Antonucci F, et al. Iliac artery stenosis or obstruction after unsuccessful balloon angioplasty: treatment with a self-expandable stent. *AJR* 1991;156:389–393.
17. Strecker E, Liermann D, Barth KH, et al. Expandable tubular stents for treatment of arterial occlusive diseases: experimental and clinical results. *Radiology* 1990;175:97–102.
18. Dorros G, Mathiak L. Direct deployment of the iliofemoral balloon expandable (Palmaz) stent utilizing a small (7.5 French) arterial puncture. *Cathe Cardiovasc Diagn* 1993;28:80–82.
19. Bjarnason H, Hunter DW, Ferral H, et al. Placement of the Palmaz stent with use of an 8-F introducer sheath and Olbert balloons. *J Vasc Intervent Radiol* 1993;4:435–439.
20. Jedwab MR, Clerc CO. A study of the geometrical and mechanical properties of a self-expanding metallic stent—theory and experiment. *J Appl Biomaterials* 1993;4:77–85.
21. Haskal ZJ, LaBerge JM, Gordon RL, Gonzales J. Response of Wallstents to dilation: therapeutic implications. *J Vasc Intervent Radiol* 1993;4:635–637.
22. Lossef SV, Lutz RJ, Mundorf J, Barth KH. Comparison of mechanical deformation properties of metallic stents with use of stress-strain analysis. *J Vasc Intervent Radiol* 1994;5:341–349.
23. Flueckiger F, Sternthal H, Klein GE, Aschauer M, Szolar D, Kleinhappl G. Strength, elasticity, and palsticity of expandable metal stents: in vitro studies with three types of stress. *JVIR* 1994;5:745–750.
24. Berry JL, Newman VS, Ferrario CM, Routh WD, Dean RH. Bulk elastic behavior of vascular stents. *J Vasc Intervent Radiol* 1995;6(1):2. (abstr.).
25. Palmaz JC. Intravascular stents: tissue–stent interactions and design considerations. *AJR* 1993;160:613–618.
26. Tanigawa N, Sawada S, Kobayashi M. Reaction of the aortic wall to six metallic stent materials. *Acad Radiol* 1995;2:379–384.
27. Hehrlein C, Zimmerman M, Metz J, Ensinger W, Kubler W. Influence of surface texture and charge on the biocompatibility of endovascular stents. *Coronary Artery Dis* 1995;6(7):581–586.
28. Barth KH. Does experimental evidence favor any of the balloon-expandable stents? Presented at the 16th annual

meeting of the Society of Cardiovascular and Interventional Radiology, San Francisco, February 16–21, 1991.

29. Fontaine AB, Spigos DG, Eaton G, et al. Stent-induced intimal hyperplasia: are there fundamental differences between flexible and rigid stent designs? *J Vasc Intervent Radiol* 1994;5:739–744.

30. Palmaz JC, Laborde JC, Rivera FJ, Encarnacion CE, Lutz JD, Moss JG. Stenting of the iliac arteries with the Palmaz stent: experience from a multicenter trial. *Cardiovasc Intervent Radiol* 1992;15:291–297.

31. Martin EC. The impact of angioplasty: a perspective. *J Vasc Intervent Radiol* 1992;3:511–514.

32. Rubenstein ZJ, Morag B, Peer A, Bass A, Schneiderman J. Percutaneous transluminal recanalization of common iliac artery occlusions. *Cardiovasc Intervent Radiol* 1987;10:16–20.

33. Pilla TJ, Peterson GJ, Tantana S, Lang ER, Wolverson MK. Percutaneous recanalization of iliac artery occlusions: an alternative to surgery in the high-risk patient. *AJR* 1984;143:313–316.

34. Ring EJ, Freiman DB, McLean GK, Schwarz W. Percutaneous recanalization of common iliac artery occlusions: an unacceptable complication rate. *AJR* 1982;139:587–589.

35. Richter GM, Roeren T, Brado M, Noeldge G. Further update of the randomized trial: iliac stent placement versus PTA—morphology, clinical success rates, and failure analysis. Presented at the 18th annual scientific meeting of the Society of Cardiovascular and Interventional Radiology, New Orleans, March 1993.

36. Pentecost MJ, Criqui MH, Dorros G, et al. Guidelines for peripheral percutaneous transluminal angioplasty of the abdominal aorta and lower extremity vessels. *Circulation* 1994;89(1):511–531.

37. Becker GJ, Palmaz JC, Rees CR, et al. Angioplasty-induced dissections in human iliac arteries: management with Palmaz balloon-expandable intraluminal stents. *Radiology* 1990;176(1):31–38.

38. White RI, Denny DF, Osterman FA, Greenwood LH, Wilkinson LA. Logistics of a university interventional radiology practice. *Radiology* 1989;170:951–954.

39. Katzen BT, Kaplan JO, Dake MD. Developing an interventional radiology practice in a community hospital: the interventional radiologist as an equal partner in patient care. *Radiology* 1989;170:955–958.

40. Hessel SJ, Adams DF, Abrams HL. Complications of angiogrpahy. *Radiology* 1981;138:273–281.

41. Murphy TP, Dorfman GS, Becker J. Use of preprocedural tests by interventional radiologists. *Radiology* 1993;186:213–220.

42. Suchman AL, Mushlin AI. How well does the activated partial thromboplastin time predict post-operative hemorrhage? *JAMA* 1986;256:750–753.

43. Turnbull JM, Buck C. The value of preoperative screening investigations in otherwise healthy individuals. *Arch Intern Med* 1987;147:1101–1105.

44. Delahunt B, Turnbull PR. How cost effective are routine preoperative investigations? *NZ Med J* 1980;1:509–513.

45. Kaplan EB, Sheiner L, Boeckmann A, et al. The usefulness of preoperative laboratory screening. *JAMA* 1985;253:3576–3581.

46. Mason JJ, Owens DK, Harris RA, Cooke JP, Hlatky MA. The role of coronary angiography and coronary revascularization before noncardiac vascular surgery. *JAMA* 1995;273:1919–1925.

47. Baron J, Mundler O, Bertrand M, et al. Dipyridamole-thallium scintigraphy and gated radionuclide angiography to assess cardiac risk before abdominal aortic surgery. *N Engl J Med* 1994;330:663–669.

48. Wesolowski SA, Martinez A, Domingo RT, et al. Indications for aortofemoral arterial reconstruction: a study of borderline risk patients. *Surgery* 1966;60:288–298.

49. Moore WS, Hall AD. Unrecognized aortoiliac stenosis. *Arch Surg* 1971;103:633–637.

50. Tetteroo E, van Engelen AD, Spithoven JH, et al. Comparison of hemodynamic and angiographic criteria for stent placement after iliac angioplasty. *Radiology* 1996;201:155–159.

51. Bonn J. Percutaneous vascular intervention: value of hemodynamic measurements. *Radiology* 1996;201:18–20.

52. Thiele BL, Strandness DE Jr. Accuracy of angiographic quantification of peripheral atherosclerosis. *Prog Cardiovasc Dis* 1983;26:223–236.

53. Sacks BA, Miller A, Gottlieb M. Fracture of an iliac artery Palmaz stent. *J Vasc Intervent Radiol* 1996;7:53–55.

54. Vorwerk D, Gunther RW. Stent placement in iliac arterial lesions: three years of clinical experience with the Wallstent. *Cardiovasc Intervent Radiol* 1992;15:285–290.

55. Schneider JR, Zwolak RM, Walsh DB, McDaniel MD, Cronenwett JL. Lack of diameter effect on short-term patency of size-matched Dacron aortobifemoral grafts. *J Vasc Surg* 1991;13:785–791.

56. Gunther RW, Worwerk D, Bohndorf K, Peters I, El-Din A, Messmer B. Iliac and femoral artery stenoses and occlusions: treatment with intravascular stents. *Radiology* 1989;172:725–730.

57. Vorwerk D, Geunther RW, Schurmann K, Wendt G, Peters I. Primary stent placement for chronic iliac artery occlusions: follow-up results in 103 patients. *Radiology* 1995;194:745–749.

58. Ravimandalam K, Rao VRK, Kumar S, et al. Obstruction of the infrarenal portion of the abdominal aorta: results of treatment with balloon angioplasty. *AJR* 1991;156;1257–1260.

59. Murphy TP, Cronan JJ, Paolella LP, Dorfman GS, Francis WW. Arterial rupture without balloon rupture during percutaneous transluminal angioplasty. *J Vasc Surg* 1987;6:528–530.

60. Murphy TP, Webb MS, Lambiase RE, et al. Percutaneous revascularization of complex iliac artery stenoses and occlusions using Wallstents: 3-year experience. *J Vasc Intervent Radiol* 1996;7:21–27.

61. Tonnesen KH, Bulow J, Holdstein, Helgstrand U. Comparison of efficacy in crossing femoropopliteal artery occlusions with movable core and hydrophilic guidewires. *Cardiovasc Intervent Radiol* 1994;17:319–322.

62. McLean GK, Cekirge S, Weiss JP, Foster RG. Stent placement for iliac artery occlusions: modified "wire-loop" technique with use of the goose neck loop snare. *JVIR* 1994;5:701–703.

63. Dotter CT, Rosch J, Seaman AJ. Selective clot lysis with low-dose streptokinase. *Radiology* 1974;111:31–37.

64. Verstraete M, Vermylen L, Donati MB. The effect of streptokinase infusion on chronic arterial occlusions and stenoses. *Ann Intern Med* 1971;74:377–382.

65. Martin M. Thrombolytic therapy in arterial thromboembolism. *Prog Cardiovasc Dis* 1979;21(5):351–374.

66. Katzen BT, van Breda A. Low dose streptokinase in the treatment of arterial occlusions. *AJR* 1981;136:1171–1178.

67. Becker GJ, Rabe FE, Richmond BD, et al. Low-dose fibrinolytic therapy. *Radiology* 1983;148:663–670.

68. Totty WG, Gilula LA, McClennan BL, Ahmed P, Sherman L. Low-dose intravascular fibrinolytic therapy. *Radiology* 1982;143:59–69.

69. Kakkasseril JS, Cranley JJ, Arbaugh JJ, Roedersheimer R, Welling RE. Efficacy of low-dose streptokinase in acute arterial occlusion and graft thrombosis. *Arch Surg* 1985;120:427–429.

70. Berni GA, Bandyk DF, Zierler E, Thiele BL, Strandness E. Streptokinase treatment of acute arterial occlusion. *Ann Surg* 1983;198(2):185–191.

71. McNamara TO, Fischer JR. Thrombolysis of peripheral arterial and graft occlusions: improved results using high-dose urokinase. *AJR* 1985;144:769–775.

72. LeBlang SD, Becker GJ, Benenati JF, Zemel G, Katzen BT, Sallee SS. Low-dose urokinase regimen for the treatment of lower extremity arterial and graft occlusions: experience in 132 cases. *JVIR* 1992;3:475–483.

73. Cragg AH, Smith TP, Corson JD, et al. Two urokinase dose regimens in native arterial and graft occlusions: initial results of a prospective, randomized clinical trial. *Radiology* 1991;178:681–686.

74. Meyerovitz MF, Goldhaber SZ, Reaghan K, et al. Recombinant tissue-type plasminogen activator versus urokinase in peripheral arterial and graft occlusions: a randomized trial. *Radiology* 1990;175:75–78.

75. Murphy TP, Webb MS, Haas RA, Lambiase RE. Thrombolysis prior to stent placement for chronic iliac artery occlusions. *Circulation* 1995;8:I–128 (abstr.).

76. Dyet JF, Nicholson AA, Gaines PA. Use of endovascular stents in the treatment of iliac occlusions without prior thrombolysis. *J Vasc Intervent Radiol* 1996;7(1suppl 2):197.

77. Sapoval MR, Chatellier G, Long AL, et al. Self-expandable stents for the treatment of iliac artery obstructive lesions: long-term success and prognostic factors. *AJR* 1996;166:1173–1179.

78. Lammer J, Pilger E, Neumayer K, Schreyer H. Intraarterial fibrinolysis: long-term results. *Radiology* 1986;161:159–163.

79. Vorwerk D, Guenther RW. Mechanical revascularization of occluded iliac arteries with use of self-expandable endoprostheses. *Radiology* 1990;175:411–415.

80. Rubenstein ZJ, Morag B, Peer A, Bass A, Schneiderman J. Percutaneous transluminal recanalization of common iliac artery occlusions. *Cardiovasc Intervent Radiol* 1987;10:16–20.

81. Blum U, Gabelmann A, Redecker M, et al. Percutaneous recanalization of iliac artery occlusions: results of a prospective study. *Radiology* 1993;189:536–540.

82. Colapinto RF, Stronell RD, Johnston WK. Transluminal angioplasty of complete iliac obstructions. *AJR* 1986;146:859–862.

83. Motarjeme A, Keifer JW, Zuska AJ. Percutaneous transluminal angioplasty of the iliac arteries: 66 experiences. *AJR* 1980;135:937–944.

84. van Andel GJ, van Erp WFM, Krepel VM, Breslau PJ. Percutaneous transluminal dilatation of the iliac artery: long-term results. *Radiology* 1985;156;321–323.

85. Simonetti G, Rossi P, Passariello R, et al. Iliac artery rupture: a complication of transluminal angioplasty. *AJR* 1983;140:989–990.

86. Murphy TP. Subintimal revascularization of chronic iliac artery occlusions. *J Vasc Intervent Radiol* 1996;7:47–51.

87. Williams DM, Brothers TE, Messina LM. Relief of mesenteric ischemia in type III aortic dissection with percutaneous fenestration of the aortic septum. *Radiology* 1990;174:450–452.

88. Slonim SM, Nyman U, Semba CP, Miller DC, Mitchell RS, Dake MD. Aortic dissection: percutaneous management of ischemic complications with endovascular stents and balloon fenestration. *J Vasc Surg* 1996;23(2):241–251.

89. Palmaz JC, Encarnicion CE, Garcia OJ, et al. Aortic bifurcation stenosis: treatment with intravascular stents. *J Vasc Intervent Radiol* 1991;2(3):319–323.

90. Long AL, Gaux JC, Raynaud AC, et al. Infrarenal aortic stents: initial clinical experience and angiographic follow-up. *Cardiovasc Intervent Radiol* 1993;16(4):203–208.

91. Diethrich EB, Santiago O, Gustafson G, Heuser RR. Preliminary observations on the use of the Palmaz stent in the distal portion of the abdominal aorta. *Am Heart J* 1993;125(2 pt 1);490–501.

92. Bosch JL, Hunink MGM. Meta-analysis of the results of percutaneous transluminal angioplasty and stent placement for aortoiliac arterial disease. Submitted to *JAMA*.

93. Rutherford RB, Becker GJ. Standards for evaluating and reporting the results of surgical and percutaneous therapy for peripheral arterial disease. *J Vasc Intervent Radiol* 1991;2:169–174.

94. Rees CR, Palmaz JC, Garcia O, et al. Angioplasty and stenting of completely occluded iliac arteries. *Radiology* 1989;172:953–959.

95. Bonn J, Gardiner GA, Shapiro MJ, Sullivan KL, Levin DC. Palmaz vascular stent: initial clinical experience. *Radiology* 1990;174:741–745.

96. Liermann D, Strecker EP, Peters J. The Strecker stent: indications and results in iliac and femoropopliteal arteries. *Cardiovasc Intervent Radiol* 1992;15:298–305.

97. Hausegger KA, Lammer J, Hagen B, et al. Iliac artery stenting: clinical experience with the Palmaz stent, Wallstent, and Strecker stent. *Acta Radiol* 1992;33(4):292–296.

98. Dyet JF, Shaw JW, Cook AM, Nicholson AA. The use of the Wallstent in aortoiliac vascular disease. *Clin Radiol* 1993;48:227–231.

99. Wolf YG, Schatz RA, Knowles HJ, Saeed M, Bernstein EF, Dilley RB. Initial experience with the Palmaz stent for aortoiliac stenoses. *Ann Vasc Surg* 1993;7(3):254–261.

100. Williams JB, Watts PW, Nguyen VA, Peterson CL. Balloon angioplasty with intraluminal stenting as the initial treatment modality in aortoiliac occlusive disease. *Am J Surg* 1994;168:202–204.

101. Cikrit DF, Gustafson PA, Dalsing MC, et al. Long-term follow-up of the Palmaz stent for iliac occlusive disease. *Surgery* 1995;118(4):608–614.

102. Henry M, Amor M, Ethevenot G, et al. Palmaz stent placement in iliac and femoropopliteal arteries: primary and secondary patency in 310 patients with 2–4 year follow-up. *Radiology* 1995;197:167–174.

103. Long AL, Sapoval MR, Beyssen BM, et al. Strecker stent implantation in iliac arteries: patency and predictive factors for long-term success. *Radiology* 1995;194:739–744.

104. Martin EC, Katzen BT, Benenati JF, et al. Multicenter trial of the Wallstent in the iliac and femoral arteries. *J Vasc Intervent Radiol* 1995;6:843–849.

105. Zollikofer CL, Antonucci F, Pfyffer M, et al. Arterial stent placement with use of the Wallstent: midterm results of clinical experience. *Radiology* 1991;179:449–456.

106. Mossad SB, Longworth DL, Olin JW. Infected pseudoaneurysm at the site of an iliac artery Palmaz stent: case report and review. *J Vasc Med Biol* 1994;5(5–6):277–281.

107. Therasse E, Soulex G, Cartier P, et al. Infection with fatal outcome after endovascular metallic stent placement. *Radiology* 1994;192:363–365.

108. Hoffman AI, Murphy TP. Septic arteritis and aneurysmal transformation of the abdominal aorta after iliac artery stent placement. *J Vasc Intervent Radiol* in press.

109. Littooy FN, Steffan G, Steinam S, et al. An 11-year experience with aortofemoral bypass grafting. *Cardiovasc Surg* 1993;1(3):232–238.

110. Hans SS. Concurrent audit of early outcome for 1,617 consecutive arterial reconstructions. *Surg Gynecol Obstet* 1993;176:382–386.

111. Schneider JR, Besso SR, Walsh DB, et al. Femorofemoral versus aortobifemoral bypass: outcome and hemodynamic results. *J Vasc Surg* 1994;19:43–57.

112. Huber TS, Harward TR, Flynn TC, et al. Operative mortality rates after elective infrarenal aortic reconstructions. *J Vasc Surg* 1995;22:287–294.

113. Erdoes LS, Bernhard VM, Berman SS. Aortofemoral graft occlusion: strategy and timing of reoperation. *Cardiovasc Surg* 1995;3(3):277–283.

114. Passman MA, Taylor LM, Moneta GL, et al. Comparison of axillofemoral and aortofemoral bypass for aortoiliac occlusive disease. *J Vasc Surg* 1996;23:263–271.

115. Brewster DC, Darling RC. Optimal methods of aortoiliac reconstruction. *Surgery* 1978;84(6):739–748.

116. Crawford ES, Bomberger RA, Glaeser DH, Salch SA, Russell WL. Aortoiliac occlusive disease: factors influencing survival and function following reconstructive operation over a twenty-five year period. *Surgery* 1981; 89(6):1055–1067.

117. Poulias GE, Polemis L, Skoutas B, et al. Bilateral aortofemoral bypass in the presence of aorto-iliac occlusive disease and factors determining results. *J Cardiovasc Surg* 1985;26:527–538.

118. Szilagyi DE, Elliott JP, Smith RF, Reddy DJ, McPharlin M. A thirty-year survey of the reconstructive surgical treatment of aortoiliac occlusive disease. *J Vasc Surg* 1986;3:421–436.

119. Sicard GA, Freeman MB, VanderWoude JC, Anderson CB. Comparison between the transabdominal and retroperitoneal approach for reconstruction of the infrarenal abdominal aorta. *J Vasc Surg* 1987;5:19–27.

120. Piotrowski JJ, Pearce WH, Jones DN, et al. Aortobifemoral bypass: the operation of choice for unilateral iliac occlusion? *J Vasc Surg* 1988;8:211–218.

121. Prendiville EJ, Burke PE, Colgan MP, Wee BL, Moore DJ, Shanik DG. The profunda femoris: a durable outflow vessel in aortofemoral surgery. *J Vasc Surg* 1992;16:23–29.

122. Vorwerk D, Gunther RW, Schurmann K, Wendt G. Aortic and iliac stenoses: follow-up results of stent placement after insufficient balloon angioplasty in 118 cases. *Radiology* 1996;198:45–48.

123. Vorwerk D, Gluenther RW, Schurmann K, Wendt G. Late reobstrucion in iliac arterial stents: percutaneous treatment. *Radiology* 1995;197:479–483.

124. Sapoval MR, Long AL, Pagny J, et al. Outcome of percutaneous intervention in iliac artery stents. *Radiology* 1996;198:481–486.

125. Johnston KW, Rae M, Hogg-Johnston SA, et al. Five-year results of a prospective study of percutaneous transluminal angioplasty. *Ann Surg* 1987;206:403–413.

126. Regensteiner JG, Hiatt WR. Medical management of peripheral arterial disease. *JVIR* 1994;5:669–677.

127. Kannel WB, Shurtleff D, National Heart and Lung Institute, National Institutes of Health. The Framingham study: cigarettes and the development of intermittent claudication. *Geriatrics* 1973;28:61–68.

128. Johnston KW. Iliac arteries: reanalysis of results in balloon angioplasty. *Radiology* 1993;186:207–212.

129. Ware JE, Sherbourne CD. The MOS 36-time short-form health survey (SF-36): I. Conceptual framework and item selection. *Med Care* 1992;30(6):473–483.

130. McHorney CA, Ware JE, Raczek AE. The MOS 36-item short-form health survey (SF-36): II. Psychometric and clinical tests of validity in measuring physical and mental health constructs. *Med Care* 1993;31(3):247–263.

131. McHorney CA, Ware JE, Lu JFR, Sherbourne CD. The MOS 36-item short-form health survey (SF-36): III. Tests of data quality, scaling assumptions, and reliability across diverse patient groups. *Med Care* 1994;32:40–66.

132. Regensteiner JG, Steiner JF, Panzer RJ, et al. Evaluation of walking impairment by questionnaire in patients with peripheral arterial disease. *J Vasc Med Biol* 1990;2:142–152.

133. Schneider JR, McHorney CA, Malenka DJ, McDaniel MD, Walsh DB, Cronenwett JL. Functinal health and well-being in patients with severe atherosclerotic peripheral vascular occlusive disease. *Ann Vasc Surg* 1993;7(5):419–428.

134. Ponte E, Cattinelli S. Quality of life in a group of patients with intermittent claudication. *Angiology* 1996;47(3):247–251.

135. Reifler DR, Feinglass J, Slavensky R, Martin GJ, Manheim L, McCarthy WJ. Functional outcomes for patients with intermittent claudication: bypass surgery versus angioplasty versus noninvasive management. *J Vasc Med Biol* 1994;5(5–6):203–211.

136. Murphy TP, Kim HM, Webb MS. Medical outcomes study of patients who have undergone treatment for intermittent claudication (abstr.). *J Vasc Intervent Radiol* 1997;8(1Part2):213.

137. Picus D. Comparing competing medical procedures: costs or charges—what should it matter? *Radiology* 1996;199:623–625.

138. Creasy TS, Fletcher EWL. Angioplasty for intermittent claudication. *Clin Radiol* 1991;43(2):81–83.

11

Chronic Iliac Occlusions: Thrombolysis, Angioplasty, Stenting

Thomas O. McNamara, M.D.

INTRODUCTORY

In the author's experience, the chronically occluded iliac artery is an excellent lesion for initial therapy with percutaneous intra-arterial thrombolysis (PIAT), followed by percutaneous transluminal angioplasty (PTA) and stent placement. Theoretically, this approach can produce the highest incidence of recanalization and the lowest incidence of distal embolization, perforation, and dissection and require the smallest number of stents. This should result in 30-day and long-term patency rates comparable to those of PTA/stenting of iliac stenoses. These benefits have been realized in the author's clinical practice, and this approach has become the standard for our treatment of chronic iliac occlusions.

This experience and approach is part of the long-standing diversity of experiences and opinions regarding treatment of chronic iliac occlusions. In contrast, PTA and/or stent therapy of a focal iliac stenosis is now regarded as standard therapy.[1]

Primary Balloon Angioplasty

A brief review of the history of interventional treatment is helpful in understanding the lack of consensus on treatment of chronic iliac occlusions. In 1964, Dotter et al published the first angioplasty of an iliac obstructive lesion.[2] It was a stenosis that was reported to be patent 14 years later. In 1979, Tegtmyer et al published the first report of a successfully recanalized iliac occlusion.[3] This encouraged others to begin to attempt to traverse and dilate these lesions. However, the increasing practice of attempting PTA for iliac occlusions was markedly slowed by a 1982 report by Ring et al.[4] They reported a success rate of traversing and satisfactorily dilating only 50% of the occlusions. They stressed that this low success rate was accompanied by a 40% incidence of clinically significant embolization to the contralateral vascular bed (two of their five successes). They concluded that this was an unacceptable compli-

cation rate yielding a poor risk/benefit ratio and recommended that chronic iliac occlusions be considered surgical lesions.

This recommendation was not universally followed. Many interventionalists continued to attempt PTA of chronic iliac occlusions. The efficacy of this approach was difficult to determine, as the reports included both stenoses and occlusions, with occlusions representing a minority of the lesions. Additionally, the reported patency rates varied widely. The best results from these combined lesion reports were 85% patency at 7.5 years[5] and 90% at 7 years.[6] One of the poorest results was a primary patency rate of 53% at 5 years.[7]

Because of the lack of uniformity of reporting standards, varying patient selection criteria, and varying long-term patency rates, an advisory committee was established by the American Heart Association. It included interventional radiologists, vascular surgeons, and cardiologists who reviewed the literature and made recommendations for the use of iliac PTA, depending on symptoms and lesion severity.[8] They recommended that most patients with limb-threatening ischemia be considered for bypass surgery and that those with intermittent claudication be considered for either conservative management or PTA.[8] They also concluded that PTA was the procedure of choice for focal stenoses of ≤3 cm and that bypass surgery was superior for stenoses of ≥5 cm and all occlusions. Similarly, the Society of Cardiovascular and Interventional Radiology rated class III (common + external) and class IV (common + external + femoral) iliac artery occlusions as unsuitable for PTA alone.[9]

Nonetheless, several investigators report reasonable results with just the use of direct guidewire traversal and PTA of chronic iliac occlusions. Colapinto et al achieved a 78% technical success rate in 64 patients[10] and Rubinstein et al reported a technical success rate of 66% in 24 patients.[11] More recently, Gupta et al reported technical success in 78% of 56 occlusions.[12]

137

The largest and most detailed analysis of the results of PTA of iliac occlusions is by Johnston.[1] In a review of 667 consecutive procedures involving PTA of iliac arteries, 83 (12%) were found to be for occlusions (presumably chronic). A total of 82 were available for follow-up at 30 days. Using an intent-to-treat approach, the success rates were 76% at 1 month, 60% at 1 year, 53% at 2 years, and 48% at 3 years. The author points out that these results include the 15 cases (18%) that were initial technical failures due to inability to traverse the occlusion with a guidewire. Excluding these cases markedly improves the results: 91% at 1 month, 73% at 1 year, 65% at 2 years, and 59% at 3 years. The author justifies excluding the failures because a complication occurred in only one case (ischemia that did not require emergency surgery). This is a 7% incidence versus 15% in the 68 occlusions that were traversed. In support of Ring's recommendation, it is of note that the incidence of complications was 13% in the 83 occlusions versus 7% in the 584 stenoses. This difference was primarily due to the higher combined incidence of worsened ischemia, distal emboli, dissection, and dye extravasation in the occlusion group (7% vs. 2%).

In view of these results, Johnston favors the use of PTA for iliac occlusions, reasoning that a successfully treated lesion has satisfactory long-term patency and that the risk of major complications associated with failure to cross the lesion is small. This is in contrast to the earlier and smaller experience of Ring et al. However, Johnston points out that patency is adversely affected by the presence of a tandem lesion that also requires PTA. In the 68 successfully traversed occlusions, the 3-year patency rate was 66% following PTA of the occlusion alone versus 17% if both an iliac occlusion and a tandem lesion were dilated. This author believes that most of the tandem lesions were probably in the superficial femoral artery (SFA), which has a much higher incidence of restenosis, and the contribution of late failure of the iliac PTA to the lower 3-year patency rate may be overestimated. Johnston does not further categorize the results relative to either length or whether the occlusion involved the common, external, or both iliac arteries. Although Johnston's results and recommendations are favorable, the fact that occlusions accounted for only 12% of the 667 treated iliac lesions indicates that interventional treatment was not regarded as the initial treatment of choice for most iliac occlusions.

Primary Stent Placement

This view is changing. Following the development of hydrophilic guidewires and stents, an increasing percentage of chronic iliac occlusions are undergoing attempted direct traversal and primary stenting. This is largely due to the published reports of Vorwerk and Guenther.[13–16] In their most recent publication (1995),

they review their experience with this approach in more than 100 patients over 6 years. They report an 81% success rate in traversing the occlusion without prior treatment with PIAT. This is consistent with the 85% successful traversal in 83 iliac occlusions reported by Johnston, 78% by Colapinto et al, and 78% by Gupta et al.[1,10,12] This is more likely to represent what one can expect than the 100% successful traversal in a small series of eight patients reported by Yedlicka et al.[17] It is noteworthy that Vorwerk et al achieved this success rate even though the mean length of the occlusions was 5.1 cm and 44/103 (43%) were graded class III and 59/103 (46%) well graded class IV (Society of Cardiovascular and Interventional Radiology criteria).[9]

As in the report by Johnston, the patency rates depend on whether they are calculated on an intent-to-treat basis versus whether the lesion was successfully traversed. Using the former, the initial technical success rate in reestablishing flow without a significant residual stenosis was only 80% (101/127) in the series of Vorwerk et al. The results are more impressive if the denominator is the number of occlusions traversed. It becomes 98% (101/103). Clearly, one must keep these differences in mind when reviewing the results of these authors.

Vorwerk and Guenther report no complications or adverse sequelae in the 24 patients (19%) in whom the efforts to cross the occlusion were unsuccessful. This is in accord with Johnston's report of one complication in 15 failed attempts at traversal (7%).[1] However, Vorwerk et al experienced an 11.6% incidence of complications in the 103 patients in whom the occlusion was successfully traversed. The complication was major in 6 of the 12 patients, requiring additional surgical or interventional treatment.

Embolization was the main complication (4.8%). To minimize embolization, the authors recommend underdilating prior to stent placement, dilating within the stent from proximal to distal, and never overdilating.[13–16] A reduction in distal embolization by the use of this technique was confirmed by Sapoval et al[18] in their treatment of 43 chronic iliac occlusions with direct traversal without prior PIAT. They had an overall incidence of distal embolism of 14%, but in their first 17 treatments, they had performed PTA prior to placement of a self-expandable Wallstent and experienced a 30% incidence of embolization versus only 4% in the ensuing 26 cases in which PTA was not performed prior to stent placement.[18] A similar finding was noted by Long et al when using the Strecker stent.[19] It is surprising that in utilizing only PTA without preceding PIAT, Johnston reports an incidence of distal embolism of only 1.4% in the successfully traversed iliac occlusions.[1] Distal embolism with PTA alone was reported to be 3.1% by Colapinto et al (4% of the traversed lesions), and 7% by Gupta et al (9% of traversed lesions).[10,12]

Sapoval et al[18] reports a higher initial success rate of 100% versus 81% by Vorwerk et al when utilizing the method of direct guidewire traversal, placement of a self-expanding Wallstent, and PTA within the stent. Their 4-year primary patency rate of 61% is based on an intent to treat and is comparable to the 59% rate reported by Vorwerk et al (including the 19% initial failures).[16]

Thrombolysis Prior to PTA Stent

The report by Sapoval et al is the only report of a large series in which the initial success rate was higher without antecedent PIAT. The initial report of PIAT prior to PTA of chronic occlusions was presented by Auster et al,[20] who cited an 88% initial success rate. They utilized a contralateral approach, used complete clot lysis as their endpoint, and followed thrombolysis with immediate PTA. These results are better now that thrombolysis and PTA can be supplemented by stent placement. Using the contralateral approach in 41 patients with chronic iliac occlusions, Motarjeme was able to recanalize 100% of the lesions.[21] He avoided traversing the lesion prior to completion of thrombolysis. There were no reocclusions within the initial 30 days, no emboli, no deaths, and no major complications.

Blum et al used the ipsilateral approach to traverse the lesion and then dissolve the clot from proximal to distal in 26 of 47 iliac occlusions. The contralateral approach was used in the other 17 patients because of inability to palpate the ipsilateral femoral pulse. The authors achieved a 98% initial success rate, but two early reocclusions reduced the 30-day patency rate to 94%. Both occlusions were retrieved by thrombolysis and stent placement. The authors experienced a 6.5% incidence of distal embolism.[22] Their series included a mixture of acute and chronic occlusions. It is interesting to speculate that the avoidance of guidewire traversal by Motarjeme and the emphasis on complete clot lysis prior to PTA stenting may account for the difference in the rates of distal embolism. Also, the lack of 30-day rethrombosis in Motarjeme's experience may have been due to the uniform placement of stents compared to the 40% placement rate by Blum et al.[22]

Hausegger et al also report improved results of recanalizing chronic occlusions by the use of PIAT prior to PTA and/or stent placement.[23] In 42 patients, they achieved a 100% incidence of recanalization. In only 6 of 42 (14%) were they able to traverse the lesion prior to PIAT. After PIAT, reestablishment of flow was achieved in 12 (28%), the occlusion was shorter in 5 (12%), and the lesion was softened sufficiently to be able to be traversed in 19 (45%) despite the lack of change in angiographic appearance. They concluded that thrombolysis facilitates traversal of a still occluded segment.

The response to thrombolysis is similar to that reported by Motarjeme.[21] Of the 41 occlusions, there was total clot lysis in 20 (50%), partial clot lysis in 9

(22%), and no change in 12 (29%). The uniform success in subsequent recanalization was explained by the thrombolysis's demonstrating the true lumen in 50% and softening the undissolved thrombus such that it offered less resistance to guidewire traversal than an intramural passage.

A similar benefit with the use of PIAT prior to recanalization of chronic iliac occlusions is cited by Henry et al.[24] In a series of 178 iliac lesions, 17 were occlusions. They were all (100%) recanalized following PIAT, and there were no emboli. The authors attribute the lack of distal emboli to pretreatment with PIAT. They report 4-year primary patency rates that were comparable for stenoses versus occlusions: 88% ± 4.2 and 76% ± 8.5, respectively. Secondary 4-year patency rates were 95% ± 2.6 for stenoses and 88% ± 5.2 for occlusions (not statistically significant). This lack of difference in the long-term patency of stenoses versus occlusions may be related to their placement of Palmaz stents in a higher proportion of the occlusions (94%) than the stenoses (10%).

Palmaz et al noted that at 50 months after stent placement, the stented occlusions had a higher cumulative patency than the stented stenoses.[25] They cautioned that a larger number of treated patients would be required to be certain of this finding, as only 13% of the lesions had been occlusions. Nonetheless, they did speculate that vessels distal to a complete occlusion may be more "protected" and relatively free of atherosclerosis. This may result in less outflow resistance, higher flow through the stent, and a diminished risk of stent thrombosis during reendothelialization (8 months). Subsequent to that, the combination of improved inflow via the stented iliac and a relatively normal outflow bed could be expected to yield the best long-term clinical result.

It is of note that Palmaz et al cautioned against placement of stents after recanalization of chronic iliac occlusions by any method that may cause wall perforation, such as laser or atherectomy.[25] They believe that this can cause pseudoaneurysm or bleeding by the stent's stretching open a defect in the wall that may have been partially or completely closed by elastic recoil.

Murphy et al utilized PIAT as the initial therapy followed by placement of Wallstents in 39 chronic iliac occlusions. The details of their infusion technique were not included in their report.[26] They achieved a 30-day success rate of 85%. The failures were due to inability to traverse and artery rupture (two). The embolization rate was low (1/39 = 3%). The embolism occurred in a patient in whom they had performed thrombolysis, PTA, and then stent placement. This prompted them to adopt the approach of Vorwerk et al, delaying adequate PTA until after placement of the Wallstent.

Murphy et al also placed Wallstents in 42 iliac arteries for diffuse stenotic disease. They did not note a significant difference in primary patency between patients treated for diffuse stenoses versus chronic occlusion. The trend, however, was toward higher patency rates in the diffuse disease group (85% versus 67% at 1 year).

They stressed that the results of their prospective study demonstrate that the indications for percutaneous treatment should be broadened beyond those suggested by the American Heart Association Advisory Committee[8] and guidelines developed by the Standards of Practice Committee of the Society of Cardiovascular and Interventional Radiology.[9] They based this conclusion on the 91% technical success rate achieved in treating lesions that were outside of those recommended for percutaneous treatment by the two committees. Specifically, the stenoses were too long, and 41% were chronic occlusions. The cumulative primary patency rates were 78% at 1 year, 53% at 2 years, and 3 years; secondary patency rates were 86% at 1 year and 82% at up to 32 months. No statistically significant difference in primary patency was observed based on lesion type, symptom severity, lesion location, or run-off status. Murphy et al also report excellent results in a group considered to be best treated with surgery because of their clinical status: patients with limb-threatening ischemia. They achieved a limb salvage rate of 98% at a mean follow-up of 14 ± 7 months.

These results were accomplished with an associated 30-day mortality rate of 1.5% and no amputations. Murphy et al argue that the issue of mortality should receive more attention when deciding on surgical versus percutaneous treatment.[26] They cite a procedure-related mortality of 3 to 5% for aortobifemoral bypass[27-31] and a procedure-related mortality rate of 0.1% for percutaneous interventions.

They also point out that primary patency rates following aortofemoral bypass surgery vary considerably, from 54% at 3 years[31] to 87% at 5 years.[28,30,31] These results are matched by the excellent secondary patency rates at 5 years following interventional treatment of chronic iliac occlusions of 77% by Murphy et al[26] and 88% by Henry et al.[24]

Secondary Patency

Henry et al make the point that the patency rate following a second intervention (percutaneous revision) is more durable than that of the primary procedure.[24] They propose that percutaneous treatment should be judged by the cumulative patency following both primary and secondary interventions. In the case of chronic iliac occlusions, the second treatment will usually be much simpler than the first, as it is usually for stenosis. In contrast, surgical revisions are often more difficult than the primary procedure and result in a lower technical success rate, more complications, and lower patency rates.

This overview of most of the pertinent literature on interventional treatment of chronic occlusions demonstrates the difficulty of utilizing published reports to arrive at an unassailable conclusion regarding patient selection, lesion selection, and treatment methodology. The author initially utilized PIAT only in acutely occluded iliac arteries and usually shunned it in treating chronic occlusions.[32]

Author's Approach

In 1990 the author began a prospective analysis of utilizing PIAT to treat chronic iliac occlusions. This preceded the availability of hydrophilic guidewires and stents but yielded excellent results (Fig. 11–1). Thus,

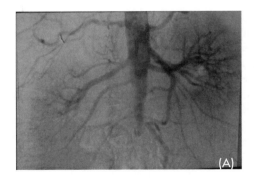
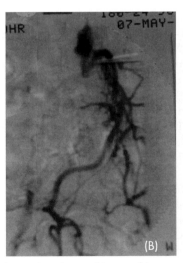
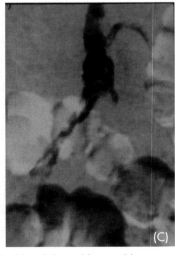

Figure 11–1. A 58-year-old white male chronic smoker with a 3-year history of impotence and disabling bilateral hip and leg claudication. (A) Initial angiogram, performed August 8, 1990, demonstrates occlusion of the aorta distal to the inferior mesenteric artery (IMA). Reconstitution of flow was at the level of the external iliac arteries. (B) Repeat angiogram 21 months later (May 7, 1991) demonstrates persistent occlusion. PIAT begun via an end-hole catheter in contact with the impenetrable proximal end of the occlusion, utilizing the transaxillary approach. (C) Follow-up angiogram after 8 hours of infusion of 60,000 IU/hr of UK demonstrates lysis of 90% of the clot in the distal aorta, 50% in the right common iliac artery (CIA), and 10% in the left CIA without reestablishment of flow.

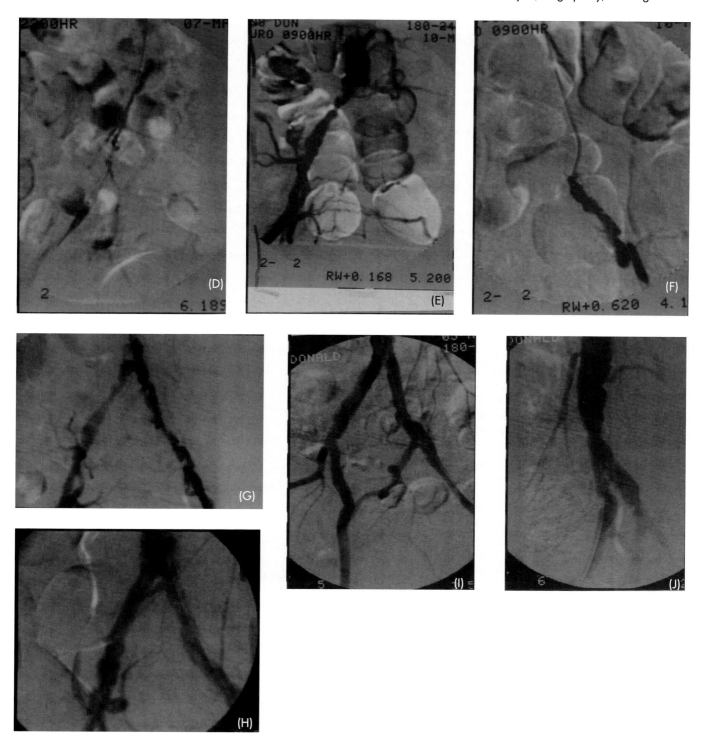

Figure 11-1. *(cont'd)*   (D) A coaxial multi-side hole infusion system (McNamara Coaxial Infusion System, Cook Catheter Co., Bloomington, IN) replaces the end hole system and is advanced into the remaining thrombus in the right CIA; the dose of UK is increased to 90,000 IU/hr. (E) Overnight infusion effects complete clot lysis and reestablishment of flow in the right CIA. (F) An end hole infusion system was used in the left CIA, as that thrombus was still difficult to traverse. Recheck after 8 hours of infusion of UK at a dose of 90,000 IU/hr demonstrates reestablishment of flow but questionable residual thrombus. (G) Overnight infusion of UK into the distal aorta at a rate of 90,000 IU/hr does not effect further lysis. Residual luminal defects are presumed to represent atheroma and organized thrombus. (H) No residual stenoses is found following kissing balloon PTA with 10-mm balloons (no stent). There are no emboli or other complications. Claudication and impotence all cleared. (I) Follow-up angiogram performed 2 years, 3 months later at the time of coronary angiography demonstrates no restenosis in the iliac system. (J) Mild stenosis in the distal abdominal aorta is noted in the lateral projection. The patient continues to be asymptomatic 6 years after recanalization (June 1, 1997) despite a 20% drop in the ankle/arm index (AAI) following exercise.

the author continues to utilize PIAT as the initial treatment for chronic iliac occlusions unless the patient is unable to tolerate being supine for 8 to 24 hours. Intolerance usually occurs in patients with chronic low back syndrome. The age, loci, length of the occlusion, and status of the runoff do not influence this approach.

Author's Technique of PIAT for Chronic Occlusions

The technique consists of using a No. 4 French micropuncture system (Cook Catheter Co., Bloomington, IN) to enter the contralateral femoral artery, inserting a Bentson 0.035 guidewire (Cook Catheter Co.), introducing and re-forming a No. 4 French McNamara contralateral catheter (Cook Catheter Co.), and placing the tip in contact with the proximal end of the occlusion. Gentle probing/tapping on the occlusion with either the Bentson or a Rosen guidewire (1.5 mm J, Cook Catheter Co.), is performed to search for a soft spot to gently embed the catheter so that the two side holes near the tip are within the clot. If none is found, an end hole infusion guidewire is advanced through the catheter and put in contact with the top of the occlusion (Fig. 11–2). Urokinase (UK) (Abbokinase, Abbott Laboratories, Abbott Park, IL) at a concentration of 2500 U/ml in either D5W or normal saline is infused at a rate of 24 ml/hr (60,000 U/hr). Concomitant heparinization is usually not administered at first.

The patient is monitored on the vascular surgery ward rather than in an intensive care unit, rests on an air mattress, and is rotated and braced in a 45° oblique position every 1 to 2 hours (to retard the development of low back pain), is on a full liquid diet, receives 75 ml/hr of parenteral fluids containing 20 mEq KCl/ 1,000 ml, has input and output monitored closely, has an indwelling bladder catheter, and receives Ancef, 1.0 g intravenously every 8 hours (to diminish the risk of urinary tract infection/sepsis). Repeat angiography is performed at 6 to 12 hours after onset of the infusion. A Rosen 1.5-mm J guidewire is advanced into the occlusion. If it advances >5 cm, the No. 4 French McNamara contralateral catheter is replaced by a multi-side hold infusion catheter (most commonly a No. 4 French Cragg-McNamara, MicroTherapeutics, Inc., San Clemente, CA) (Fig. 11–1).

With advancement into the occlusion, a coaxial system may be utilized. This usually consists of a No. 5.5 French Balkins sheath (Cook Catheter Co.) plus a multi-side hole No. 4 or 5 French catheter. The dose of UK is then increased to 36 ml/hr, with 12 ml/hr via the sheath (proximal end of the original occlusion) and 24 ml/hr directly into the remaining thrombus, for a total dose of 90,000 U/hr. The infusion is then supplemented by intra-arterial heparin at a dose of 700 to 1000 U/hr, sufficient to effect an activated partial thromboplastin time of 1.5 times baseline. The heparin is also delivered via the sheath. The infusion continues overnight. The patient is not given a bolus of either UK or heparin, and every effort is made to avoid fragmenting or dislodging the clot. Thus, neither pulse spray nor lacing is performed.

In the morning, the inner catheter is further advanced if clot lysis has progressed, but the distal portion of the occlusion remains. The infusion is then resumed, and the patient is returned in the afternoon for PTA and stent placement regardless of persistent occlusion. If complete clot lysis is demonstrated in the morning or sooner, then immediate PTA and stent placement are performed (Fig. 11–2). The anatomy will dictate if this is done contralaterally or ipsilaterally. If no change is noted after 24 hours of infusion, attempts are made to traverse the lesion using hydrophilic guidewires and catheters. Both contralateral and ipsilateral approaches will be used if necessary. Following successful traversal of an uncovered stenosis or residual occlusion, the lesion will be underdilated by 2 mm. Then a stent will be placed and dilated to the estimated normal size for that vessel segment.

At this time, we use the Wallstent for long external iliac occlusions and the Palmaz stent for all other lesions. The Palmaz stent is usually introduced on a No. 4.8 French Olbert catheter (Boston Scientific, Watertown, MA) via a No. 6 or 7 French sheath. Subsequent PTA by high-pressure balloons on either No. 5 or 6 French shafts is then accomplished. Careful inspection is performed to be certain of excellent wall contact, and every effort is made to ensure continuous stent contact with the wall. The sheath(s) is then removed, a Vasoseal is introduced into the tract, and heparin and UK are discontinued. The patient is immobilized for 4 hours and then allowed to go home if desired.

Author's Results

In our prospective series of 21 consecutively treated chronic iliac occlusions, the UK infusion effected 95% clot lysis and reestablishment of flow in 9 (43%), partial lysis (shortening) without reestablishment of flow in 7 (33%), and no change in 5 (24%). Our impression was that all of the residual occlusions were softer following PIAT. Occlusions that had been impenetrable could be traversed with a guidewire that originally would not enter the lesion. We achieved successful PTA/stent results in 100% of the completely lysed occlusions, in 100% of those with partial lysis, and in 60% of those that were only softened. This yielded a 30-day patency rate of 90%. No distal emboli occurred, and there were no deaths at (30 days).

Some of these lesions were treated prior to the availability of stents. The only common iliac reocclusion occurred in a patient who did not have a stent. Two external iliac reocclusions occurred, even though both patients had Wallstents placed following the initial

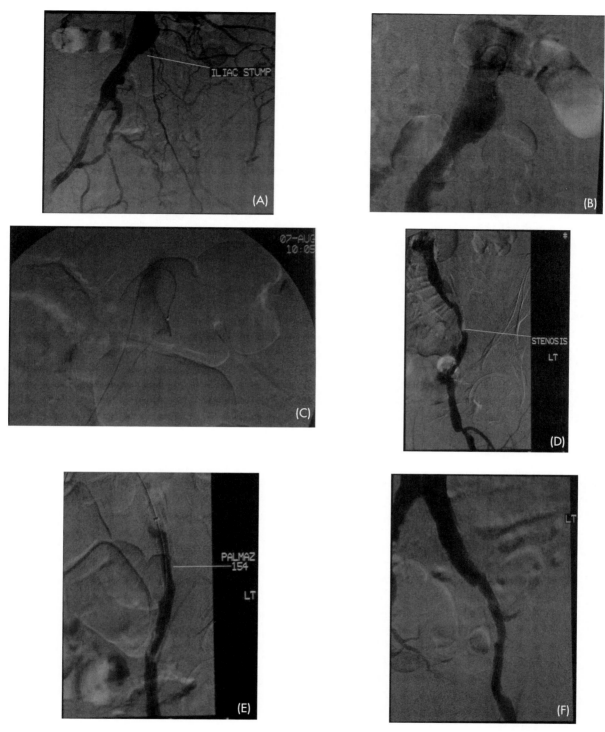

Figure 11–2. A 60-year-old black male chronic smoker presents with left foot rest pain 8 weeks following the sudden onset of left leg numbness, coolness, pain, and disappearance of the left femoral pulse. (A) Initial angiogram demonstrates complete occlusion of both the left common iliac artery (CIA) and the external iliac artery (EIA). A residual "stump" at the proximal end of the occlusion indicates that the underlying stenosis is not at the origin of the CIA. (B) A No. 4 French shepherd's hook catheter is re-formed in the aorta (McNamara Contralateral Infusion Catheter, Cook Catheter Co.). (C) The infusion catheter is gently wedged into the proximal end of the occlusion, and UK is begun at dose of 90,000 IU/hr. (D) Reestablishment of flow and 95% clot lysis are demonstrated 7 hours after the onset of PIAT. There is severe stenosis in the proximal EIA and residual thrombus in the distal EIA. The patient complains of severe low back pain due to chronic lumbar disc disease. Therefore, PIAT is terminated. (E) A Palmaz 154 stent is placed via a No. 7 French contralateral sheath (Balkins sheath, Cook Catheter Co.) and dilated to 7 mm. The sheath is pulled. The patient is maintained on IV heparin overnight and discharged in the morning on 325 mg/day of aspirin. (F) A follow-up angiogram 4 months later, at the time of treatment of the right leg, demonstrates persistent patency and interval endogenous fibrinolysis of the residual thrombus. The left leg is asymptomatic.

thrombolysis and PTA. Several of the initially treated lesions have remained patent and the patients asymptomatic despite the absence of stents (Fig. 11–1).

Some of the original patients have returned with symptoms and a new stenosis. They have been retreated with primary stent placement (Fig. 11–3). None have gone on to occlude. The assisted primary patency at 5 years is 81% (based on intent to treat).

An argument is often made that PIAT is too time-consuming, expensive, and dangerous.[12,16] Motarjeme examined the duration of the procedure, the fluoro-

scopy time, and the success rate relative to the effects of PIAT.[21] He demonstrated 100% success following PIAT compared to the usual 80% when direct guidewire traversal is used without PIAT. He also demonstrated that the total procedure (fluoroscopy/radiology) time was less if PIAT was effective. Total fluoroscopy time was 34 minutes for lesions that responded completely, 50 minutes for those that underwent partial lysis, and 52 minutes for those that softened but did not dissolve. Thus, PIAT increases the initial technical success rate and reduces the fluoros-

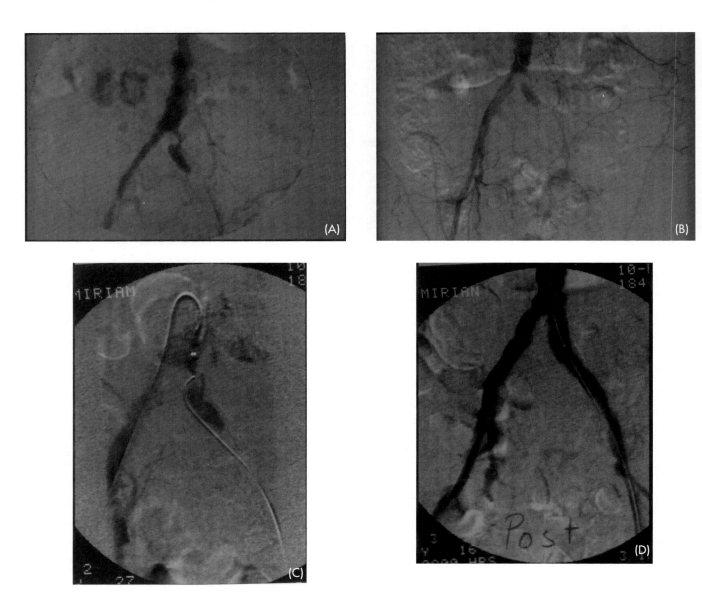

Figure 11–3. A 68-year-old white female former smoker with hypertension and hyperlipidemia (cholesterol = 660 mg/dl) presents with a 3-year history of mild right calf and severe left hip and leg claudication (resting left AAI = 0.3). (A) Initial angiogram at another hospital demonstrated occlusion of the distal left CIA and SFA (March 21, 1990). Attempts to traverse the occlusion failed using both the contralateral and ipsilateral approaches (March 21, 1990). The patient refused surgery. (B) A repeat angiogram 23 months later (February 10, 1992) prior to attempted PIAT demonstrates persistent occlusion, which was firm and impenetrable to a nonhydrophilic guidewire. (C) Following 8 hours of infusion of UK at a dose of 60,000 IU/hr, the short occlusion was softer and easily traversed. (D) PTA using 8-mm diameter kissing balloons effected brisk flow with no residual stenosis.

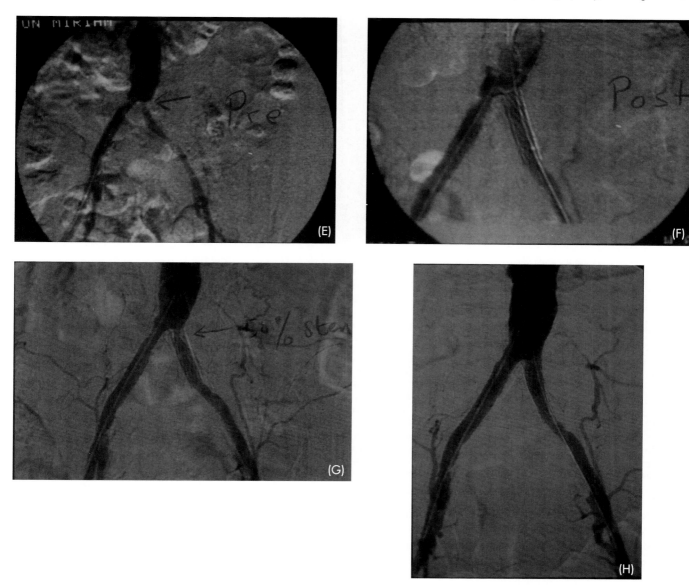

Figure 11–3. *(cont'd)* (E) Mild recurrent left leg claudication and a drop in the resting AAI from 0.79 to 0.60 occurred at 1 year 3 months. A repeat angiogram (May 6, 1993) demonstrates continued patency but restenosis at the origin of the left CIA. (F) A Palmaz 294 stent was placed and dilated to 8 mm, with restoration of normal caliber and brisk flow. (G) Recurrence of left leg claudication and a 0.20 drop in resting AAI after 20 months occurs. A repeat angiogram demonstrates stenosis within the proximal end of the stent. The patient had poorly controlled hypertension and remained moderately hyperlipidemic (cholesterol = 290 mg/dl). (H) After kissing balloon angioplasties with 10-mm balloons, the caliber and flow are normal. More aggressive measures were instituted to control blood pressure and to lower cholesterol. The patient remained asymptomatic and experienced no deterioration in AAI 2 years 5 months later (June 1, 1997).

copy time and radiation exposure for both patient and the interventionalist. It also reduces the number of stents, which counterbalances the cost of the drug.

In our experience, the average hospital stay was 2 days. This is the time usually reported for the direct guidewire traversal method because of the practice of anticoagulating with IV heparin for 24 to 48 hours posttreatment.[14–17,18,33]

Some have suggested that lysis be reserved for those occlusions that cannot be traversed.[12] In the author's experience, the use of PIAT following unsuccessful attempts to advance a hydrophilic guidewire has been associated with significant retroperitoneal bleeding (Fig. 11–4). Palmaz has had a similar experience (personal communication). This can be explained by the presumed mechanism of tiny perforations from the hydrophilic guidewire slowly leaking when exposed to the thrombolytic agent. This was the only major complication in the author's series.

Summary

In summary, a growing number of techniques have made it possible to treat most chronic iliac occlusions

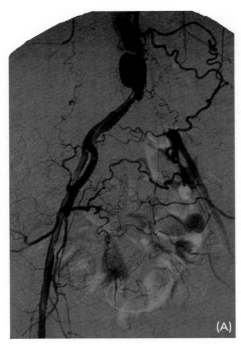

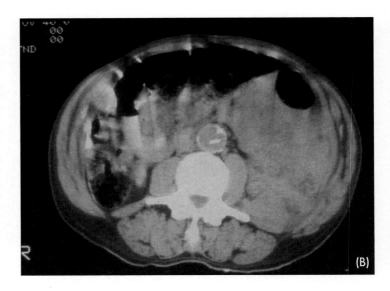

Figure 11–4. A 54-year-old hypertensive, chronically smoking white female with a 2-year history of moderate left hip and leg claudication. (A) Initial angiogram demonstrates occlusion of the left CIA and stenosis of the right CIA. Because of a history of lumbar disc disease, avoiding prolonged immobilization during PIAT was desirable. Attempts were made to traverse the occlusion from the contralateral approach using both regular and hydrophillic guidewires. Following failure of multiple attempts at traversal, PIAT was begun with a contralateral infusion catheter in contact with the proximal end of the occlusion. UK was infused at a rate of 60,000 IU/hr. Concomitantly, heparin was administered via the same catheter at a rate of 800 U/hr because of the stenosis in the origin of the right CIA and the resultant risk of the development of pericatheter thrombus. (B) The patient developed hypotension, tachycardia, and pain in the left flank 9 hours after the onset of PIAT. An emergency computed tomography scan demonstrates a large left retroperitoneal hematoma. The infusion catheter can be seen in the distal aorta. PIAT was terminated, the patient was transferred to the intensive care unit, and 5 units of blood were given. She experienced an uneventful recovery.

percutaneously and achieve a high initial technical success rate, a high 30-day patency rate, and high secondary or assisted primary 3- to 5-year patency. The best approach is the subject of controversy. In the author's experience, the sequence of PIAT, PTA, and stent placement has yielded excellent initial success (90%), with a short hospitalization (2 days), no instances of distal emboli, no deaths, a 5% complication rate, and an 81% assisted primary patency rate (no occlusion) at 5 years. These results are better than those reported in most series utilizing direct guidewire traversal and primary stent placement. They are not as good as those reported by some other investigators who utilize PIAT as the initial treatment for chronic occlusions.[21,22] They are better than those reported from series in which PIAT was used for a short time at a high dose without complete clot lysis as the endpoint.[34] Once one embarks on PIAT, it may be best to infuse for 24 hours, as old clot lyses more slowly and less completely than acute thrombus. Otherwise, one may have a lower incidence of traversal and a higher incidence of embolism than we experienced and that has been reported by Motarjeme and Blum.[21,22] Irrespective of the method, the percutaneous approaches now rival bypass surgery.

REFERENCES

1. Johnston KW. Iliac arteries: reanalysis of results of balloon angioplasty. *Radiology* 1993;186:207–212.
2. Dotter CT, Frische LH, Judkins MP, et al. The "nonsurgical" treatment of iliofemoral arteriosclerotic obstruction. *Circulation* 1964;30:654–670.
3. Tegtmeyer CJ, Moore TS, Chandler JG, et al. Percutaneous transluminal dilation of a complete block in the right iliac artery. *AJR* 1979;133:532–535.
4. Ring EJ, Freiman DB, McLean GK, et al. Percutaneous recanalization of common iliac artery occlusions: an unacceptable complication rate. *AJR* 1982;139:587–589.
5. Tegtmyer CJ, Hartwell GD, Selby JB, et al. Results and complications of angioplasty in aortoiliac disease. *Circulation* 1991;83 (suppl 2):I53–I60.
6. van Andel GJ, van Erp WFM, Krepel VM, et al. Percutaneous transluminal dilatation of the iliac artery: long-term results. *Radiology* 1985;156:321–323.
7. Johnston KW, Rae M, Hogg-Johnston SA, et al. 5-Year results of a prospective study of percutaneous transluminal angioplasty. *Ann Surg* 1987;206:403–413.
8. Pentecost MJ, Crigui MH, Dorros G, et al. Guidelines for peripheral percutaneous transluminal angioplasty of the abdominal aorta and lower extremity vessels. *Circulation* 1994;89:511–531.
9. Standards of Practice Committee of the Society of Cardiovascular and Interventional Radiology. Guidelines for

percutaneous transluminal angioplasty. *Radiology* 1990; 177:619–626.

10. Colapinto RF, Stronell RD, Johnston WK. Transluminal angioplasty of complete iliac obstructions. *AJR* 1986; 146:859–862.

11. Rubinstein ZJ, Morag B, Peer A, et al. Percutaneous transluminal recanalization of common iliac artery occlusions. *Cardiovasc Intervent Radiol* 1987;10:16–20.

12. Gupta AK, Ravmandalam K, Rao VRK, et al. Total occlusion of iliac arteries: results of balloon angioplasty. *Cardiovasc Intervent Radiol* 1993;16:165–177.

13. Vorwerk D, Guenther RW. Mechanical revascularization of occluded iliac arteries with use of self-expandable endoprostheses. *Radiology* 1990;175:411–415.

14. Vorwerk D, Guenther RW, Keulers P, et al. Surgical and percutaneous management of contralateral thrombus dislodgement following stent placement and dilatation of iliac artery occlusions: technical note. *Cardiovasc Intervent Radiol* 1991;14:134–136.

15. Vorwerk D, Guenther R. Stent placement in iliac artery lesions: three years of clinical experience with the Wallstent. *Cardiovasc Intervent Radiol* 1992;15:285–290.

16. Vorwerk D, Guenther RW, Schurman K, et al. Primary stent placement for chronic iliac artery occlusions: follow-up results in 103 patients. *Radiology* 1995;194:745–749.

17. Yedlicka JW, Ferral H, Bjarnason H, et al. Chronic iliac artery occlusions: primary recanalization with endovascular stents. *JVIR* 1994;5:843–847.

18. Sapoval MR, Chatellier G, Long AL, et al. Self-expandable stents for the treatment of iliac artery obstructive lesions: long-term success and prognostic factors. *AJR* 1996; 166:1173–1179.

19. Long AL, Sapoval MR, Beyssen BM, et al. Strecker stent implantation in iliac arteries: patency and predictive factors for long-term success. *Radiology* 1995;194:739–744.

20. Auster M, Kadir S, Mitchell S, et al. Iliac artery occlusion: management with intrathrombus streptokinase infusion and angioplasty. *Radiology* 1984;153:385–388.

21. Motarjeme A. Thrombolysis prior to stenting in chronic iliac artery occlusions. Presented at the American Roentgen Ray Society annual meeting, Boston, MA, May 7, 1997.

22. Blum U, Gabelmann A, Redecker M, et al. Percutaneous recanalization of iliac artery occlusions: results of a prospective study. *Radiology* 1993;189:536–540.

23. Hausegger KA, Lammer J, Klein G, et al. Perkutane rekanalisation von beckenarterien verschlussen: lyses fibrinolyse, PTA, stents. *Fortschr Roentgenstr* 1991;155:550–555.

24. Henry M, Amor M, Ethevenet G, et al. Palmaz stent placement in iliac and femoropopliteal arteries: primary and secondary patency in 310 patients with 2–4 year follow-up. *Radiology* 1995;197:167–174.

25. Palmaz JC, Laborde JC, Rivera FJ, et al. Stenting of the iliac arteries with the Palmaz stent: experience from a multicenter trial. *Cardiovasc Intervent Radiol* 1992;15:291–297.

26. Murphy TP, Webb MS, Lambiase RE, et al. Percutaneous revascularization of complex iliac artery stenoses and occlusions with use of Wallstents: three-year experience. *JVIR* 1996;7:21–27.

27. Piotrowski JJ, Pearce WH, Jones DN, et al. Aorto-femoral bypass: the operation of choice or unilateral iliac occlusion. *J Vasc Surg* 1988;8:211–218.

28. Poulias GE, Polemis L, Skoutas B, et al. Bilateral aorto-femoral bypass in the presence of aorto-iliac occlusive disease and factors determining results: experience and long term follow-up with 500 consecutive cases. *J Cardiovasc Surg (Torino)* 1985;26:527–538.

29. Brewster DC, Darling RC. Optimal methods of aortoiliac reconstruction. *Surgery* 1978;84:739–748.

30. Crawford ES, Bomberger RA, Glaeser DH, et al. Aortoiliac occlusive disease: factors influencing survival and function following reconstructive operation over a twenty-five year period. *Surgery* 1981;90:1055–1067.

31. Szilagyi DE, Elliott JP, Smith RF, et al. A thirty-year survey of the reconstructive surgical treatment of aortoiliac occlusive disease. *J Vasc Surg* 1986;3:421–436.

32. McNamara TO. Thrombolytic therapy for iliac artery occlusions. In Kadir, ed. Kadir, S. *Current Practice of Interventional Radiology*. Philadelphia, C Decker; 1991:301–306.

33. Martin EC, Katzen BT, Benenati JF, et al. Multicenter trial of the Wallstent in the iliac and femoral arteries. *JVIR* 1995;6:843–849.

34. Rees CR, Palmaz JC, Garcia O, et al. Angioplasty and stenting of completely occluded iliac arteries. *Radiology* 1989;172:953–959.

12

Endovascular Repair of Occlusive Disease of the Aorta and Iliac Arteries

Michael L. Marin, M.D.
Frank J. Veith, M.D.

Aortofemoral bypass has proven over the years to be durable and effective for the revascularization of ischemic lower extremities, demonstrating good long-term patency and acceptable procedural morbidity and mortality.[1–6] However, cardiopulmonary failure and other perioperative complications will continue to occur as increasingly older patients with occlusive disease undergo surgery. In addition, graft thrombosis of at least one limb of an aortobifemoral reconstruction occurs in as many as 10 to 20% of patients during long-term follow-up. The risk of operative complications may be somewhat greater after secondary procedures.[2–4] Patients presenting with limb-threatening ischemia and tissue necrosis frequently have multilevel occlusive disease that often requires an infrainguinal bypass after the aortoiliac reconstruction to achieve tissue healing. Such extensive, multilevel revascularizations may further increase the operative morbidity and mortality in this population of medically high-risk patients.

Alternative interventions to open aortic procedures have been sought to reduce morbidity and costs and to improve the outcome. Percutaneous balloon angioplasty of the iliac vessels, with or without intravascular stent support, has proven to be an effective technique for treating focal disease in the common iliac artery.[7–14] Unfortunately, diffuse disease involving multiple segments of the aorta, iliac, and femoral arteries has compromised the results of these catheter-based approaches.[14,15] For example, recurrent stenoses at the sites of previous interventions for diffuse arterial occlusive disease, with a return of clinical symptoms, have made these endovascular techniques unsatisfactory for treating long-segment disease in the iliac and femoropopliteal arteries.

An alternative approach, which extends the potential of existing endovascular modalities for arterial occlusive disease, combines angioplasty with endovascular grafts (intravascular stents linked to prosthetic grafts) to bridge long, diffuse arterial occlusive disease.[16] These devices were initially conceptualized by Dotter[17] and subsequently tested in a variety of experimental models.[18–21] Variations in endovascular graft designs have resulted in devices for treating simple and complex aortic aneurysms, peripheral artery aneurysms, long, diffuse arterial occlusive disease, and traumatic arterial injuries.[22–32] This chapter will review the Montefiore Medical Center experience with endovascular grafts for treating 42 long-segment aortoiliofemoral artery occlusions.

METHODS

Patients

Forty-two patients with limb-threatening ischemia secondary to aortoiliac and femoropopliteal occlusive disease have been treated at the Montefiore Medical Center in New York with endovascular grafts in a project that began in February 1992. There were 20 men and 22 women, whose ages ranged from 45 to 89 years (mean, 65 years). Ten patients had severe ischemic rest pain, and the remaining 32 presented with ischemic tissue necrosis. Most of these patients had one or more coexisting medical problems, including severe coronary artery disease, renal insufficiency, or chronic obstructive pulmonary disease. Pulse volume recordings, ankle/brachial indices, and aortography with femoropopliteal and tibial runoff views were performed in all patients prior to and after each intervention.

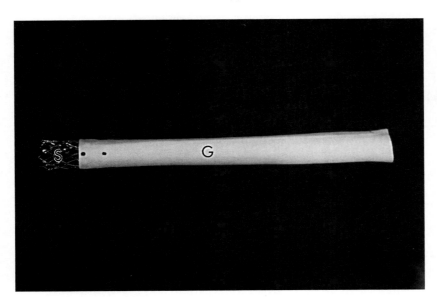

Figure 12–1. Endovascular stented graft used for aortoiliac reconstruction. A Palmaz stent (S) is sutured to the overlying PTFE graft (G) with four diametrically opposed PTFE sutures. No distal stent is seen attached to the graft because in each case the distal end of the endovascular graft was endoluminally suture-anastomosed to an appropriate outflow vessel.

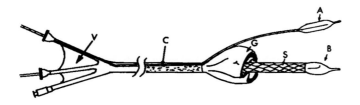

Figure 12–2. Introducer/delivery catheter used for delivery and deployment of endovascular stented grafts for aortoiliac reconstruction. Each introducer catheter is equipped with two balloons. Balloon A functions as a mechanism to form a tapered tip to the catheter system (see details in text). Balloon B functions to deploy an overlying Palmaz stent. With expansion of balloon B, the endovascular graft (G) becomes firmly fixed to the underlying arterial wall. (C, delivery catheter sheath; V, hemostatic valve mechanism.)

Endovascular Stented Graft Devices

The endovascular stented grafts (ESGs) used for treating aortoiliac occlusive disease were composed of Palmaz balloon expandable stents (30 mm) (Johnson and Johnson Interventional Systems, Warren, NJ) and 6-mm polytetrafluoroethylene (PTFE) thin-walled grafts (W.L. Gore and Associates, Flagstaff, AZ). Each stent was attached to the proximal end of the PTFE graft by four CV–6-0 PTFE sutures (W.L. Gore and Associates), so that one-half of the stent protruded from the end of the graft (Fig. 12–1). The stent and graft combination was then mounted on an 8 mm × 3 or 4 cm angioplasty balloon (Blue Max or PMT, Meditech Corporation, Watertown, MA). The entire balloon, stent, and graft complex was then wrapped around a second balloon catheter shaft ("tip balloon") and inserted into a delivery sheath, so that the stent portion of the device was 2 cm from the distal delivery sheath tip (Fig. 12–2). One-half of the 6 mm × 4 cm tip balloon was adjusted so that it protruded from the distal portion of the delivery sheath. When inflated, the tip balloon occluded flow from the sheath tip, allowing sheath pressurization and providing a smooth, tapered transition to the end of the delivery sheath (Fig. 12–2). Other configurations of this delivery system were also used, including a single shaft with two balloons or two balloons linked to one another by a small fenestration in the shaft of the tip balloon. This hole in the tip balloon catheter accepted

the tip of the stent deployment balloon. The complete endovascular graft and delivery system were prepared on a separate sterile table in the operating room during each procedure.

Operative Technique

All procedures were performed using an open dissection and exposure of the femoral arterial access site. This approach allowed for repair of diseased femoral arteries when necessary. Based on the overall condition of the patient at the time of the procedure and the extent of the expected procedure below the inguinal ligament, either general (9[22%]), epidural (30 [71%]), or local (3 [7%]) anesthesia was selected. One of two potential techniques for arterial recanalization was used to create a wide tract within the wall of the diseased iliac arteries. When the contralateral iliac artery was patent, canalization was carried out by means of a contralateral percutaneously inserted guidewire "up and over" the aortic bifurcation. This approach permitted a prograde dissection plane to be developed within the occluded arterial wall (see Fig. 12–3). This technique allows for maximal control of arterial inflow, should arterial perforation occur, and ensures that the initiation of the recanalization process is within the true arterial lumen. When the up and over approach was not technically feasible (contralateral occlusion present), retrograde recanalization of the diseased

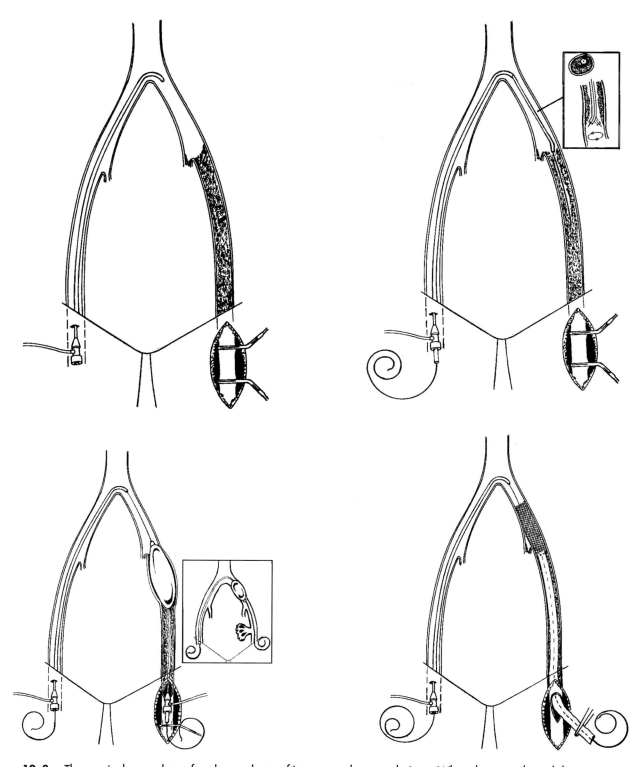

Figure 12–3. The surgical procedure of endovascular grafting: up and over technique. When the contralateral iliac artery is patent, recanalization is carried out by means of a contralateral, percutaneously inserted guidewire, up and over the aortic bifurcation, developing a prograde arterial wall dissection plane. This technique allows for maximal control of arterial inflow and ensures that the recanalization process begins within the native arterial lumen. (Reprinted from Ref. 16 with permission.)

artery was performed (see Fig. 12–4). Recanalizations were performed through an occluded artery in 34 patients and through a diffusely stenotic but patent ves-sel in 8 patients. Each arterial recanalization was accomplished with a 0.035-inch hydrophilic guidewire directed by means of an angled catheter. Thirty-nine of

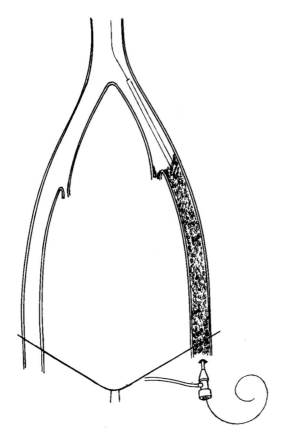

Figure 12–4. The surgical procedure of endovascular grafting: retrograde technique. When the up and over approach was not technically feasible, retrograde recanalization was used. (Reprinted from Ref. 16 with permission.)

42 patients were successfully recanalized using one of the above techniques. Those patients who could not be successfully recanalized underwent extra-anatomic bypasses.[3] Two additional patients in whom the endovascular grafts thrombosed within 24 hours, requiring revision, were also considered technical failures.

Following successful wire passage, each iliac artery was dilated along the entire length of the diseased vessel using an 8-mm-diameter angioplasty balloon. A previously prepared endovascular graft system was then inserted over a guidewire into the newly created tract within the arterial wall. Once the device was fluoroscopically located at the predetermined site, the sheath was partially retracted, permitting proximal stent deployment. The introducer sheath was then completely withdrawn, allowing the redundant portion of the distal end of the endovascular graft to emerge from the access vessel arteriotomy. The distal end of the endovascular graft was then endoluminally or extraluminally anastomosed, using one of the techniques illustrated in Figure 12.5. Multilevel occlusive disease was frequently treated with an infrainguinal bypass extension (using PTFE or reversed saphenous vein) which originated from the site of the arteriotomy used for the endovascular graft insertion (Fig. 12–6).

An intraoperative completion angiogram was performed at the conclusion of each endovascular graft procedure. In 8 of the 39 patients (20%), midgraft stenoses from either inadequate graft expansion, underlying vessel tortuosity, or extraluminal compression of the prosthesis were detected. All these lesions were successfully corrected by balloon dilatation of the narrowed graft segment and, in four patients, by the insertion of an additional intragraft balloon expandable stent.

ESGs originated from the aorta (5) or the common iliac artery (34) and were inserted into the common femoral or deep femoral artery using endovascular anastomoses. ESG lengths ranged from 16 to 30 cm (mean, 21 cm).

RESULTS

Technical success in arterial recanalization was achieved in 39 of the 42 iliac arteries (93%) (Fig. 12–5A,B). Two additional patients, who experienced acute graft thrombosis and who required conversion to a standard operative alternative, were also considered technical failures, resulting in a total technical failure rate of 12%. Following endovascular aorto-iliofemoral reconstruction and, in some instances, supplementary conventional infrainguinal surgical bypass, ankle/brachial indices improved significantly ($p < 0.05$) from a mean of 0.39 to 0.76, and the thigh pulse volume recordings improved from a mean amplitude of 9.75 mm to a mean of 37.8 mm. The 18-month primary and secondary cumulative life table patency rates for all

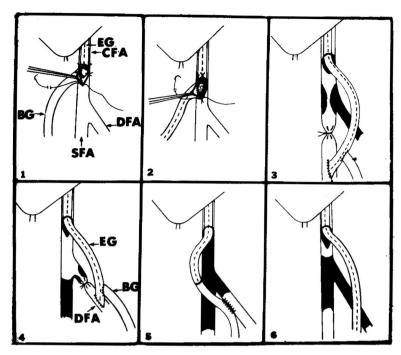

Figure 12–5. The distal end of the endovascular graft can be anastomosed to the patent distal arterial tree in several ways. (1) Type I: an endoluminal anastomosis to the femoral artery is performed, and a separate proximal anastomosis of the distal extravascular graft is performed to the femoral anteriotomy. (2) Type II: the intravascular anastomosis and proximal anastomosis of the distal extravascular graft are included in a single anastomotic closure. (3) Type III: the stented graft is brought out through the femoral arteriotomy and anastomosed to the patent distal superficial femoral artery. From this site, a distal extension or a crossover femorofemoral extension can be performed if necessary. (4) Type IV: the endovascular graft is brought out through the femoral arteriotomy and anastomosed to the patent distal profunda femoris artery. An extension to the distal arterial tree or to the contralateral femoral artery can be performed from this graft if necessary. (5) Type V: the end of the endovascular graft is brought out through the femoral arteriotomy, and a distal graft extension is anastomosed end-to-end to this graft, side-to-side to the patent distal profunda artery, and extended further to the distal arterial tree. (6) Type VI: the endovascular graft is brought out through the femoral arteriotomy. It can bypass multiple levels of occlusive disease and be anastomosed distally to the popliteal or tibial arteries if all femoral vessels are occluded. (EG, endovoascular graft; BG, distal bypass graft; SFA, superficial femoral artery; DFA, deep femoral artery; CFA, common femoral artery.) (Reprinted from Ref. 16 with permission.)

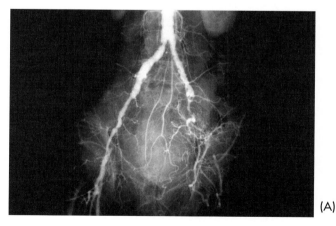

(A)

Figure 12–6. A 62-year-old woman was admitted with limb-threatening ischemia of the left lower extremity. (A) A pelvic anteriogram showed diffuse iliac disease. (B) The left iliac artery occlusion was corrected using an endovascular stented graft extending from the proximal common iliac artery to the common femoral artery. This graft was extended to the popliteal artery. (Reprinted from Ref. 16 with permission.)

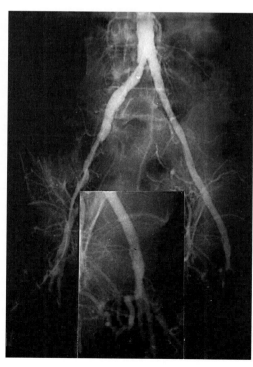

(B)

ESGs were 89% (± 9 SE) and 100%, respectively. Limb salvage was achieved in 94% of the patients at 24 months (± 8 SE).

Minor complications, including lymphocele and groin hematomas, occurred in four instances (10%). One patient sustained an uncomplicated subendocardial myocardial infarction. One patient died of heart failure following an endovascular aortoiliac bypass procedure, resulting in a procedural mortality rate of 2%.

SUMMARY

Occlusive disease of the aorta, iliac arteries, and femoral arteries may be responsible for limb-threatening ischemia, particularly when multiple levels of the arterial system are involved. The combined treatment of severe aortoiliac and infrainguinal disease using standard techniques may be hazardous or contraindicated in patients with multiple previous reconstructions and/or severe comorbid medical illnesses. Endovascular aortoiliac grafts, often in combination with conventional surgical infrainguinal bypasses, are a technically feasible and potentially safe option for the treatment of limb-threatening aorto-iliofemoral occlusive disease and have demonstrated encouraging early patency. Long-term follow-up will be necessary prior to widespread application of this technique.

REFERENCES

1. Brewster DC, Darling RC. Optimal methods of aortoiliac reconstruction. *Surgery* 1978;8:739.
2. Szilagyi DE, Elliott JP Jr, Smith RF, Reddy DJ, McPharlin M. A thirty-year survey of the reconstructive surgical treatment of aortoiliac occlusive disease. *J Vasc Surg* 1986;3:421.
3. Brothers TE, Greenfield LJ. Long-term results of aortoiliac reconstruction. *JVIR* 1990;1:49.
4. Nevelsteen A, Wouters L, Suy R. Long-term patency of the aortofemoral Dacron graft. A graft limb related study over a 25-year period. *J Cardiovasc Surg* 1991;32:174.
5. Poulias GE, Doundoulakis N, Prombonas E, et al. Aortofemoral bypass and detriments of early success and late favourable outcome. Experience with 1000 consecutive cases. *J Cardiovasc Surg* 1992;33:664.
6. Rutherford RB. Aortobifemoral bypass, the gold standard: technical considerations. *Semin Vasc Surg* 1994;7:11.
7. Johnston KW, Rae M, Hogg-Johnston SA, et al. 5-Year results of a prospective study of percutaneous transluminal angioplasty. *Ann Surg* 1987;206:403.
8. Martin EC. Percutaneous therapy in the management of aortoiliac disease. *Semin Vasc Surg* 1994;7:17.
9. Tegtmeyer CJ, Hartwell GD, Selby JB, Robertson R Jr, Kron IL, Tribble CG. Results and complications of angioplasty in aortoiliac disease. *Circulation* 1991;83(suppl 1):I-53.
10. Liermann D, Strecker EP, Peters J. The Strecker stent: indications and results in iliac and femoropopliteal arteries. *Cardiovasc Intervent Radiol* 1992;15:298.
11. Palmaz JC, Laborde JC, Rivera FJ, Encarnacion CE, Lutz JD, Moss JG. Stenting of the iliac arteries with the Palmaz stent: experience from a multicenter trial. *Cardiovasc Intervent Radiol* 1992;15:291.
12. Hausegger KA, Cragg AH, Lammer J, et al. Iliac artery stent placement: Clinical experience with a Nitinol stent. *Radiology* 1994;190:199.
13. Vorwerk D, Gunther RW. Stent placement in iliac arterial lesions: three years of clinical experience with the Wallstent. *Cardiovasc Intervent Radiol* 1992;15:285.
14. Johnston KW. Iliac arteries: reanalysis of results of balloon angioplasty. *Radiology* 1993;186:207.
15. Laborde JC, Palmaz JC, Rivera FJ, Encarnacion CE, Picot MC, Dougherty SP. Influence of anatomic distribution of atherosclerosis on the outcome of revascularization with iliac stent placement. *JVIR* 1995;6:513.
16. Marin ML, Veith FJ, Sanchez LA, et al. Endovascular aortoiliac grafts in combination with standard infrainguinal arterial bypasses in the management of limb-threatening ischemia: preliminary report. *J Vasc Surg* 1995;22:316.
17. Dotter CT. Transluminally-placed coilspring endarterial tube grafts. Long-term patency in canine popliteal artery. *Invest Radiol* 1969;4:329.
18. Balko A, Piasecki GJ, Shah DM, Carney WI, Hopkins RW, Jackson BT. Transfemoral placement of intraluminal polyurethane prosthesis for abdominal aortic aneurysm. *J Surg Res* 1986;40:305.
19. Mirich D, Wright KC, Wallace S, et al. Percutaneously placed endovascular grafts for aortic aneurysms: feasibility study. *Radiology* 1989;170:1033.
20. Laborde JC, Parodi JC, Clem MF, et al. Intraluminal bypass of abdominal aortic aneurysm: feasibility study. *Radiology* 1992;184:185.
21. Chuter TAM, Green RM, Ouriel K, Fore WM, DeWeese JA. Transfemoral endovascular aortic graft placement. *J Vasc Surg* 1993;18:185.
22. Marin ML, Veith FJ, Cynamon J, et al. Initial experience with transluminally placed endovascular grafts for the treatment of complex vascular lesions. *Ann Surg* 1995;222:449.
23. Parodi J, Palmaz J, Barone HD. Transfemoral intraluminal graft implantation for abdominal aortic aneurysms. *Ann Vasc Surg* 1991;5:491.
24. Parodi JC. Endovascular repair of abdominal aortic aneurysms and other arterial lesions. *J Vasc Surg* 1995;21:549.
25. May J, White G, Waugh R, Yu W, Harris J. Treatment of complex abdominal aortic aneurysms by a combination of endoluminal and extraluminal aortofemoral grafts. *J Vasc Surg* 1994;19:924.
26. Scott RAP, Chuter TAM. Clinical endovascular placement of bifurcated graft in abdominal aortic aneurysm without laparotomy. *Lancet* 1994;343:413. Letter to the Editor.
27. Marin ML, Veith FJ, Panetta TF, et al. Transfemoral stented graft treatment of occlusive arterial disease for limb salvage: a preliminary report. *Circulation* 1993;88(4):I-11. Abstract.
28. Cragg AH, Dake MD. Percutaneous femoropopliteal graft placement. *JVIR* 1993;4:455.
29. Marin ML, Veith FJ, Lyon RT, Cynamon J, Sanchez LA. Transfemoral endovascular repair of iliac artery aneurysms. *Am J Surg* 1995;170:179.
30. Marin ML, Veith FJ, Panetta TF, et al. Transfemoral endoluminal stented graft repair of a popliteal artery aneurysm. *J Vasc Surg* 1994;19:754.
31. Marin ML, Veith FJ, Panetta TF, et al. Transluminally placed endovascular stented graft repair for arterial trauma. *J Vasc Surg* 1994;20:466.
32. Volodos NL, Shekhanin VE, Karpovich IP, Troian VI, Gur'ev IuA. Self-fixing synthetic prosthesis for endoprosthetics of the vessels. *Vestn Khir (Russia)* 1986;137:123.

13

The Results of Surgical Treatment of Infrainguinal Occlusive Disease

Michael Belkin, M.D.
Magruder C. Donaldson, M.D.
Anthony D. Whittemore, M.D.

GENERAL PRINCIPLES OF REPORTING AND INTERPRETATION OF RESULTS

Interpretation of the results of infrainguinal arterial reconstructive surgery reported in the literature has historically been complicated by lack of a common language and uniform statistical techniques. Recognition of this problem led to the formation of an ad hoc committee of the International Society for Cardiovascular Surgery and Society for Vascular Surgery (ISCVS/SVS) that developed suggested standards for reports dealing with lower-extremity ischemia. The report of this committee was published in 1986 and has served as a useful framework for evaluating the quality of reports within the vascular surgery literature.[1] Nonetheless, several recommendations of that committee proved cumbersome and have not been widely adopted. The committee, for example, suggested that chronic ischemia be divided into six separate categories ranging from mild claudication (1) to major tissue loss (6). Despite the recognition that the indications for a particular procedure may vary widely, and that the indications from series to series may differ, most authors have broadly divided the indications for surgery into procedures for disabling claudication versus those for limb-threatening ischemia. The limb-threatening ischemia indication is generally subdivided into procedures performed for ischemic rest pain and those performed for tissue loss. Despite the simplicity of this classification and the general understanding of the terminology, there is much subjectivity and room for interpretation in this form of classification. The term *disabling claudication* may vary from an inability to perform one's job to difficulty walking nine holes of golf. Similarly, symptoms of rest pain

may be confused with other chronic pain syndromes including neuropathy or arthritis. Even tissue ulceration may be mistakenly attributed to ischemia when neuropathy is the true etiology. Most studies in the literature provide objective data from the vascular laboratory to help classify the extent of vascular impairment.

Graft patency rates are generally reported as *primary* and *secondary*. A graft is considered to have *primary patency* if, from the time of implantation, it has remained continuously patent, without the need for thombectomy, thrombolysis, surgical revision, transluminal dilation, or any other intervention on the graft itself. Some authors consider grafts as primarily patent when thrombectomy and revision are required with 48 hours of surgery. Still others consider separately grafts that require some form of revision while still patent to have "primary assisted patency" or "primary revised patency." A graft is considered to have secondary patency if it remains patent after some form of intervention to restore and maintain patency. For example, a bypass graft that undergoes successful thrombolysis and vein patch angioplasty after vein graft thrombosis is considered to have suffered a primary failure but to be secondarily patent. Secondary patency rates should not be confused with primary patency rates achieved after secondary (ie, reoperative) operations. Successful limb salvage is defined as preservation of the limb in the absence of a major amputation. When necessary, toe and transmetatarsal amputations are generally considered part of successful limb salvage. Unfortunately, many reports are confounded by including patients who underwent surgery for claudication (not a limb salvage procedure) in their calculations of limb salvage rates. In general, only operations performed for limb salvage indications should be included in these calculations.

As suggested by the standards committee of the ISCVS/SVS, most authors have adopted life table methods for reporting the results of graft patency, limb salvage, and patient survival rates. The life table evaluation is the best available technique for evaluating a series of patients who were operated on at different times and were followed for varying intervals. This technique also facilitates the evaluation of patients who have been followed to various endpoints, including graft failure, limb loss, death, lost to follow-up, and time-censored patients. Despite the universal recognition of the value of this technique, review of the vascular surgery literature will reveal frequent indiscretions and abuses of this statistical technique.[2,3] The most common deficiency is "front end loading," whereby large numbers of patients are followed for short intervals and only a minority of patients have long-term follow-up, so that patency curves are extended to intervals where there are few grafts and high standard errors. The recommendations of the ISCVS/SVS reporting standards committee include very detailed definitions and instructions for calculating, comparing, and reporting of life tables to standardize the literature and prevent misrepresentation.[1] A recent survey of the vascular literature, however, revealed that only a small minority of papers adhered to the proposed guidelines.[2,4,5]

VARIABLES INFLUENCING OPERATIVE RESULTS

Accurate interpretation of the results of any series of infrainguinal arterial reconstructions requires a clear understanding of the surgical technique and the conditions under which the procedures were performed. Among the most important factors to be considered are the conduit employed, the proportion of reoperative or secondary operations, the distribution of the distal anastomotic sites, and the extent of comorbidity.

The most important factor among these various determinants of success is the conduit employed. In most situations, autogenous vein provides a more durable conduit for infrainguinal arterial reconstruction than does a prosthetic graft. Nonetheless, some series have combined autogenous and prosthetic grafts. In either the in situ or reversed configuration, greater saphenous vein is generally superior to other autogenous veins including arm, lesser saphenous, and composite vein grafts. Many studies include a variety of vein graft types, and many reports do not differentiate between primary and secondary bypass operations, despite the clear difference in long-term results.[6] In

addition, the quality and caliber of vein utilized are important but not easily documented variables. Technical considerations also confound accurate comparison of concurrent reports. Variations in methods of vein preparation, magnification, experience of the surgical team, and intraoperative assessment on completion of the bypass occurs. While arteriography on completion has undoubtedly reduced the number of technical complications resulting in early graft failure, both intraoperative duplex scanning and angioscopy are being utilized with increasing frequency and may favorably influence the ultimate result.

The extent of significant comorbidity also influences the ultimate outcome. The high incidence of coronary artery disease increases the risk of perioperative cardiac morbidity and mortality, as well as long-term patient survival. The presence of diabetes has not significantly altered patency and limb salvage rates compared to those observed in nondiabetics. Patients with mild renal insufficiency and threatened limbs achieve graft patency rates comparable to those of patients with normal renal function, but they sustain higher operative mortality and diminished survival. Those with end-stage renal disease, however, especially diabetics, demonstrate lower patency and significantly poorer survival.[7] The relatively recent recognition that a significant number of our patients harbor a variety of hypercoagulopathies, most commonly antiphospholipid syndrome (APS) and heparin-induced platelet aggregation (HIPA), represents another example of significant comorbidity that may affect the outcome of bypass results.[8]

Postoperative management of these patients and their risk factors has a major impact on long-term graft patency. Persistent use of tobacco is associated with a significant reduction in both graft patency and limb salvage rates compared to patients who stop smoking following reconstruction. The role of chronic anticoagulation is currently under investigation among patients undergoing autogenous reconstruction in a cooperative study. It has been shown to enhance the primary patency of long prosthetic grafts and is commonly used after secondary intervention for a failed graft. Aggressive postoperative graft surveillance with serial duplex scans is an important adjunct in maintaining graft patency. It has been repeatedly shown that repair of a vein graft or perianastomotic stenosis prior to graft thrombosis provides satisfactory, sustained patency of approximately 80% after 5 years. In contrast, similar intervention for recently thrombosed grafts, necessitating initial catheter thrombectomy or thrombolysis, yields 20 to 30% patency rates. Variations in postoperative surveillance protocols, therefore will significantly alter the secondary patency results and overall limb salvage among series.

Table 13-1.   Infrainguinal Reconstruction with Autogenous Vein

Author	Year	Number of Limbs	Operative Mortality	5-Year Cumulative Graft Patency		Limb Salvage	% of Patients
				Primary	Secondary		
Taylor[9]	1990	516	1%	75%	80%	90%	28%
Bergamini[10]	1991	361	3%	63%	81%	86%	57%
Donaldson[4]	1991	440	2%	72%	83%	84%	66%
Leather[11]	1992	1688	3%	70%	81%	92%	58%
Weighted Average		3005	2%	70%	81%	90%	54%

Table 13-2.   Weighted Average Primary Graft Patency Rates Associated with Infrainguinal Reconstruction Utilizing Autogenous Vein

Site of Distal Anastomosis	Source	Total Number of Limbs	5-Year Cumulative Patency Rates	
			Primary	Secondary
Popliteal Above-knee	Donaldson[4] Taylor[9]	155	75%	83%
Below-knee	Donaldson[4] Taylor[9] Bergamini[10] Leather[11]	952	74%	83%
Intrapopliteal	Donaldson[4] Taylor[9] Bergamini[10] Leather[11]	1843	67%	78%

RESULTS OF INFRAINGUINAL ARTERIAL RECONSTRUCTION WITH AUTOGENOUS VEIN

As mentioned above, autogenous vein is the optimal conduit for infrainguinal arterial reconstruction. The collective patency rates from four of the larger series of infrainguinal bypasses performed with autogenous vein are shown in Table 13.1.[4,9–11] Five year primary patency rates ranged from 63-75% with a weighted average of 70%. Five year secondary patency rates were remarkably similar ranging from 80-83%. All series demonstrated excellent limb salvage rates ranging from 84-92% at five years. Conversely, five year patient survival rates varied markedly between series ranging from 28-66% (weighted average 54%). Although comparable in many respects, there are important differences between these four studies. For example, the study of Taylor et. al. include only reversed vein grafts while the others are comprised of in situ saphenous vein grafts. The studies of Bergamini and Leather had a higher percentage of procedures performed for limb salvage and more distal outflow vessels than did the series of Donaldson and Taylor. The impact of outflow level on the five year patency rates is shown in Table 13-2.

Although the patency rates were higher for bypasses to the popliteal artery, the differences are rather modest due to improved results associated with bypasses to more distal outflow vessels. The use of the in situ bypass technique, in particular, has greatly improved our ability to successfully perform very distal bypasses, utilizing veins as small as 2.5 mm in diameter. Bypasses to the inframalleolar level have become commonplace with reported results similar to those achieved with femoral-tibial reconstructions. Pomposelli et. al. recently reviewed their results with 384 consecutive bypasses to the dorsalis pedis artery and reported 5 year primary and secondary patency rates of 68 and 82%, respectively.[12]

As vascular surgeons have become increasingly aggressive in performing limb salvage surgery, wider experience has been gained with a variety of alternative autogenous vein conduits. Reported primary patency rates associated with arm vein have ranged from 40% at three years to 50% after five years, with secondary patency rates approached 60% after 5 years, and limb salvage rates were as high as 82%. The lesser saphenous vein is another useful autogenous conduit for infrainguinal arterial reconstruction. A report by

Chang et al from Albany documented a 55% 3-year primary patency rate and a 73% 3-year secondary patency rate after 69 consecutive bypasses with lesser saphenous vein.[13]

As more secondary bypasses to more distal outflow vessels are being undertaken, patients are increasingly encountered who have insufficient greater saphenous vein (ipsilateral or contralateral) with which to complete the reconstructive operation. A variety of useful strategies have evolved to facilitate vascular reconstruction in these patients. These include adjunctive endovascular techniques, "short" bypass grafts based on more distal inflow vessels, and bypass grafts to more proximal outflow vessels that, although suboptimal, are often satisfactory for limb salvage. Equally important, however, is the construction of composite vein grafts made up of spliced segments of autogenous vein to create a conduit of sufficient length to complete the reconstruction. These conduits are often partially or totally constructed from ectopic venous segments. In our experience, 36% of the grafts were composed of greater saphenous/greater saphenous vein grafts, 11% of greater saphenous/arm vein grafts, 15% of greater saphenous/lesser saphenous vein grafts, and 38% of arm/arm vein grafts.[14] The two general indications for a composite vein graft are to optimize an otherwise flawed solitary venous conduit or to create a venous conduit of adequate length. The results of four of the larger series from the literature are shown in Table 13.3.[9,14–16]

The management of patients with a failed arterial reconstruction is one of the major challenges facing the vascular surgeon. Often these patients have recurrent ischemia and require secondary bypass to maintain limb salvage. Scarring from previous surgery and a lack of autogenous vein are among the many problems these patients present. By definition, patients requiring secondary bypass have failed previous infrainguinal reconstructions and therefore tend to include those who have more severe atherosclerosis, those who form more virulent intimal hyperplasia, those with hypercoagulable states, and those with small or poor-quality autogenous vein. These factors may have contributed to the early failure of the primary bypass graft and place the second graft at risk. It is therefore not surprising that the results of secondary operations are uniformly inferior to those of primary procedures. The results we obtained in a consecutive series of 300 secondary bypass operations are described in Table 13.4 (A–H).[6] As can be seen, the results of secondary operations performed with autogenous vein were superior to those completed with prosthetic grafts (A). Early primary graft failure (<30 days) suggested a poor prognosis for the secondary bypass as well (B). The results of secondary bypasses with autogenous vein improved significantly between 1975 and 1984 and between 1985 and 1993 (C). The distal outflow level did not affect the overall results (D). However, bypasses completed with greater saphenous vein were superior to those completed with alternative vein (E). The small number of patients who underwent surgery for disabling claudication did remarkably well (G). Despite recent improvements achieved with secondary bypass grafts, the results remain inferior to those noted after primary bypass operations (H). Compared to secondary operations, primary operations had superior 5-year primary (65.1% vs 49.5%), 5-year secondary (79.7% vs 59.1%), and 5-year limb salvage (91.3% vs 72.4%) rates.

RESULTS OF INFRAINGUINAL ARTERIAL RECONSTRUCTION WITH PROSTHETIC GRAFTS

The short- and long-term results of infrainguinal bypass and polytetrafluoroethylene (PTFE) grafts have been less satisfactory than those achieved with autogenous vein, and the differences have been most pronounced in bypasses to the tibial level[17–29] As shown in Table 13.5, infrapopliteal reconstruction with PTFE provides an average 5-year patency rate of 14%, rendering autogenous vein from nearly any source the preferred conduit. In contrast, PTFE in the femoropopliteal position provides 5-year patency rates averaging 40%, less discrepant from those obtained with autogenous vein. As is true of vein conduits, superior results are achieved with reconstructions performed for claudication as opposed to limb salvage. This finding is most pronounced for above-knee reconstructions, where overall primary patency rates achieved in claudicants range from 42 to 68% at 5 years and average 63%.

Table 13–3. Collected Results of Composite Autogenous Vein Grafts

Author	Number of Grafts	Secondary Patency Rate	Interval (years)	Limb Salvage	Interval (years)
Chang[15]	184	61%	4	92%	3
Harris[16]	54	74%	1	82%	1
Taylor[9]	70	83%	2	—	—
Belkin[14]	66	77%	3	86%	3

Table 13–4. life Table Analysis Secondary Infrainguinal Reconstruction

	Graft Type or Indication for Surgery	No. of Grafts	5-Year Primary Patency (%)	5-Year Secondary Patency (%)	5-Year Limb Salvage (%)	%-Year Patient Survival (%)
A	Prosthetic grafts	87	25.3 ± 5.7	27.4 ± 6.1	53.5 ± 7.5	71.5 ± 6.7
	Autogenous grafts	213	43.2 ± 4.6	51.5 ± 4.6	58.7 ± 5.5	72.6 ± 4.7
	p value		$p = 0.007$	$p = 0.001$	$p = 0.23$	$p = 0.45$
B	Early primary graft failure	44	27.2 ± 7.7*	29.8 ± 8.3*	43.9 ± 10*	81.4 ± 10.7*
	Late Primary graft failure	169	51.5 ± 4.9*	61.1 ± 4.7*	74.9 ± 4.4*	75.2 ± 4.6*
	p value		$p = 0.017$	$p = 0.003$	$p = 0.004$	$p = 0.3$
C	Autogenous bypass, 1975–84	59	28.8 ± 6.3	38.3 ± 6.3	40.4 ± 7.6	73.8 ± 7.6
	Autogenous bypass, 1985–93	154	49.5 ± 6.3	59.1 ± 5.8	72.4 ± 6.6	74.4 ± 4.8
	p value		$p = 0.01$	$p = 0.017$	$p = 0.001$	$p = 0.24$
D	Popliteal outflow	43	44.5 ± 9.7	53.8 ± 9.4	62.8 ± 12.5	N/A†
	Tibial outflow	111	51.4 ± 8.1	60.9 ± 7.4	78.2 ± 5.7	N/A†
	p value		$p = 0.295$	$p = 0.281$	$p = 0.174$	—
E	Greater saphenous vein[1]	79	60.4 ± 7.1	68.5 ± 6.0	77.8 ± 7.4	N/A†
	Alternative vein[2]	75	35.0 ± 11.0	48.3 ± 10.5	54.2 ± 11.8	N/A†
	p value		$p = 0.020$	$p = 0.090$	$p = 0.046$	—
F	Arm vein[3]	46	46.4 ± 9.2*	56.5 ± 8.1*	65.4 ± 8.0*	N/A†
	Lesser saphenous vein[4]	34	54.7 ± 9.9*	54.7 ± 9.9*	55.0 ± 14.1*	N/A†
	p value		$p = 0.268$	$p = 0.417$	$p = 0.261$	—
G	Claudication	35	63.8 ± 9.2	75.8 ± 8.1	87.4 ± 7.1	85.2 ± 6.9
	Limb salvage	178	45.1 ± 7.7	52.3 ± 7.9	66.6 ± 9.5	72.8 ± 5.5
	p value		$p = 0.079$	$p = 0.048$	$p = 0.056$	$p = 0.09$
H	Primary autogenous bypass	435	65.1 ± 4.2	79.7 ± 3.3	91.3 ± 4.3	75.1 ± 4.3
	Secondary autogenous bypass	154	49.5 ± 6.3	59.1 ± 5.8	72.4 ± 6.6	74.4 ± 4.8
	p value		$p = 0.020$	$p = 0.001$	$p = 0.003$	$p = 0.456$

* Follow-up interval is 4 years for these groups.
† N/A = not applicable for comparsion.
[1] Greater saphenous vein graphs include in situ, nonreversed, translocated, and reversed grafts.
[2] Alternative vein grafts include arm vein grafts, lesser saphenous vein grafts, and composite vein grafts.
[3] Includes arm vein and arm vein composite vein grafts.
[4] Includes lesser saphenous vein and lesser saphenous vein composite vein grafts.

The variation from series to series seen in Table 13.5 largely reflects differences in patient populations and patient selection for surgery. A prosthetic bypass to a compromised popliteal artery with single-vessel runoff cannot be expected to provide the durability of a similar bypass to a relatively disease-free popliteal artery with two- or three-vessel runoff. Most published series represent the summation of some combination of these extremes, yet a preponderance of one or the other will shift overall patency rates to the higher or lower end of the range accordingly.

Recent experience with Dacron and umbilical vein grafts for infrainguinal reconstruction is more limited. Rosenthal et al compared Dacron and PTFE for femoropopliteal bypass and found similar results, with 5-year primary patency rates of 67% and 65%, respectively.[27] The experience with umbilical vein grafts has been similar, with 5-year patency rates of 60 to 81% reported for above-knee popliteal bypasses.[19,30] Aneurysmal degeneration of umbilical vein grafts has been a significant problem during long-term follow-up. Dardik and colleagues reported aneurysmal degeneration in 36%

and noted dilatation in an additional 21% of cases at 5 years of follow-up.[31]

FUNCTIONAL OUTCOME AFTER INFRAINGUINAL ARTERIAL RECONSTRUCTION

Vascular surgeons have historically judged the results of infrainguinal arterial reconstruction based on patency rates, limb salvage rates, and, in some cases, maintenance of hemodynamic improvement. More recently, we have begun to focus on the objective measurement of functional patient outcomes after infrainguinal surgery, with greater emphasis placed on physical function and comfort, role function, and general health perception. A small early study by Albers et al employed Spitzers' QL INDEX to assess quality of life in a series of patients, 3, 6, and 12 months after treatment for ischemic lesions of the foot. This index is based on occupational status, activities of daily living, perception of own health, support structure, and outlook on life. Not surprisingly, patients who had limb salvage

Table 13–5. Infrainguinal Reconstruction with PTFE

| | | 5-Year Primary Patency Rate (%) | | | | | | | |
| | | AK and BK | | AK | | Femoropopliteal AK Claudication | | Infrapopliteal | |
Author	Year	(N)	Patency	(N)	Patency	(N)	Patency	(N)	Patency
Hobson[22]	1985	(80)	22%					(41)	12%
Charlesworth[23]	1985	(134)	24%	(53)	39%				
Tilanus[24]	1985	(24)	37%						
Sterpetti[25]	1985			(90)	58%	(41)	76%		
Veith[17]	1986	(171)	38%	(91)	38%			(98)	12%
Whittemore[18]	1989	(279)	37%	(182)	42%	(64)	62%	(21)	12%
Patterson[26]	1990			(138)	54%				
Prendeville[20]	1990			(114)	42%	(44)	57%		
Rosenthal[27]	1990					(100)	65%		
Davies[28]	1992			(48)	63%				
Alders[19]	1992			(49)	39%	(41)	42%		
Quinones-Baldrich[21]	1992	(294)	59%	(219)	61%	(110)	68%	(28)	22%
Pevec[29]	1992	(85)	27%						
Weighted Average		(1067)	40%	(984)	50%	(400)	63%	(202)	14%

Abbreviations: AK, above-knee; BK, below-knee.

through either conservative management or revascularization had a significantly improved outcome compared to those undergoing immediate or delayed amputation.[32] A larger study was recently reported by Gibbons et al, including 156 patients undergoing infrainguinal reconstruction for limb-threatening ischemia who were assessed with questionnaires prior to treatment and after 6 months of follow-up.[33] The questionnaires focused on general health status, activities of daily living, social activity, mental well-being, and a vitality scale adopted from the SF-36 Health Survey. At 6 months of follow-up, improved mental well-being, vitality, and activities of daily living were documented. These patients with better functional status and better general well-being at baseline showed more improvement than patients with poorer baseline status. Despite the documented improvements in well-being and function, however, only 45% of patients reported that they were "back to normal" at 6 months. This was attributed to the poor general health status of many of these patients and their significant comorbidity (84% had diabetes mellitus and 83% had cardiac problems).

CONCLUSIONS

One of the major achievements of vascular surgery over the past three decades has been steady improvement in the results of infrainguinal arterial reconstruction. These advances are attributable to a number of factors including technical improvements, better perioperative management, better risk factor modification, superior graft surveillance, and, finally, improved reporting standards. Ischemic limbs that formerly required amputation are now often salvaged through aggressive limb-saving operations. Nonetheless, these efforts are expensive and may be associated with significant morbidity and even mortality. Careful scrutiny of the functional outcomes and cost effectiveness of these procedures will be required in the future to justify these operations and continue our progress. The results of infrainguinal surgery must be continuously updated to serve as a benchmark against which the results of evolving endovascular techniques should be compared.

REFERENCES

1. Rutherford RB, Flanigan DP, Gupta SK, et al. Suggested standards for reports dealing with lower extremity ischemia. *J Vasc Surg* 1986;4:80–94
2. Myers KA. Reporting standards for evaluating intervention. *Cardiovasc Surg* 1995;3:455–461
3. Underwood CJ, Faragher EB, Charlesworth D. The uses and abuses of life-table methods in vascular surgery. *Br J Surg* 1984;71:496–498.
4. Donaldson MC, Mannick JA, Whittemore AD. Femoral-distal bypass with in situ greater saphenous vein: long-term results using the Mills valvulotome. *Ann Surg* 1991;213:457–465.
5. Harrington ME, Maringtom EB, Schanzer H, et al. The dorsalis pedis bypass—moderate success in difficult situations. *J Vasc Surg* 1992;409–416
6. Belkin M, Conte MS, Donaldson MC, et al. Preferred strategies for secondary infrainguinal bypas: lessons learned from 300 consecutive reoperations. *J Vasc Surg* 1995;21:282–295.

7. Whittemore AD, Donaldson MC, Mannick JA. Infrainguinal reconstruction for patients with chronic renal insufficiency. *J Vasc Surg* 1992;17:32–39.

8. Donaldson MC, Weinberg DS, Belkin M, et al. Screening the hypercoagulable states in vascular practice: a preliminary study. *J Vasc Surg* 1990;11:825–831.

9. Taylor LM, Edwards JM, Porter JM. Present status of reversed vein bypass grafting: five-year results of a modern series. *J Vasc Surg* 1990;11:193–206.

10. Bergamini TM, Towne JB, Bandyk DF, Seabrook GR, Schmitt DD. Experience with in situ saphenous vein bypass during 1981 to 1989: determinant factors of lonterm patency. *J Vasc Surg* 1991;13:137–149.

11. Leather RP, Fitzgerald K. Personal communication from Vascular Data Registry, Department of Surgery, Albany Medical College, October 19, 1992.

12. Pomposelli FB, Marcaccio EJ, Gibbons GW, et al. Dorsalis pedis arterial bypass: durable limb salvage for foot ischemia in patients with diabetes mellitus. *J Vasc Surg* 1995:21:375–384.

13. Chang BB, Paty PSK, Shah DM, Leather RP. The lesser saphenous vein: an appreciated source of autogenous vein. *J Vasc Surg* 1992:15:152–157.

14. Belkin M, Donaldson MC, Whittemore AD. Composite autogenous vein grafts. *Semin Vasc Surg* 1995;:8:202–208.

15. Chang BB, Darling RC, Bock DEM, et al. The use of spliced vein bypass for infrainguinal arterial reconstruction. *J Vasc Surg* 1995;21:403–412.

16. Harris RW, Andros G, Salles-Cunha SX, et al. Totally autogenous venovenous composite bypass grafts: salvage of the almost irretrievable extremity. *Arch Surg* 1986;121:1128–11320.

17. Veith FJ, Gupta SK, Ascer E, et al. Six-year prospective multicenter randomized comparison of autologous saphenous vein and expanded polytetrafuoroethylene graft in infrainguinal arterial reconstruction. *J Vasc Surg* 1986;3:104–114.

18. Whittemore AD, Kent KC, Donaldson MC, et al. What is the proper role of polytetrafluoroethylene grafts in infrainguinal reconstruction? *J Vasc Surg* 1989;10:299–305.

19. Aalders GJ, van Vroonhoven TJM. PTFE versus HUV in above-knee femoropopliteal bypass. Six year results of a randomized clinical trail. *J Vasc Surg* 1992;16:816.

20. Prendiville EJ, Yeager A, O'Donnell TF, et al. Long-term results with the above-knee popliteal expanded polytetrafluoroethylene graft. *J Vasc Surg* 1990;11:517–524.

21. Quinones-Baldrich WJ, Prego AA, Ucelay-Gomez R, et al. Long-term results of infrainguinal revascularization with polytetrafluoroethylene: a ten-year experience. *J Vasc Surg* 1992;16:209–217.

22. Hobson RW II, Lynch TG, Zafar J, et al. Results of revascularization and amputation in severe lower extremity ischemia: a five-year clinical experience. *J Vasc Surg* 1985;2:174–185.

23. Charlesworth PM, Brewster DC, Darling RC, Robison JG, Hallet JW. The fate of polytetrafluoroethylene grafts in lower limb bypass surgery: a six-year follow-up. *Br J Surg* 1985;72:896–899.

24. Tilanus HW, Obertop H, Van Urk H. Saphenous vein or PTFE for femoropopliteal bypass. A prospective randomized trail. *Ann Surg* 1985;202:780–782.

25. Sterpetti AV, Schultz RD, Feldhaus RJ, Peetz DJ Jr. Seven-year experience with polytetrafluoroethylene as above-knee femoropopliteal bypass graft. Is it worthwile to preserve the autologous saphenous vein? *J Vasc Surg* 1985;2:907–912.

26. Patterson RB, Fowl RJ, Kempczinski RF, Gewirtz R, Shukla R. Preferential use of ePTFE for above-knee femoropopliteal bypass grafts. *J Vasc Surg* 1990;4:338–343.

27. Rosenthal D, Evans D, McKinsey J, et al. Prosthetic above-knee femoropopliteal bypass for intermittent claudication. *J Cardiovasc Surg* 1990;31:462–468.

28. Davies MG, Feeley TM, O'Malley MK, et al. Infrainguinal polytetrefluoroethylene grafts: saved limbs or wasted effort? A report on ten years experience. *Ann Vasc Surg* 1991;5:519–524.

29. Pevec WC, Darling RC, L'Italien GJ, Abbott WM. Femoropopliteal reconstruction with knitted, nonvelour Dacron versus expanded polytetrafluoroethylene. *J Vasc Surg* 1992;16:60-65.

30. McCollum C, Kenchington G, Alexander C, et al. PTFE or HUV for femoropopliteal bypass: a multi-center trail. *Eur Vasc Surg* 191;5:435–443.

31. Dardik H, Miller N, Dardik A, et al. A decade of experience with the glutaraldehyde-tanned human umbilical cord vein graft for revascularization of the lower limb. *J Vasc Surg* 1988;7:336–346.

32. Albers M, Fratezi AC, De Luccia N. Assessment of quality of life of patients with severe ischemia as a result of infrainguinal arterial occlusive disease. *J Vasc Surg* 1992;16:54–59.

33. Gibbons GW, Burgess AM, Guadagnoli E, et al. Return to well-being after infrainguinal revascularization. *J Vasc Surg* 1995;21:35–45.

14

The Role of Duplex Surveillance in the Management of Infrainguinal Bypass Grafts

Brad L. Johnson, M.D.
Dennis F. Bandyk, M.D.

Duplex scanning has been established as the standard method for postoperative surveillance of lower extremity revascularization procedures and may also improve intraoperative surgical technique. While it is accepted by most vascular surgeons as a method of maximizing graft patency and limb salvage, a number of issues such as testing intervals, correlation of hemodynamic and ultrasound results, point of intervention determination, and repair method (ie, surgery vs. balloon angioplasty) are not clearly delineated. Prior to duplex scanning, the history and physical exam, ankle-brachial index (ABI), and angiography were used to follow infrainguinal bypass grafts. Although angiography provides a clear anatomic picture of the graft with detection of abnormalities, it is costly and invasive and does not provide hemodynamic information. The symptomatic history and physical exam continue to play a role, yet they often fail to change prior to thrombosis of the bypass.[1] With the addition of postoperative duplex scanning, graft patency and limb slavage have improved, with an associated decrease in patient morbidity[2] Failure to repair a stenotic graft leads to increased failure, as demonstrated by Grigg et al and Moody et al, with a 21% and 23% incidence of graft thrombosis in stenotic grafts not repaired, respectively.[3,4]

Conversely, graft surveillance programs have resulted in assisted-primary patency rates of 82% to 93% at 5 years compared to 30% to 50% secondary patency rates of thrombosed vein grafts.[5,6] Now that the clinical benefit of duplex scan monitoring of infrainguinal bypass grafts has been demonstrated, research efforts have been directed toward identifying the proper scanning interval and criteria for intervention. The many variables that influence the interval of duplex scan surveillance and the timing of intervention will be discussed

to construct a practical algorithm that can be applied by the practicing vascular surgeon. Also, a brief discussion is provided on intraoperative duplex scanning, its role in the improvement of intraoperative surgical technique and decision making, and its effect on the postoperative surveillance program.

GRAFT FAILURE: MECHANISMS AND TEMPORAL OCCURRENCE

Essential to establishing an efficient surveillance protocol is a basic understanding of graft failure causes and temporal occurrence (see Chapter 18). Early perioperative failure (<30 days) is most commonly due to technical error or occasional graft thrombosis resulting from a hypercoagulable syndrome or platelet aggregation. Technical errors involve anastomotic stricture/intimal flaps, suture stenosis of the conduit, retained valves in the in situ or nonreversed vein conduits, adjacent inflow or outflow artery stenoses, graft entrapment/torsion, or retained thrombus. These errors are preventable with the use of intraoperative graft monitoring via angiography, angioscopy, or duplex scan. While angiography, the most commonly utilized modality, is quick and easy to interpret, it does not provide any hemodynamic information important in long-term graft surveillance. It also fails to detect 10% of retained valve leaflets or platelet aggregation with associated turbulent flow and can lead to unnecessary repair of strictures that have no effect on graft hemodynamics.[7] Angioscopy can better identify retained valve sites and quantify anastomotic or vein graft strictures, but it also does not provide hemodynamic information. Intraoperative duplex scanning provides not only anatomic assessment of the graft and

163

inflow and outflow vessels, but also hemodynamic information that assists in planning long-term graft surveillance. It detects graft anatomic problems, which, if hemodynamically insignificant, do not need repair. Platelet aggregation, though rare, is detectable with the newer high-resolution intraoperative scan heads. Disadvantages include the expense and availability of the duplex scanner, slight increase in operative time (approximately 15 minutes), and proper interpretation of findings. These disadvantages are greatly outweighed by the decreased incidence of an immediate return to the operating room for graft thrombosis and the hemodynamic information (useful in postoperative graft surveillance) provided.[8]

From 30 days to 2 years postoperatively, the most common cause of graft stenosis is myointimal hyperplasia within the vein conduit or at the anastomotic sites. These lesions occur in 11 to 33% of all saphenous vein grafts, with approximately 75% developing within the first year.[9–11] Recent work in our institution suggests that in situ vein conduits, especially those with normal intraoperative duplex scans, have different incidences of myointimal hyperplasia. Ten percent of in situ saphenous vein grafts with normal intraoperative duplex scans failed or required revision compared to 28% of reversed vein grafts, 20% of nonreversed vein grafts, and 32% of spliced vein grafts. Also, reversed vein bypasses tended to develop more multiple or diffuse areas of myointimal hyperplasia. Most postoperative vein graft stenoses and thromboses occurred in patients with abnormal intraoperative duplex scans demonstrating mild to moderate lesions that progressed, rather than inadequate runoff.[12] Progression

of atherosclerotic disease leads to most graft stenoses more than 2 years following surgery. Lesions can develop within the graft or, more commonly, in adjacent arteries. Lesions that develop in adjacent arteries usually decrease flow within the graft. Therefore, this etiology should be considered if graft surveillance demonstrates a continual decrease in graft velocities throughout the entire conduit without any evidence of graft stenoses. Aneurysmal degeneration within the vein conduit (Fig. 14–1) or at the anastomotic site, while rare, can lead to occlusion or distal embolization. Usually this is detected on routine postoperative surveillance scans, but it should be suspected when graft failure occurs following a previously normal duplex scan imaged only at intermittent sites.

HEMODYNAMICS

A clear understanding of normal graft hemodynamics during the first year postimplantation is one of the keys to a successful graft surveillance program. Factors that affect the blood flow within grafts include the type of conduit, inflow and outflow arteries, prior degree of limb ischemia, and hemodynamic status of the patient. Peak systolic velocities usually exceed 40 cm/sec in vein conduits 3 to 6 mm in diameter. Velocities less than this should lead one to suspect inflow or outflow disease, with low diastolic flow more indicative of poor runoff. Exceptions include arm vein conduits, large varicose vein conduits, or bypasses to isolated tibial or popliteal segments. Bypasses to inframalleolar arteries may have velocities less than 40 cm/sec, but they have been found to average 59 cm/sec compared to tibial

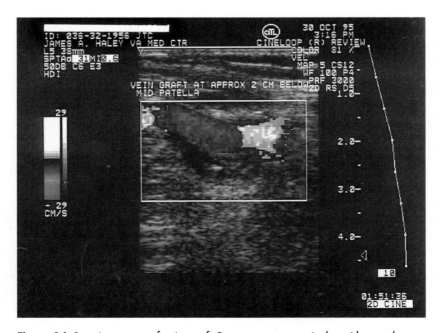

Figure 14–1. Aneurysm of vein graft 2 years postoperatively, with mural thrombus along the posterior wall that resulted in distal arterial embolization.

(77 cm/sec) and popliteal (71 cm/sec) insertion sites.[13] Therefore, peak systolic velocities less than 40 cm/sec do not always predict graft failure, but they are a guide to intervals of graft follow-up and the possible need for adjuncts such as anticoagulation, jump grafts, or distal arteriovenous fistulae. More important, a graft with normal velocities that progressively decrease may indicate impending graft failure. If the graft has no stenotic lesions, then arterial inflow or outflow problems should be suspected and evaluated by angiography. High peak systolic velocities (>150 cm/sec) usually occur as a step-up in stenotic areas but may be present along the entire vein graft or extended segments, indicating a narrow conduit (<3 mm) or a sclerotic vein. Intensive early graft surveillance will be required in these grafts, with possible replacement of the involved area.

Duplex waveform analysis following graft implantation depends on the degree of limb ischemia, runoff vessels, and, rarely, the hemodynamic state of the patient. Patients with critical limb ischemia will develop a hyperemic state associated with vessel vasodilatation, low resistance, and increased diastolic flow within the graft. Over a period of days to weeks, a biphasic waveform will convert a normal arterial triphasic waveform. Taylor et al believe that failure of the graft to convert from a biphasic to a triphasic waveform predicts poorer graft patency.[9] Fifty-four of 63 (86%) grafts that had persistence of the biphasic waveform beyond 3 months developed a stenosis or occlusion. The difference in the development of stenoses and occlusion among grafts that converted to a triphasic waveform when compared to those that remained biphasic was highly significant by chi square analysis ($p < 0.001$). Taylor et al were unable to explain the mechanism for this.

Another infrequent occurrence that we are currently studying is the observation of bypass grafts with waveforms having minimal diastolic flow by intraoperative scan even after the use of intragraft papaverine injection. This has occurred mainly in patients with end-stage renal disease who have severe peripheral atherosclerosis and may be attributable to their rigid, calcified vessel walls, although this remains speculative.

Three characteristic waveform patterns are associated with graft stenosis or pending graft occlusion. *Type I* is the biphasic waveform, with an associated ABI of 0.4 to 0.7, which occurs in more than 50% of abnormal grafts. This is especially true in grafts that on prior scans had a triphasic waveform and converted to biphasic with a drop the ABI. *Type II* is the monophasic waveform, occurring in approximately 40% of grafts with stenoses (Fig. 14–2). Most are asymptomatic, with ABIs ranging from 0.7 to 0.9 and graft stenoses classified as 50 to 75% by duplex scan and arteriography. *Type III* is the staccato waveform, found in 6% of abnormal grafts and associated with a high-grade distal outflow stenosis. This represents backward and forward flow within the conduit and poor progression of blood flow distally. It may lead to poor visualization of the graft by angiography. The combination of velocity measurements, spectral analysis, and ABIs, especially when analyzed sequentially, provides the most comprehensive understanding of graft hemodynamics in terms of predicting outcome.

INTRAOPERATIVE DUPLEX SCANNING

Intraoperative duplex scanning is being increasingly performed as more vascular surgeons acquire familiar-

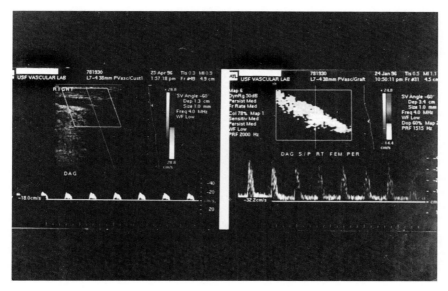

Figure 14–2. Duplex scan on the left showing a monophasic waveform that in a scan 3 months earlier (depicted on the right) had demonstrated a biphasic waveform.

Table 14–1. Bypass Surveillance Protocol: Representative Patient

	PAG	HT	AK	BK	DAG
Intraop*	65	70	70	120	100
PO 7 days†	60	65	68	110	95
PO 6 wks†	55	75	70	120	90
PO 3 mo†	60	65	70	130	100
PO 6 mo†	60	75	75	130	95
PO 9 mo†	55	70	70	150	90
PO 12 mo†	25	30	40	300	35
PO 13 mo†	60	70	75	90	100

Note: Depiction of center stream velocities (cm/sec) at different sites of the graft. Note the decrease in graft flow velocities with increased peak systolic velocity at the below-knee site at 12 months, which returned to normal following balloon angioplasty. PO, postoperative interval; PAG, proximal anastomotic graft; HT, high thigh; AK, above-knee; DAG, distal anastomotic graft.
*Entire bypass scanned.
†Center stream velocities at different sites.

ity with its use and duplex scan heads are specifically designed for operating room use. It provides hemodynamic information as well as anatomic imaging of the infrainguinal bypass graft. It has the ability to determine graft defects and inflow and outflow vessel abnormalities that can result in early graft failure. The use of intraoperative scanning has resulted in an early (<30 day) graft thrombosis rate of only 1.2% (4 of 334 bypasses) at our institution, clearly increasing graft patency and decreasing patient morbidity and hospital stay. Our protocol of intraoperative scanning includes the use of papaverine (30 to 60 mg) injected directly into the vein to augment flow and increase the sensitivity of the study. The entire graft is then imaged, and any color flow abnormalities are Doppler sampled to detect stenosis. Peak systolic velocity is recorded at the proximal and distal anastomoses, three to four graft segments, and inflow and outflow vessels. In addition, in situ saphenous vein grafts are imaged to detect graft vein side branches with the graft occluded distally and the Doppler probe placed proximally, looking for continued diastolic flow. Those graft segments that demonstrate a peak systolic velocity of more than 150 cm/sec or a velocity ratio ($V = \mathrm{PSV}_{\mathrm{at\ lesion}}/\mathrm{PSV}_{\mathrm{proximal}}$) greater than 2.5 undergo immediate operative repair (PSV, peak systolic velocity). Low flow states and platelet aggregation are also detected and appropriate measures taken to prevent graft failure. Furthermore, baseline hemodynamic data are acquired, which will guide postoperative surveillance and possible intervention for infrainguinal bypass graft abnormalities.

TIMING OF SURVEILLANCE AND CRITERIA FOR INTERVENTION

The graft surveillance protocol and criteria for intervention are still evolving. The time interval depicted in Table 14–1 is the one currently used in our vascular surgery department, yet it may vary depending on the patient's clinical situation. Bypass grafts that develop stenotic sites not requiring intervention are duplex scanned at 1- to 2-month intervals to establish stabilization or progression of the lesion(s). Recent research in our institution suggests that in situ vein bypasses that are normal on a duplex scan 6 months postoperatively require less frequent surveillance. In cases in which the duplex scan was judged to have no significant anatomic or hemodynamic abnormality, 11 (10%) of 111 in situ vein bypasses failed or required revision during follow-up compared to 31 (28%) of 109 reversed vein bypasses ($p < 0.001$); chi square = 12.0). During the first postoperative year, reversed vein bypasses were revised more frequently than in situ bypasses for duplex-identified stenosis or unexpected thrombosis. Only 5 (4%) of 131 in situ vein bypasses required revision or failed more than 6 months postoperatively. Accordingly, the intensity of our graft surveillance is now based on graft type and on the results of intraoperative duplex scans (Table 14–2).

The value of graft surveillance of prosthetic conduits is controversial. Most studies suggest that it is not beneficial,[14,15] although Calliagaro et al reported that duplex scanning is more sensitivity than other modalities for predicting the falure of prosthetic grafts.[16] Duplex scanning had a sensitivity of 81% versus 24% for grafts followed by clinical symptoms, ABI, and ankle pulse volume recordings. Calliagaro et al found that 48% of stenoses were located at anastomtic sites, 38% at inflow or outflow arteries, and 14% within the graft. Yet failure of a prosthetic graft is not as detrimental as vein graft occlusion because prosthetic grafts can easily be replaced, so that the cost of an intensive surveillance program may not be justified. One could derive from this that prior to discharge from the hospital, a limited graft study of only adjacent inflow and outflow arteries and anastomotic sites, as well as determination of midstream graft flow, would be adequate surveillance for

Table 14–2. Rank Order Listing of Vein Bypass Graft Types Relative to the Intensity (Frequency) of Postoperative Duplex Surveillance

Type of Vein Bypass	Relative Need for Duplex Surveillance
	Intensive surveillance (every 1–3 months)
Modified reversed vein bypasses	
Alternative vein bypasses	
Reversed vein bypasses	
Nonreversed vein bypasses	
In situ saphenous vein bypass	
In situ vein bypasses with normal intraoperative duplex scan	
	Infrequent surveillance (every 6–12 months)

prosthetic grafts. Furthermore, documentation of low flow (<45 cm/sec) has led us to recommend anticoagulation in an attempt to decrease prosthetic graft thrombosis. Currently, we obtain a baseline duplex scan postoperatively to document residual lesions or low graft flow, with limited duplex studies at 3 months followed by repeat scans at 6-month intervals. While the hemodynamic classification of graft stenoses is well established (Table 14–3), criteria for intervention are less clear. Following detection of graft abnormality, lesions with a PSV or less than 300 cm/sec with no change in ABI are followed at 6-week intervals (Fig. 14–3). Approximately 30% to 35% of these moderate flow-restricting lesions will resolve and 10 to 20% will remain stable. Those lesions with a PSV greater than 300 cm/sec, velocity ratio above 3.5, or ABI decrease below 0.2 are studied by arteriography or proceed directly to surgery. Following balloon angioplasty or

operative repair, the initial graft surveillance protocol is resumed.

SUMMARY

The optimal graft surveillance program should utilize an early postoperative scan (<7 days following surgery) followed by an intense surveillance protocol within the first year. Initial visualization of the entire graft and adjacent inflow and outflow arteries with determination of peak systolic flow and areas of stenosis, along with ABI, is the first step. However, the key to a successful program is accumulation of further data, with attention to changes in graft hemodynamics and a comprehensive knowledge of how they affect graft patency. Further research should be directed toward increasing efficiency by identifying those grafts that require less frequent surveillance, better criteria for corrective intervention, and which lesions are amenable to balloon angioplasty rather than direct surgical repair (see Chapter 18). Until then, aggressive surveillance, especially in the early postoperative period (<1 year), is essential to maximizing long-term graft patency.

Table 14–3. Classification of Graft Stenosis

Diameter Reduction	Velocity Ratio (Vr) and Velocity Spectra
<20% stenosis	Vr <1.5, mild spectral broadening in systole, peak systolic velocity <150 cm/sec
20–50% stenosis	Vr 1.5–2.5, spectral broadening throughout systole, no change in waveform configuration across stenosis, peak systolic velocity <150 cm/sec
50–75% stenosis	Vr >2.5, severe spectral broadening in systole with reversed flow components, peak systolic velocity >150 cm/sec
>75% stenosis	Vr >3.5, end-diastolic flow velocity in "flow jet" >100 cm/sec, peak systolic flow velocity >300 cm/sec

REFERENCES

1. Barnes RW, Thompson BW, MacDonald CM, et al. Serial noninvasive studies do not herald postoperative failure of femoropopliteal or femorotibial bypass grafts. *Ann Surg* 1989;210:486–494.
2. Bandyk DF, Bergamini TM, Towne JB, et al. Durability of vein graft revision: the outcome of secondary procedures *J Vasc Surg* 1991;13:200–210.
3. Grigg MJ, Nicolaides AN, Wolfe JHN. Femorodistal graft stenoses. *Br J Surg* 1988;75:737–740.
4. Moody AP, Gould DA, Harris PL. Vein graft surveillance improves patency in femoropopliteal bypass. *Eur J Vasc Surg* 1990;4:117–120.

Abnormal Graft Surveillance Algorithm

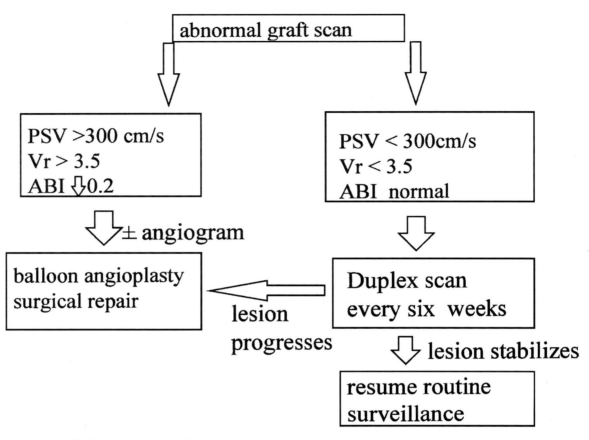

Figure 14–3.   Algorithm for management of abnormal vein graft scans.

5. Donaldson MC, Mannick JA, Whittemore AD. Causes of primary graft failure after in situ saphenous vein bypass grafting *J Vasc Surg* 1991;13:137–149.
6. Bergamini TM, Towne JB, Bandyk DF, et al. Experience with in situ saphenous vein bypass during 1981 to 1989. Determinant factors of long-term patency. *J Vasc Surg* 1991;13:137–149.
7. Bush HL, Corey CA, Nabseth DC. Distal in situ saphenous vein grafts for limb salvage—increased operative flow and postoperative patency. *Am J Surg* 1983:145:542–548.
8. Bandyk D, Mills JL, Gahtan V, et al. Intraoperative duplex scanning of arterial reconstructions: fate of repaired and unrepaired defects. *J Vasc Surg* 1994;20:426–433.
9. Taylor PR, Wolfe JHN, Tyrrell MR, et al. Graft stenosis—justification for 1-year surveillance. *Br J Surg* 1990;77(10):1125–128.
10. Mills JL, Bandyk D, Gahtan V, et al. The origin of infrainguinal vein graft stenosis: a prospective study based on duplex surveillance. *J Vasc Surg* 1995;21:16–25.

11. Mills JL, Fujitani RM, Taylor SM. The characteristics and anatomic distributionof lesions that cause reversed vein graft failure: a five-year prospective study. *J Vasc Surg* 1993;17(1):195–206.
12. Bandyk DF, Johnson BL, Gupta AK, et al. Nature and management of duplex abnormalities encountered during vein bypass grafting. *J Vasc Surg* 1996:24:430–438.
13. Belkin M, Mackey WC, Maclaughlin R, et al. The variation in vein graft flow velocity with luminal diameter and outflow level. *J Vasc Surg* 1992;15:991–999.
14. Lawlike NJ, Hanel KC, Hunt J, et al. Duplex scan surveillance of infrainguinal prosthetic bypass grafts. *J Vasc Surg* 1994;20:637–41.
15. Lundell A, Lindblad B, Berqvist D, et al. Femoropopliteal-cural graft patency is improved by an intensive surveillance program: a prospective randomized study. *J Vasc Surg* 1995;13:26–34.
16. Calligaro KD, Musser DJ, Chen AY, et al. Duplex ultrasonography to diagnose failing arterial prosthetic grafts. *Surgery* 1996;120(3):455–459.

15

Femoropopliteal Angioplasty and Stents: Patient Selection and Results

Robert R. Murray, Jr., M.D.
James D. Lutz, M.D.

Femoropopliteal percutaneous transluminal angioplasty (PTA) was first described by Dotter and Judkins in 1964.[1] This original coaxial catheter (Dotter) technique was further improved with the introduction of a new double-lumen balloon catheter technique by Gruntzig and Hopff in 1974 for the treatment of peripheral arterial disease (PAD).[2,3] Since then, balloon catheter PTA has become widely accepted by patients and the medical community for the treatment of PAD.

Although thousands of patients have experienced femoropopliteal PTA and many articles have been written about it, there has been much confusion and controversy concerning patient selection and outcome. This was due to failure to provide rigorous statistical analysis and the absence of standards for evaluating and reporting results initially. To address this problem, standards were adopted and later modified in 1993 to allow a more meaningful comparison of the various treatment modalities for patients with femoropopliteal PAD.[4,5] Also, practice guidelines have been developed for femoropopliteal PTA to encourage a more uniform application of this technique.[6,7] The adoption of these standards and guidelines has helped to further our understanding of conventional PTA, particularly as it relates to other endovascular procedures and bypass surgery. To date there have been too few long-term prospective, randomized studies comparing femoropopliteal PTA and surgery.[8,9] The Society of Cardiovascular and Interventional Radiology's (SCVIR) national registry and larger multicenter trials will help to clarify and solidify our understanding in the future.

PATIENT CLASSIFICATION AND PTA GUIDELINES

The diagnosis of femoropopliteal PAD can be established with a thorough history and physical exam. Appropriate noninvasive hemodynamic testing is confirmatory and helps to document and quantify the severity of ischemia. The patient is then stratified in terms of the severity of chronic limb ischemia[5] (Table 15–1). The Fontaine classification or grade is more popular in Europe than in the United States, where most patients are categorized (0 to 6) largely based on the efforts of the Society for Vascular Surgery, the North American Chapter of the International Society for Cardiovascular Surgery, and the SCVIR.[4,5] The seven-category system allows a more thorough analysis of the patient mix and aids in clinical assessment of treatment outcomes.

After appropriate clinical evaluation and categorization of the patient's ischemia, angiography is performed for those who have either failed medical management for debilitating claudication or have critical ischemia. It is important to describe fully all vascular lesions, especially to compare the results of various endovascular and surgical techniques. Lesions are described on the following bases:

1. Location and type
   Eccentric or concentric
   Calcified or noncalcified
   Focal of diffuse
   Occlusion or stenosis
2. Length of lesion
   Less than 2 cm

Table 15–1. Clinical Criteria for Categories of Chronic Limb Ischemia

Grade (Fontaine Classification)	Category	Clinical Description	Noninvasive Laboratory Description
	0	Asymptomatic, no hemodynamically significant occlusive disease	Normal results of treadmill/stress test*
I	1	Mild claudication	Treadmill exercise completed, postexercise AP greater than 50 mm Hg but more than 25 mm Hg less than normal
	2	Moderate claudication	Symptoms between those of categories 1 and 3
	3	Severe claudication	Treadmill exercise cannot be completed, postexercise AP less than 50 mm Hg
II	4	Ischemic rest pain	Resting AP of 40 mm Hg or less, flat or barely pulsatile ankle or metatarsal plethysmographic tracing, toe pressure less than 30 mm Hg
III	5	Minor tissue loss, nonhealing ulcer, focal gangrene with diffuse pedal ischemia	Resting AP of 60 mm Hg or less, ankle or metatarsal plethysmographic tracing flat or barely pulsatile, toe pressure less than 40 mm Hg
	6	Major tissue loss extending above transmetatarsal level, functional foot no longer salvageable	Same as for category 5

Source: Modified from Rutherford RB, Flannigan DP, Gupta SK, et al. Suggested standards for reports dealing with lower extremity ischemia. *J Vasc Surg* 1986:4:80–94.
Abbreviation: AP, ankle pressure.
*Five minutes at 2 mph on 12-degree incline.

2 to 5 cm
5 to 10 cm
More than 10 cm
3. Status of run-off
Good (two- to three-vessel)
Poor (zero- to one-vessel)[5,7]

Objective hemodynamic evaluation consists of determining the resting ankle/brachial index (ABI) at a minimum, with pulse-volume recording, Doppler waveform analysis, and exercise ABI as deemed appropriate.[5]

For patients with significant lifestyle-limiting claudication or critical ischemia, the angiographic appearance is a major determinant of whether the patient is a candidate for PTA or bypass. It is not the sole determinant, however; other factors such as technical success rate, short- and long-term durability, risk of complications, operator skill, and patient preference must be considered. The American Heart Association (AHA) Task Force guidelines for femoropopliteal PTA were published with input from councils on cardiovascular radiology, arteriosclerosis, cardiothoracic and vascular surgery, clinical cardiology, epidemiology, and prevention [7] (Table 15–2). These guidelines, however, must be applied individually to fit the unique clinical circumstance of each patient. For physicians to apply these guidelines more effectively and for patients to make informed decisions concerning percutaneous or surgical options, a thorough understanding of the results and risks of femoropopliteal PTA is needed. A discussion of the technique of femoropopliteal angioplasty is beyond the scope of this chapter, but it is presented in detail elsewhere.[10,11]

PATIENT SELECTION

The AHA guidelines were developed based on results from available literature and experience, with emphasis on seccess rate and patency. Becker et al summarized many reports on femoropopliteal PTA from the 1970s and 1980s (4304 procedures), noting an initial patency of 81% and a 2-year patency of 67%.[12] Many of these early reported patency rates are not applicable to today's standards because of improvement in balloon and guidewire technology, advances in pharmacologic adjunctive agents, and increased operator experience. Also, more strict and uniform practice guidelines and reporting standards have been widely adopted. The remainder of this chapter emphasizes data from the more recent experience, particularly with respect to long-term patency.

It has been shown that many factors influence short- and long-term patency following femoropopliteal PTA (Table 15–3). These may be divided into *clinical* and *anatomic* factors based on the angiogram. Of the clinical factors, the mode of presentation (claudication vs critical ischemia) has been shown to strongly influence patency. Patients presenting with claudication have a more benign overall disease process than those presenting with critical ischemia (limb salvage). Claudicants are more apt to have successful early and late clinical PTA patency (Table 15–4). Hunink et al showed that for patients undergoing PTA for stenotic lesions, claudicants had better 5-year patency than those with criti-

Table 15–2.   AHA Task Force Guidelines for femoropopliteal Angioplasty

	Definition	Appropriate Vascular Lesion
Category 1	Lesion for which PTA alone is the procedure of choice. PTA of these lesions will have a high technical success rate and will generally provide complete relief of symptoms or normalization of pressure gradients.	1. Single stenosis up to 5 cm in length and not at origin of SFA or distal portions of popliteal artery. 2. Single occlusion up to 3 cm in length not at origin of SFA or distal portion of popliteal artery.
Category 2	Lesions that are well suited to PTA. Treatment will provide complete relief or significant improvement in symptoms, pulses, or pressure gradients. Includes lesions that will be treated by procedures to be followed by surgical bypass to treat multilevel disease	1. Single stenosis 5–10 cm in length not involving the distal popliteal artery. 2. Single occlusion 3–10 cm in length not involving the distal popliteal artery. 3. Stenosis up to 5 cm in length that is heavily calcified. 4. Multiple lesions (stenoses or occlusions) each less than 3 cm in length. 5. Single or multiple lesions in which there is no continuous tibial runoff to improve inflow for distal surgical bypass.
Category 3	Lesions that may be treated with PTA but that, beacuse of disease extent, location, or severity have a significantly lower chance of initial technical success or long-term benefit than if treated with bypass. PTA may be performed, generally because of patient risk factors or lack of suitable bypass material.	1. Single occlusion 3–10 cm in length involving distal popliteal artery. 2. Multiple focal lesions, each 3–5 cm in length; may be heavilty calcified. 3. Single lesion (stenoses or occlusion) more than 10 cm in length.
Category 4	Extensive disease in which PTA has a limited role because of the low technical success rate or small long-term benefit. In very-high-risk patients or in those for whom no surgical procedure is applicable, PTA may have some use.	1. Complete common femoral artery SFA occlusions. 2. Complete popliteal and proximal trifurcation occlusions. 3. Severe diffuse disease with multiple lesions and no intervening normal vascular segments.

Abbreviation: SFA, superficial femoral artery.

Table 15–3.   Factors Associated with PTA Results

Favorable	Unfavorable
Claudication	Critical ischemia
Stenosis	Occlusion
Short lesion	Long lesion
Good runoff	Poor runoff
Palpable pulse after PTA	No palpable pulse after PTA
Concentric lesion	Eccentric lesion
No residual stenosis	Residual stenosis

Table 15–4.   Femoropopliteal PTA Patency (%)

	Claudiants			Critical Ischemia		
	1 mo	1 yr	3 yr	1 mo	1 yr	3 yr
Adar[13]	89.1	69.8	62.4	76.8	50.3	43.1
Johnston[14]	93.1			72.0		
Stanley[15]	75			54		

cal ischemia (55% vs 29%).[16] They reported 5-year patency for occlusions of 36%.[16]

Risk factors such as smoking, hyperlipidemia, and hypertension have not specifically been associated with a poor femoropopliteal PTA outcome. Diabetes mellitus has been shown by some to reduce long-term patency,[17] but these results have not been universally confirmed.[14,18–20] It is more probable that some diabetic populations present with more advanced PAD (ie, critical ischemia or very poor runoff), which decreases long-term patency.

The patency rate is also determined to some extent by the anatomic characteristics of the patient's atherosclerotic disease. The type of lesion dilated (stenosis or occlusion) may play a role in long-term durability. A statistically significant difference was noted between patients treated for stenosis vs. occlusion.[14,16,19,21] The stenotic group showed better long-term patency; however, this may be due in part to a confounding variable. Most technical failures occur due to inability to cross a lesion successfully, which is more difficult in patients with complete occlusion.[17] It has been shown that if an occlusion can be traversed and dilated, its long-term patency is similar to that of stenotic lesions.[17,22,23]

Patients with long, stenotic arterial segments tend to have worse patency than those with short segment involvement. Although long occlusions may show worse patency than short occlusions,[15,23] it is often difficult to determine which portion of an occlusion is due to underlying atherosclerotic disease as opposed to superimposed thrombus. This may represent a negative selection bias against PTA. While a recent report showed improved technical success and improved long-term patency (including both stenotic and occlusive lesions),[24] others have shown that PTA of long, diffuse stenoses (>7 cm) had the poorest long-term patency.[18,25] Careful patient selection and clear short-term objectives (eg, ulcer healing) appear prudent.

Good runoff (two or three crural vessels to the ankle)[14,15,18,21,22] and palpable peripheral pulses after the procedure[17] are associated with significantly better long-term clinical patency than poor runoff. Concentric lesions also show better long-term patency than eccentric ones.[22,23] The presence of a residual stenosis after PTA is associated with worse patency and may be due to vascular recoil or underdilatation.[17]

It should be noted that regardless of the patient's clinical presentation or lesion morphology, most clinical failures are seen in the first year after PTA.[8,13,18,21-23,26] Restenosis due to intimal hyperplasia occurs within months after PTA, whereas progression of atherosclerosis is probably a more important cause 9 months or more after PTA.[27] Patients who experience the best long-term results with PTA (ie, claudicant, short concentric stenosis, good runoff) also tend to have less aggressive restenosis or slower progression of atherosclerosis in general. Characteristics that are favorable for femoropopliteal PTA have been discussed, but there have been few studies adequately comparing PTA to surgical bypass as an option for revascularization.

PTA VERSUS SURGERY

After a patient with femoropopliteal occlusive disease fails conservative therapy, the principal revascularization options are PTA and surgical bypass. The only long-term prospective, randomized studies comparing surgery and femoropopliteal PTA for patients with chronic limb ischemia (categories 2 to 5) showed no significant difference between the surgical bypass or PTA group of patients[8,9] (Table 15–5). Randomized patients were acceptable candidates for either procedure and had angiographic evidence of significant stenosis or occlusion.

Hunink and colleagues developed a model to evaluate patency results, quality-adjusted life expectancy, lifetime costs, and cost effectiveness ratios for patients undergoing PTA versus bypass surgery.[28] They analyzed 26 reports published after 1985 including those on 4800 PTAs and 4511 surgeries. It was shown that initial treatment with PTA was more effective and saved lifetime expenditures compared to surgery for *patients with claudication* due to femoropopliteal disease (stenosis or occlusion) and for *patients with chronic critical ischemia* due to femoropopliteal stenosis. Bypass surgery was more effective for those with critical ischemia due to occlusion.

Long-term patency in patients presenting with chronic critical ischemia is most likely not as important as achieving a specific clinical goal (eg, ulcer healing) because these patients usually have severe generalized atherosclerosis and resultant high comorbidity and mortality rates.[29] Patients initially presenting with an ankle-arm index ≤0.3 had a 36% survival rate at 6 years; 57% of the deaths were related to vascular causes.[30] Several series have reported an overall patient survival for this group ranging from 70% at 1 year[31] to 57% at 5 years (excluding 5.2% operative mortality).[32] Blair et al showed these patients to have a 2.3 times greater risk of death than amputation during the reporting period.[33]

It has been shown that a high restenosis rate in this group of patients does not necessarily mean a high clinical failure rate, especially for patients with ulceration or tissue loss. Ray et al reported a 6-month restenosis rate of 55% but a recurrent ulceration rate of only 12.5%.[34] Thus, the second European Consensus Document on Chronic Critical Leg Ischemia recommends PTA as the first option for this group of patients when possible, even though they may eventually require surgery.[35] They estimate that PTA may be applicable to as many as 25% of patients presenting with chronic critical ischemia.

Because bypass surgery is more effective for lesions that are unfavorable to treatment with PTA, the two methods of revascularization should be viewed as complementary rather than competitive. Bypass surgery is more effective in treating long-segment, diffuse stenosis or occlusion particularly involving the origin of

Table 15–5. Randomized PTA versus Surgery[8]

	Bypass		PTA	
	Patency	Limb Survival	Patency	Limb Survival
Claudication	57.7	85.1	59.5	92.7
Rest pain	56.3	59.7	52.5	90.9

Note: Median follow-up period was 4 years.

the superficial femoral artery or distal popliteal artery and trifurcation. For those who are candidates for either PTA or surgery, the results are comparable.[8,9] However, it is very important to note that the procedures and consequence of failure are not equivalent. Patients undergoing PTA may avoid the pain, expense,[36] longer hospital stay,[9,37] and longer postprocedural convalescence of surgical bypass. They would also save autogenous vein for possible future revascularization, especially coronary bypass. Frail patients who are poor surgical risks may benefit from the less invasive nature of PTA.

As a consequence of a failed *attempt* at revascularization with PTA, most patients' clinical status[38–40] or subsequent successful surgical bypass[33] is not negatively impacted. Also, patients are usually no worse off clinically if there is a restenosis or reocclusion after successful PTA. Most restenoses occur in the same segment and are similar in appearance to the primary lesion.[26,34,41] It should be noted that not all clinical PTA failures are due to restenosis of the original lesion. A surprising number of patients (8 to 14%) in fact showed the prior PTA site to be patent angiographically; clinical worsening was due to disease progression elsewhere.[26,42] Repeat PTA is thought to have a risk and an outcome similar to those of the initial PTA,[17,22,38] although a recent study disputes this.[41] For patients with chronic critical ischemia, limb salvage is not significantly different for those initially treated with PTA compared to surgical bypass.[33] Therefore, the patient's clinical status and possible revascularization options are not significantly worse as a result of a failed PTA attempt.

The usual benign clinical course following failed PTA contrasts to that of the less favorable course following failed surgical bypass. For patients treated with bypass surgery, careful follow-up evaluation is important to identify early graft failure before thrombosis occurs.[43,44] Repeat surgery is almost always indicated to maintain the patency of occluded grafts, whether preceded by thrombolysis or thrombectomy.[45] The 5-year patency of 28% for thrombosed grafts treated with thrombectomy and revision is disappointing.[46] Some surgeons avoid revision of failed bypass grafts and advocate placement of a second venous graft for optimum results (5-year limb salvage, 90%).[47] Thus the patient's clinical status is usually worse as a result of a graft stenosis (PTA or revision) or an occlusion (thrombolysis, thrombectomy, revision, or repeat bypass) compared to failed PTA.

COMPLICATIONS

The overall complication rate for *diagnostic arteriography* in patients with claudication or critical ischemia is approximately 2%; patients with congestive heart failure and those using furosemide have been shown to be at greater risk than others.[48] It is difficult to arrive at a consensus on the historical complication rate of femoropopliteal PTA, as reported from numerous institutions, because of differences in patient selection, procedure technique, and the variability of reporting complications. Accordingly, standards were developed for reporting PTA complications, as they were for reporting patency.[4,5]

Complications are categorized as procedure related (within 24 hours of the procedure) or nonprocedure related. Deaths occurring within 30 days of PTA are considered surgical mortality. Uniform reporting standards now allow comparison of complication risk among various revascularization procedures if patient populations are similar. It should be emphasized that failure to pass an obstruction or dilate a lesion is considered a technical failure and not a procedural complication.

Differences in patient population influence the risk of complication. Elderly patients (>65 years old) and those presenting with critical ischemia have a significantly increased risk of complications.[16,49,50] Hunink et al showed that more patients presenting with critical ischemia experienced a systemic ($N = 10$) complication as opposed to a local vascular complication ($N = 2$).[16] This is likely due to the more diffuse disease present in patients with critical ischemia and resultant coronary and cerebrovascular comorbidity.

The complications reported from several recent articles on femoropopliteal PTA are shown in Table 15–6. This table demonstrates great variability in the total complication rate (3.6 to 14.4%), as well as variability in the mix of complications. Complications such as hematoma, dissection, thrombosis, and embolization were more consistently reported than others, particularly nonprocedure-related complications. Hopefully, future reports will show more uniformity.

The incidence of peripheral vascular complications associated with PTA (including femoropopliteal PTA) has been published and may serve as a guideline to institutions where PTA is performed.[7] Each institution should keep data on complications as part of a continuing quality improvement program.[6]

It is difficult to determine the consequence of reported complications. Most likely not every reported hematoma required surgical evacuation or transfusion, or altered the level or length of postprocedure observation. Pseudoaneurysm formation (symptomatic and asymptomatic) has been detected by sonography in as many as 18.5% of patients undergoing antegrade femoral catheterization for PTA, but this rate was reduced to 0.9% by increasing the manual compression at least 5 minutes after local bleeding stopped.[52] The consequences of a pseudoaneurysm may be less significant, as some are now successfully treated noninvasively with ultrasound-guided compression repair. Suboptimal or

Table 15–6.   Femoropopliteal PTA: Percentage of Complications

Complications	A (Ref. 9)	B (Ref. 14)	C (Ref. 15)	D (Ref. 16)	E (Ref. 17)	F (Ref. 22)	G (Ref. 23)	H (Ref. 25)	I (Ref. 39)	J (Ref. 51)
Procedure Related										
Hematoma/hemorrhage	7.50	8.60	1.50	0.80		1.20	1.80	1.50	2.90	1.50
Thrombosis	3.80		2.50		2.60	0.60	1.20	1.50	1.50	
Embolization				0.80	1.20	1.20	2.40	2.00	10.00	3.00
Pseudoaneurysm		0.40	1.00			0.60				1.50
A-V fistula			0.50		0.60					1.50
Renal failure				2.40				0.50		
Other	1.90	3.60	0.50		3.80		0.60	1.00		0.80
Nonprocedure Related										
Pneumonia				0.80						
CHF				0.80						
Arrhythmia				2.40						
MI				2.40						
Total	13.20	12.60	6.00	10.40	8.20	3.60	6.00	6.50	14.40	8.30
30-day mortality	0.00	0.40	2.00	0.80	1.40	1.00	?	?	?	1.00

Abbreviations: A-V, arteriovenous; CHF, congestive heart failure; MI, myocardial infarction.

failed PTA results may be improved by adjunctive endovascular procedures. Many of the reported embolizations have been successfully treated percutaneously with intra-arterial thrombolysis. Patients experiencing significant acute dissections or occlusions may be candidates for endoprostheses.

FEMOROPOPLITEAL STENTS

Several vascular endoprostheses have been or are being investigated for implantation in the femoropopliteal arteries.[53–58] Both covered and uncovered stents have been developed. Covered-stent systems are in the early stages of investigation, primarily in Europe; the fact that they are being tested for this indication is testimony to the failure of current uncovered stents to improve revascularization results in the femoropopliteal arteries.

Preliminary investigations of uncovered femoropopliteal stents have shown unfavorable risk-reward ratios and have been largely abandoned. A European single-center prospective study showed conventional femoropopliteal PTA to have a 1-year primary patency rate (65%) equivalent to that of femoropopliteal Wallstents' secondary patency rate (69%).[56] The study also found early, clinically significant restenosis in the stent group (38%) and, more important, early thrombosis requiring thrombolysis/thrombosuction (19%). A Food and Drug Administration-sponsored phase II multicenter U.S. trial of femoropopliteal Wallstents showed 61% primary and 84% secondary clinical patency at 1 year, with 49% primary and 72% secondary patency at 2 years.[55] Importantly, a 16.7% major complication rate was reported. This compares unfavorably to both iliac stenting (4.3% rate of major complications in the same study) and conventional femoropopliteal PTA. Because of the lack of benefit over conventional PTA and the increased risk of complications, most clinicians reserve stent placement in the femoropopliteal system to compassionate use for suboptimal PTA results including dissection, thrombosis, or recoil in high-risk surgical patients. Randomized, prospective studies have not been performed to document the efficacy of femoropopliteal stenting and would be necessary before routine bailout stenting could be routinely advocated.

CONCLUSION

Conventional femoropopliteal PTA has been shown to be durable and cost effective for selected patients. Those who benefit most from PTA usually have short-segment disease. Even though PTA is less durable in patients with critical ischemia, they may have comorbidity that precludes surgery and PTA may be an alternative. PTA is usually complementary to infrainguinal bypass and should provide options that can maximize the treatment of patients with femoropopliteal vascular disease.

REFERENCES

1. Dotter CT, Judkins MP. Transluminal treatment of arteriosclerotic obstruction description of a new technic and a preliminary report of its application. *Circulation* 1964;30:654–670.
2. Gruntzig A, Hopf H. Perkutane Rekanalisation Chronisccher Arterieller Verschlusse mit einem neven Dilatationskatheter. Modifikation der Dotter-Technik. *Dtsch Med Wochenschr* 1974;99:2502–2505.
3. Gruntzig A, Kumpe DA. Technique of percutaneous transluminal angioplasty with the Gruntzig balloon catheter. *AJR* 1979;132:547–552.
4. Rutherford RB, Becker GJ. Standards for evaluating and reporting the results of surgical and percutaneous therapy for peripheral arterial disease. *JVIR* 1991;2:169–174.
5. Ahn SS, Rutherford RB, Becker GJ, et al. Reporting standards for lower extremity arterial endovascular procedures. *J Vasc Surg* 1993;17:1103–1107.
6. Spies JB, Bakal CW, Burke DR, et al. Angioplasty standard of practice. *JVIR* 1992;3:269–271.
7. Pentecost MJ, Criqui MH, Dorros G, et al. Guidelines for peripheral percutaneous transluminal angioplasty of the abdominal aorta and lower extremity vessels. *Circulation* 1994;89(1):511–531.
8. Wolf, GL, Wilson SE, Cross AP, et al. Surgery of balloon angioplasty for peripheral vascular disease: a randomized clinical trial. *JVIR* 1993;4:639–648.
9. Holm J, Arfvidsson B, Jivegard L, et al. Chronic lower limb ischaemia. A prospective randomized controlled study comparing the 1-year results of vascular surgery and percutaneous transluminal angioplasty. *Eur J Vasc Surg* 1991;5:517–522.
10. Kadir S, ed. *Current Practice of Interventional Radiology.* Philadelphia: BC Decker; 1991.
11. Darcy MD, La Berge JR, eds. *Peripheral Vascular Interventions.* Society of Cardiovascular and Interventional Radiology Syllabus, 1994.
12. Becker GJ, Katzen BT, Dake MD. Noncoronary angioplasty. *Radiology* 1989;170:921–940.
13. Adar R, Critchfield GC, Eddy DM. A confidence profile analysis of the results of femoropopliteal percutaneous transluminal angioplasty in the treatment of lower extremity ischemia. *J Vasc Surg* 1989;10:57–67.
14. Johnston KW. Femoral and popliteal arteries: reanalysis of results of balloon angioplasty. *Radiology* 1992;183:767–771.
15. Stanley B, Teague B, Raptis S, et al. Efficacy of balloon angioplasty of the superficial femoral artery and popliteal artery in the relief of leg ischemia. *J Vasc Surg* 1996;23:679–685.
16. Hunink MGM, Donaldson MC, Meyerovitz MF, et al. Risks and benefits of femoropopliteal percutaneous balloon angioplasty. *J Vasc Surg* 1993;17:183–194.
17. Capek P, MeLean GK, Berkowitz HD. Femoropopliteal angioplasty factors influencing long-term success. *Circulation* 1991;83(suppl I):I-70–I-80.
18. Stokes KR, Strunk HM, Campbell DR, et al. Five-year results of iliac and femoropopliteal angioplasty in diabetic patients. *Radiology* 1990;174:977–982.
19. Becquemin JP, Cavillon A, Haiduc F. Surgical transluminal femoropopliteal angioplasty: multivariate analysis outcome. *J Vasc Surg* 1994;19:495–502.
20. Jeans WD, Cole SEA, Horrocks M, et al. Angioplasty gives good results in critical lower limb ischemia. A 5-year follow-up in patients with known ankle pressure and dia-

betic status having femoropopliteal dilatations. *Br J Radiol* 1994;67:123–128.

21. Jeans WD, Armstrong S, Cole SEA, et al. Fate of patients undergoing transluminal angioplasty for lower-limb ischemia. *Radiology* 1990;177:559–564.

22. Matsi PJ, Manninen HI, Vanninen RL, et al. Femoropopliteal angioplasty in patients with claudication: primary and secondary patency in 140 limbs with 1–3 year follow-up. *Radiology* 1994;191:727–733.

23. Krepel, VM, Van Andel GJ, van Erp WFM, et al. Percutaneous transluminal angioplasty of the femoropopliteal artery: initial and long-term results. *Radiology* 1985; 156:325–328.

24. Murray JG, Apthorp LA, Wilkins RA. Long-segment (≥10 cm) femoropopliteal angioplasty: improved technical success and long-term patency. *Radiology* 1995;195:158–162.

25. Murray RR, Hewes RC, White RI, et al. Long-segment femoropopliteal stenoses: is angioplasty a boon or a bust? *Radiology* 1987;162:473–476.

26. Vroegindeweij D, Tielbeek AV, Buth J, et al. Recanalization of femoropopliteal occlusive lesions: a comparison of long-term clinical, color duplex US, and arteriographic follow-up. *JVIR* 1995;6:331–337.

27. Phillips-Hughes J, Kandarpa K, Restenosis: pathophysiology and preventive strategies. *JVIR* 1996;7:321–333.

28. Hunink MGM, Wong JB, Donaldson MC, et al. Revascularization for femoropopliteal disease: a decision and cost-effectiveness analysis. *JAMA* 1995;274(2):165–171.

29. Criqui MH, Langer RD, Fronek A, et al. Mortality over a period of 10 years in patients with peripheral arterial disease. *N Engl J Med* 1992;326(6):381–386.

30. Howell MA, Colgan MP, Seeger RW, et al. Relationship of severity of lower limb peripheral vascular disease to mortality and morbidity: a six-year follow-up study. *Vasc Surg* 1989;9:691–697.

31. Matsi PJ, Manninen HI, Suhonen MT, et al. Chronic critical lower limb ischemia: prospective trial of angioplasty with 1–36 months follow-up. *Radiology* 1993;188:381–387.

32. Dawson I, van Bockel H, Brand R. Late nonfatal and fatal cardiac events after infrainguinal bypass for femoropopliteal occlusive disease during a thirty-one year period. *J Vasc Surg* 1993;18:249–260.

33. Blair JM, Gewertz BL, Moosa H, et al. Percutaneous transluminal angioplasty versus surgery for limb-threatening ischemia. *J Vasc Surg* 1989;9:698–703.

34. Ray SA, Minty I, Buckenham TM, et al. Clinical outcome and restenosis following percutaneous transluminal angioplasty for ischaemic rest pain or ulceration. *Br J Surg* 1995;82:1217–1221.

35. Second European consensus document on chronic critical leg ischemia. *Circulation* 1991;84 (suppl 4):IV-1–IV-26.

36. Hunink MGM, Cullen KA, Donaldson MC. Hospital costs of revascularization procedures for femoropopliteal arterial disease. *J Vasc Surg* 1994;19:632–641.

37. Varty K, Nydahl S, Butterworth P, et al. Changes in the management of critical limb ischaemia. *Br J Surg* 1996;83:953–956.

38. Kalman PG, Johnston KW. Outcome of a failed percutaneous transluminal dilatation. *Surgery, Gynecology & Obstetrics* 1985;161:43–46.

39. Morgenstern BR, Getrajdman GI, Laffey KJ, et al. Total occlusions of the femoropopliteal artery: high technical success rate of conventional balloon angioplasty. *Radiology* 1989;172:937–940.

40. London NJM, Varty K, Sayers RD, et al. Percutaneous transluminal angioplasty for lower-limb critical ischaemia. *Br J Surg* 1995;82:1232–1235.

41. Treiman GS, Ichikawa L, Treiman RL, et al. Treatment of recurrent femoral or popliteal artery stenosis after percutaneous transluminal angioplasty. *J Vasc Surg* 1994;29:577–587.

42. Matsi PJ, Manninen HI. Impact of different patency criteria on long-term results of femoropopliteal angioplasty: analysis of 106 consecutive patients with claudication. *JVIR* 1995;6:159–163.

43. Sanchez LA, Gupta SK, Veith FJ, et al. A ten-year experience with one hundred fifty failing or threatened vein and polytetrafluoroethylene arterial bypass grafts. *J Vasc Surg* 1991;14:729–738.

44. Belkin M, Donaldson MC, Whittemore AD, et al. Observations on the use of thrombolytic agents for thrombotic occlusion of infrainguinal vein grafts. *J Vasc Surg* 1990;1:289–296.

45. Graor RA, Risius B, Young JR, et al. thrombolysis of peripheral arterial bypass grafts: surgical thrombectomy compared with thrombolysis. *J Vasc Surg* 1988;7:347–355.

46. Cohen JR, Mannick JA, Couch NP, et al. Recognition and management of impending vein-graft failure: importance for long-term patency. *Arch Surg* 1986;121:758–759.

47. Edwards JE, Taylor LM, Porter JM. Treatment of failed lower extremity bypass grafts with new autogenous vein bypass grafting. *J Vasc Surg* 1990;11:136–145.

48. Egglin TKP, O'Moore PV, Feinstein AR, et al. Complications of peripheral arteriography: a new system to identify patients at increased risk. *J Vasc Surg* 1995;22:787–794.

49. Belli AM, Cumberland DC, Knox AM, et al. The complication rate of percutaneous peripheral balloon angioplasty. *Clin Radiol* 1990;41:380–383.

50. Hasson JE, Acher CW, Wojtowycz M, et al. Lower extremity percutaneous transluminal angioplasty: multifactorial analysis of morbidity and mortality. *Surgery* 1990;108:748–754.

51. Matsi PJ, Manninen HI, Soder HK, et al. Percutaneous transluminal angioplasty in femoral artery occlusions: primary and long-term results in 107 claudicant patients using femoral and popliteal catheterization techniques. *Clin Radiol* 1995;50:237–244.

52. Katzenschlager R, Ugueluoglu A, Ahmadi A, et al. Incidence of pseudoaneurysm after diagnostic and therapeutic angiography. *Radiology* 1995;195:463–466.

53. White GH, Liew SCC, Waugh RC, et al. Early outcome and intermediate follow-up of vascular stents in the femoral and popliteal arteries without long-term anticoagulation. *J Vasc Surg* 1995;21:270–281.

54. Henry M, Amor M, Etherenot G, et al. Palmaz stent placement in iliac and femoropopliteal arteries: primary and secondary patency in 310 patients with 2–4 year follow-up. *Radiology* 1995;197:167–174.

55. Martin EC, Katzen BT, Benenati JF, et al. Multicenter trial of the Wallstent in the iliac and femoral arteries. *JVIR* 1995;6:843–849.

56. Do D, Triller J, Walpoth BH, et al. A comparison study of self-expandable stents vs balloon angioplasty alone in femoropopliteal artery occlusions. *Cardiovasc Int Radiol* 1992;15:306–312.

57. Rousseau HP, Raillat CR, Joffre FG, et al. Treatment of femoropopliteal stenoses by means of self-expandable endoprostheses: midterm results. *Radiology* 1989;172:961–964.

58. Sapoval MR, Long AL, Raynaud AC, et al. Femoropopliteal stent placement: long-term results. *Radiology* 1992;184:833–839.

16

Tibial Angioplasty

Curtis W. Bakal, M.D., M.P.H.
Jacob Cynamon, M.D.

Dotter and others described infrapopliteal angioplasty using tapered catheters, but they achieved mixed results.[1–5] Subsequent commercial availability of Gruentzig-type balloon catheters enabled stenoses to be dilated to larger diameters than the arteriotomy sites and resulted in practical, safe iliac angioplasty techniques. However, for about a decade after the Gruentzig-type balloons became available,[6] their large size and stiffness precluded their use in the tibial distribution. During this decade, data on femoropopliteal angioplasty performed on mixed populations of claudicants and limb salvage patients were being accumulated.[7–11] Some of these studies strongly suggested that the presence of poor calf runoff distal to the femoropopliteal angioplasty site would negatively influence the durability and clinical efficacy of the femoropopliteal percutaneous transluminal angioplasty (PTA); however, this runoff could not be effectively treated interventionally or even surgically during this period.[9–11] In the mid-1980s, small-diameter balloons and steerable guidewires were introduced, as were vasodilators such as nifedipine. Thus, interventional radiologists were able to extend angioplasty techniques from the iliac and femoral arteries to the distal popliteal and infrapopliteal arteries. This advance was facilitated by the subsequent availability and growing use of thrombolytic agents, digital fluoroscopy with road mapping, and nonionic contrast material.[12–14] Reversed or in situ saphenous venous bypasses to the tibial or pedal vessels were now becoming more routine in vascular surgical practice.[15] Many vascular surgeons supported the use of distal angioplasty because increasing surgical skills with distal bypass could potentially "rescue" failed PTAs and because many patients with calf vessel occlusive disease were poor surgical candidates with increased risk due to comorbid conditions such as diabetes and coronary artery disease. Because

the complications of tibial angioplasty might have potentially dire consequences, most vascular radiologists and surgeons have reserved tibial angioplasty for limb salvage situations.[3,16] However, a minority have advocated distal PTA for use in patients with moderate to severe claudication to increase the effectiveness and durability of femoropopliteal PTA.[17] Beliefs about potentially dire consequences of distal angioplasty have not been borne out by the literature, however; thus, the minority of clinicians advocating tibial angioplasty for claudication seem to have gained a larger following in recent years. The use of tibial PTA in clinical practice seems to have grown enormously over the past 5 or 6 years. Over a dozen authors have reported their results with infrapopliteal angioplasty in peer-reviewed journals since 1988, when the first reports of small vessel balloon angioplasty appeared.[1–27] These reports include over 800 patients. The efficacy of infrapopliteal PTA has been influenced heavily by improvements in technique and appears to be very dependent on appropriate patient selection. In experienced hands, the procedure seems to be relatively safe in difficult patients, with only two procedure-related deaths reported in the literature.

In centers experienced in treating limb salvage patients, surgical bypass and angioplasty, including tibial angioplasty, are often used together to manage these patients. For example, at Montefiore,[28,29] tibial angioplasty has been used as an integral component of treatment in over 2000 limb salvage patients, and amputation rates decreased from 49 to 14%. Tibial angioplasties represent about one-quarter of all peripheral angioplasties at our institution. The recognition that infrapopliteal angioplasty is an effective tool is evidenced by the presence of vascular surgeons on many of the published tibial angioplasty series and the continued referral of patients for the procedure.

177

ANGIOPLASTY TECHNIQUE

Infrapopliteal angioplasty must be preceded by a high-quality diagnostic arteriogram that visualizes the entire vascular tree from the aortoiliac segments down to the pedal arch. Ideally, aspirin should be started the night before the angioplasty and should be continued throughout the postprocedure period. Prior to the procedure, careful assessment of cardiac status and control of hypertension is necessary. IV hydration should be given, and renal function should be monitored and maximized. Of course, dedicated personnel are needed to monitor the patient during the procedure with continuous electrocardiographic monitoring and frequent vital sign checks. The use of IV sedation mandates the use of pulse oximetry and nasal oxygen.[30,31] Cardiac and antihypertensive medicines should be given the night before the procedure. The patients are generally given either nothing by mouth or a clear liquid diet. If a patient is diabetic, the insulin dose needs to be adjusted.

We administer sublingual nifedipine and reserve intra-arterial nitroglycerin for the rare patient in whom spasm is noted during or immediately after the angioplasty. Transcatheter boluses of nitroglycerin (100 to 200 μg) delivered to the PTA site are usually effective in breaking such spasm. Others use intra-arterial nitroglycerin more liberally during tibial PTA. Some use boluses of intra-arterial verapamil.

Infrapopliteal angioplasty is best accomplished via an antegrade puncture and using a sidearm sheath. In selected patients with straightforward proximal tibial stenoses, angioplasty can be performed from the contralateral femoral artery; in such cases, an over-the-top sheath should be used. A liberal heparin bolus [7000 units intra-arterially (IA)] is given before crossing the target lesion, and this initial dose should be supplemented if the procedure is prolonged. During the procedure, active monitoring of activated clotting time or partial thromboplastin times should be undertaken and heparin should be supplemented as needed. We generally do not give protamine to reverse the effect of heparin; this is especially true in diabetics, in whom cross-reactions with NPH insulin can occur. The introducer sheath is removed after the heparin effect has diminished (eg, activated clotting time below 200 seconds). Brown et al noted that intraprocedural thrombosis rates decreased after heparin doses during angioplasty were increased.[14,18] We prefer to dilate proximal lesions first and work distally, from the femoropopliteal artery through the tibial vessels[17,23] (Fig. 16–1). For tibial angioplasties, 0.014- to 0.018-inch steerable guidewires and low-profile balloons, generally with hydophilic coatings, are currently state of the art. Although we use cut film arteriography for most of our peripheral runoff studies, long-leg changer (BCM Industries, Montreal, Canada), digital arteriography and fluoroscopy are extremely valuable and should be used routinely during infrapopliteal PTA. Digital fluoroscopy with last image hold and road mapping decreases radiation exposure to the operator and patient, and allows precise catheter and wire tracking. It also allows use of relatively small volumes and dilute concentrations of contrast agents, decreasing contrast-related pain and complication rates and enhancing patient tolerance and cooperation.

After the procedure, careful fluid and vital sign monitoring with bed rest is mandatory, and clinical and noninvasive follow-up should be obtained. In patients with tissue loss, if immediate, noninvasive and clinical follow-up (eg, distal pulses) do not show significant improvement, then either repeat angioplasty (if thought to be of possible benefit) or surgical bypass should be instituted soon afterward. Patients with infection and tissue loss need to be treated aggressively, so a technically insufficient angioplasty should not be allowed to linger, as it is unlikely to improve with time if left alone.

Patients must be monitored for occult hemorrhage after any procedure, especially after antegrade punctures, which have a higher propensity to bleed into the thigh or retroperitoneum. These hemorrhages can be delayed and can present suddenly; they are potentially disastrous in patients with poor cardiac reserve. Serial hematocrits and urine output should be monitored, and vital sign checks should be done frequently. Oliguria can be a sign of contrast-related acute tubular necrosis, but it may also be the only sign of hypovolemia due to occult retroperitoneal hemorrhage. We have seen two such cases; in both, the blood pressure and pulse rate were stable (taken supine). If there is any suspicion of occult bleeding, an immediate non-contrast computed tomography (CT) study should be performed, scanning from the pelvis through the upper thigh.

RESULTS

Techniques for performing tibial angioplasty have improved with time, and these techniques are associated with better results. We experienced a threefold increase in technical success, from 29 to 86%, when small vessel balloons replaced Dotter-type dilating catheters in the mid-1980s.[16] Patient selection and operator experience, given the currently high state of technology, is the key to maximizing patient benefit.

The technical success rate, as reported in the literature by various authors, ranges from 86 to 100%. Dilatation of occlusions appears to be slightly less successful than dilatation of stenoses.[13] Other anatomic factors that adversely influence technical success include long lesion length, poor runoff distal to the angioplasty site, severe cracking or occlusive flaps, residual stenosis, and ostial location.[16,20] Because tibial angioplasty is per-

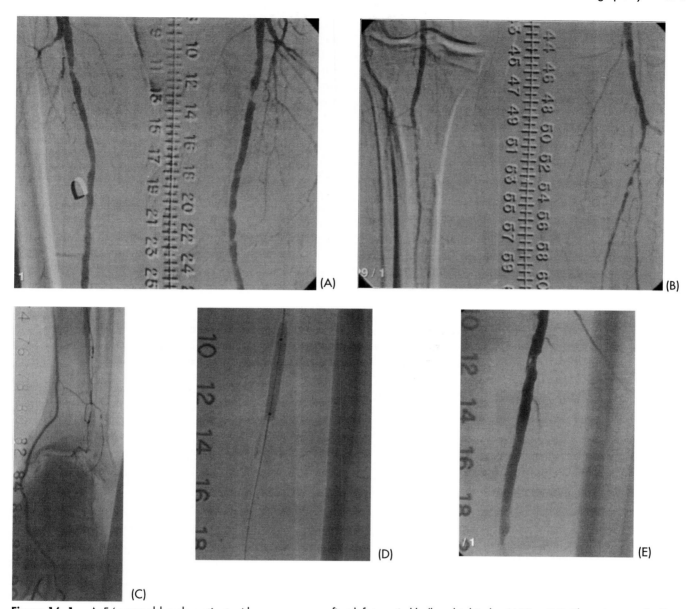

Figure 16–1. A 54-year-old male patient with a gangrenous first left toe. Ankle/brachial index (ABI) = 0.3. There is a markedly diminished left popliteal pulse, and there are no pedal pulses. There is a focal pinpoint stenosis of the left midsuperficial femoral artery (A). There is also occlusion of the anterior tibial artery, and severe diffuse disease of the tibioperoneal and peroneal arteries (B), and a moderate proximal stenosis of the proximal posterior tibial artery, with continuity of the posterior tibial artery to the foot (C). The superficial femoral artery lesion was angioplastied, with a very good result (D, E), together with augmentation of the popliteal pulse and restoration of a good posterior tibial pulse. A repeat ABI obtained on the operating table was now 0.8, and there was excellent augmentation of baseline pulse volume recording. On the basis of the pulses and the results of noninvasive studies, we elected to forego the planned dilatation of the posterior tibial artery. The patient experienced good healing following the proximal angioplasty.

formed predominantly in a limb salvage population, most patients undergoing angioplasty have multilevel disease, poor distal runoff, and a predominance of longer lesions, once again emphasizing the need for appropriate anatomic selection of patients. Multisegment disease is usually femoropopliteal and tibioperoneal; concomitant iliac and tibioperoneal distribution of significant disease is decidedly rare. In our own experience, 73% of patients either underwent a con-

current femoropopliteal artery angioplasty (52%) or had undergone previous femoropopliteal bypass grafting (21%), and virtually all had three-vessel tibial disease.[16] Only 20 to 30% of limb salvage patients have tibial occlusive disease focal enough (<5 cm) to make them good candidates for tibial angioplasty.[23]

Complications of tibial angioplasty have been reported in 2 to 11% of patients, with the most frequent being puncture site hematomas and vessel occlusions. Complications appear to occur more frequently during combined attempts at lysing closed surgical bypass grafts and dilating tibioperoneal lesions[18] or in treating long, complex lesions. Conversely, some embolic or occlusive complications that were reported in earlier patient series would currently be treated with transcatheter lysis and would no longer be classified as such. Two deaths have been reported in the over 800 patients reported in published series of patients.

While many tibial angioplasty series have included claudicators, several important series studied patients for limb salvage only[16,23,24] and other clinicians have treated these patients separately in their outcome analyses.[19,21,25] Overall, about 60 to 65% of patients appear to benefit clinically at 1- to 2-year follow-up, but in appropriately selected patients with focal disease and good tibial runoff distal to the targeted sites, an 80 to 85% clinical success rate appears to be the norm.[1–27] We found that angioplasty of lesions proximal to diffusely diseased or obstructed runoff all failed within 11 months; however, if angioplasty restored straight-line flow to the foot, we saw a 97% initial response rate and an 80% clinical success rate at 24 months.[17,32] (Figs. 16–2, 16–3). This clinical durability was seen in diabetics as well as in nondiabetics in whom straight-line flow to the foot was restored. Varty et al increased their 2-year success rate by closely following patients with fail-

ing angioplasties and repeating angioplasties on the majority of patients who needed them.[19]

The primary goals of tibial angioplasty in the limb salvage population are to avoid a major amputation and to salvage a functioning foot. Restoring hemodynamic patency at the PTA site is a secondary objective. In an important minority of patients, delayed closure of the tibial angioplasty site after tissue healing results in continued limb salvage, with no need for further intervention, because critically ischemic lesions may not recur. This is similar in concept to continued limb salvage occurring after closure of surgical grafts.[33,34] Thus, patency rates might justifiably lag behind limb salvage rates after angioplasty, as they can after surgical bypass.[17,19,25,29,34]

CLINICAL ADVANTAGES OF INFRAPOPLITEAL ANGIOPLASTY

Because of its relative noninvasiveness, we believe that tibial angioplasty should be utilized in all patients with appropriate clinical indications and amenable anatomy. In experienced hands, tibial angioplasty almost never precludes the performance of a subsequent bypass graft or alters previously planned surgery.[33] Precluding a potential or planned surgical option was reported in only two cases in the literature.[35] Failed angioplasty

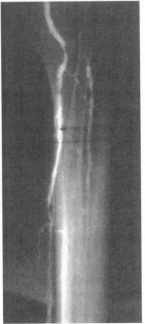
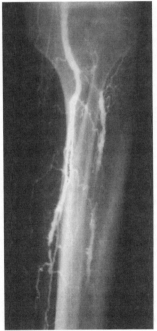

(A)   (B)

Figure 16–2.   A 70-year-old male with severe three-vessel tibial occlusive disease and gangrene in the left foot. (A) Tight focal stenosis of the tibioperoneal trunk, occlusion of the anterior and posterior tibial arteries, and severe disease and occlusion of the midperoneal artery. (B) Successful angioplasty of the focal tibioperoneal lesion. This angioplasty was unable to restore straight-line flow to the foot. The patient underwent an amputation 11 days after the procedure. We now know that angioplasty of such lesions proximal to occluded outflow is of little clinical benefit, and we would no longer select this type of anatomy for tibial PTA.

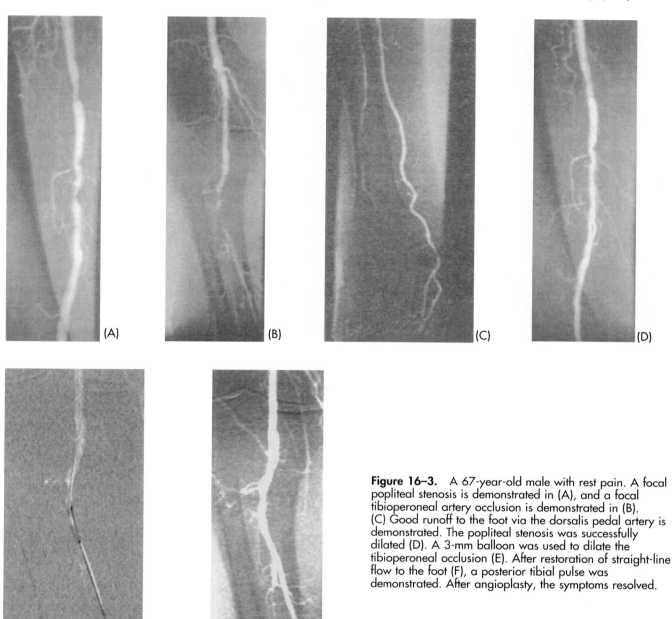

Figure 16–3. A 67-year-old male with rest pain. A focal popliteal stenosis is demonstrated in (A), and a focal tibioperoneal artery occlusion is demonstrated in (B). (C) Good runoff to the foot via the dorsalis pedal artery is demonstrated. The popliteal stenosis was successfully dilated (D). A 3-mm balloon was used to dilate the tibioperoneal occlusion (E). After restoration of straight-line flow to the foot (F), a posterior tibial pulse was demonstrated. After angioplasty, the symptoms resolved.

usually is limited to occlusion, reocclusion, or restenosis of the target segment, without destruction of the collaterals, inflow segments, or outflow segments; distal embolization occurs rarely and can be treated with lysis and suction embolectomy. PTA is a relatively noninvasive way to treat a very sick group of patients, many of whom have had myocardial infarction, contralateral amputation, or stroke, and it may often be accomplished quickly and relatively inexpensively at the time of diagnostic angiography. PTA also potentially spares vein for future use in the peripheral or coronary circu-

lation, which is an important consideration in patients who can be expected to undergo repeat revascularization attempts in the same or contralateral limb and who have a high likelihood of coronary artery disease comorbidity.[16,20,28,36,37] We have used infrapopliteal angioplasty to restore outflow effectively in failing distal bypass grafts (Fig. 16–4) and have also used it (very rarely) when overlying soft tissue infection has precluded a surgical anastomosis (Fig. 16–5). In our opinion, repeat angioplasty performed to enhance secondary patency is underutilized; it is relatively noninva-

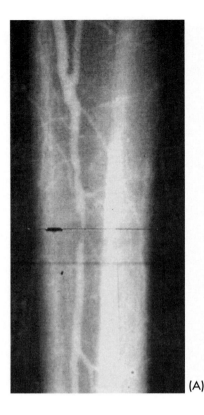
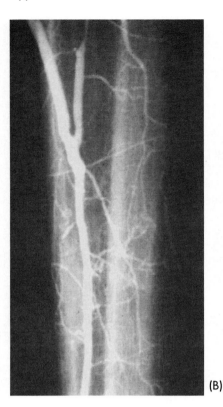

(A) (B)

Figure 16–4. Peroneal artery stenosis distal to a failing femoroperoneal saphenous vein bypass graft. (A) A focal lesion approximately 4 cm distal to the distal anastomosis of the graft and (B) restoration of outflow after angioplasty are demonstrated. These types of patients are usually preselected for favorable anatomy and respond well to angioplasty because bypass grafts are usually placed into patent and continuous runoff segments and close postsurgical surveillance detects relatively early focal disease.

Figure 16–5. A 57-year-old diabetic female with progressing cellulitis of the dorsum of the right foot and absent pedal pulses. Tibial occlusive disease precluded adequate healing of this soft tissue infection and also precluded placement of a dorsalis pedal anastomosis. Three focal stenoses were noted in the distal anterior tibial artery (A). After angioplasty, the dorsalis pedal pulse was restored (B), and subsequently the foot healed.

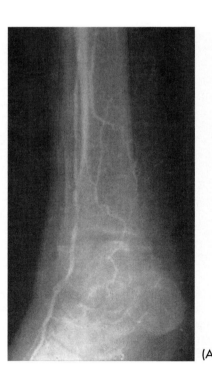
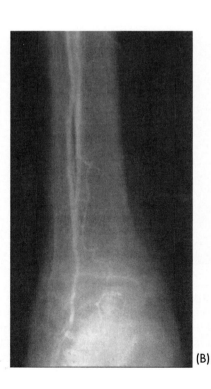

(A) (B)

sive and inexpensive compared to surgery. For these reasons, even if PTA rates are found to be somewhat lower than surgical patency rates, PTA is still acceptable to patients, to referring physicians and surgeons, and to vascular radiologists. There are problems with angioplasty in general and with angioplasty, particularly of the tibial vessels, that affect its efficacy, both real and perceived. These problems include the following:

1. Poor patient selection and stratification. Many of the published series have included patients with diffuse disease and poor tibial runoff.[12,16,17,20,21] These studies often fail to stratify for lesion length and runoff status. Thus, these aggregate results do not describe the better outcomes that are seen in appropriately selected patient subgroups. We now know that improving inflow to collaterals by angioplasty in the absence of straight-line flow to the foot will not help most limb salvage patients,[16] but unfortunately, this knowledge was not disseminated before data were accumulated for many of the published tibial angioplasty studies.

2. Choice of patient subgroups for heroic tibial angioplasty. Patients undergoing tibial angioplasty are not like iliac angioplasty patients, who traditionally have been chosen for more focal and less serious disease than patients undergoing bypass. Interventional radiologists are often referred patients for tibial angioplasty who are poor surgical candidates.[16,17,20,22] The ability to help patients who are not good surgical candidates with less invasive technology is one of the great advantages of PTA. This group of poor surgical candidates includes three very different subsets of patients. The first are patients who are too sick for surgery because of their poor medical status, not because of adverse surgical anatomy. Angioplasty is an attractive and appropriate option in this subset. A second group of poor surgical candidates referred for angioplasty consists of a small group of patients who have absent or adverse anatomy for bypass; these patients may have focal occlusive disease but lack good saphenous vein or, in very rare cases, may have infection in potential anastomotic sites. This patient population is also appropriate for angioplasty. The third subset of these poor surgical candidates are adversely selected and should be inappropriate candidates for angioplasty. These are patients with poor surgical anatomy who have no options for surgical bypass because they have very diffuse or advanced occlusive disease and no identifiable good distal anastomotic sites. As we know now, these patients derive almost no enduring clinical benefit, yet vascular radiologists have been loath to turn them away and some surgeons continue to refer them because the only other option is amputation. This is precisely the group that we think will do poorly with angioplasty, yet an undefined but probably substantial number of these patients have been included in published series of femoropopliteal and infrapopliteal angioplasties.[35] These are desperate cases who may have very advanced diabetes, often with end-stage renal disease (ESRD). In fact, ESRD patients compose about 8% of our limb salvage population and, historically, a higher proportion of our tibial angiopalsty patient population. Interventional radiologists may attempt a "Hail Mary" play in such poorly selected patients, but these attempts most often fail. In the past, we performed many such heroic angioplasties (believing that they would probably not succeed) because the remaining options were so poor. These cases negatively skew our aggregate outcome statistics and will probably not stand up to close scrutiny in this era of cost-effective, monitored medical care. Similarly, ESRD patients have never been stratified separately in the literature on distal angioplasty and undoubtedly exert a similar negative effect on PTA efficacy for any aggregate series of patients.[38]

The importance of restoring straight-line flow to the foot has been emphasized above, and while we and others have looked at the presence or absence of straight-line flow to the foot (ie, to the proximal foot) as a prognostic indicator, it is probable that the status of the pedal arch—not analyzed in infrainguinal angioplasty series—also affects the outcome of tibial angioplasty. Whereas most patients with limb salvage indications have intact or partial pedal arches, allowing reconstitution of straight-line flow down and through the pedal arch by tibial angioplasty, about 20% may have frankly occluded pedal arches.[39] The destruction of the pedal arch is probably more pronounced in patients with ESRD; these patients may fare poorly due to local metabolic factors even with patent bypass grafts and PTA sites.[38,40,41] It is possible that these patients may account for a substantial proportion of those noted by Fraser et al[42] and others in whom angiographic patency exceeds limb salvage.

3. Maintenance and definition of patency. Repeat angioplasty can extend the durability of the initial dilatation,[19] but PTA has clearly been underutilized for restenosis. Interventional radiologists, who often serve as consultants to surgeons,[43] do not often get the go-ahead to reintervene, so post-PTA occlusion or restenosis often means either surgical bypass or amputation rather than a repeat angioplasty. Primary and secondary patency curves in tibial angioplasties approximate each other because only a small fraction of patients appear to undergo repeat angioplasty for failure.[17,22] By contrast, vascular surgeons routinely can and do reoperate when needed. They have also learned that intense postprocedure surveillance with early reintervention (surgical or percutaneous), if necessary, substantially improves the durability of their bypasses.[28,44] Although there is evidence suggesting that duplex ultrasound imaging is sensitive in detecting restenosis and, along with clinical and other noninvasive follow-up, could be very useful in augmenting PTA durability,[45] surveillance after angioplasty is probably not as vigorous or frequent as surveillance after bypass grafting.

There is also an inherent bias in the definition of patency that tends to undervalue PTA relative to surgery: failing or failed bypass grafts salvaged by angioplasty augment primary assisted or secondary surgical patency. However, if angioplasty is deemed to be failing and a surgical bypass is performed, the PTA is necessarily defined as a failure.[35] Because restenoses are rarely redilated, this means that primary assisted or secondary patency rates for bypass grafts are compared with angiographic recurrences or clinical failures that have not been retreated percutaneously.

SUMMARY

In conclusion, infrapopliteal artery angioplasty is an effective technique for treating patients with distal atherosclerotic occlusive disease. It has been utilized primarily in limb salvage patients with multisegment disease. Appropriate anatomic selection of patients is key to maximizing the benefit of this technique.

REFERENCES

1. Dotter CT, Judkins MP. Transluminal treatment of arteriosclerotic obstruction. Description of a new technic and a preliminary report of its application. *Circulation* 1964;30:654–670.
2. Sprayregen S, Sniderman KW, Sos TA, Vieux U, Singer A, Veith FJ. Popliteal artery branches: percutaneous transluminal angioplasty. *AJR* 1980;135:945–950.
3. Greenfield A. Femoral, popliteal, and tibial arteries: percutaneous transluminal angioplasty. *AJR* 1980;135:927–935.
4. Starck EE, McDermott J, Crummy AB, Heydwolf AV. Angioplasty of the popliteal and tibial arteries. *Semin Intervent Radiol* 1984;4:269–277.
5. Tamura S, Sniderman KW, Beinart C, Sos TA. Percutaneous transluminal angioplasty of the popliteal artery and its branches. *Radiology* 1982;143:645–648.
6. Gruentzig A, Hopff H. Perkutane rekanalizaton chronischer arteniellar. Verschlusse mit einem nuen Dilatationkatheter. Modifikation der Dotter-Technik. *Dtsch Med Wochenschr* 1974;99:2502–2505.
7. Capek P, McLean GK, Berkowitz HD. Femoropopliteal angioplasty, factors influencing long-term success. *Circulation* 1991;83(suppl I):I-70–I-80.
8. Hewes RC, White RI, Murray RR. Long term results of superficial femoral artery angioplasty. *AJR* 1986;146:1025–1029.
9. Johnston KW, Rae M, Hogg-Johnston SA, et al. Five-year results of a prospective study of percutaneous transluminal angioplasty. *Ann Surg* 1987;206:403–413.
10. Johnston KW. Femoral and popliteal arteries: reanalysis of results of balloon angioplasty. *Radiology* 1992;183:767–771.
11. Stokes KR, Holger HM, Campbell DR, Gibbons GW, Wheeler HG, Clouse ME. Five-year results of iliac and femoropopliteal angioplasty in diabetic patients. *Radiology* 1990;174:977–982.
12. Casarella WJ. Percutaneous transluminal angioplasty below the knee: new techniques, excellent results. *Radiology* 1988;169:271–272.
13. Schwarten DE, Cutcliff WB. Arterial occlusive disease below the knee: treatment with percutaneous transluminal angioplasty performed with low-profile catheters and steerable guide wires. *Radiology* 1988;169:71–74.
14. Brown KT, Schoenberg NY, Moore ED, Saddenkni S. Percutaneous transluminal angioplasty of infrapopliteal vessels: preliminary results and technical considerations. *Radiology* 1988;169:75–78.
15. Veith FJ, Gupta SK, Ascer E. Femoral, popliteal and tibial occlusive disease. In: Wilson SE, Veith FJ, Hobson RW, Williams RA, eds. *Vascular Surgery: Principles and Practice.* New York: McGraw-Hill; 1987:353–375.
16. Bakal CW, Sprayregen S, Scheinbaum K, Cynamon J, Veith FJ. Percutaneous transluminal angioplasty of the infrapopliteal arteries: results in 53 patients. *AJR* 1990;154:171–174.
17. Horvath W, Oertl M, Haidinger D. Percutaneous transluminal angioplasty of crural arteries. *Radiology* 1990;177:565–569.
18. Brown KT, Moore ED, Getrajdman GI, Saddekni S. Infrapopliteal angioplasty: long-term follow-up. *JVIR* 1993;4:139–144.
19. Varty K, Bolia A, Naylor AR, Bell PRF, London NJM. Infrapopliteal percutaneous transluminal angioplasty: a safe and successful prcoedure. *Eur J Vasc Endovasc Surg* 1995;9:341–345.
20. Matsi PJ, Manninen HI, Suhonen MT, Pirinen AE, Soimakallio S. Chronic critical lower-limb ischemia: prospective trial of angioplasty with 1–36 months follow-up. *Radiology* 1993;188:381–387.
21. Wagner HJ, Starck EE, McDermott JC. Infrapopliteal percutaneous transluminal revascularization: results of a prospective study on 148 patients. *J Intervent Radiol* 1993;8:81–90.
22. Bull PG, Mendel H, Hold M, Schlegl A, Denck H. Distal popliteal and tibioperoneal transluminal angioplasty: long-term follow-up. *JVIR* 1992;3:45–53.
23. Schwarten DE. Clinical and anatomical considerations for nonoperative therapy in tibial disease and the results of angioplasty. *Circulation* 1991;83(suppl I):I-86–I-90.
24. Saab MH, Smith DC, Aka PK, Brownlee RW, Killeen JD. Percutaneous transluminal angioplasty of tibial arteries for limb salvage. *Cardiovasc Intervent Radiol* 1992;15:211–216.
25. Sivananthan UM, Browne TF, Thorley PJ, Rees MR. Percutaneous transluminal angioplasty of the tibial arteries. *Br J Surg* 1994;81:1282–1285.
26. Wack C, Wolfle KD, Loeprecht H, Tietze W, Bohndorf K und. Perkutane ballondilatation bei isolierten Lasionen der Unterschenkelarterien mit kritischer Beinischamie. *VASA* 1994;23:30–34.
27. Bolia A, Sayers RD, Thompson MM, Bell PRF. Subintimal and intraluminal recanalization of occluded crural arteries by percutaneous balloon angioplasty. *Eur J Vasc Surg* 1994;8:214–219.
28. Veith FJ, Gupta SK, Wengerter KR, et al. Changing arteriosclerotic disease patterns and management strategies in lower-limb-threatening ischemia. *Ann Surg* 1990;212:402–414.
29. Veith FJ, Gupta SK, Samson RH, et al. Progress in limb salvage by reconstructive arterial surgery combined with new or improved adjunctive procedures. *Ann Surg* 1981;194:386.
30. *ACR Standards for Use of Intravenous Conscious Sedation* Reston, VA: American College of Radiology; 1996.

31. Spies JB, Bakal CW, Burke DR, et al. Standards for diagnostic arteriography in adults. *J Vasc Intervent Radiol* 1993;4:385–395.

32. Bakal CW, Cynamon J, Sprayregen S, et al. Infrapopliteal artery angioplasty—follow-up and factors influencing clinical response in 53 patients. Presented at the SCVIR 17th annual meeting of the Washington, DC, April 1992.

33. Veith FJ, Panetta TF, Wengerter KR, et al. Femoropopliteal tibial occlusive disease. In: Veith FJ, Hobson RW, Williams RA, Wilson SE, eds. *Vascular Surgery. Principles and Practice,* 2nd ed. New York: McGraw Hill; 1994;421–446.

34. Veith FJ, Gupta SK, Ascer E, et al. Six year prospective multicenter randomized comparison of autologous saphenous vein and expanded polytetrafluoroethylene grafts in infrainguinal internal reconstructions. *J Vasc Surg* 986;3:104–114.

35. Bakal CW, Cynamon J, Spraryregen S. Infrapoplitela angioplasty: what we know. *Radiology* 1996;200:36–42.

36. Criqui MH, Langer RD, Fronek A, et al. Mortality over a period of 10 years in patients with peripheral arterial disease. *N Engl J Med* 1992;326:381–386.

37. Jeans WD, Armstrong S, Cole SEA, Horrocks M, Baird RN. Fate of patients undergoing transluminal angioplasty for lower-limb ischemia. *Radiology* 1990;177:559–564.

38. Cynamon JC, Parisi A, Bakal CW, Sprayregen S, Epstein SB, Veith FJ. Balloon angioplasty severely diseased infrapopliteal arteries. Abstract. Orlando, FL: American Roentgen Ray Society; 1992.

39. Karacagil S, Almgrren B, Bowald S, Eriksson I. Arterial lesions of the foot vessels in diabetic and non-diabetic patients undergoing lower limb revascularisation. *Eur J Vasc Surg* 1989;3:239–244.

40. Sanchez LA, Goldsmith J, Rivers SP, Panetta TF, Wengerter KR, Veith FJ. Limb salvage surgery in end stage renal disease: is it worthwhile? *J Cardiovasc Surg* 1992;33:344–348.

41. Edwards JM, Taylor LM, Porter JM. Limb salvage in end-stage renal disease (ESRD). Comparison of modern results in patients with and without ESRD. *Arch Surg* 88;123:1164–1168.

42. Fraser SCA, Al-Kutoubi MA, Wolfe JNA. Angioplasty of the infrapopliteal vessels: the evidence. *Radiology* 1996;200:33–36.

43. White RI Jr. Status of admitting privileges for university-affiliated diagnostic radiology departments. *Radiology* 1990;175:391–392.

44. Green RM, McNamara J, Ouriel K, DeWeese JA. Comparison of infrainguinal graft surveillance techniques. *J Vasc Surg* 1990;11:207–215.

45. Vroegindewij D, Tielbeck AV, Buth S, et al. Recanalization of a femoropopliteal occlusive lesions: a comparison of long term clinical, color duplex US, and arteriographic follow-up. *JVIR* 1995;6:331–337.

17

Current Status of Atherectomy: Options, Patient Selection, and Results

Samuel S. Ahn, M.D.,
Blessie Concepcion, B.Sc.

The application of catheter-based endovascular systems has revolutionized the treatment of peripheral vascular disease by providing less invasive methods to enhance or replace conventional vascular reconstructive procedures. For example, pecutaneous transluminal angioplasty (PTA) has facilitated treatment of patients who are poor surgical candidates with disabling claudication or limb-threatening ischemia. However, the limitations of PTA in calcified, eccentric, or occlusive lesions, and the incidence of restenosis, led to the concept of mechanically ablating and removing obstructing plaque under direct vision.

Atherectomy is the selective removal of atheroma from diseased arteries, either percutaneously or through a small arteriotomy remote from the diseased site. The concept of *debulking* plaque is designed to address the limitations of balloon angioplasty. Such an appealing alternative has led to the development and investigation of at least 12 different atherectomy devices. Although early clinical results have been promising, results beyond 6 months have been disappointing. Nevertheless, atherectomy has been shown to enhance the immediate results in treating short lesions, with eccentric stenoses or hard, calcified plaque. Recently, atherectomy has been found effective in treating recurrent infrainguinal bypass graft stenoses and may be useful in treating failing hemodialysis access grafts.

This chapter will discuss three atherectomy devices that have undergone extensive clinical investigations and are currently available. A promising new atherectomy catheter, the OmniCath, will also be discussed. These devices are characterized by their process of cutting atheroma within the arterial wall and then removing the excised plaque. Extirpative or directional atherectomy shaves or slices atheroma and directly removes the excised plaque from the vessel with a collection chamber. Extirpative catheters include the Simpson AtheroTrack, the Transluminal Extraction Catheter, and the new OmniCath. Ablative or rotational atherectomy utilizes a high-speed rotary device that pulverizes atheroma into microparticles small enough to be aspirated or removed through the reticuloendothelial system. The Auth Rotablator is an ablative catheter. For detailed operational information, the reader is referred to *The ISCVS/SVS Handbook on Endovascular Procedures*.[1]

DESCRIPTION OF ATHERECTOMY DEVICES

Simpson AtheroTrack

The Simpson AtheroTrack (Mallinckrodt Medical, Inc., St. Louis, MO) is the new and improved model of the Simpson AtheroCath. The AtheroTrack offers both over-the-wire and fixed-wire shaft designs to facilitate the introduction to complex or simple stenotic lesions by providing more maneuverability in steering the catheter. The catheter has a housing unit composed of a cutter within a longitudinal opening on one side and a balloon attached on the opposite side. Inflation of the balloon at 20 to 40 psi engages the atheroma against a 20-mm cutter window. Then the cutter slices the plaque at 2000 rpm while simultaneously pushing the excised particles into a collection chamber. The catheter also has a tip guard with a hemostasis valve to protect its wire tip. The proximal assembly consists of a balloon inflation port, a flush port, and an adapter spline for the drive cable connector. A small lever attached to the cable allows the operator to lock the cutter in places before advancing it manually. The AtheroTrack catheter is available in 7, 8, 9, 10, and 11 Fr. sizes.

Transluminal Extraction Catheter

The Transluminal Extraction Catheter (TEC) (InterVentional Technologies, Inc., San Diego, CA) is a semiflexible, torque-controlled catheter with a rotating, cone-shaped cutter that tracks over a central guidewire. The cone has openings on the distal tip and the catheter itself is hollow, so the particles resulting from atherectomy can be suctioned out of the vessel and collected in a separate collecting chamber (125 mL). The cone-shaped cutter rotates at 700 rpm and leaves relatively large (1 mm) particles. Suction is applied from the proximal port to aspirate the particles into the collecting chamber and thus minimize embolic complications. Continuous heparin irrigation via the introducer sheath's sidearm is required to maintain efficiency in the aspiration of excised particles. The catheter is currently available in 6, 7, 8, 9, 10, 12, and 14 Fr. sizes.

OmniCath

The OmniCath (American BioMed, Inc., Georgetown, TX) is a new extirpative atherectomy device currently approved by the Food and Drug Administration for investigational use only. It is a radiopaque, torqueable, braided catheter with a hollow cylindrical housing at the distal end. This housing unit contains the cutter within a longitudinal window on one side and a unique unibody tripod composed of an extendible wire configuration on the opposite side. The internal beveled cutter spins at 11,000 rpm and is stabilized by an axial guide or track when making a cut. The cutter is activated by hand and rotated by a battery-powered motor via a hollow drive shaft. An idler shaft covers a 2-cm section of the drive shaft at the distal end to minimize or eliminate the potential for tissue wrapping or binding onto the shaft. The rotating cutter passes back and forth across the lesion, shaving off thin segments of the atheromatous particles with each pass. The atheromatous debris is collected in the housing unit and continuously aspirated through a removal port at the proximal end of the catheter. A radiopaque gold dot just beyond the distal end of the window enhances operative visualization of the device.

An atraumatic deflector wire pad braces the cutter assembly securely against the obstructive lesion and allows continuous distal perfusion during atherectomy. This anchoring system can be adjusted and thus can regulate the depth of cut by its degree of extension. The extended anchoring wire can withhold a maximum pressure of 27 psi. This mechanism is designed to prevent injury to the vessel wall (ie, perforation) and thus reduce the likelihood of acute closure and restenosis.

Auth Rotablator

The Auth Rotablator (Boston Scientific Corp., Natick, MA) is a flexible, catheter-deliverable atherectomy device with a variably sized, football-shaped metal burr on the distal tip. The burr is studded with multiple diamond chips (22 to 45 µm in size) that function as multiple microknives. The burr comes in various sizes, ranging from 1.25 to 6.0 mm in diameter. Progressively larger burrs are used incrementally during the recanalization process until a satisfactory lumen is obtained. The burr rotates at 100,000 to 200,000 rpm and tracks along a central guidewire. The guidewire must first traverse the lesion before rotational atherectomy can proceed. The high-speed rotation allows the diamond microchips to preferentially attack hard, calcified atheroma while leaving the surrounding elastic soft tissue of normal arterial wall intact. The device leaves a smooth, polished intraluminal surface and no intimal flaps.

Similar to PTA, atherectomy is associated with a low rate of morbidity and mortality, minimal blood loss, and less pain and faster recovery compared to conventional surgical revascularization. The technical and clinical success of atherectomy devices depends on patient selection, as well as characteristics of the obstructing plaque.

PATIENT SELECTION

Although the results are inferior to those achieved with the conventional bypass procedure, atherectomy may be a reasonable alternative for patients with severe, disabling claudication or limb-threatening ischemia who are considered poor surgical candidates due to associated comorbidity. Furthermore, atherectomy can be performed as an adjunct to a standard revascularization procedure to improve inflow or outflow while minimizing the operative risk in these patients.

Currently, conventional bypass grafting remains the gold standard of treatment for patients with severe, disabling claudication or limb-threatening ischemia. However, the patient with significant infrainguinal disease and without adequate autogenous vein for bypass grafting may benefit from atherectomy. Some investigators have advocated endovascular intervention in high-risk patients with less advanced disease and without any suitable vein to prevent or delay the progression of atherosclerosis and thus the need for subsequent surgical treatment, although the appropriateness of this approach is unproven!

CHARACTERISTICS OF OBSTRUCTED LESIONS

Type of Lesion: Stenosis versus Occlusion

Stenotic lesions are amenable to treatment by atherectomy. Any of the atherectomy devices described above can be used to remove enough of the atherosclerotic plaque so that the stenotic lesion becomes hemodynamically insignificant or permits another endovascular intervention such as PTA to be subsequently performed. However, the debulking of plaque does not prevent or reduce the likelihood of restenosis. On the contrary, the restenosis rate of atherectomy is similar to, if not worse than, that observed after conventional PTA.

Complete occlusions are generally not appropriate for treatment by atherectomy. Previous clinical studies demonstrated a high technical failure rate due to the inability to cross the lesion first with a guidewire, as well as poor short- and long-term patency. Some investigators have reported successful recanalization of total occlusions by using hydrophilic guidewires such as the Glidewire (Medi-Tech Boston Scientific Corp., Natick, MA) to cross the lesion, followed by balloon angioplasty, directional atherectomy, and/or laser angioplasty.[2] However, complications associated with atherectomy in treating such lesions include perforation, embolization, and immediate rethrombosis. Surgical bypass grafting is still the gold standard for complete occlusions.

Length of Lesion: Short versus Long

Short stenoses (<5 cm) are the most favorable lesions for treatment by atherectomy using any of the devices listed above. However, the most appropriate endovascular therapeutic option for these lesions remains PTA. Atherectomy becomes an acceptable alternative only if the stenotic lesions are complex, that is, eccentric and/or calcified, and not amenable to conventional angioplasty.

Long stenotic lesions (>5 cm) are amenable to atherectomy if a guidewire can be passed successfully across the lesion first. This over-the-wire technique minimizes the risk of perforation when the atherectomy catheter traverses the lengthy lesion. The Auth Rotablator can be used to recanalize lengthy stenoses; directional atherectomy catheters, on the other hand, such as the Simpson AtheroTrack or the new Omni-Cath, may take too long to do so. Atherectomy may be a reasonable alternative to treat long lesions in patients considered poor surgical candidates because long lesions tend to be complex and less amenable to percutaneous balloon angioplasty, although these patients need to be aware that they may obtain only short-term benefit from this intervention. For acceptable surgical candidates, bypass grafting still remains the first-line treatment for patients with long stenotic lesions.

Short and long complete occlusions are generally not amenable to treatment by atherectomy, although some workers believe that hydrophilic guidewires can offer a solution to this limitation. Furthermore, initial treatment with lytic therapy may lyse an occluding thrombus and thus convert a total occlusion into a short stenosis.

Location

Iliac Artery

The optimal endovascular intervention for iliac artery stenoses is PTA. Atherectomy can be used as an adjunct to balloon angioplasty to expand further the diameter of the vessel lumen and obtain a final angiographic result of <25% residual stenosis. Any of the previously described atherectomy devices can be used for this purpose, although one should be aware of the increased risk of major retroperitoneal hemorrhage from perforation in this region. The passage of a guidewire across the iliac artery lesion is crucial in keeping the atherectomy catheter intraluminal; conversely, passage of the guidewire in a subintimal plane can lead to a dissection or perforation, necessitating emergent surgical intervention.

Femoral/Popliteal Arteries

The results of PTA in the treatment of infrainguinal lesions have been suboptimal, and any of the atherectomy catheters can be used in this region. However, selection of the appropriate catheter should be based on the length of the lesion and the characteristics of the plaque. Accurate characterization of the obstructing plaque can be performed using a variety of modalities, such as ankle/brachial indices and segmental Doppler pressure measurements, as well as imaging modalities such as angioscopy, angiography, Duplex scanning, and intravascular ultrasound (see Chapter 5).

Tibial Artery

Because most of the obstructive lesions in this region are complex (ie, diffuse, calcified) and not ideally amenable to PTA, atherectomy may be a reasonable alternative. Because of its flexibility, the only atherectomy device that can be used to safely recanalize short stenotic lesions in the tibial region is the Auth Rotablator. Although the results are inferior to those achieved with distal lower extremity bypass grafting, atherectomy is particularly suitable for patients with no suitable vein conduit, or as an adjunct to more proximal bypass grafting to improve outflow.

Runoff Vessels

As with most endovascular procedures, the status of the runoff vessels is an important variable in predicting the probability of a successful atherectomy. Obviously, atherectomy of a stenotic lesion with good distal runoff (graded 2 or 3) will be associated with the most favorable results. As noted above, atherectomy of a distal artery stenosis can be performed in conjunction with surgical revascularization, or another endovascular procedure, to improve outflow and thus increase the likelihood of clinical success.

Recurrent Stenosis

Failing Lower Extremity Bypass Grafts

It is suggested that patients with failing lower extremity bypass grafts should be treated with atherectomy, rather than PTA, because graft failure is caused predominantly by intimal hyperplastic tissue not ideally amenable to balloon angioplasty. Secondary infrainguinal saphenous vein bypass graft patency following balloon angioplasty has been disappointingly low, and surgical revision (ie, vein patch angioplasty, interposition graft) conveys a higher risk of morbidity. Directional atherectomy has been proven to be safe and effective in treating synthetic and vein bypass graft stenoses in the anastomotic and intragraft areas[3,4] Furthermore, some investigators advocate early endovascular intervention in asymptomatic patients with noninvasive documentation of graft stenosis before graft thrombosis occurs.

Failing Arteriovenous Hemodialysis Access Grafts

Directional atherectomy can also be used to treat recurrent stenotic hemodialysis access fistulas. As in failing lower extremity bypass graft stenoses, fibromuscular intimal hyperplasia is the most common cause of failure in these conduits. Results with balloon angioplasty are also poor, and each surgical revision is associated with a decreasing likelihood of long-term success.[5,6] Preliminary studies utilizing atherectomy show promising results, although further follow-up is necessary.

CHARACTERISTICS OF PLAQUE

Eccentric Atheroma

Eccentric stenoses are ideally suited for atherectomy. The Simpson Athero Track and the new OmniCath device can successfully recanalize this type of plaque. Hard, eccentric plaque is best treated with the Auth Rotablator due to its differential cutting ability without disrupting the normal arterial wall diametrically opposite the plaque site. The TEC, on the other hand, does not offer any particular advantage in treating eccentric lesions.

Diffusely Disease

Diffusely diseased stenotic arteries can be recanalized by atherectomy alone or in conjunction with balloon angioplasty. These lesions tend to be complex and long, so this approach should be considered only in poor surgical candidates. The Rotablator can be used to recanalize these lengthy stenoses because directional atherectomy would take too long to achieve successful recanalization. However, patients should be aware of the limited patency associated with this approach.

Calcified Atheroma

Calcified plaque is ideally suited for rational atherectomy because PTA may fail to crack the lesion. The Rotablator can effectively pulverize this type of atheroma because of its differential cutting ability, and directional atherectomy can penetrate such lesions, albeit not as effectively.

Intimal Hyperplasia

As previously mentioned, atherectomy is a better alternative than balloon angioplasty to treat intimal hyperplasia, which is a primary cause of recurrent stenoses. However, successful atherectomy does not prevent intimal hyperplasia from recurring in these lesions. Atherectomy may simply extend the patency of the failing lower extremity bypass or hemodialysis access graft.

Rubbery Plaque

Rubbery plaque is amenable to directional atherectomy catheters. The opposing balloon of the Simpson Athero Track and the anchoring deflector wire pad of the OmniCath function to secure such rubbery plaque into their respective cutting windows. Other alternatives such as the Rotablator or balloon angioplasty simply deflect the rubbery plaque, which then bounces right back.

RESULTS

Simpson AtheroTrack

Several clinical studies using the Simpson atherectomy device to treat peripheral arterial occlusive disease have documented high initial success rates, varying from 80% to 100% (Table 17.1).[7–16] Graor and Whitlow[10] achieved <20% residual stenosis in 100% of lesions ≤5 cm and in 93% of lesions >5 cm, primarily due to the pretreatment of occluded lesions with urokinase. However, other investigators have reported suboptimal intermediate patency results at 6 to 24 months (Table 17.1). In the treatment of infrainguinal lesions, Lugmayr et al[13] and Vroegindewij et al[14] reported patencies of 42% and 35% at 2 years, respectively, which are similar to those previously reported for balloon angioplasty.[17–19]

Table 17–1. Literature Review Using the Simpson Atherectomy Device to Treat Peripheral Occlusive Disease

Study	No. of Patients	No. of Lesions	Technical Success	Primary Patency		
				6 Mo	12 Mo	24 Mo
Simpson et al[7]	61	136	87%	69%	NA	NA
Polnitz et al[8]	60	94	82%	99%	72%	NA
Hinohara et al[9]	100	195	90%	83%	NA	NA
Graor & Whitlow[10]	106	106	100% lesions ≤5 cm	NA	93%	88.4%
			93% lesions >5 cm	NA	86%	73%
Dorros et al[11]	126	213	99%	45%	NA	NA
Kim et al[12]	77	85	92%	94%	86%	86%
Lugmayr et al[13]	94	132	95%	NA	69%	42%
Vroegindewij et al[14]	38	38	92%	84%	42%	35%
Savader et al[15]	61	136	80%	NA	76%	58%
Wildenhain et al[16]	75	84	92%	NA	78%	57%

Abbreviation: NA, not available.

Adjunctive balloon angioplasty is required in some cases to facilitate the passage of the atherectomy catheter or to increase the final lumen diameter. In such cases, Kim et al[12] tried to compare the results of the Simpson device with those of balloon angioplasty in both iliac and infrainguinal lesions. They compared lesions ($n = 68$) treated with atherectomy alone with lesions ($n = 17$) treated with both atherectomy and supplemental balloon angioplasty. Lesions treated with the Simpson device alone achieved patencies of 92%, 84%, and 84%, respectively, and patencies of 78%, 67%, and 57% at 1, 2, and 3 years, respectively, were obtained with the lesions treated by combined atherectomy and balloon angioplasty. In such a study, it is difficult to delineate the influence of each treatment modality. In a more appropriate prospective randomized clinical study, Vroegindewij et al[14] recently reported 2-year cumulative patency rates of 35% in lesions ($n = 38$) treated with Simpson atherectomy alone compared to 56% in lesions ($n = 35$) treated by balloon angioplasty. Although this cumulative patency difference was found not to be statistically significant, the study noted that atherectomy was associated with a significantly lower patency rate than balloon angioplasty among patients with a lesion length of 2 cm or more.

Recently, the Simpson atherectomy catheter has been found to be effective in treating recurrent infrainguinal bypass graft stenoses. Dolmatch et al[3] reported a 92% technical success rate in treating 18 lower extremity bypass grafts (11 PTFEs, 7 autologous saphenous veins) with 23 areas of anastomotic stenosis. Graft patency was 88%, with a mean follow-up of 14 months. Additionally, to evaluate the long-term results of Simpson atherectomy, Porter et al[4] performed 52 procedures (atherectomy alone in 42, atherectomy plus balloon angioplasty in 10) to treat 67 stenoses (28 anastomotic, 39 intragraft) in 44 infrainguinal vein grafts.

They reported a 96% technical success rate by reducing the average diameter stenosis of 81% (range, 50% to 99%) before treatment to 11% (range, 0% to 30%) after treatment. Postintervention primary patency was 83%, 80%, and 80% at 1, 2, and 3 years, respectively. These results suggest that Simpson atherectomy is effective and more durable than PTA in this clinical setting, and its results may be comparable to the results associated with surgical revision.[20,21]

The Simpson atherectomy catheter has also been used to treat failing hemodialysis access fistulas. In their initial experience, Zemel et al[5] reported a 77% technical success rate using the Simpson device to treat stenotic hemodialysis fistulas in 13 patients. Gray et al[6] reported an 83% technical success rate and a 50% patency rate at 6 months in treating hemodialysis access conduits with 12 intragraft stenoses. These investigators claim that the Simpson atherectomy device is safe and effective in the treatment of recurrent stenotic hemodialysis access fistulas. Further clinical investigation with a larger study population is currently indicated to evaluate the intermediate- and long-term efficacy of this treatment modality.

Complications and Limitations

The Simpson atherectomy device is relatively safe. The most frequent complications associated with it include hematoma caused by bleeding at the atherectomy entry site, pseudoaneurysm, and distal embolization. Graor and Whitlow[10] reported seven cases of hematoma that required major intervention, including one patient who also developed a pseudoaneurysm. Kim et al[12] attributed the 11 cases of hematoma in their study to the bulky 7 Fr. to 12 Fr. vascular sheaths used and reported three cases of pseudoaneurysm that required surgical repair. Distal embolic problems were also noted, which required surgical intervention in severe cases and urokinase infusion or no treatment if clinically insignificant.

Savader et al[15] stated that Simpson atherectomy has a patency similar to that reported for balloon angioplasty in the treatment of femoral and popliteal artery lesions but also a high complication rate of 42.8%, including 15 (21.4%) major and 15 (21.4%) minor complications. The major complications included four puncture-site hematomas attributed to the use of 9 Fr. or larger sheaths (these patients subsequently underwent vessel repair and/or an extended hospital stay); seven distal embolic episodes treated with aspiration embolectomy and/or urokinase therapy; two cases of contrast-induced renal failure that required rehydration or dialysis; one pseudoaneurysm that required surgical repair; and a thrombosed arterial lesion within 24 hours treated conservatively. All 15 minor complications were puncture-site hematomas that required no treatment. This complication rate is higher than that associated with conventional PTA.[17–19]

One of the main limitations of the Simpson atherectomy device is its failure to reduce the rate of restenosis. At 6 months, Simpson et al[7] reported a restenosis rate of 36%, Polnitz et al[8] reported rates of 24% and 11% for concentric and eccentric lesions, respectively; and Dorros et al[11] reported a 55% recurrence rate. In the treatment of recurrent infrainguinal bypass graft stenosis, Dolmatch et al[3] reported a 26% restenosis and reocclusion rate, although Porter et al[4] noted only a 12% restenosis rate in treating vein graft stenosis.

The other significant limitation of the Simpson device is its relative ineffectiveness in treating long, diffusely diseased segments and long, totally occluded lesions. Polnitz et al[8] observed restenosis at 1 year of 7% among vessels with short ≤5 cm stenoses and 14% in vessels with complex >5 cm lesions. Dorros et al[11] reported a 100% recurrence rate in superficial femoral artery lesions ≥10 cm and a rate of 59% among lesions <10 cm in length. Furthermore, Vroegindewij et al[14] found that their treated lesions of 2 cm or more were associated with a significantly lower patency rate at 1 year (14%) compared to the lesions less than 2 cm in length (50%).

Transluminal Extraction Catheter

Much less experience has been reported using the TEC device in the treatment of peripheral arterial occlusive disease, and the results are difficult to interpret. Wholey and Jarmolowski[22] and Myers et al[23] reported initial technical success rates of 92% and 86%, respectively, and immediate clinical success rates of 90% and 79%, respectively. However, Wholey and Jarmolowski provided 6-month follow-up for only 50 of the 95 patients, and only 16 patients had undergone repeat angiography. Myers et al reported patency rates of 80% for lesions ≤5 cm in length and 64% for lesions >5 cm

in length at 6 months, although adjunctive balloon angioplasty was performed in 76% of all treated lesions.

Complications and Limitations

Complications associated with the TEC device have not been reported in detail. Wholey and Jarmolowski[22] reported only two (2%) thrombotic complications, which were subsequently treated with urokinase infusion. Meyers et al[23] reported a 6% complication rate in treating primarily long, complex lesions including two deaths, catheter fracture requiring removal and replacement in two cases, thromboembolism in two cases, and puncture-site bleeding in three cases.

Restenosis and reocclusion are the primary limitations of the TEC device. Of the 16 patients who underwent repeat angiography during follow-up, Wholey and Jarmolowski[22] found restenosis in four (25%) patients at 3 months and reocclusion in four patients whose lesions were >8 cm in length. Myers et al[23] reported restenosis in 26 (18%) and reocclusion in 51 lesions (35%) at 6 months of follow-up.

OmniCath

Preliminary clinical data using the OmniCath device for peripheral atherectomy have not been published, but animal data have been reported by Mazur et al.[24] Concentric and eccentric lesions were induced in the bilateral external iliac arteries of 10 miniature swines and subsequently underwent atherectomy with the OmniCath device. Five swines were sacrificed 3 days after the atherectomy procedure and the other five at 6 weeks. Histologic sections of the 3-day-old atherectomized lesions showed that the depth of cuts ranged from partial plaque removal to nearly full luminal thickness of the artery. Histologic sections of the 6-week atherectomized lesions revealed a minimal healing response. No evidence of vessel wall injury or significant neointimal proliferation at the anchoring wire deployment sites was found. Angiography revealed 20% luminal narrowing in one lesion at 6 weeks. In evaluating a prototype of the device in microswines, Sapoval et al[25] determined its maneuverability to be satisfactory but its aspiration apparatus inefficient. The OmniCath device underwent several modifications before use in humans.

Complications and Limitations

Mazur et al[24] reported spasm at the atherectomy site in most of the animals, and Sapoval et al[25] reported arterial ruptures in three of four animals. Human clinical trials are currently warranted to determine the safety and efficacy of the OmniCath device in the treatment of peripheral arterial occlusive disease.

Table 17–2. Literature Review Using the Auth Rotablator Device to Treat Peripheral Occlusive Disease

Study	No. of Patients	No. of Lesions	Technical Success	Immediate Clinical Success	Primary Patency		
					6 Mo	12 Mo	24 Mo
Dorros et al[26]	43	82	95%	88%	NA	NA	NA
Ahn et al[27]	20	42	93%	72%	66%	47%	12%
White et al[28]	17	18	94%	94%	82%	NA	NA
CRAG[29]	72	107	89%	77%	47%	31%	18.6%
Henry et al[30]	150	212	97%	85%	NA	NA	NA
Myers & Denton[31]	34	36	94%	92%	68%	60.7%	NA

Abbreviation: NA, not available.

Auth Rotablator

Clinical studies have documented promising technical and immediate clinical success with the Auth Rotablator (Table 17.2).[26–31] However, half of these series reported a follow-up of only 6 months, and patencies obtained at this time interval were suboptimal, ranging from 47% to 82%. Furthermore, 1-year patency rates were substantially poorer (31% to 61%).[27,29,31]

Ahn et al[27] performed atherectomy with the Auth Rotablator in 20 patients with claudication, ulcer or gangrene, rest pain, or an asymptomatic failing graft. Twenty-five lesions were treated; 20 lesions had 50% to 95% stenoses, and 5 lesions were complete occlusions. Although the technical success rate was 93%, the in-hospital success rate was only 72% because of complications that developed in 17 (68%) of 25 cases. The cumulative 2-year patency rate was a dismal 12%.

The Collaborative Rotablator Atherectomy Group[29] (CRAG) reported their experience with the Auth Rotablator on a multicenter trial. Technical angiographic success (<25% residual lumen) was achieved in 70 of 79 limbs (89%) and in 82 of 107 arteries (77%). In addition to the nine technical failures, in-hospital thrombosis occurred in nine limbs, resulting in an in-hospital success rate of 77% (61 of 79 limbs). Furthermore, complications occurred in approximately half of the patients, and half of them subsequently underwent an urgent or emergent surgical procedure within 30 days. Six of these patients underwent amputation, two of which were associated with the device. Late failure was observed in 32 limbs within 15 to 41 months, four of which also resulted in an amputation. The 2-year cumulative patency rate was a most disappointing 18.6%.

Complications and Limitations

In addition to the poor intermediate and long-term results discussed above, peripheral atherectomy with the Auth Rotablator currently has limited application because of several complications associated with the device. Significant early thrombosis occurs not infre-

quently. Ahn et al[27] reported five in-hospital cases of vessel thrombosis (25%), although four were associated with hypercoagulable states. The CRAG[29] reported nine cases of early thrombosis (11%), and two subsequently led to amputation. Henry et al[30] correlated the 12 thromboses (8%) in their series with a number of factors, including dissection, elastic recoil, intimal flaps, lengthy lesion, residual stenosis, or vasospasm. In addition, arterial spasm was found in 23% of cases by Dorros et al[26] and 11% by Henry et al,[30] most often in small distal arteries. This has been attributed to the use of large burrs, long rotational sequences, and/or rotational speed.

Gross hemoglobinuria without any clinical sequelae was found in 63% of the cases by Dorros et al,[26] in 20% of the cases by Ahn et al,[27] and in 13% of the cases by the CRAG.[29] These complications were transient and developed in lesions that required larger burrs and prolonged rotational sequences.

Contrary to previous studies using a canine model,[32] the atherectomized particles are not always small enough to pass safely through the reticuloendothelial system. Indeed, the rate of embolic complications was 20% in the series of Ahn et al,[27] 10% on the CRAG study,[29] and 1% in the report of Henry et al.[30] Three of the eight embolic events reported by the CRAG resulted in cutaneous necrosis and one in toe amputation.

Like all other atherectomy devices, the Auth Rotablator was also reported to cause dissections, perforations, and puncture-site hematomas.[26–30] Similarly, late restenosis and reocclusion is a significant limiting factor of the Auth Rotablator. Although most of the residual lumens achieved were less than 20%, Ahn et al[27] reported restenosis in 45% (9 of 20) and reocclusion in 80% (4 of 5) within 18 months. Intimal hyperplasia was believed to be the causative factor in these cases. The CRAG[29] reported late restenoses and reocclusions in 40% (32 of 79 limbs) during long-term follow-up of 15 to 41 months. Recently, Henry et al[30] reported a 24% restenosis rate, mostly in lesions ≥7 cm in length.

CONCLUSION

All atherectomy devices that have undergone clinical investigation have failed to reduce the incidence of restenosis, which occurs in association with other endovascular procedures such as PTA. Despite actual removal, debulking, and even polishing of the plaque, the invariable arterial wall trauma still induces intimal hyperplasia, which subsequently results in restenosis. Until the problem of restenosis can be solved, atherectomy will be limited to those instances in which balloon angioplasty may be ineffective or contraindicated. Such instances might include the presence of hard, eccentric, and/or calcified lesions that are difficult to dilate and the presence of intimal hyperplastic, recurrent, stenotic lesions in the failing lower extremity bypass graft and hemodialysis access site.

REFERENCES

1. In: Ahn SS (ed): *ISCVS/SVS Handbook on Endovascular Procedures.* RG Landes Bioscience, 1996;
2. Pieczek AM, Langevin RE, Razvi S, Rosenfield K. Successful percutaneous revascularization of 180/190 (95%) consecutive peripheral arterial total occlusions using hydrophilic ("Glide") wire. *Circulation* 1992;86(suppl 1):I-704. Abstract.
3. Dolmatch BL, Gray RJ, Horton KM, Rundback JH, Kline ME. Treatment of anastomotic bypass graft stenosis with directional atherectomy: short-term and intermediate results. *J Vasc Intervent Radiol* 1995;6:105–113.
4. Porter DH, Rosen MP, Skillman JJ, Kent KC, Kim D. Long term results with directional atherectomy of vein graft stenoses. *J Vasc Surg* in press.
5. Zemel G, Katzen BT, Dake MD, Benenati JF, Lempert TE, Moskowitz L. Directional atherectomy in the treatment of stenotic dialysis access fistulas. *J Vasc Intervent Radiol* 1990;1:35–38.
6. Gray RJ, Dolmatch BL, Buick MK. Directional atherectomy treatment for hemodialysis access: early results. *J Vasc Intervent Radiol* 1992;3:497–503.
7. Simpson JB, Selmon MR, Robertson GC, et al. Transluminal atherectomy for occlusive peripheral vascular disease. *Am J Cardiol* 1988;61:96–101.
8. Polnitz A, Nerlich A, Berger H, Hofling B. Percutaneous peripheral atherectomy. *J Am Coll Cardiol* 1990;15:628–688.
9. Hinohara T, Selmon MR, Robertson GC, Braden L, Simpson JS. Directional atherectomy: new approaches for treatment of obstructive coronary and peripheral vascular disease. *Circulation* 1990;81(suppl IV):IV-79–IV-91.
10. Graor R, Whitlow P. Transluminal atherectomy for occlusive peripheral vascular disease. *J Am Coll Cardiol* 1990;15:1551–1558.
11. Dorros G, Iyer S, Lewin R, Zaitoun R, Mathiak L, Olson K. Angiographic follow-up and clinical outcome of 126 patients after percutaneous directional atherectomy (Simpson AtheroCath) for occlusive peripheral vascular disease. *Cathet Cardiovasc Diagn* 1991;22:79–84.
12. Kim D, Gianturco LE, Porter DH, et al. Peripheral directional atherectomy: 4-year experience. *Radiology* 1992;183:773–778.
13. Lugmayr H, Pachinger O, Deutsch M. Long term results of percutaneous atherectomy in peripheral arterial occlusive disease. *Rofo Fortschr Geb Rontgenstr Neuen Bildgeb Verfahr* 1993;158:532–535.
14. Vroegindewij D, Tielbeek AV, Buth J, Schol FPG, Hop WCJ, Landman GH. Directional atherectomy vs. balloon angioplasty in segmental femoropopliteal artery disease: 2-year follow-up with color flow duplex scanning. *J Vasc Surg* 1995;21:255–269.
15. Savader SJ, Venbrux AC, Mitchell SE, et al. Percutaneous transluminal atherectomy of the superficial femoral and popliteal arteries: long term results in 48 patients. *Cardiovasc Intervent Radiol* 1994;17:312–318.
16. Wildenhain PM, Wholey MH, Jarmolowski CR, Hill KL. Infrainguinal directional atherectomy: long-term follow-up and comparison with percutaneous transluminal angiopolasty. *Cardiovasc Intervent Radiol* 1994;17:305–311.
17. Johnston KW, Rae M, Hogg-Johnston SA, et al. five-year results of a prospective study of percutaneous transluminal angioplasty. *Ann Surg* 1987;206:403–413.
18. Samson RH, Sprayregen S, Veith F, et al. Management of angioplasty complications, unsuccessful procedures and early and late failures. *Ann Surg* 1984;199:234–240.
19. Stanley B, Teague B, Raptis S, Taylor DJ, Berce M. Efficacy of balloon angioplasty of the superficial femoral artery and popliteal artery in the relief of leg ischemia. *J Vasc Surg* 1996;23:679–685.
20. Perler BA, Osterman FA, Mitchell SE, et al. Balloon dilatation versus surgical revision of infra-inguinal autogenous vein graft stenoses: long-term follow-up. *J Cardiovasc Surg* 1990;31:656–661.
21. Whittemore AD, Donaldson MC, Polak JF, Mannick JA. Limitations of balloon angioplasty for vein graft stenosis. *J Vasc Surg* 1991;14:340–345.
22. Wholey MH, Jarmolowski CR. New reperfusion devices: the Kensey catheter, the atherolytic reperfusion wire device, and the transluminal extraction catheter. *Radiology* 1989;172:947–952.
23. Myers KA, Denton MJ, Devine TJ. Infrainguinal atherectomy using the transluminal endarterectomy catheter: patency rates and clinical success for 144 procedures. *J Endovasc Surg* 1994;1:61–70.
24. Mazur W, Ali NM, Rodgers GP, Schulz DG, French BA, Raizner AE. Directional atherectomy with the OmniCath: a unique new catheter system. *Cathet Cardiovasc Diagn* 1994;31:79–???.
25. Sapoval MR, Gaux JC, Bruneval P, Peronneau P. Animal evaluation of the prototype OmniCath atherectomy catheter. *Cardiovasc Intervent Radiol* 1994;17:226.
26. Dorros G, Iyer S, Zaitoun R, Lewin R, Cooley R, Olson K. Acute angiographic and clinical outcome of high speed percutaneous rotational atherectomy (Rotablator). *Cathet Cardiovasc Diagn* 1991;22:157–166.
27. Ahn SS, Eton D, Yeatman LR, Deutsch LS, Moore WS. Intraoperative peripheral rotary atherectomy: early and late clinical results. *Ann Vasc Surg* 1992;6:272–280.
28. White CJ, Ramee SR, Escobar A, Jain S, Collins TJ. High speed rotational ablation (Rotablator) for unfavorable lesions in peripheral arteries. *Cathet Cardiovasc Diagn* 1993;30:115–119.
29. The Collaborative Rotablator Atherectomy Group: Peripheral atherectomy with the Rotablator: a multicenter report. *J Vasc Surg* 1994;19:509–515.

30. Henry M. Amor M, Ethevenot G, Henry I, Allaoui M. Percutaneous peripheral atherectomy using the Rotablator: a single center experience *J Endovasc Surg* 1995;2:51–66.

31. Myers KA, Denton MJ. Infrainguinal atherectomy using the Auth Rotablator: patency rates and clinical success for 36 procedures. *J Endovasc Surg* 1995:2:67–73.

32. Ahn SS, Auth D, Marcus D, Moore WS. Removal of focal atheromatous lesions by angioscopically guided high-speed rotary atherectomy. Preliminary experimental observations. *J Vasc Surg* 1988;7:292–300.

18

PTA of Infrainguinal Bypass Graft Stenoses: Patient Selection and Results

Henry D. Berkowitz, M.D.

The long-term success of infrainguinal bypass grafts depends on meticulous surgery followed by an equally meticulous program of postoperative surveillance to detect and treat new stenotic lesions that threaten graft patency. There is now general agreement that, excluding intraoperative technical problems, the development of stenotic lesions in the graft conduit and/or contiguous arteries is the most common cause of postoperative graft thrombosis. It appears that most lesions develop within the first postoperative year. The current emphasis on diagnosis and repair of these stenotic, "failing" grafts represents a significant change in postoperative management and is largely responsible for the improved long-term results in contemporary reports.

The most common method of repairing a stenotic graft is to replace or bypass the stenotic segment with a short length of a new graft. This procedure is highly successful and has a low recurrence rate. The role of percutaneous transluminal angioplasty (PTA) as an alternative to surgery has been somewhat controversial, and only a few reports include enough cases to allow meaningful statistical analyses of patency. Although satisfactory results compared to those of surgery are reported in some studies when proper selection criteria are used, there is a high recurrence rate and more repeat interventions are required. The controversy surrounding PTA involves the relative benefit of avoiding surgery, which can be technically demanding, with a less invasive procedure, which is more likely to require reintervention.

This chapter will review the incidence, appearance times, and location of stenotic graft lesions. The information pertains primarily to vein grafts, although some data on PTFE grafts will also be presented. The diagnostic laboratory tests used to detect the failing graft will be described, and the criteria and rationale for using PTA as the primary treatment for a stenotic graft will be presented, based on the author's experience as well as on published data from other centers.

INCIDENCE

Graft stenosis is an inclusive term that refers to the combined problem of strictures within the graft conduit, as well as within the inflow and outflow arteries. The large variation in the reported incidence of graft stenosis, 8 to 35% (median, 21%), is related to many factors such as graft type, duration of follow-up, and the tests used for diagnosis.[1-13] The majority of the stenotic lesions are diagnosed within the first postoperative year (range, 36 to 77%), but new lesions have been identified up to 10 years after surgery.[3,10,11] In one study, grafts that were patent for at least 4.5 years had a 50% incidence of significant abnormalities discovered by duplex ultrasonography. Many of these abnormalities were focal stenoses in grafts that had been revised previously, but aneurysms and generalized atherosclerosis were also seen.[10]

Because most stenotic grafts are discovered during the first 1 to 2 years after surgery, follow-up examinations at 3-month intervals are required. After 2 years, the intervals can be lengthened to 6 to 12 months, but the examinations should be continued indefinitely to detect the additional 20 to 30% of mature grafts that may become strictured.

Compared to vein grafts, stenotic polytetrafluoroethylene (PTFE) grafts are prone to spontaneous occlusion even when noninvasive studies are normal, and therefore information on the incidence of PTFE graft stenosis is limited. The high (24%) incidence reported by O'Donnell et al[8] was obtained from an analysis of grafts that were already occluded, and the low (3%) incidence reported by Ascer et al[9] reflected a policy of not obtaining repeat arteriograms in patients with suspected graft stenosis if they remained asymptomatic.

ANATOMIC DISTRIBUTION OF LESIONS

Approximately 75% of stenotic vein graft lesions are found within the graft conduit and only 25% in the contiguous arteries.[1–6,13,14] It is convenient to group lesions according to their position in the proximal, middle, or distal third of the graft. Strictures found in the proximal and distal third of the graft are further subdivided into anastomotic and juxta-anastomotic segments. Reversed veins have the smallest graft diameter located in the proximal third of the bypass, while the small end of the in situ graft is found distally. Stenotic lesions in the proximal graft, particularly the juxta-anastomotic segment, are the most common lesions found in reversed veins.[15,16] They are usually short, concentric, fibrous constrictions probably caused by smooth muscle proliferation, and their microscopic appearance is consistent with intimal hyperplasia. The lesions are commonly found immediately distal to the "cobra head" of the proximal anastomosis. Conversely, in situ grafts develop relatively more stenoses in the distal rather than the proximal third of the graft, where the graft is narrowest,[17] although most in situ graft stenoses develop in the middle third of the conduit. These lesions are usually short, web-like stenoses at the site of venous valves that may have been incompletely excised during insertion of the graft or became hypertrophic later. Anastomotic strictures are the third major type of graft lesion, and are found at both anastomoses as well as at the anastomosis between spliced vein segments. They are frequently long, tapering stenoses and may be less amenable to PTA than other lesions.

Lesions in the contiguous arteries develop later than those within the graft.[3,10,11] These lesions are composed predominantly of atherosclerotic plaques that form de novo, but because some are located immediately adjacent to an anastomosis, it is believed that clamp trauma during bypass surgery may be an important etiology.

In contrast to vein grafts, PTFE grafts develop stenotic lesions almost exclusively in the outflow artery and at the distal anastomosis.[8]

DIAGNOSIS OF FAILING GRAFTS

Stenotic or failing grafts should be suspected whenever recurrent symptoms or changes in distal pulses are discovered during follow-up examinations. Because in a significant percentage of cases even severely stenotic grafts may not be associated with symptoms, and because distal pulses may still be present,[3,4,11,18] these grafts may only be detected with vascular laboratory tests. Hemodynamic measurements based on Doppler-derived ankle/brachial indexes (ABI) and segmental plethysmography (PVR)[19,20] were the original tests used for this purpose. A drop in ABI >0.1 to 0.2 on serial measurements can identify 60% of stenotic grafts when a >50% diameter-reducing stenosis is present.[7,15] Serial measurements of PVR that show a >5-mm decrease in amplitude at the ankle can identify 79% of grafts that have a >60% diameter-reducing stenosis. The combination of the two studies was 90% accurate in one report.[15]

The measurement of Doppler-derived graft velocity measurements at selected sites within the graft has proved more sensitive than the pure hemodynamic measurements described above in identifying graft stenoses (see Chapter 14). The subcutaneous position of in situ grafts makes them readily accessible for velocity measurements. Bandyk et al[7] reported that a single velocity measurement of <45.0 cm/sec correctly identified 96% of stenoses. Subsequent reports have broadened the velocity indicators to include high (>120.0 to 300.0 cm/sec) and low (<30.0 cm/sec) velocity parameters.[4,5,16,21] Color flow Doppler scanning has extended the use of velocity measurements by facilitating examination of the entire graft. Peak systolic velocities are measured at the point of maximum stenosis and at normal adjacent segments, and a velocity ratio ($Vr = V^{stenosis}/V^{normal}$) is calculated. The Vr has been correlated with degrees of graft stenosis and varies from >2.0 for a >50% diameter-reducing stenosis to >6.0 for a >80% diameter-reducing stenosis.[5,12,21]

The justification for discovering and repairing graft stenoses is based on the fundamental assumption that a stenotic graft will eventually occlude. However, until recently, there were no prospective studies that followed stenotic grafts without repairing them. Idu et al[4] found that 57% of grafts with a 50 to 69% stenosis and 100% of grafts with a 70 to 99% stenosis occluded during 5 years of follow-up if the stenosis was not revised, while only 10% of similar grafts occluded if they were revised. Green et al[22] followed grafts using duplex velocity and serial ABI measurements over 2 years. They reported that if both ABI and Doppler measurements were abnormal, 66% of the grafts were thrombosed when examined 3 months later, but only 4% were occluded if the ABI was normal. Mattos et al[5] utilized a Vr >2.0 to identify grafts with a >50% diameter-reducing stenosis. Twenty-six percent of the nonrevised grafts occluded by 48 months compared to only 8% of the revised grafts. Moody et al[18] obtained angiograms 2 to 36 months after the initial bypass in a group of asymptomatic patients and repeated them after a mean interval of 13 months. Severe strictures (>66% narrowing) were found in 12% of the grafts on the first arteriogram, and 50% of these grafts became occluded, or more severely stenotic, by the second examination. It seems clear that stenotic grafts with >50% diameter-reducing stenoses are susceptible to thrombosis, and the risk increases with the severity of stenosis.

PERCUTANEOUS BALLOON ANGIOPLASTY

Surgical revision of stenotic vein grafts has been associated with 5-year cumulative graft patency ranging from 85 to 92%.[16] While simple excision or patch angioplasty of a localized lesion in a subcutaneous graft is readily accomplished, a surgical procedure can be technically demanding for lesions that occur near an anastomosis or in a reversed vein graft located in a deep anatomic plane.

The treatment of vein graft lesions by PTA was initially reported in 1979.[23] While the author has continued to use PTA as the preferential initial therapy for treating graft lesions, other centers have reported less than satisfactory results. Therefore, PTA has not been uniformly accepted as an alternative to surgery.

PTA is most successful when treating short-segment lesions in otherwise normal graft conduits. The author has preferentially surgically revised graft stenoses longer than 5.0 cm and has reserved PTA for grafts with short (<5.0 cm) stenoses. In fact, in a previous publication,[15] 73% of the 72 graft lesions revised by PTA were actually <2.0 cm long. Although dilation of a long, irregular stenosis is technically feasible, rapid restenosis occurs in a high percentage of cases, and surgical repair using short interposition or bypass grafts provides the best long-term treatment for these lesions.[7,16] Published reports that have demonstrated the greatest success in treating lesions with PTA have also stressed the importance of selecting short (<1.5–5.0-cm) segmental graft lesions for dilatation.[15] Berkowitz et al[15] reported PTA of 72 stenotic vein grafts that contained lesions <5.0 cm long, and the 5-year primary assisted patency was 80%. Sanchez et al[25] reported a 66% primary patency at 24 months for 41 vein grafts revised by PTA if the grafts had a minimum diameter of 3.0 mm and contained only a single lesion that was less than 1.5 cm long. Fifty-four grafts that did not meet these criteria had a 24-month patency rate of only 17%. London et al[26] used PTA to revise 28 stenotic vein grafts, including 94% with stenoses that were <2.0 cm long, and the 42-month secondary graft patency rate was 69%.

The data showing poor results after PTA may be related more to adverse case selection than to inherent problems with the technique. Whittemore and associates[27] reported an 18% primary patency rate 5 years after PTA in 54 stenotic vein grafts. However, there were multiple factors that may have predisposed these grafts to fail after PTA. Twenty percent of the grafts were initially thrombosed and required lysis before the stenotic lesion was revised, 56% of the grafts had long, irregular stenoses, and 65% required simultaneous revision of multiple lesions. Only the subgroup of grafts

with a single lesion had a significantly better 36-month primary patency rate of 59% compared to the other grafts. Perler et al[28] used PTA to treat 19 stenotic grafts, and recurrent lesions developed in 67%. Repeating the PTA provided little benefit, and the 36-month secondary patency rate was only 27%. No analysis of the results based on multiplicity or length of the treated lesions was provided.

Vein grafts are not a completely homogeneous group, and bypass patency will depend on the particular type of vein used. The term *alternate vein* has been coined to differentiate grafts composed of cephalic, lesser saphenous, and spliced veins from grafts composed of a single segment of greater saphenous vein. Donaldson et al[29] reported a 79% 5-year cumulative secondary patency in 447 grafts constructed with saphenous veins compared to a 49% patency in 138 alternate veins. These differences in graft patency suggest that the results after revising stenotic grafts also depend on the type of the underlying vein graft.

The author's vascular registry now includes 155 stenotic vein grafts composed of 127 (82%) greater saphenous grafts and 28 (18%) alternate vein grafts. The veins were used primarily as reversed grafts (82%), and 18% were placed in situ. PTA was used to revise 76% (118 of 155) grafts with a single short (<5.0 cm) stenosis, including 100 saphenous vein grafts (Table 18–1), and surgical revision was used for the other 24%, which contained multiple or long (>5.0 cm) stenoses. The cumulative primary patency following PTA was only 15% at 5 years because 42% of the grafts required a secondary revision. Primary patency calculations include both revision and occlusion as patency endpoints (Fig. 18–1). However, the cumulative primary assisted patency was 68% 5 years following PTA because this calculation considers only occlusion as an endpoint for graft patency. PTA was clearly more successful with saphenous vein grafts (Fig. 18–2), and the

Table 18–1. Location of Stenotic Lesions and Graft Patency After PTA in 100 Saphenous Vein Grafts

Location of Stenosis	No. of Lesions	5-Year Patency* (%)
Inflow artery	20	80
Proximal anastomosis	14	54
Proximal juxta-anastomosis	28	80
Midgraft	9	89
Distal anastomosis	10	70
Distal juxta-anastomosis	10	57
Outflow artery	9	67
Total	100	

* Five-year cumulative primary assisted patency.
S.E. > 10% for all patencies at 5 years.

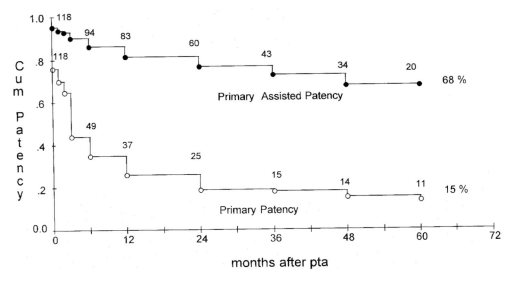

Figure 18–1. Cumulative patency after PTA of 118 stenotic saphenous plus alternate vein grafts. Comparison of primary versus primary assisted patency. S.E. ± 0.03 primary and 0.06 primary assisted patency at 5 years.

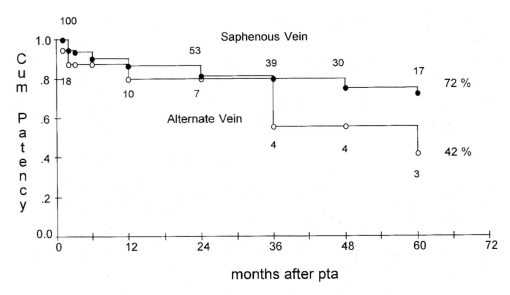

Figure 18–2. Cumulative primary assisted patency after PTA of 100 saphenous versus 18 alternate stenotic vein grafts. Saphenous vein S.E. ± 0.06 at 5 years, alternate vein S.E. > 0.10 after 6 months. $P < 0.33$ (ns) Wilcoxon (Gehan) statistic.

5-year primary assisted patency rate of 72% was nearly twice the 42% patency achieved in treating alternate vein grafts. Surgical revision proved equally successful in both types of vein grafts; patency of 65% and 66% were found in the 27 saphenous and 10 alternate vein grafts, respectively. Thirty-eight percent of the surgically revised grafts required a secondary revision, similar to the 42% incidence after PTA (Table 18–2).

A possible explanation for the inferior results after revision of alternate vein grafts with PTA may be related to the finding that 50% of these grafts were composed of spliced vein segments, with strictures at the vein–vein anastomoses. This suggests that suture line strictures may be resistant to balloon dilatation. This conclusion has been reinforced by the observation that PTA of a stenotic proximal or distal anastomosis, even in a saphenous vein graft, had a poor late patency (Table 18–1).

The most common lesion revised by PTA was a proximal juxta-anastomotic stenosis, which was found in 28% of the grafts (Table 18–1). The 5-year cumulative patency following PTA of these grafts was 80%. PTA also resulted in excellent patency for inflow arterial and midgraft lesions (Table 18–1). These three lesions

Table 18–2. Graft Revisions After Initial PTA in 118 Stenotic Saphenous and Alternate Vein Grafts

Graft Revision Procedures	PTA	Surgery	Total Revisions	Revisions per Graft	No. of Grafts	% of Grafts	
First	118*		118	1	69	58	
Second	28	21	49	2	29	25	
Third	8	12	20	3	16	14	42%
Fourth	2	2	4	4	4	3	
Total	38	35	191		118	100	

*118 PTA − 35 secondary surgical revisions = 83 grafts (72%) treated exclusively by PTA.

taken as a group comprised 57% of the revised saphenous vein grafts and had a combined 80% primary assisted patency 5 years after PTA, while the other grafts with lesions in the proximal and distal anastomoses, distal juxta-anastomotic, and outflow arteries had a combined 61% cumulative patency. However, there were small numbers of grafts in each group and large standard errors.

Cumulative primary assisted patency of the original 100 saphenous grafts revised by PTA was 80% at 5 years, which was essentially equal to the 76% patency of 548 saphenous grafts that did not undergo any graft revision (Fig. 18–3). These results are quite comparable to published results of surgically revised grafts. Bandyk et al[7] revised 83 stenotic, predominantly in situ vein grafts. Twenty-seven percent required a secondary revision, and the 5-year primary assisted patency was 85%. In a series of 100 revised vein grafts reported by Nehler et al, secondary revisions were required in only 13%

and the 5-year primary assisted patency of the original grafts was 92%.[16] This value is considerably higher than the 77 to 82% femoropopliteal patency and the 74 to 82% femorotibial patency of vein bypass grafts currently reported by this group.

The major disadvantage of PTA is the large number of recurrences that require one or more secondary revisions. An analysis of recurrent strictures after PTA (Table 18–2) indicated that 42% of 118 vein grafts required a secondary revision for recurrent stenosis, while 58% were successfully managed by a single PTA. Two revisions were required in 25%, three revisions were required in 14%, and four revisions were required in 3% of the 118 saphenous and alternate vein grafts initially treated by PTA. In total, 72% (83 of 118) of the grafts were managed exclusively by PTA and only 28% required a surgical revision.

The potential attractiveness of PTA over surgery is that it requires a short hospital stay, usually overnight,

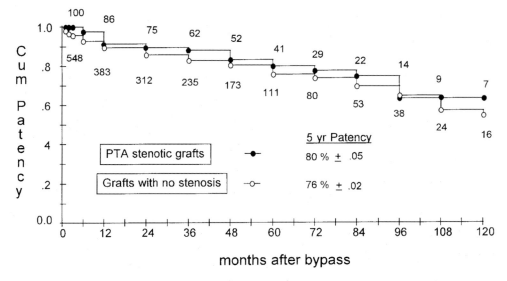

Figure 18–3. Cumulative primary assisted patency of 100 stenotic saphenous grafts treated with PTA versus 548 saphenous grafts with no diagnosis of stenosis. S.E. < 0.10 out to 108 months for both groups. P < 0.17 (ns) Wilcoxon (Gehan) statistic.

has minimal morbidity and mortality, and can easily be repeated. Although recurrences after PTA are common, the 27% secondary revision rate after surgical repair reported by Bandyk et al[7] is not very different from the 30% (26) and 42% (author's series) rates found after PTA. Surgery for these lesions is often referred to almost casually as minor, but this is true mainly for in situ graft lesions that are subcutaneous and easily accessible, except for the anastomotic area. The repair of lesions in perianastomotic areas or in grafts placed in anatomic tunnels may be formidable, and longer hospitalization and more resources are required.

PTA of stenotic graft lesions results in long-term patency comparable to that of surgical revision, provided that certain principles are followed. Only short (<5.0 cm and preferably <2.0 cm) stenoses should be dilated, and grafts with multiple lesions should be excluded. The best results are obtained with grafts composed of a single segment of greater saphenous vein. Midgraft, proximal juxta anastomotic, and inflow arterial stenoses appear to be more favorable candidates for PTA than proximal, distal, and vein–vein anastomotic lesions.

REFERENCES

1. Szilagyi DE, Elliott JP, Hagemn JH, et al. Biologic fate of autogenous vein implants as arterial substitutes: clinical, angiographic and histopathologic observations in femoro-popliteal operations for atherosclerosis. *Ann Surg* 1973;178:232–244.
2. Sladen JG, Gilmore JL. Vein graft stenosis: characteristics and effect of treatment. *Am J Surg* 1981;141:549–553.
3. Berkowitz HD, Greenstein S, Barker CF, et al. Late failure of reversed vein bypass grafts. *Ann Surg* 1989;210:782–786.
4. Idu MM, Blankenstein JD, De Grier P, et al. Impact of color-flow duplex surveillance program on infrainguinal vein graft patency: a five-year experience. *J Vasc Surg* 1993;17:42–53.
5. Mattos MA, Van Bemmelen PS, Hodgson KJ, et al. Does correction of stenosis identified with color duplex scanning improve infrainguinal graft patency? *J Vasc Surg* 17:54–66.
6. Mills JL, Fujitani RM, Taylor SM. The characteristics and anatomic distribution of lesions that cause reversed vein graft failure: a five-year prospective study. *J Vasc Surg* 1993;17:195–206.
7. Bandyk DF, Bergamini TM, Towne JB, et al. Durability of vein graft revision: the outcome of secondary procedures. *J Vasc Surg* 1991;13:200–210.
8. O'Donnell TF, Mackey W, McCullough JL, et al. Correlation of operative findings with angiographic and noninvasive hemodynamic factors associated with failure of polytetrafluoroethylene grafts. *J Vasc Surg* 1984;1:136–148.
9. Ascer E, Collier P, Gupta SK, et al. The importance of distal outflow site and operative technique in determining outcome. *J Vasc Surg* 1987;5:298–310.
10. Reifsnyder T, Towne JB, Seabrook GR, et al. Biologic characteristics of long-term autogenous vein grafts: a dynamic evolution. *J Vasc Surg* 1993;17:207–217.
11. Erickson CA, Towne JB, Seabrook GR, et al. Ongoing vascular laboratory surveillance is essential to maximize long-term in situ saphenous vein bypass patency. *J Vasc Surg* 1996;23:18–27.
12. Grigg MJ, Nicolaides AN, Wolfe JHN. Detection and grading of femorodistal vein graft stenosis: duplex velocity measurements compared with angiography. *J Vasc Surg* 1988;8:661–666.
13. Leather RP, Shah DM, Chang BB, et al. Resurrection of the in situ saphenous vein bypass: 1000 cases later. *Ann Surg* 1988;208:435–442.
14. Mills JL, Harris J, Tyalor LJR, et al. The importance of surveillance of distal bypass grafts with duplex scanning: a study of 379 reversed vein grafts. *J Vasc Surg* 1990;12:379–389.
15. Berkowitz HD, Fox AD, Deaton DH. Reversed vein graft stenosis: early diagnosis and management. *J Vasc Surg* 1992;15:130–142.
16. Nehler MR, Moneta GL, Yeager RA, et al. Surgical treatment of threatened reversed infrainguinal vein grafts. *J Vasc Surg* 1994;20:558–565.
17. Mills JL, Bandrk DF, Gahtan V, et al. The origin of infrainguinal vein graft stenosis: a prospective study based on duplex surveillance. *J Vasc Surg* 1995;21:16–25.
18. Moody P, DeDossart LM, Douglas HM, et al. Asymptomatic strictures in femoro-popliteal vein grafts. *Eur J Vasc Surg* 1989;3:389–392.
19. Berkowitz HD, Hobbs CL, Roberts B, et al. Value of routine vascular laboratory studies to identify vein graft stenosis. *Surgery* 1981;90:971–979.
20. Sampson RH, Gupta SK, Veith FJ, et al. Evaluation of graft patency utilizing ankle-brachial pressure index and ankle pulse volume recording amplitude. *Am J Surg* 1984;147:786–787.
21. Sladen JG, Reid JDS, Cooperberg PL, et al. Color flow duplex screening of infrainguinal grafts combining low and high velocity criteria. *Am J Surg* 1989;158:107–112.
22. Green RM, McNamara J, Ouriel K, et al. Comparison of infrainguinal graft surveillance techniques. *J Vasc Surg* 1990;11:207–215.
23. Alpert JR, Ring EJ, Berkowitz HD, et al. Treatment of vein graft stenosis by balloon catheter dilation. *JAMA* 1979;242:2769–2771.
24. Sanchez LA, Gupta SK, Veith FJ, et al. A ten year experience with one hundred fifty failing or threatened vein and PTFE arterial bypass grafts. *J Vasc Surg* 1991;14:729–738.
25. Sanchez LA, Suggs WD, Marin ML, et al. Is percutaneous balloon angioplasty appropriate in the treatment of graft and anastomotic lesions responsible for failing vein bypasses? *Am J Surg* 1994;168:97–101.
26. London NJM, Sayers RD, Thompson MN, et al. Interventional radiology in the maintainence of infrainguinal vein graft patency. *Br J Surg* 1993;80:187–193.
27. Whittemore AD, Donaldson MC, Polak JF, et al. Limitation of balloon angioplasty for vein graft stenosis. *J Vasc Surg* 1991;14:340–345.
28. Perler BA, Ostermon FA, Mitchell SE, et al. Balloon dilation versus surgical revision of infrainguinal autogenous vein graft stenosis: Long-term follow-up. *J Cardiovasc Surg* 1990;31:656–661.
29. Donaldson MC, Whittemore AD, Mannick JA, et al. Further experience with an all autogenous tissue policy for infrainguinal reconstruction. *J Vasc Surg* 1993;18:41–48.

19

Atheroembolism: Diagnosis and Management of the Blue Toe Syndrome

Richard R. Keen, M.D.
James S.T. Yao, M.D., Ph.D.

The diagnosis and management of atheroembolization from distal arteries is one of the more difficult clinical problems that the vascular specialist encounters.[1] The diagnosis of atheroembolism is often delayed because many physicians fail to recognize the unique clinical features. When patients first present with the painful, tender, discolored fingers or toes characteristic of atheroembolism, palpable extremity pulses are often still present. This classic physical finding of the blue toe syndrome along with palpable distal pulses, although paradoxical, is characteristic of atheroembolism. Unless the physician is familiar with atheroembolization, the normal axial pulses lead to a missed diagnosis and subsequent delay of therapeutic intervention.[2]

The morbid course of untreated atheroembolism is brought out by the historical recognition of atherosclerotic embolization as a pathologic event. The earliest reports of embolic events where the proximal arteries were found to be the sources of artery-to-artery emboli were based on autopsy studies. The link between severely diseased atherosclerotic aorta and visceral atheroemboli was first recognized by Flory in 1945, when he observed that autopsy cases in which the abdominal aorta had the most extensive atherosclerosis also has the largest number of visceral and muscular atheroemboli.[3] Flory's hypothesis that atheroembolism was due to atherosclerotic plaque was tested by removing and solubilizing human aortic atheroma and injecting this slurry into rabbit ear veins. This experiment reproduced pulmonary lesions in rabbits that were identical to the visceral and muscular lesions found in humans with atheroembolization.

Untreated atheroembolism is characterized by high rates of recurrent embolic episodes leading to tissue loss, multiple organ failure, and death. The natural history of untreated extremity atheroembolism was reported by Karmondy et al in 1976.[4] They observed that the nonoperative treatment of the "blue toe syndrome" (unilateral lower extremity ischemia due to emboli originating from a superficial femoral artery lesion) resulted in recurrent embolic events in four of five patients (80%) and limb loss in three of five patients.

The prognosis of untreated atheroembolism arising from an aortic source is even more dismal. Among patients in whom the thoracic or abdominal aorta was the embolic source and who did not undergo operative intervention for atheroembolic disease, Hollier et al reported a 5-year survival of less than 10%.[5]

PHYSICAL FINDINGS OF MICROEMBOLI AND MACROEMBOLI

The presence of atherosclerotic arterial-to-arterial emboli is suspected by the characteristic appearance of the limb. Atheroembolism presents as microscopic emboli (pulses intact) or macroemboli (pulse deficit); a combination of micro- and macroemboli also can occur. Microemboli consist of either fibrinoplatelet aggregates or cholesterol crystals that occlude arteries 100 to 200 μm in diameter. Microemboli lodged in terminal digital arterioles and subcutaneous tissues cause dermal cyanosis and the characteristic blue discoloration adjacent to areas of well-perfused skin (Fig. 19–1A). Focal areas of ischemia that are mixed with normally perfused skin can lead to the diffuse, web-like patterns of erythematous and violaceous skin discoloration characteristic of livedo reticularies (Fig. 19–1B). Noninvasive arterial Doppler studies are useful in confirming extremity ischemia, and in particular, the use

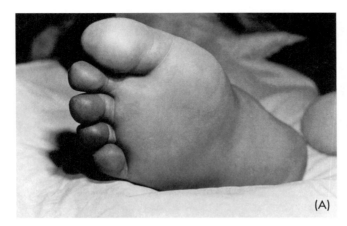
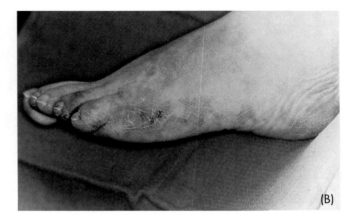

Figure 19–1.   Blue toes (A) and livedo reticularis (B) are characteristic of extremity atheroemboli.

of digital systolic pressure to establish the diagnosis of digital ischemia.

Microscopic atheroemboli cause exquisite pain and tenderness in the extremity that differs markedly from the characteristic physical findings seen with chronic lower extremity ischemic rest pain. In the absence of infection, chronic lower extremity ischemic rest pain is seldom associated with tenderness. Blue toes and livedo reticularis often are misdiagnosed as vasculitis, dermatitis, or vasospasm, especially in a setting of microembolization and palpable extremity pulses. Cholesterol microembolization triggers a vasculitic-type inflammatory response in the surrounding arterial wall that is characterized by inflammatory foreign body giant cells, granulocyte inflammation, and necrotizing angiitis.[6,7] A skin biopsy may help to establish the diagnosis of cholesterol embolization.

Aneurysm of the aorta or of major arteries such as subclavian and popliteal arteries also can present with embolization. However, in these cases, the events tend to be microembolic and more protean, as the progressive obliteration of the distal extremity arterial circulation is relatively silent. Microemboli from subclavian and popliteal artery aneurysms do not elicit the same degree of extremity pain and hyperesthesia found with microemboli from other sources. One possible explanation is the difference in the embolic debris. Subclavian, axillary, and popliteal artery aneurysms tend to embolize luminal thrombus, while emboli from other atherosclerotic sources consist more commonly of some cholesterol plaque that triggers the inflammatory response.

NORTHWESTERN UNIVERSITY EXPERIENCE

In recent years, we have undertaken a study in patients with atheroembolization. The following summarizes our experience in the treatment of these patients.[1,2]

Patient Demographics

Our patients with atheroembolism ranged in age from 32 to 90, with a mean age of 62 ± 11 years. Risk factors included smoking in 74%, hypertension in 46%, and diabetes in 22% of patients. Our patient population was 70% male and 30% female.

Location of Embolization

Isolated microemboli occurred in 45% of all cases, and combined micro- and macroemboli were present in 16% of patients. Macroscopic atheroemboli alone occurred less frequently (39% of cases), and presented with the findings of acute arterial occlusion and extremity ischemia.[2] At the time of clinical presentation or intervention, these macroemboli often cannot be distinguished from emboli of cardiac origin. Recognizing atherosclerotic macroemboli and differentiating them from emboli of a cardiac source requires a thorough evaluation of potential embolic sources.

The most common targets of atheroemboli were the lower extremities. (Fig. 19–2). Atheroemboli lodged in the renal arteries in 11% of patients. Eosinophilia is pathognomonic of renal atheroembolism and helps differentiate renal atheroembolism from muscle injury and myoglobin release as the cause of renal insufficiency following massive atheroembolism.[8]

Sources of Atherosclerotic Emboli

We reviewed 141 patients with atherosclerotic emboli to the lower or upper extremities treated at Northwestern University over a 12-year period,[2] and observed that the infrarenal aorta was responsible for the majority of atheroembolic events. Among 107 patients with lower extremity atheroembolism, aortoiliac occlusive disease was the embolic source in 52%, small aortic aneurysms were responsible in 20% (Fig. 19–3), lower extremity stenoses in 11% (Fig. 19–4), a shaggy thoracoabdominal aorta in 8%, degenerating bypass grafts in 7%, and

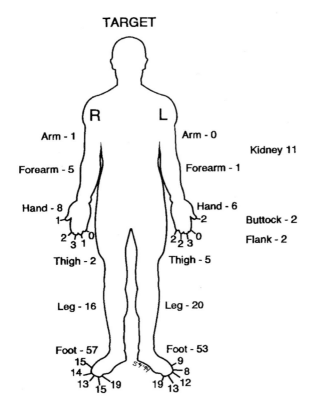

TARGET

Figure 19–2. Presenting targets of atheroembolic events in 100 patients treated with an operation directed at the source of atheroemboli. (Reprinted from Ref. 2 with permission.)

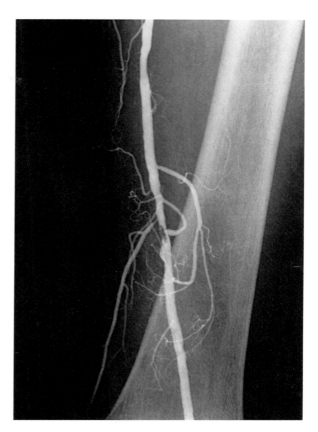

Figure 19–4. Characteristic superficial femoral artery atheroembolic lesion responsible for blue toe syndrome. (Reprinted from Ref. 2 with permission.)

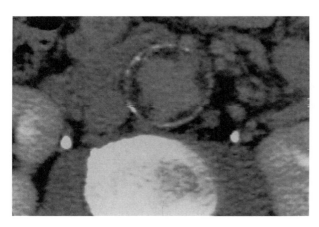

Figure 19–3. Star-shaped thrombus in small (3.7-cm) abdominal aortic aneurysm that presented with embolization, leading to transmetatarsal and above-knee amputation. A characteristic operative finding in aneurysms that embolized was irregular, complex thrombus overlying ulcerative aortic plaque. (Reprinted from Ref. 2 with permission.)

lower extremity arterial aneurysms in 2%. The sources of the atheroemboli among the 100 patients who eventually underwent operative treatment are depicted in Figure 19–5.

Our findings differed from those of Karmody et al, who reported that 23 (74%) of 31 patients with atheroemboli had a source below the inguinal ligament, because atherosclerotic disease proximal to the inguinal ligament accounted for more than 80% of all lower extremity emboli in our series. The reason for this difference is not clear, but it may be due to patient demographics or the smaller number of patients in the study of Karmody et al.[4] In our patients, the mean size of infrarenal aortic aneurysms that embolized was only 3.5 ± 0.8 cm. A higher mean blood flow velocity in small aortic aneurysms seems to be the most likely explanation for why smaller aneurysms embolize, while larger aneurysms usually do not.[5] In our series of 21 aortic aneurysms responsible for embolic events, only 1 aneurysm was larger than 4.5 cm.

Upper extremity atheroembolism occurs less frequently than atheroemboli to the lower extremities. Thirty of 141 patients with atheroembolism had a source in the upper extremity arteries[1] (Fig. 19–6).

SOURCE

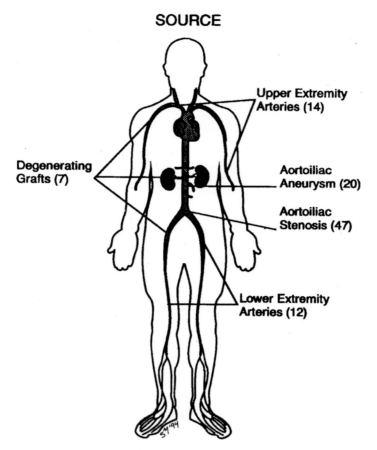

Figure 19–5. Source of atheroemboli in 100 patients treated with an operation undertaken to eliminate the source of emboli. (Reprinted from Ref. 2 with permission.)

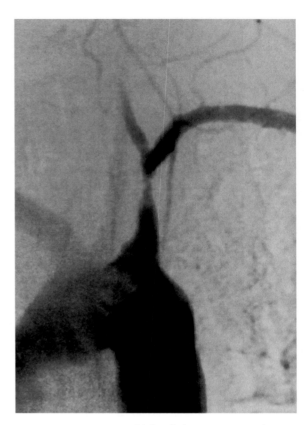

Figure 19–6. Proximal left subclavian stenosis that presented with microemboli to the fingers. (Reprinted from Ref. 2 with permission.)

However, other atheroembolism complicates a high proportion of cases of upper extremity ischemia. Mesh and Yao observed that atheroembolism occurred in 70% of upper extremity aneurysms.[9] Thoracic outlet syndrome arterial abnormalities were responsible for approximately half of the cases of upper extremity emboli.[2,10]

Diagnostic Technique to Identify the Embolic Source

The initial examination of the patient's extremity pulses determines the most appropriate diagnostic strategy to localize the embolic source. The majority of patients with atheroembolism (55%) have a pulse deficit on presentation,[2] and among patients who present with a new pulse deficit, arteriography with extremity runoff is the first localizing study undertaken. Arteriography is the most common and often the only diagnostic test needed to confirm and localize an atheroembolic source. Arteriography usually can both localize the source of the macroembolus that has caused the pulse deficit and provide the road map needed to plan any further radiologic or operative intervention.

Caution must be exercised when performing arteriography in patients with atheroemboli because the risk of a procedure-related embolic shower is significant[11] (Fig. 19–7). Therefore, among patients with atheroemboli who require arteriography, an axillary or brachial approach should be seriously considered. Atherosclerotic plaques that embolize are, by their nature, unstable, and the risk of material embolizing when a guidewire catheter is passed over the responsible lesion is increased compared to arterial plaques that have not embolized. In our series, in fact, arteriography precipitated the initial atheroembolic episode in 17% of the patients.[2]

The strategy for obtaining imaging studies in the other 45% of patients who present with microembolization alone (where the axial pulses are intact) is different. Specifically, among patients with palpable distal pulses and livedo reticularis or blue toes, a contrast-enhanced computed tomography (CT) scan of the abdominal aorta is the first study performed.[12] Because the aorta is the most common source of the microscopic atheroemboli that cause livedo reticularis and blue toes, abdominal aortic contrast-enhanced CT can

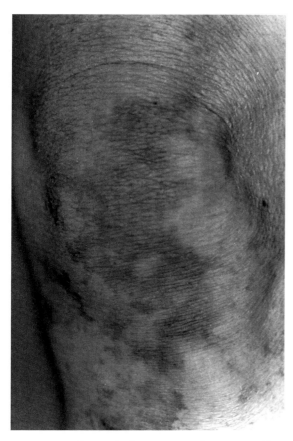

Figure 19–7. Atheroembolic events can be triggered by arteriography and balloon angioplasty. Livedo reticularis of the popliteal region was observed following iliac artery balloon angioplasty and atheroembolism through the profunda femoral artery runoff.

localize the source of the emboli as either aortoiliac occlusive disease, a small aortic aneurysm, or a shaggy abdominal aorta. In cases of shaggy abdominal aorta, a contrast-enhanced CT scan of the thoracic aorta also should be obtained to delineate the extent of intrathoracic disease. Contrast-enhanced CT usually provides enough detail of the thoracic and abdominal aortic lumens to localize the responsible atherosclerotic lesion. Intravenous contrast is essential to delineate the intra-arterial thrombus. CT scans of the thoracic and abdominal aortas are usually obtained in separate settings in order to have optimal timing of the contrast bolus. The characteristic finding of CT scan in atheroembolization is the star-shaped lumen of the aorta (Fig. 19–3), and the contrast-enhanced CT scan is often the only test necessary prior to operating on patients with microembolization.

Duplex ultrasonagraphy is useful for confirming extremity arterial lesions that appear suspicious on arteriography. Confirming elevated flow velocities through high-grade stenoses in iliac, femoral, or popliteal arteries, or identifying small aneurysms on B-mode ultrasound imaging, can confirm or exclude lesions that are questionable sources of emboli on extremity arteriography.

If the CT scan demonstrates an ulcer or a thrombus in the thoracic aorta, either transesophageal echocardiography or magnetic resonance imaging can be used to confirm these findings. Renal insufficiency is a fairly common finding in patients with shaggy aorta because of prior renal atheroemboli. In these patients, transesophageal echocardiography provides an ideal technique to evaluate the thoracic arch and the descending aorta.[13] Three-dimensional CT may prove useful as this technology further develops, but we have not used it to date.

Management of Atheroembolization

The best medical treatment for atheroemboli has not improved the outcome when compared to historical cases of untreated atheroembolism. Kempczinski observed that recurrent embolic episodes occurred in three of four patients with atheroemboli of aortic origin who were treated with aspirin or warfarin.[14] The poor outcome of patients who do not undergo operative treatment for atheroembolism has led to our philosophy of thoroughly searching for the atheroembolic source and performing operative intervention to prevent further embolic events.[2]

Operations undertaken to manage atheroembolism include procedures both to eliminate the atheroembolic source and to treat the extremity ischemia. The treatment of ischemic complications of atheroemboli proceeds simultaneous with the workup to localize the embolic source. Profound extremity ischemia is temporized with intravenous heparin anticoagulation that will decrease the incidence of further embolic events, increase extremity perfusion by acting as a vasodilator,[15] and limit thrombotic complications distal to the emboli. Thrombolytic therapy has proven especially useful for managing embolic complications of upper and lower extremity aneurysms,[16] but the role of thrombolytic therapy in treating embolic complications for more proximal sources, including the abdominal aorta, is not known. Evidence suggesting a poor outcome and an increased risk from the use of thrombolytic therapy for the treatment of cholesterol embolism is supported by reports of atheroembolization aggravated or initiated by thrombolytic therapy.[17]

Operations performed to treat embolic sources include direct arterial replacement with autogenous or prosthetic bypass grafts, local endarterectomy and patch, and extra-anatomic arterial reconstruction with exclusion of the proximal source.[18] Among our 141 patients with either upper or lower extremity or visceral atheroemboli, 25 did not undergo operations because of medical unfitness or patient refusal. Of the 116 patients who underwent operations, 86 had operations for visceral and lower extremity atheroemboli and 30

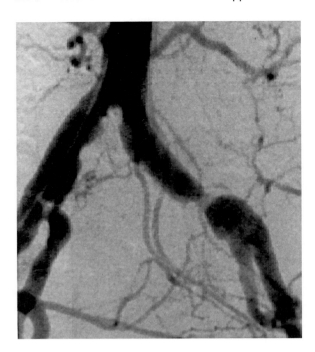

Figure 19–8. Common iliac artery stenosis in a patient who presented with livedo reticularis of the toes had elevated iliac artery velocities by duplex imaging consistent with a high-grade stenosis. This lesion was treated by iliac endarterectomy and patch angioplasty. (Reprinted from Ref. 2 with permission.)

had operations for upper extremity emboli. Atheroemboli secondary to complications of the thoracic outlet syndrome were reported in a separate study.[10] Among 100 patients who underwent operations to treat an atheroembolic source, 14 presented with nonthoracic outlet, upper extremity atheroemboli and 86 with lower extremity or visceral atheroemboli.

Aortic operations were required in 57 patients. Three distinct patterns of aortic iliac disease were observed: aortoiliac occlusive disease, small aortic aneurysms without aneurysmal involvement of the iliac arteries, and small aortic aneurysms with iliac occlusive disease. Aortofemoral bypass was performed in 26 patients, aortoiliac bypass in 10 patients, aortic tube bypass in 16 patients, and aortic endarterectomy and patch in 5 patients. Isolated iliac occlusive disease (Fig. 19–8) was treated by endarterectomy and patch angioplasty in 6 patients, while infrainguinal reconstructions were undertaken in 17 patients, including common femoral artery endartectomy and patch, superficial femoral or popliteal artery endarterectomy and patch, repair of pseudoaneurysms, and femoropopliteal and femorotibial bypasses. Both autogenous and prosthetic patches and grafts were used for these reconstructions. Extra-anatomic reconstructions including axillofemoro-femoral bypass and femorofemoral-femoral bypass were undertaken in six patients. In total, 78% of embolic sources required bypass procedures, while 22% of patients had focal disease successfully treated with local endarterectomy and patch angioplasty.

The 30-day operative mortality was 4%. A total of seven operation-related deaths occurred in the first 6 months following these operations. All deaths occurred in patients undergoing operation for proximal embo-

lic sources, with no mortality in the 31 patients with upper extremity or infrainguinal lesions. The cumulative survival probabilities were 89% at 1 year, 83% at 3 years, and 73% at 5 years (Fig. 19–9), and are clearly superior to the 9% survival at 5 years in Hollier's series of patients who did not undergo operation.[5] Retrospective review revealed that all seven deaths within 6 months of operation occurred among 12 patients who had major suprarenal aortic thrombus noted on preoperative CT scanning that was not removed at the time of operation.

Renal atheroembolization necessitating hemodialysis was a factor contributing to mortality in six of these seven patients. Temporary or permanent hemodialysis was required in 10 of 11 patients with renal emboli. Other major morbidities seen with atheroembolism included intraoperative embolization (Fig. 19–10) and limb loss. Intraoperative emboli occurred in seven patients and led to deterioration of renal function in three. Major postoperative leg amputations were required in 9 patients and toe amputations in 10 patients, but many of these amputations were due to preexisting ischemia from the initial embolic event.

Recurrent emboli occurred in five patients from 1 to 8 months after operation. In each of these patients, residual suprarenal aortic disease not treated at the primary operation was observed in retrospect. This suprarenal disease was characterized on CT scan as irregular, shaggy thrombus in an aorta of normal diameter. Among the five patients who had recurrent embolic episodes, four were receiving warfarin at the time of the recurrence. Only 1 of 82 patients not receiving warfarin after the operation had recurrent embolic events, suggesting that warfarin anticoagulation was associated

Surgical Treatment of Atheroemboli

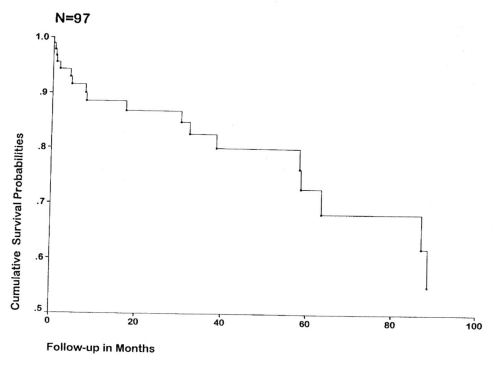

Figure 19–9. Cumulative survival probabilities for patients who underwent operations to treat the source of atheroemboli. Ninety-seven patients were available for follow-up at a mean interval of 32 months. Survival probabilities were 89% ± 4%, 83% ± 5%, and 73% ± at 1, 3, and 5 years, respectively. (Reprinted from Ref. 2 with permission.)

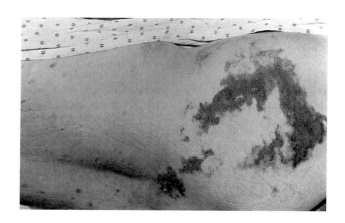

Figure 19–10. "Trash can": intraoperative embolization to the buttock via the internal iliac artery. (Reprinted form Ref. 12 with permission.)

with recurrent emboli. This finding does not necessarily indicate that warfarin caused the emboli, as the patients at greatest risk appeared to be the ones treated with warfarin anticoagulation, although other authors have reported that warfarin initiates atheroembolism.[19,20]

Operations for atheroemboli can be performed with low overall morbidity and mortality on the vast majority of patients. The subgroup of patients who have a higher risk are those with a shaggy aorta—extensive atherosclerosis and intraluminal thrombus that extends proximal to the suprarenal abdominal aorta or into the descend-

ing thoracic aorta (Fig. 19–11). The higher morbidity and mortality rates in this subgroup appear to be due to the higher risk of visceral and renal atheroemboli in addition to lower extremity emboli, as well as to the difficulty of direct operative intervention to eliminate the embolic source and halt further embolic events.

Recurrent emboli appear secondary to untreated aortic disease and suggest the need to completely eliminate both the suprarenal and infrarenal sources of emboli if direct aortic repair is undertaken in these highest-risk patients. Another option is extra-anatomic reconstruction with axillofemorofemoral bypass graft-

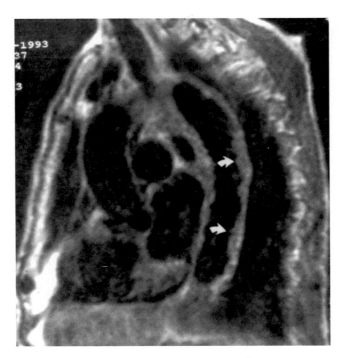

Figure 19–11. Magnetic resonance image demonstrates severe atherosclerosis of the descending thoracic aorta (arrows) in a 79-year-old man who presented with blue toes and renal insufficiency 6 months after aortobifemoral bypass. Transesophageal echocardiography revealed that this plaque was mobile. (Reprinted from Ref. 1 with permission.)

ing. Whether suprarenal aortic thromboendarterectomy, extra-anatomic reconstruction, or observation has the best long-term outcome for this group of patients with extensive disease is not known.

Percutaneous transluminal angioplasty (PTA) has been used successfully to treat focal stenoses of extremity arteries not associated with atheroembolic events. Although the limited extent of disease in most extremity lesions responsible for atheroemboli makes them appear to be technically attractive PTA candidates, lesions that are the source of emboli do not seem appropriate for balloon angioplasty because the nature of the underlying disease process, with plaque instability, may predispose to angionasty-induced embolization.

REFERENCES

1. Keen RR, Yao JST. Experience in the management of atherosclerotic emboli. In: Yao JST, Pearce WH, eds. *The Ischemic Extremity*. Norwalk, CT: Appleton & Lange; 1995:313–323.
2. Keen RR, McCarthy WJ, Pearce WH, et al. Surgical management of atheroembolization. *J Vasc Surg* 1995;21:773–781.
3. Flory CM. Arterial occlusions produced by emboli from eroded aortic atheromatous plaques. *Am J Pathol* 1945;21:549–565.
4. Karmody AM, Powers SR, Monaco VJ, et al. "Blue-toe" syndrome: an indication for limb salvage surgery. *Arch Surg* 1976;3:1263–1268.
5. Hollier LH, Kazmier FJ, Ochsner J, et al. "Shaggy" aorta syndrome with atheromatous embolization to visceral vessels. *Ann Vasc Surg* 1991;5:439–444.
6. Richards AM, Elliot RS, Kanjuh VI, et al. Cholesterol embolism: a multiple disease masquerading as polyarteritis nodosa. *Am J Cardiol* 1965;5:696–707.
7. Cappiello RA, Espinoza LR, Adelman H, et al. Cholesterol embolism: a pseudovasculitic syndrome. *Semin Arthritis Rheum* 1989;18:240–246.
8. Kasinath BSM, Corwin HL, Bidani AK, et al. Eosinophilia in the diagnosis of atheroembolic renal disease. *Am J Nephrol* 1987;7:137–177.
9. Mesh CL, Yao JST. Upper extremity bypass: five-year follow-up. In: Yao JST, Peace WH, eds. *Long-term Results in Vascular Surgery*. Norwalk, CT: Appleton & Lange; 1993:353–365.
10. Durham JR, Yao JST, Pearce WH, Nuber GM, McCarthy WJ. Arterial injuries in the thoracic outlet syndrome. *J Vasc Surg* 1995;21:57–70.
11. Gaines PA, Kennedy A, Moorehead P, Cumberland DC, Welsh CL, Rutley MS. Cholesterol embolization: a lethal complication of vascular catheterization. *Lancet* 1988; 1:168–170.
12. Keen RR, Yao JST. Aneurysms and embolization: detection and management. In: Yao JST, Peace WH, eds. *Aneurysms: New Findings and Treatments*. Norwalk, CT: Appleton & Lange; 1994:305–313.
13. Wiet SP, Pearce WH, McCarthy WJ, Joob AW, Yao JST, McPherson DD. Utility of transesophageal echocardiography in the diagnosis of disease of the thoracic aorta. *J Vasc Surg* 1994;20:613–620.
14. Kempczinski RF. Lower-extremity arterial emboli from ulcerating atherosclerotic plaques. *JAMA* 1979;241:800–810.
15. Sternberg WC III, Sobel M, Makhoul R. Heparinoids with low anticoagulant potency atenuate post-ischemic endothelial cell dysfunction. *J Vasc Surg* 1995;21:477–483.
16. Giddings AEB. Influence of thrombolytic therapy in the management of popliteal aneurysms. In: Yao JST, Pearce WH, eds. *Aneurysms: New Findings and Treatments*. Norwalk, CT: Appleton & Lange; 1994:493–508.
17. Bhardwjah M, Goldweit R, Erlebacher J, et al. Tissue plasminogen activator and choelsterol crystal embolization. *Ann Intern Med* 1989;11:687–688.
18. Friedman SG, Krishnasastry KV. Eternal iliac ligation and axillary-bifemoral bypass for blue toe syndrome. *Surgery* 1994;115:27–30.
19. Bruns FJ, Segel DP, Adler S. Case report: control of cholesterol embolization by discontinuation of anticoagulant therapy. *Am J Med Sci* 1978;275:105–108.
20. Hyman BT, Landas SK, Ashman RF, et al. Warfarin-related purple toes syndrome and cholesterol microembolization. *Am J Med* 1978;82:1233–1237.

20

The Diabetic Foot

Cameron M. Akbari, M.D.[1]
Frank B. Pomposelli, Jr, M.D.[2]

Diabetes mellitus afflicts as many as 13 million people nationally, or 5.2% of the U.S. population, and more than 65,000 new cases are diagnosed annually.[1] Foot problems are the most common cause of hospitalization in diabetic patients, with an annual health care cost of over $1 billion.[2] Diabetes accounts for half of all the lower extremity amputations in the United States, and it has been estimated that the relative risk of amputation is 40 times greater in people with diabetes.[1,3] Moreover, up to 50% of diabetic amputees will undergo a second leg amputation within 5 years of the initial amputation. Diabetic foot ulceration will affect 15% of all diabetic individuals during their lifetime, with a 3% annual incidence and a 10% prevalence rate in patients with diabetes, and is clearly a significant risk factor in the pathway to limb loss.[4]

Given these staggering numbers, the U.S. Department of Health and Human Services has set a goal of a 40% reduction in diabetic amputation rates by the year 2000.[5] Central to achieving this goal is a clear understanding of the pathogenesis and treatment of foot problems in patients with diabetes mellitus.

PATHOGENESIS

The principal pathogenic mechanisms in diabetic foot disease are neuropathy and ischemia. Acting synergistically and seldom alone, they contribute to the sequence of tissue necrosis, ulceration, and ultimately gangrene (Fig. 20–1). Reduced resistance to infection among diabetic patients increases the complexity of the disease. Prevention and treatment of diabetic foot problems should be tailored to the pathogenic factors.

Vascular Disease

Ischemia is a fundamental consideration in the evaluation of the diabetic foot. Many diabetic foot problems have been erroneously ascribed to small-vessel disease, a common misconception implying that an occlusive lesion exists at the arteriolar level.[6] This belief originated from retrospectively examined amputation specimens demonstrating periodic acid–Schiff-positive staining in the arterioles[7]; however, subsequent prospective staining and arterial casting studies demonstrated the absence of an arteriolar occlusive lesion.[8,9] The term *small-vessel disease* should be abandoned because it encourages attempts at arterial reconstruction and propagates the misconception of an arteriolar occlusive lesion.[10]

Atherosclerosis is accelerated in diabetes mellitus and is the cause of ischemia in both diabetic and nondiabetic patients. One notable difference between these populations is the pattern and location of the occlusive lesion. Diabetic patients are more likely to have occlusive disease affecting the infrageniculate, or tibial, arteries. However, in spite of the extensive infrapopliteal disease, the foot arteries are often spared,[11] a finding that allows successful arterial bypass to these distal vessels. Conversely, the superficial femoral or popliteal artery is less likely to be affected by the occlusive process in the diabetic patient, allowing these vessels to serve as the origin of arterial bypass grafts (inflow source).

Nonocclusive microcirculatory (capillary and arteriolar) dysfunction is another important problem in the diabetic patient. Autonomic neuropathy leads to an increased arteriovenous shunt in the diabetic foot, with concomitant increase in skin temperature and metabolic demand but inefficient tissue perfusion. Similarly, postural vasoconstriction is impaired in the presence of neuropathy, which leads to increased transmural pressure in the microcirculation and capillary structural damage.[12] This abnormality is characterized by basement membrane thickening and may theoretically

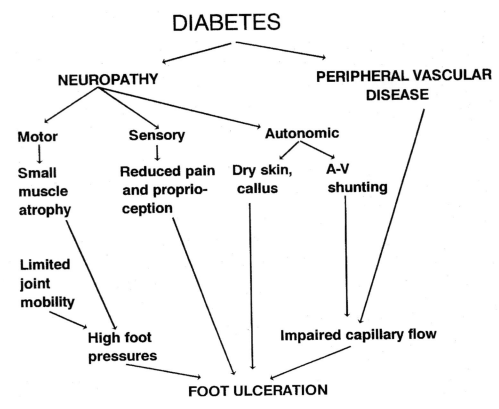

Figure 20–1. The pathogenesis of foot ulceration in the diabetic patient. A-V, arteriovenous. (Reprinted from Ref. 22 with permission.)

impair the migration of leukocytes and the hyperemic response following injury, thereby increasing the susceptibility of the diabetic foot to infection.[13,14] Although resting total skin microcirculatory flow is similar in both diabetic and nondiabetic patients, capillary blood flow is reduced in diabetes, indicating a maldistribution that may result in functional ischemia of the skin.[15] The net result of these changes is an inability to vasodilate and achieve maximal blood flow following injury.

Diabetes also affects the axon reflex. Normally, stimulation of the nociceptive C fibers causes the secretion of active peptides, such as substance P, which directly and indirectly (through mast cell release of histamine) cause vasodilation. This neurogenic vasodilatory response is impaired in diabetic patients, further reducing the hyperemic response when it is most needed, during conditions of injury and inflammation.[16]

Neuropathy

Neuropathy is a common complication of diabetes, afflicting as many as 50 to 60% of all patients,[17,18] and is present in over 80% of diabetic patients with foot lesions.[5] These complications are broadly classified as focal and diffuse neuropathies. The latter are more common and include the autonomic and chronic sen-

sorimotor polyneuropathies implicated in foot ulceration. A combination of metabolic and microvascular defects has been proposed in the pathogenesis of diabetic neuropathy, such as decreased nitric oxide production, decreased nerve myoinositol concentration, and glycosylated neural proteins.[19–21]

Sensorimotor neuropathy initially involves the distal lower extremities, progresses centrally, and tends to be symmetrical. Sensory nerve fiber involvement leads to loss of the protective sensation of pain, whereas motor fiber loss results in small muscle atrophy in the foot. Consequently, the metatarsals are flexed, with a prominence of the metatarsal heads and clawing of the toes. This results in the development of abnormal pressure points on the plantar bony prominences, without protective sensation, and subsequent high foot pressures and ulceration. As noted above, loss of sympathetic tone causes increased arteriovenous shunting and inefficient nutrient flow. Moreover, autonomic denervation of the sweat glands and anhidrosis leads to cracking of dry skin, with a predisposition to skin breakdown and ulceration.[22]

Diabetic neuropathy may also lead to the development of osteoarthropathy, or the Charcot foot. Continued ambulation on an insensate joint causes further joint instability, loss of joint architecture, and ultimately bone and joint destruction. This destructive process promotes increased bone blood flow and concomitant resorption and softening of normal bone, which in turn leads to further bone destruction.[23] While ischemia often coexists in the non-Charcot neuropathic foot, adequate circulation is needed for osteoarthropathy to develop, so that ischemia is a rare component of the Charcot process.[22,24]

DIAGNOSIS

The clinical spectrum of diabetic foot disease ranges from a superficial ulcer in a neuropathic foot to extensive gangrene with ischemia and life-threatening sepsis. Because the former may rapidly progress to a potentially limb- or life-threatening infection, particularly in an ischemic limb, a thorough evaluation for infection and ischemia should be routinely performed in these patients.

Infection

Diabetic foot infection may result from a simple puncture wound, a neuropathic ulcer, the nail plate, or from the interdigital web space. Untreated cellulitis can lead to bacterial spread along tendon sheaths, progressing to advanced deep space plantar infection, destruction of the interosseous fascia, and spread to the dorsum of the foot.[25] The subsequent edema elevates compartmental pressures and further impairs capillary blood flow and recovery.

Classical signs of infection, such as erythema and pain, are often absent in the infected diabetic foot, as a consequence of neuropathy, leukocyte abnormalities, and microneurovascular dysfunction.[26] Even among patients with deep abscesses, fever, chills, and leukocytes may be absent in up to two-thirds of cases, with hyperglycemia frequently the sole presenting sign.[27] A lack of sensation in the foot, along with an absence of typical signs of infection, often leads to delayed recognition of the problem by both patient and physician. Encrusted and heavily calloused areas should be unroofed and the wound thoroughly inspected to determine the extent of involvement,

The majority of infections are polymicrobic, with the most common pathogens being staphylococci, enterococci, and streptococci. Anaerobes and gram-negative bacilli are also commonly cultured.[28] Cultures from the ulcer surface may be misleading. Therefore, swabs should not be taken from the superficial surface of the ulcer, but rather should be obtained from the base of an ulcer or the depths of an abscess after debridement.[5,29]

Osteomyletitis is a common sequela of diabetic foot ulceration. Bone biopsy–proven osteomyelitis may be demonstrated in almost 70% of benign-appearing ulcers, emphasizing the need for a high index of suspicion in dealing with this complication.[30] Radiographic evaluation for osteomyelitis may include plain radiographs, a three-phase bone scan (utilizing technetium-99 and gallium-67 isotopes), labeled leukocyte scans, CT scans, and magnetic resonance imaging. Although leukocyte scanning appears to be the most sensitive modality,[31] indiscriminate use of these tests is both costly and, in our experience, often unnecessary.

A more cost-effective approach involves the use of a sterile probe to detect bone in an open ulcer.[32] Because this test has a positive predictive value of nearly 90%, osteomyelitis should be presumed if bone is palpated on probing, thus rendering other specialized and expensive radiographic tests unnecessary.

Ischemia

Assessment of arterial perfusion is critical in the diabetic foot. Noninvasive arterial tests have several limitations in the presence of diabetes. Medial arterial calcification occurs frequently in diabetic patients, and calcification of the tibial arteries results in noncompressible vessels and an artifactual elevation of the ankle/brachial pressure index. Less extensive calcification in the toe vessels supports the use of toe systolic pressures as a more reliable indicator of arterial flow to the foot.[33] The use of toe pressures is often limited by the proximity of the foot ulcer to the cuff site, but it is still a valuable addition to the evaluation of foot ischemia in the diabetic patient.

Pulse volume recordings may also be of value in diabetic patients because they are unaffected by medial calcification. Limitations of this technique include the presence of ulceration, which precludes forefoot cuff placement, and peripheral edema, which often accompanies the infectious process. An occasional patient with near-normal tracings and a non-healing ulcer will be found to have significant and correctable distal arterial occlusion by arteriography.[34]

Transcutaneous oxygen tension ($TcPO_2$) measurements are also unaffected by medial calcification, and recent reports have noted its reliability in predicting the success of diabetic foot ulcer healing.[35] Its use is limited, however, by a lack of equipment standardization, user variability, and a large "gray area" of values in which healing is unpredictable. In addition, $TcPO_2$ measurements are actually higher in diabetic patients with foot ulcers than in the nondiabetic population, which further confounds the ability to predict ischemia in these patients.[36]

The limitations of noninvasive vascular testing emphasize the continued importance of a thorough bedside evaluation and sound judgment. We continue to believe that the most important aspect of the physical exam is the status of the foot pulses. In simplest terms, it can be assumed that occlusive disease is present if the foot pulses are not palpable. This finding alone is an indication for contrast arteriography in the clinical setting of tissue loss, poor healing, or gangrene, even if neuropathy and/or infection may have been the antecedent cause of skin breakdown or ulceration. Concern about contrast-induced renal dysfunction in the presence of diabetes should not mitigate against performance of a high-quality angiogram of the entire lower extremity circulation. Several prospective sudies have documented that the incidence of contrast nephropathy is not higher in the diabetic patient without preexisting renal disease, even with the use of ionic contrast agent.[37-41] The more costly nonionic agents should therefore be reserved for the diabetic patient with compromised renal function. Even among these patients, however, the risk of contrast nephropathy should not contraindicate the use of arteriography.

Because the foot vessels are often patent in the diabetic patient, even when the crural arteries are occluded, it is essential that arteriograms not be terminated at the midtibial level. The complete infrapopliteal circulation should be evaluated, including the foot vessels, and digital subtraction techniques have significantly improved visualization of these distal vessels. Both anteroposterior and lateral foot views should be included to obtain a complete assessment of all stenosis and occlusions. Excessive plantar flexion should be avoided, as this may interrupt flow in the dorsalis pedis artery and impede visualization.

TREATMENT

Treatment should be aimed at the pathogenic factors outlined above. In general, this can be broken down into a few simple guidelines[42]:

1. Prompt control of infection.
2. Complete non–weight bearing of the involved extremity.
3. Evaluation for ischemia.
4. Prompt arterial reconstruction once active infection has resolved.
5. Secondary procedures, such as further debridement, toe amputations, local flaps, and even free flaps, may then be carried out separately in the fully vascularized foot.

Control of Infection

The method of treatment of the infected diabetic foot depends on the severity of the infection.[43] Superficial infections may be treated on an outpatient basis with oral antibiotics (pending culture results), provided that there is no systemic toxicity, the patient is compliant, and, most important, there is no evidence of deeper infection. Our first choice of agents is a first- or second-generation cephalosporin, which has excellent activity against staphylococcus and streptococcus. Weight bearing is avoided until healing is achieved. Once the patient is ambulatory, modified footwear to protect high-pressure and ulcer-prone areas should be prescribed.

Patients with deeper infections involving tendon or bone, or with infections that represent a threat to limb and life, require prompt hospitalization, complete bed rest, and correction of systemic abnormalities. Given the polymicrobial nature of these infections, broad-spectrum intravenous antibiotics should be started and then tailored according to the culture results. Abscess and deep sepsis mandate immediate incision and drainage of all infected tissue planes. Beause of the coexisting neuropathy, this can often be done at the bedside, particularly for localized infections. More extensive infection, however, should be drained in the operating room. Incisions should be longitudinal and should extend the length of the entire abscess to promote dependent drainage. Involved tendons, bones, or joints should be removed. The use of drains and small stab incisions is mentioned only to be condemned. Surgical dressings should be kept simple, consisting of gauze sponges moistened with saline or dilute one-quarter strength providone-iodine solutions. Full-strength astringents and solutions, hot compresses, and whirlpools are not used.

Evaluation for ischemia may begin once the infection has started to resolve and signs of systemic toxicity have disappeared. The decision to perform arteriography and vascular reconstruction should be made during this period, which is usually no longer than 5 to 7 days. Further delays may compromise the opportunity to salvage the foot.[44]

Arterial Reconstruction

The goal of arterial reconstruction is to obtain maximum perfusion to the foot. Ideally, we try to restore a palpable foot pulse, particularly in situations involving extensive gangrene or tissue loss.

Proximal bypass to the popliteal or tibioperoneal arteries may restore foot pulses. More often, however, because of the pattern of occlusive disease in the diabetic patient, bypass grafting to the popliteal or even tibial arteries cannot accomplish this goal due to the presence of more distal obstructive disease. Similarly, although excellent results have been reported with peroneal artery bypass,[45] the peroneal artery is not in continuity with the foot vessels and may not provide maximal flow to the foot to achieve healing.

Autogenous vein grafting to the dorsalis pedis artery represents a technical advance that provides durable and effective salvage.[46] The principal indication for the pedal graft is the absence of other vessels with continuity to the foot, particularly in cases with tissue loss. Dorsalis pedis bypass is unnecessary when a more proximal bypass will restore foot pulses, and it should not be done if the dorsum of the foot is extensively infected.

The distal location of the dorsalis pedis artery theoretically necessitates a long venous conduit, which may not be available. However, if the popliteal or distal superficial femoral artery is used as an inflow site, a shorter length of vein may be used, with excellent long-term patency.[47] This is particularly true in the diabetic patient due to the pattern of atherosclerotic disease. In the Deaconess Hospital experience with 384 pedal bypasses over a 7-year period, 60% of grafts utilized a distal inflow site, usually the popliteal artery.[48] This avoids dissection in the groin and upper thigh, a common location for wound complications. In addition, the shorter length of saphenous vein obviates the need for distal extension of the vein harvest incision, parallel to the one required to expose the dorsalis pedis artery, thus avoiding the resultant skin bridge, which may occasionally become ischemic from tension after closure.

Other technical details include the use of a longitudinal rather than a transverse incision in dissecting the dorsalis pedis artery, so that adequate proximal and distal exposure may be obtained. If the saphenous vein needs to be exposed to the foot and a skin bridge is created, avoidance of tunneling the vein graft through the skin bridge is important. Foot and distal leg wounds should be closed with fine plastic surgical technique rather than skin staples. The vein graft to the dorsalis pedis artery can be prepared as an in situ, reversed, or nonreversed vein graft, with no significant difference in outcome.[49]

Active infection in the foot is not a contraindication to dorsalis pedis bypass, provided that the infectious process is controlled and surgical incisions or anastomoses are not placed in infected tissues (Fig. 20–2). At the Deaconess Hospital, the results of 56 vein bypasses to the dorsal pedal artery in patients with ischemic foot lesions complicated by infection were reviewed.[50] Included in this group were 15 patients with severe gangrene, osteomyelitis, and/or deep space abscess of the forefoot or heel. The average interval between hospital admission and bypass surgery was 10 days. Although there was a 12% wound infection rate, the primary graft patency was 92% at 36 months' follow-up. Importantly, this aggressive approach to revascularization in the ischemic and infected foot resulted in a limb salvage rate of 98% at the end of 3 years.

We have performed dorsalis pedis bypass grafts on 367 patients over an 8-year period at the Deaconess Hospital.[48] Tissue loss was an indication for surgery in almost 85% of these patients. The actuarial primary, secondary patency, and limb salvage rates were 68%, 82%, and 87%, respectively, at 5 years' follow-up. A closer examination of the data reveals the underlying reasons for this success. The preoperative arteriogram was able to demonstrate the dorsalis pedis artery in 93% of extremities. In the remaining cases in which no artery was seen but an audible Doppler signal was present, arterial bypass was successful in 57%, empha-

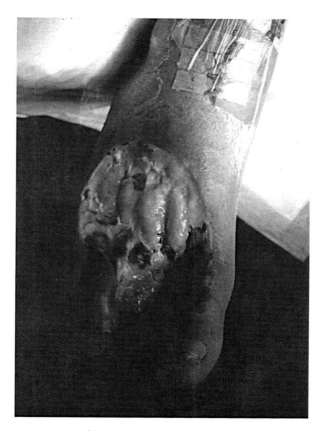

Figure 20–2. This patient presented with extensive infection requiring open toe amputation, drainage, and debridement of the distal dorsal foot. Following control of the infection, a dorsal pedis bypass graft was performed successfully.

sizing that blind exploration is reasonable, especially when amputation is the only other option.

Secondary Procedures Following Revascularization

Following successful revascularization, a variety of secondary procedures are possible in the diabetic foot to enhance limb salvage. Extensive tissue loss may be treated by either local flap coverage or free tissue transfer, which will allow ambulation in many cases.[51] In the patient with underlying bony structural abnormalities causing recurrent ulceration, metatarsal head resection or osteotomy may be performed to preserve the forefoot and prevent recurrent ulceration.[52]

SUMMARY

This systemic approach to diabetic foot disease has resulted in improved limb salvage among diabetic patients. Since 1984, there has been a significant reduction in every category of amputation at the Deaconess Hospital, with an increase in the number of patients undergoing arterial reconstruction[53] (Fig. 20–3). Concomitant with this reduction in amputation rates has been a greater application of the dorsalis pedis bypass graft. Improved knowledge of the pathophysiology of

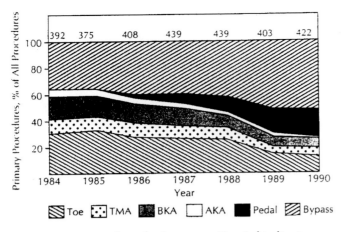

Figure 20–3. Data from the Deaconess Hospital indicating a fall in every category of major amputation, with an increase in the number of bypass operations. TMA, transmetatarsal amputation; BKA, below-knee amputation; AKA, above-knee amputation. (Reprinted from Ref. 53 with permission.)

diabetic foot disease, combined with an aggressive and orderly treatment plan, will lead to a continued reduction in amputation rates and improved limb salvage among diabetic patients.

REFERENCES

1. *Diabetes: 1993 Vital Statistics.* American Diabetes Association; 1993.
2. Grunfeld C. Diabetic foot ulcers: etiology, treatment, and prevention. *Adv Intern Med* 1991;37:103–132.
3. Nathan DM. Long-term complications of diabetes mellitus. *N Engl J Med* 1993;328:1676–1685.
4. Reiber GE, Boyko EJ, Smith DG. Lower extremity foot ulcers and amputations in diabetes. In: National Diabetes Data Group, ed. *Diabetes in America.* 2nd ed. Washington, DC: National Institutes of Health, 1995:409–428.
5. Caputo GM, Cavanagh PR, Ulbrecht JS, Gibbons GW, Karchmer AW. Assessment and management of foot disease in patients with diabetes. *N Engl J Med* 1994; 331:854–860.
6. LoGerfo FW, Coffman JD. Vascular and microvascular disease of the foot in diabetes. *N Engl J Med* 1984; 311:1615–1619.
7. Goldenberg SG, Alex M, Joshi RA, Blumenthal HT. Nonatheromatous peripheral vascular disease of the lower extremity in diabetes mellitus. *Diabetes* 1959;8:261–273.
8. Strandness DE Jr, Priest RE, Gibbons GE. Combined clinical and pathologic study of diabetic and nondiabetic peripheral arterial disease. *Diabetes* 1964;13:366–372.
9. Conrad MC. Large and small artery occlusion in diabetics and nondiabetics with severe vascular disease. *Circulation* 1967;36:83–91.
10. Logerfo FW. Vascular disease, matrix abnormalities, and neuropathy: Implications for limb salvage in diabetes mellitus. *J Vasc Surg* 1987;5:793–796.
11. Menzoian JO, LaMorte WW, Paniszyn CC, et al. Symptomatology and anatomic patterns of peripheral vascular disease: differing impact of smoking and diabetes. *Ann Vasc Surg* 1989;3:224–228.
12. Flynn MD, Tooke JE. Diabetic neuropathy and the microcirculation. *Diabet Med* 1995;298–301.
13. Flynn MD, Tooke JE. Aetiology of diabetic foot ulceration: a role for the microcirculation? *Diabet Med* 1992;8:320–329.
14. Rayman G, Williams SA, Spencer PD, et al. Impaired microvascular hyperaemic response to minor skin trauma in Type I diabetes. *Br Med J* 1986;292:1295–1298.
15. Jorneskog G, Brismar K, Fagrell B. Skin capillary circulation severely impaired in toes of patients with IDDM, with and without late diabetic complications. *Diabetologia* 1995; 38:474–480.
16. Parkhouse N, LeQueen PM. Impaired neurogenic vascular response in patients with diabetes and neuropathic foot lesions. *N Engl J Med* 1988;318:1306–1309.
17. The DCCT Research Group. Factors in the development of diabetic neuropathy: baseline analysis of neuropathy in the feasibility phase of the Diabetes Control and Complications Trial (DCCT). *Diabetes* 1988;37:476–481.
18. Dyck PJ, Kratz KM, Karnes JL, et al. The prevalence by staged severity of various types of diabetic neuropathy, retinopathy, and nephropathy in a population-based cohort: the Rochester Diabetic Neuropathy Study. *Neurology* 1993;43:817–824.
19. Stevens MJ, Feldman EL, Greene DA. The aetiology of diabetic neuropathy: The combined roles of metabolic and vascular defects. *Diabet Med* 1995;12:566–579.
20. Pfeifer MA, Schumer MP. Clinical trials of diabetic neuropathy: Past, present, and future. *Diabetes* 1995;44:1355–1361.
21. Stevens MJ, Dananberg J, Feldman EL, Lattimer SA, Sima A, Greene D. The linked roles of nitric oxide, aldose reductase and Na^+/K^+ ATPase in the slowing of nerve conduction in the streptozotocin diabetic rat. *J Clin Invest* 1994;94:853–859.
22. Young MJ, Veves A, Boulton AJM. The diabetic foot: aetiopathogenesis and management. *Diabetes Metab Rev* 1993;9:109–127.
23. Frykberg RG, Kozak GP. The diabetic Charcot foot. In: Kozak GP, Campbell DR, Frykberg RG, Habershaw GM, eds. *Management of Diabetic Foot Problems.* 2nd ed. Philadelphia: WB Saunders; 1995:88–97.
24. Edelman SV, Kosofsky EM, Paul RA, et al. Neuroosteoarthropathy (Charcot's joints) in diabetes mellitus following revascularization. Three case reports and a review of the literature. *Arch Intern Med* 1987;147:1504–1508.
25. Bridges RM Jr, Deitch EA. Diabetic foot infections: pathophysiology and treatment. *Surg Clin North Am* 1994; 74:537–555.
26. Mills JL, Beckett WC, Taylor SM. The diabetic foot: consequences of delayed treatment and referral. *South Med J* 1991;84:970–974.
27. Gibbons GW. Diabetic foot sepsis. *Semin Vasc Surg* 1992;5:244–248.
28. Wheat LJ, Allen SD, Henry M. Diabetic foot infections: bacteriologic analysis. *Arch Intern Med* 1986;146:1935–1940.
29. Lipsky BA, Percoraro RE, Wheat LJ. The diabetic foot: soft tissue and bone infection. *Infect Dis Clin North Am* 1990;4:409–432.
30. Newman LG, Waller J, Palestro CJ, et al. Unsuspected osteomyelitis in diabetic foot ulcers: diagnosis and monitoring by leukocyte scanning with Indium In 111 oxyquinoline. *JAMA* 1991;266:1246–1251.
31. Newman LG, Waller J, Palestro CJ, et al. Leukocyte scanning with 111 In is superior to magnetic resonance imaging in diagnosis of clinically unsuspected osteomyelitis in diabetic foot ulcers. *Diabetes Care* 1992;15:1527–1530.

32. Grayson ML, Gibbons GW, Balogh K, et al. Probing to bone in infected pedal ulcers: a clinical sign of underlying osteomyelitis in diabetic patients. *JAMA* 1995; 273:721–723.

33. Young MJ, Adams JE, Anderson GF, et al. Medial arterial calcification in the feet of diabetic patients and matched non-diabetic control subjects. *Diabetologia* 1993;36:615–621.

34. Pomposelli FB Jr. Noninvasive evaluation of the arterial system in the diabetic lower extremity. In: Kozak GP, Campbell DR, Frykberg RG, Habershaw GM, eds. *Management of Diabetic Foot Problems.* 2nd ed. Philadelphia: WB Saunders; 1995:138–148.

35. Ballard JL, Eke CC, Bunt TJ, et al. A prospective evaluation of transcutaneous oxygen measurements in the management of diabetic foot problems. *J Vasc Surg* 1995;22:485–492.

36. Wyss CR, Matsen FA III, Simmons CW, et al. Transcutaneous oxygen tension measurements on limbs of diabetic and nondiabetic patients with peripheral vascular disease. *Surgery* 1984;95:339–346.

37. D'Elia JA, Gleason RE, Alday M, et al. Nephrotoxicity from angiographic contrast material: a prospective study. *Am J Med* 1982;72:719–725.

38. Mason RA, Arbeit LA, Giron F. Renal dysfunction after arteriography. *JAMA* 1985;253:1001–1004.

39. Parfrey PS, Griffiths SM, Barrett BJ, et al. Contrast material–induced renal failure in patients with diabetes mellitus, renal insufficiency, or both. A prospective controlled study. *N Engl J Med* 1989;321:395–397.

40. Schwab SJ, Hlatky MA, Pieper KS, et al. Contrast nephrotoxicity: a randomized controlled trial of a nonionic and ionic contrast agent. *N Engl J Med* 1989;320:149–153.

41. Gussenhoven MJ, Ravensbergen J, van Bockel JH, et al. Renal dysfunction after angiography; a risk factor analysis in patients with peripheral vascular disease. *J Cardiovasc Surg* 1991;32:81–86.

42. Pomposelli FB Jr, LoGerfo FW. Dorsalis pedis bypass in diabetic patients. In: Yao JST, Pearce WH, eds. *The Ischemic Extremity: Advances in Treatment.* Norwalk, CT: Appleton & Lange; 1995:289–294.

43. Gibbons GW. The diabetic foot: Amputations and drainage of infection. *J Vasc Surg* 1987;5:791–793.

44. Pomposelli FB Jr, LoGerfo FW. Distal reconstructions to the dorsal pedis artery in diabetic patients. *Adv Vasc Surg* 1994;2:41–58.

45. Plecha EJ, Seabrook, GR, Bandyk DF, et al. Determinants of successful peroneal artery bypass. *J Vasc Surg* 1993;17:97–106.

46. Pomposelli FB Jr, Jepsen SJ, Gibbons GW, et al. Efficacy of the dorsal pedis bypass for limb salvage in diabetic patients: short-term observations. *J Vasc Surg* 1990; 11:745–752.

47. Veith FJ, Gupta SK, Samson RH, et al. Superficial femoral and popliteal arteries as inflow sites for distal bypasses. *Surgery* 1981;90:980–990.

48. Pomposelli FB Jr, Marcaccio EJ, Gibbons GW, et al. Dorsalis pedis arterial bypass: durable limb salvage for foot ischemia in patients with diabetes mellitus. *J Vasc Surg* 1995;21:375–384.

49. Pomposelli FB Jr, Jepsen SJ, Gibbons GW, et al. A flexible approach to infrapopliteal vein grafts in patients with diabetes mellitus. *Arch Surg* 1991;126:724–729.

50. Tannenbaum GA, Pomposelli FB Jr, Marcaccio EJ, et al. Safety of vein bypass grafting to the dorsal pedal artery in diabetic patients with foot infections. *J Vasc Surg* 1992;15:982–990.

51. Cronenwett JL, McDaniel MD, Zwolak RM, et al. Limb salvage despite extensive tissue loss: free tissue transfer combined with distal revascularization. *Arch Surg* 1989;124:609–615.

52. Rosenblum BI, Pomposelli FB Jr, Giurini JM, et al. Maximizing foot salvage by a combined approach to foot ischemia and neuropathic ulceration in patients with diabetes. *Diabetes Care* 1994;17:983–987.

53. LoGerfo FW, Gibbons GW, Pomposelli FB Jr, et al. Trends in the care of the diabetic foot: expanded role of arterial reconstruction. *Arch Surg* 1992;127:617–621.

21

The Diagnosis and Management of Buerger's Disease

Elizabeth A. Forsyth, M.D.
Anton N. Sidawy, M.D.

In 1908, Leo Buerger presented his findings following pathologic examination of 11 amputation specimens from patients afflicted with limb ischemia and gangrene.[1] Although the condition was initially described by Winiwater in 1879,[2] it was the study by Buerger that provided the clinical and histologic criteria to distinguish the disorder he termed *thromboangiitis obliterans* (*TAO*). In his original series, Buerger observed that the disease predominantly affected young men with a history of tobacco use in a segmental pattern of thrombotic vascular occlusion. Although the existence of TAO as a distinct entity has been questioned by Wessler and others,[3–5] strict adherence to the classic diagnostic guidelines clearly delineates Buerger's disease as an important form of thrombo-occlusive vasculitis.

ETIOLOGY

Although the underlying mechanism of TAO remains unknown, several possible etiologies have been proposed. While evidence is available in support of each hypothesis, the causation is most likely multifactorial.

Tobacco Use

The close association between habitual tobacco use and TAO suggests a causal relationship, although this has not been definitively demonstrated. In a 1991 study by Matsushita et al,[6] cotinine, a major metabolite of nicotine, was measured to ascertain the degree of patient tobacco use. Of the 10 patients found to have high levels of cotinine (more than 50 ng per milligram of creatinine), 7 experienced exacerbation of their ischemic symptoms. Although a specific inciting factor has not been elucidated, these findings indicate that the level

of disease activity correlates with the continuation of tobacco use. The rarity of this diagnosis among nonsmokers further supports the role of tobacco use in the development of TAO.[7,8]

Inherited Factors

The prevalence of TAO in Eastern Europe, the Mediterranean, and the Orient may indicate the existence of a genetic predisposition.[9–10] Several investigators[12–14] demonstrated an increased frequency of human leukocyte antigen (HLA) of haplotype antigens A9 and B5 in patients affected by Buerger's disease. However, these findings were not confirmed in another report.[15] In another study, Papa et al identified a statistically significant increase in the incidence of HLA–DR4 among TAO patients in comparison to nonsmokers. In this study population, no evidence to support an increased frequency of HLA-A or -B antigens was observed.[15] These disparate findings indicate that while a genetic component may be involved in the development of Buerger's disease, the exact contribution of hereditary factors remains undefined.

Immune Response

The potential role of an autoimmune phenomenon in TAO has been postulated by some investigators.[16,17] Adar et al found that patients with TAO exhibited a heightened cell-mediated sensitivity to human collagen types I and III, which are normal constituents of the vessel wall.[16] While this physiologic responce may explain the inflammatory reaction characteristic of Buerger's disease, further studies are needed to identify features of the autoimmune response associated with TAO that are distinct from those present in other immunologic disorders such as systemic lupus erythematosus and rheumatoid arthritis.[18]

Other Factors

Pietraszek et al found impaired platelet serotonin uptake and an increased concentration of free serotonin in patients with Buerger's disease compared to age-matched controls.[19] Alterations in blood viscosity have also been described in patients with Buerger's disease.[20] For example, Szendro et al reported that hematocrit values and fibrinogen levels were higher in patients with Buerger's disease compared to controls. In contrast, the erythrocyte filterability index was lower. However, when washed erythrocytes from these patients were incubated with control plasma of blood type AB, the filterability index improved. These findings suggest that patients suffering from Buerger's disease show an abnormality in factors affecting blood viscosity.[20]

INCIDENCE

Geographic Distribution

TAO is a relatively uncommon disorder. However, even within this small patient population, there is significant risk stratification based on geographic location. In North America a surge of new cases of TAO was seen from the late 1930s to the early 1950s,[21] but over the past four decades there has been a sharp decline in the diagnosis. This trend is illustrated by the Mayo Clinic experience. Records from 1947 reveal the prevalence rate of Buerger's disease to be 104 per 100,000 patient registrants at that institution. By 1976 the incidence of TAO among Mayo Clinic patients had declined to 9.9 per 100,000 admissions, reflecting a more than 10-fold decrease in the diagnosis.[22] Overall, Buerger's disease represents less than 1% of all patients presenting with severe peripheral ischemia in the United States. In contrast, TAO is responsible for approximately 5% of such cases in the Mediterranean and Eastern Europe and may exceed 16% in the Orient.[23]

Sex

TAO is classically described as a disease that preferentially affects young men.[24] In Buerger's landmark publication, all subjects were male. In a subsequent series of 500 patients, Buerger reported only two cases among women, for an overall incidence of 0.2%.[25] Despite the continued male predominance among patients with TAO, reports have documented an increase in the incidence among women.[26] Lie et al presented a thorough clinical pathologic analysis of 12 women afflicted with Buerger's disease.[22] In Olin et al's investigation of 112 patients with TAO, 23% of the study population were female.[27] While this change in demographics is not completely understood, it may reflect the increase in habitual tobacco use among women.[28]

PATHOLOGY

TAO characteristically afflicts medium- and small-caliber arteries and veins in the distal aspect of both upper and lower extremities. Involvement of more proximal vessels has also been reported.[29,30] In addition, a rare case of Buerger's disease affecting a saphenous vein used for coronary bypass was reported in a male patient who continued to smoke after the cardiac bypass operation.[31] While the inflammatory lesion of Buerger's disease is not pathognomonic, its evolution does produce several features that are distinctive for the disorder.[32] Confirmation of the diagnosis is partially based on the characteristic microscopic appearance of these lesions. The histologic findings are utilized to classify the lesions as acute, subacute, or chronic.

Acute Phase

The presence of multiple, small microabcesses within fresh thrombus is indicative of an acute lesion. An abundance of polymorphonuclear leukocytes within the core of the microabscess is a frequent finding. In addition, multinucleated gaint cells are often closely associated with the punctate abscesses[22,23] (Fig. 21–1). The vessel wall contains the elements of a chronic inflammatory response producing a picture of panarteritis. However, the vasculitis that occurs in TAO is unusual because of the maintenance of vessel wall architecture and lack of wall necrosis.[2,7]

Subacute Phase

This stage of lesion development is typified by the disappearance of the microabscess. Epithelial nodules are present within the organizing thrombus, which is surrounded by a small number of giant cells.[33] Intact internal elastic lamellae are usually found in the artery and the vein[22] (Fig. 21–2). Unlike the acute lesion, the vessel wall demonstrates only minimal inflammatory changes.

Chronic Phase

The final phase in the formation of this occlusive lesion involves recanalization of the organized thrombus. Concurrently, fibroblasts migrate to the periphery of the vessel and, with the deposition of collagen, produce extensive fibrosis.[2,7] In conjunction with these nonspecific features, dramatic revascularization of the vessel wall occurs, as evidenced by penetration of the vasa vasora through the media[22] (Fig. 21–3).

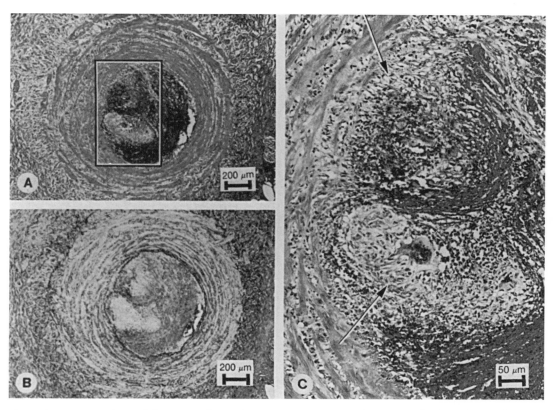

Figure 21-1.   Histology of the acute phase of TAO. (A, B) Sequential sections of a digital vein of the foot stained with H & E and elastic van Gieson stains (×40), respectively. The lumen is occluded with an inflammatory thrombus, with celluar infiltrate of the vessel wall. (C) Higher magnification (×200) of the boxed area in (A), showing microabscesses (arrows) with giant cells. (Reprinted from Ref. 22 with permission.)

CLINICAL FEATURES

Lower Extremity Disease

While the occlusive lesions of Buerger's disease are not found exclusively in the lower extremity, the classic pattern of distribution involves the infragenicular vasculature.[34] The most common presenting complaint is pain out of proportion to the objective findings.[23] Physical examination reveals strong femoral pulses and distal pulses that are diminished or absent. Further evaluation demonstrates the presence of foot claudication due to ischemia of the plantar muscles, a finding that is essentially pathognomonic for TAO.[34,35] Progression of the disease process results in the development of trophic changes. In Olin et al's study of 112 patients, 46 had evidence of lower extremity ischemic ulceration at the time of diagnosis.[27] Although seen less frequently, TAO of the lower extremity may be indicated by other abnormalities, such as sensory disturbances and thrombophlebitis. Patients with Buerger's disease may rarely have occlusive disease of the aorta and its branches such as the celiac[36,37] or renal arteries.[38] A microcirculatory lesion was also described as an early feature in the feet of patients with Buerger's disease.[39] These abnormalities, found using intra-arterial injection of the radioisotopes thallium-201 chloride and 99m-Tc macroaggregated human serum albumin, were fixed lesions that were not reversible with sympathectomy.[39]

Upper Extremity Disease

Upper extremity ischemia may be the only manifestation of Buerger's disease or it may occur concomitantly with lower extremity disease. TAO of the upper extremity preferentially affects the distal vasculature, while the subclavian, axillary, and brachial arteries remain free of disease. Initial complaints affecting this region are usually confined to numbness, discoloration, and rest pain.[40] Clinically, TAO of the upper limb may be indicated by a positive Allen's test, which suggests ulnar artery occlusion. Tissue loss secondary to ulceration and gangrene occurs in approximately 5% of patients with upper limb involvement.[40]

Thrombophlebitis Migrans

This term refers to the recurrent venous thrombosis frequently found in association with Buerger's disease. The vessels involved are usually superficial; however, deep vein thrombosis does occur. Initially, the veins

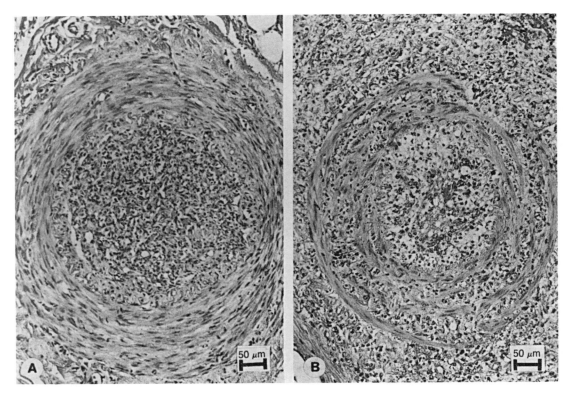

Figure 21-2. Early organization of occlusive thrombus, with an inflammatory cell infiltrate characterizing the subacute phase of TAO in a digital artery (A) and a vein (B). (Reprinted from Ref. 22 with permission.)

appear tense and are easily palpable, but as the disease progresses, vasodilation occurs and the veins appear tortuous.

DIAGNOSIS

Although no absolute criteria exist, a constellation of clinical features, supported by typical histologic and radiographic findings, provide the physician with adequate guidelines with which to make a confident diagnosis.

Clinical Features

The most important clinical features of TAO include (1) a history of cigarette smoking, (2) onset of symptomatology prior to 50 years of age, (3) distribution of occlusive lesions in the infragenicular vascular tree, (4) involvement of the upper extremity or the presence of phlebitis migrans, and (5) absence of other known atherosclerotic risk factors.[34] Although these characteristics do not have significant predictive value when considered individually, their presentation in combination strongly suggests the diagnosis of Buerger's disease.

Histopathologic Findings

As previously stated, microscopic examination of the occlusive lesion does not reveal a hallmark feature her-

alding the diagnosis of Buerger's disease. However, histologic support for the diagnosis of TAO can be observed in the acute phase of lesion development. The formation of microabscesses within fresh thrombus and infiltration of the vessel wall by mediators of inflammation provide the best pathologic evidence for Buerger's disease.[33]

Digital Plethysmography

Because Buerger's disease preferentially involves small and medium-sized vessels, digital plethysmography may be helpful in confirming the diagnosis. In patients with occlusion of the digital arteries, the plethysmogram typically demonstrates a flattening of the pulse wave and disappearance of the dicrotic notch.[41,42] While these findings are not specific for TAO, this modality provides a relatively inexpensive and noninvasive means of quantifying the severity of disease.

Arteriography

The radiographic characteristics of Buerger's disease were originally detailed by McKusick et al.[33] In addition to noting that the most frequently involved vessels were of small or medium caliber, they found that the occlusive process was segmental rather than disseminated throughout the length of the vessel; the luminal surface of the artery proximal to the lesion appeared

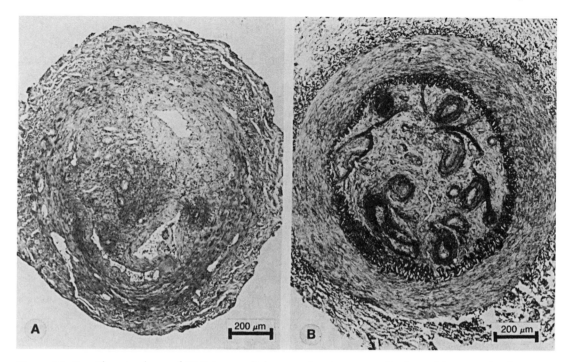

Figure 21–3. Chronic phase of TAO in a radial artery showing recanalization of the organized thrombus with vascularization of the media. (A) H & E stain; (B) Elastic van Gieson stain. (Reprinted from Ref. 22 with permission.)

smooth in contrast to the intimal irregularity seen in association with atherosclerosis; and the authors described the collateral circulation as having a "tree roots" or "spider legs" configuration, with its origin about the point of abrupt occlusion (Fig. 21–4).[33] Others have confirmed that these features are indicative, if not diagnostic, of Buerger's disease.[7,43]

DIFFERENTIAL DIAGNOSIS

The argument challenging the existence of TAO as a distinct disease process was fueled by its close similarity to several previously described disorders. Each of the following pathologies should be considered when evaluating a patient with peripheral occlusive disease.

Atherosclerosis Obliterans

Differentiation of TAO from atherosclerosis obliterans was a diagnostic challenge for early clinicians. However, with further study of both disease processes, several salient points of distinction have been uncovered. For example, although tobacco has been implicated as a causative agent in both atherosclerosis and Buerger's disease, several other comorbid conditions such as diabetes mellitus, hypercholesterolemia, and hypertension have been linked to atherosclerosis but are not associated with TAO. Similarly, although both disorders have a higher incidence in the male population, atherosclerosis generally afflicts persons more than 50 years of age while Buerger's disease has an earlier

onset. Additionally, TAO has been shown to involve the distal circulation of both the upper and lower extremities in a segmental pattern, in contrast to atherosclerosis, which affects the arteries of the lower limb in a diffuse manner.[7]

Collagen Vascular Disease

Collagen vascular diseases such as systemic lupus erythematosus, rheumatoid arthritis, and scleroderma preferentially affect women. However, with the increasing incidence of TAO in the female population, Buerger's disease should be considered in any young woman presenting with limb ischemia. Both disorders produce occlusion of the distal vasculature; however, collagen vascular diseases have associated clinical features such as sclerodactyly, arthritis, and gastrointestinal involvement that are rarely found in conjunction with TAO.[34] In addition, specific autoantibodies have been found in the circulation of patients afflicted with collagen vascular diseases, whereas no single serologic marker has been identified for Buerger's disease.[44,45] The availability of such routine serologic screening examinations simplifies the potential diagnostic dilemma in determining the cause of peripheral ischemia among women.

Takayasu's Arteritis

Although TAO and Takayasu's arteritis are both characterized by the development of inflammatory occlu-

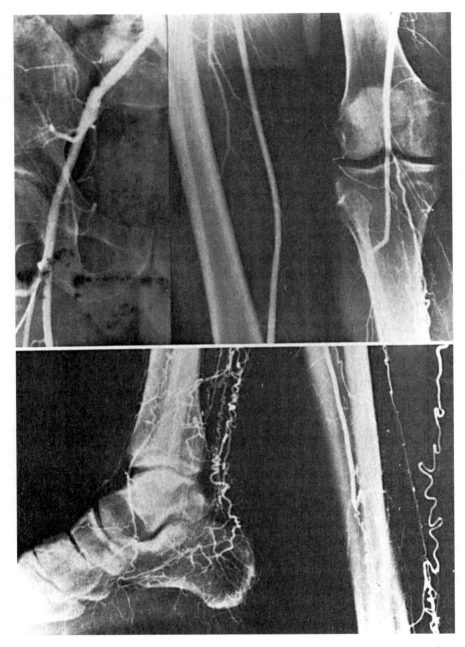

Figure 21–4. A 34-year-old male with TAO showing tibioperoneal occlusion and the corkscrew appearance of the collateral vessels. Proximal arteries are normal. (Reprinted from Ref. 41 with permission.)

sive lesions, the distribution of disease in these two disorders is quite different. Takayasu's arteritis affects the aorta and its major branches, with only rare involvement of the lower extremity.[40] In patients with TAO of the upper extremity, differentiation from Takayasu's arteritis may be based on the presenting symptomatology. Although skin discoloration and sensory abnormalities occur in both disorders, trophic changes occur more frequently among patients with Buerger's disease. In TAO the lesions occur in the small vessels of the wrist as well as in the digital arteries, whereas Takayasu's arteritis is characterized by lesions of the aortic arch, subclavian arteries, and proximal axillary arteries.[40] (See Chapter 24).

Popliteal Artery Entrapment

This condition also occurs in young males. The entrapment of the popliteal artery may lead to complete thrombosis and occlusion, with signs of acute ischemia. Biplane dynamic arteriography is helpful in diagnosing this condition.[46,47] (See Chapter 22).

TREATMENT

Despite intense research, there is no curative therapy for Buerger's disease. Therefore, the clinician's efforts must be focused on arresting the progression of disease and treating its symptoms.

Abstinence from Tobacco Use

The habitual use of tobacco products has been clearly linked to exacerbation of TAO.[7,9,48,49] Cessation of smoking is the only effective means of halting disease progression.[34] The importance of this lifestyle factor was demonstrated by Mills et al in their review of 26 patients with the diagnosis of Buerger's disease.[41] Specifically, five patients who quit smoking suffered no further tissue loss as a result of TAO, whereas all eight patients who continued to use tobacco products subsequently underwent major amputation procedures.[41] Total smoking abstinence is necessary for the success of any other intervention.

Conservative Management

Because multiple distal vessels are frequently involved in Buerger's disease, initial therapy should be conservative. The goal is to promote blood flow through collateral circulation in an effort to alleviate the ischemia produced by the occlusive lesions.

Physical Therapy

In addition to improving mobility and retarding muscle atrophy, physiotherapy may increase blood flow to the affected limb. While the augmentation of blood flow reduces the degree of ischemia, an added advantage may be an increase in the amount of neovascularization found at points of occlusion. This hypothesis is supported by the work of Ratschow, who demonstrated that an acceleration in blood velocity also facilitates the development of collateral circulation.[50] Therefore, walking exercise benefiting the ischemic lower extremity acts as a cornerstone in the medical management of patients with TAO.

Pharmacologic Therapy

Because intravenous administration of vasoactive substances can result in unwanted systemic manifestations, the best route for delivery of these agents is via intra-arterial infusion. This technique allows the clinician to target the collateral vasculature for vasodilation.

Prostaglandins have played a critical role in the management of patients with Buerger's disease. Their beneficial effect in the treatment of this pathologic process has been attributed to the pharmacologic properties of vasodilation and decreased platelet aggregation. Two agents that have received the most attention are prostaglandin E_1 (PGE_1) and prostacyclin (PGI_2). The effectiveness of PGE_1 in the management of ischemic ulcers was demonstrated by Shionoya et al. In their series of 255 patients, there were 40 extremities with disease that was not amenable to surgical intervention. Following continuous intra-arterial infusion of PGE_1 for a mean period of 44 days, ulcers were healed in 30% of the limbs and improved in 52%.[51] Equally encouraging results were reported in a randomized trial of PGE_1 treatment conducted by Sakaguchi and coworkers.[52]

Although PGI_2 shares the pharmacologic features that are responsible for the therapeutic benefit of PGE_1, its chemical instability precludes its use in the clinical setting. However, the development of prostacyclin derivatives has provided an alternative to PGE_1 infusion. One trial evaluated the efficacy of Iloprost, a prostacyclin analogue, in comparison to low-dose aspirin. In a randomized prospective study, 133 patients with pain secondary to critical ischemia received either Iloprost or aspirin for 28 days. At the conclusion of the experimental period, 85% of patients in the Iloprost treatment arm experienced relief of their ischemic pain in contrast to only 17% of patients in the aspirin therapy group. In addition, of the 133 patients with Buerger's disease, 98 presented with lower extremity ulceration. The administration of Iloprost produced complete resolution of leg ulcers in 35% of patients compared to a healing rate of 13% among patients treated with aspirin.[53] Similarly, Nizankowski et al found that the treatment of ischemic ulcers with the intra-arterial infusion of a prostacyclin derivative was beneficial in a randomized trial of 30 patients.[54] These data reflect the important position of prostanoids in the therapeutic regimen of patients with TAO.

In a 38-year-old male smoker diagnosed with Buerger's disease with symptoms of hand and foot ischemia, Palomo et al reported regression of symptoms using nifedipine in addition to smoking cessation.[55] Another case report suggested the beneficial effect of nifedipine in combination with antiplatelet therapy and complete cessation from tobacco use.[56] Because these case reports included smoking cessation and other modalities in addition to nifedipine use, the beneficial effect of the drug itself cannot be confirmed. However, calcium channel blockers such as nifedipine may be beneficial in treating the symptoms of TAO through peripheral vasodilatation.

Thrombolysis and Angioplasty

These techniques have not been used frequently in the setting of Buerger's disease. A case report was published by Hodgson and colleagues in England detailing the successful use of streptokinase to lyse a popliteal artery thrombus in a 24-year-old man. The popliteal artery was then found to have long segment of stenosis, which was balloon dilated. Angioplasty of an anterior tibial artery lesion was not successful. However, the patient obtained good symptomatic relief of the severe foot pain and paraesthesia. He remained symptoms free 2 years after the procedure. Of note, the patient stopped smoking after the procedure, which probably contributed to the success of this technique.[57] In another case of upper extremity ischemia due to Buerger's disease, urokinase and angioplasty were used successfully, with symptomatic relief.[58] However, the use of thrombolytic agents is generally limited to treatment of an acute thrombotic event. While the use of these medications may prove to be effective in select situations, there is no evidence to support the widespread administration of thrombolytics in the chronic management of Buerger's disease.

Surgical Management

Patients who fail to improve under conservative management are referred for evaluation as potential surgical candidates. When considering a patient for operative intervention, a surgeon may take one of two possible approaches based on the patient's symptomatology. If the primary complaint involves discoloration and trophic changes of the skin, sympathetic denervation should be employed to improve cutaneous circulation. However, if the presentation is one of rest pain or tissue loss, the feasibility of arterial reconstruction should be vigorously investigated.

Regional Sympathectomy

Interruption of sympathetic innervation eliminates vascular tone and produces vasodilation. The resultant increase in blood flow is particularly beneficial in patients who experience cold sensitivity or who have evidence of limited or superficial skin ulceration.[34] Sympathectomy does not improve circulation to muscles and is therefore not indicated in the treatment of intermittent claudication.[59] Excision of the sympathetic chain from L2 to L4 is performed through a retroperitoneal approach for patients with lower extremity involvement. Patients whose symptoms are localized to the upper extremity are treated with removal of T2, T3, and the lower third of the stellate ganglion. This procedure is carried out via a posterior approach to include Kuntz's nerve in the resection. It can be done thoracoscopically, with very good results and decreased morbidity.[60] Although sympathectomy does not alter the natural history of Buerger's disease, it does produce significant improvement in symptoms with minimal side effects. In their series of 266 patients with TAO, Shionoya et al reported that 128 sympathectomies were performed for treatment of trophic changes to the skin in 72% and cold sensitivity of Raynaud's phenomenon in 28%.[61] The outcome was considered satisfactory by the majority of patients who underwent the procedure. Similar results were obtained in a series of lumbar sympathectomies reviewed by Nakata et al.[62] In summary, this technique provides symptomatic relief to a specific group of patients by selectively altering vascular tone, thereby increasing blood flow through preexisting collateral vessels.

Thromboendarterectomy

This procedure is limited to patients with involvement of vessels above the knee. In using this technique, it is important to identify the cleavage plane that allows removal of the entire inflammatory process. Failure to eliminate all evidence of inflammation may result in recurrence of the disease process in the revascularized segment and is thought to be responsible for many of the early failures of thromboendarterectomy.[63]

Reconstructive Surgery

Arterial reconstruction has become the most frequently used technique for limb salvage.[34] The specific procedure employed is determined by the location of the involved segment.

Aortoiliac occlusion is a rare complication of TAO. However, when it is present, synthetic grafts are utilized to restore arterial flow from the proximal aorta to the lower extremity. The results of aortofemoral bypass in Buerger's disease are very good, with cumulative patency rate of 88.2%, and are superior to the results of aortoiliac or iliofemoral bypass.[30] These results were also found to depend on the patency of the profunda femoris artery, which should be assessed preoperatively with angiography.[34] Occlusion of the femoral, popliteal, or crural arteries is much more common in patients with Buerger's disease. If the superficial femoral artery is occluded and the popliteal artery is free of disease and is in continuity with an infragenicular vessel, a femoropopliteal bypass should be performed. Conversely, if the popliteal artery is occluded, a bypass graft from the femoral system to one of the crural arteries is indicated. When available, the autologous greater saphenous vein should be employed as graft material in infrapopliteal bypass procedures for optimal results.[30] Cessation of smoking has been associated with improved patency of these bypasses (73.3% vs. 64.8%).[30] An additional factor that predicts early graft failure is the quality of the distal runoff. Adequate flow is indicated by good visualization of a complete pedal arch, which should be evaluated radiographically.[64] However, Yano and colleagues reported a 5-year cumulative patency rate of 77.3% using autogenous vein bypasses to isolated tibial and peroneal arteries segments more than 12 cm in length.[65] Among patients in whom the tibial and peroneal arteries are occluded, with patency of inframalleolar vessels, autogenous vein bypasses to the dorsalis pedis or plantar arteries can be performed, with a considerable limb salvage rate, especially in patients who have stopped smoking.[66] Autogenous vein bypass to collateral arteries has also been reported as a novel technique for limb salvage in patients with no named patent vessels.[67]

Occlusion of forearm arteries occurs in patients with TAO who have upper extremity involvement. The preferred technique in these cases is in situ bypass utilizing either the cephalic or basilic vein.[34]

Amputation

When conservative management and surgical limb salvage procedures fail, amputation of necrotic tissue is necessary to prevent systemic infection and preserve a functional limb. Overall, the amputation rate in several large series ranges from 20 to 30% of patients with documented Buerger's disease.[7,27,41] The vast majority of these cases occur in patients who continue to smoke cigarettes, emphasizing the strong relationship between tobacco use and the severity of TAO.

PROGNOSIS

Formerly, it was widely believed that a diagnosis of Buerger's disease denoted a diminished life expectancy. This notion was partially based on the increased incidence of amputation procedures in this patient group. However, later studies refuted this hypothesis by demonstrating that the mortality rate in patients with TAO is similar to that in age-matched controls.[68,69]

SUMMARY

TAO is a thrombo-occlusive disorder that affects medium-sized and small vessels of the distal circulation. This disease process preferentially strikes young men with a history of habitual tobacco use. Although the etiology remains unknown, substantial data suggest that hereditary factors or autoimmunity may have a role in the development of the characteristic occlusive lesion. Histologic examination of the acute inflammatory lesion reveals the presence of multifocal microabscesses that are distinctive for Buerger's disease. Such lesions are found in both the upper and lower extremities and produce symptoms of ischemia. In addition to this clinical presentation, the diagnosis of TAO is supported by the typical angiographic findings which include the appearance of collaterals described as having a "tree root" or "spider legs" configuration. Absolute smoking cessation is essential in the management of these patients. Conservative therapy utilizing exercise and pharmacologic agents should be the initial approach. If symptoms remain intractable, surgical intervention warrants consideration. Sympathectomy and arterial reconstruction are the two approaches that have produced the greatest benefit. Although no cure is currently available, the natural history of Buerger's disease is relatively benign, with a life expectancy comparable to that of the general population, although progressive disease is associated with a significant incidence of amputation.

REFERENCES

1. Buerger L. Thromboangiitis obliterans: a study of the vascular lesions leading to presenile spontaneous gangrene. *Am J Med Sci* 1908;136:567–580.
2. Von Winiwater F. Ueber eine eigenthumliche form von endarteritis und endophlebitis mit gangran des fusses. *Arch Klin Chir* 1879;23:202–226.
3. Wessler S, Ming S, Gurewich V, Freiman D. A critical evaluation of thromboangiitis obliterans: the case against Buerger's disease. *N Engl J Med* 1960;262:1149–1156.
4. Gore I, Burrows S. A reconsideration of the pathogenesis of Buerger's disease. *Am J Clin Pathol* 1958;29:319–330.
5. Fisher C. Cerebral thromboangiitis: including a critical review of the literature. *Medicine* 1957;36:169–209.
6. Matsushita M, Shionoya S, Matsumoto T. Urinary cotinine measurement in patients with Buerger's disease—effects of active and passive smoking on the disease process. *J Vasc Surg* 1991;14:53–58.
7. Jurgens J. Thromboangiitis obliterans (Buerger's disease, TAO). In: Juergens J, Spittell J, Fairbain J (eds): *Peripheral Vascular Disease.* Philadelphia: WB Saunders; 1980:468–491.
8. Vink M. Symposium on Buerger's disease. *J Cardiovasc Surg* 1970;14:1–51.
9. Mozes M, Cahansky G, Doitsch V, Adar R. The association of atherosclerosis and Buerger's disease: a clinical and radiological study. *J Cardiovasc Surg* 1970;11:52–59.
10. Shionoya S, Ban I, Nakata Y, Matsubara J, Shinjo K. Diagnosis, pathology, and treatment of Buerger's disease. *Surgery* 1974;75:695–700.
11. Inada K, Iwashima Y, Okada A, Matsumoto K. Nonatherosclerotic segmental arterial occlusion of the extremity. *Arch Surg* 1974;108:663–37.
12. McLoughlin G, Hesby C, Evans C, Chapman D. Association of HLA-A9 and HLA-B5 with Buerger's disease. *Br Med J* 1976;2:1165–1166.
13. Ohtawa T, Juji T, Kawano N, Mishima Y, Tohyama H, Ishikawa K. HLA antigens in thromboangiitis obliterans. *JAMA* 1974;230:1128–.
14. De Moerloose P, Jeannet M, Mirimanoff P, Bouvier C. Evidence for an HLA-linked resistance gene in Buerger's disease. *Tissue Antigens* 1979;14:169–173.
15. Papa M, Bass A, Adar R, et al. Autoimmune mechanisms in thromboangiitis obliterans (Buerger's disease): the role of tobacco antigen and the major histocompatibility complex. *Surgery* 1992;111:527–531.
16. Adar R, Papa M, Halpern Z, et al. Cellular sensitivity to collagen in thromboangiitis obliterans. *N Engl J Med* 1983;308:1108–1116.
17. Spittel J. Thromboangiitis obliterans: an autoimmune disorder? *N Engl J Med* 1983;308:1157–.
18. Steffen C. Consideration of pathogenesis of rheumatoid arthritis as collagen autoimmunity. *Immunoforsh* 1970;139:219–227.
19. Pietraszek MH, Choudhury NA, Baba S, et al. Serotonin as a factor involved in pathophysiology of thromboangiitis obliterans [see comments]. *Int Angiol* 1993;12:9–12.

20. Szendro G, Golcman L, Cristal N. Study of the factors affecting blood viscosity in patients with thromboangiitis obliterans. A preliminary report. *J Vasc Surg* 1988;7:759–762.

21. Lie JT. The rise and fall and resurgence of thromboangiitis obliterans (Buerger's disease). *Acta Pathol Jpn* 1989;39:153–158.

22. Lie JT. Thromboangiitis obliterans (Buerger's disease) in women. *Medicine (Balt)* 1987;66:65–72.

23. Wheeler H. Thromboangiitis obliterans (Buerger's disease) in women. In: Sabiston D (ed): *Textbook of Surgery*. 1988:1637–1640.

24. Wong J, Lam ST, Ong GB. Buerger's disease—a review of 105 patients. *Aust NZ J Surg* 1978;48:382–387.

25. Buerger L. *The Circulatory Disturbances of the Extremities Including Gangrene, Vasomotor, and Trophic Changes*. Philadelphia: WB Saunders; 1924:

26. Leavitt RY, Bressler P, Fauci AS. Buerger's disease in a young woman. *Am J Med* 1986;80:1003–1005.

27. Olin JW, Young JR, Graor RA, Ruschhaupt WF, Bartholomew JR. The changing clinical spectrum of thromboangiitis obliterans (Buerger's disease). *Circulation* 1990;82:IV3–IV8.

28. Remington P, Forman M, Gentry E, Marks J, Hogelin G, Trowbridge F. Current smoking trends in the United States the 1981–1983 behavior risk factor surveys. *JAMA* 1985;2553:2975–2978.

29. Shionoya S, Ban I, Nakata Y, Matsubara J, Hirai M, Kawai S. Involvement of the iliac artery in Buerger's disease (pathogenesis and arterial reconstruction). *J Cardiovasc Surg (Torino)* 1978;19:69–76.

30. Izumi Y, Sasajima T, Inaba M, Morimoto N, Goh K, Kubo Y. Results of arterial reconstruction in Buerger's disease. *Nippon Geka Gakkai Zasshi* 1993;94:751–754.

31. Lie JT. Thromboangiitis obliterans (Buerger's disease) in a saphenous vein arterial graft. *Hum Pathol* 1987;18:402–404.

32. Dible J. The pathology of limb ischemia. In: Edinburgh: Oliver and Boyd; 1966:79–96.

33. McKusick V, Harris W, Ottensen O, Goodman R, Shelley W, Bloodwell R. Buerger's disease: a distinct clinical and pathologic entity. *JAMA* 1962;181:5–12.

34. Shionoya S. Buerger's disease: diagnosis and management. *Cardiovasc Surg* 1993;1:207–214.

35. Hirai M, Shinonoya S. Intermittent claudication in the foot and Buerger's disease. *Br J Surg* 1978;65:210–213.

36. Sobel RA, Ruebner BH. Buerger's disease involving the celiac artery. *Hum Pathol* 1979;10:112–115.

37. Broide E, Scapa E, Peer A, Witz E, Abramowich D, Eshchar J. Buerger's disease presenting as acute small bowel ischemia. *Gastroenterology* 1993;104:1192–1195.

38. Gomi T, Ikeda T, Yuhara M. Renovascular hypertension due to Buerger's disease. *Jpn Heart J* 1978;19:308–314.

39. Nishikimi N, Sakurai T, Shionoya S, Oshima M. Microcirculatory characteristics in patients with Buerger's disease. *Angiology* 1992;43:312–319.

40. Mishima Y. Arterial insufficiency of the upper extremity with special reference to Takayasu's arteritis and Buerger's disease. *J Cardiovasc Surg (Torino)* 1982;23:105–108.

41. Mills JL, Taylor LM Jr, Porter JM. Buerger's disease in the modern era. *Am J Surg* 1987;154:123–129.

42. Mills JL, Friedman EI, Taylor LM Jr, Porter JM. Upper extremity ischemia caused by small artery disease. *Ann Surg* 1987;206:521–528.

43. Szilagyi D, DeRusso F, Elliott J. Thromboangiitis obliterans: clinico-angiographic correlation. *Arch Surg* 1964;88:824–835.

44. Gulati S, Singh K, Thusoo T, Saha K. Immunological studies in thromboangiitis obliterans (Buerger's disease). *J Surg Res* 1979;27:287–293.

45. Gulati SM, Saha K, Kant L, Thusoo TK, Prakash A. Significance of circulatory immune complexes in thromboangiitis obliterans (Buerger's disease). *Angiology* 1984;35:276–281.

46. Love JW, Whelan TJ. Popliteal artery entrapment syndrome. *Am J Surg* 1965;109:620–624.

47. Greenwood LH, Hallett JW Jr, Yrizarry JM, Robison JG, Brown SB. The angiographic evaluation of lower-extremity arterial disease in the young adult. *Cardiovasc Intervent Radiol* 1985;8:183–186.

48. Abramson D, Zayas A, Canning J, Edinburgh J. Thromboangiitis obliterans: true clinical entity. *Am J Cardiol* 1963;12:107–118.

49. Silbert S. Etiology of thromboangiitis obliterans. *JAMA* 1945;129:5–9.

50. Ratschow M. Kritisches zu atiologie und grundlagen einer konservativen therapie periphere durchblutungstorungen. *Langenbecks Arch Klin Chir* 1959;292:188–197.

51. Shionoya S. *Buerger's Disease: Pathology, Diagnosis, and Treatment*. Nagoya: University of Nagoya Press; 1990:225–229.

52. Sakagushi S, Kusaba M, Mishima Y. A multi-clinical, double-blind study with PGE$_1$ (cyclodextrin clathrate) in patients with ischemic ulcer of the extremities. *Vasa* 1978;7:263–266.

53. Fiessinger JN, Schafer M. Trial of iloprost versus aspirin treatment for critical limb ischaemia of thromboangiitis obliterans. The TAO Study. *Lancet* 1990;335:555–557.

54. Nizankowski R, Krolikowski W, Bielatowicz J. Prostacyclin for ischemic ulcers in peripheral arterial disease. *Thromb Res* 1985;37:21–28.

55. Palomo Arellano A, Gomez Tello V, Parilla Herranz P, Castilla Plaza A, Marcos Sanchez F, Duran Perez-Navarro A. Buerger's disease starting in the upper extremity. A favorable response to nifedipine treatment combined with stopping tobacco use. *An Med Interna* 1990;7:307–308.

56. O'Dell JR, Linder J, Markin RS, Moore GF. Thromboangiitis obliterans (Buerger's disease) and smokeless tobacco. *Arthritis Rheum* 1987;30:1054–1056.

57. Hodgson TJ, Gaines PA, Beard JD. Thrombolysis and angioplasty for acute lower limb ischemia in Buerger's disease. *Cardiovasc Intervent Radiol* 1994;17:333–335.

58. Lang EV, Bookstein JJ. Accelerated thrombolysis and angioplasty for hand ischemia in Buerger's disease. *Cardiovasc Intervent Radiol* 1989;12:95–97.

59. Hirai M, Kawai S, Shionoya S. Effect of lumbar sympathectomy on muscle circulation in dogs and patients. *Nagoya J Med Sci* 1975;37:71–77.

60. Ishibashi H, Hayakawa N, Yamamoto H, Nishikimi N, Yano T, Nimura Y. Thoracoscopic sympathectomy for Buerger's disease: a report on the successful treatment of four patients. *Surg Today* 1995;25:180–183.

61. Shionoya S, Ban I, Nakata Y, Matsubara J, Hirai M, Kawai S. Surgical treatment of Buerger's disease. *J Cardiovasc Surg (Torino)* 1980;21:77–84.

62. Nakata Y, Suzuki S, Kawai S, et al. Effects of lumbar sympathectomy on thromboangiitis obliterans. *J Cardiovasc Surg* 1975;16:415–425.

63. Shionoya S, Ban I, Nakata Y, Matsubara J, Hirai M. Vascular reconstruction in Buerger's disease. *Br J Surg* 1976;63:841–846.

64. Shionoya S, Matsubara J, Hirai M. Measurement of blood pressure, blood flow, and flow velocity in arterial reconstruction of lower extremity. *Angiology* 1983;34:244–256.

65. Yano T, Shionoya S, Ikezawa T, et al. Indication of femorotibial and femoroperoneal bypass for Buerger's disease. *Nippon Geka Gakkai Zasshi* 1989;90:1110–1116.

66. Sasajima T, Kubo Y, Izumi Y, Inaba M, Goh K. Plantar or dorsalis pedis artery bypass in Buerger's disease. *Ann Vasc Surg* 1994;8:248–257.

67. Shindo S, Kamiya K, Suzuki O, Kobayashi M, Tada Y. Collateral artery bypass in Buerger's disease: report of a novel procedure. *Surg Today* 1995;25:92–95.

68. Hussein EA, el Dorri A. Intra-arterial streptokinase as adjuvant therapy for complicated Buerger's disease: early trials. *Int Surg* 1993;78:54–58.

69. Nielubowicz J, Rosnowski A, Pruszynski B, Przetakiewicz Z, Potemkowski A. Natural history of Buerger's disease. *J Cardiovasc Surg (Torino)* 1980;21:529–540.

22

Popliteal Entrapment and Adventitial Cystic Disease

Norman M. Rich, M.D., F.A.C.S.

An extensive literature attests to the ongoing challenge that popliteal vascular entrapment and adventitial cystic disease poses in both diagnosis and therapy.[1-42] While the number of cases of popliteal vascular entrapment and popliteal arterial adventitial cystic disease do not approximate that of popliteal vascular trauma, these two relatively rare and unusual lesions are being recognized with increasing frequency. Initial case reports have been replaced with more extensive reviews for both popliteal vascular entrapment and adventitial cystic disease of the popliteal artery.

Intermittent claudication is not an infrequent complaint among our increasingly aging population, with a high prevalence of arteriosclerosis obliterans. In contrast, however, relatively young male athletes present with popliteal vascular entrapment and men in their mid-40s with adventitial cystic disease of the popliteal artery, although these conditions are being increasingly identified in women. Yao and associates made a valuable contribution by describing measurements of ankle systolic pressure in arterial disease affecting the lower extremities in their work in 1969,[42] and Barnes and Strandness outlined physiologic parameters suggesting isolated popliteal arterial lesions in 1972.[2] Darling and colleagues[10] and McDonald and coworkers,[33] with the latter group at Walter Reed Army Medical Center, attempted to correlate noninvasive testing with the angiographic diagnosis of popliteal vascular entrapment in the mid-1970s.

This chapter will outline the development of our understanding of these two lesions and summarize their current clinical status.

POPLITEAL VASCULAR ENTRAPMENT

Historical Perspective

It is always interesting to identify the observations of a medical student. It was T.P.A. Stuart, while attending medical school in Edinburgh in 1879, who dissected the amputated leg of a 64-year-old man and reported that the popliteal artery

> passes almost vertically downwards internally to the inner head of the gastrocnemius. It reaches the bottom of the space by turning round the inner border of that head, and then passes downwards and outwards beneath it. . . .[39]

It was recognized that this anomaly had not been recorded previously, nor has there been any subsequent challenge to this claim.

Although an article appeared in the French literature in 1925, it was nearly 80 years after Stuart's observation that notice in the English-speaking world was given by Hamming in 1959 at Leyden University in the Netherlands.[24] He reported an anomaly similar to that described by Stuart in a 12-year-old boy in Leyden, providing the first broadly recognized clinical identification of this anomaly involving the popliteal artery. Hamming credited the initial report of Stuart, and he also acknowledged that Chambardel-Dubreuil in 1925 had described a case in which the popliteal artery was separated from the popliteal vein by an accessory slip of the gastrocnemius muscle. It remains widely recognized nearly 40 years later that Hamming's case represents the first successful clinical treatment of complications associated with popliteal arterial entrapment. Servello at the University of Padua in Italy in 1962 described a finding similar to that outlined by Hamming's case.[38] He evaluated complaints of a 28-year-old Italian farmer and made his diagnosis based on Hamming's article. He also noted a small aneurysm of the popliteal artery distal to the anomalous area. Additional reports by Hall in 1961[22] and 1964,[23] as well as by Carter and Eban in 1964,[7] further clarified our understanding of this condition. However, the term *popliteal artery entrapment syndrome* was used for the first time by Love and Whelan in 1965 when they reported two unusual cases at Walter Reed General Hospital.[32] A subsequent case report by Rich and Hughes in 1967 emphasized for the first time that the popliteal vein, as well as the popliteal artery, could be involved in a variety of anomalies, and that these anomalies frequently involved an abnormal attachment of the medial head of the gastrocnemius muscle[35] (Fig. 22–1). Increasingly, this lesion has been recognized by military surgeons throughout the world who have had a specific interest in these challenging lesions associated with abnormal lateral attachment of the medial head of the gastrocnemius muscle, accessory muscle slips, and other associated anatomic variants causing external popliteal compression. Nonmilitary colleagues including di Marzo and coworkers in Italy have added a recent extensive civilian experience.[12,13]

Incidence and Pathophysiology

The anatomic variant resulting in popliteal vascular entrapment is being recognized with increasing frequency. The 1979 report from Walter Reed Army Medical Center identified popliteal vascular entrapment in 14 extremities between 1966 and 1979.[36] In a similar report from the Letterman Army Medical Center in 1989,[8] 20 extremities were involved in 12 patients, and 8 of the 12 had bilateral entrapment.

International interest and documentation have also been associated with popliteal vascular entrapment, particularly in Europe and Japan. Biemans and van Bockell in 1977 published an extensive review of 58 patients with documented cases with the same clinical signs and symptoms described in the literature since the first case report from the Netherlands in 1959 by Hamming.[3] Subsequently, Ferrero and associates provided an extensive review of the management of 84 patients with popliteal vascular entrapment syndrome.[18] The article included seven cases from their personal experiences observed in Turin from a total of 35 popliteal artery occlusions that were treated surgically. From South Africa, Gaylis described two patients with popliteal artery entrapment syndrome in 1972,[20] and Gaylis and Rosenberg described a bilateral case the following year.[21] From Japan, Inada and associates reported the case of a patient with bilateral popliteal artery entrapment and stated that there were 10 re-

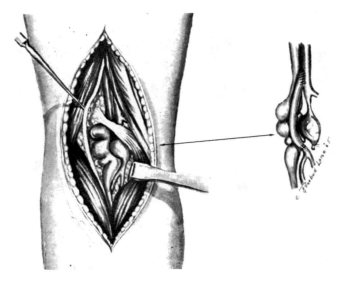

Figure 22–1. The drawing shows entrapment with formation of aneurysms in both the popliteal artery and the popliteal vein caused by an accessory slip of the gastrocnemius muscle (left). Arterial reconstruction by autogenous greater saphenous vein bypass with ligation of the popliteal arterial aneurysm was successful (right). The accessory slip of muscle was incised near its insertion to release the entrapment of both the artery and vein. (Reprinted from Ref. 35 with permission.)

ports in the Japanese literature. Ikeda and associates expanded the study to 18 cases in Japan in their report in 1981.[26] From Greece, Bouhoutsos and Goulios expanded their series from their original report of 1977 of popliteal artery entrapment in a young Greek soldier.[4–6] In Italy, di Marzo and associates have written extensively about their rapidly expanding civilian experience.[12,13]

An unusual variant of vascular entrapment in a patient following injury to the lower extremity was described by Evans and Bernhard.[17] No anatomic variants or compressive bands were found in their patient, who presented with compression of both the popliteal artery and vein. It was their impression that this form of popliteal vascular entrapment was caused by massive edema of the heads of the gastrocnemius muscle. An acquired type of popliteal artery entrapment was presented by Baker and Stoney.[1] Their unusual variant was associated with arterial bypass surgery. The list continues to expand with the emphasis of physiological entrapment reported by Rignault in 1985.[37]

While entrapment of the popliteal vein was overlooked initially, Connell reported the first isolated entrapment of the popliteal vein in 1978,[9] which added to the initial report in 1967 identified previously by Rich and Hughes in which both the popliteal artery and vein were entrapped.[35] Subsequent reports, including those from Italy, Japan, and the United States, have identified an increasing recognition of popliteal venous entrapment.

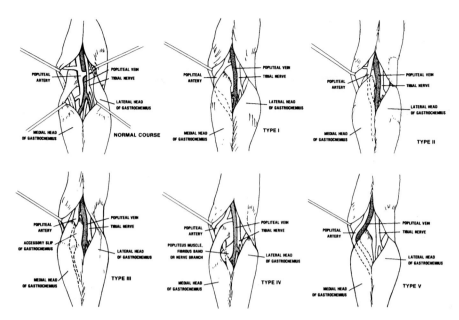

Figure 22–2. The normal course of the neurovascular bundle in the popliteal fossa from the posterior approach is compared with four generally accepted types of anomalies involving entrapment of the popliteal artery that are usually associated with abnormal configuration of the medial head of the gastrocnemius muscle. Classification, however, does not satisfy all anatomic variants. Empirically, type IV was expanded to include a branch of the tibial nerve as a structure compressing the popliteal artery, and type V was added to emphasize that the popliteal vein can be entrapped with the artery in all four types. (Reprinted from Ref. 36 with permission.)

Several classification systems have been proposed to describe the anatomic variants associated with entrapment of the popliteal artery and vein. An early classification system in 1970 by Insua and associates[27] was modified subsequently by Delaney and Gonzalez.[11] The classification was expanded by Ferrero and associates to include a total of 10 lesions. Figure 22–2 graphically depicts the five lesions in a system that was helpful in understanding the presentation in 14 extremities with popliteal vascular entrapment treated at Walter Reed Army Medical Center.[36]

External compression of the popliteal artery has resulted in a variety of changes ranging from poststenotic dilatation to true aneurysm formation. Progression to thrombosis has also occurred in the popliteal artery at the site of entrapment. Midpopliteal arterial occlusion from this localized area of thrombosis is an important diagnostic sign. Extensive collateral arterial development is frequently seen. Aneurysmal changes have occurred in the popliteal vein that is entrapped, as well as in the popliteal artery.

Several unresolved issues involving the segment of the popliteal artery in the entrapped area and the segment immediately distal to the area of entrapment remain. For example, it is not clear whether a true aneurysm will develop after release of the entrapment. Long-term follow-up of patients who have had operative correction will be helpful in answering this important question.

Clinical Presentation

Popliteal vascular entrapment should be considered in any active individual who develops calf claudication with strenuous exercise. While this has been seen most frequently in young men, an increasing number of lesions are being recognized in young, athletic women. The diagnosis of these lesions has been made increasingly in long-distance runners. Also, an increasing number of middle-aged patients have been diagnosed with popliteal vascular entrapment, who have presented with either a popliteal arterial aneurysm or popliteal artery occlusion. Bilaterality of these lesions is being documented with increasing frequency. Venous entrapment can be associated with lower extremity swelling and/or superficial varicosities.

Diagnosis

The patient's history should lead to a suspicion of the anomaly of popliteal vascular entrapment. The noninvasive techniques noted above, and most recently including the use of color flow duplex, may be required to establish a definitive diagnosis. Angiography continues to provide the classic finding of medial deviation of the popliteal artery (Fig. 22–3). Because

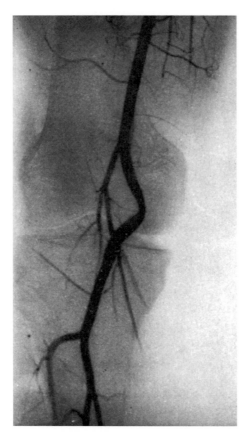

Figure 22–3. From the posteroanterior view, angiography of the left popliteal artery demonstrates abnormal medial deviation caused by an accessory slip of the medial head of the gastrocnemius muscle with the foot in neutral position. External compression was accentuated with the foot in both dorsal flexion and plantar flexion. (Reprinted from Ref. 36 with permission.)

there are a variety of possible anatomic variants, this classic finding may not be seen. Also, there might be segmental occlusion of the midpopliteal artery and/or aneurysmal formation. Contrast in the venous system may identify venous entrapment, occlusion, or aneurysmal change.

Management

Operative intervention is indicated to prevent the complications associated with popliteal vascular entrapment. Release of entrapping anomalies has become widely accepted. Early intervention should reduce the likelihood of threats to the lower extremity such as thrombosis and/or distal emboli, as well as stenotic dilatation that may progress to true aneurysm formation.

The first successful clinical management of popliteal arterial entrapment was reported in 1959 by Hamming, who used an S-shaped posterior incision in the popliteal fossa. Although many contemporary surgeons prefer the medial approach to the popliteal artery, the

posterior approach has been the choice at Walter Reed Army Medical Center, as outlined in a review of 14 lesions. Bilateral lesions may be repaired simultaneously, as in three patients at Walter Reed, to limit the anesthetic risk to a single induction. No associated postoperative complications occurred with this approach. The S-shaped incision allows identification of the variety of possible anomalies responsible for popliteal vascular entrapment, ranging from abnormal insertion of the medial head of the gastrocnemius muscle to accessory muscles slips to a variety of abnormal bands, as well as adequate exposure for repair of the arterial aneurysmal and thrombotic complications. The medial incision may not allow easy identification of these varied anomalies. It can be argued that the exact pathology identified remains moot because the patient's problems associated with midpopliteal thrombosis or popliteal aneurysm formation can be appropriately treated surgically by autogenous greater saphenous vein bypass through the medial approach. Fortunately, transection of the anomalous gastrocnemius muscle, accessory muscle, fibrous bands, and similar external compressing anomalies manages the majority of these cases successfully. Autogenous venous tissue, such as the greater saphenous vein, can be used as patch grafts or bypass conduits when necessary.

POPLITEAL ARTERIAL ADVENTITIAL CYSTIC DISEASE

Historical Perspective

Ejrup and Hiertonn provided the first description of adventitial cystic disease of the popliteal artery in Sweden in 1954.[15] Hiertonn had made a transverse incision in the middle of a thickened area of the popliteal artery in a patient to find a mass filled with gelatinous material. Mucoid degeneration of the media was the tentative diagnosis. Hiertonn et al reported four cases of cystic degeneration of the popliteal artery in 1957.[25] They described "clear, jelly-like material similar in appearance to that seen in a ganglion." They added that "the specimen looked like a sausage and was 7 cm in length" and "the lumen was compressed by an intramural cyst containing jelly under high tension." They made reference to a publication by Atkins and Key in 1946, describing what was adventitial probably cystic disease of the external iliac artery. Similar adventitial cystic degeneration has been identified in a variety of arteries, although it appears that the popliteal artery has been most frequently involved with this lesion.

In 1961, Ishikawa et al noted an important diagnostic sign when they observed that the normal distal pulsations were obliterated with flexion of the patient's knee.[28] On straightening of the knee, the pulses immediately returned to normal. Jaquet and Meyer-Burgdorff stated that the cyst might present as a localized stenosis that allowed distal arterial flow only at the peak of systolic pressure.[30] In 1963, Eastcott made a similar observation and suggested that an arterial murmur within the popliteal fossa was an important sign in establishing the proper diagnosis in the young, athletic nonsmoker with intermittent claudication due to a popliteal artery stenosis created by arterial adventitial cystic disease.[14] In 1967, Taylor and colleagues added the important observation that "the sudden onset of symptoms in our case may have been due to the floor of the superficial cyst giving away, resulting in the extrusion of the contents into the dissection plane of the vessel, so forming an internal projection which constricted the lumen."[41] Again, the analogy to ganglia was made, as the cysts were degenerative described as cysts containing collagenous material and possibly resulting from previous trauma. While the actual cause of adventitial cystic disease of the popliteal artery remains unknown, it is being recognized with increasing frequency.

Incidence and Etiology

Although still relatively uncommon, there has been an increasing number of reports of arterial adventitial cystic disease of the popliteal artery in recent years. In 1979, Flanigan and his colleagues reported the findings of their corrrespondence center concerning arterial adventitial cystic disease at Northwestern University.[19] They reviewed the history and findings in 115 cases around the world, and their reference remains a classic review of this problem. The authors noted that approximately 50% of the cases came from continental Europe (56 of the 115 cases), with an additional 12 cases from Scandinavia and 14 cases from Great Britain. There were 13 cases in both North America and Australia. Cystic adventitial disease of the popliteal artery predominantly affects men. The age range is 11 to 70 years, with a mean age of 42 years.

The etiology is uncertain, although three theories have been proposed. One theory is that of repetitive trauma, which could cause degeneration of the arterial wall and cystic degeneration of the adventitia. Because the lesion has been described in children, the trauma theory appears unlikely. A second theory is that of a generalized body disorder, implying that the adventitial degenerative process is a mucinous or myxomatous condition. However, follow-up has not documented the development of these cysts contralaterally, and generalized connective tissue disorders have not appeared in patients who have been followed. A third theory assumes that developmental inclusion of mucin-secreting cells within the adventitia of the artery allows a cyst to develop within the adventitia. Numerous reports evaluating ganglia have noted a similarity to adventitial cyst disease. It has been thought either that there can be enlargement of the capsular synovial cyst that could develop along a genicular artery to involve the adventitia of the popliteal artery or that synovial rests can be sequestered into the arterial wall during development. This might help explain why the cyst can be entirely adventitial and encapsulated or more involved, which will not allow enucleation.

Pathophysiology

The contents of these cysts have been extensively studied. Endo and colleagues isolated and identified proteohyaluronic acid for the cyst of cystic mucoid degeneration.[16] Leaf performed amino acid analysis of the protein present in adventitial cystic disease of the popliteal artery.[31] Chemical and histologic analyses indicate that ganglia and adventitial cysts are quite similar, with both involving mucoproteins and mucopolysaccharides.

Men in their fourth decade are most frequently identified as having cystic adventitial disease of the popliteal artery. The sudden onset of symptoms in all patients, however, is probably caused by rapid change in the cyst that has been developing for a long time. The cyst produces a stenosis while preserving patency of the popliteal artery. Intracystic pressure may exceed that of the adjacent artery, causing occlusion, with or without thrombosis. Claudication without severe ischemia is a common finding because of the development of collateral circulation.

Clinical Findings

Sudden onset of claudication that is quite limiting in a man in his mid-40s is the typical presentation of a patient with cystic adventitial disease of the popliteal artery. Occasionally, there may be an ischemic neuropathy associated with the sudden onset of claudication. Popliteal and pedal pulses may be present if there is only a stenosis. A bruit may be heard over the popliteal fossa. Popliteal and pedal pulses may be absent, however, if thrombosis of the popliteal artery has occurred. Because stenosis is more frequent than occlusion, popliteal and pedal pulses may disappear during acute knee flexion, with immediate restoration of pulsations on straightening of the knee. The patient may have experienced the sudden onset of cramping pain in the calf, followed later by typical intermittent claudication with the development of good collateral circulation during the progressive stenosis of the popliteal artery.

Diagnostic Evaluation

Clinical evaluation with the knee in the neutral and flexed positions, noninvasive blood flow laboratory tests assessing flow by both pressure measurements and waveform analysis, and ultrasound and color flow duplex evaluation can aid in the clinical diagnosis. Angiography, as emphasized by Sutton in 1962, is an important diagnostic test.[40] Angiography may outline a smooth wall stenosis, usually in the midportion of the popliteal artery, which extends from 1 to 8 cm in length, or there may be evidence of a localized complete occlusion of this portion of the popliteal artery, with the remainder of the lower extremity arterial anatomy appearing normal. A smooth taper to the lesion may be concentric and described as "hourglass" in shape or it may be described as a "scimitar sign" when the artery tapers above and below the cyst (Fig. 22–4). Lateral and anteroposterior views are important to ensure that the lesion is not missed. Angiographic findings should be characteristic and diagnostic.

Management

Optimal treatment is provided by surgical intervention. Conservative surgical approaches including aspiration or enucleation have been successful in eradicating the arterial occlusion in some patients. Consequently, surgical procedures have been divided into nonresectional and resectional techniques. Nonresectional techniques have been used mainly when the occlusion is incomplete. Enucleation or evacuation is the most frequent approach. Once thrombosis has occurred, however,

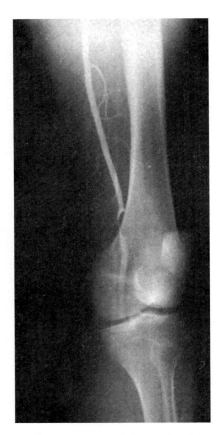

Figure 22–4. This angiogram of the popliteal artery reveals smooth tapering above and below the cyst that created severe stenosis of the popliteal artery. This "scimitar sign" is diagnostic for adventitial cystic disease of the popliteal artery. (Reprinted from Ref. 34 with permission.)

resection and segmental replacement with an autogenous venous interposition graft has been utilized most frequently. A review by Flanigan and his colleagues emphasized the high degree of success possible when properly selected approaches are utilized.[19] Hiertonn has been particularly interested in the long-term follow-up of autogenous vein grafts used for arterial reconstruction when segmental techniques have been required.[25] Also, it is important to note that recurrent occlusions due to cysts have been treated successfully by needle aspiration of various amounts of gelatinous material. Advocates of this approach of simple evacuation of the cyst by aspiration emphasize a relatively high degree of success.

The S-shaped posterior incision in the popliteal fossa or a medial popliteal incision can be used to approach the lesion. The popliteal artery is usually found to be enlarged and sausage-shaped. Adhesions may bind the cystic adventitial structure to the adjacent vein or to the posterior aspect of the joint capsule. The cyst is usually unilocular, although an occasional cyst may be multilocular with septa. Fluid is usually crystal clear and may vary from yellow to currant jelly in color, depending on the amount of recent or old hemorrhage that has occurred. Arterial patency is usually restored with incision into the cyst followed by evacuation of the cystic contents. Resection and arterial reconstruction may be required.

SUMMARY

Thought to be rare until approximately 25 years ago, popliteal vascular entrapment and popliteal arterial adventitial cystic disease are being recognized with increasing frequency. Knowledge of these lesions is mandatory in evaluating patients, particularly younger patients in the nonarteriosclerotic age group who are non-smokers. These diagnoses should be suspected in athletic individuals with the sudden onset of intermittent claudication.

REFERENCES

1. Baker WH, Stoney RJ. Acquired popliteal entrapment syndrome. *Arch Surg* 1972;105(5):780–781.
2. Barnes RW, Strandness DE Jr. Isolated popliteal artery occlusion: physiologic observations and management. *Vasc Surg* 1972;6(3):103–113.
3. Biemans RG, van Bockel JH. Popliteal artery entrapment syndrome. *Surg Gynecol Obstet* 1977;144(4):604–609.
4. Bouhoutsos I. Popliteal artery entrapment syndrome. Reports of 29 cases. *Vasc Surg* 1980;14:365–374.
5. Bouhoutsos I, Daskalakis E. Muscular abnormalities affecting the popliteal vessels. *Br J Surg* 1981;68:501–506.
6. Bouhoutsos I, Goulios A. Popliteal artery entrapment: Report of a case. *J Cardiovasc Surg* 1977;18(5):481–484.
7. Carter AE, Eban R. A case of bilateral developmental abnormality of popliteal arteries and gastrocnemius muscles. *Br J Surg* 1964;51:518–522.

8. Collins PS, McDonald PT, Lim RC. Popliteal artery entrapment: an evolving syndrome. *J Vasc Surg* 1989; 10:484–489.

9. Connell J. Popliteal vein entrapment. *Br J Surg* 1978; 65(5):351.

10. Darling RC, Buckley CJ, Abbott WM, et al. Intermittent claudication in young athletes: popliteal artery entrapment syndrome. *J Trauma* 1974;14:543–552.

11. Delaney TA, Gonzalez LL. Occlusion of popliteal artery due to muscular entrapment. *Surgery* 1971;69:97–101.

12. di Marzo L, Cavallaro A, Sciacca V, et al. Diagnosis of popliteal artery entrapment syndrome: the role of duplex scanning. *J Vasc Surg* 1991;13:434–438.

13. di Marzo L, Cavallaro A, Sciacca V, Mingoli A, Stipa S. Natural history of entrapment of the popliteal artery. *J Am Coll Surg* 1994;178:553–556.

14. Eastcott HHG. Cystic myxomatous degeneration of popliteal artery. *Br Med J* 1963;2:1270.

15. Ejrup B, Hiertonn T. Intermittent claudication. Three cases treated by free vein graft. *Acta Chir Scand* 1954; 108:217–230.

16. Endo M, Tamura S, Minakuchi S, et al. Isolation and identification of proteohyaluronic acid from a cyst of cystic mucoid degeneration. *Clin Chim Acta* 1973;47:417–424.

17. Evans WE, Bernhard V. Acute popliteal artery entrapment. *Am J Surg* 1971;121:739–740.

18. Ferrero R, Barile C, Buzzacchino A, et al. La sindrome da costrizione dell'arteria poplita. *Minerva Cardioangiol* 1978;26:389–410.

19. Flanigan DP, Burnham SJ, Goodreau JJ, Bergan JJ. Summary of cases of adventitial cystic disease of the popliteal artery. *Ann Surg* 1979;189:165–175.

20. Gaylis H. Popliteal artery entrapment syndrome. *S Afr Med J* 1972;46(3):1071–1075.

21. Gaylis H, Rosenberg B. The popliteal artery entrapment syndrome: a bilateral case. *S Afr J Surg* 1973;11(2):51–54.

22. Hall KV. Anomalous insertion of the medical gastrocnemic head, with circulatory complications. *Acta Pathol Microbiol Scand* 1961;148(S):53–58.

23. Hall KV. Intravascular gastrocnemius insertion. *Acta Chir Scand* 1964;128:193–196.

24. Hamming JJ. Intermittent claudication at an early age, due to an anomalous course of the popliteal artery. *Angiology* 1959;10:369–371.

25. Hiertonn T, Lindberg K, Rob C. Cystic degeneration of the popliteal artery. *Br J Surg* 1957;44:348.

26. Ikeda M, Iwase T, Ashida K, Tankawa H. Popliteal artery entrapment syndrome: report of a case and study of 18 cases in Japan. *Am J Surg* 1981;141(6):726–730.

27. Insua JA, Young JR, Humphries AW. Popliteal artery entrapment syndrome. *Arch Surg* 1970;101:771–775.

28. Ishikawa K, Mishima Y, Kobayashi S. Cystic adventitial disease of the popliteal artery. *Angiology* 1961;12:357–366.

29. Iwai T, Sato S, Muraoka Y, et al. Popliteal vein entrapment (compression) syndrome caused by an anomalous muscle belonging to the medial head of the gastrocnemius muscle: report on two surgical cases. *Jpn J Phlebol* 1991;2(1):99–103.

30. Jaquet GH, Meyer-Burgdorff G. Arterielle durchblutungstorung infolge cystischer degeneration der adventitia. *Der Chirurg* 1960;31:481.

31. Leaf G. Amino-acid analysis of protein present in a popliteal artery cyst. *Br Med J* 1967;3:415.

32. Love JW, Whelan TJ. Popliteal artery entrapment syndrome. *Am J Surg* 1965;109:620–624.

33. McDonald PT, Easterbrook JA, Rich NM, et al. Popliteal artery entrapment syndrome: clinical common noninvasive and angiographic diagnosis. *Am J Surg* 1980; 139:318–325.

34. Rich NM. Popliteal entrapment and adventitial disease in the Monograph. *Surg clin N Amer* 1982;62:449–465.

35. Rich NM, Hughes CW. Popliteal artery and vein entrapment. *Am J Surg* 1967;113:696–698.

36. Rich NM, Collins GJ Jr, McDonald PT, et al. Popliteal vascular entrapment. *Arch Surg* 1979;114:1377–1384.

37. Rignault DP, Pailler JL, Lunel F. The "functional" popliteal entrapment syndrome. *Int Angiol* 1985;4:1–3.

38. Servello M. Clinical syndrome of anomalous position of the popliteal artery: differentiation from juvenile arteriopathy. *Circulation* 1962;26:885–890.

39. Stuart TPA. A note on a variation in the course of the popliteal artery. *J Anat Physiol* 1879;13:162–165.

40. Sutton D. *Arteriography*. Edinburgh: E. and S. Livingstone; 1962.

41. Taylor H, Taylor RS, Ramsay CA. Cyst of popliteal artery. *Br Med J* 1967;4:109–110.

42. Yao JST, Hobbs JT, Irvine WT. Ankle systolic pressure measurements in arterial disease affecting the lower extremities. *Br J Surg* 1969;56:676–679.

23

Diagnosis and Management of Raynaud's Syndrome

Robert B. McLafferty, M.D.
James M. Edwards, M.D.
John M. Porter, M.D.

Raynaud's syndrome (RS) is a clinical condition manifested by episodic attacks of digital ischemia caused by closure of the small arteries and arterioles of the most distal parts of the extremities in response to cold or emotional stress. Classically, these attacks last for 10 to 30 minutes, affect the digits of the hands more frequently than the feet, and are characterized by intense pallor followed by cyanosis and rubor on rewarming. A subset of patients do not have this "triple-color" response but do have one or more color changes accompanied by numbness and/or aching. Patients with severe hand ischemia, rest pain, and digital ulceration due to fixed arterial obstruction also have vasospasm of varying levels.

In 1862, Maurice Raynaud gave the first description of 25 patients with finger ischemia, presumably from digital artery vasospasm.[1] His patients had varying degrees of intermittent digital pallor and cyanosis frequently associated with localized finger gangrene. Raynaud proposed that sympathetic hyperactivity was the cause as all of these patients had normal wrist pulses and in some patients, large artery patency at autopsy. It is now evident that many if not all of these patients had unrecognized far advanced small artery occlusive disease in addition to episodic vasospasm.

At the turn of the century, Hutchinson challenged Raynaud's vasospastic hypothesis.[2] He observed the association of a variety of disease processes such as arteriosclerosis, scleroderma, and heart failure, with episodic digital ischemia and gangrene. He coined the term *Raynaud's phenomenon* and applied it to episodic digital vasoconstriction occurring with a wide group of diverse diseases. Approximately 30 years later, Allen

and Brown recognized that episodic digital artery vasoconstriction could occur in the presence or absence of a variety of associated diseases, most of which, interestingly, cause digital artery occlusion.[3] They proposed a classification schema in which patients with benign idiopathic episodic vasoconstriction not associated with a systemic disease were designated as having Raynaud's disease and those fulfilling similar clinical criteria in the presence of an associated disease were designated as having Raynaud's phenomenon. Rigid diagnostic criteria were created in an attempt to categorize patients as having Raynaud's disease or phenomenon, as patients with Raynaud's phenomenon were noted to have a distinctly worse prognosis.

Since 1932, natural history studies have contributed to a better understanding of RS. Allen and Brown's approach, although appealing in theory, did not take into account changing clinical patterns, such as the late appearance of a connective tissue disease that would necessitate reclassification of the patient from disease to phenomenon. Lewis and Pickering reported that most of their patients had a benign course.[4] Gifford and Hines described patients who developed the diagnosis of an associated disease long after the onset of typical benign symptoms of RS.[5] Similarly, deTakats and Fowler astutely noted that a long period of clinical observation may pass before an associated disease became manifest.[6] The failure of Allen and Brown's classification was due in part to the inability, by present day standards, to identify associated diseases in their early stages. These findings have been confirmed by our own clinical experience in following over 1000 of these patients prospectively for over 25 years.[7-14] We use the term *Raynaud's syndrome* to describe patients with cold or emotionally induced episodic digital ischemia and realize that significant number, regardless of the severity of ischemic symptoms, will develop an associated disease.

EPIDEMIOLOGY

Although the exact prevalence of RS in the general population is unknown, approximations are possible based on geographic location. It is estimated that 20 to 25% of people who reside in damp, cool climates such as the Pacific Northwest, Denmark, and England are affected by RS. A study by Olsen and Nielson found that 22% of women between the ages of 21 and 50 in Copenhagen reported symptoms of RS.[15] Studies by Porter et al in the Pacific Northwest found that 30% of individuals selected at random described symptoms suggestive of RS.[7–9] In contrast, Mariq and colleagues conducted a population-based survey in South Carolina and found the prevalence of RS to be 5.1% in females and 3.5% in males.[16]

The majority of patients afflicted with RS are women, comprising 70 to 90% of all patients reported. It is important to note that the majority of patients reported in the literature with RS have symptoms severe enough to seek medical attention. It is unclear how many patients have mild symptoms and do not seek medical attention. It is likely that patients with mild symptoms greatly outnumber those who seek medical attention. Thus it is impossible to know with certainty that conclusions drawn in the literature on RS are equally applicable to the larger group with minimal symptoms.

PATHOPHYSIOLOGY

Classic attacks of RS are caused by closure of palmar and digital arteries resulting in cessation of capillary perfusion and stimulated usually by cold or emotional stress. Eventually the capillaries and venules then reflexly dilate secondary to accumulation of by-products of anaerobic metabolism. With time, the arterial spasm subsides and a trickle of blood enters the dilated capillary bed, where it quickly desaturates with resultant cyanosis. Subsequently, rubor develops due to reactive hyperemia as more blood flows into the capillaries. The attack subsides as arterial spasm ends and baseline arterial flow returns.

The biochemical mechanisms responsible for the vasoconstriction of RS have been the subject of considerable research for more than a century. Sir Thomas Lewis in the 1920s and 1930s repeatedly demonstrated that these attacks could not be blocked with local anesthesia applied to autonomic and somatic nerves, thus disproving Maurice Raynaud's hypothesis of sympathetic hyperactivity.[4,17] From these findings, he concluded that a "local vascular fault" was responsible for the physiologic changes taking place in response to cold exposure exclusive of sympathetic innervation.

Our studies lead us to conclude that there are two distinct pathophysiologic mechanisms responsible for RS. We have termed these mechanisms *obstructive* and *spastic*. Obstuctive RS occurs in the presence of diffuse arterial obstruction, either large artery disease proximal to the wrist or the palmar and digital arteries. This results in a decrease in the intraluminal distending pressure. An attack occurs when arterial closure is produced by the normal vasoconstrictive response to cold or emotional stimuli overcoming the decreased intraluminal pressure.

Patients with vasospastic RS appear to have an abnormally forceful vasoconstrictive response to cold, which results in digital artery closure. In contrast to the relatively straightforward quantitative relationship surrounding obstructive RS, vasospastic RS remains poorly understood. Angiographic and plethysmographic studies demonstrate complete digital artery closure after cold exposure despite a previous normal finger systolic blood pressure and the absence of significant obstruction.[15,18,19] Krahenbuhl and associates determined that at a critical temperature, precipitous digital artery closure occurred.[18] With simultaneous finger cooling and measurement of digital artery blood pressure, an abrupt decline in systolic blood pressure to unmeasurable levels was observed when the temperature reached about 28°C (Fig. 23–1).

Although the exact cause of vasospastic RS is unknown, experimental observations suggest that there may be some merit in Lewis' "local vascular fault." Coffman and Cohen examined finger blood flow before and after cooling in patients with and without RS.[20,21] Normal fingers subjected to hypothermia showed a decrease in arteriovenous shunt flow without alterations in nutrient capillary flow. In contrast, patients with RS exhibited reduced shunt flow and capillary nutrient flow. Pretreatment of these patients with reserpine, a sympathetic blocking agent, significantly increased capillary flow at room temperature and after cooling. These findings suggest that adrenergic neuroeffector activity may be enhanced and therefore play a major role in the pathophysiology of RS.

The fundamental concept that a receptor population may be altered in sensitivity or number in RS remains an active area of research. We and others have demonstrated alteration in alpha-2-adrenoreceptor activity in patients with RS. Other factors have been implicated in the pathophysiology of vasospastic RS, including abnormal serum proteins,[22] alterations in blood viscosity,[23] elevated serotonin levels,[24] altered shear stress,[25,26] and abnormalities in vasoactive peptides such as calcitonin and endothelin.[27–30]

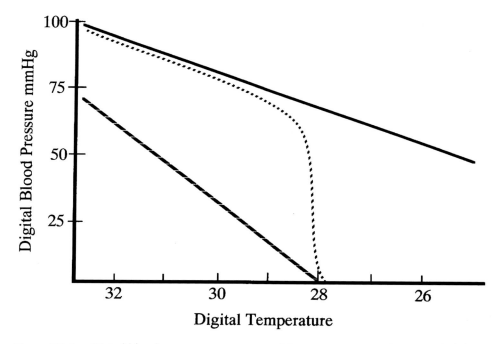

Figure 23–1. Digital blood pressure response to cold exposure in normal patients (solid line), patients with vasospastic Raynaud's syndrome (dotted line), and patients with obstructive Raynaud's syndrome (dashed line).

ASSOCIATED DISEASES

Many seemingly unrelated diseases are associated with RS (Table 23–1). The majority of these have small artery obstruction of the distal extremities as part of the disease process. Interestingly, it appears local patient referral patterns likely have a significant influence on the frequency of an associated disease in patients with RS. In the early years of our Raynaud's Clinic we were referred only severely symptomatic patients, and 80% of them were found to have an associated autoimmune disease.[31] As awareness increased, more patients with milder symptoms were referred, reducing the fraction of associated diseases to 60%. This percentage approximates the experience of other referral centers, and similarly, about 40% of patients with RS have the idiopathic variety caused by vasospasm alone.[7–9,31]

Approximately one-third of patients with RS and a connective tissue disorder have scleroderma. The remainder suffer from a variety of autoimmune disorders including rheumatoid arthritis, mixed connective tissue disorder, systemic lupus erythematosus, and Sjogren's syndrome. A significant number of patients do not fit the pattern of a classically defined syndrome but present with abnormal serologic tests and may have evidence of end organ involvement. These patients are classified as having undifferentiated connective tissue disease.

Numerous arterial diseases may be associated with obstructive RS including atherosclerosis, Buerger's disease, and embolization from a subclavian artery lesion or thoracic outlet syndrome.[32–34] Various myeloproliferative disorders such as leukemia, polycythemia rubra vera, and myeloid metaplasia may be associated with digital artery obstruction and RS.[35,36] Likewise, disorders associated with hyperviscosity such as multiple myeloma or cryoglobulinemia may result in digital ischemia.[37] Occupational exposure to chronic vibration for long periods of time may cause digital artery occlusion and obstructive RS.[38] Other causes of RS include various drugs,[39–42] endocrine abnormalities,[43] and the long-term sequelae from frostbite injury.[49] Table 23–2 is our most recently tabulated series of 1089 patients whom we have prospectively followed in our Raynaud's Clinic for over 20 years.[14]

CLINICAL PRESENTATION

RS consists of episodic coldness of the digits precipitated by cold exposure or emotional stimuli. Color changes such as pallor, cyanosis, and/or rubor typically occur and are often associated with mild pain, paresthesias, and numbness. Severe pain with attacks is distinctly unusual in the absence of digital ulceration. Occasionally, the presenting complaint may be persistent cyanosis, digital ulceration, and severe pain in a patient who has had long-standing RS.[9] Alternatively, asymptomatic patients may present with acute onset of digital gangrene and go on to develop chronic RS after resolution of the initial ischemic symptoms.[31–33] It is important to note that vasospasm alone never causes

Table 23–1.   Disorders Associated with Raynaud's Syndrome

Autoimmune connective tissue diseases
  Dermatomyositis
  Henoch-Schonlein purpura
  Hepatitis B antigen—induced vasculitis
  Mixed connective tissue disease
  Polyarteritis nodosa
  Polymyositis
  Reiter's syndrome
  Rheumatoid arthritis
  Scleroderma—CREST syndrome
  Sjogren's syndrome
  Systemic lupus erythematosus
  Undifferentiated connective tissue disease

Hypersensitivity angiitis
  (rapid-onset vascular occlusion)

Myeloproliferative disorders
  Leukemia
  Myeloid metaplasia
  Polycythemia rubra vera
  Thrombocytosis

Circulating globulins
  Cold agglutinins
  Cryoglobulinemia
  Malignancy
  Macroglobulinemia
  Multiple myeloma

Obstructive arterial diseases
  Atherosclerosis
  Buerger's disease

Peripheral embolization
  Atherosclerosis
  Thoracic outlet syndrome

Environmental conditions
  Repetitive trauma
  Vibration injury
  Cold injury

Drug induced (without arteritis)
  Ergots
  Beta blockers
  Oral contraceptives

Miscellaneous
  Chronic renal failure
  Drug-induced vasculitis
  Vinyl chloride disease
  Polyneuropathy
  Neurofibromatosis
  Endocrine disorders

Table 23–2.   Associated Disorders in 1089 Patients with Raynaud's Syndrome (Oregon Health Sciences University, 1970–1995)

Autoimmune diseases		260
Scleroderma	95	
Undifferentiated connective tissue disease	24	
Mixed connective tissue disorder	23	
Systemic lupus erythematosus	17	
Sjogren's syndrome	16	
Rheumatoid arthritis	9	
Positive serology	106	
Other diseases		301
Atherosclerosis	46	
Trauma	44	
Hematologic abnormalities	42	
Carpal tunnel syndrome	35	
Frostbite	32	
Buerger's disease	28	
Vibration	21	
Hypersensitivity angiitis	18	
Hypothyroidism	13	
Cancer	13	
Erythromyalgia	8	
No associated disease		498
Total		1089

ischemic digital ulceration, a condition that always implies palmar and digital artery obstruction.

CLINICAL AND LABORATORY EVALUATION

As always, the history and physical examination are important in determining the source of the patient's problem. Subsequent diagnostic tests are directed toward quantification of the degree of ischemia and identification of associated disorders. The history should include inquiries regarding arthralgia, dysphagia, xerostomia, or xeropthalmia that may suggest a connective tissue disorder. Other important questions include a history of occupational vibration exposure, symptoms of large artery occlusive disease, prior trauma, or a history of malignancy. The physical exam is frequently unremarkable but specific attention should be directed to the presence of digital ulcerations, quality of peripheral pulses, evidence of prior tissue loss, or joint changes. The skin on the face and hands should be examined for telangiectasias, rashes, thinning, or tightening indicating the presence of scleroderma.

Laboratory examination varies, depending on the initial clinical suspicions. The minimal baseline evaluation required for all patients with RS includes a complete blood count with differential, chemistry profile, urinalysis, erythrocyte sedimentation rate, serum rheumatoid factor, and antinuclear antibody titer. The latter three tests are most helpful in establishing the diagnosis of rheumatoid arthritis, scleroderma, systemic lupus erythematosus, and mixed connective tissue disease. In selected patients additional laboratory testing may be indicated depending on the results of screening tests (Table 23–3). A radiograph of the hand may also aid in the diagnosis of a connective tissue disorder by the presence of tuft resorption, calcinosis, or arthritis.

Table 23–3. Laboratory Evaluation of Raynaud's Syndrome

Baseline Tests (Routine)	Adjunctive Tests (in Selected Patients)
Complete blood count	Serum protein electrophoresis
Chemistry profile	Anti-native DNA antibody
Erythrocyte sedimentation rate	Extractable nuclear antibody
	HEP-2 antinuclear antibody
Urinalysis	Cryoglobulins
Rheumatoid factor	Complement levels
Antinuclear antibody	Hepatitis B screen
	Anticentromere antibody

VASCULAR LABORATORY AND ARTERIOGRAPHIC EVALUATION

Vascular laboratory documentation is usually not essential in making the diagnosis of RS in most patients. Objective testing may provide critical adjuvant information for some patients in ruling out large artery disease, evaluating symptomatic patients without digital color changes, providing information for medicolegal claims, and quantitating results of treatment.

The primary vascular laboratory tests to detect distal small artery obstruction and thus differentiate vasospastic from obstructive RS are digital blood pressures and analysis of photoplethysmographic (PPG) digital waveforms. When well performed, these tests are as accurate as arteriography in detecting arterial obstruction.[13,44] Digital pressures 20 torr or more below wrist pressures combined with the presence of obstructive PPG waveforms establish the diagnosis of significant palmar and/or digital artery obstruction. Another finding associated with RS is a peaked pulse on digital waveform.[45] Representative tracings of normal, vasospastic (peaked pulse), and obstructive waveforms are shown in Figure 23–2. It is important to note that if the digital arteries are occluded beyond the proximal phalanx (ie, distal to cuff placement) or if only one digital artery is occluded, digital pressures and waveforms may appear normal. The measurement of digital pressures will allow the differentiation of distal ischemia caused by proximal large artery disease from primary occlusive disease of the palmar and digital arteries. If large artery occlusive disease in the upper extremity is suspected, segmental pressure measurements should be performed. In the case of isolated distal occlusive disease of the hand, particularly if only one side is involved, duplex scanning may be indicated to seek a source of emboli such as subclavian artery aneurysm. Duplex scanning may also assist in the diagnosis of pseudoaneurysms after arterial catheterization, ulnar artery aneurysms, Takayasu's disease, and congenital arterial abnormalities.[46–52]

The other group of vascular laboratory tests central to the diagnosis of RS involves cold challenge testing.

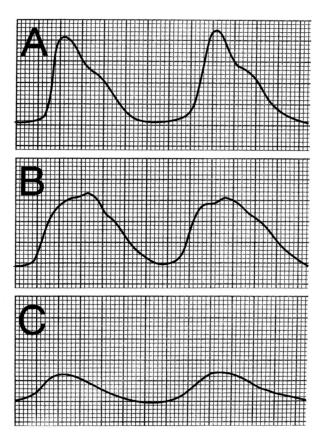

Figure 23–2. Representative waveforms of (A) normal PPG, (B) peaked pulse PPG associated with vasospastic Raynaud's syndrome, and (C) obstructive digital PPG.

Normal individuals have less than a 20% drop in digital artery pressure in response to cold.[53,54] Patients with vasospastic RS follow a similar curve of digital artery reduction until a critical temperature threshold is reached at which abrupt arterial closure occurs. Patients with obstructive RS parallel normal curves at a lower level with cooling and digital artery closure usually occurs once a sufficient level is reached (Fig. 23–1).

The most sensitive and specific test currently available for the diagnosis of RS is the occlusive digital hypothermic challenge test described by Nielsen and Lassen.[55] A specifically designed machine determines the decrease in digital pressure at various temperatures. (Fig. 23–3). Our vascular laboratory examined 100 patients and determined the test to be 87% specific and 90% sensitive, with an overall accuracy of 92% compared to the clinical diagnosis.[56] Interestingly, no investigator has shown conclusively that the magnitude of the pressure drop corresponds to the severity of RS. This test can objectively diagnose the majority of patients with cold-induced RS.

Other diagnostic tests, routine and experimental, have been used but none appear to equal the accuracy of the digital hypothermic challenge test. These

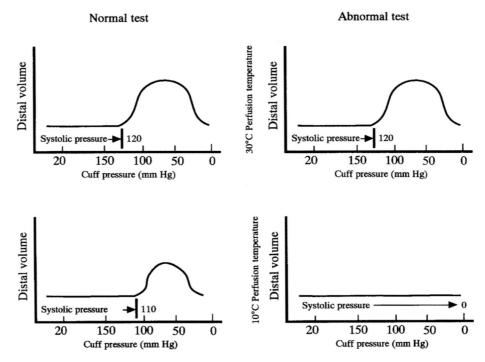

Figure 23–3. Normal response (left) and positive response (right) for vasospasm with the digital hypothermic challenge test.

include the hand ice water immersion test,[20] cold challenge testing with laser Doppler,[57] thermal entrainment,[58] digital thermography,[59] venous occlusion plethysmography, digital artery caliber measurement,[60] and other tests measuring digital blood flow.[61] The Nielson test and digital plethysmography have almost entirely replaced the need for hand arteriography in diagnosing RS. We recommend upper extremity arteriography only in patients suspected of having large artery disease. Typically, these patients have unilateral hand involvement or absence of pulses on examination.

TREATMENT

Currently, no curative treatment is available for patients with RS and palliation remains the primary goal. Most patients' symptoms range from mild to moderate and respond well to avoiding cold and tobacco and wearing gloves. Certain pharmacologic agents such as oral contraceptives,[39] beta-adrenergic blocking agents,[40,41] and ergotamine agents[62,63] should be avoided, as they have been reported to exacerbate RS.

A few patients will be sufficiently symptomatic to require pharmacologic intervention. Vasospastic RS generally responds much more favorably to treatment than does obstructive RS. Calcium channel blockers are the mainstay of treatment for symptomatic RS. Nifedipine, 30 mg orally at bedtime in the sustained release form or as 10 mg three times a day, is our first-line

treatment.[64,65] Improvement in vasospastic symptoms has been shown with controlled prospective trials.[66–68] Diltiazem appears to be less effective. For those patients who respond incompletely to a calcium channel blocker, the addition of prazosin may provide further relief.

Sympatholytic agents were formerly the mainstay of pharmacologic therapy of RS. Oral reserpine, guanethidine, methyldopa, isoxsuprine, phenoxybenzamine, and prazosin were widely used in an attempt to blunt vasospasm.[10,69–71] Typically, high doses were required if single agents were used, which resulted in a high incidence of side effects. Combination therapy with lower doses has reduced side effects. One regimen still used on occasion is guanethadine, 10 mg daily, and 1 to 2 mg of prazosin per day.[72]

Treatment of patients with obstructive RS and associated digital ulceration is more difficult. Infusion of Prostaglandin E_1 and prostacyclin I_2, both of which are potent vasodilators and inhibitors of platelet aggregation have been tried.[73–75] In placebo-controlled, double-blind studies, the intravenous administration of iloprost, a stable analogue of prostacyclin I_2, demonstrated decreased frequency of Raynaud's attacks and increased frequency of ulcer healing.[76,77] The disadvantage of iloprost and the prostaglandins is that they must be given intravenously. Currently, iloprost in an oral preparation is undergoing clinical trials with encouraging early results.[78]

Sympathectomy for vasospastic RS and ischemic digital ulceration associated with small artery occlusive disease has met with mixed results. Cervicothoracic sympathectomy has been performed and rates of response vary, depending on the surgical series.[79–82] In general, symptomatic recurrence seems to follow an initial period of improvement. Sympathectomy can also be performed locally on the digital arteries by stripping the adventitia and dividing the terminal sympathetic nerve branches with the aid of a surgical microscope.[83] These reports are anecdotal, and controlled clinical trials essential to compare this mode of therapy with other types of treament are conspicuously absent. We do not recommend cervicothoracic sympathectomy.

Unconventional therapies with or without sympathectomy for patients with RS and ischemic ulceration have reported healing rates of 80 to 85%. We treated 100 consecutive patients with conservative therapy without sympathectomy.[72] Our regimen consisted of gentle soap and water scrubs, debridement of necrotic tissue, removal of the nail to facilitate drainage of infection, administration of culture-specific antibiotics, and delayed length-conserving digital amputation. With this simple approach, complete healing without recurrence was achieved in 88% of patients. This no doubt reflects the natural history of the condition irrespective of therapy. In our experience, recurrent digital ulcers occur with connective tissue disorders, most often scleroderma. There is some evidence, albeit weak, that the hemorrheologic agent pentoxifylline may aid in the healing of digital ulcers. We give our patients 400 mg three times a day until the ulcer is healed.

SUMMARY

RS consists of episodic digital pallor or cyanosis frequently associated with mild discomfort or numbness. Attacks are usually induced by cold exposure or emotional stress. Approximately 20 to 30% of people in cool damp climates are affected. Although not mutually exclusive, two distinct pathophysiologic mechanisms appear to be responsible for RS. Some patients have normal appearing unobstructed digital arteries yet display an exaggerated vasospastic response to cold stimuli. For the majority of patients with vasospastic RS, the condition represents little more than a nuisance. Other patients have palmar and/or digital artery obstruction and decreased perfusion pressure to the digits. A normal vasospastic response to cold causes a vasospastic attack in these patients with diminished digital artery pressure. Patients with obstructive RS are more likely to have an associated disease, most often autoimmune in nature. There is no cure for RS and treatment is directed to relieving symptoms. The majority of individuals are adequately treated by cold and tobacco avoidance. For the remainder, calcium channel blockers, specifically nifidipine, result in symptom-

atic improvement in approximately 50%. There is no evidence that sympathectomy has any long-term benefit. Occasional patients develop digital ulcers and gangrene. Almost all of these patients respond well to conservative therapy consisting of local cleansing, antibiotics, and limited debridement. On balance, RS continues to be a challenging clinical entity with a wide spectrum of severity.

REFERENCES

1. Raynaud M. On local asphyxia and symmetrical gangrene of the extremities. In: *Selected Monographs*. London: New Syndeham Society; 1888:
2. Huthinson J. *Raynaud's Phenomena*. Med Circa Press 1901;123:403.
3. Allen EV, Brown GE. Raynaud's disease: a critical review of minimal requisities for diagnosis. *Am J Med Sci* 1932;1983:187.
4. Lewis T, Pickering GW. Observations upon maladies in which the blood supply to the digits ceases intermittently or permanently and upon bilateral gangrene of the digits; observations relevant to so-called Raynaud's disease. *Heart* 1933;15:7.
5. Gifford RW Jr, Hines EA Jr. Raynaud's disease among women and girls. *Circulation* 1957;16:1012.
6. deTakats G, Fowler EF. Raynaud's phenomenon. *JAMA* 1962;179:99.
7. Porter JM, Bardana EJ, Baur GM, et al. The clinical significance of Raynaud's syndrome. *Surgery* 1976;80:756.
8. Porter JM, Friedman EI, Mills JL Jr. Raynaud's syndrome: current concepts and treatment. *Med Tribune Therapaeia* 1988;29:23.
9. Porter GM, Rivers SP, Anderson CJ, et al. Evaluation and management of patients with Raynaud's syndrome. *Am J Surg* 1981;142:183.
10. Rivers SP, Porter JM. Clinical approach to Raynaud's syndrome. *Vasc Diagn Ther* 1983;4:15.
11. River SP, Porter JM. Raynaud's syndrome and upper extremity small artery occlusive disease. In: Wilson SE, Vieth FJ, Hobson RW, et al, eds. *Vascular Surgery: Principles and Practice*. New York: McGraw-Hill; 1987:696.
12. Rivers SP, Porter JM. Management of Raynaud's syndrome. In: Bergan JJ, ed. *Clinical Surgery International*. New York: Churchill Livingstone; 1984:185.
13. McLafferty RB, Edwards JM, Taylor LM Jr, et al. Diagnosis and long-term clinical outcome in patients diagnosed with hand ischemia. *J Vasc Surg*, 1995;22:361.
14. Landry GJ, Edwards JM, McLafferty RB, et al. Long-term outcome of Raynaud's syndrome in a prospectively analyzed cohort. *JVS* 1996;23:76.
15. Olsen N, Nielson SL. Prevalence of primary Raynaud's phenomena in young females. *Scand J Clin Lab Invest* 1978;37:761.
16. Mariq HR, Weinrich MC, Keil JE, et al. Prevalence of Raynaud's phenomena in the general population. *J Chronic Dis* 1986,39:423.
17. Lewis T. Experiments relating to the peripheral mechanism involved in spastic arrest of the circulation of the fingers, a variety of Raynaud's disease. *Heart* 1929,15:7.
18. Krahenbuhl B, Nielson SL, Lassen NA. Closure of the digital arteries in high vascular tone states as demonstrated by measurement of systolic blood pressure in the finger. *Scand J Clin Lab Invest* 1977;37:71.

19. Rosch J, Porter JM, Gralino BJ. Cryodynamic hand angiography in the diagnosis and management of Raynaud's syndrome. *Circulation* 1977;55:807.

20. Coffman JD. Total and nutritional blood flow in the finger. *Clin Sci* 1979;42:243.

21. Coffman JD, Cohen AS. Total and capillary blood flow in the finger in Raynaud's phenomena. *N Engl J Med* 1971;285:259.

22. Tietjen GW, Chien S, Leroy C, et al. Blood viscosity, plasma proteins, and Raynaud's syndrome. *Arch Surg* 1975;110:1343.

23. Goyle KG, Dormandy JA. Abnormal blood viscosity in Raynaud's phenomena. *Lancet* 1976;1:1317.

24. Halpern A, Kuhn PH, Shaftel HE, et al. Raynaud's phenomena and seratonin. *Angiology* 1960;11:151.

25. Nerem RM. Vibration-induced arterial shear stress: The relationship to Raynaud's phenomenon of occupational origin. *Arch Environ Health* 1973;26:105.

26. Schmid-Schonbein H. Critical closing pressure or yield shear stress as the cause of disturbed peripheral circulation? *Acta Chir Scand* 1976;465(suppl):10.

27. Bunker CB, Terenghi G, Springall DR, et al. Deficiency of calcitonin gene-related peptide in Raynaud's phenomena. *Lancet* 1990;336:1530.

28. Fyhrquist F, Saijonmaa O, Metsarinne K, et al. Raised plasma endothelin-1 concentration following cold pressor test. *Biochem Biophys Res Commun* 1990;169:217.

29. Shawket S, Dickerson C, Hazelman B, et al. Prolonged effect of CGRP in Raynaud's patients: a double-blind randomized comparison with prostacyclin. *Br J Clin Pharmacol* 1991;32:209.

30. Zamora MR, O'Brien RF, Rutherford RB, et al. Serum endothelin-1 concentrations and cold provocation in primary Raynaud's phenomena. *Lancet* 1990;336:1144.

31. Porter JM, Snider RL, Bardana EJ, et al. The diagnosis and treatment of Raynaud's syndrome. *Surgery* 1975;77:11.

32. Mills JL, Taylor LM Jr, Porter JM. Buerger's disease in the modern era. *Am J Surg* 1987;154:123.

33. James EC, Kuhn NT, Fedde CW. Upper limb ischemia resulting from arterial thromboembolism. *Am J Surg* 1979;137:739.

34. Schmidt FE, Hewitt RL. Severe upper limb ischemia. *Arch Surg* 1980;115:1188.

35. O'Donnell JR, Keaveny TV, O'Connell LG. Digital arteritis as a presenting feature of malignant disease. *Ir J Med Sci* 1980;149:326.

36. Baur GM, Porter JM, Bardana EJ, et al. Rapid onset of hand ischemia of unknown etiology: clinical evaluation and follow-up of ten patients. *Ann Surg* 1977;186:184.

37. Gorevic PD. Mixed cryoglobulinemia: clinical aspects and long-term follow-up of 40 patients. *Am J Med* 1980;68:287.

38. James PB, Galloway RW. Arteriography of the hand in men exposed to vibration. In: Taylor W, Pelmear PL, eds. *Vibration White Finger in Industry*. London: Academic Press; 1975:31.

39. Eastcott HHG. Raynaud's disease and the oral contraceptive pill. *Br Med J* 1976;2:447.

40. Frolich ED, Tarayi RC, Dutson MP. Peripheral arterial insufficiency as a complication of beta-adrenergic blocking therapy. *JAMA* 1969;208:2471.

41. Marshall AJ, Roberts CJC, Barritt DW. Raynaud's phenomenon as a side effect of beta-blockers in hypertension. *Br Med J* 1976;1:1498.

42. Teutsch C, Lipton A, Harvey A. Raynaud's phenomenon as a side effect of chemotherapy with vinblastine and bleomycin for testicular carcinoma. *Cancer Treat Rep* 1977;61:925.

43. Blunt RJ, Porter JM. Raynaud's syndrome. *Semin Arthritis Rheum* 1981;11:282.

44. Homgren K, Baur GM, Porter JM. The role of digital photophethysmography in the evaluation of Raynaud's syndrome. *Bruit* 1981;5:19.

45. Sumner DS, Strandness DE. An abnormal finger pulse associated with cold sensitivity. *Ann Surg* 1972;175:294.

46. Ackerstaff RGA, Hoeneveneld H, Slowikowski JM, et al. Ultrasonic duplex scanning in atherosclerotic disease of the innominate, subclavian, and vertebral arteries. A comparative study with angiography. *Ultrasound Med Biol* 1984;10(4):409.

47. Grosveld WJHW, Lawson JA, Eikelboom BC, et al. Clinical hemodynamic significance of innominate artery lesions evaluated by ultrasonography and digital angiography. *Stroke* 1988;19:958.

48. Thomas VC, Roder HU, Moser GH, Diagnostiche wertigkeit der angiodynographie bei pulsierenden raumforderungen. *Fortschr Rontgenstr* 1989;150:454.

49. Koman LA, Bond MG, Carter RE, et al. Evaluation of upper extremity vasculature with high resolution ultrasound. *J Hand Surg* 1985;10A:249.

50. Reed AJ, Fincher RME, Nichols FT. Case report: Takayasu arteritis in a middle aged caucasian woman: clinical course correlated with duplex ultrasonography and angiography. *Am J Med Sci* 1989;298:324.

51. Guzzetti A, Bellotti R. Usefulness of Doppler echocardiography in the diagnosis of upper thoracic outlet syndrome. *Chir Ital* 1988;40:152.

52. Merlob P, Schonfield A, Ovadia Y. Real-time echo-Doppler duplex scanner in the evaluation of patients with Poland sequence. *Eur J Obstret Gynecol Reprod Biol* 1989;32:103.

53. Carter SA. The effects of cooling on toe systolic pressures in subjects with and without Raynaud's syndrome in the lower extremities. *Clin Physiol* 1991;11;253.

54. Carter SA, Dean E, Kroegor EA. Apparent finger systolic pressures during cooling in patients with Raynaud's syndrome. *Circulation* 1988; 77(5):988.

55. Nielson SL, Lassen NA. Measurement of digital blood pressure after local cooling. *J Appl Physiol* 1977;43:907.

56. Gates KH, Tyburczy JA, Zupan T, et al. The noninvasive quantification of digital vasospasm. *Bruit* 1984;8:34.

57. Brain SD, Petty RG, Lewis JD, et al. Cutaneous blood flow responses in the forearms of Raynaud's patients induced by local cooling and intradermal injections of CGRP and histamine. *Br J Clin Pharmacol* 1990;30:853.

58. Lafferty K, de Trafford JC, Roberts VC, et al. Raynaud's phenomena and thermal entrainment: an objective test. *Br Med J* 1983;286:290.

59. Chucker R, Fowler RC, Molomiza T, et al. Induced temperature gradients in Raynaud's disease measured by thermography. *Angiology* 1971;22:580.

60. Singh S, de Trafford JC, Baskerville PA, et al. Digital artery caliber measurement—a new technique of assessing Raynaud's phenomena. *Eur J Vasc Surg* 1991;5:199.

61. Yao JST, Gourmos C, Papathanasiou K, et al. A method for assessing ischemia of hands and fingers. *Surg Gynecol Obstet* 1972;135:373.

62. Graham MR. Methylsergide for prevention of headache: experience in five hundred patients over three years. *N Engl J Med* 1964;271:67.

63. Henry LG, Blockwood JS, Cowley JE, et al. Ergotism. *Arch Surg* 1975;110:929.

64. Kahan A, Weber S, Amor B, et al. Nifedipine and Raynaud's phenomenon. *Ann Intern Med* 1981;94:546. Letter.
65. Murdoch D, Brogden RN. Sustained release nifedipine formulations. *Drugs* 1991;41:737.
66. Gjorup KG, Kelback H, Hartling OJ, et al. Controlled double blind trial of the clinical effect of nifedipine in the treatment of idiopathic Raynaud's phenomenon. *Am Heart J* 1986;111:742.
67. Rodeheffer RJ, Rommer JA, Wigley F, et al. Controlled double-blind trial of nifedipine in the treatment of Raynaud's syndrome. *Vasc Diagn Ther* 1983;4:15.
68. Smith CD, McKendry RJR. Controlled trials of nifedipine in the treatment of Raynaud's phenomenon. *Lancet* 1982;2:1299.
69. Varadi DP, Lawrence AM. Suppression of Raynaud's phenomenon by methyldopa. *Arch Intern Med* 1969;124:13.
70. Wesseling H, denHeeten A, Wouda AA. Sublingual and oral isoxsuprine in patients with Raynaud's phenomenon. *Eur J Clin Pharmacol* 1981;20:329.
71. Waldo R. Prazosin relieves Raynaud's vasospasm. *JAMA* 1979;241:1037.
72. Porter JM, Taylor LM Jr. Limb ischemia caused by small artery disease. *World J Surg* 1983;7:326.
73. Szczeklik A, Cryglewski RJ, Nizankowski R, et al. Prostacyclin therapy in peripheral arterial disease. *Thromb Res* 1980;19:191.
74. Clifford PC, Martin MFR, Dieppe PA, et al. Prostaglandin E1 infusion for small vessel ischemia. *J Cardiovasc Surg* 1983;24:503.
75. Clifford PC, Martin MFR, Shedden EJ, et al. Treatment of vasospastic disease with prostaglandin E1. *Br Med J* 1980,2:1031.
76. Kyle MV, Wise RA, Seibold JR, et al. Placebo controlled study showing therapeutic benefit of iloprost in the treatment of Raynaud's phenomenon. *J Rheumatol* 1992;19:1403.
77. Wigley FM, Seibold JR, et al. Intravenous iloprost treatment of Raynaud's phenomenon and ischemic ulcers secondary to systemic sclerosis. *J Rheumatol* 1992;19:1407.
78. Belch JJF, Capell HA, Cooke ED. Oral iloprost as a treatment for Raynaud's syndrome: a double blind multicentre placebo control study. *Ann Rheum Dis* 1995;54:197.
79. Dale WA. Occlusive arterial lesion of the wrist and hand. *J Tenn Med Assoc* 1964;57:402.
80. Gifford RW Jr, Hines EA Jr, Craig WM. Sympathectomy for Raynaud's phenomenon: follow-up study of 70 women with Raynaud's disease and 54 women with secondary Raynaud's phenomenon. *Circulation* 1958;17:5.
81. Hall KV, Hillestad LK. Raynaud's phenomenon treated with sympathectomy; a follow-up study of 28 patients. *Angiology* 1960;11:186.
82. Johnston ENM, Summerly R, Birnstingly M. Prognosis in Raynaud's phenomenon after sympathectomy. *Br Med J* 1978;1:962.
83. Flatt AE. Digital artery sympathectomy. *J Hand Surg* 1980;5:550.

24

Clinical Presentation and Natural History of Takayasu's Arteritis and Other Inflammatory Arteritides

David B. Hellmann, M.D.
John A. Flynn, M.D.

OVERVIEW

The vasculitides, a heterogeneous group of uncommon disorders in which inflammatory cells infiltrate and damage blood vessels, are among the greatest diagnostic and therapeutic challenges in medicine.[1] Vasculitis often presents initially with nonspecific signs of inflammation that unfold over weeks to months. Eventually, however, the diagnosis usually can be suspected from bedside clues and then confirmed by biopsy or angiography. Whereas only several decades ago vasculitis was a relentlessly progressive, fatal disease, today most patients with vasculitis can be helped and some even cured.

Classification of Vasculitis

Because the causes of most forms of vasculitis are unknown, the vasculitides have been classified by their clinicopathologic features[1] (Table 24–1). Important classification variables include the typical host (eg, young women in Takayasu's arteritis), the types of vessels affected (eg, large arteries in Takayasu's arteritis, small muscular arteries in polyarteritis), the nature of the inflammatory infiltrate (eg, granulomatous inflammation in Wegener's granulomatosis), the typical target organs (eg, the upper and lower respiratory tracts and kidneys in Wegener's granulomatosis), and other disease associations (eg, the association of Churg Strauss vasculitis with asthma).[1]

Pathogenesis and Etiology

Although the etiology of most forms of vasculitis is not known, the pathogenesis involves both humoral and cellular immunity.[1] Animal models have shown that deposition of circulating immune complexes in blood vessels can produce vasculitis. Perhaps the best example of immune complex disease in humans is polyarteritis nodosa associated with hepatitis infection.[2,3] Approximately 20 to 50% of patients with polyarteritis nodosa have active hepatitis B or C or both. In mounting an immune response to the hepatitis virus, the patient forms circulating immune complexes that provoke a cascade of events. The inflammatory process begins with deposition of the complexes in vessels, which activates complement and generates chemotactic fragments (C3a and C5a), continues with recruitment of inflammatory cells, and ends with activated polymorphonuclear cells releasing oxygen radicals and lysoenzymes that destroy the vessel wall. Cellular immunity appears to play an important role in some diseases, especially Takayasu's arteritis and giant cell arteritis.[4–6] Both disorders are characterized by granulomatous inflammation, a process known to require T-cell help. The mechanisms or antigens driving these diseases have not yet been identified. Wegener's granulomatosis, a disease associated with a novel group of autoantibodies (the antineutrophil cytoplasmic antibodies) and characterized by granulomatous inflammation, may involve both humoral and cellular immune responses.[5]

Prognosis and Treatment

In the absence of treatment, most forms of systemic vasculitis cause death from progressive tissue infarction.[1,5] Medical therapy attempts to halt the inflammation with corticosteriods, immunosuppressive drugs, or both.

Table 24–1.   Vasculitis: Classification and Selected Clinical Features

Type of Vasculitis	Typical Host	Vessels	Target Tissues
Takayasu's arteritis	20 yo woman	Aorta and main branches	Heart, brain, skeletal muscle
Polyarteritis nodosa	40 yo IV drug abuser	Small muscular arteries	Kidney, nerve, gut, heart
Wegener's granulomatosis	40 yo man	Small and medium-sized arteries; veins	Sinus, lung, kidney
Temporal (giant cell) arteritis	>60 yo woman or man	Large, elastic arteries	Eye
Primary angiitis of the central nervous system	48 yo woman	Arterioles, capillaries	Brain
Hypersensitivity vasculitis*	20–50 yo woman or man	Capillaries, venules	Skin, kidney, gut, nerve
Vasculitis with connective tissue disease (eg, SLE,† rheumatoid arthritis)	35 yo woman with SLE	Like polyarteritis nodosa or hypersensitivity vasculitis	
Churg-Strauss syndrome	45 yo man with chronic asthma	Like Wegener's granulomatosis	Skin, lung, kidney
Lymphomatoid granulomatosis	50 yo man or woman	Like polyarteritis nodosa	Skin, lung, brain
Buerger's disease	35 yo male heavy smoker	Arterioles, veins	Skin, digits, muscles
Cogan's syndrome	50 yo man or woman	Aorta, arterioles	Eye, cochlea, heart
Behcet's syndrome	25 yo woman	Arterioles, veins	Mouth, genitals, eye, brain
Vasculitis associated with malignancy	70 yo man or woman with lymphoma	Capillaries, veins	Skin
Relapsing polychondritis	45 yo man or woman	Arterioles	Ear, trachea, eye

*Includes serum sickness, Henoch-Schönlein purpura, and cryoglobulinemia.
†Systemic lupus erythematosus.
Source: Modified from Ref. 1, Table 3.5-1, p. 216, with permission.

Complications of inflammation or scarring of large vessels may require surgery or other interventions. Aortic regurgitation and renal artery stenosis are two complications in Takayasu's arteritis that are discussed below.

TAKAYASU'S ARTERITIS

Clinical Presentation

Takayasu's arteritis is a form of vasculitis that affects the aorta and its primary branches and occurs most frequently in young women.[4,7] Onset occurs, on average, in the late twenties but may be as early as age 7 or as late as the seventh decade of life.[4,7] Histologically, the involved vessels show evidence of a panarteritis that may include granulomatous as well as lymphocytic infiltration. Pronounced intimal thickening develops in the setting of continued inflammation. This can lead to narrowing and eventual obliteration of the arterial lumen. Inflammation of these large arteries can also result in arterial dilatation, with subsequent aneurysm formation. Patients can present with systemic manifestations of inflammation (such as fever), with symptoms of localized vascular insufficiency (such as arm claudication or new-onset hypertension), or with both[4,7,8] (Table 24–2).

Patients may be a clinical mystery at first, presenting with constitutional symptoms such as weight loss or fever for months before they develop telltale bruits,

unequal blood pressures, or loss of pulses. Up to half of the patients develop muscle and joint symptoms such as myalgia, arthralgia, or arthritis[4,7,8] (Table 24–2).

Many patients have no systemic symptoms but present instead with signs and symptoms of vascular insufficiency of the involved large arteries. This may take the form of claudication, which most commonly occurs in the upper extremities. The term *pulseless disease* has been applied to this condition to describe the absence of radial or ulnar pulses that can be a presenting feature. New-onset hypertension is seen in almost half of the patients as a result of renal ischemia secondary to narrowing of the aorta or renal artery.[7] Postural dizziness is also a feature and reflects carotid artery involvement. Rarely, this can lead to central nervous system ischemia with stroke or to visual symptoms from retinal ischemia. Cardiac disease may take one of two forms. The first, which may develop in up to 10% of patients, is coronary artery involvement with ischemic heart disease. The second form, which has been reported to occur in up to 20% of patients, is aortic root dilatation with progression to aortic regurgitation. Acute dissection of the aorta has been described but is a rare event. Takayasu's arteritis is one of the rare forms of vasculitis that can involve pulmonary arteries.[7] In contrast to polyarteritis, Takayasu's arteritis usually spares vessels supplying the mesentery and peripheral nerves. Physical examination may demonstrate de-

Table 24–2. Clinical Features of Takayasu's Arteritis in Two Series

	NIH Series*	Mayo Series†
Demographics		
Number of patients	60	32
Percent female	81%	97%
Age of onset, median (range)	25 (7–64)	31 (15–48)
Delay in diagnosis (months)	10	18
Constitutional symptoms		
Fever	30%	42%
Weight loss	25%	36%
Myalgia/arthralgia	50%	56%
Vascular findings		
Extremity claudication	65%	45%
Hypertension	41%	40%
Bruits	80%	94%
Angiographic findings		
Aortic lesions	80%	65%
Stenotic lesions	96%	84%
Aneurysms	30%	27%

*From Ref. 7.
†From Ref. 4.

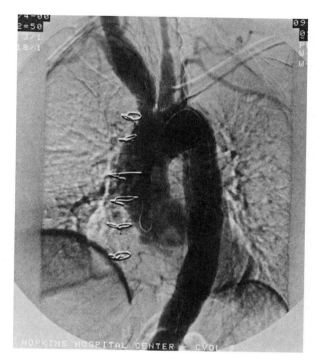

Figure 24–1. Left anterior-oblique digital subtraction aortogram in a 44-year-old woman with Takayasu's arteritis showing marked dilation of the brachiocephalic and proximal right common carotid arteries. The left common carotid also demonstrates fusiform dilation, with occlusion of the artery just distal to its origin. The edges of the contrast margin of the descending thoracic aorta are irregular, indicating the effects of mural inflammation. The patient had previously undergone an aortic valve replacement.

creased or absent pulses within an extremity, and there may be asymmetric blood pressure measurements. New bruits may be heard over the carotid and subclavian arteries or the abdominal aorta.

Diagnostic Evaluation

Diagnosis may be difficult in the initial stages of constitutional symptoms and before arterial manifestations become clinically evident. The cause of these symptoms is usually appreciated only with the recognition of associated vascular insufficiency. During the inflammatory phases of the disease, several laboratory parameters may be abnormal. These can include a normochromic normocytic anemia, an elevated sedimentation rate, and possibly an increase in gamma globulin production.[4,7,8] No specific serologic markers are identified in this condition.

Definitive diagnosis is generally established by arteriography.[4,7,8] Arteriographic changes are typically most pronounced in the region of the aortic arch and its primary branches and are typically multifocal. At least two-thirds of patients have abnormal radiographic findings in the aortic arch. The most common angiographic lesions are long, smooth, tapering arterial stenotic segments. Less frequently, these lesions show irregularity or frank occlusion of the lumen. Aneurysmal dilatations are seen in roughly one-fourth of patients (Figs. 24–1 and 24–2). Magnetic resonance (MR) images do not provide the level of detail of angiogrpahy.[9] However, MR has the ability to reveal thickening of the vessel wall,

which may be the only demonstrable abnormality in the early stages of the disease[3] (Fig. 24–3). Furthermore, because MR is relatively noninvasive, it can be easily repeated, thereby providing useful follow-up information. Sonography does not image the aorta well, but it can reveal vessel wall thickening and blood flow changes in the carotid and renal arteries.[10,11]

Natural History and Prognosis

As with polyarteritis, a high mortality rate occurs in patients with untreated disease.[4,7,8] This is typically due to congestive heart failure in the setting of profound aortic insufficiency or coronary ischemia. The clinical variables that convey an increased risk of mortality include severe hypertension and marked aortic insufficiency. Two North American series however, indicate a rather favorable prognosis.[4,7] Reported 5-year survival was 90%.[4,7] However, there is significant associated morbidity with functional impairment, resulting in permanent disability in half of the patients in one of these series.

Treatment

Two key issues must first be addressed in the management of Takayasu's arteritis. First, one must determine

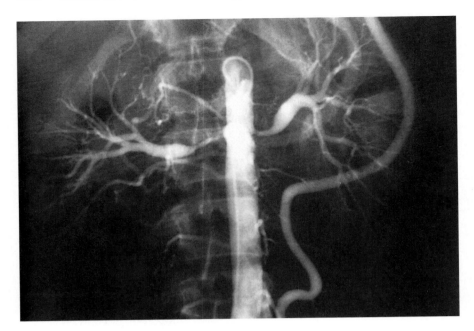

Figure 24–2. Flush anterior-posterior abdominal aortogram demonstrating bilateral proximal renal artery stenoses in a patient with Takayasu's arteritis. There is minimal aortic irregularity adjacent and slightly inferior to the left renal artery. Note the large, serpiginous left colic branch of the inferior mesenteric artery providing collateral flow to the superior mesenteric distribution.

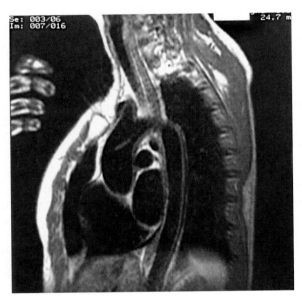

Figure 24–3. Parasagittal MR image showing thickening of the wall of the thoracic aorta in a 19-year-old girl with Takayasu's arteritis. The arteriogram of this area was normal. (Courtesy of Scott J. Savader, M.D.)

whether there is ongoing inflammation that requires immunosuppressive therapy. Second, one must assess whether there is vascular involvement that requires intervention.

In the absence of tissue biopsy, inflammation is difficult to judge absolutely, but it is assumed to be present if the patient has systemic symptoms, an unexplained elevated erythrocyte sedimentation rate, or rapidly progressing vascular abnormalities. In this setting, corticosteroids should be used and are extremely effective in suppressing the constitutional symptoms associated with this inflammatory condition. Corticosteroids may also help arrest, and rarely reverse, the arterial insufficiency (Fig. 24–4). If the patient has no evidence of ongoing vascular inflammation, the disease is probably burned out and corticosteroids are not required. Treatment focuses on vascular intervention only in the setting of critical vascular involvement.

Rarely, patients are critically ill from the ongoing inflammation, with evidence of end-organ ischemia. In these cases, high-dose corticosteroids should be used acutely in a pulse fashion. By this method, corticosteroids (solumedrol, up to 1000 mg/day parenterally) are given for 2 to 3 days. Following this course of treatment, prednisone is given orally in a dose of 1 mg/kg/day.[4,7,8] Fortunately, the majority of patients are not acutely ill. In these cases, prednisone may be initiated orally in a dose of 1 mg/kg/day. Initially, this therapy alone induces remission in two-thirds of patients. The dosage is tapered over a period of at least 6 months. If relapse is evident during this time or if remission was not initially achieved with steroids alone, then a second immunosuppressive medication such as oral methotrexate,[6] azathioprine, or cyclophosphamide should be added. In roughly half of the patients, the disease is controlled with corticosteroids alone.

Vascular intervention is not required for most stenotic lesions because most of these lesions are not clinically important. For example, a modest subclavian stenosis, which is asymptomatic, should simply be followed clinically. Even when mild arm claudication is present, symptoms may improve over time. However, among patients with evidence of critical vascular ischemia unresponsive to medical therapy, further intervention may be required. The clinical situations that most commonly warrant this are uncontrollable

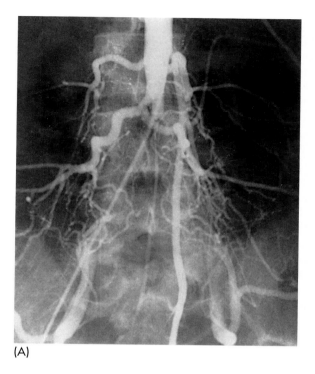

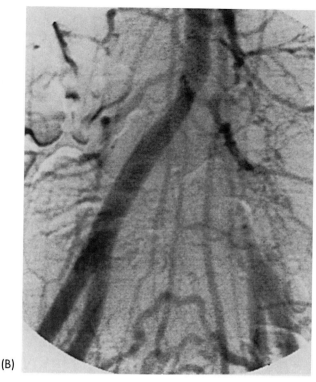

Figure 24–4. Initial and follow-up aortograms of 16 year old woman with Takayasu's arteritis. (A) A right transfemoral abdominal aortogram taken shortly after disease onset, demonstrating segmental occlusion of the distal aorta and both iliac arteries. Large lumbar collaterals are present. (B) An intravenous digital subtraction aortogram performed 18 months after corticosteroid therapy, showing a patent, but slightly narrowed, distal aorta and widely patent right common, external and internal iliac arteries. The left common iliac artery remains occluded. (Figures and legend reprinted from Hellmann D, Hardy K, Lindenfeld S, Ring E: Takayasu's aortitis associated with crescentic glomerulonephritis. *Arthritis Rheum* 1987;30:451–454, with permission.

hypertension or renal insufficiency from renal artery or aortic stenosis, severe aortic regurgitation, and ongoing coronary ischemia. Repair of these lesions can be accomplished either through percutaneous transluminal angiopalsty (PTA), surgical revascularization, or aortic valve replacement.[12–14] Ideally, this should be done after the acute arterial inflammation is suppressed with medication. However, the acuity of the situation may require urgent intervention.

PTA is most commonly performed for stenoses involving the aorta and renal arteries. Balloon angioplasty appears to be safe and modestly effective for treatment of these stenotic lesions. Initial success with these procedures is obtained in 85 to 95% of patients.[11–13] Long-term follow-up shows that restenosis can occur in up to 30% of patients up to 2 years after the procedure. The variables that increase the risk of restenosis of the renal artery include (1) proximal stenosis of the renal artery, (2) coexistent abdominal aortic disease, and (3) noncompliant stenoses that require prolonged balloon inflation. Restenosis following PTA of aortic lesions most often occurs after treatment of segments longer than 4 cm.[14]

Surgical revascularization should be considered for patients with diffuse vascular disease that is not amendable to angioplasty or for those who fail angioplasty. Vascular structures unaffected by inflammation are the preferred sites for anastomosis, with autologous grafts showing a higher success rate than synthetic conduits. In one large series, long-term graft patency was 70%.[8]

POLYARTERITIS NODOSA

Clinical Presentation

Polyarteritis nodosa (PAN), the prototype of systemic necrotizing vasculitis, can strike at any age but usually affects individuals in the fourth or fifth decade.[1–3,15] Men are affected twice as often as women. Approximately 20 to 50% of patients develop polyarteritis nodosa in the setting of active hepatitis B or C infection, so the disease is more common in intravenous drug users and in patients receiving chronic hemodialysis. The etiology of polyarteritis in patients without hepatitis is unknown. In contrast to Takayasu's aortitis, polyarteritis chiefly affects the small muscular arteries,

Table 24–3. Clinical Clues to the Diagnosis of Polyarteritis Nodosa

General
Multisystemic disease
Subacute onset
Prominent inflammation
Pain: arthralgia, myalgia, neuralgia

Specific
Neurologic
Peripheral nervous system: mononeuritis multiplex
Central nervous system: headache, encephalopathy,
multifocal strokes
Skin: palpable purpura, ulcers, livedo reticularis, nodules
Renal: hypertension, proteinuria, hematuria,
glomerulonephritis
Gastrointestinal: "abdominal angina," bleeding,
gangrene, perforation
Ocular: scleritis
Sudden, critical end-organ damage: testicular infarction,
myocardial infarction

Source: Reprinted from Ref. 1, Table 2.5-2, p. 217, with permission.

especially those of the kidney, peripheral nerve, skin, gastrointestinal tract, and heart.[1–3,15]

The general clues that suggest that a patient has polyarteritis nodosa include a *multisystemic disease* that unfolds *subacutely* over weeks or months, features signs of *inflammation*, and causes *pain*[1] (Table 24–3). Initially, nonspecific symptoms including malaise, fever, weight loss, arthralgia, and myalgia predominate. Weeks to months later, the patient usually develops more specific clues to the diagnosis of PAN (Table 24–3). Of these, the most helpful are mononeuritis multiplex and cutaneous manifestations of vasculitis.

Mononeuritis multiplex, a peripheral neuropathy in which named nerves are infarcted one at a time, is probably the most specific sign that a patient has PAN.[1,16,17] Mononeuritis multiplex affects the lower extremities slightly more often than the upper ones. Peroneal and tibial nerve infarctions are most common. Infarction of cranial nerve is less common; thoracic nerve roots are rarely involved. In about 50% of patients, proximal limb pain precedes by 12 to 24 hours the development of the neurologic deficit. The neuropathy almost always causes a painful sensory deficit and produces weakness in two-thirds of cases. Occasionally, the motor deficits may be so extensive that the patient is unable to walk or use the hands.

The diagnosis of mononeuritis multiplex can usually be made based on the history and physical examination. A few patients may require electromyelography to demonstrate the characteristic pattern of multifocal axonal neuropathy. Although in theory mononeuritis multiplex has a varied differential diagnosis, in practice it is almost always a sign of vasculitis if diabetes and multiple compression injuries have been excluded.

The skin is another excellent source of clues to the diagnosis of PAN.[2,3] While cutaneous vasculitis occurs in only 30% of patients with PAN, its ease of detection makes it a better clue than some visceral organs that are more commonly but less obviously involved. Palpable purpura, nodules, periungual infarcts, digital ischemia, ulcers, and livedo reticularis are easily recognizable clues suggesting the diagnosis.

PAN can produce important signs and symptoms in other organ systems.[15] Although at autopsy renal disease is readily and universally detected in PAN, during life renal disease must be inferred form the new onset of hypertension, nocturia, renal insufficiency, or red cell casts in the urine. Gastrointestinal involvement may manifest as abdominal pain, especially intestinal angina, in which abdominal pain from ischemia develops 20 to 60 minutes after eating. Hemorrhage, diarrhea, or cholecystitis-like symptoms from infarction of the gallbladder are other gastrointestinal manifestations. Rarely, patients present with collapse or an acute abdomen from rupture of a microaneurysm in the liver, kidney, or pancreas. Cardiac involvement can cause myocardial infarction or diffuse myocarditis resulting in congestive heart failure. Testicular infarction may mimic torsion of the testicle. Central nervous system disease is less common except as a complication of uncontrolled hypertension. Ocular manifestations include scleritis. Pulmonary disease rarely develops in PAN.

Laboratory test results are nonspecific but usually show mild normochromic, normocytic anemia, mild leukocytosis, thrombocytosis, and an elevated erythrocyte sedimentation rate.[15] Liver function tests are often normal or only minimally elevated even in the face of active hepatitis B or hepatitis C. Renal insufficiency, proteinuria, and hematuria may also develop. Less than one-third of patients have a positive rheumatoid factor or hypocomplementemia.

Natural History

If untreated, 88% of patients with PAN will die within 5 years.[15] Corticosteroids increase the 5-year survival rate to 50%. With combination corticosteroid and immunosuppressive therapy, the 5-year survival rate increases to 75%. Death most commonly results from renal failure, heart failure, or infectious complications of immunosuppressive therapy. About 50% of the patients with mononeuritis multiplex will improve, though the improvement may take 6 to 24 months and may be incomplete.[16] Risk factors for a poor prognosis are renal disease and gastrointestinal involvement. In the presence of renal and gastrointestinal disease, 5-year survival is less than 50%. In the absence of these risk factors, 5-year survival with medical therapy is greater than 80%.

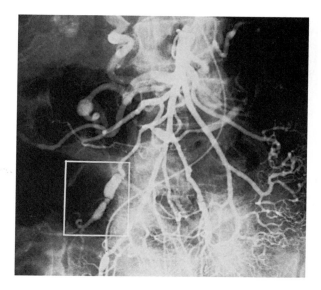

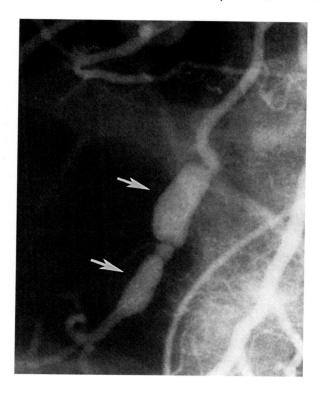

Figure 24–5. (A) PAN. Mesenteric arteriogram shows multiple diagnositc aneurysmal dilatations, two of which are magnified (arrows) in the detail panel (Reprinted from Ref. 1, Figure 3.5-1, p. 218, with permission.)

Diagnostic Evaluation

Sutton's law—"go where the money is"—applies well to PAN. If the patient has a painful muscle or an involved sural nerve, then biopsy of these sites is 66% sensitive and 100% specific for the diangosis.[18] If muscle or nerve is not involved clinically, the sensitivity of biopsy drops to 33%. Instead of using blind biopsy of an asymptomatic muscle or nerve, one should perform visceral angiography, which has 66% sensitivity in detecting the characteristic microaneurysms of PAN (Fig. 24–5). The hepatic artery may be involved even when liver function tests are normal. Renal involvement is more common in patients who are hepatitis B positive and in those with hypertension and clinical renal disease. Angiography may entail additional risk, especially if the patient already has some degree of renal insufficiency. To avoid fatal hemorrhage from ruptured microaneurysms, percutaneous renal biopsy should be avoided unless an arteriogram has already excluded renal microaneurysms. Biopsy of purpuric lesions usually demonstrates only leukocytoclastic vasculitis, which can complicate any form of vasculitis including some that are limited to the skin and not associated with visceral disease. If the patient has cutaneous nodules, biopsy is more likely to show a true arteritis.

Treatment

The treatment of polyarteritis is usually medical. Conventional therapy begins with prednisone, 1 mg/kg/day, and cyclophosphamide, 2 mg/kg/day po.[3,15] The prednisone is continued for 1 to 2 months and then tapered, while the cyclophosphamide is continued for up to 12 months after remission is induced. In controlled trials, the addition of cyclophosphamide did not improve survival but did reduce the risk of relapse. The risk and toxicities of cyclophosphamide—including a 2.4-fold increased risk of all malignancies (with an even higher risk of bladder cancer, lymphoma, and skin cancer), hemorrhagic cystitis, infection, and gonadal failure—may limit its use.[5]

For patients with polyarteritis secondary to hepatitis B, antiviral therapy may now be the treatment of choice.[2] With conventional therapy, hepatitis B–associated PAN will improve, but almost all patients become chronic carriers and are susceptible to complications of chronic hepatitis B, including cirrhosis, variceal bleeding, liver failure, and hepatoma. A French group has shown that in these patients, prednisone used for 2 weeks to control inflammation, accompanied by plasmapheresis to remove immune complexes, followed by antiviral therapy with agents such as alpha-2b-interferon, achieves 70% 10-year survival rates and cures the hepatitis B infection in 20 to 30% of patients.[2]

The most common reason for surgery in PAN is for suspected intestinal gangrene or perforation. Intestinal infarction usually occurs after weeks of abdominal pain. However, less than 50% of patients give a classic history of intestinal angina with postprandial exacerbation of pain. The usual signs of peritonitis may be muted or absent in patients taking corticosteroids and immunosuppressive therapy. The platelet count may be particularly valuable, as it is usually high in active polyarteritis nodosa but falls below normal once the bowel perforates or develops gangrene. Infarction of the gallbladder may mimic cholecystitis, and may be both a reason for surgery and the mechanism by which the diagnosis of PAN is first made.

Surgery is also performed when patients present with shock and intra-abdominal or retroperitoneal hemorrhage from rupture of a microaneurysm. The most common site of rupture is the kidney. Hepatic and parapancreatic ruptures have also been described.

Vascular surgeons may be asked to consult on patients experiencing of intestinal or digital ischemia. Intestinal ischemia short of infarction is best treated medically with bowel rest, total parenteral nutrition, and immunosuppressive therapy. The vascular disease is usually too diffuse to be amenable to endovascular interventions. Digital ischemia is also best treated medically, although sympathectomy or amputation may be warranted in some cases.

REFERENCES

1. Hellmann BD. Vasculitis. In Stobo JD, Hellmann DH, Ladenson PW, Petty BG, and Traill TA, eds. *The Principles and Practice of Medicine.* 23rd ed. Norwalk, CT: Appleton & Lange, 1996;215–221.
2. Guillevin L, Lhote F, Cohen P, et al. Polyarteritis nodosa related to hepatitis B virus. A retrospective study with long-term observation of 41 patients. *Medicine* 1995; 74:238–253.
3. Guillevin L, Lhote F, Gayraud M, et al. Prognostic factors in polyarteritis nodosa and Churg-Strauss syndrome: a prospective study in 342 patients. *Medicine* 1996; 75:17–28.
4. Hall S, Barr W, Lie JT, Stanson AW, Kazmier FJ, Hunder GG. Takayasu arteritis: a study of 32 North American patients. *Medicine* 1985;64:89–99.
5. Hoffman GS, Kerr GS, Leavitt RY, et al. Wegener granulomatosis: an analysis of 158 patients. *Ann Intern Med* 1992;116:488–498.
6. Hoffman GS, Leavitt RY, Kerr GS, Rottem M, Sneller MC, Fauci AS. Treatment of glucocorticoid-resistant or relapsing Takayasu arteritis with methotrexate. *Arthritis Rheum* 1994;37:578–582.
7. Kerr GS, Hallahan CW, Giordano J, et al. Takayasu arteritis. *Ann Intern Med* 1994;120:919–929.
8. Lupi-Herrera E, Sanchez-Torres G, Marcushamer J, Mispireta J, Horwitz S, Vela JE. Takayasu's arteritis. Clinical study of 107 cases. *Am Heart J* 1977;93:94–103.
9. Tanigawa K, Eguchi K, Kitamura Y, et al. Magnetic resonance imaging detection of aortic and pulmonary artery wall thickening in the acute stage of Takayasu arteritis: improvement of clinical and radiologic findings after steroid therapy. *Arthritis Rheum* 1992;35:476–480.
10. Maeda H, Handa N, Matsumoto M, et al. Carotid lesions detected by B-mode ultrasonography in Takayasu's arteritis: "macaroni sign" as an indicator of the disease. *Ultrasound Med Biol* 1991;17:695–701.
11. Buckley A, Southwood T, Culham G, Nadel H, Malleson P, Petty R. The role of ultrasound in evaluation of Takayasu's arteritis. *J Rheumatol* 1991;18:1073–80.
12. Rao SA, Mandalam KR, Rao VR, et al. Takayasu arteritis: initial and long-term follow-up in 16 patients after percutaneous transluminal angioplasty of the descending thoracic and abdominal aorta. *Radiology* 1993;189:173–179.
13. Sharma S, Sexena A, Talwar KK, Kaul U, Mehta SN, Rajani M. Renal artery stenosis caused by nonspecific arteritis (Takayasu disease): results of treatment with percutaneous transluminal angioplasty. *Am J Radiol* 1992;158:417–422.
14. Tyagi S, Kaul UA, Nair M, Sethi KK, Arora R, Khalilullah M. Balloon angioplasty of the aorta in Takayasu's arteritis: initial and long-term results. *Am Heart J* 1992;124:876–882.
15. Cupps TR, Fauci AS. Systemic necrotizing vasculitis of the polyarteritis nodosa group. In: Smith LH Jr, ed. *The Vasculitides* (vol XXI). Philadelphia: WB Saunders; 1981:26–49.
16. Hellmann DB, Laing TJ, Petri M, Whiting-O'Keefe O, Parry GJ. Mononeuritis multiplex: the yield of the evaluation for occult rheumatic diseases. *Medicine* 1988; 67:145–153.
17. Hellmann DB. Mononeuritis multiplex. In: Klippel JH, Dieppe UK, eds. *Rheumatology.* Baltimore: CV Mosby; 1994:6-26.2–6-26.5.
18. Albert DA, Rimon D, Silverstein MD. The diagnosis of polyarteritis nodosa. I. A literature-based decision analysis approach. *Arthritis Rheum* 1988;31:1117–1134.

Section 2

Acute Peripheral Arterial Occlusive Disease

25

The Surgical Management of Acute Limb Ischemia: Limb Salvage, Morbidity, and Mortality

Robert C. Allen, M.D.
Ramin Beygui, M.D.
Thomas J. Fogarty, M.D.

Acute extremity ischemia is the sudden onset of peripheral arterial occlusion that may threaten both life and limb. This is vividly illustrated by the high amputation, morbidity, and mortality rates seen in the past prior to the advent of more modern surgical techniques.[1] Yet, despite advances in both diagnostic and therapeutic approaches, the management of acute limb-threatening ischemia remains an area of controversy. Surgical therapy remains the primary mode of treatment, especially in patients with an obvious embolic event or advanced limb-threatening ischemia.

ETIOLOGY

There are two principal categories, thrombotic and embolic, that together account for more than 90% of all cases of acute limb ischemia. This specifically excludes traumatic and iatrogenic etiologies. A metanalysis of reported series indicates a thrombotic etiology in 59% and embolization in 41% of the cases.[2] These numbers are blurred by the inability to distinguish embolus from thrombosis in at least 15 to 30% of cases and by the varied means used by authors in the past to differentiate an embolus from in situ thrombosis of an atherosclerotic vessel.[3,4] The term *thromboembolism* is frequently used and exemplifies the vague categorization presented in numerous reports. The separation of causation into embolic versus thrombotic categories is important, as each has markedly different clinical implications and therefore treatment strategies. The reported cases of thrombotic limb ischemia reveal acute occlusion of a bypass graft in 50 to 60% of patients and of native artery in 40 to 50%.[4–7]

Table 25–1 summarizes the more important etiologies of acute limb ischemia. The sources of emboli are divided into cardiac and noncardiac etiologies. Cardiac sources account for 75 to 85% of the cases of acute embolic limb ischemia.[2,8,9] Tumor embolus (cardiac myxomas) and paradoxical embolus (deep venous thrombosis) are rare causes of acute limb ischemia. Another important etiology is aortic dissection because in 30 to 50% of cases the dissection may extend to compromise extremity flow.[10]

Arterial emboli are almost always of cardiac etiology and are a reflection of underlying cardiac pathology. The cardiac disease process has, however, changed in recent years from rheumatic heart disease to atherosclerosis in the majority of patients. Atrial fibrillation

Table 25–1. Etiologies of Acute Limb Ischemia

Embolic: (41%)	Cardiac (atrial fibrillation, myocardial infarction, valve vegetation, aneurysm)	80%
	Atherosclerotic occlusive disease plaque	5%
	Peripheral aneurysm (abdominal aorta, femoral, popliteal)	5%
	"Cryptogenic" source	5%
	Paradoxical (deep venous thrombosis)	1%
	Tumor (atrial myxoma)	1%
Thrombotic: (59%)	Peripheral bypass graft (saphenous vein, synthetic)	55%
	Atherosclerotic occlusive disease	45%
	Peripheral aneurysm (abdominal aorta, femoral, popliteal)	1%
	Nonatherosclerotic vascular lesions	1%

and acute myocardial infarction are the two most important risk factors for peripheral arterial emboli from cardiac sources. Other cardiac sources of peripheral emboli include left ventricular aneurysm following myocardial infarction and valvular disease. Proximal ulcerated atherosclerotic lesions and peripheral aneurysms account for 5 to 10% of arterial emboli in the extremities. Interestingly, despite the present sophistication of diagnostic testing, in approximately 5% of patients the embolic source cannot be found after extensive evaluation. These *cryptogenic* emboli highlight the limitations of present diagnostic testing. The peripheral extremity vessels are involved in 70 to 80% of arterial embolic events, and the incidence in the lower extremities is four to five times higher than in the upper extremities.[8,11] The common femoral bifurcation is the most frequent site of embolic occlusion. Meta-analysis of reported cases reveals the following distribution: femoral arteries (43%), iliac arteries (18%), aortic saddle emboli (16%), popliteal arteries (15%), carotid arteries (13%), upper extremities (9%), and visceral and renal arteries (7%).[2,11]

However, the most common cause of acute limb ischemia today is in situ thrombosis of stenotic atherosclerotic vessels. Native arterial thrombosis results in varying degrees of limb ischemia that is dependent on the degree of collateral circulation development. The insidious occlusion of a very stenotic atherosclerotic lesion may result in only mild clinical symptoms, while thrombosis due to plaque rupture or hemorrhage into the wall of a vessel with only a moderate stenosis will typically result in more severe symptoms due to the lack of collateral circulation. Thrombosis of peripheral aneurysms may also result in acute limb-threatening ischemia, and in fact peripheral aneurysms are more likely to thrombose than rupture. For example, popliteal aneurysms frequently present with thrombosis or embolization and limb ischemia, but rupture is unusual. Saphenous vein and synthetic bypass grafts may acutely thrombose, and the etiology depends on the time interval from the primary procedure. Technical errors account for early graft thrombosis, with neointimal hyperplasia occurring during intermediate follow-up and progressive atherosclerosis later. Several nonatherosclerotic diseases can also result in acute limb ischemia, including fibromuscular dysplasia, adventitial cystic disease, and various inflammatory arteritides. Finally, hypercoagulable states may precipitate limb ischemia in extremities with otherwise normal vessels.

CLINICAL PRESENTATION

Acute arterial occlusion of an extremity may result in varying degrees of limb ischemia. The classical presentation is described by the ''five Ps'': pulselessness, pain, pallor, paresthesia, and paralysis. These signs and symptoms typically occur in the following order: pain, pallor, sensory loss, and motor loss. Pulselessness is often difficult to assess, as the prior status of peripheral pulses may be unknown, and pulsations may still be transmitted through fresh thrombus. The pain is a severe, steady ache below the level of the occlusion, and is progressively worse farther distally in the extremity. The pain is not relieved by dependency. The limb is pale, and the lack of color may be especially noticeable in comparison to the contralateral extremity, sometimes progressing to a white, waxy, ''cadaveric'' appearance. Numbness and paresthesias are early warning signs of nerve dysfunction. Advanced ischemia is noted by the progressive loss of sensory and then motor function. Sensation is best assessed by testing light touch and is the best guide to extremity viability.[8,12] Paralysis is first suggested by the loss of fine movements in the foot, and suggests advanced ischemia with both neural and muscle involvement. Irreversible ischemia is suggested by the presence of profound anesthesia and muscle rigor. The Ad Hoc Committee on Reporting Standards (Society for Vascular Surgery/International Society for CardioVascular Surgery) recommended the clinical categories of acute limb ischemia found in Table 25–2.[13] These clinical categories help define and standardize the degree of limb ischemia, and therefore the timing and modality of treatment. The examiner should not rely too heavily on Doppler signals, as they may not accurately reflect tissue viability, especially in patients with long-standing peripheral vascular disease. The anatomic location of the arterial occlusion can often be determined by careful physical examination. The level of temperature demarcation is usually ''one joint'' distal to the point of occlusion. For example, a femoral occlusion will demarcate at or just above the knee level.

DIAGNOSIS

The diagnosis of acute limb ischemia is determined by a careful history and physical examination. This will also frequently lead to the discovery of the etiology of extremity arterial occlusion, which is essential for guiding treatment. The major differential diagnosis is embolus versus thrombosis. A history of arrhythmias, myocardial infarction, or cardiovascular instrumentation is indicative of acute embolic ischemia. In contrast a history of claudication, peripheral aneurysms, or the presence of an arterial bypass graft suggests thrombo-

Table 25–2. Clinical Categories of Acute Limb Ischemia

Clinical Category	Capillary Return	Muscle Weakness	Sensory Loss	Doppler Signals
Viable	Intact	None	None	Audible
Threatened	Slow	Mild	Mild	Inaudible
Irreversible	Absent	Profound	Profound	Inaudible

Source: Reprinted form Ref. 13, p. 80, with permission.

sis as the cause of acute limb ischemia. Careful physical examination to assess pulses, the presence of capillary refill, and the degree of neurologic deficit helps to determine the level of arterial occlusion and the severity of ischemia. The use of a hand-held continuous-wave Doppler instrument allows the examiner to assess distal perfusion and to determine the ankle/brachial index (ABI).

Duplex scanning may be used to image the extremity vessels directly and may help to distinguish embolus from thrombus, determine the location and extent of obstruction, and diagnose proximal ulcerated plaques or peripheral aneurysms. In equivocal patients, contrast arteriography is an important diagnostic tool in differentiating embolus from thrombosis (Table 25–3, Figs. 25–1 and 25–2) and is essential in assessing patients with thrombotic occlusion for planning operative intervention. In contrast, a preoperative angiogram is rarely

necessary for embolic disease and only serves to prolong limb ischemia time.

INITIAL MANAGEMENT

The initial management of limb-threatening ischemia should be aimed at limiting further thrombus formation and determining the necessity and timing of possible surgical intervention. Past dogma dictated a "golden period" of 4 to 6 hours for intervention, but the physiologic status of the limb is much more important than any arbitrary time period. The viable acutely ischemic limb requires urgent treatment, whereas the threatened extremity demands emergent intervention. Irreversible limb ischemia should be treated with primary amputation, as limb revascularization is ultimately futile and will result in reperfusion injury, with the potential life-threatening sequelae of hyperkalemia, acidosis, arrhythmias, and death.

Table 25–3. Angiographic Findings: Embolus Versus Thrombosis

Embolus	Thrombosis
Minimal atherosclerosis	Occlusive disease with plaques and stenoses
Sharp cutoff with "reversed miniscus" sign	Tapering vessels with irregular occlusion
Multiple filling defects in different arterial beds	Single or multiple areas of stenoses/occlusion
Few collateral vessels	Well-developed collateral circulation
Located at arterial bifurcations	Specific locations (adductor canal)

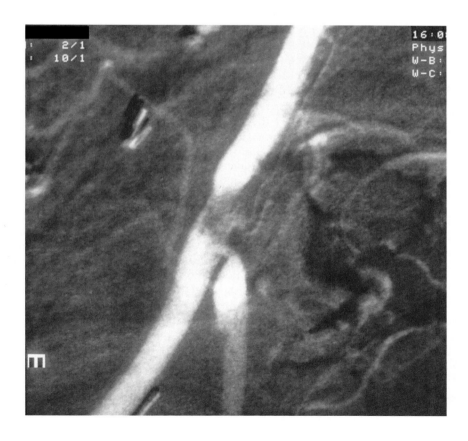

Figure 25–1. Angiogram demonstrating an embolus at the right common iliac artery bifurcation. Note the normal-appearing vessels and absence of collateral circulation.

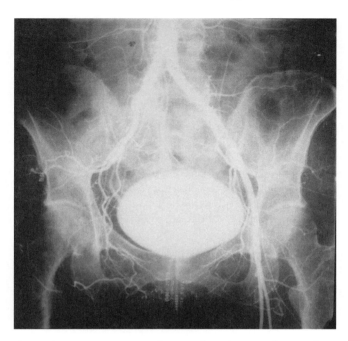

Figure 25–2. Angiogram showing thrombotic occlusion of right iliac vessels with abundant collaterals and diffuse atherosclerotic disease.

Patients with viable extremities should be initially treated with a heparin bolus (5000 to 10,000, 100 U/Kg IV) and placed on intravenous heparin to maintain the activated partial thromboplastin time at 1.5 to 2 times the control value. This will prevent further clot propagation and maintain patent collateral circulation. A metanalysis of the outcome of acute limb ischemia demonstrates a reduction in mortality and increased limb salvage when preoperative heparin therapy is initiated prior to Fogarty catheter thromboembolectomy.[2,9,14,15]

Initial laboratory studies should include electrolytes, blood urea nitrogen and creatinine, complete blood count, prothrombin time/activated partial thromboplastin time, arterial blood gas, creatine phosphokinase, and urine myoglobin. A 12-lead electrocardiogram should be obtained to diagnose arrhythmias and myocardial ischemia.

Treatment of acidosis and alkalization of the urine is initiated using intravenous sodium bicarbonate, and mannitol is used to reduce the risk of renal failure due to myoglobinuria and ischemic limb reperfusion.

SURGICAL TREATMENT

The timing and method of surgical treatment for acute limb ischemia are greatly dependent on the etiology (embolic versus thrombotic) and severity of the limb ischemia. Embolic patients with a threatened limb are usually more emergent due to the lack of collateral circulation. In contrast, patients with arterial thrombosis and a viable but ischemic limb require preoperative

angiography. There is, however, considerable variation, and each case must be carefully evaluated to determine the best course of treatment.

Acute Arterial Embolus

Most cases of acute embolic arterial occlusion are best treated by emergent thromboembolectomy using a Fogarty embolectomy catheter.[3,14,15] This can frequently be accomplished via a transfemoral approach with a local anesthetic and intravenous sedation. Aortic saddle emboli can be removed using bilateral groin approaches. A No. 4 or No. 5 Fogarty embolectomy catheter is usually appropriate for thromboembolectomy of the distal aorta and iliac arteries. If the transfemoral catheter-based thromboembolectomy is unsuccessful due to the presence of intrinsic aortic lesions, then transperitoneal or retroperitoneal exposure of the aorta under general anesthesia is required. Iliofemoral thromboembolectomy can be accomplished using a No. 4 or No. 3 Fogarty embolectomy catheter. Exposure of common femoral, superficial femoral, and profunda femoris arteries allows passage of a balloon catheter into each artery through an arteriotomy of the common femoral artery. Proximal popliteal artery thromboembolectomy can usually be accomplished using a transfemoral groin exposure.

Occlusion of the distal popliteal artery and its branches may require exposure of the below-knee popliteal artery and proximal tibial vessels to allow individual branch thromboembolectomy. The balloon catheter preferentially enters the peroneal artery in 90% of cases when passed blindly from a transfemoral approach.[16] A No. 3 or No. 2 balloon catheter is used to thromboembolectomize the popliteal artery and, individually, the anterior tibial, posterior tibial, and peroneal arteries. Alternatively, this may be accomplished via the transfemoral approach using fluoroscopic guidance with adjunctive use of a guidewire and the "thru-lumen" Fogarty embolectomy catheter or by slightly "bending" the tip of the conventional Fogarty embolectomy catheter (Fig. 25–3). The thru-lumen Fogarty catheter may also be used to infuse thrombolytic agents into the distal extremity arteries to assist in opening small vessels.

Exposure of the posterior and anterior tibial arteries at the ankle may be required if the distal tibial branches are occluded. This allows manipulation of the balloon catheter beyond the area of obstruction. A transverse arteriotomy of the distal tibial vessel may be required if simple manipulation of the distal tibial artery fails to allow the passage of the balloon catheter introduced through the below-knee popliteal artery arteriotomy. A No. 2 balloon catheter is passed distally via a transverse arteriotomy in the distal tibial vessel at the ankle level, followed by the infusion of thrombolytic agents. The distal transverse arteriotomy is

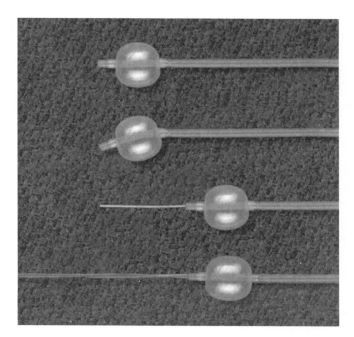

Figure 25–3. The conventional Fogarty catheter (above) may be directed by gently bending and shaping the tip of the catheter. The Fogarty thru-lumen balloon catheter (below) allows adjunctive guidewire use and distal infusion.

closed with interrupted 7-0 Prolene suture. The need for concomitant fasciotomy must be individualized, but early operative intervention will minimize the necessity for compartmental decompression.

Fogarty thromboembolectomy for embolic disease is very effective, but proper technique is essential. Balloon inflation and catheter retraction should be performed by the same surgeon to provide tactile feedback to reduce the risk of injury to the artery. Inflation of the balloon should begin as the catheter is being withdrawn to avoid overdistention and injury to the vessel wall. Saline should be used for balloon inflation, as it provides better feedback for proper inflation pressure. However, air is the preferred inflation medium in the No. 2 and No. 3 Fogarty catheters. A transverse arteriotomy is used during thromboembolectomy procedures for embolic occlusions if minimal atherosclerosis is present. It is then closed primarily at the termination of the procedure. Conversely if significant atherosclerosis is present, a vertical arteriotomy is utilized and then closed with a patch at the termination of the case. It is essential to asses the adequacy of the revascularization following the thromboembolectomy. Backbleeding and failure to recover any further distal thrombus are unreliable predictors of adequate revascularization.[8,14,17] Doppler evaluation of the distal pulses and clinical evaluation of the distal extremity perfusion are essential to assess the completeness of the procedure. Completion angiography or angioscopy is a helpful adjunct to ensure an adequate thromboembolectomy and limb salvage because 35 to 40% of thromboembo-

lectomies have been shown to be incompelte.[18] It is also imperative to address the underlying cardiac condition and continue anticoagulation in the postoperative period.

Acute Thrombotic Occlusion

Acute thrombosis of a native artery or a bypass graft frequently requires more extensive arterial reconstruction to restore adequate perfusion. Fortunately, the majority of acute thrombotic occlusions present with a viable ischemic extremity and therefore are able to undergo initial arteriography followed by urgent intervention. It is preferable to avoid emergency operative interventions in this patient population. Thrombolysis may be useful in identifying the underlying lesion that led to the thrombosis. It is essential to ascertain the underlying etiology of the thrombosis because thrombolysis as the sole treatment for thrombotic limb ischemia is associated with a very high rate of rethrombosis.[18,19] In certain cases, such as thrombosis of a popliteal artery aneurysm, thrombolysis may improve the outflow, thus making the bypass conduit more likely to remain patent.[20]

A conventional Fogarty balloon embolectomy catheter is quite effective in removing fresh clots within an artery, but removal of old thrombus with concurrent atherosclerosis, or thrombus within a synthetic graft, may require the use of new modifications of the Fogarty balloon catheter. One such variation is the latex-covered adherent clot catheter (ACC), which is used for removing adherent thrombus from diseased atherosclerotic native vessels, areas of anastomosis, and synthetic bypass grafts (Fig. 25–4). The ACC allows a more vigorous thrombectomy to be performed without increased risk of vessel injury. It is inserted in its low-profile mode and retracted in its expanded mode to remove more tenacious thrombus. Similarly, a graft thrombectomy catheter (GTC) uses stiffer, shorter, non-latex-covered spirals, making it suitable for graft thromboembolectomy (Fig. 25–5). This allows for even more vigorous clot removal than can be attained with the ACC and is specifically designed for use in thrombosed synthetic grafts. For example, a thrombosed suprainguinal synthetic bypass graft (ie, aortofemoral bypass limb occlusion) may be thrombectomized using GTC. If successful, thrombectomy of an aortofemoral bypass (AFB) graft and possible revision of the outflow, if needed, is a much simpler operation than revision of the entire AFB graft. These specialized thrombectomy catheters (ACC and GTC) may allow in situ thrombosis to be treated via a minimally invasive approach and avoid open endarterctomy or bypass grafting. Patients with graft thrombosis, especially prosthetic conduits, are usually best approached via the distal anastomosis.

Thrombosis of an infrainguinal autogenous bypass graft usually requires placement of a new graft. When

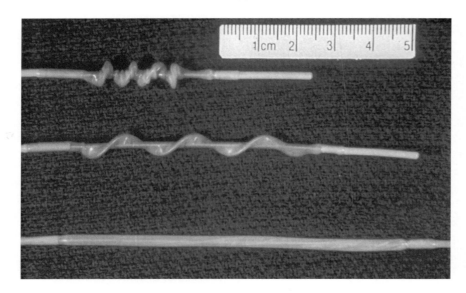

Figure 25–4. The ACC allows more vigorous clot removal but minimizes vessel injury due to the latex coating on the end of the catheter.

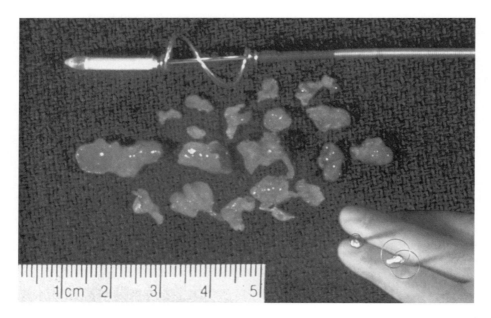

Figure 25–5. The GTC is specifically designed for use in prosthetic grafts and the extraction of mature thrombus, pannus, or pseudointima.

acute graft thrombosis is recognized within a few days of the event, thrombolysis may help delineate the underlying graft lesion that resulted in acute thrombosis. Identified isolated lesions may be amenable to local surgical treatment (ie, endarterectomy, patch angioplasty), thus preserving the bypass conduit. Graft thrombosis presenting in a delayed manner or diffusely diseased grafts are best managed by the placement of a new bypass graft. An autogenous vein graft, preferably greater saphenous vein, is the conduit of choice. In the absence of a suitable autogenous saphenous vein or arm veins, a polytetrafluoroethylene (PTFE) graft may be used as the bypass conduit. Ultimately, the type of reconstruction performed for acute limb ischemia depends on multiple factors including the anatomic site of disease, the overall medical condition of the patient, and the conduit available for possible bypass

grafting. The adjunctive use of intraoperative thrombolytics and the necessity for a fasciotomy must also be considered in patients with extensive thrombosis and possible compartment syndrome.

SURGICAL RESULTS

Acute Arterial Embolus

The surgical management and outcome of acute limb ischemia secondary to embolic disease were significantly changed with the introduction of the Fogarty embolectomy catheter in 1963.[21] Multiple studies have documented the dramatic decrease in morbidity and mortality and the increased limb salvage rate.[22,23] Present results show a limb salvage rate of 80 to 95%, with a mortality rate varying from 5 to 20%.[2,11,14,15] These differences reflect the heterogeneity of the

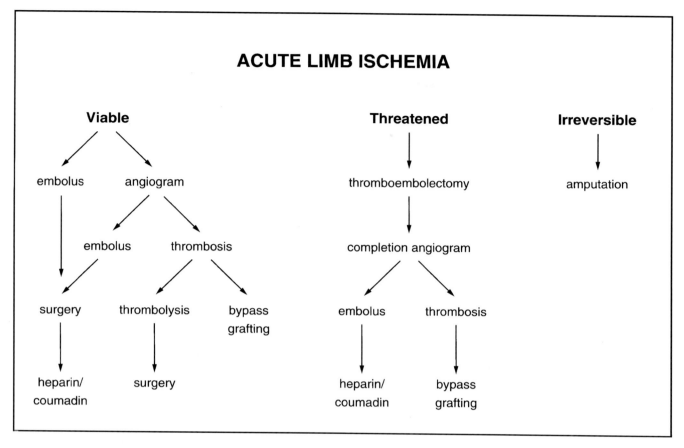

Figure 25–6. Flow diagram for the treatment of acute limb ischemia. A careful history and physical examination are the key to initial evaluation and treatment, allowing urgent or emergent intervention.

patients in the various series in terms of variables such as comorbidities, site of embolus, and degree of ischemia. However, the most significant factor in all series that directly accounts for the continued high mortality rate is the extent of the underlying cardiac disease.[8,11,14,22]

Acute Thrombotic Occlusion

The results of surgical intervention in acute thrombotic limb ischemia are also quite variable, but a definite trend toward improved outcomes has been achieved with continued improvements in diagnostic, operative, and medical management.[2,24,25] The variability in outcome is due to the numerous confounding factors including extent of peripheral vascular disease, anatomic location of the disease process, comorbidities, and degree of ischemia at the time of presentation.[2,24,25] Overall, the surgical results among patients with thrombotic limb ischemia in comparison to patients with embolic disease tend to show a decreased mortality rate but a lower rate of limb salvage. This reflects the relative reduction in the degree of associated coronary artery disease and the increased incidence of peripheral vascular disease in this patient

cohort. Limb salvage rates are 70 to 87%, with mortality rates of 3 to 20%.[2,24,25] The severity of limb ischemia at presentation has been shown to be the best predictor of limb salvage in this patient group.[8,24,26]

SUMMARY

Patients with embolic limb ischemia are effectively and safely treated with balloon catheter thromboembolectomy. Perioperative heparin therapy reduces the mortality and improves limb salvage. Preoperative arteriography is an important diagnostic tool in patients with acute thrombosis of native atherosclerotic vessels or bypass grafts. Thrombolytic agents may help identify the culprit lesion and therefore reduce the magnitude of surgery in patients with mild to moderate ischemia. However, thrombolysis is only an adjunct to definitive surgical treatment in our experience. Surgical revascularization, especially with the advent of more minimally invasive approaches, remains the treatment of choice for acute thrombotic limb ischemia. The algorithm for surgical management of acute limb ischemia is summarized in Figure 25–6.

REFERENCES

1. Blaisdell RW, Steele M, Allen RE. Management of acute lower extremity arterial ischemia due to embolism and thrombosis. *Surgery* 1978;84:822–834.

2. Mills JL, Porter JM. Acute limb ischemia. In: Porter JM, Taylor LM Jr, eds. *Basic Data Underlying Clinical Decision Making in Vascular Surgery.* St Louis: Quality Medical; 1994:134–136.

3. Fogarty TJ. Management of arterial emboli. *Surg Clin North Am* 1979;59:749–759.

4. Jivegaard L, Holm J, Shersten T. The outcome in arterial thrombosis misdiagnosed as arterial embolism. *Acta Chir Scand* 1986;152:251–256.

5. Cambria RP, Abbott WM. Acute arterial thrombosis of the lower extremity: its natural history contrasted with arterial embolism. *Arch Surg* 1984;119:784–787.

6. McPhail NV, Fratesi SJ, Barger GG. Management of acute thromboembolic limb ischemia. *Surgery* 1983;93:381–385.

7. Meier GH, Brewster DC. Acute arterial thrombosis. In: Bergan JJ, ed. *Vascular Surgical Emergencies.* Orlando, FL: Grune & Stratton; 1987;499–515.

8. Brewster DC. Acute peripheral arterial occlusion. *Cardiol Clin* 1991;9:497–513.

9. Elliott JP, Hageman JH, Szilagyi E, et al. Arterial embolization: problems of source, multiplicity, recurrence, and delayed treatment. *Surgery* 1980;88:833–845.

10. Fann JI, Sarris GE, Mitchell RS, et al. Treatment of patients with aortic dissection presenting with peripheral vascular complications. *Ann Surg* 1990;212:705–713.

11. Brewster DC, Chin AK, Hermann GD, Fogarty TJ. Arterial thromboembolism. In: Rutherford RB, ed. *Vascular Surgery.* Philadelphia: WB Saunders; 1995:647–667.

12. Perry MO. Acute limb ischemia. In: Rutherford RB, ed. *Vascular Surgery.* Philadelphia: WB Saunders; 1995:641–647.

13. Rutherford RB, Flanigan DP, Gupta SK, et al. Suggested standards for reports dealing with lower extremity ischemia. *J Vasc Surg* 1986;4:80–94.

14. Panetta T, Thompson JE, Talkington CM, et al. Arterial embolectomy: A 34-year experience with 400 cases. *Surg Clin North Am* 1986;66:339–353.

15. Dale WA. Differential management of acute peripheral arterial ischemia. *J Vasc Surg* 1984;1:269–278.

16. Short D, Vaughn GD, Jachimzyk J, et al. The anatomic basis for the occasional failure of the transfemoral balloon catheter thromboembolectomy. *Ann Surg* 1979;190:555–556.

17. Beard JD. Embolectomy and operative thrombolysis for acute ischemia of the lower limb. In: Greenhalgh RM, Hollier LH, eds. *Emergency Vascular Surgery.* London: WB Saunders; 1992:411–424.

18. Plecha FR, Pories WJ. Intraoperative angiography in the immediate assessment of arterial reconstruction. *Arch Surg* 1972;105:902–907.

19. Faggioli GL, Peer RM, Pedrini L, et al. Failure of thrombolytic therapy to improve long-term vascular patency. *J Vasc Surg* 1994;19:289–297.

20. Carpenter JP, Barker CF, Roberts B, et al. Popliteal artery aneurysms: current management and outcome. Vol. 19, No. 1. *J Vasc Surg.* 1994:65–73.

21. Fogarty TJ, Cranley JJ, Krause RJ, et al. A method for extraction of arterial emboli and thrombi. *Surg Gynecol Obstet* 1963;116:241–244.

22. Abbott WM, Maloney RD, McCabe CC, Lee CE, Wirthlin LS. Arterial embolism: a 44 year perspective. *Am J Surg* 1982;143:460–464.

23. Baxter-Smith D, Ashton F, Slaney G. Peripheral arterial embolism. *J Cardiovasc Surg* 1988;33:453–457.

24. Yeager RA, Moneta GL, Taylor LM Jr, Hamre DW, McConnell DB, Porter JM. Surgical management of severe acute lower extremity ischemia. *J Vasc Surg* 1992;15:385–393.

25. Edwards JE, Taylor LM, Porter JM. Treatment of failed lower extremity bypass grafts with new autogenous vein bypass grafting. *J Vasc Surg* 1990;11:136–145.

26. Felix WR, Sigel B, Gunther L. The significance for morbidity and mortality of Doppler-absent pedal pulses. *J Vasc Surg* 1987;5:849–855.

26

Antithrombotic and Antiplatelet Therapy: Practical Pharmacologic Considerations

Sophie M. Lanzkron, M.D.
William R. Bell, M.D.

Pharmacologic therapy is a useful adjunct to the surgical and endovascular treatment of arterial disease. However, the decision to initiate antithrombotic therapy must take into account the risks of thrombosis and hemorrhage. Therefore, a basic understanding of each drug's indications, mechanisms of action, and methods used to monitor its therapeutic effects is paramount in diminishing these risks. This chapter will review these issues as they apply to the most commonly used antithrombotic and antiplatelet agents, as well as some of the newer agents available to treat and prevent thrombotic events.

ANTIPLATELET AGENTS

Aspirin

The antiplatelet activity of aspirin is related to its ability to impair prostaglandin synthesis, specifically prostaglandin H synthase. This enzyme is required for the first step in prostaglandin synthesis, the conversion of arachidonate to prostaglandin H_2. Prostaglandin H synthase is present in two isoenzymes: type I, found in platelets and most other tissues, and type II. Aspirin irreversibly acetylates a portion of the type 1 isoenzyme, causing loss of its cyclo-oxygenase activity. It is this loss that leads to the decreased formation of a variety of vasoactive substances, including thromboxane A_2, prostaglandin E_2, and prostacyclin. Inhibition of thromboxane A_2 formation, which normally causes platelet aggregation, is believed to be the mechanism by which aspirin exerts its antiplatelet affects.[1] Because platelets are not equipped for RNA synthesis, they are unable to replenish the acetylated enzyme with a functional prostaglandin H synthase. This explains the prolonged effect (7 to 10 days) of one dose of aspirin on platelet function, which corresponds to the average life span of the platelet. There is a gradual recovery of platelet function over this time period due to the release of new, unaffected, non-acetylated platelets from the bone marrow.[2]

The indications for the use of aspirin in the treatment of vascular disorders have been widely studied. In 1994 the Antiplatelet Trialists' Collaboration published a review of randomized trials in which antiplatelet therapy was compared to control or in which one antiplatelet regimen was compared to another in maintaining vascular patency.[3] They concluded that antiplatelet therapy significantly decreased the risk of vascular occlusions in patients with coronary artery grafts, peripheral artery disease, and hemodialysis shunts.[3] They also found a significant decrease in the number of patients developing postoperative pulmonary embolisms when treated with antiplatelet agents.[4] In high-risk patients, the use of medium-dose aspirin therapy (75 to 325 mg/day) has been shown to decrease mortality from all vascular causes by one-sixth.[5] Additionally, low-dose aspirin therapy (75 mg/day) has been found to reduce the number of immediate (within 1 week) postoperative neurologic events following carotid surgery.[6] The issue of the optimum dose of aspirin was also addressed by the Antiplatelet Trialists' Collaboration. They were unable to find any evidence that high doses (160 to 325 mg/day) of aspirin were more efficacious than medium doses (75 to 325 mg/day) in preventing thrombosis.[5]

There are several important side effects of aspirin therapy, including renal dysfunction and hypertension.

Supported in part by NIH Research Grant HL 36260 from the NHLBI of the National Institutes of Health, Bethesda, MD.
W.R.B. is the Hubert E. and Anne E. Rogers Scholar in Academic Medicine and the Edyth Harris Lucas–Clara Lucas Lynn Professor Hematology—The Johns Hopkins University School of Medicine.

These effects are not commonly seen because at low doses the effect of aspirin on renal synthesis of vasodilatory prostaglandins is minimal.[1] Gastrointestinal side effects, however, are quite common. These range from mild gastric erosions to frank ulcers and can lead to hemorrhage. These bleeding events have been shown to be dose dependent[7,8] but even at lower doses (75 mg/day) the risk of gastrointestinal bleeding is higher than in controls.[9] Fatalities from hemorrhage with aspirin use have been reported.[10] The risk of bleeding with the use of aspirin has also been evaluated in the perioperative setting. In a Veterans Administration cooperative study, patients given aspirin 12 hours prior to coronary artery bypass surgery had a significantly increased rate of postoperative bleeding and required reoperation for control of bleeding more often than patients in a control group.[11] When aspirin was given immediately after surgery, no increase in bleeding was demonstrated, and early graft patency was improved compared to that of patients who received no aspirin.[12]

The management of patients who have received aspirin and require surgery or are bleeding is relatively straightforward. Ideally, any patient who is going to surgery should stop taking aspirin 7 to 10 days prior to the procedure. However, if that is not possible, measurement of a template bleeding time can be useful. If the bleeding time is markedly prolonged that is, more than 10 to 12 minutes, then a platelet transfusion may be necessary. Replacement of approximately 25% of the patient's total platelet mass with normal platelets, should restore near-normal platelet function.

Dipyrimadole

Dipyrimadole is a platelet adhesion inhibitor whose mechanism of action is not clearly defined. Aspirin and dipyrimadole have been evaluated together in several studies.[11,13,14] In one report, dipyrimadole with aspirin, at a dose of 225 mg/day, decreased the frequency of saphenous vein graft closure compared to placebo.[14] In randomized studies, dipyridamole plus aspirin has been shown to be at least equivalent to,[15] or better than,[14] aspirin alone in improving graft patency. The side effects of dipyrimadole are minor, tend to be transient, and can be treated symptomatically.

Indobufen

Although both aspirin and indobufen exert their antiplatelet effects by blocking platelet cyclooxygenase, indobufen does so in a reversible manner. Therefore, its effect is short-lived, with normal platelet function returning within 24 hours after discontinuation of drug therapy. In randomized studies, indobufen, at doses of 200 mg twice a day, was shown to be as effective as aspirin and dipyrimidole in maintaining graft patency and was associated with fewer bleeding complications.[16,17] It also significantly improved walking distances in patients with intermittent claudication[18] and reduced the risk of ischemic events in patients with heart disease[19] compared to placebo-treated patients. These studies suggest a side effect profile similar to that of aspirin. Given its short half-life, stopping indobufen 1 day prior to surgery should be sufficient to avoid bleeding complications. If this is not possible, an evaluation for platelet transfusion therapy should be performed, as previously described for aspirin.

Ticlopidine

Ticlopidine is a thienopyridine derivative that has been shown to impair the aggregation of platelets in response to a variety of stimuli including adenine diphosphate, epinephrine, thrombin, collagen, and arachidonic acid.[20] It has also been shown to inhibit shear-induced platelet aggregation, which is thought to be a mechanism of thrombosis in stenotic arteries.[21] After administration, the inhibition of aggregation is delayed for 24 to 48 hours.[17] The half-life of ticlopidine after repeat dosing is 4 to 5 days. Ticlopidine has been demonstrated to reduce the frequency of stroke[17] and is therefore approved for the treatment of patients with cerebral ischemia. When tested against placebo, ticlopidine, at a dose of 250 mg twice daily, has been shown to significantly decrease the frequency of graft occlusion within the first 6 months after coronary artery bypass surgery.[22] Additionally, it has been associated with improved walking ability and ankle systolic blood pressure, as well as with a decrease in vascular complications, among patients with intermittent claudication.[23-25]

The most serious side effect of ticlopidine is severe reversible neutropenia, which occurs in about 1.0% of patients. Isolated thrombocytopenia has also been reported, and more recently, several case reports in the literature have clearly demonstrated an association between the use of ticlopidine and the development of thrombotic thrombocytopenic purpura-hemolytic uremic syndrome.[26-29] Therefore, the patient's blood counts must be closely monitored, with a complete blood count performed every 2 weeks for the first 3 months of therapy.[30] Given its side effect profile, ticlopidine can only be recommended at this time for the prevention of stroke in patients who are intolerant of aspirin. The drug can be monitored by measuring the bleeding time. Little is known about reversing its activity. Among healthy subjects receiving ticlopidine, 1-deamino-(8-D-arginine)-vasopressin (DDAVP) decreases the bleeding time,[21] but whether this decreases clinical bleeding is unknown.

Platelet Glycoprotein IIB/IIIa Inhibition

Glycoprotein IIB/IIIa (GP IIb/IIIa) is a platelet membrane receptor. It plays an important role in platelet aggregation. When activated, GP IIb/IIIa undergoes a conformational change that allows it to bind to fibrinogen[31] and then cross-link adjacent platelets, forming a platelet plug. In 1985 Coller et al produced a murine monoclonal antibody against GP IIb/IIIa called 7E3 and in a canine model demonstrated the antithrombotic effect of this drug.[32] Inhibition of platelet function is dose dependent, with maximum inhibition seen at doses of 0.25 to 0.30 mg/kg.[33]

In humans studies, the uses of 7E3 in conjunction with heparin and aspirin can reduce the incidence of myocardial infarction in patients with unstable angina.[34] In the EPIC trial, a randomized study comparing 7E3 with placebo in 2099 patients undergoing coronary angioplasty or athrectomy, a significant decrease in ischemic complications was seen in patients who received a bolus injection (0.25 mg/kg) or a bolus injection with a 12-hour infusion (10 μg/min) of the drug,[35] although there was an increase in bleeding complications in the treatment group. On further evaluation, it was demonstrated that among patients who underwent emergent coronary artery bypass surgery (2.8% of patients enrolled in the study), no significant difference in bleeding complications was observed in the patients who received 7E3 versus those who received aspirin, heparin, or placebo.[36] Additional studies are required to fully assess the bleeding risk with this agent.

Other Antiplatelet Agents

Prostaglandin E_1 (PGE$_1$) increases platelet cyclic AMP levels, which inhibits platelet function.[37] In clinical studies in patients with peripheral vascular disease, PGE$_1$ (40 μg over 2 hours two times a day), in combination with exercise, increased the symptom-free walking distance by 604% during a 4-week period of treatment.[38] This was a significant increase compared to either exercise alone or exercise in combination with intravenous pentoxifylline. The effects of the drug decreased over time, but at 1 year there was still a 149% increase in walking distance compared to baseline. Other studies, however, have failed to show any long-term beneficial effect from PGE$_1$ therapy treatment in peripheral vascular disease.[39]

Pentoxifylline is a methylxanthine with weak antithrombotic activity and is approved for use in patients with intermittent claudication. The data from randomized studies with respect to its clinical usefulness are inconclusive.[39] Picotamide is an antiplatelet agent that inhibits the enzyme thromboxane synthase, thereby blocking the conversion of prostaglandin H_2 (PGH$_2$) to thromboxane A_2,[39] as well as acting as an antagonist of the thromboxane A_2 receptor.[40] In a randomized study, picotamide reduced cardiovascular complications, compared to placebo, in patients with peripheral vascular disease.[40]

Dextran (low molecular weight dextran) is a branched polysaccharide composed of glucose units with a molecular mass between 65,000 and 80,000 daltons. Although its mechanism of action is not clear, its effects appear to be mediated by alterations in platelet membrane function. Although it has been shown to improve lower extremity graft patency for the first week after surgery, compared to no antiplatelet therapy,[41] the effect is short-lived.

ANTITHROMBOTIC AGENTS

Unfractionated Heparin

Unfractionated heparin is mixture of polysaccharides ranging in molecular mass from 3,000 to 30,000 daltons. Its anticoagulant effect is mediated primarily by its binding to antithrombin III. Once bound, heparin accelerates the inhibitory effects of antithrombin III on thrombin, as well as on other factors in the coagulation cascade including factors IXa, Xa, XIa, and XIIa.[42] This inhibitory activity blocks thrombin generation. Without the ability to produce thrombin, no fibrin is generated and therefore no new clot is formed. The half-life of heparin is less than 90 minutes. Consequently, the best method of administration, to ensure constant levels of anticoagulation, is by the intravenous route. Subcutaneous injection is usually reserved for prophylaxis and is not used for active therapy.

The indications for the use of heparin can be divided into two categories. The first is to prevent progression and propagation of existing thrombi, as in the treatment of deep vein thrombosis, pulmonary embolism, arterial thrombosis, and as adjunctive therapy in patients with acute myocardial infarction. The second major use of heparin is for prophylaxis against the formation of thrombosis in high-risk patients, such as those with atrial fibrillation, prolonged bed rest, or during and after cardiovascular surgery.

The test most commonly used for monitoring the adequacy of heparin therapy is the activated partial thromboplastin time (aPTT). For routine therapy, the aPTT is usually kept between 1.5 and 2.0 times normal baseline values. The major complication seen with heparin therapy is hemorrhage. A recent review of the risks associated with heparin therapy demonstrated that, when it is used alone, the rate of bleeding is less than 5%.[43] When it is used in combination with thrombolytic therapy, however, an increase in intracranial bleeding has been seen.[43,44] With discontinuation of heparin therapy, the anticoagulant effects diminish significantly within 90 minutes. If reversal of anticoagulation is needed more emergently, protamine sulfate, at a dose of 1 mg/100 units of unfractionated heparin, will normalize the aPTT. The side effects of protamine sulfate are significant, including hypotension and anaphylaxis. Given these side effects and the short half-life of heparin, protamine reversal therapy is usually reserved for episodes of life-threatening hemorrhage or in a controlled setting, such as the operating room.

Low Molecular Weight Heparin (LMWH)

LMWHs are portions of unfractionated heparin that retain the ability to bind to antithrombin III. LMWHs have a longer half-life than unfractionated heparin because of their lower affinity for heparin-binding proteins and endothelial cells.[45] The anticoagulant response to weight-adjusted doses is less variable with LMWH than with unfractionated heparin.[45] This, along with its longer half-life, allows the medication to be given subcutaneously once or twice daily without the need for laboratory monitoring.

Most of the experience with LMWHs has been in the prevention of deep vein thrombosis (DVT). LMWHs have been shown to significantly decrease (60 to 90%) the risk of DVT, compared to placebo, in high-risk patients.[45] Other studies have demonstrated that LMWH is at least as effective as unfractionated heparin in preventing DVT in patients after cardio-vascular accident (CVA)[46] and following hip surgery.[47] One study demonstrated the effectiveness of LMWH over warfarin in decreasing the incidence of DVT in postsurgical patients.[48] However, a higher risk of bleeding was seen in the LMWH-treated group.[48] Two recent studies have shown that LMWH can be used to treat proximal DVT at home as successfully as it is treated with unfractionated heparin in a hospital.[49,50] These studies, however, excluded patients with complicated medical problems.

As with unfractionated heparin, the major complication of LMWH therapy is bleeding. Because LMWH has a longer half-life than unfractionated heparin, discontinuation of therapy may not be sufficient to limit excessive bleeding. In a recent study examining the ability of protamine to reverse the anticoagulant effect of LMWH, a significant impairment in coagulation remained despite the administration of the recommended dose of protamine.[51] Further studies are necessary to confirm the usefulness and safety of LMWH before it can be recommended for routine use in cases of acute thrombosis.

Hirudin

Hirudin is produced from the salivary glands of the European leech. This agent is a specific inhibitor of thrombin and, unlike heparin, does not require a cofactor for activity. The half-life of hirudin is about 1 hour and, as with heparin, the adequacy of therapy can be monitored by measuring the aPTT.[52] Hirudin has been shown to produce more consistent levels of anticoagulation when compared with heparin.[53] This agent has been used in a number of studies of patients with unstable angina undergoing percutaneous transluminal coronary angioplasty and with acute coronary syndromes. However, earlier studies had to be stopped, and the dose of hirudin adjusted, because of the increase in bleeding complications.[52,54]

Hirulog

Hirulog was designed based on the structure of hirudin. Because it forms only a transient complex with thrombin, it has a shorter half-life than hirudin.[52] In a large, randomized study of the safety of hirulog versus heparin, hirulog was shown to have a better safety profile, with fewer hemorrhagic events than heparin.[55] It appears to be as effective as heparin in decreasing the ischemic complications in patients undergoing angioplasty for postinfarct angina.[56] These direct antithrombins, hirudin and hirulog, are relatively new agents that will require further study before they become part of the mainstream therapy for treatment of thrombosis.

Warfarin

Warfarin is a vitamin K antagonist. It interferes with the cyclic interconversion of vitamin K epoxide to vitamin K to vitamin KH_2 and then back to vitamin K epoxide. Without the reduced form of vitamin K, posttranslational carboxylation of glutamate residues on vitamin K–dependent proteins does not occur. There are several vitamin K–dependent coagulant proteins including prothrombin (Factor II), factors VII, IX, and X and the anticoagulant proteins C and protein S. Because factor VII has the shortest half-life, the therapeutic effect of warfarin is primarily seen by measuring the prothrombin time (PT). To standardize the degree of anticoagulation with warfarin, the international normalized ratio (INR) was developed. The INR uses a correction factor, the international sensitivity index (ISI), to account for the variability in the different tissue thromboplastins used to perform the PT assay. The formula to calculate INR is

$$INR = (PT\ ratio)^{ISI}$$

The American College of Chest Physicians recommends using the INR to manage patients receiving warfarin therapy.[57]

Warfarin therapy has been shown to be effective in the prophylaxis of DVT in postoperative patients.[58–60] Two studies have shown that mini-dose warfarin, 1 mg a day, is ineffective in preventing thrombosis in patients undergoing orthopedic surgery.[61,62] The recommended range of INR for the prevention of venous thrombosis is between 2.0 and 3.0. Additionally, this level of anticoagulation is recommended for the treatment of patients with established thrombosis after initial treatment with heparin, for chronic atrial fibrillation, for prosthetic heart valves, and after acute myocardial infarction to prevent peripheral arterial embolism.[57,63]

Several studies have looked at the risk of bleeding in patients receiving oral anticoagulation.[64–66] Two of these studies were performed before INRs were used routinely, and therefore the PT ratio was employed (where PT ratio = patient's PT/control).[65,66] Both studies showed a significant increase in bleeding in patients whose PT ratio was greater than 2.0. Other risk factors for increased bleeding while taking warfarin include older age (>65 years) and a history of CVA or other comorbid conditions.[64,65] The risk of bleeding appears to be highest in the first month of therapy and decreases thereafter.[64,65] To reverse warfarin's anticoagulation effect in nonemergent situations, AquaMEPHYTON (vitamin K_1) can be given subcutaneously or intravenously at a dose of 10 mg. If given intravenously, the drug must be administered slowly. Reversal with vitamin K therapy will make subsequent reinstitution of warfarin anticoagulation more difficult. Therefore, any patient with a strong indication for anticoagulation must be maintained on intravenous heparin. If the patient receiving warfarin anticoagulation is acutely bleeding or requires emergent surgery, the effects of warfarin can be temporarily reversed with the use of fresh frozen plasma (FFP). FFP will supply the necessary carboxylated coagulation factors. The effect of FFP, however, lasts for only 2 to 3 hours, and therefore repeat infusions may be required.

THROMBOLYTICS

Thrombolytics function, in general, by converting plasminogen to plasmin, which in turn digests fibrin into fibrin degradation products, thereby dissolving thrombi. The mode of action of each lytic agent is slightly different. Streptokinase (SK) binds to plasminogen in the circulation, as well as in the thrombus, and undergoes an autocatalytic reaction to activate plasminogen.[67] Anisoylated plasminogen activator complex (APSAC) is a derivative of the SK–plasminogen complex.[67] Urokinase (UK) binds preferentially to plasminogen in the thrombus and promotes the conversion of plasminogen to plasmin.[67] Tissue plasminogen activator (r-TPA) may weakly bind to fibrin and thus localize to the thrombus, where the bound fibrin increases the conversion of plasminogen to plasmin.[67] Each of these thrombolytic agents can be monitored with the thrombin time. Because all of the coagulation proteins are affected, bleeding may potentially complicate treatment with all of these agents.[68]

Thrombolytic therapy has become the standard of care for the treatment of myocardial infarction. In a large trial (GUSTO) that compared SK with subcutaneous heparin, SK with intravenous heparin, r-TPA with intravenous heparin and a combination of SK, r-TPA, and intravenous heparin, the r-TPA group was found to have a marginally significant decrease in mortality when compared to the other groups.[44] However, there was an increase in hemorrhagic strokes in the r-TPA group. The overall benefit did, however, favor the r-TPA group, with an additional 10 lives saved per 1000 treated in the r-TPA group compared with any of the SK regimens. The use of thrombolytics in peripheral artery occlusion has also been extensively studied (see Chapters 28, 29).

Thrombolytic therapy is monitored by detecting the degradation of fibrinogen and fibrin, tests that assess the activity of the fibrinolytic system. Due to its simplicity as well as its rapid turnaround time, the thrombin time is one of the most useful techniques for monitoring fibrinolytic activity.[69] After a baseline thrombin time measurement is made and thrombolytic therapy instituted, a repeat thrombin time should be performed. Four to 6 hours after the initiation of thrombolytic therapy, a level that is prolonged 1.5 to 5.0 times the baseline value is considered adequate. The thrombin time should be monitored every 12 hours thereafter as long as therapy continues. No test available at this time has been shown to correlate the level of fibrinolytic activity with thrombolytic efficacy or with the frequency of hemorrhagic complications.[69]

There are two absolute contraindications to the use of thrombolytic therapy: (1) active bleeding and (2) central nervous system conditions occurring within 1 to 2 months. The central nervous system conditions includes infarction, hemorrhage, trauma, surgery, and primary or metastatic neoplastic disease.[70] R-TPA is contraindicated in any patient who has ever experienced a central nervous system condition of any type. Relative contraindications include surgery or internal trauma with 10 days, gastrointestinal ulcers, subacute bacterial endocarditis, atrial fibrillation with intracardiac thrombi, severe hypertension, pregnancy or the first 10 days postpartum, hepatorenal insufficiency, progressive cavitating lung disease, and an allergy to thrombolytic agents.

As previously mentioned, bleeding can complicate treatment with all thrombolytic agents, the greatest magnitude of bleeding occurring with the use of r-TPA. Most bleeding occurs at sites of vascular puncture, but hemorrhage can occur anywhere. As with the other short-acting agents, when bleeding occurs, initial therapy should be to discontinue the thrombolytic agent. The duration of the coagulopathy will depend on the agent given and the biochemical status of the patient. The reversal of thrombolytic therapy is based on the ability to restore the normal coagulation proteins that were degraded by the lytic agent, specifically fibrinogen. If the patient is bleeding and the fibrinogen concentration is less than 75 to 100 mg/dL, cryoprecipitate or FFP should be administered. The goal of this therapy is to obtain a fibrinogen concentration of at least 100 mg/dL. One bag of cryoprecipitate will raise the fibrinogen concentration by 5 to 7 mg/dL in a 70-kg patient. Antifibrinolytic agents may also be helpful in decreasing bleeding in patients after thrombolytic therapy, especially if emergent surgery is required. Aprotinin, a serine protease inhibitor and an antifibrinolytic agent, has been shown to decrease perioperative blood loss in emergent surgeries after thrombolytic therapy.[71-73] Other antifibrinolytic agents, such as epsilon-aminocaproic acid (EACA) and tranexamic acid, are thought to have a mode of action similar to that of aprotinin and are less expensive. A meta-analysis of prophylactic treatment to prevent bleeding in patients after cardiovascular surgery demonstrated no benefit of aprotinin over EACA in preventing bleeding.[74] A randomized study comparing the efficacy of these different agents has yet to be done. For adult patients who bleed after thrombolytic therapy or who are to go to the operating room emergently, a loading dose of 5 g of EACA given with cryoprecipitate is followed by 2 g every 4 hours until bleeding has ceased. Disseminated intravascular coagulation is a contraindication to the use of antifibrinolytic agents, as the administration of these agents may result in vascular thrombosis. Previous concerns that the use of antifibrinolytics with vascular surgery might increase the risk of graft thrombosis have not been realized.[74,75]

REFERENCES

1. Patrono C. Aspirin as an antiplatelet drug. *N Engl J Med* 1994;330:1287–1293.
2. Roth G, Calverley DC. Aspirin, platelets, and thrombosis: theory and practice. *Blood* 1994;83:885–898.
3. Antiplatelet Trialists' Collaboration. Collaborative overview of randomized trials of antiplatelet therapy—II: maintenance of vascular graft patency or arterial patency by antiplatelet therapy. *Br Med J* 1994;308:159–168.
4. Antiplatelet Trialists' Collaboration. Collaborative overview of randomized trials of antiplatelet therapy—III: reduction in venous thrombosis and pulmonary embolism by antiplatelet prophylaxis among surgical and medical patients. *Br Med J* 1994;308:235–246.
5. Antiplatelet Trialists' Collaboration. Collaborative overview of randomized trials of antiplatelet therapy—I: prevention of death, myocardial infarction, and stroke by prolonged antiplatelet therapy in various categories of patients. *Br Med J* 1994;308:81–106.
6. Linblad B, Persson NH, Takolander R, et al. Does Low Dose Acetylsalicylic acid prevent stroke after carotid surgery? A double blind, placebo-controlled randomized trial. *Stroke* 1993;24:1125–1128.
7. Slattery J, Warlow CP, Shorrock CJ, et al. Risks of gastrointestinal bleeding during secondary prevention of vascular events with aspirin—analysis of gastrointestinal bleeding during the UK-TIA Trial. *Gut* 1995;37:509–511.
8. Roderick PJ, Wilkes HC, Meade TW. The gastrointestinal toxicity of aspirin: an overview of randomized controlled trials. *Br J Clin Pharmacol* 1993;35:219–226.
9. Stalnikowicz-Darvasi R. Gastrointestinal bleeding during low-dose aspirin administration for prevention of arterial occlusive events. A critical analysis. *J Clin Gastroenterol* 1995;21:13–16.
10. Lekstrom JA, Bell WR. Aspirin in the prevention of thrombosis. *Medicine* 1991;70:161–178.
11. Sethi GK, Copeland JG, Goldman S, et al. Implications of preoperative administration of aspirin in patients undergoing coronary artery bypass grafting. *J Am Coll Cardiol* 1990;15:15–20.
12. Gavaghan TP, Gebski V, Baron DW. Immediate postoperative aspirin improves vein graft patency early and late after coronary artery bypass graft surgery. A placebo controlled, randomized study. *Circulation* 1991;83:1526–1533.
13. Stein PD, Dalen JE, Goldman S, et al. Antithrombotic therapy in patients with saphenous vein and internal mammary artery bypass grafts. *Chest* 1995;108:424S–430S.
14. Sanz G, Pajarón A, Algería E, et al. Prevention of early aortocoronary bypass occlusion by low-dose aspirin and dipyridamole. *Circulation* 1990;82:765–773.
15. Mulder BJM, Van Der Doef RM, Van Der Wall EE, et al. Effect of various antithrombotic regimens (aspirin, aspirin plus dipyridamole, anticoagulants) on the functional status of patients and grafts one year after coronary artery bypass grafting. *Eur Heart* 1994;15:1129–1134.
16. Rajah SM, Rees M, Walker D, et al. Effects of antiplatelet therapy with indobufen or aspirin-dipyridamole on graft patency one year after coronary artery bypass grafting. *J Thorac Cardiovasc Surg* 1994;107:1146–1453.
17. Hirsh J, Dalen JE, Fuster V, et al. Aspirin and other platelet-active drugs. *Chest* 1994;108:247S–257S.
18. Tonnesen KH, Albuquerque P, Baitsch G, et al. Doubleblind, controlled, multicenter study of indobufen versus placebo in patients with intermittent claudication. *Int Angiol* 1993;12:371–377.
19. Fornaro G, Rossi P, Mantica PG, et al. Indobufen in the prevention of thromboembolic complications in patients with heart disease. A randomized, placebo-controlled, double-blind study. *Circulation* 1993;87:162–164.
20. Di Minno G, Cerbone AM, Mattioli PL, et al. Functionally thrombasthenic state in normal platelets following the administration of ticlopidine. *J Clin Invest* 1985;75:328–338.
21. Cattaneo M, Lombardi R, Bettega D, et al. Shear-induced platelet aggregation is potentiated by desmopressin and inhibited by ticlopidine. *Arterioscler Thromb* 1993;13:393–397.
22. Limet R, David J, Magotteaux, et al. Prevention of aortacoronary bypass graft occlusion: beneficial effect of ticlopidine on early and late patency rates of venous coronary bypass grafts: A double-blind study. *J Thorac Cardiovasc Surg* 1987;94:773–783.
23. Balsano F, Coccheri A, Libertti G, et al. Ticlopidine in the treatment of intermittent claudication: a 21-month double-blind trial. *J Lab Clin Med* 1989;114:84–91.
24. Arcan JC, Blanchard J, Boissel JP, et al. Multicenter double blind study of ticlopidine in the treatment of intermittent claudication and the prevention of it complications. *Angiology* 1988;39:802–809.
25. Janzon L, Bergqvist J, Boberg, M, et al. Prevention of myocardial infarction and stroke in patients with intermittent claudication; effects of ticlopidine. Results from STIMS, the Swedish Ticlopidine Multicentre Study. *J Intern Med* 1990;227:301–308.
26. Page Y, Tardy B, Zeni F, et al. Thrombotic thrombocytopenic purpura related to ticlopidine. *Lancet* 1991;337:774–776.
27. Kovacs MJ, Soong PY, Chin-Yee IH. Thrombotic thrombocytopenic purpura associated with ticlopidine. *Ann Pharmacother* 1993;27:1060–1061.
28. Ellie E. Durrieu C, Besse P, et al. Thrombotic thrombocytopenic purpura associated with ticlopidine. *Stroke* 1992;23:922–923.

29. Capra R, Marciano N, Fieni F. Cerebral hemorrhage and thrombotic thrombocytopenic purpura during ticlopidine treatment; case report. *Acta Neurol Belg* 1992;92:83–87.

30. *1995 Physicians Desk Reference*, Section 5. 49th ed. Montvale, NJ: Medical Economics Data Production Company; 1995:2489.

31. Coutré S, Leung L. Novel antithrombotic therapeutics targeted against platelet glycoprotein IIb/IIIA. *Annu Rev Med* 1995;46:257–265.

32. Coller BS, Folts JD, Scudder LE, et al. Antithrombotic effect of a monoclonal antibody to the platelet glycoprotein IIB/IIIa receptor in an experimental animal model. *Blood* 1985; 68:783–786.

33. Simoons ML, de Boer MJ, van den Brand MJ, et al. Randomized trial of a GPIIb/IIIa platelet receptor blocker in refractory unstable angina. European Cooperative Study Group. *Circulation* 1994;89:596–603.

34. The EPIC Investigators: Use of a monoclonal antibody directed against the platelet glycoprotein IIb/IIIa receptor in high risk coronary angioplasty. *N Engl J Med* 1994;330:956–961.

35. Boehrer JD, Kereiakes DJ, Navetta FI, et al. Effects of profound platelet inhibition with c7E3 before coronary angioplasty on complications of coronary bypass surgery. *Am J Cardiol* 1994;74:1166–1170.

36. Bhattacharya S, Jordan R, Machin S, et al. Blockade of the human platelet GPIIb/IIIa receptor by a murine monoclonal antibody Fab fragment (7E3): potent dose-dependent inhibition of platelet function. *Cardiovasc Drugs Ther* 1995;9:665–675.

37. Harker LA, Fustre V. Pharmacology of platelet inhibitors. *J Am Coll Cardiol* 1986;8:21B–32B.

38. Scheffler P, de la Hamette D, Gross J, et al. Intensive vascular training in stage IIb of peripheral arterial occlusive disease; the additive effects of intravenous prostaglandin E₁ or intravenous pentoxifylline during training. *Circulation* 1994;90:812–822.

39. Clagett GP, Krupski WC. Antithrombotic therapy in peripheral arterial occlusive disease. *Chest* 1995;108:431S–443S.

40. Balsano F, Violi F, and the ADEP Group: Effect of picotamide on the clinical progression of peripheral vascular disease; a double-blind placebo-controlled study. *Circulation* 1993;87:1563–1569.

41. Rutherford RB, Jones DN, Bergentz SE, et al. The efficacy of dextran 40 in preventing early postoperative thrombosis following difficult lower extremity bypass. *J Vasc Surg* 1984;1:765–773.

42. Rosenberg RD, Bauer KA. The heparin-antithrombin system: a natural anticoagulant mechanism. In: Coleman RW, Hirsh J, Marder VJ, Salzman EW, eds. *Hemostasis and Thrombosis: Basic Principles and Clinical Practice*. Philadelphia: JB Lippincott; 3rd ed. 1994:839.

43. Levine NL, Raskob G, Landefeld S, et al. Hemorrhagic complications of anticoagulant treatment. *Chest* 1995;108:276S–290S.

44. The GUSTO Investigators: An international randomized trial comparing four thrombolytic strategies for acute myocardial infarction. *N Engl J Med* 329:673–682.

45. Hirsh J, Levine MN. Low molecular weight heparin. *Blood* 1992;79:1–17.

46. Turpie AG, Gent M, Cote R, et al. A low-molecular-weight heparinoid compared with unfractionated heparin in the prevention of deep vein thrombosis in patients with acute ischemic stroke. A randomized, double-blind study. *Ann Intern Med* 1992;117:353–357.

47. Levine MN, Hirsh J, Turpie AG, et al. Prevention of deep vein thrombosis after elective hip surgery. A randomized trial comparing low molecular weight heparin with standard unfractionated heparin. *Ann Intern Med* 1991;114:545–551.

48. Hull R, Raskob G, Pineo G, et al. A comparison of subcutaneous low-molecular-weight heparin with warfarin sodium for prophylaxis against deep-vein thrombosis after hip or knee implantation. *N Engl J Med* 1993;329:1370–1376.

49. Levine M, Gent M, Hirsh J, et al. A comparison of low-molecular-weight heparin administered primarily at home with unfractionated heparin administered in the hospital for proximal deep-vein thrombosis. *N Engl J Med* 1996;334:677–681.

50. Koopman MMW, Prandoni P, Piovella F, et al. Treatment of venous thrombosis with intravenous unfractionated heparin administered in the hospital as compared with subcutaneous low-molecular-weight heparin administered at home. *N Engl J Med* 1996;334:682–687.

51. Wolz M, Weltermann A, Nieszpaur-Los M, et al. Studies on the neutralizing effects of protamine on unfractionated and low molecular weight heparin (Fragmin) at the site of activation of the coagulation system in man. *Thromb Haemost* 1995;73:439–443.

52. Verstraete M, Zoldhelyi P. Novel antithrombotic drugs in development. *Drugs* 1995;49:856–884.

53. Cannon CP, Braunwald E. Hirudin: initial results in acute myocardial infarction, unstable angina and angioplasty. *J Am Coll Cardiol* 1995;25:30S–37S.

54. The GUSTO Investigators. Randomized trial of intravenous heparin versus recombinant hirudin for acute coronary syndromes. *Circulation* 1994;90:1631–1637.

55. Bittl JA. Comparative safety profiles of hirulog and heparin in patients undergoing coronary angioplasty. *Am Heart J* 1995;130:658–665.

56. Bittl JA, Strony J, Brinker JA. Treatment with Bivalrudin (hirulog) as compared with heparin during coronary angioplasty for unstable angina or postinfarction angina: hirulog angioplasty study investigators. *N Engl J Med* 1995;333:754–759.

57. Hirsh J, Dalen JE, Deykin D, et al. Oral anticoagulants; mechanism of action, clinical effectiveness, and optimal therapeutic range. *Chest* 1995;108:231S–246S.

58. Poller L, Mckernan A, Thomson JM, et al. Fixed minidose warfarin: a new approach to prophylaxis against venous thrombosis after major surgery. *Br Med J* 1987;295:1309–1312.

59. Powers PJ, Gent M, Jay RM, et al. A randomized trial of less intense postoperative warfarin or aspirin therapy in the prevention of venous thromboembolism after surgery for fractured hip. *Arch Intern Med* 1989;149:771–774.

60. Francis CW, Pellegrini VD Jr, Marder VJ, et al. Comparison of warfarin and external pneumatic compression in prevention of venous thrombosis after total hip replacement. *JAMA* 1992;267:2911–2915.

61. Dale C, Gallus A, Wycherley A, et al. Prevention of venous thrombosis with minidose warfarin after joint replacement. *Br Med J* 1991;303:224.

62. Fordyce MJ, Baker AS, Staddon GE. Efficacy of fixed minidose warfarin prophylaxis in total hip replacement. *Br Med J* 1991;303:219–220.

63. Altman R, Rouvier J, Gurfinkel E, et al. Comparison of two levels of anticoagulant therapy in patients with substitute heart valves. *J Thorac Cardiovasc Surg* 1991;101:427–431.

64. Landefeld CS, Goldman L. Major bleeding in outpatients treated with warfarin: incidence and prediction by factors known at the start of outpatient therapy. *Am J Med* 1989;87:144–152.

65. Hylek EM, Singer DE. Risk factors for intracranial hemorrhage in outpatients taking warfarin. *Ann Intern Med* 1994;120:897–902.

66. Fihn SD, McDonell M, Martin D, et al. Risk factors for complications of chronic anticoagulation; a multicenter study. *Ann Intern Med* 1993;118:511–520.

67. Ludlam CA, Bennett B, Fox AA, et al. Guidelines for the use of thrombolytic therapy. *Blood Coag Fibrin* 1995;6:273–285.

68. Califf RM, Topol EJ, et al. Bleeding during thrombolytic therapy for acute myocardial infarction: mechanisms and management. *Ann Intern Med* 1989;111:1010–1022.

69. Bell WR. Laboratory monitoring of thrombolytic therapy. *Clin Lab Med* 1995;15:165–178.

70. Bell WR. Hemostasis and thrombosis. In: Hoffman R, Benz EJ Jr, Shattil SJ, Furie B, Cohen HJ, Silberstein LE, eds. *Hematology: Basic Principles and Practice.* 2nd ed. New York: Churchill Livingstone; 1995:1824.

71. Van Doorn CA, Munsch CM, Cowan JC. Cardiac rupture after thrombolytic therapy: the use of aprotinin to reduce blood loss after surgical repair. *Br Heart J* 1992;67:504–505.

72. Efstratiadis T, Munsch C, Crossman D, et al. Aprotinin used in emergency coronary operation after streptokinase treatment. *Ann Thorac Surg* 1991;52:1320–1321.

73. Alajmo F, Calamai G. High-dose aprotinin in emergency coronary artery bypass after thrombolysis. *Ann Thorac Surg* 1992;54:1022. Letter.

74. Fremes SE, Wong BI, Lee E, et al. Metaanalysis of prophylactic drug treatment in the prevention of postoperative bleeding. *Ann Thorac Surg* 1994;58:1580–1588.

75. Daily PO, Lamphere JA, Dembitsky WP, et al. Effect of prophylactic epsilon-aminocaproic acid on blood loss and transfusion requirements in patients undergoing first-time coronary artery bypass grafting: a randomized, prospective, double-blind study. *J Thorac Cardiovasc Surg* 1994;108:99–108.

27

Hypercoagulability Syndromes: What the Interventionalist Needs to Know

Timothy K. Liem, M.D.
Donald Silver, M.D.

Hypercoagulable conditions have been recognized in association with venous thrombotic disorders since 1965.[1] Their association with arterial thrombotic conditions has been identified in the last decade. The vascular surgeon, interventional radiologist, and vascular medicine specialist should be familiar with the common thrombophilic states: their modes of presentation, diagnostic tests, and indications for therapy.

NORMAL ANTITHROMBOTIC MECHANISMS

The normal anticoagulant state is maintained by a variety of plasma proteins that inhibit thrombus formation or enhance the dissolution of formed thromboses. These include antithrombin III (AT III), protein C, protein S, thrombomodulin, heparin cofactor II, tissue factor pathway inhibitor, and plasminogen. The mechanisms are depicted in Figure 27–1.

AT III inactivates thrombin and coagulation factors IXa, Xa, XIa, and XIIa. Its ability to inactivate thrombin is enhanced more than 1000-fold when heparin is present. AT III, stimulated by heparan sulfates on the endothelial surface, has a low level of activity that regulates thrombin activity during normal conditions. Thrombin is also inactivated by thrombomodulin (TM), a glycoprotein expressed on the endothelium of all organs with the exception of the brain.

The TM–thrombin complex is a potent activator of protein C. Protein C and protein S are vitamin K–dependent factors synthesized in the liver. Activated protein C (APC), with its cofactors protein S and factor V, inactivates factor Va and factor VIIIa. Heparin cofactor II, synthesized by the liver, inactivates thrombin via a mechanism independent of AT III. Heparin cofactor II is activated by heparin, dermatan sulfate, and endothelial heparan sulfate. Unlike AT III, heparin cofactor II is specific for thrombin.

An extrinsic coagulation pathway regulator, tissue factor pathway inhibitor (TFPI), has recently been identified. It binds to the tissue thromboplastin–factor VIIa–calcium complex, inhibiting activation of factor X to Xa and factor IX to IXa. TFPI is released from endothelial cells in response to heparin.

Unlike the anticoagulant proteins listed above, the plasminogen–plasmin system cleaves cross-linked and non-cross-linked fibrin to inactive fibrin degradation products (FDP). Under normal conditions, trace amounts of tissue plasminogen activator (t-PA) and urokinase activate plasminogen. t-PA is synthesized in endothelial cells; urokinase is synthesized in the kidney. The plasminogen–plasmin system is regulated by the short half-life of t-PA and by plasminogen activator inhibitors 1 and 2 (PAI-1, PAI-2).

THROMBOPHILIC STATES IN VENOUS DISEASE

The prevalence of congenital and acquired hypercoagulable states in studies of unselected consecutive patients with deep vein thrombosis has ranged from 2.1% to 40%.[2-5] The more common abnormalities identified were decreases in protein C and protein S and increased resistance to activated protein C (APC-R). AT III and plasminogen deficiencies occur less commonly (0.7% to 1%).[2,3] Lupus anticoagulants were found in 2.2% to 9.2% of patients with venous thrombosis. The majority of these patients had no clinical criteria for systemic lupus erythematosus.[2,4] The reported incidence of fibrinolytic abnormalities, excluding inherited plasminogen deficiencies, varies substantially

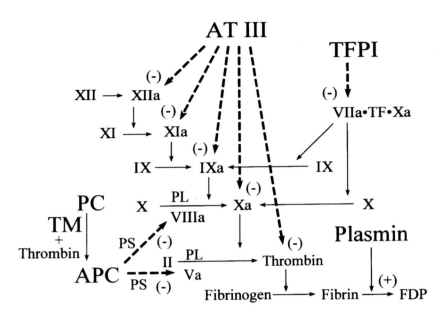

Figure 27–1. Normal antithrombotic mechanisms. AT III, antithrombin III; TFPI, tissue factor pathway inhibitor; TM, thrombomodulin; PC, protein C; APC, activated protein C; PS, protein S; PL, phospholipid.

(15% to 33%).[2,4,6] A critical analysis of euglobulin fibrinolytic activity, t-PA, and PAI found that levels of these substances have significant day-to-day variations, which do not correlate with the incidence of venous thrombosis.[2]

Patients who develop venous thrombosis at an early age and those with recurrent thrombosis have a higher incidence of identifiable anticoagulant protein abnormalities. In one study, protein C deficiencies were found in 8.1% of patients with venous thromboembolism who were younger than 41 years, whereas older patients had an incidence of only 1.2%.[7] This finding agrees with another study of young patients (<45 years) with venous thrombosis, in whom the incidence of combined protein C and protein S deficiency was 9%.[8] Eight percent of patients with recurrent thrombosis have been found to have either protein C or protein S deficiency.[9]

Patients with hypercoagulable states may present with venous thromboses in unusual locations. Inherited protein S, protein C, and AT III deficiencies have been found in association with mesenteric venous thrombosis. Acquired causes of thrombophilia such as anticardiolipin antibody and myeloproliferative disorders also may present in a similar manner. Thrombosis of the cavernous sinus, veins draining the femur (Legg-Perthes disease), and penile vein (priapism) also have been described in association with thrombophilic states.

Recent interest has focused on the role of APC-R in patients with idiopathic venous thromboses. APC-R is most often caused by a mutation in the factor V gene, during which Arg506 is replaced with Gln, thus making activated factor V resistant to digestion by activated protein C. APC-R in control populations has a prevalence of 3% to 7%.[5,10,11] However, its prevalence in

patients with venous thrombosis is 19.5% to 40%.[5,10] APC-R may confer a 5- to 10-fold increased risk of thrombosis. Some families with multiple genetic defects (protein C deficiency and APC-R) seem to be at even greater risk of venous thrombosis.[12]

THROMBOPHILIC STATES IN ARTERIAL DISEASES

The prevalence of hypercoagulable states in arterial thrombotic disorders is less well defined. Numerous case reports have described arterial thromboembolic disease in association with protein C, protein S, and AT III deficiencies. Other retrospective reviews have identified additional associations with heparin-induced thrombocytopenia, lupus anticoagulant, antiphospholipid antibodies, hyperaggregable platelets, heparin cofactor II deficiency, and decreased t-PA release.[13–18]

A recent retrospective communitywide survey found a 15% prevalence of hypercoagulability in young patients (<40 years old) with lower extremity ischemia. This number probably underestimates the true incidence in these young patients. AT III deficiency was the most commonly diagnosed disorder. Deficiencies of protein C, protein S, heparin cofactor II, and t-PA release were also detected. In addition, thrombophilia was found to be highly predictive of amputation and early surgical failure.[18] Another retrospective analysis of patients with lupus anticoagulants who underwent vascular procedures revealed a 50% incidence of postoperative thrombotic complications. As in the above study, this hypercoagulable condition was predictive of eventual amputation.[15]

Other studies, both retrospective and prospective, have found the prevalence of thrombophilic states in arterial disease to range from 8% to 40%.[19,20] The wide variation in prevalence appears to be related to the design of the studies. The cohorts selected for study varied from an entire vascular surgical practice to only young adults with lower extremity ischemia. The anti-coagulant protein levels were measured preoperatively in some studies,[21,22] whereas in others they may have been measured soon after surgery or many years post-operatively, and therefore may not be accurate indica-tors of congenital thrombophilia. Acquired AT III, protein C, and protein S deficiencies are known to occur after surgery and trauma. A significant number of patients initially found to have an anticoagulant pro-tein deficiency postoperatively subsequently were found to have normal levels on repeat study.

Recently, APC resistance has been described in patients with arterial occlusive disease. Ouriel and colleagues identified APC resistance in approximately 5% to 14% of patients with arterial occlusive and aneurysmal dis-ease. The prevalence might have been higher if patients with acute limb ischemia were included. In addition, patients with APC resistance were at greater risk of infrainguinal graft failure.[23] We have had sev-eral patients with arterial graft thromboses who had functional protein S deficiencies.

DETECTION AND MANAGEMENT OF COMMON THROMBOTIC CONDITIONS

A congenital or acquired thrombophilic condition should be suspected when venous and/or arterial thrombosis occurs in young patients, in unusual loca-tions, and with frequent recurrences. Other factors that should stimulate the search for a hypercoagulable con-dition include a family history of venous thrombo-embolism, recurrent thrombosis despite adequate anticoagulation, and early failure of a technically sound arterial reconstruction. The presence of other throm-bogenic or cardiovascular risk factors should not deter the investigation of a hypercoagulable state.

The evaluation of these patients includes a careful history and physical examination; a complete blood count, prothrombin time, and partial thromboplastin time; testing for APC-R, and for deficiencies of AT III, protein C, and protein S; and testing for the presence of antiphospholipid antibodies, lupus anticoagulant, and heparin-associated antibodies. If these are found to be normal, other less common thrombophilic condi-tions can be sought (eg, decreased heparin cofactor II, decreased or abnormal plasminogen, increased plasmi-nogen activator inhibitor-1, or increased or abnormal fibrinogen, homocystinemia, and lipoprotein A excess).

AT III

AT III is measured via functional assays which deter-mine the amount of thrombin that is inhibited. Mild overestimations may occur due to the presence of hep-arin cofactor II, α1-antitrypsin, or α2-macroglobulin.

The normal plasma concentration of AT III is approxi-mately 150 µg/mL, and the normal range of activity is 80% to 120%. Certain disease states are associated with acquired AT III deficiency, such as cirrhosis, nephrotic syndrome, and disseminated intravascular coagulation. Oral anticoagulants have a variable effect on AT III lev-els; on AT III levels; Heparin, L-asparaginase, and oral contraceptives may decrease AT III levels.

Therapeutic options for AT III deficiency include heparin and long-term warfarin. AT III concentrates, fresh frozen plasma, or cryoprecipitates are sometimes required as adjuvant therapy. The primary treatment for acute thrombotic events is heparin, although higher doses are often required. Heparin administration in AT III–deficient patients has been found to decrease the AT III level and increase its clearance. However, the incidence of recurrent deep vein thrombosis in AT III–deficient patients treated with heparin and then war-farin is no higher than the incidence in patients with normal AT III activity.

AT III concentrates may be used as an adjunct to heparin therapy in acute thrombotic events and as thrombotic prophylaxis for AT III–deficient patients in high-risk situations such as parturition and surgery. Therapeutic AT III concentrates should be adminis-tered to obtain at least 80% of normal AT III activity. The units required can be calculated from the follow-ing equation:

$$\text{Units required (IU)} = \frac{[\text{desired} - \text{baseline ATIII level}] \times \text{weight (kg)}}{1.4}$$

Although long-term warfarin therapy in asymptomatic patients is debatable, it should be offered to patients with a history of thrombotic episodes. Patients with AT III deficiency and pregnancy have been managed suc-cessfully with the daily administration of subcutaneous unfractionated or low molecular weight heparin.[24,25]

Protein C and Protein S

The normal concentration of protein C is 2 to 6 µg/mL, while that of protein S is 25 µg/mL. Protein C deficiency can be established using functional or immu-nologic assays. Heterozygous protein C–deficient patients usually have about 50 to 60% of normal ac-tivity. As with detection of AT III deficiency, certain factors (eg, cirrhosis, disseminated intravascular coagu-lation) may obscure an accurate diagnosis of protein C or protein S deficiency. The timing of the laboratory assessment in acute thromboembolic disease is critical because acute thrombosis and warfarin therapy can decrease protein C and protein S concentrations. Pro-tein C assays are best performed several weeks after resolution of the thrombotic event and 2 to 4 weeks after discontinuation of warfarin therapy.

Protein S exists either as free protein S (30 to 40%) or bound to the complement pathway protein, C4b-binding protein. Only free protein S can act as cofactor for APC. Protein S deficiency has been categorized according to whether the plasma concentration of total protein S, the free component, or the functional protein S activity is decreased. Accurate diagnosis of protein S deficiency requires measurement of total, free, and bound protein S. It has been recognized recently that patients with type II or functional protein S deficiency (normal total and free protein S, decreased protein S activity) may have been misdiagnosed. The majority of patients in this category actually have APC resistance.

A variety of conditions can predispose to acquired protein C and protein S deficiency. These include liver failure, surgery, adult respiratory distress syndrome, disseminated intravascular coagulation, and warfarin theapy. Besides its activity as a complement protein, C4b-binding protein is also an acute phase reactant. Acute inflammatory conditions that increase the level of C4b-binding protein may lead to free protein S deficiency and a tendency toward thrombosis.

Heterozygous protein C deficiency occurs with a prevalence of 1 in 200 to 1 in 300 in the general population; however, the incidence of thromboembolic events is much lower. Long-term treatment of asymptomatic patients with protein C deficiency is not indicated. However, prophylactic heparin anticoagulation for patients at higher risk (surgery, pregnancy, etc.) is indicated.

Protein C–deficient patients with acute thrombosis should be treated with fibrinolytic agents and/or heparin. Lifelong warfarin therapy is indicated but should be initiated only while the patient is receiving heparin. The initial administration of warfarin may reduce protein C and protein S concentrations even further, resulting in a temporary hypercoagulable state that may contribute to recurrent thrombosis, and warfarin-induced skin necrosis. The management of patients with protein S deficiency is similar to that for protein C deficiency.

Antiphospholipid Antibodies

Antiphospholipid antibodies (APA) are a related group of immunoglobulins that include lupus anticoagulants and anticardiolipin antibodies. The lupus anticoagulants are a group of antibodies that prolong phospholipid-dependent coagulation reactions in vitro: prothrombin time, activated partial thromboplastin time (aPTT), and dilute Russell's viper venom time (dRVVT). In vivo, lupus anticoagulants and a variety of other antiphospholipid antibodies are associated with a syndrome including recurrent venous (occasionally arterial) thrombotic complications, repeated fetal loss, and/or thrombocytopenia.

Detection of antiphospholipid antibodies, including lupus anticoagulants, has been hampered by nonstandardized assay systems and a heterogeneous population of antibodies (IgG, IgM, IgA). Patients suspected of having the antiphospholipid syndrome should be studied with the aPTT and dRVVT and tested for anticardiolipin antibodies with specific enzyme immunoassays for IgG, IgA, and IgM. The modified dRVVT is the most sensitive and specific test for lupus anticoagulants. High antiphospholipid titers generally have a stronger association with thromboembolic events. Low titers are often transient and can be induced by a variety of clinical situations such as medication use, infections, and malignant and nonmalignant diseases.

Asymptomatic patients with antiphospholipid antibodies can either be observed or treated with life-long low-dose aspirin. In patients with a history of thromboembolic complications, long-term warfarin therapy significantly reduces the incidence of recurrent thrombosis. Warfarin should be continued as long as the antibodies persist. In addition, high-intensity warfarin (international normalized ratio ≥3) is significantly more effective than low-intensity warfarin.[26] Other forms of therapy include heparin anticoagulation during pregnancy, immunosuppressive agents, and intravenous immunoglobulin.

Heparin-Induced Thrombocytopenia

Type I heparin-induced thrombocytopenia (HIT) is caused by idiosyncratic, clinically insignificant platelet aggregation in the presence of heparin that is not immune mediated. Type II HIT is caused by IgG and IgM antibodies that are specific for heparin. Type II HIT occurs in approximately 3 to 5% of patients receiving heparin therapy. The heparin–immunoglobulin complex causes platelet activation, the release reaction, and platelet aggregation. Antibodies usually can be detected by days 4 to 15 of heparin therapy and have persisted for up to 13 years. Type II HIT usually presents with the triad of decreasing platelet counts, heparin resistance, and new or progressive thromboembolic events.

HIT antibodies can be detected by measurement of platelet aggregation,[14] C-serotonin release, and enzyme immunoassays for platelet-associated IgG. Other, less commonly performed assays involve platelet factor 3 availability, complement fixation, and hemagglutination. The most sensitive and specific assay is for[14] C-serotonin release, but it is quite labor intensive and requires several hours to perform. The platelet aggregation assay is a more widely used test and has comparable sensitivity (88%) and specificity (82 to 100%) if the proper platelet donor and heparin concentrations are used.

Management of type II HIT includes discontinuation of heparin and use of alternative anticoagulants. Warfarin has been used with success but requires several days to achieve full anticoagulation. In the interim, low molecular weight heparin (LMWH) may be used in some patients with HIT because 25 to 61% of patients with type II HIT who react with beef or pork heparin in vitro, will not cross-react with a LMWH.[27] Ancrod is a defibrinogenating agent derived from the Malayan pit viper that has been used with success in HIT patients. However, it is not yet approved for use in the United States. Aspirin, dipyridamole, and dextran are minimally effective antithrombotic agents in patients with HIT. Other "antithrombotics," such as hirudin, thrombin inhibitors, and glycoprotein IIb/IIIa inhibitors, are being evaluated in the management of the HIT syndrome. We have found that HIT thromboses are relatively resistant to lysis with urokinase.

Activated Protein C Resistance

Assays for APC-R have been introduced recently. These tests are based on the prolongation of the aPTT or prothrombin time in the presence of APC. It is still unclear which tests and which reagents are optimal. Factors such as pregnancy, protein S deficiency, and the presence of a lupus anticoagulant may decrease the specificity of such assays.[28]

Data regarding the management of patients with APC-R are incomplete. Asymptomatic patients who are homozygous for APC-R and those with combined defects (eg, protein C or protein S deficiency) are at much higher risk of thrombosis.[12] At a minimum, they should receive anticoagulant prophylaxis in high-risk situations such as pregnancy and surgery. It is not known whether they should receive long-term or lifelong therapy. Heterozygous and homozygous patients with thromboembolic events should be offered lifelong warfarin therapy.

Abnormalities of the Fibrinolysis

Less common thrombophilic conditions include decreased or abnormal plasminogen, decreased t-PA, and increased PAI. Functional and immunologic assays are available for plasminogen, t-PA, and PAI. The fibrinolytic system should be evaluated several months after the acute thrombotic event because plasminogen activity is frequently decreased during acute thromboses. In addition, PAI is an acute phase reactant and may be elevated during surgery, trauma, and acute thromboembolism. Long-term warfarin therapy may decrease the incidence of recurrent thromboembolism in patients with abnormalities of the fibrinolytic system.

Conclusion

Patients with thrombophilic conditions are at increased risk of venous and arterial thromboembolic events. The vascular interventionist should be familiar with the common congenital and acquired thrombophilic conditions, their frequency, and their modes of presentation. A successful outcome in patients with these disorders depends on the ability to recognize and manage the hypercoagulable state.

REFERENCES

1. Egeberg O. Inherited antithrombin deficiency causing thrombophilia. *Thromb Diathes Haemorr* 1965;13:516–530.
2. Malm J, Laurell M, Nilsson IM, Dahlback B. Thromboembolic disease—critical evaluation of laboratory investigation. *Thromb Haemost* 1992;68:7–13.
3. Heijboer H, Brandjes DPM, Buller HR, Sturk A, ten Cate JW. Deficiencies of coagulation-inhibiting and fibrinolytic proteins in outpatients with deep-vein thrombosis. *N Engl J Med* 1990;323:1512–1516.
4. Doig RG, O'Malley CJ, Dauer R, McGrath KM. An evaluation of 200 consecutive patients with spontaneous or recurrent thrombosis for primary hypercoagulable states. *Am J Clin Pathol* 1994;102:797–801.
5. Svensson PJ, Dahlback B. Resistance to activated protein C as a basis for venous thrombosis. *N Engl J Med* 1994;330:517–522.
6. Nilsson IM, Ljungner H, Tengborn L. Two different mechanisms in patients with venous thrombosis and defective fibrinolysis: low concentration of plasminogen activator or increased concentration of plasminogen activator inhibitor. *Br Med J Clin Res Ed* 1985;290:1453–1456.
7. Broekmans AW, van del Linden IK, Veltkamp JJ, Bertina RM. Prevalence of isolated protein C deficiency in patients with venous thrombotic disease and in the population. *Thromb Haemost* 1983;50:350. Abstract.
8. Gladson CL, Scharrer I, Hach V, Beck KH, Griffin JH. The Frequency of type I heterozygous protein S and protein C deficiency in 141 unrelated young patients with Venous Thrombosis. *Thromb Haemost* 1988;59:18–22.
9. Broekmans AW, van der Linden IK, Jansen-Koeter Y, Bertina RM. Prevalence of protein C (PC) and protein S (PS) deficiency in patients with thrombotic disease. *Thromb Res* 1986; Cited, volume unknown (suppl VI):135. Abstract. Cited by Malm J, Laurell M, Nilsson IM, Dahlback B. Thromboembolic disease—critical evaluation of laboratory investigation. *Thromb Haemost* 1992;68:7–13.
10. Rosendaal FR, Koster T, Vandenbroucke JP, Reitsma P. High risk of thrombosis in patients homozygous for factor V leiden (activated protein C resistance). *Blood* 1995;85:1504–1508.
11. Beauchamp NJ, Daly ME, Hampton KK, Cooper PC, Preston FE, Peake IR. High prevalence of a mutation in the factor V gene within the U.K. population: relationship to activated protein C resistance and familial thrombosis. *Br J Haematol* 1994;88:219–222.
12. Dahlback B. Inherited thrombophilia: resistance to activated protein C as a pathogenic factor of venous thromboembolism. *Blood* 1995;85:607–614.
13. Kapsch D, Silver D. Heparin-induced thrombocytopenia with thrombosis and hemorrhage. *Arch Surg* 1981;116:1423–1427.
14. O'Donnell TF, Carvalho ACA, Colman RW, Clowes GH Jr. Platelet function abnormalities in a family with recurrent arterial thrombosis. *Surgery* 1978;83:144–150.
15. Ahn SS, Kalunian K, Rosove M, Moore WS. Postoperative thrombotic complications in patients with the lupus anti-

coagulant: increased risk after vascular procedures. *J Vasc Surg* 1988;7:749–756.

16. Eason JD, Mills JL, Beckett WC. Hypercoagulable states in arterial thromboembolism. *Surg Gynecol Obstet* 1992; 174:211–215.

17. Levy PJ, Gonzalez FM, Rush DS, Haynes JL. Hypercoagulable states as an evolving risk for spontaneous venous and arterial thrombosis. *J Am Coll Surg* 1994;178:266–270.

18. Levy PJ, Hornung CA, Haynes JL, Rush DS. Lower extremity ischemia in adults younger than forty years of age: a community-wide survey of premature atherosclerotic arterial disease. *J Vasc Surg* 1994;19:873–881.

19. Allaart CF, Aronson DC, Ruys T, et al. Hereditary protein S deficiency in young adults with arterial occlusive disease. *Thromb Haemost* 1990;64:206–210.

20. Ray SA, Rowley MR, Loh A, et al. Hypercoagulable states in patients with leg ischemia. *Br J Surg* 1994;81:811–814.

21. Eldrup-Jorgensen J, Flanigan DP, Brace L, et al. Hypercoagulable states and lower limb ischemia in young adults. *J Vasc Surg* 1989;9:334–341.

22. Donaldson MC, Weinberg DS, Belkin M, Whittemore AD, Mannick JA. Screening for hypercoagulable states in vascular surgical practice: a preliminary study. *J Vasc Surg* 1990; 11:825–831.

23. Ouriel K, Green RM, DeWeese JA, et al. Activated protein C resistance: prevalence and implications in peripheral vascular disease. *J Vasc Surg* 1996;23:46–52.

24. Gillis S, Shushan A, Eldor A. Use of low molecular weight heparin for prophylaxis and treatment of thromboembolism in pregnancy. *Int J Gynaecol Obstet* 1992;39:297–301.

25. Brandt P. Observations during the treatment of antithrombin-III deficient women with heparin and antithrombin concentrate during pregnancy, parturition, and abortion. *Thromb Res* 1981;22:15–24.

26. Khamashta MA, Cuadrado MJ, Mujic F, et al. The management of thrombosis in the antiphospholipid-antibody syndrome. *N Engl J Med* 1995;332:993–997.

27. Kikta MJ, Keller MP, Humphrey PW, et al. Can low molecular weight heparins and heparinoids be safely given to patients with heparin-induced thrombocytopenia syndrome? *Surgery* 1993;114:705–710.

28. Vasse M, Leduc O, Borg JY, Chretien MH, Monconduit M. Resistance to activated protein C: evaluation of three functional assays. *Thromb Res* 1994;76:47–59.

28

Thrombolytic Therapy for Occluded Arteries and Grafts: Patient Selection and Results

Kenneth Ouriel, M.D.

Ischemic symptoms due to peripheral arterial occlusion are traditionally grouped into two categories: non-limb-threatening ischemia (claudication) and limb-threatening ischemia (rest pain, ischemic ulceration, or gangrene). The severity of symptoms following occlusion of a peripheral artery or bypass graft is dependent on the adequacy of the collateral circulation.[1] In the absence of prior occlusive disease, typically seen in the patient presenting with an acute occlusion, collaterals are virtually absent and the leg becomes acutely ischemic, with pain, pallor, paresthesia, and coolness below the level of the occlusion. Acute limb ischemia is therefore characterized by presentation with a well-defined onset, generally within 14 days, whereas chronic ischemic symptoms are more insidious in onset and it is frequently impossible for the patient to identify the time of onset with precision.

The results of therapy for peripheral arterial occlusion are dependent on the severity of ischemia. Among patients with chronic occlusive disease, for example, DeWeese and Rob reported a 5-year patency rate of 74% among patients undergoing saphenous vein femoropopliteal bypasses for claudication versus 42% in patients with limb-threatening ischemia.[2] Similarly, Jivegard et al observed a correlation between the severity of ischemia and the perioperative mortality rate associated with surgical revascularization in the setting of acute ischemia.[3] With these considerations in mind, Rutherford et al published a grading scheme for acute limb ischemia.[4] This classification system attempts to standardize the severity of ischemia and thus allow the rational comparison of data from different studies. The criteria were adopted by the Society of Vascular Surgery and the North American Chapter of the International Society for Cardiovascular Surgery, and have been dubbed the *SVS/ISCVS criteria*. Limbs may be sub-categorized into one of these gradations of ischemia using the SVS/ISCVS criteria. The least severe category includes limbs without limb-threatening symptoms, generally with claudication alone (category I). The middle category includes limbs that are threatened but can still be salvaged by therapeutic intervention (category II). The final category identifies those limbs with irreversible ischemia where therapeutic interventions can be predicted to be futile (category III). Most studies evaluating operative or thrombolytic treatment modalities for acute ischemia have generally included patients with SVS/ISCVS category II ischemia that is, threatened but not irreversibly so.

THERAPEUTIC OPTIONS

The primary therapeutic objective in the setting of peripheral arterial occlusion is the restoration of blood flow through recanalization of the occluded native artery or bypass graft (thrombectomy or thrombolysis) or through placement of a (new) bypass graft around the occlusive process. Surgical intervention in the setting of acute limb ischemia consists of balloon catheter thromboembolectomy following the introduction of the device by Fogarty et al in 1963.[5] Although balloon catheter thromboembolectomy remains appropriate for embolic problems, many have advocated placement of a new bypass graft conduit for all other etiologies. At present, surgery remains the standard form of therapy against which alternative modalities must be compared. Although open surgical techniques are safe and highly efficacious in the setting of chronic peripheral arterial occlusion, operation for acute occlusion has been associated with a high rate of amputation and mortality, in large measure as a result of the compromised medical status of this patient subgroup. Blaisdell et al were one of the first groups to identify the high rate of morbid-

Table 28–1. Morbidity and Mortality Rates Associated with Surgical Treatment of Acute Lower Limb Ischemia

Author	Year	Etiology	Amputation	Death
Blaisdell[6]	1978	Embolism, thrombosis	30%*	25%*
Jivegard[3]	1986	Embolism, thrombosis	16%*	18%*
Edwards[31]	1990	Graft thrombosis	6%**	23%†

*In-hospital data.
†Six-month actuarial data.

Table 28–2. Secondary Treatment Modalities Utilized Following Successful Thrombolysis

Clinical Scenario Following Thrombolysis	Therapeutic Alternatives
Complete dissolution of arterial embolus	Long-term anticoagulation
Open graft without a residual lesion	Long-term anticoagulation
Solitary lesion in saphenous vein graft	Surgical patch angioplasty Balloon dilatation
Multiple lesions in saphenous vein graft	Replacement of some or all of the graft
Atherosclerotic stenosis of native artery, short	Surgical endarterectomy Balloon dilatation Bypass grafting
Atherosclerotic stenosis of native artery, long	Bypass grafting

ity and mortality associated with surgical intervention for acute limb ischemia.[6] They suggested that immediate operative intervention be delayed and that the patient be treated with high-dose heparin therapy until stabilization was achieved. Although this therapeutic strategy never became fully accepted, later studies by such investigators as Jivegard et al[3] and Yeager[7] have confirmed the high mortality associated with surgical intervention (Table 28–1).

Thrombolytic Therapy

Thrombolytic dissolution of the occluding fibrin-platelet thrombus has been employed as an alternative to surgery. Plasminogen activators such as streptokinase, urokinase, and recombinant tissue plasminogen activator have been administered directly into the thrombus through a catheter-directed approach. Thrombolytic therapy provides two potential advantages over standard surgical methods. First, the obstructing thrombus or thromboembolus may be ameliorated using techniques less invasive than open operation. Second, patency of the original conduit or native artery may be restored, thus obviating the need to place a new bypass graft.

Despite the potential advantages of thrombolysis, a clinically successful outcome often requires endovascular or open surgical treatment of stenotic lesions unmasked after clot dissolution and thought to be the causative etiology of the occlusive event (Table 28–2). Thrombolytic techniques should not be strictly considered a replacement modality for open surgical repair, although this is possible and appropriate in a minority

of cases (Fig. 28–1). For example, successful thrombolysis of an occluded vein graft is likely to uncover a stenotic lesion responsible for the failure of the conduit.[8] This stenosis may then be treated by a surgical technique such as patch angioplasty or an endovascular modality such as balloon angioplasty (Fig. 28–2). Only in rare cases of embolic events or prosthetic graft occlusion will thrombolysis be sufficient as the sole intervention (Fig. 28–1).

The evaluation of novel treatment modalities, such as thrombolysis, must include the careful evaluation of early and long-term follow-up data. Primary outcome measures such as limb salvage and patient mortality must be assessed and compared with the results of standard therapy. Potential benefits, such as a reduction in the frequency and magnitude of required interventions and a decrease in the cost of treatment, are relevant secondary endpoints that become important once equivalence in the primary outcome measures has been proven.

In the United States, patients with peripheral arterial occlusion are frequently admitted under the direct care of a vascular surgeon as the primary decision maker. Nevertheless, the optimal treatment of these patients should be multidisciplinary, involving the interventionalist in a direct role and occasionally cardiologists, hematologist, and vascular medicine specialist.

Following admission, diagnostic arteriography is performed by the interventionalist, who reviews the diagnostic arteriogram and confers with the vascular surgeon about the most appropriate management of

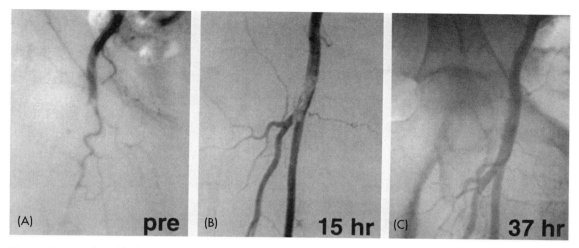

Figure 28–1. This elderly woman presented with a classic history of a right femoral embolus originating from the left atrium. She had decreased sensation and a mottled, cool foot. Although open operative procedures are usually indicated for localized femoral emboli without significant propagation, this series of arteriograms documents complete resolution with intra-arterial urokinase thrombolysis. (A) The pretreatment diagnositc film documents obstruction of common femoral outflow into the superficial femoral and profunda trunks. (B) After 15 hours of intra-arterial urokinase therapy the fresh, propagated thrombus was dissolved, leaving the older embolic material from the heart. The limb was restored to viability at this point. (C) After 37 hours, complete dissolution was achieved and pedal pulses were restored.

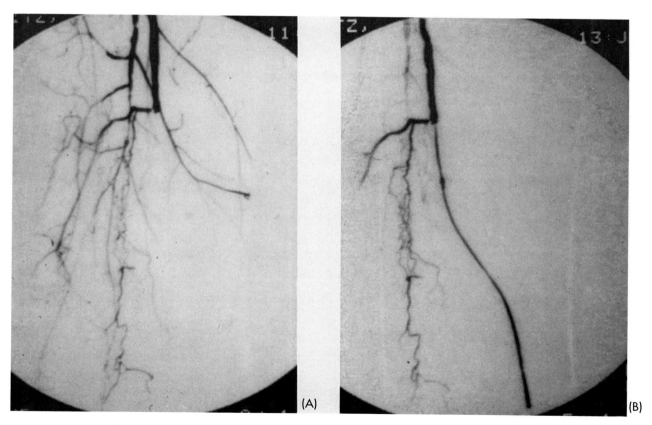

Figure 28–2. (A) This patient presented with an occluded superficial femoral to posterior tibial reversed saphenous vein graft inserted 3 years earlier. (B) After 6 hours of intra-arterial urokinase thrombolysis, the vein graft was completely open, revealing a long, stenotic proximal segment that required interposition of a 15-cm length of saphenous vein from the contralateral thigh.

the patient, including immediate surgery, thrombolysis, or an endovascular intervention such as balloon angioplasty, stenting, or atherectomy. If a thrombolytic strategy is elected, interplay between the interventionalist and vascular surgeon is continuous and ongoing. Decisions regarding termination of the thrombolytic infusion and the performance of subsequent surgical or endovascular interventions should be made by the vascular surgeon in collaboration with the interventionalist.

Clinical Trials of Thrombolysis for Peripheral Arterial Occlusion

Thrombolysis for peripheral arterial occlusion was not attempted until the mid-1950s, despite the discovery of streptokinase over two decades previously by Tillett and Garner.[9] Lack of purity of the agents was an early problem, forcing Tillett to limit its use to extravascular disease processes, specifically the dissolution of loculated hemothoraces.[10] Despite Tillett's initial experience with the intravascular administration of varying doses of streptokinase in 11 volunteer subjects,[11] Cliffton and Grossi were the first to report the use of thrombolytic agents to treat intravascular thrombus using a combination of streptokinase and plasminogen to generate plasmin.[12] Cliffton and Grossi assumed that the exogenous plasmin was the substance responsible for dissolution of the thrombus. Later studies, however, would reveal that excess streptokinase in the preparation was the active agent, converting endogenous fibrin-bound plasminogen to plasmin.[13]

Anecdotal experiences predominated in the three decades that followed the initial clinical reports, using both systemic[14–18] and intra-arterial[19–21] thrombolytic routes of administration to address peripheral arterial thrombosis. Dotter et al popularized the use of catheter-directed thrombolysis with streptokinase, reporting success rates superior to those achieved with systemic administration with what they termed "selective, low-dose therapy."[22]

These anecdotal experiences were followed by retrospective reports. Investigators such as Hess et al,[20] McNamara and Fischer,[23] and Graor et al[21] reported their individual experiences with large numbers of patients, and with remarkable results. Urokinase became the agent of choice for peripheral arterial occlusion,[1] with thrombolytic success rates of more than 80% and patient mortality rates of less than 10%.

Prior to the 1990s, however, there existed no randomized comparison of thrombolysis with standard surgical intervention. The need for a prospective comparison became clear with the publication of several reports with poorer thrombolytic success rates than originally reported.[24–26] Although a randomized trial of rt-PA versus surgical thrombectomy was reported in the

European literature,[27] its small size (only 20 patients) precluded meaningful conclusions.

A randomized trial of intra-arterial urokinase versus surgical intervention was reported by the Rochester group in 1994.[28] This adequately powered study enrolled 114 patients with severe, limb-threatening acute limb ischemia. Decreased in-hospital cardiopulmonary complications and a corresponding improvement in patient survival were achieved in the urokinase group. There was no difference in the rate of amputation, with limb salvage in approximately 80% of the patients (Table 28–3). The date must be viewed with caution, however, as the study population comprised a subgroup with very recent onset (mean, less than 24 hours' duration) and very severe ischemia (mean ankle/brachial index 0.04).

Shortly after the publication of the Rochester trial, the Surgery or Thrombolysis for Ischemia of the Lower Extremity (STILE) report appeared.[29] The STILE trial was a multicenter, randomized comparison of rt-PA, urokinase, and operation in patients with nonembolic lower extremity ischemia of less than 6 months' duration. In other words, the study included both acute and chronic peripheral arterial occlusions. The trial documented a death or amputation rate of 38% in patients who presented within 2 weeks of the onset of symptoms compared with 10% among patients presenting after 2 weeks. No mortality differences were noted.

The STILE trial utilized a composite index of adverse clinical outcomes as the primary study endpoint. This outcome measure included the objective and clinically relevant outcomes of death and amputation, as well as measures such as renal failure and wound complications—events less directly associated with the thrombolytic procedure. In addition, "ongoing ischemia" was added to the list of adverse events included as the major endpoint, a measure that is subjective and difficult to assess. In fact, a benefit in the composite index was detected by the safety committee of the STILE trial and forced the premature termination of the study, despite a lack of differences in limb-salvage or mortality among the groups. However, among patients who presented with ischemic symptoms of less than 14 days' duration, there was a lower ampu-

Table 28–3. Results of the Rochester Trial of Urokinase Versus Operation in the Initial Treatment of Patients with Limb-Threatening Peripheral Arterial Occlusion

	Amputation Rate		Mortality Rate	
	30 Days	12 Months	30 Days	12 Months
Urokinase (57)	9%	18%	12%	16%
Operation (57)	14%	18%	18%	58%
	n.s.	n.s.	n.s.	$p = 0.01$

Source: Ref. 28.

tation rate and a shorter duration of hospitalization associated with thrombolysis. There were no significant differences in outcome when patients treated with rt-PA were compared to those treated with urokinase.

These observations have been instrumental in the formulation and design of subsequent thrombolytic trials. The most objective and clinically relevant endpoints when studying peripheral arterial ischemia are limb salvage and patient survival. Benefits of one form of therapy over another are likely to be realized, however, only in study populations with a sufficiently high event rate (eg, the Rochester study).

The study of Thrombolysis or Peripheral Arterial Surgery (TOPAS) is the most recently completed thrombolytic trial, comparing recombinant urokinase (r-UK) with operative intervention in the treatment of peripheral arterial occlusions less than or equal to 14 days in duration.[30] The TOPAS trial was originally designed to mimic the Rochester study. As such, the sample sizes were chosen based on event rates observed in the Rochester study. As the TOPAS trial progressed, however, it became evident that the patients enrolled differed substantially from those entered into the Rochester trial. The morality and amputation rates were significantly lower in TOPAS, so that there was little chance of achieving differences in the primary endpoint between the two treatment groups. Moreover, publication of the Rochester data created investigator bias toward thrombolysis for acutely ischemic extremities. Specifically, investigators were unwilling to randomize those patients who would benefit the most from thrombolysis—the medically compromised subpopulation with recent onset of severly ischemic symptoms.

The most important secondary endpoint in the TOPAS trial was the quantification of the severity of vascular interventions over a 6-month follow-up. Interventions were ranked through deliberations by a committee of vasuclar practitioners, ranging from lowest severity (medical or thrombolytic intervention alone) to open surgical procedures, amputation, and death. Although no differences were detected with regard to amputation or death, a significant benefit in lowering the requirement for open surgical interventions was observed in the thrombolytic group. The fact that the need for invasive interventions was lower in the thrombolytic group over the duration of follow-up attested to the durability of thrombolytic interventions in the TOPAS trial.

The secondary benefit of lowering the magnitude of invasive interventions is an outcome that is likely to be of great importance to patients. It is appropriate to rely on secondary endpoints only when the primary endpoints are equivalent between treatment groups, and a preliminary overview of the TOPAS data suggested that the primary endpoint of amputation-free survival was equivalent in the r-UK and surgical groups. A thorough statistical analysis, however, detected a small probability that the two treatments were not equivalent. It is conceivable that this probability is small enough, and the secondary endpoint differences are great enough, that r-UK therapy is likely to be of benefit to individuals with acute limb ischemia. The TOPAS data suggested that overall clinical results may be superior in patients with bypass graft occlusions compared to those with native artery occlusions, with no significant differences observed in patients with suprainguinal versus infrainguinal occlusions. There were no differences in results with regard to the duration of the occlusion up to a maximum of 14 days.

The results of clinical trials of thrombolysis versus operation are dependent on the skill of the clinical management team in interventional and surgical techniques and on the patient selection criteria defining the composition of the study population. Although the STILE trial has been criticized on the basis of poor thrombolytic technical results, and specifically due to failure to successfully cannulate the thrombus in a significant percentage of patients, it is likely that differences in selection criteria is the most significant factor accounting for differences in study results.

Medically compromised patients with recent onset of severe ischemia comprise the subpopulation most likely to benefit from thrombolytic interventions because the perioperative mortality rate has been high in this subgroup,[6,28,31] presumably due to the inability of these patients to tolerate open surgical interventions without adequate preparation. Exlcusion of this subgroup from randomization would bias the results against thrombolysis, as was probalby observed in the TOPAS trial. In a similar manner, inclusion of patients with chronic ischemia is likely to bias the results against thrombolysis. This phenomenon was observed in the STILE because, as noted above, the benefit of thrombolysis was observed only after subgroup analyses were performed, with post hoc stratification into acute and chronic ischemia subgroups.

Given the data generated by the three adequately powered comparisons of thrombolysis and operation, it is unlikely that new comparative trials will be possible. Investigator sentiment is such that preconceived notions regarding the most appropriate form of therapy render patient acquisition difficult. Subsequent trials are likely to be directed at an evaluation of newer thrombolytic agents and strategies rather than comparisons with operation. Thus, the data presently available may represent the only opportunity to critically compare thrombolysis and operation for peripheral arterial occlusion.

REFERENCES

1. McNamara TO, Bomberger RA, Merchant RF. Intra-arterial urokinase as the initial therapy for acutely ischemic lower limbs. *Circulation* 1991;83(suppl I): I-106–I-119.
2. DeWeese JA, Rob CG. Autogenous venous grafts 10 years later. *Surgery* 1977;82:775–782.
3. Jivegard L, Holm J, Schersten T. Acute limb ischemia due to arterial embolism or thrombosis: influence of limb ischemia versus pre-existing cardiac disease on postoperative mortality rate. *J Cardiovasc Surg* 1988;29:32–36.
4. Rutherford RB, Flanigan DP, Gupta SK, et al. Suggested standards for reports dealing with lower extremity ischemia. *J Vasc Surg* 1986;4:80–94.
5. Fogarty TJ, Cranley JJ, Drause RJ, Strasser ES, Hafner CD. A method for extraction of arterial emboli and thrombi. *Surg Gynecol Obstet* 1963;116:241–244.
6. Blaisdell FW, Steele M, Allen RE. Management of acute lower extremity arterial ischemia due to embolism and thrombosis. *Surgery* 1978;84:822–834.
7. Yeager RA, Moneta GL, Taylor LM, Jr, Hamre DW, McConnell DB, Porter JM. Surgical management of severe acute lower extremity ischemia. *J Vasc Surg* 1992;15:385–393.
8. Ouriel K, Shortell CK, Green RM, DeWeese JA. Differential mechanisms of late failure of autogenous and prosthetic bypass conduits. In press.
9. Tillett WS, Garner RL. The fibrinolytic activity of hemolytic streptococci. *J Exp Med* 1933;58:485–502.
10. Tillett WS, Sherry S. The effect in patients of streptococcal fibrinolysin (streptokinase) and streptococcal desoxyribonuclease on fibrinous, purulent, and sanguinous pleural exudations. *J Clin Invest* 1949;28:173–190.
11. Tillett WS, Johnson AJ, McCarty WR. The intravenous infusion of the streptococcal fibrinolytic principle (streptokinase) into patients. *J Clin Invest* 1955;34:169–185.
12. Cliffton EE, Grossi CE. Investigations of intravenous plasmin (fibrinolysin) in humans; physiologic and clinical effects. *Circulation* 1956;14:919.
13. Alkjaersig N, Fletcher AP, Sherry S. The mechanism of clot dissolution by plasmin. *J Clin Invest* 1959;38:1086–1095.
14. Marder VJ. The use of thrombolytic agents: choice of patient, drug administration, laboratory monitoring. *Ann Intern Med* 1979;90:802–812.
15. Sherry S, Fletcher AP, Alkjaersig N. Developments in fibrinolytic therapy for thromboembolic disease. *Ann Intern Med* 1959;50:560–570.
16. Camiolo SM, Thorsen S, Astrup T. Fibrinogenolysis and fibrinolysis with tissue plasminogen activator, urokinase, streptokinase-activated human globulin, and plasmin. *Proc Soc Exp Biol Med* 1971;138:277–280.
17. Sharma GVRK, Cella G, Parisi AF, Sasahara AA. Thrombolytic therapy. *N Engl J Med* 1982;306:1268–1276.
18. Martin M. Thrombolytic therapy in arterial thromboembolism. *Prog Cardiovasc Dis* 1979;21:351–374.
19. McNicol GP, Douglas AS. Treatment of peripheral vascular occlusion by streptokinase perfusion. *Scand J Clin Lab Invest* 1964;16(suppl 78):23–29.
20. Hess H, Ingrisch H, Mietaschk A, Rath H. Local low-dose thrombolytic therapy of peripheral arterial occlusions. *N Engl J Med* 1982;307:1627–1630.
21. Graor RA, Risius B, Young JR, et al. Low-dose streptokinase for selective thrombolysis: systemic effects and complications. *Radiology* 1984;152:35–39.
22. Dotter CT, Rosch J, Seaman AJ. Selective clot lysis with low-dose streptokinase. *Radiology* 1974;111:31–37.
23. McNamara TO, Fischer JR. Thrombolysis of peripheral arterial and graft occlusions: improved results using high-dose urokinase. *Am J Roentgenol* 1985;144:769–775.
24. Sicard GA, Schier JJ, Totty WG, et al. Thrombolytic therapy for acute arterial occlusion. *J Vasc Surg* 1985; 2:65–78.
25. Ricotta JJ. Intra-arterial thrombolysis. A surgical view. *Circulation* 1991;83:120–121.
26. Ricotta JJ, Green RM, DeWeese JA. Use and limitations of thrombolytic therapy in the treatment of peripheral arterial ischemia: results of a multi-institutional questionnaire. *J Vasc Surg* 1987;6:45–50.
27. Nilsson L, Albrechtsson U, Jonung T, et al. Surgical treatment versus thrombolysis in acute arterial occlusion: a randomised controlled study. *Eur J Vasc Surg* 1992; 6:189–193.
28. Ouriel K, Shortell CK, DeWeese JA, et al. A comparison of thrombolytic therapy with operative revascularization in the treatment of acute peripheral arterial ischemia. *J Vasc Surg* 1994;19:1021–1030.
29. The STILE Investigators. Results of a prospective randomized trial evaluating surgery versus thrombolysis for ischemia of the lower extremity. The STILE trial. *Ann Surg* 1994;220:251–268.
30. Ouriel K, Veith FJ, Sasahara A, Marder VJ. Thrombolysis or peripheral arterial surgery: Phase I results. *J Vasc Surg.* 1996;23:64–75.
31. Edwards JE, Taylor LMJ, Porter JM. Treatment of failed lower extremity bypass grafts with new autogenous vein bypass grafting. *J Vasc Surg* 1990;11:136–145.

29

Pulse-Spray Pharmacomechanical Thrombolysis: Principles, Technique, Indications, and Results

Joseph J. Bookstein, M.D.

As thrombolytic methodology continues to improve, pharmacologic dissolution of pathologic thrombus has become a widely accepted clinical adjunct. Early thrombolytic methods employed intravenous administration of the fibrinolytic agent streptokinase (SK), and later two-chain urokinase (UK), but results were inconsistent and required prolonged infusions.[1,2] Subsequent methods began to exploit the potential of selective catheter infusion adjacent to[3] or within[4,5] thrombus, using SK,[3] UK[4,6] or tissue plasminogen activator (tPA).[7]

None of the above methods proved highly satisfactory. Our initial (early 1980s) results after selective thrombolysis were typical of that era. Using SK for treatment of thromboembolism of lower extremity arteries or grafts, or thrombosed hemodialysis access grafts,[8,9] technical success was achieved in 75% of attempts, lysis times were 24 to 72 hours (average, 38 hours), and major or minor hemorrhagic complications occurred in over 30% of cases. Prompted by these unsatisfactory results, an experimental program was initiated in our research laboratory to exploit more fully the potential of selective pharmacologic thrombolysis. Specifically, we sought to identify and exploit variables that would maximize thrombolytic speed, consistency, safety, and efficiency. The results of our initial laboratory work led to the development of a clinical methodology termed *pulse-spray pharmacomechanical thrombolysis (PSPMT)*. Since then, some or all of the principles and methods of PSPMT have been incorporated into the thrombolytic regimen at many institutions.

SCIENTIFIC BACKGROUND FOR PSPMT

The principles and rationale for PSPMT are derived from the following in vivo and in vitro experimentation, supplemented by clinical experience. In addition,

histologic observations of thrombus have also influenced our methodology.

1. In an in vitro model, no relative advantage of SK, UK, or tPA with regard to speed or amount of lysis could be demonstrated, using equimolar concentrations approximating those used clinically for selective infusions.[10]
2. Inflow of plasminogen-containing plasma proved unnecessary for complete thrombolysis. In vitro thrombus aged 2 hours contained sufficient plasminogen for total lysis, and lysis progressed almost linearly with time.[10]
3. A marked increase (10- to 1000-fold) in the concentration of UK or tPA accelerated thrombolysis moderately. However, raising the concentration of SK beyond 10^{-5} molarity proved counterproductive and resulted in markedly diminished lysis.[10] This paradoxical effect is attributable to preferential conversion of intrathrombic plasminogen by SK to an SK-plasminogen activator. The activator, in turn, activates any residual plasminogen, but little residual plasminogen may remain in the presence of highly concentrated SK.
4. Maceration of clot during exposure to a fibrinolytic agent significantly augmented the rate of lysis, presumably by increasing the area of interface between clot and lytic agent.[10] Maceration plus a high concentration of UK or tPA had additive effects.
5. Thrombolysis is associated with strong procoagulant effects, and concurrent rethrombosis occurs during thrombolysis.[11-14] Admixture of fibrinolytic agent with an antithrombin agent such as heparin[15] or argatroban,[16] or admixture with an antiplatelet agent such as prostaglandin E_1 (PGE_1),[17] significantly accelerated PSPMT, presumably by inhibiting

concurrent rethrombosis. Furthermore, admixture of these agents accelerated thrombolysis more effectively than did systemic administration. Prior in vitro evaluation showed no interference by heparin with the fibrinolytic activity of UK and only slight interference with that of tPA.[18]

6. The procoagulant effects of thrombolysis have been explained, at least in part, by the following laboratory observations:
   a. With digestion of fibrin, fibrin-degradation-products (FDP) that are bound to thrombin are released. The FDP-bound thrombin is active and can activate coagulation.[11,12]
   b. Thrombin and plasmin are released during thrombolysis; both are extremely potent platelet activators.[13]
   c. The high-velocity jet associated with the pulse-spray is a potent platelet activator[19] and has powerful procoagulant effects that can be largely inhibited by heparin.[20]

7. Histologic studies of thrombus indicate various structural elements that influence clot lysability. One such element consists of bands of dense fibrin known as *lines of Zahn*.[21] These lines are thought to be attributable to condensations of platelet-rich (fibrin-rich) thrombus. Platelet-rich thrombus is relatively lysis resistant[22] for many reasons:
   a. Platelets release factor XIII, which
      (1) stimulates cross-linking of fibrin. Cross-linked fibrin is 30 to 50% more lysis resistant than non-cross-linked fibrin[23];
      (2) accelerates cross-linking of alpha-2 antiplasmin to fibrin[24]; and
      (3) promotes cross-linking of fibronectin to fibrin,[25] thus facilitating intrathrombic migration of fibroblasts.
   b. Platelets release a number of other factors that inhibit lysis, such as plasminogen activator inhibitor-1 and alpha-2-antiplasmin.
   c. Platelets promote clot retraction, which impairs fibrinolysis, perhaps by sheltering binding sites for tPA[26] or UK.

Another structural element that probably influences clot lysability is a surface clot membrane or skin.[27] This membrane too seems to be secondary to dense accumulations of fibrin-rich thrombus, perhaps secondary to periods of increased platelet adhesion and activation on the clot surface. These membranes have been shown to block diffusion of molecules as small as 8 kD, far smaller than the UK or tPA molecule.[28]

Gross and histologic examinations of clots have also frequently demonstrated a nidus of platelet-rich "white" thrombus at the head of the clot. We have found that such a nidus is almost invariably present at the arterial–graft anastomosis in thrombosed polytetrafluoroethylene (PTFE) hemodialysis grafts. This small plug is composed of dense fibrin accumulations and is therefore quite resistant (but not totally resistant) to pharmacologic lysis.

TECHNIQUE

The basic item needed for pulse-spray injection is a catheter with multiple side openings, preferably extremely fine side slits, in combination with a tip-occlusion arrangement (Angiodynamics, Inc., Queensbury, NY). Multiple side slits over a length of up to 30 cm enable a moderately penetrating, nearly equivolume spray over that active length. Powerful pulsed small-volume injections can be obtained via a tuberculin syringe. The usual arrangement of the catheter and occluding guidewire, tuberculin syringe, reservoir syringe, and adaptors is indicated in Figure 29–1.

TECHNICAL PRINCIPLES AND RATIONALE

Based on the scientific observations noted above, the technical principles and rationale of PSPMT are as follows:

1. Penetrating intrathrombic injections of fibrinolytic spray are used, thus macerating the clot and augmenting the interactive surface area, mechanically penetrating and bypassing lysis-resistant surface membranes and lines of Zahn.
2. Injection is intrathrombic, isolating thrombolytic agents from circulating inhibitors, minimizing dilution of the fibrinolytic agent, reducing dosage requirements, and minimizing systemic effects.
3. Small pulse volumes (0.2 mL) are critical to minimize embolization. The pulse rate is two per minute. In arteries or bypass grafts, pulsed treatment of a 1- to 2-cm distal plug is often delayed for the first 10 to 15 minutes in a further attempt to minimize embolization.
4. Whenever possible, the entire clot (except for the distal plug) is treated simultaneously to minimize lysis times. If the thrombus is longer than the active length of the catheter, the catheter's position is alternated at about 10- to 15-minute intervals to prevent rethrombosis of one segment while the adjacent segment is treated. When treating thrombosed hemodialysis access grafts, two catheters are required to allow simultaneous treatment of the entire graft and both anastomoses, and to allow access for balloon angioplasty to both anastomoses (Fig. 29–1B).
5. Concentrated agent, usually 25,000 units/mL UK, is used to increase the rate of thrombolysis.
6. Heparin is mixed with the fibrinolytic agent to achieve the maximal intrathrombic anticoagulant effect and systemic aspirin is given for its antiplatelet effect. In addition, 1000-2000 units of heparin

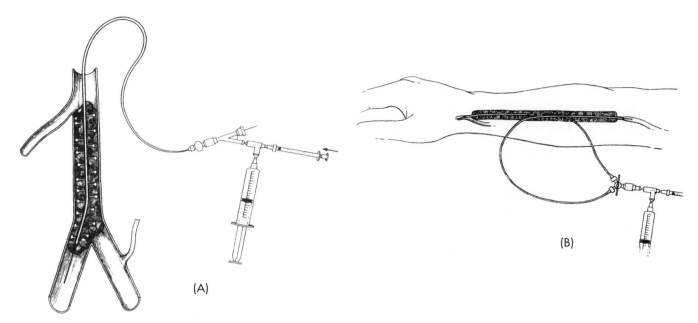

Figure 29–1.   Diagrammatic depiction of pulse-spray technique via the pulse-spray system. (A) Arrangement for thrombolysis of thrombus in a native artery or bypass graft. Multislit catheter, reservoir syringe, tuberculin-type pulse-syringe, valved adapter mechanism, and Y-connector are illustrated. Note the multiple side slits within the thrombus. Because almost all the resistance to flow is via these tiny slits, the amount of fluid issuing through the slits is little affected by whether or not they are located entirely within in thrombus or whether some may be above or below the thrombus. (B) Arrangement for thrombolysis of dialysis graft thrombosis. Two catheters are used, along with one (as illustrated) or more (commonly two) injection assemblies. Use of two systems allows simultaneous treatment of the entire thrombus, as well as later access for angioplasty of both anastomoses and the entire graft.

are given IV. The activated clotting time (ACT) may be monitored via a Hemotec device (Hemotec, Englewood, CO) to maintain ACT at about 250 to 300 seconds during PSPMT. Caveat: for overnight infusions, an ACT of 250 to 300 seconds is excessive, and the heparin dose should be adjusted to maintain the partial thromboplastin time (PTT) at only about twice control values.

7. Lysis is continued until *lytic stagnation* is observed. Lytic stagnation refers to initial lysis followed by insignificant further lysis on angiograms obtained at 30- to 60-minute intervals (see below).

8. Small amounts of residual clot that may persist after lytic stagnation are macerated by balloon compression.

9. Transluminal angioplasty, atherectomy or stents are used on completion of lysis, as needed, for underlying stenoses. What about stents? They are much more commonly used than atherectomy devices. Atherectomy devices have been relegated to the realm of niche tools.

Lytic Stagnation

Ideally, PSPMT is continued until the vascular luminal caliber is fully restored. Atherosclerotic is a disease, not a pathologic entity amenable to lysis. Atherosclerotic plaque, organized thrombus, neointimal hyperplasia, and dissection can cause persistent luminal compro-

mise, making it difficult to know when to terminate lysis. We have tended to rely on the principle of lytic stagnation (Fig. 29–2). When partial luminal compromise persists after initial partial clearing, we perform angiograms after administration of each 250,000-unit ampule of UK, that is, at about 30-minute intervals. When no change is apparent between interval arteriograms, lytic stagnation is said to have been achieved, indicating that thrombolysis may be terminated and balloon angioplasty initiated. This practice significantly diminishes the time required for PSPMT. When this principle was employed, the incidence of peripheral embolization was 19% in a group of 21 cases recently reported,[29] a frequency comparable to that achieved wiith other reported thrombolytic methods. Most emboli were clinically silent. Dependence on the principal of lytic stagnation appears quite safe *except* when the residual mural material is largely intraluminal and exophytic.

Related to the principle of lytic stagnation is our management of the fibrin-rich ''white-clot'' nidus, described above, which usually is present at the proximal extent of thrombosed hemodialysis access grafts, as well as bypass grafts and sometimes native arterial thromboses. Rather than incur the time, expense, and risk of prolonged pharmacologic lysis of these generally small but highly lysis-resistant clot fragments, we usually crush them with an angioplasty balloon. In dialysis grafts, balloon maceration is usually applied

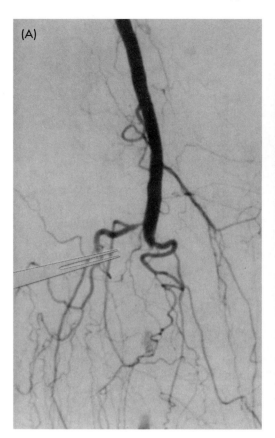
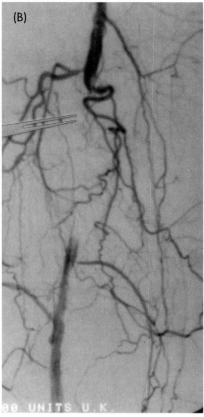
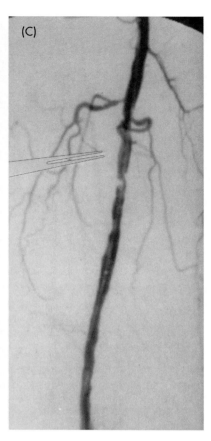

Figure 29–2.   Demonstration of the principle of lytic stagnation after 58 minute lysis time. (A) Thrombosis of superficial femoral and popliteal arteries of approximately 2 weeks' duration. (B) After passage of the pulse-spray system and 20 minutes of pulsing with 250,000 units of UK, there is no significant change. (C) After another 20 minutes of pulsing with an additional 250,000 units of UK, there is moderate patency and good blood flow.

after only about 10 minutes of lysis; in peripheral bypass grafts or native arteries, a longer trial of PSPMT is offered, and residual small, lysis-resistant foci are usually crushed only after about 1.5 hours. Observation of lack of change in these foci over a period of 20 to 30 minutes of PSPMT, so-called lytic stagnation is a key clinical indicator for termination of thrombolysis and initiation of balloon angioplasty.

Value of Noting Traversability of the Vascular Obstruction

Performance of PSPMT requires the catheter to enter, if not totally traverse, obstructive thrombus. Red cell–rich thrombus, along with clot membrane and lines of Zahn, is generally easily punctured by a catheter and/or guidewire. For this reason, vascular obstructions that are traversable by a catheter and/or guidewire usually indicate unorganized and lysable clot, while obstructions that cannot be traversed usually indicate unlysable material such as organized thrombus or atherosclerotic plaque. This guideline is fallible, however. The white nidus often present at the proximal end of thrombus can be quite resistant to instrument passage; perseverance is required before it can be concluded that an

obstruction is composed of unlysable, nontraversable material. Of 15 cases in the report of Smith et al[30] in which a fibrinolytic infusion was tried proximal to an impassable obstruction, lysis that enabled subsequent intrathrombic catheter placement was observed in 7, and complete lysis was obtained in 3.

On the other hand, we have had a number of cases in which the catheter passed across occlusions that were primarily due to organized thrombus or atherosclerotic plaque in which the amount of lysable thrombus was minimal. This occurred most frequently in patients with chronic occlusion of the iliac artery. Most of these iliac occlusions can eventually be traversed with perseverance and use of a variety of technical maneuvers. In such cases, the difficulty of initial catheter passage throughout the length of an obstruction is an important clue to the low likelihood of clinically successful lysis, and in most such cases transluminal recanalization requires angioplasty and stenting. Dissection is another cause of catheter-traversable but unlysable arterial obstruction.

A word about the age of thrombus. Conventional wisdom teaches that thrombi over a given age (eg, 1 month) are not lysable. We have found, however, par-

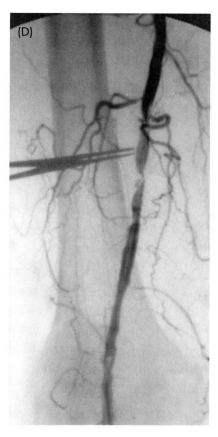

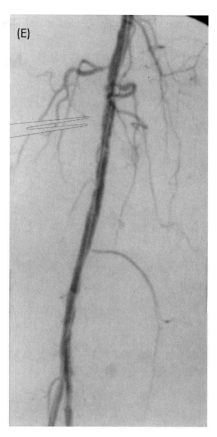

29–2 (cont)   (D) After a third 20-minute period involving the use of a third 250,000-unit ampule of UK, there is no significant further change. At this point, the criteria of lytic stagnation were met and transluminal angioplasty was performed to eliminate residual luminal narrowing, presumed to represent primarily underlying atherosclerosis and/or lysis-resistant or organized thrombus. (E) Final appearance after angioplasty with a 5 mm balloon. There was good flow and good popliteal pulse. Clinical response was excellent, and has persisted to the present, 8 months post-treatment.

ticularly when using PSPMT, that older thrombi lyse nearly as rapidly as young ones so long as they are at least partially catheter traversable. Of course, thrombi become progressively less catheter traversable as they organize with age, but in general, a trial of catheter passage is justified in a chronic symptomatic vascular thrombus or embolus that is otherwise suitable for PSPMT, regardless of the duration of occlusion.

PSPMT in Conjunction with Infusion Therapy

PSPMT may be used in conjunction with conventional thrombolytic infusion. Particularly in recent years, patients that present in the late afternoon or evening are often treated initially with PSPMT until flow and partial patency have been achieved, and then sent to the ward for overnight infusion of UK at a rate of 60,000 to 120,000 units/hr. Although some flow is initially reestablished promptly by such a regimen, the benefit of PSPMT is blunted when it is used in this manner because of the greater required dose of UK, longer total infusion times, and higher costs incurred through use of the intensive or intermediate care unit.

PSPMT can also prove very useful *after* conventional infusion. For example, if residual luminal compromise persists after overnight infusion, one additional 250,000-unit ampule of UK may be given by PSPMT to rapidly determine the lysability of residual material. If no change is observed, the criterion of lytic stagnation will have been fulfilled, and angioplasty may be performed if indicated. In such a case, the residual luminal compromise would be considered to represent unlysable material such as atherosclerotic plaque or organized thrombus.

RESULTS

Most of our clinical experience with PSPMT has been obtained in patients with thrombosed PTFE hemodialysis access grafts, thrombosed PTFE or venous bypass grafts, or thrombosed native arteries of the pelvis or lower extremities. Technical results at the time of last compilation are indicated in Table 29–1. Thrombolysis with UK was performed in 351 patients in whom arterial or graft occlusion was catheter negotiable. The results indicated in Table 29–1 are based on the situa-

Table 29–1. Pulse-Spray Pharmacomechanical Thrombolysis with UK (331 Successful Lyses/339 Attempts [98%])

Classification	n	Time to Pulse or Flow (min)	Total Lysis Time (min)	Units UK (thousands)
Successful lysis	331			
Dialysis graft	253	18 ± 14	33 ± 19	325 ± 131
Native artery	55	43 ± 44	87 ± 41	546 ± 222
Bypass graft	23	48 ± 47	118 ± 69	607 ± 227

Table 29–2. UK Pulse-Spray Pharmacomechanical Thrombolysis: Complications in 351 Attempts

Complications: 29 (8%)
Additional therapy required in 16 (5%)

10—hemorrhage
  0 intracranial hemorrhages
  0 requiring transfusion
  4 moderate-sized groin hematomas, no Rx
  1 large flank hematoma prolonging hospitalization
  1 large groin hematoma requiring evacuation
  1 gastrointestinal hemorrhage not requiring transfusion
  1 nosebleed
  2 extravasations from dialysis graft requiring discontinuation of lysis

14—distal emboli (9 in arterial or bypass grafts, 5 to hand or foot in dialysis grafts
  7 lysed
  2 removed optionally during bypass for other reasons
  1 elective embolectomy of the dorsalis pedis artery
  1 embolectomy of the posterior tibial artery
  3 no treatment required

2—sepsis from lysis of infected bypass graft

1—pseudoaneurysm of arm vein after angioplasty

1—heart failure due to overhydration during continued infusion

1—sheared catheter fragment

tion at the conclusion of PSPMT and angioplasty, and exclude 12 cases of thrombosed bypass graft in which PSPMT was followed by overnight infusion before angioplasty. Tables 29–1 and 29–2 exclude 27 patients treated with tPA, although results were similar to those of UK[31]. Table 29–2 includes the 12 thrombosed bypass grafts in which UK PSPMT was followed by UK infusion, as well as light failures.

Of the eight technical failures, four occurred in patients with thrombosed hemodialysis access grafts and four in thrombosed native arteries or arterial bypass grafts. Failure in the patients with thrombosed arteries or bypass grafts was due to intramural passage in one case, difficult but eventually successful passage through organized thrombus in two cases, and diffuse spasm of a venous bypass graft in one case. The causes of technical failure in the four failed dialysis grafts were inability to access the entire length of clotted vessel in two patients and hypercoagulability in two.

The complications in cases treated with UK are indicated in Table 29–2. In addition to these complications, approximately 20% of our patients have developed shaking chills secondary to the UK. Such rigors disappear within 1 to 2 minutes after treatment by intravenous injection of 25 mg meperidine. In nine instances (eight cases), persistent material after PSPMT was obtained for histologic analysis via biopsy with an atherectomy catheter, biopsy forceps, or operation. In each instance, the material was either lysis resistant (four cases) or totally nonlysable (five cases). Histologic examination demonstrated platelet-rich (potentially lysable) thrombus (three cases), thrombus with a lysis-resistant membrane (one case) (Fig. 29–3), fibrous organized tissue (two cases), suture material from prior vascular surgery (one case), prior patch-graft material and fibrous tissue (one case), and organizing thrombus containing granulation tissue (one case).

Intermediate and Long-Term Results

In a prior analysis,[32] primary 12-month patency after PSPMT of thrombosed hemodialysis access grafts was 26%, and 12-month secondary patency was 51%. In another group of patients studied for the effect of long-term aspirin administration following thrombolysis of

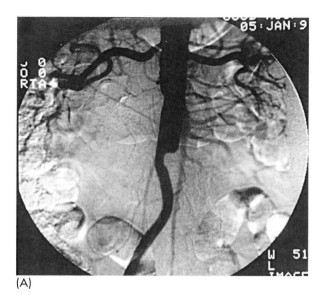

(A)

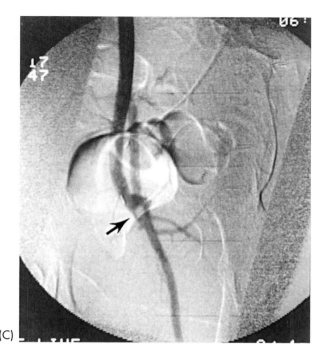

(C)

(B)

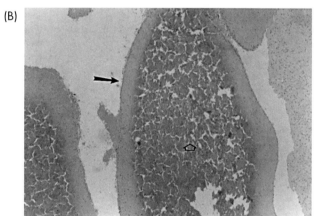

Figure 29–3. Demonstration of fibrin-rich surface clot membrane, one of the causes of lysis-resistant material. (A) Recently thrombosed limb of an aortobifemoral graft. (B) Following 75 minutes of pulse-spray thrombolysis with 750,000 units of UK, the graft was completely patent except for a small amount of residual material at the distal anastomotic site (arrow). This material oscillated with the pulse. There was no change after a further overnight conventional infusion of 1,000,000 units of UK (not shown). Although this small amount of residual material could have been treated by balloon angioplasty, its mobile nature and concern about embolization, as well as the desire to know its composition, prompted operative removal. (C) Histologic examination nicely demonstrates a fibrin-rich membrane (solid arrow) surrounding a red cell–rich clot (hollow arrow). These fibrin-rich membranes are relatively (but probably not absolutely) lysis resistant. Fibrin-rich, presumably lysis-resistant lines of Zahn may also be found within thrombus. Puncture of these membranes and lines by a multi–side slit catheter helps overcome the barrier imposed by these structures to diffusion of thrombolytic material within thrombus. This case also demonstrates the usual futility of continued conventional infusion of a thrombolytic agent when material proves resistant to pulse-spray.

access grafts, the 6- and 12-month primary patency rates increased to 60% and 40%, respectively, in patients receiving aspirin compared with 21% and 7%, respectively, in a control group that did not receive aspirin.[33] We continue to recommend long-term aspirin administration following transluminal therapy for dysfunctional hemodialysis access grafts.

In our reported series of patients with thrombosed PTFE bypass grafts,[34] 40 were referred with intent to treat by PSPMT. In three cases the occlusion proved impassable by catheter, and thrombolysis was attempted by conventional infusion only, with technical failure in each case. Of the 37 treatments in which PSPMT could be used because the thrombus was traversable, technical success was obtained in each case. UK was used in 35 grafts and tPA in 2. In 25 patients treated by PSPMT alone, the mean lysis time was 118 minutes and the dose of UK (23 cases only) was 607,000 units. In 12 patients, conventional infusion of 60,000 to 120,000 units of UK per hour was instituted after a short period of PSPMT and before lytic stagnation had been demonstrated. In this group, the mean lysis time was 13.5 hours and the mean dose of UK was 1,230,000 units, a time and dose considerably greater than those required with PSPMT alone but less than the 2 million units of UK over 18 to 24 hours still usually required after thrombolysis by conventional infusion.[4,35,36]

Lesions believed to contribute to graft occlusion were revealed in 35 of 37 cases. Twenty of these contributory lesions were treated by balloon angioplasty, and 12 grafts were surgically revised or replaced. Primary patency was 28% at 30 months and secondary patency was 46% at 18 months, results comparable to those of series of patients managed exclusively by surgery.[37–39] We concluded that thrombolysis of thrombosed bypass grafts is worthwhile because (1) along with transluminal angioplasty, it may provide long-term patency without operation and (2) it reveals the underlying anatomy and causative lesions, enabling more rational determination of conservative, surgical, or transluminal management.

Although the technical success rate of PSPMT is very high, evaluation of its clinical value is difficult, confounded as it is in our series by nonrandomized patient selection, adjunctive surgical and transluminal procedures, and the variability of the natural progression of atherosclerosis. There is no reason to believe that successful recanalization by PSPMT is associated with either a better or worse long-term benefit than recanalization by conventional infusion thrombolysis. In a prior article,[40] the intermediate and long-term efficacy of PSPMT in patients with thrombosed native peripheral arteries was reported. PSPMT was technically successful in 47/48 treated patients. Seventeen patients in this group (36%) then underwent an operative procedure. Early operation was avoided in approximately one-third of cases, and in one-half of these, arterial patency persisted for 3 to 28 months. In the remaining cases, the postlysis arteriogram usually provided information critical to rational patient management.

Results in Venous Thrombosis

We have used PSPMT effectively in several cases of freshly thrombosed transjugular intrahepatic portosystemic shunt (TIPS). After about 20 minutes of PSPMT, flow has been reestablished and residual thrombus has been removed by clot displacement using an occlusion balloon. We have also used PSPMT in a few venous thromboses involving the upper extremity. Initial partial patency was achieved rapidly, that is, within ~1 to 2

hours. However, complete lysis often, though not invariably, required more time than arterial or bypass thrombosis. The reasons for the somewhat prolonged lysis times of venous thrombosis are not known, but larger clot volumes and absence of forceful pulsations or rapid flow are suspected contributing factors. While the use of lytic stagnation as an index for terminating lysis and initiating angioplasty still seems applicable in venous thrombolysis, overnight infusion is required frequently before lytic stagnation can be ascertained.

Results of PSPMT Reported by Others

A few reports have appeared from other institutions describing the results of the pulse-spray methodology. In general, these results indicate significant acceleration of thrombolysis compared to conventional infusion methods, although they do not quite match our own results with regard to speed or consistency of lysis. Kandarpa et al[41] reported an approximately twofold increase in the amount of lysis at 1 hour in a rabbit model after pulsatile infusion compared to constant infusion. However, in a prospective randomized clinical study,[42] little difference was noted between groups that had pulsatile infusion or conventional infusion, and in neither group did the lysis times approach the speed of ours, namely, about 90 to 120 minutes in peripheral arteries and bypass grafts. In a commentary on this article,[43,44] our group explained the disparate results by differences in technique, primarily the fact that Kandarpa et al did not depend on lytic stagnation as an endpoint for lysis, did not mix heparin with the thrombolytic agent, and for most of the pulse-spray treatment period treated only the upper portion of thrombus.

Mewissen et al[45] treated eight patients with thromboses of the lower extremity using a modified pulse-spray regimen. Mean lysis time was reduced to 48 minutes and the mean dose of UK to 500,000 units.

In a prospective, randomized study of 18 patients with peripheral arterial thrombosis, Yusuf et al[46] found that the average lysis time after high-dose pulse-spray with tPA was 195 minutes compared to 1390 minutes when tPA was infused by conventional low-dose methods. The authors attributed much of the difference in lysis times to pulsing itself rather than to the difference in dosage.

To my knowledge, only two reports of the use of PSPMT in the venous system have appeared to date.[47,48] In one case, a combination of methods was used by Robinson and Teitelbaum,[47] and the contribution of pulsing in that case was indeterminate. In the case report by Hansen et al,[48] pulse-spray with UK proved effective in rapidly reducing caval and right iliac vein thrombus, even though that thrombus had progressed during conventional infusion. The left iliac thrombus, which was not treated with pulse-spray, remained unchanged.

INDICATIONS AND CONTRAINDICATIONS

Because of the many advantages of PSPMT, including rapidity, safety, consistency, efficacy, convenience, cost reduction, dose reduction, and patient and physician acceptance, PSPMT is almost always the method initially employed at our institution. Thus, at our institution, the indications for PSPMT are synonymous with the indications for thrombolysis itself. In addition to commonly accepted indications, such as severely symptomatic acute thrombosis of a lower extremity artery or bypass graft, PSPMT has enabled expansion of the indications to include almost all symptomatic peripheral vascular thrombotic occlusions, provided that the thrombus is readily catheter traversable. Thus PSPMT may be indicated regardless of the age of the thrombus, the location (upper or lower extremity, hand or foot, aorta, viscera), structure (artery, vein, vein graft, synthetic graft, bypass graft, hemodialysis access graft), cause of thrombus (embolus, spontaneous in situ thrombus from atherosclerosis, iatrogenic thrombus from catheterization, angioplasty, or thrombolysis), recent minor operation, recent prior thrombolysis, and amount of thrombotic material (except that peripheral arterial occlusions less than 1 to 2 cm long may be treated by angioplasty alone). Contrary to prevailing practice at many institutions, the speed of PSPMT allows application in some patients with critical ischemia and mild neurologic and/or motor impairment, so long as frank gangrene or totally irreversible ischemia is not present.

Some specific indications for PSPMT, and commentary, include the following:

1. Thrombosed hemodialysis access grafts. These patients are generally referred directly to the vascular interventionalist, and are usually treated the same day by thrombolysis and angioplasty. The duration of thrombolysis itself is now only about 15 minutes, usually followed by balloon compression and dislodgment of a lysis-resistant, fibrin-rich white thrombus at the arterial anastomosis and transluminal angioplasty of a venous anastomotic stenosis.

2. Iliac artery occlusions, either thrombotic or embolic. If the occlusion is traversable, PSPMT is usually attempted before angioplasty and/or stenting. If marked resistance to passage of the guidewire and/or catheter is encountered throughout the length of the occlusion, we now tend to proceed directly to angioplasty and/or stenting.

3. Infrainguinal arterial thrombotic occlusions longer than 1 to 2 cm, prior to angioplasty, and infrainguinal emboli. Although concern had existed regarding production of additional emboli from thrombolysis of an embolic occlusion, this concern has proved unfounded, particularly in view of the speed of thrombolysis and the dosage reduction enabled by PSPMT methodology.

4. Thrombosed axillofemoral, pelvic, or infrainguinal bypass grafts. Although results may be better in grafts that have been in place for more than 12 months, or in PTFE rather than vein grafts, these predictive indices are fallible,[34] and a trial of PSPMT is usually indicated.

5. Symptomatic thrombosis or embolism occurring during angiography or transcatheter therapy.

6. Visceral arterial thrombosis prior to angioplasty, or visceral embolism, or renal vein thrombosis of native or transplanted kidneys.

7. Symptomatic upper extremity venous occlusions unresponsive to heparin. If these are caused by the presence of a venous access device, a trial of thrombolysis with the device in place is often warranted unless there is infection.

8. Phlegmasia cerulea dolens or severely symptomatic lower extremity venous thrombosis.

9. Pulmonary artery embolism in patients with impending cardiovascular collapse.

10. To our knowledge PSPMT has not yet been reported in coronary artery occlusion.

11. Miscellaneous applications: (a) one iatrogenic basilar artery embolus, (b) several thrombosed TIPS treated at our institution, and (3) one dural sinus thrombosis.

Contraindications to PSPMT, and commentary, include the following:

1. General contraindications to thrombolysis, such as recent major trauma, recent major abdominal or thoracic surgery, pregnancy or recent delivery, recent stroke or the presence of intracranial neoplasm, severe hypertension, or bleeding diathesis. These contraindications are in general only relative, and the risk of hemorrhagic complications must be weighed against the risk of alternative or no therapy, keeping in mind the usual speed, safety, and efficacy of PSPMT and the usual need for only relatively small doses of UK. We have, for example, performed PSPMT in recent surgical fields without serious hemorrhage.

2. When even partial passage into an obstructed segment cannot be achieved, pulse-spray is technically impossible. In such cases, a simple infusion of UK may be tried for a few hours, but in our experience, such trials are almost uniformly unrewarding.

3. When a thrombosed graft appears to be infected. We have lysed two infected bypass grafts. Both patients survived despite the development of acute bacteremia.

4. Unavailability of an experienced interventional team, particularly in severe emergency situations.

5. Irreversible ischemia with gangrene and total motor and sensory denervation.
6. Marked hypercoagulability, particularly in patients with underlying neoplasm, is often associated with poor results because of a strong tendency toward rethrombosis.

The only exception to almost exclusive use of PSPMT for thrombolysis might be in a patient with very distal and widespread thromboembolic obstruction, where an intrathrombic catheter position might not be obtainable or practical in all areas. Also, as stated above, patients with native arterial thromboembolic occlusions are now frequently treated initially by PSPMT until flow is achieved, but then, for logistic reasons are sent to the intensive or intermediate care unit for further conventional infusions.

FUTURE DIRECTIONS

Although almost all thrombi can now by lysed by PSPMT, lysis times remain somewhat longer than desired. There seems to be no theoretical limit to the speed of pharmacologic thrombolysis, however, and consistent thrombolysis within a few minutes may become feasible in the not too distant future. The current average requirement of over 1.5 hours for PSPMT of arteries or bypass grafts is probably attributable to a number of factors. Rate of diffusion is probably one limiting factor, and the pharmaceutical industry should work to design a more diffusible fibrinolytic molecule, perhaps by reducing the molecular size. Concurrent rethrombosis certainly plays a role, and newer, more effective antithrombin agents such as hirudin[12] or antiplatelet agents such as monoclonal antibody against the $GPII_b/III_a$ platelet receptor[49] may counteract this limitation. Several investigators[50,51] are evaluating the feasibility of plasminogen enrichment during thrombolysis or the use of antibodies against alpha-2-plasmin inhibitor.[52] We are continuing to evaluate these and other adjuncts in association with PSPMT using our rabbit inferior vena cava thrombosis model.

PSPMT has already yielded important advantages over conventional selective infusion thrombolysis. Nevertheless, the duration of thrombolytic therapy continues to concern many physicians. Venous thrombolysis generally requires days rather than hours of treatment, occasionally even at our own institution. More powerful thrombolytic methods can be expected to further augment the therapeutic ratio, applicability, and clinical acceptance of this valuable therapeutic modality.

REFERENCES

1. Martin M. Thrombolytic therapy in arterial thromboembolism. *Prog Cardiovasc Dis* 1979;21:351–374.
2. The Urokinase Pulmonary Embolism Trial: A national cooperative study. *Circulation* 1973;47(suppl 2):1–108.
3. Dotter CT, Rosch J, Seaman AJ. Selective clot lysis with low-dose streptokinase. *Radiology* 1974;111:31–37.
4. McNamara TO, Fischer JR. Thrombolysis of peripheral arteries and bypass grafts: improved results using high dose urokinase *AJR* 1985;144:769–775.
5. Hess H, Mietaschk A, Bruecki R. Peripheral arterial occlusions: a 6-year experience with local low-dose thrombolytic therapy. *Radiology* 1987;163:753–758.
6. van Breda A, Katzen BT, Deutsch AS. Urokinase versus streptokinase in local thrombolysis. *Radiology* 1987;165:109–111.
7. Meyerovitz MF, Goldhaber SZ, Reagan K, et al. Recombinant tissue-type plasminogen activator versus urokinase in peripheral arterial and graft occlusions: a randomized trial. *Radiology* 1990;175:75–78.
8. Mori KW, Bookstein JJ, Heeney DJ, et al. Selective streptokinase infusion: clinical and laboratory correlates. *Radiology* 1983;148:676–682.
9. Rodkin RS, Bookstein JJ, Heeney DJ, et al. Streptokinase and transluminal angioplasty in the treatment of acutely thrombosed hemodialysis access fistulae. *Radiology* 1983;149:425–428.
10. Bookstein JJ, Saldinger E. Accelerated thrombolysis. In vitro evaluation of agents and methods of administration. *Invest Radiol* 1985;20:731–735.
11. Bloom AL. The release of thrombin from fibrin by fibrinolysis. *Br J Haematol* 1962;8:129–133.
12. Mirshahi M, Soria J, Soria C, et al. Evaluation of the inhibition by heparin and hirudin of coagulation activation during r-tPA-induced thrombolysis. *Blood* 1989;74:1025–1030.
13. Penny WE, Ware JA. Platelet activation and subsequent inhibition by plasmin and recombinant tissue-type plasminogen activator. *Blood* 1992;79:91–98.
14. Gulba DC, Bartheis M, Westhoff-Bleck, M et al. Increased thrombin levels during thrombolytic therapy in acute myocardial infarction: relevance for the success of therapy. *Circulation* 1991;83:937–944.
15. Valji K, Bookstein JJ. Efficacy of adjunctive intrathrombic heparin with pulse spray thrombolysis in rabbit inferior vena cava thrombosis. *Invest Radiol* 1992;27:912–917.
16. Valji K, Bookstein JJ. Benefit of the direct thrombin inhibitor Argatroban during pulse spray thrombolysis in experimental thrombosis. *JVIR* 1995;6:91–95.
17. Valji K, Bookstein JJ. Effects of intrathrombic administration of prostaglandin E_1 during pulse-spray thrombolysis with tissue-type plasminogen activator in experimental thrombosis. *Radiology* 1993;186:873–876.
18. Bookstein JJ, Valji K. Pulse-spray pharmacomechanical thrombolysis. Updated clinical and laboratory observations. *Semin Intervent Radiol* 1992;9:174–181.
19. Bernstein EF, Marzec U, Johnston GG. Structural correlates of platelet functional damage by physical forces. *Trans Am Soc Artif Intern Organs* 1977;23:617–625.
20. Bookstein JJ, Arun K. Experimental investigations of hypercoagulant conditions associated with angiography. *JVIR* 1995;6:197–204.
21. Freiman DG. The structure of thrombi. In: Colman RW, Hirsh J, Marder VJ, Salzman EW, eds. *Hemostasis and Thrombosis: Basic Principles and Clinical Practice.* Philadelphia and Toronto: JB Lippincott; 1982, pp. 766–780.
22. Jang I-K, Gold HK, Ziskind AA, et al. Differential sensitivity of erythrocyte-rich and platelet-rich arterial thrombi to lysis with recombinant tissue-type plasminogen activator. *Circulation* 1989;79:920–928.
23. Francis CW, Marder VJ. Increased resistance to plasmic degradation of fibrin with highly crosslinked α-polymer

chains formed at high factor XIII concentration. *Blood* 1988; 71:1361–1365.

24. Reed GL, Matseuda GR, Haber E. Fibrin-fibrin and alpha 2-antiplasmin-fibrin cross linking by platelet factor XIII increase the resistance of platelet clots to fibrinolysis. *Thromb Haemost* 1991;68:881–887.

25. Mosher DF. Cross-linking of cold-insoluble globulin by fibrin-stabilizing factor. *J Biol Chem* 1975;250:6614–6621.

26. Kunitada S, FitzGerald GA, Fitzgerald DJ. Inhibition of clot lysis and decreased binding of tissue-type plasminogen-activator as a consequence of clot retraction. *Blood* 1992;79:1420–1427.

27. Galanakis DK. Anticoagulant albumin fragments that bind to fibrinogen/fibrin: possible implications. *Semin Thromb Hemost* 1992;18:44–52.

28. Loike JD, Silverstein R, Cao L, et al. Activated platelets form protected zones of adhesion on fibrinogen and fibronectin-coated surfaces. *J Cell Biol* 1993;121:945–955.

29. Valji K, Bookstein JJ, Roberts AC, Sanchez RB. Lytic stagnation: an endpoint for pulse-spray pharmacomechanical thrombolysis of occluded peripheral arteries and bypass grafts. *Radiology* 1993;188:389–394.

30. Smith DC, McCormick MJ, Jensen DA, et al. Guide wire traversal test: retrospective study of results with fibrinolytic therapy. *JVIR* 1991;2:339–342.

31. Bookstein JJ, Valji K. Pulse-spray pharmacomechanical thrombolysis. Updated clinical and laboratory observations. *Semin Intervent Radiol* 1992;9:174–181.

32. Valji K, Bookstein JJ, Roberts AC, et al. Pharmacomechanical thrombolysis and angioplasty in the management of clotted hemodialysis grafts: early and late clinical results. *Radiology* 1991;178:243–247.

33. Abedon SI, Le H, Valji K, et al. Effect of aspirin on hemodialysis graft patency. *Radiology* 1993;189(P):175.

34. Hye RJ, Turner C, Valji K, et al. Is thrombolysis of occluded popliteal and tibial bypass grafts worthwhile? *J Vasc Surg* 1994;20:588–597.

35. LeBlang SD, Becker GJ, Benenati JF, et al. Low-dose urokinase regimen for the treatment of lower extremity arterial and graft occlusions: experience in 132 cases. *JVIR* 1992;3:475–483.

36. Sullivan KL, Gardiner GA, Kandarpa K, et al. Efficacy of thrombolysis in infrainguinal bypass grafts. *Circulation* 1991;83(suppl)I-99–I-105.

37. Green RM, Ouriel K, Ricotta JJ, et al. Revision of failed infrainguinal bypass grafts: principles of management. *Surgery* 1986;100:646–653.

38. Ascer E, Collier P, Gupta SK, Veith FJ. Re-operation for polytetrafluoroethylene bypass failure: the importance of

distal outflow site and operative technique in determining outcome. *J Vasc Surg* 1987;5:298–310.

39. Quinones-Baldich WJ, Prego A, Ucelay-Gomez R, et al. Failure of PTFE infrainguinal revascularization: patterns, management alternatives and outcome. *Ann Vasc Surg* 1991;5:163–169.

40. Valji K, Roberts AC, Davis GB, Bookstein JJ. Pulse-spray thrombolysis of arterial and bypass graft occlusions. *AJR* 1991;156:617–621.

41. Kandarpa K, Drinker PA, Singer SJ, Caramore D. Forceful pulsatile local infusion of enzyme accelerates thrombolysis: in vivo evaluation of a new delivery system. *Radiology* 1988;168:739–744.

42. Kandarpa K, Chopra PS, Aruny JE, et al. Intraarterial thrombolysis of lower extremity occlusions: prospective, randomized comparison of forced periodic infusion and conventional slow continuous infusion. *Radiology* 1993;188:861–867.

43. Bookstein JJ, Valji K, Roberts AC. Pulsed versus conventional thrombolytic infusion techniques. *Radiology* 1994;193:318-320.

44. Bookstein JJ, Valji K, Roberts AC. Intrathrombic administration of lytic agents. *Radiology* 1994;193:324.

45. Mewissen MW, Minor PL, Beyer GA, Lipchik EO. Symptomatic native arterial occlusions: early experience with "over-the-wire" thrombolysis. *JVIR* 1990;1:43–47.

46. Yusuf WS, Whitaker SC, Gregson RH, et al. Prospective randomized comparative study of pulse spray and conventional local thrombolysis. *Eur J Vasc Endovasc Surg* 1995;10:136–141.

47. Robinson DL, Teitelbaum GP. Phlegmasia cerulea dolens: treatment by pulse-spray and infusion thrombolysis. *AJR* 1993;160:1288–1290.

48. Hansen ME, Miller GL, Starks KC. Pulse-spray thrombolysis of inferior vena cava thrombosis complicating filter placement. *Cardiovasc Intervent Radiol* 1994;17:38–40.

49. Coller BS. Blockade of platelet GPIIb/IIIa receptors as an antithrombic strategy. *Circulation* 1995;92:2373–2380.

50. Stoughton J, Ouriel K, Shortell CK, et al. Plasminogen acceleration of urokinsase thrombolysis. *J Vasc Surg* 1994;19:298–305.

51. Sakharov DV, Rijken DC. Superficial accumulation of plasminogen during plasma clot lysis. *Circulation* 1995; 92:1883–1890.

52. Sakata Y, Eguchi Y, Mimuro J, et al. Clot lysis induced by a monoclonal antibody against alpha2-plasmin inhibitor. *Blood* 1989;24:2692–2697.

30

Percutaneous Thromboembolectomy: Indications, Techniques, and Results

Sally Mitchell, M.D.

The management of acute thrombosis, whether of arteries or veins or bypass grafts of arteriovenous (AV) dialysis grafts, is evolving. From heparinization and development of collaterals to surgical Fogarty balloon thromboembolectomy, the management eventually developed into catheter-directed thrombolytic therapy for most non-limb-threatening acute arterial thromboses. The application of catheter-directed thrombolytics in venous thromboses has lagged behind the arterial applications but has recently enjoyed widespread enthusiasm. For AV dialysis grafts, catheter-directed thrombolytics or Fogarty balloon mechanical declotting have been widely used.

Thrombolytic therapy can be a time-consuming and expensive effort, especially when intensive care monitoring is required. In addition, the risk of developing a systemic thrombolytic state and bleeding complications reduce the therapeutic potential of thrombolytic therapy.

In addition, the time required to reopen the occluded vessels must be considered. If the limb is severely threatened, immediate thrombectomy is required. Because thrombolytics may take 24 to 48 hours or longer, a more urgent treatment may be required.

In 1963, Fogarty et al[1] wrote of "A Method for Extraction of Arterial Emboli and Thrombi." This technique was to aid removal of emboli and thrombi at some distance from the arteriotomy by using what we now call the *Fogarty balloon catheter.* Surgical success with this catheter is good. However, the procedure is not visually guided, vascular damage can occur, and clot removal may be incomplete. In 1972, Greep et al[2] described the use of a Dormia basket after the Fogarty balloon could recover no more clot, and in almost all instances, additional thrombus was removed. In 1986, Zimmerman et al[3] described the percutaneous and fluoroscopically guided use of a 3F Fogarty balloon to remove clot through a 9F sheath in three patients after angioplasty. All three had had distal embolization after percutaneous transluminal angioplasty (PTA), and embolectomy was successful in all three. Nonetheless, even with visual guidance, the lack of control of the clot as it was pulled proximally into larger and branching vessels left room for development of improved devices for thromboembolectomy.

Percutaneous manual aspiration of thromboemboli is useful as an adjunct to angioplasty or atherectomy. Aspiration before angioplasty may help avoid peripheral embolization of clot (Fig. 30–1). Aspiration of clot after PTA can avoid the use of thrombolytics or shorten their use. Aspiration of atheroma after angioplasty or after atherectomy can avoid surgical embolectomy or compromised outflow (Fig. 30–2). Percutaneous aspiration thromboembolectomy may be useful as an adjunct to thrombolytics for fast removal of clot.

This technique requires a sheath in place to remove the aspiration catheter under suction. The sheath works best with a removable hub so that clot trapped below the hemostasis valve can be removed easily (Fig. 30–3). Specialty sheaths for this purpose have been developed[4–6] (Table 30–1). [If regular sheaths are used (Fig. 30–4), the sheath side arm must be aspirated for clot. If there is no blood flow, the sheath must be cut off below the side arm and exchanged for a new sheath. This procedure must be repeated with each aspiration pass.] Sheaths used for aspiration thrombectomy can be short, requiring a long traverse of blood vessel with clot trailing from the catheter tip. Or sheaths can be long to protect side branches from clot breaking loose. One disadvantage of withdrawing clot into a sheath is the mismatch in size, possibly allowing clot to shear off between the sheath and the vessel wall (Fig. 30–5). To avoid this, a "Tulip sheath" (Fig. 30–6) was developed[4,5] to expand to the vessel side wall during clot withdrawal (Table 30–1).

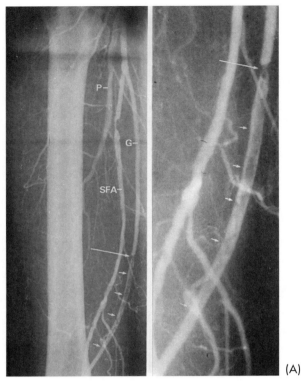
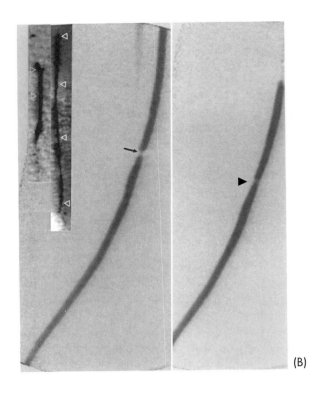

Figure 30–1. (A) Right lower extremity arteriogram with magnified view in a 50-year-old white male. He had undergone right femoral-posterior tibial vein graft 6 months earlier for popliteal and trifurcation occlusion. He has now been admitted for pain in the right toes and a diminished right posterior tibial pulse. Angiogram shows profunda (P), diseased native superficial femoral artery (SFA) (which occludes at popliteal), and a femoral posterior tibial vein graft (G). Note the severe stenosis in the graft (long arrow), probably at a valve site. Below the stenosis is fresh clot trailing for about 10 cm (short arrows). (B) Graft angiogram after manual aspiration of clot with a 5F nontapered catheter. All of the clot was removed (open white arrowheads); (see inset), leaving underlying valve stenosis (black arrow). After angioplasty with a 5-mm balloon, the lumen was markedly improved (arrowhead) and the pulse was strongly palpable.

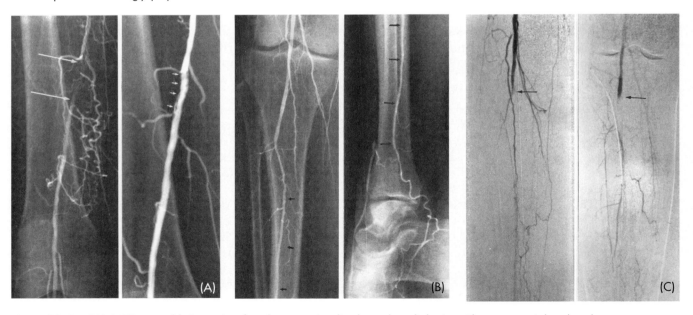

Figure 30–2. (A) A 73-year-old Caucasian female, a non-insulin-dependent diabetic, with severe peripheral and coronary vascular disease. Arteriogram showed a 2-cm-long occlusion of the distal superficial femoral artery before angioplasty (long arrows), with good patency after angioplasty (short arrows). (B) Runoff before angioplasty shows single-vessel runoff via peroneal (arrows) on an anterior view below the knee (left) and on a lateral view at the ankle (right). (C) Runoff after angioplasty shows an early and a later view of a digital angiogram from the level of the knee joint to just above the ankle. The tibioperoneal trunk is occluded with stasis in the popliteal artery (arrow).

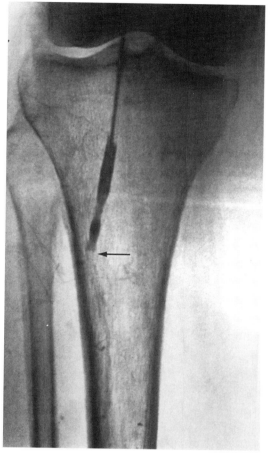

(D)

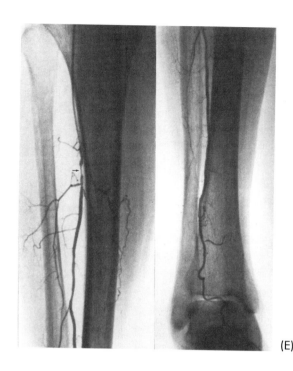

(E)

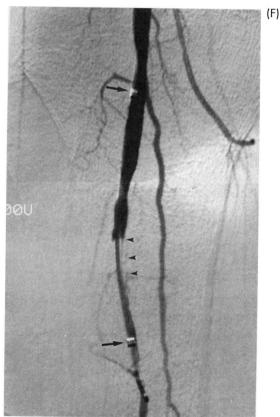

(F)

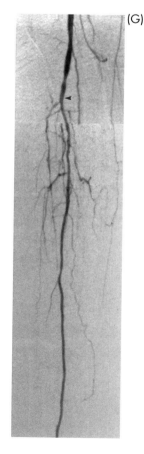

(G)

Figure 30–2 (cont'd)   (D) Catheter injection in the distal popliteal artery shows abrupt, straight cutoff of contrast material (arrow). (E) Obstruction crossed with a guidewire and a 5F catheter. Contrast injection shows peroneal runoff intact, with some proximal guidewire spasm (arrow) but no distal occlusions. (F) Urokinase infusion catheter (arrows) placed across the obstruction (arrowheads). The presumed focal clot was pulse sprayed with 250,000 U urokinase, with no change. We then placed a 5F nontapered catheter to the filling defect and aspirated manually with a 50-cc syinge. When the catheter was removed, there was no clot in it. However, the sheath was occluded. The top of the sheath, with its hemostasis valve and side arm, were removed. There was good flow in the distal part of the sheath, which was then exchanged for a new one. The old sheath sidearm was flushed, and a piece of plaque was found. (G) After aspiration of plaque, a digital subtraction angiogram shows a patent tibioperoneal trunk at the site of a previous embolic occlusion (arrowhead). Runoff via the peroneal trunk remained good. Follow-up showed an increase in the ankle/brachial index (ABI) from 0.5 to 0.85 on the right, with good resolution of pain. Six-month follow-up showed an ABI of 1.0, with good waveforms to the feet and palpable pulses.

Table 30–1. Sheaths Developed for Manual Percutaneous Aspiration Thromboembolectomy

Reference	Sheath Name	Company	Description	Catheter Size	Sheath Size	Adv/Disadv	Study	Results
Vorwerk et al[4]	Tulip sheath	Schneider Europe, Zurich, Switzerland	•54-cm-long outer catheter •Coaxial inner catheter to which a 60 x 8 mm Wallstent with 1-cm taper is attached •Inner diameter (ID) of inner catheter is 4.5F to allow 3F and 4F Fogarty catheters	9F and 10F	9F and 10F with removable hemostasis valve	Open weave allows flow when sheath expanded	In vitro	Successful, with no peripheral embolization
Vorwerk et al[5]	Tulip sheath						In vivo sheep	Successful retrievals
Weigele et al[6]	Intimax	Applied Vascular Devices, Laguna Hills, CA	•Self-expanding sheath made from silicone and a polyester braid	•3- to 3.3-mm outer diameter (OD) when collapsed •6- to 8-mm OD when expanded •5- to 7-mm ID when fully expanded	9F or 10F	When it expands, blood flow is occluded	Two patients: 74-year-old female with atheromatous plaque in Common Femoral Artery after PTA Female with displaced coil in Common Iliac Artery	

Table 30–2. Catheters Developed for Manual Percutaneous Aspiration Thromboembolectomy

Reference	Catheter Name	Company	Description	Catheter Size	Sheath Size	Adv/Disadv	Study	Results
Sniderman et al[7]	One-handed clot aspiration valve set (OCAVS)	Cook, Europe	•80-cm 8.5F NT catheter with straight or curved tip •Clear Plexiglas clot reception chamber with 8.5F ID for catheter to pass through	8.5F	40 cm 9F	•No hemostasis valve for clot to get caught behind •Physician can see clot as it is being removed	Case report of one patient	Acute embolus to left trifurcation successfully removed
	Thrombus aspiration catheter sets	Cook, Australia	•Sheath with removable check-flow adaptor •Nontapered aspiration catheter	6F, 7F, 8F or 9F	Same			

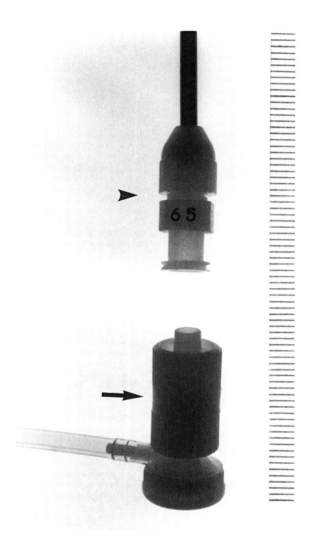

Figure 30–3.   Removable hub (arrow) on a 6.5F sheath (Cook, Australia) (arrowhead). This allows repeated removal of the valve and clearing of clot caught in the valve during percutaneous aspiration.

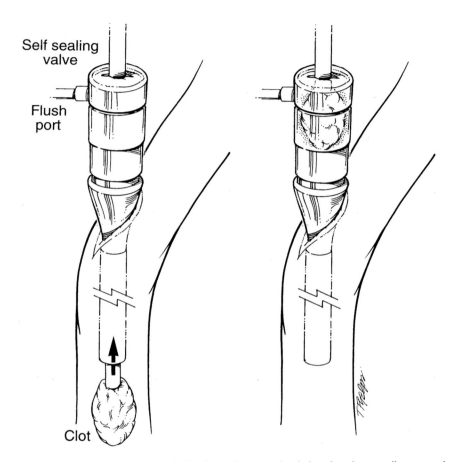

Self sealing
valve

Flush
port

Clot

Figure 30–4.   Manual aspiration of clot through a standard sheath. Clot usually is caught at the hemostasis valve, requiring one to cut off the sheath below the valve and exchange it for a new one.

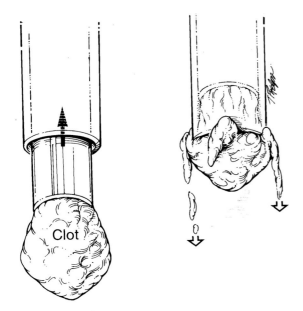

Figure 30–5. One disadvantage of hand aspiration of clot is that the clot diameter may be too large to allow it to be pulled into the sheath, dislodging the clot or shearing fragments off.

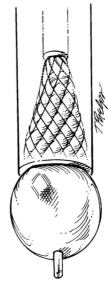

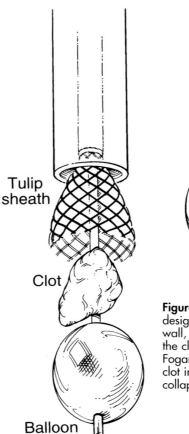

Figure 30–6. A Tulip sheath designed to expand to the vessel wall, allowing one to capture all of the clot during hand aspiration. The Fogarty balloon helps to hold the clot in place as the tulip sheath collapses into the outer sheath.

The development of more thin-walled, large-lumen catheters has made aspiration of larger amounts of clot per pass more feasible. Although a 5F non-tapered catheter may be all that is necessary to remove small amounts of clot or even atheroma (Figs. 30–1 and 30–2), sheaths and catheters of 7F and 8F or larger may be more useful for larger atheromas or larger amounts of clot. Two catheter/sheath sets have been developed specifically for manual aspiration thromboembolectomy[7] (Table 30–2).

The published clinical results of percutaneous manual aspiration thromboemblectomy (MPAT) are outlined in Table 30–3. Four centers[8–11] have evaluated their results with a total of 76 patients. The catheter/sheath sets used have ranged from 5F to 8F. All have stressed the advantage of the removable hemostasis valve on the sheath to avoid sheath changes for occluded sheaths. The reported locations in which MPAT has been useful have been mostly in the lower extremity. MPAT has also been used in lower extremity grafts and in a couple of patients in the superior mesenteric artery (SMA) and renal arteries. MPAT has been used alone or in combination with urokinase, as well as after PTA/atherectomy. Success has been defined as improved by angiography immediately

(81%) and clinically improved in short-term follow-up (93%) in one series.[10] Reported success rates have ranged from 81% to 100% (Table 30–3).

In recent years, development of new catheters and assessment of some atherectomy catheters have begun in an effort to achieve more rapid yet safe removal of clot in arteries, veins, and dialysis grafts. These mechanical percutaneous thromboembolectomy devices are outlined in Tables 30–4 to 30–8.

The simplest device is a small Dormia basket with a leading floppy wire.[12] This basket is used to trap clot, which is then removed through an 8F or 9F sheath with a removable hemostasis valve.

The other devices are more complex, with most having a rotating part within a catheter[13–24] (Table 30–4, Fig. 30–7). The rotating devices are either a flexible wire, a wire fitted with a propeller tip or blender tip, or a rotating spiral. The rotating part is used either to wind large amounts of clot mechanically around a wire and remove it manually or to break up clot, which is then aspirated. One device (Kensey device)[22] breaks up the clot without removal. The Amplatz thrombectomy device (Microvena, White Bear Lake, MN)[13–19] breaks up the clot into small fragments, which the authors initially recommended be aspirated.[14] (Fragment embo-

Table 30-3. Clinical Articles on Manual Percutaneous Aspiration Thromboembolectomy

Reference	Authors	Devices/Catheters Used	Sheaths Used	Number of Patients	Success	Locations of Thromboemboli
Ref. 8	• Cleveland et al • Sheffield, England	• 50-cc syringe • 5F or 7F Van Andel* with tip cut off. • Judkins R.† • Cook single-handed aspiration set.‡	5F or 7F with removable hemostasis valve	21 patients total: 14 post PTA 1 post atherectomy 6 with urokinase (UK)	• Atherectomy and PTA patients 87% (13/15) • UK patients 100% (6/6)	• SFA • Popliteal • Trifurcation
Ref. 9	• Murray et al. • San Francisco, CA	• 5F or 8F catheter • 50-cc syringe	8F sheath (15–50 cm) with removable hemostasis valve	8 patients total: 5 post PTA or with UK 3 as sole procedure	• PTA and UK patients 60% (3/5) • HPAT only 100% (3/3)	• Iliac • PFA • SFA • Popliteal • Trifurcation • Fem-pop graft
Ref. 10	• Starck et al • Frankfurt, Germany and University of Wisconsin, Madison	• 50-cc syringe • Minimally tapered, thin-walled catheter	8F sheath up to 80 cm long with removable hemostasis valve	41 patients total: 14 HPAT only 12 UK + HPAT 9 PTA + HPAT 10 UK, PTA, + HPAT	• 81% were improved by angiographic criteria 50–100% • 93% were clinically improved in early follow-up	• Renal • SMA • External iliac • SFA • PFA • Popliteal • Trifurcation • Tibial vessels • Bypass grafts
Ref. 11	Sniderman et al. Cornell, NY	• 8F nontapered catheter • 50-cc syringe	8F sheath Either exchanged sheath for new one when it occluded with clot or used a removeable hub	6 patients	83% (5/6)	• Popliteal • Trifurcation

*Cook, Inc.; Bloomington, Indiana
†Mallinkrodt Medical, St. Louis, Mo.
‡Cook, Inc.; Bloomington, Indiana

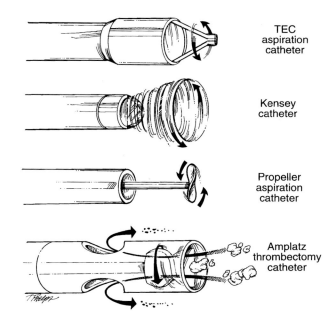

TEC
aspiration
catheter

Kensey
catheter

Propeller
aspiration
catheter

Amplatz
thrombectomy
catheter

Figure 30–7. Schematic drawing of four rotational thrombectomy devices described in more detail in the text.

lization was controlled by a blood pressure cuff inflated downstream until all fragments were aspirated manually.) Subsequent recommendations were that the clot is sufficiently liquefied so as to not require post-thombectomy aspiration.[13,17] The rotational wires[20–22] wind the clot fibrin around the wire. This is then removed from the catheter and the fibrin removed by hand. The transluminal extraction catheter (TEC),[23] rotative spiral aspiration,[22] and Cook[24] aspiration thrombectomy systems employ constant aspiration during clot fragmentation. The RAT system is a ball-tipped spiral that winds fibrin around itself and also aspirates debris. The TEC and Cook systems have blades or propellers that break up the clot into fragments that are then aspirated. The TEC system was developed for atherectomy. There is one case report[23] of its use as a thrombectomy device (Table 30–4).

In 1991, Schmitz-Rode and Gunther[25] compared five rotational atherectomy devices (Table 30–5). The devices were tested in vitro in model circuits with femoral artery and pulmonary artery flow conditions. The femoral artery model had wall-adherent 5-day-old thrombotic occlusion with 4 g of clot, 10 cm long and 7 mm diameter, with perfusion at a rate of 350 cc/min. The pulmonary model had free-floating thrombi weighing 10 g in a 12-mm-diameter branched tube, with perfusion at a rate of 1500 cc/min. The study provides an interesting assessment of several variables (1) nonaspirating versus aspirating, (2) slow versus fast rotation effect on clot maceration, (3) treatment duration effect on clot maceration, (4) adherent versus free-floating

clot, (5) small versus large clot burden, and (6) strong suction versus minimal suction devices.

Results showed that with the nonaspirating devices (Kensey and Bildsoe), an increase in treatment duration from 30 to 60 seconds and an increase in rotation speed from 40,000 to 80,000 rpm decreased the percentage of larger particles (>1000 µm) in the effluent. This decrease was most dramatic in the pulmonary model. All devices performed well in the superficial femoral artery (SFA) model with the percentage of larger particles ranging from 0.81% to 1.72%.

In the pulmonary model, there was a much larger range in the percentage of large particles (1.78% to 10.27%). In this evaluation, the Kensey catheter performed best (1.78%) and the Bildsoe catheter performed worst (10.27%). This result may be explained by the fact that the Kensey catheter has a stronger suction vortex than the Bildsoe catheter. This difference allows clot fragments to recirculate for further fragmentation. Also, with larger quantities of clot, the Bildsoe catheter became obstructed by fibrin wrapping around the propeller and housing. The three aspirating rotational devices evaluated also developed fibrin wrapping, which was least with the Gunther device, more with the propeller aspiration device, and most with the loop aspiration device. Of the aspirating devices, the suction vortex was best with the propeller aspiration device. The other aspirating devices had a negligible hydrodynamic effect because of their low speed of rotation. Of the five catheters, the Kensey and propeller aspiration devices had the strongest suction effect on clot recirculation into the cutting device.

Another interesting point elucidated in this study was that the amount of blood volume aspirated in the clinical application of rotating aspiration devices approximated 110 cc in the femoral region and 210 cc in the pulmonary.

There are four rheolytic or hydrodynamic thrombectomy devices[26–35] (Tables 30–6 and Fig. 30–8). The Hydrolyzer works by a retrograde jet of saline injected by a conventional angiographic injector. The injection port of the catheter connects to a port that turns 180 degrees at the tip of the end hole–occluded catheter. This jet is directed at a large exhaust or discharge lumen. The high-velocity jet of saline crosses within the catheter but just under a large side hole in the catheter near the tip. This jet causes low pressure to occur inside the side hole, drawing clot into the catheter. The clot is then broken up further by the jet and pushed into the exhaust lumen. Extra suction on the exhaust seems not to be required, although some rheolytic thrombectomy devices employ it.

In addition to this central jet, the early Angiojet device (Table 30–6) had four, six, or eight jets oriented retrograde and radially around the catheter. These radial jets were oriented retrograde in order not to

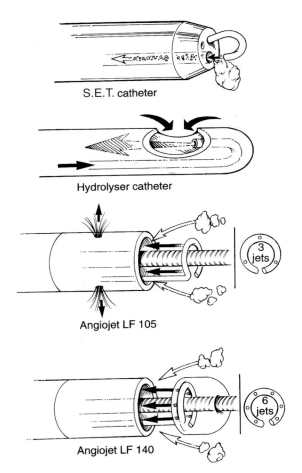

Figure 30–8.   Schematic drawing of four rheolytic thrombectomy devices described in more detail in the text.

damage the lateral vessel wall. These jets create a vortex that draws clot into the catheter side hole. In addition, there is probably some direct clot fragmentation by these jets. The Angiojet underwent some changes between 1992 and 1996, as detailed in Tables 30–6 and 30–7. The current Model F105 has three retrograde high-pressure jets and three perpendicular low-pressure jets. The LF 140 has six retrograde jets of higher pressure, with a tapered and more flexible catheter. The side jets were removed. Also, there is a cap over the distal catheter that may be less traumatic (Fig. 30–8). One advantage of the Angiojet system is that it is isovolumetric. In other words, the amount of fluid entering is equal to the amount being removed with the clot. The Angiojet is now FDA approved for use in dialysis fistula grafts.

An advantage of the hydrodynamic devices is that the catheter can be small and flexible, with some being as small as 4F or 5F (Tables 30–6 and 30–7). This S.E.T. (Successful Extraction of Thrombus) catheter is another rheolytic thrombectomy catheter whose clinical investigation is beginning in the United States. This catheter is a three-lumen device. The inflow lumen turns 180 degrees to inject saline toward the outflow

lumen. There is a dedicated guidewire lumen. The catheters can range from 4F to 10F. The U.S. trials will use the 6F for dialysis grafts and the 8F or 6/8F in peripheral vessels.

A recent article[36] (Table 30–7) compared the Hydrolyzer and Angiojet hydrodynamic devices. As they had done with rotational devices[25] (Table 30–5), the authors compared these two hydrodynamic devices. The Angiojet was superior in having fewer large particles embolizing distally (1.8% compared to 4.8% with the Hydrolyzer). Clot removal was equal in the in vitro venous model. In the arterial model, the Hydrolyzer performed better, possibly because of its 7F size versus the 5F used in the Angiojet. When the Hydrolyzer was used within a 7F multipurpose catheter to guide the thrombectomy device, thrombus removal improved in both venous and arterial models and was fairly equal.

In a study of vessel wall reaction to the Hydrolyzer device versus the Fogarty balloon, van Ommen et al[37] showed significant intimal thickening with the Fogarty balloon 3 weeks after use. The Hydrolyzer saline jets had no effect on the vessel wall.

In an extension of their previous work,[27] Reekers, et al[28] evaluated the Hydrolyzer in a total of 28 patients with acute infrainguinal arterial thrombosis, 5 of whom had subacute worsening of their claudication and 23 of whom had acute ischemia with rest pain. Fresh thrombus (mean age, 12 days) was found in native arteries in 11 patients (9 superior femoral artery/popliteal and 2 popliteal femoral artery) and in bypass grafts in 17 (eight vein grafts and nine synthetic or composite). [Of the 17 grafts, 14 were >1 year old. Of the eight vein grafts, one was a femoro-popliteal (fem-pop) above knee, two were fem-pop below the knee and 5 were fem-distal grafts. Of the nine synthetic grafts, two were fem-pop above the knee, two were fem-pop below the knee, and five were fem-distal.] Their results showed a technical success in clearing 90% of the clot in 23/28 patients (82%): 8/11 native vessels (73%) and 15/17 grafts (88%). The initial clinical success was achieved in 17/28 patients (61%): 8/11 native vessels (73%) and 9/17 grafts (53%). Thirty-day success was achieved in 14/28 patients (50%): 8/11 native vessels (73%) and 6/17 grafts (35%).

The authors attributed the lower graft success rate to the poor outflow of the grafts and to the fact that 40% of the grafts were beyond repair after removal of the clot. Because of the limitations of the 7F catheter to vessels 5 mm or larger in diameter, the thrombosuction procedure was used for debulking in some patients, with thrombolysis used for residual clot in the runoff vessels. The thrombosuction procedure was quick, lasting for approximately 15 minutes.

Devices[22,38] that oscillate in the longitudinal direction either just within the tip of a catheter or even extending a few millimeters from the tip of the catheter have been developed (Table 30–8). This "jackhammer" probe motion may also be combined with a slight rotational motion. These oscillating metal probes are moved by an ultrasound device or an electric motor. Clot is removed rapidly, and the debris is aspirated. The electric motor–driven device is more flexible than the ultrasound one, does not have the thermal problems of the ultrasound device, and has fewer embolic particles. These experimental devices have been evaluated only in vitro.

The ideal mechanical thromboembolectomy device would be flexible, low profile, very effective at complete aspiration, atraumatic to the vessel wall, able to lyse or fragment all clot, and inexpensive. Of all the devices being evaluated, the rotational devices have been used most often. In the United States, the Amplatz thrombectomy device was recently FDA approved for thrombosed dialysis grafts. The hydrodynamic devices are the smallest in profile, the most flexible, and seem to offer good clinical results, with removal of clot from native vessel.[28] The Angiojet (Possis Medical, Minneapolis, MN) has also been recently FDA approved for thrombosed dialysis grafts. The electric motor–driven oscillating probe seems to show more promise than the ultrasound-driven device in early experimental studies.

As for simple manual aspiration, this is even more productive today, now that manufacturers have developed thin-walled, low-profile catheters. The importance of aspirating the sheath side arm after catheter aspiration clot removal cannot be stressed enough. A removable hub and side arm make exchange of a clot-filled hub easier than changing the whole sheath.

The major clinical objectives of percutaneous mechanical or manual aspiration thromboembolectomy in the peripheral arteries include (1) removal of thromboembolic or atheroscleroembolic fragments complicating angioplasty or atherectomy; (2) removal of clot before administration of urokinase to quickly decrease the clot burden, during urokinase infusion to aid catheter adjustment and to quicken thrombolysis, or after urokinase infusion to completely rid the vessel of embolized clot rather than waiting for urokinase to lyse it; (3) aspiration of clot in thrombolytic treatment failures; and (4) rapid removal of fresh clot in the acutely ischemic leg as an alternative to surgical thromboembolectomy.

Percutaneous mechanical aspiration thromboembolectomy would provide a great advantage in restoring flow to clotted dialysis fistula grafts. Although thrombolytics can help, they are time-consuming in these patients, who may require repeated procedures. Several other techniques and devices have been developed for mechanical thrombectomy without aspiration of debris. Indeed, even the Amplatz device, which is now FDA approved as a mechanical thrombectomy device for dialysis fistulas, does not aspirate the debris, although it does liquefy the clot to a large extent.

A mechanical thromboembolectomy device that would work for pulmonary embolectomy would also be extremely valuable. The current FDA approved device, the Pulmonary Embolectomy Catheter (Medi Tech Corp., Watertown, MA), is an IOF single lumen catheter with a 5mm or 7mm diameter cup that is threaded on the tip. The catheter is steerable when used with the control handle. This system is introduced through a venotomy under local anesthesia, steered into the pulmonary artery, and then removed during syringe suction to withdraw the pulmonary embolus.

Another device that has been tested for removal of pulmonary emboli experimentally in vitro and in vivo is an impeller basket catheter.[39] This is a flexible 7F hollow metal spiral with a four-wire basket near the tip. On the metal spiral in the center of the basket is a small blade that rotates at 100,000 rpm. This is placed through a 9F guiding catheter. The clot is broken into tiny fragments that are washed away with the blood flow. This device does not aspirate the debris. In vivo results showed >90% clot fragmentation to particle size <10 μm in diameter. In vivo results showed safe and effective fragmentation of pulmonary emboli in dogs. Fragmentation was rapid, occurring within 10 seconds. Limited steerability did not allow complete fragmentation beyond the main and central pulmonary branches. Other investigators have tried the Kensey catheter for pulmonary embolus fragmentation in dogs. However, the potential for pulmonary artery wall damage or perforation requires a device that protects the thin vascular wall during fragmentation of clot. This is the purpose of the wire basket surrounding the rotating blade in the impeller basket thrombectomy catheter.

Recently, Uflacker et al[13] reported on the use of the Amplatz thrombectomy device for treating massive pulmonary emboli. Five patients underwent mechanical thromboembolectomy using the Amplatz device through a 10F multipurpose guiding catheter. With the use of ventilation/perfusion scans and pulmonary angiography to assess pulmonary perfusion, one patient was markedly improved, three were moderately improved, and one experienced no change. One patient developed hemoptysis due to reperfusion syndrome.[40] All patients had elevated plasma free hemoglobin after the procedure, which returned to normal by 24 hours with no clinical sequelae.

An ideal device for pulmonary aspiration thromboembolectomy would be a flexible, relatively low-profile system that would safely fragment the clot and aspirate the fragments. These are the same criteria required for the arterial system, but the catheter size requirements would, of course, be less stringent.

Table 30–4. Rotational Thrombectomy Devices

Reference	Catheter Name	Company	Description	Catheter Size	Sheath Size	Rotation Speed	Aspiration of Debris?
Uflacker et al[13]	Amplatz thrombectomy device	Microvena	• 120-cm catheter • 5-mm-long distal cylinder • Impeller inside metal cap	8F	10F guiding catheter	150,000 rpm	No
Tadavarthy et al[14]	Amplatz thrombectomy device	Microvena Corporation, White Bear Lake, MN	• 100-cm catheter with distal 1-cm metal cylinder • Cylinder has end hole and two side holes • "Blender" blades on a drive shaft within metal cylinder • Air motor rotates blades	8F	8F	150,000 rpm	• Not by device. Clot is aspirated into metal capsule, macerated by rotating blades, and expelled through side ports back into blood vessel. BP cuff placed distally. • After fragmentation, authors used an 8F guiding catheter with 0.072" ID (Schneider USA, Plymouth, MN) and hand aspiration of debris.
John et al[15]	Amplatz thrombectomy device	Microvena	As above	8F	9F	150,000 rpm	As above
Johnson and Murphy[16]	Amplatz thrombectomy device	BMV Medical, Burbage, Leicestershire, U.K.	As above	8F	8F	100,000 rpm	No
Yasui et al[17]	Amplatz thrombectomy device, recirculation version	Microvena	• 8F rapidly spinning helical screw propeller • Screw and bearing housed in 8F short metal capsule • Rest as above	8F		100,000 rpm	No
Coleman et al[18]	Amplatz thrombectomy device	Microvena	As above	8F	8F or 9F	150,000 rpm	As above
Blidsoe et al[19]	Amplatz thrombectomy device	Prototype	36 cm long Simple propeller	8F	N/A	10,000 to 80,000 rpm	No
Dewhurst et al[20]	Rotational thrombectomy device	Univ. of Washington	Rotating 0.016-inch stainless steel wire core covered with helical coil spring	8F guide catheter	9F	5000 rpm	No; manual removal of clot wrapped around wire
Ritchie et al[21]	Rotational thrombectomy device	Prototype, Seattle, WA	• Blunt platinum tip 0.025 inch in diameter and 0.08 inch long • Bonded onto 0.008-inch flexible steel wire • Air-driven motor rotates the wire • Coaxial inside 4F Teflon catheter	4F alone or coaxial in 8F guiding catheter	Same as catheter	4000 rpm	No; fibrin must be removed mechanically after it winds around wire
Schmitz-Rode et al[22]	Trac-Wright catheter (Kensey)	Dow Corning, Wright/Theratek, Miami Lakes, FL	• Rotating cam attached to an internal rotation wire, which is connected to external drive system • Cam is relatively blunt to avoid vessel damage	8F	N/A	100,000 rpm	No
Schmitz-Rode et al[22]	RAT device	Angiomed AG, Karlsruhe, Germany	• Ball-tipped spiral • Length, 30 mm • Diameter 6F • Rotates within 8F aspiration catheter	8F	N/A	2000 rpm	Yes
Matsumoto et al[23]	TEC	Interventional Technologies San Diego, CA	• 2 triangular cutting blades mounted on rotating torque tube • Advances over 0.014-inch wire.	5–14F	Same as catheter	700 rpm	Yes
Guenther et al[24]	Aspiration Thrombectomy System	Cook, Europe Bjaeverskov, Denmark	• 7F and 10F Teflon catheters with rotating coaxial impeller-tipped wire • 80 cm long	7F and 10F	Same as catheter	500–1000 rpm	Yes

Study Size and Type	Results	Clot Removal Rate	Rate of Effluent Particles >100 µm	Adv/Disadv
5 patients with massive pulmonary embolus	• 1 markedly improved perfusion • 3 moderately improved perfusion • 1 no change	Approximately 7 to 8 minutes required for thrombectomy device activation	N/A	• FDA approved for dialysis grafts • 1 patient with hemoptysis from reperfusion • Faster perfusion than with UK
14 patients: 10 grafts 2 native arteries 2 veins	• 10 complete successes • 2 partial successes • 2 failures	Thrombectomy time 2–3 minutes, with aspiration to follow	N/A	• Device broke up clot, but fragments were then aspirated by hand. • Blades recessed in metal cylinder to avoid vessel wall damage • Authors no longer aspirate debris because debris is minimal
Case report 21-y F with liver trauma Inferior vena cava (IVC) clot	Success in clearing IVC clot.	20 minutes to clear thrombus	N/A	
Case report 78-y M thrombosed polytetrafluoroethylene fem-pop graft x 5 months	• Success in clearing graft clot • Anastomotic PTA required • Patent on 1 month follow-up	N/A	N/A	Able to remove organized thrombus
• In vitro • Human clot 4 and 10 days old	• All postthrombectomy particles <1000 µm. • Particle size and number decreased with longer time of maceration and fresher clot	• 99.2% of 4-day-old clot after 60 seconds • 98.8% of 10-day-old clot after 60 seconds	Particles 500–1000 µm were measured	
• Phase I clinical trials • 5 patients: 2 occluded PTFE femoral grafts 3 occluded SFAs	• Successful complete removal of clot in 2 PTFE grafts and 1 native SFA • Partial clot removal in 2 SFA patients, both with a more fibrous, probably older thrombus	• Time required for thrombus maceration; 63–138 seconds	N/A	
• In vitro • Clot containing tubes	More complete clot dissolution with faster rotation speeds	• 50% without rotation in 2 minutes • 95% at 10,000 rpm in 2 minutes • 95% at 60,000 rpm in 27 seconds • 97% at 80,000 rpm in 10 seconds	N/A	
• 14 swine • In vivo in coronaries	• Successful recanalization in 13/14 (93%) animals • Less reocclusion compared to PTA	N/A	N/A	
• In vitro • In vivo, canine femoral artery	• In vitro, force required to penetrate clot reduced 5× by rotation • Fibrin selectively extracted from clot • In vivo, patency restored in 91% of patients	• One to 3 passes to remove SFA clot • Total clot removal in 32% • Partial clot removal in 59%	N/A	• One arterial perforation • Only the fibrin is removed
In vitro dialysis graft study		95%	3.6%	• Risk of native vessel wall perforation due to extension of rotating cam beyond guide catheter tip • High effluent particle rate: >100 µm
In vitro dialysis graft study		• 51% • Takes 5 minutes	0%	Partial obstruction of rotating spiral with fibrin strands
Case report: 75-y man Occluded R SFA popliteal, trifurcation following incomplete thrombolysis	• Restoration of patency in all vessels. • AAI = 1.0	N/A	N/A	FDA approved as atherectomy device
3 patients: SFA Popliteal Dialysis fistula	Successful in all three	N/A	N/A	Impeller tip stays within guiding catheter while rotating so that vessel wall damage is avoided

Table 30–5.   Summary of Comparison Study of Five Rotating Thrombectomy Devices

Catheter	Company	Description	French Size	Aspiration of Debris?	Treatment Duration	Rotation Speed
Kensey[22] (Table 30–4)	Cordis Corp., Miami Lakes, FL	• Blunt rotating cam • Driven by internal torsion drive wire	8F	No; saline injected at 20 cc/min	30 seconds and 60 seconds	40,000 rpm and 80,000 rpm
Bildsoe[19] (Table 30–4)	Prototype to Microvena's Amplatz thrombectomy device	• High-speed torsion wire-driven propeller rotates in metal housing with two side holes • Metal housing 10 mm long; outer diameter 8F; inner diameter 2.2 mm • Side holes 3.3 mm long and 1.5 mm wide • Propeller 2.0 mm diameter; blades angled 30 degrees	8F	No; saline injected at 20 cc/min	30 seconds and 60 seconds	40,000 rpm and 80,000 rpm
Propeller aspiration device		• Propeller similar to that of Bildsoe device • Rotates within large-bore catheter tip	8F; ID 2.1 mm	Yes; negative pressure of –600 mm Hg	N/A	40,000 rpm and 80,000 rpm
Gunther aspiration device[24] (Table 30–4)	Cook, Europe, Bjaeverskov, Denmark	• Wire-driven impeller (small paddle with a blade; 1.2 mm in diameter) • Rotates within large-bore catheter tip	8F; ID 2.1 mm	Yes; negative pressure of –600 mm Hg	N/A	500 rpm
Loop aspiration device		• Wire-driven loop made of flat profile spring steel • Rotates within catheter tip	8F; ID 2.1 mm	Yes; negative pressure of –600 mm Hg	N/A	500 rpm

Source: Reference 25.

Effluent Particles SFA 10–100 μm	SFA 100–1000 μm	SFA >1000 μm	Pulmonary 10–100 μm	Pulmonary 100–1000 μm	Pulmonary >1000 μm	Fibrin Obstruction	Vortex Suction
0.5%	1.3%	2.5%	0.5%	2.6%	8.6%	N/A	• Long distal extension
0.5%	1.3%	1.1%	0.5%	2%	1.78%		• Strong suction vortex
N/A	N/A	N/A	0.5%	2%	30.4%	Fibrin wrapped around propeller and eventually obstructed housing when treating large quantities of clot	• Short distal extension
N/A	N/A	1.25%	0.5%	2%	10.27%		• Suction of clot not as good
N/A	N/A	N/A	N/A	N/A	N/A	Rotating wire was wrapped in fibrin along its entire length; fibrin obstruction occurred less than with the loop device but more than with the Gunther device.	• Long distal extension
<0.1%	<0.1%	.81%	<0.1%	<0.1%	4.72%		• Strong suction vortex
<0.1%	<0.1%	1%	<0.1%	<0.1%	4.66%	Fibrin coated the wire but left enough gap to allow sufficient suction	• Negligible hydrodynamic effect due to low-speed rotation
<0.1%	<0.1%	1.72%	<0.1%	<0.1%	5.97%	Fibrin stretched around loop eye and caused significant obstruction	• Negligible hydrodynamic effect due to low-speed rotation

Table 30–6. Rheolytic Thrombectomy Devices

Reference	Catheter Name	Company	Description	Catheter Size	Sheath Size	Infusion Speed
van Ommen et al[26]	Hydrolyzer	Cordis Europe. Roden, the Netherlands	• Nylon catheter with two lumens: 0.6-mm narrow injection channel and wide discharge channel • Injection channel connects to conventional injector with saline • End hole-occluded catheter • Injection channel turns 180 degrees and injects into discharge lumen • Jet of saline crosses within catheter and under large side hole in catheter • High-velocity jet causes low pressure inside side hole (Venturi effect)	7F 65, 80, 100, and 135 cm long	7F sheath or 9F guiding catheter	3 cc/sec at 500–600 psi
Reekers et al[27]	Hydrolyzer	As above	As above	As above	As above	3 cc/sec at 750 psi
Reekers et al[28]	Hydrolyzer	As above	As above	As above	As above	4 cc/sec at 750 psi
Douek, et al[31]	Rheolytic Thrombectomy Catheter	NIH prototype	• Catheter with three lumens: latex balloon inflation lumen, high-pressure infusion lumen, and large lumen for particle evacuation • Balloon is inflated proximally to hold fragmented debris from retrograde loss • High-pressure infusion lumen divides into seven distal jets: one is 120 μm in diameter and turns 180 degrees to direct at evacuation lumen; Six jets are 60 μm in diameter each and turn 145 degrees back to radially inject back toward the proximal catheter and 40 degrees out	• 6F over the wire; • guidewire passed through evacuation lumen when pump is inactive	6F	0.2 cc/sec at 11,000 psi
Yamauchi et al[29,30]	Saline-jet aspiration thrombectomy catheter	Clinical Supply Co. Hajima, Japan	• Over-the-wire design • Standard angiographic injector	12F		8 cc/sec

Aspiration of Debris?	Study Type and Size	Results	Clot Removal Rate	Rate of Effluent Particles >100 μm	Adv/Disadv
Thrombus is sucked into side hole by pressure differential, fragmented by the jet of saline, and discharged through wide channel without adding extra suction	9 goats: Clot created in 18 arteries and 29 veins Thrombectomy performed 1, 4, or 8 days later	Successful recanalization in all arteries and veins	• Residual non-obstructing thrombus in 2 arteries (11%) • Residual non-obstructing thrombus in 16 veins (55%)	N/A	An over-the-wire system is apparently available, although the tested device was not
As above	7 patients: 4 SFA 3 popliteal	Success in 7/7 (100%)	1 cm/sec	No clinical embolization	
As above	28 patients: Acute infrainguinal arterial thrombosis 11 native arteries 17 grafts	• Technical success: native 73%, graft 88% • Clinical success: native 73%, graft 53% • 30-day success: native 73%, graft 35%	1 cm/sec	N/A	• Unable to use for vessels <5 mm • Can use conventional angiographic injector
Yes; 6 radial jets create vortex that carries particles into catheter; radial jets also fragments clot; central jet further fragments particles and pushes debris into evacuation lumen; external pump provides suction on evacuation lumen	In vitro 11 clots 20 collgen gels	95% fragmentation into particles measuring 0.8 μm 5% of fragments >40 μm. Older thrombus not as well fragmented	0.9 cm/sec	5% >40μm	• Fast fragmentation of clot • Fragments diameter 5× larger than catheter • Small amounts of fluid required for large thrombi
Yes.	• IVC thrombus removed in 39-y male	• No damage to IVC wall • Successfully recanalized			• Catheter can be steamed into any curve • No hemolysis

Table 30–6. Cont.

Reference	Catheter Name	Company	Description	Catheter Size	Sheath Size	Infusion Speed
Drasler et al[32]	Rheolytic Thrombectomy Catheter Angiojet	Possis Medical Co., Minneapolis, MN	• 4F to 6F dual-lumen catheter. • Small lumen to inflate balloon and contains high-pressure tubing to jets • 4 to 8 jets sized 25–50 μm oriented retrograde; one directed at exhaust lumen, others directed radially. • Exhaust lumen is also guidewire lumen	5F to 14F available	4–6F	50 cc/min saline at 10,000 to 15,000 psi
Vicol et al[33]	S.E.T.	DeWitt Group International, San Diego, CA	• Three-lumen device • Inflow lumen turns 180 degrees at tip and directs saline jet at outflow lumen • Venturi effect created, which pulls thrombus in • Thrombus is fragmented and removed via outflow lumen • Dedicated guidewire lumen • Uses conventional angiographic injector	10F, 8F, 6F, 5F 65 to 124 cm in length	Same as catheters	850 psi
Vicol and Dalichau[34]	S.E.T.	As above	As above	As above	As above	As above
Hopfner et al[35]	S.E.T.	As above	As above	As above	As above	As above

Aspiration of Debris?	Study Type and Size	Results	Clot Removal Rate	Rate of Effluent Particles >100 µm	Adv/Disadv
Yes; external pump and jet directed at exhaust lumen provide removal of debris	• in vitro clot in tubing and grafts • in vivo 6-y canine with PTFE grafts.	• Successful lysis of in vitro clot • Success in vivo, with no vessel damage	Approximately 0.2 cm/sec	N/A	• Small caliber and flexible • Can use in vessels 2 mm or larger • FDA approved for dialysis grafts • Requires special drive unit and single-use pump set with the catheter
• No added suction • Clot is removed via outflow lumen	19 pigs: Extremity artery thromboemboli created Acute and chronic clot removed	• Complete removal of clot • No vessel wall damage		Distal micro-embolization in 10.6% due to 8F prototype used in this study	• Can use conventional angiographic injector • Dedicated guidewire lumen
As above	10 adult goats: 13 venous segments thrombosed and aged 12 days	• Complete thrombus removal in 12 of 13 segments • No complications			
As above	3 patients with femoro-popliteal thrombo-embolic obstruction	• All obstruction could be removed • Some older clot needed hand aspiration thromb-ectomy • Underlying atherosclerotic disease treated with PTA			

Table 30–7. Summary of Comparison Study of Two Hydrodynamic Thrombectomy Devices

Catheter	Company	Description	Guiding Catheter	Injection Pressure	Catheter Length
Hydrolyzer	Cordis Europa, Roden, the Netherlands	• 7F double-lumen catheter • 6-mm oval side hole • Injection channel 0.6 mm • Exhaust lumen 1 mm	9F	• 750 psi • 4 cc/sec saline • Injection via standard angiographic injector	80–100 cm
Angiojet F 105	Possis Medical, Minneapolis, MN	• 5F double-lumen catheter • Three side holes near end that direct water jets perpendicularly with low pressure (1–2 psi) • Three high-pressure jets (1000 psi) at tip of catheter are directed retrograde to create Venturi effect	7–8F (0.080-inch ID)	• Three low-pressure jets, 1–2 psi • Three high-pressure jets, 1000 psi • Injection via special drive unit and pump	105 cm
Angiojet LF 140	Possis Medical Minneapolis, MN	• 5F tapered to 3F • Six retrograde high-pressure (2500 psi) jets • No side jets	7–8F (0.080-inch ID)	• 2500 psi	140 cm

Source: Reference 36.

Guidewire	Particle Aspiration	Embolized Thrombus Particles In Effluent: 10–100 μm	100–1000 μm	>1000 μm	Thrombus Removal Rate: Venous Model	Venous with 7F Multipurpose Guiding Catheter	Arterial Model	Arterial with 7F Multipurpose Guiding Catheter
0.46 mm– 0.63 mm	Yes; negative pressure of 230–380 mm Hg	0.9%	1.5%	4.8%	88%	95%	65%	81%
0.46 mm (.014–.018 in.)	Yes; negative pressure of 230–380 mm Hg	0.6%	1%	1.8%	85%	97%	49%	89%
(.014–.018 in.)	Yes							

Table 30–8.   Oscillating Thrombectomy Devices

Reference	Catheter Name	Company	Description	Catheter Size	Speed of Clot Removal	Aspiration of Debris
Schmitz-Rode et al[22]	US-OAT (ultrasound driven, oscillating, ball-tipped probe aspiration thrombectomy) device	Prototype	• Ball-tipped metal probe attached to a transducer that oscillates probe longitudinally with 30-μm amplitude at 27 kHz • Probe protrudes 4 mm from catheter tip • Probe 1-mm diameter • Ball-tip 1.8-mm diameter	8F	1 minute	Yes; Y adaptor allows intermittent suction from proximal catheter
Schmitz-Rode et al[38]	US-OAT	As above	• Non-ball-tipped probe operated 1 mm inside tip of catheter • Ball-tipped probe operated while protruding 4 mm from catheter tip	7–9F	80–240 seconds for 100 g of clot, with faster times for larger catheters	Yes
Schmitz-Rode et al[22]	EM-OAT (electric motor driven, oscillating probe aspiration thrombectomy) device	Prototype	• 0.5-mm-diameter probe oscillated by electric motor into longitudinal (1.3-mm amplitude) and rotational (25 degree angle) oscillations at 40 Hz • Straight and curved (20 degrees for 10 mm) tip probes tested.	8F	1 minute	Yes

Study Size and Type	Results	Clot Removal Rate	Rate of Effluent Particles >100 µm	Adv/Disadv
In vitro dialysis graft study		73%	0.6%	• Complex equipment is much more expensive than EM-OAT • Stiffer than EM probe and therefore harder to go around curves • US-driven probe can heat up
• In vitro aspiration of clot from petri dish • In vitro aspiration of clot from silicone and glass tubes	• Oscillating ultrasound (US) probe during aspiration through large catheter helped avoid catheter occlusion by thrombus compared to simple aspiration • Aspiration was sufficient to cool the US probe, making flushing with cool saline unnecessary, thereby decreasing effluent fragments • Decreased downstream particles with US aspiration compared to simple aspiration alone	Same for ball-tipped and non-ball-tipped probes	• US + flushing; 20% fragments >10 µm • Aspiration alone: 6% fragments >10 µm • US + aspiration: 3% fragments >10 µm	• Not flexible
In vitro dialysis graft study		68–88%	• 0% for straight tip • <0.1% for angled tip	• More flexible than US- driven probe • No thermal side effects

In summary, aspiration thromboembolectomy can be done by manual aspiration or by using mechanical devices. The mechanical devices are currently in a state of development but show promise for the future management of thromboembolism. In time, rotational (Fig. 30–7), oscillating, or rheolytic (Fig. 30–8) thromboembolectomy may be the primary mode of thrombus removal, with urokinase reserved for secondary cleanup of clot. This may result in expedited flow restoration, whether in the peripheral vasculature, in dialysis grafts, or in the pulmonary arteries. There is much room for development in this area: in device development, in preclinical research, and in clinical applications.

REFERENCES

1. Fogarty TJ, Cranley JJ, Krause RJ, et al. A method for extraction of arterial emboli and thrombi. *Surg Gynecol Obstet* 1963;116:241–244.
2. Greep JM, Aleman PJ, Jarrett F, Bast TJ. A combined technique for peripheral arterial embolectomy. *Arch Surg* 1972;105:869–874.
3. Zimmerman JJ, Cipriano PR, Hayden WG, Fogarty TJ. Balloon embolectomy catheter used percutaneously. *Radiology* 1986;158:260–262.
4. Vorwerk D, Guenther RW, Clerc C, Schmidt-Rode T, Imbert C. Percutaneous embolectomy: in vitro investigations of the self-expanding Tulip sheath. *Radiology* 1992;182:415–418.
5. Vorwerk D, Gunther RW, Schurmann K, Schmitz-Rode T, Biesterfeld S. Percutaneous balloon embolectomy with a self-expanding Tulip sheath: In vivo experiments. *Radiology* 1995;197:153–156.
6. Weigele JB, Sheline ME, Cope C. Expandable intravascular catheter: percutaneous use for endoluminal retrievals. *Radiology* 1992;185:604–606.
7. Sniderman KW, Kalman PG, Quigley MJ. Percutaneous aspiration embolectomy. *J Cardiovasc Surg* 1993;34:255–257.
8. Cleveland TJ, Cumberland DC, Gaines PA. Percutaneous aspiration thromboembolectomy to manage the embolic complications of angioplasty and as an adjunct to thrombolysis. *Clin Radiol* 1994;49:549–552.
9. Murray JG, Brown AL, Wilkins RA. Percutaneous aspiration thromboembolectomy: a preliminary experience. *Clin Radiol* 1994;49:553–558.
10. Starck EE, McDermott JC, Crummy AB, et al. Percutaneous aspiration thromboembolectomy. *Radiology* 1985;156:61–66.
11. Sniderman KW, Bodner L, Saddekni S, et al. Percutaneous embolectomy by transcatheter aspiration. *Radiology* 1984;150:357–361.
12. Gunther RW, Vorwerk D. Minibasket for percutaneous embolectomy and filter protection against distal embolization: technical note. *Cardiovasc Intervent Radiol* 1991;14:195–198.
13. Uflacker R, Strange C, Vujic I. Massive pulmonary embolism: preliminary results of treatment with the Amplatz thrombectomy device. *JVIR* 1996;7:519–528.
14. Tadavarthy SM, Murray PD, Inampudi S, et al. Mechanical thrombectomy with the Amplatz device: human experience. *JVIR* 1994;5:715–724.
15. John TG, Chalmers N, Redhead DN, et al. Case report: inferior vena caval thrombosis following severe liver trauma and perihepatic packing—early detection by intraoperative ultrasonography enabling treatment by percutaneous mechanical thrombectomy. *Br J Radiol* 1995;68:314–317.
16. Johnson JN, Murphy GJ. Mechanical graft thrombectomy: a new technique for unblocking long-standing graft thrombosis. *Br J Surg* 1994;81:50.
17. Yasui K, Qian Z, Nazarian GK, et al. Recirculation-type Amplatz clot macerator: determination of particle size and distribution. *JVIR* 1993;4:275–278.
18. Coleman CC, Krenzel C, Dietz CA, et al. Mechanical thrombectomy: results of early experience. *Radiology* 1993;189:803–805.
19. Bildsoe MC, Moradian GP, Hunter DW, et al. Mechanical clot dissolution: new concept. *Radiology* 1989;171:231–233.
20. Dewhurst TA, Bruneau R, Titus B, et al. Percutaneous rotational thrombectomy reduces acute reocclusion in an animal model of acute coronary thrombosis. *Cathet Cardiovasc Diagn* 1993;30:120–126.
21. Ritchie JL, Hansen D, Vracko R, Auth DC. Mechanical thrombolysis: a new rotational catheter approach for acute thrombi. *Circulation* 1986;73(5):1006–1012.
22. Schmitz-Rode T, Pfeffer JG, Bohndorf K, Gunther RW. Percutaneous thrombectomy of the acutely thrombosed dialysis graft: in vitro evaluation of four devices. *Cardiovasc Intervent Radiol* 1993;16:72–75.
23. Matsumoto AH, Sarosi MG, Selby JB, Tegtmeyer CJ. Thromboembolectomy with the transluminal extraction catheter (TEC) as an adjunct to thrombolysis. *JVIR* 1992;3:491–495.
24. Guenther RW, Vorwerk D. Aspiration catheter for percutaneous thrombectomy: clinical results. *Radiology* 1990;175:271–273.
25. Schmitz-Rode T, Gunther RW. Percutaneous mechanical thrombolysis: a comparative study of various rotational catheter systems. *Invest Radiol* 1991;26:557–563.
26. van Ommen V, van der Veen FH, Daemen MJ, et al. In vivo evaluation of the hydrolyser hydrodynamic thrombectomy catheter. *JVIR* 1994;5:823–826.
27. Reekers JA, Kromhout JG, van der Waal K. Catheter for percutaneous thrombectomy: first clinical experience. *Radiology* 1993;188:871–874.
28. Reekers JA, Kromhout JG, Spithoven HG, et al. Arterial thrombosis below the inguinal ligament: percutaneous treatment with a thrombosuction catheter. *Radiology* 1996;198:49–53.
29. Yamauchi T, Furui S, Irie T, et al. Saline-jet aspiration thrombectomy catheter. *AJR* 1993;161:401–404.
30. Yamauchi T, Furui S, Katoh R, et al. Acute thrombosis of the inferior vena cava: treatment with saline-jet aspiration thrombectomy catheter. *AJR* 1993;161:405–407.
31. Douek PC, Gandjbakhche A, Leon MB, et al. Functional properties of a prototype rheolytic catheter for percutaneous thrombectomy. *Invest Radiol* 1994;29:547–552.
32. Drasker WJ, Jenson ML, Wilson GJ, et al. Rheolytic catheter for percutaneous removal of thrombus. *Radiology* 1992;182:263–267.
33. Vicol C, Dalichau H, Kohler J, et al. Performance of indirect embolectomy aided by a new developed flush-suction catheter system. Forty-seven experimental embolectomy procedures in test animals. *J Cardiovasc Surg* 1994;35(3):193–200.
34. Vicol C, Dalichau H. Recanalization of aged venous thrombotic occlusions with the aid of a rheolytic system; an experimental study. *Cardiovasc Intervent Radiol* 1996;19(4):255–259.

35. Hopfner W, Vicol C, Bohndorf K, et al. Percutaneous transluminal hydrodynamic thrombectomy—the initial results (review). Rofo. Fortschritte Auf Dem Gebiete Der Rontgenstrahlen und Der Neuen Bildgebenden Verfahren 1996;164(2):141–145. (In German).

36. Bucker A, Schmitz-Rode T, Vorwerk D, Gunther RW. Comparative in vitro study of two percutaneous hydrodynamic thrombectomy systems. *JVIR* 1996;7:445–449.

37. van Ommen VG, van der Veen FH, Geskes GG, et al. Comparison of arterial wall reaction after passage of the hydrolyser device versus a thrombectomy balloon in an animal model. *JVIR* 1996;7:451–454.

38. Schmitz-Rode T, Gunther RW, Muller-Leisse C. US-assisted aspiration thrombectomy: in vitro investigations. *Radiology* 1991;178:677–679.

39. Schmitz-Rode T, Gunther RW. New device for percutaneous fragmentation of pulmonary emboli. *Radiology* 1991;180:135–137.

40. Schimokawa S, Uehara K, Toyohira H, et al. Massive endobronchial hemorrhage after pulmonary embolectomy. *Ann Thorac Surg* 1996;61:1241–1242.

31

Intraoperative, Intra-arterial Thrombolytic Therapy

Anthony J. Comerota, M.D., F.A.C.S.

Intra-arterial delivery of plasminogen activators is an important adjunct in the treatment of patients with acute limb ischemia. Initially, intra-arterial thrombolysis was reserved for patients who were not operative candidates or prior to taking the patient to the operating room. The principle of intra-arterial thrombolytic therapy is based on the activation of fibrin-bound plasminogen to promote clot/thrombus dissolution and significant clot lysis has been observed in most patients prior to the development of a systemic fibrinolytic response[1] Distal acute arterial emboli have also been successfully lysed with short infusions of intra-arterial catheter-directed lytic agents, without bleeding complications.[2] These clinical observations indicated that the direct intra-arterial infusion of lytic agents could dissolve blood clots within a short period of time without a significant risk of bleeding complications.

These observations are important in light of the observation of residual intra-arterial thrombi following both clinical and experimental balloon catheter thromboembolectomy for acute arterial occlusion. For example, Greep et al[3] showed that almost all patients treated with standard balloon catheter technique had additional thrombus removed with a modified wire basket catheter retrieval system. Angiographic studies demonstrated that 36% of patients had residual thrombus extracted following the best attempts at balloon catheter thromboembolectomy for acute arterial occlusion.[4] Such data were subsequently corroborated in an experimental study demonstrating that 85% of dogs had angiographically demonstrable residual thrombi following balloon catheter thromboembolectomy.[5] The existence of residual thrombi following the surgeon's best attempt at mechanical removal provides a strong rationale for administering thrombolytic agents in the operating room. Moreover, in the intraoperative set-

ting, the careful use of lytic agents with a short half-life might minimize or avoid a systemic lytic effect that persists after wound closure.

LABORATORY BACKGROUND

Experimentally, canine hindlimb ischemia for more than 6 hours produces arteriolar thrombosis.[6] This extensive degree of thrombotic occlusion indicates that simple mechanical thrombectomy does not restore perfusion to nutrient vessels even if patency is restored to the main arteries.

In a controlled canine hindlimb perfusion study, Quinones-Baldrich et al[5] demonstrated that thrombolysis following the best attempt at balloon catheter thromboembolectomy produced significantly improved angiographic results and a marked trend toward improved perfusion compared with control limbs. Belkin et al,[7] in an isolated limb ischemic muscle preparation, demonstrated that urokinase (UK) infusion salvaged more ischemic muscle compared to a control group. Additionally, significantly less injury, as demonstrated by reperfusion edema, was noted in the lytic group compared to the control group. This study also demonstrated a trend toward improved blood flow with a lytic infusion. Therefore, experimental animal models confirm the clinical observations that balloon catheter thromboembolectomy frequently leaves residual thrombus. These models also demonstrate that arteriolar perfusion can be restored, tissue salvaged, and reperfusion injury reduced with the judicious intra-arterial administration of lytic agents.

CLINICAL RESULTS

Despite an isolated early report indicating that the use of intraoperative streptokinase (SK) was associated with significant bleeding complications,[8] subsequent experience has shown that intraoperative intra-arterial thrombolysis is valuable in the management of patients with acute limb ischemia. Quiones-Baldrich et al[9] reported five patients with angiographically documented residual thrombi following balloon catheter thrombectomy who were treated with intra-arterial SK over a 30-minute period. All five patients had successful lysis without bleeding complications.

Norem et al[10] demonstrated that the infusion of SK following their best attempts at mechanical thrombectomy allowed retrieval of additional thrombus. After balloon catheter thromboembolectomy, intra-arterial SK was infused in the operating room. Following a short waiting period, a repeat balloon catheter thrombectomy yielded additional thrombus removal, and all patients demonstrated angiographic improvement. Similar findings occurred with the administration of UK.[11]

Parent et al[12] treated 28 patients with acute ischemia and residual thrombus following balloon catheter thrombectomy. Seventeen patients had operative arteriograms demonstrating thrombi. Of those 17, 15 had successful lysis when treated with intraoperative thrombolytic therapy. Both SK and UK were found to be equally effective, indicating a success rate of 85% with SK and 91% with UK (p = N.S.). However, bleeding complications were significantly greater with SK compared to UK (29% vs 5%; $p < 0.05$). Patients treated with SK had significantly greater fibrinogen depletion (p = 0.054), and in 43% of SK-treated patients the fibrinogen level fell to less than 100 mg%, whereas this occurred in only 5% of the patients treated with UK ($p < 0.05$).

Intraoperative, intra-arterial thrombolytic therapy is part of the routine operative care of patients with acute limb ischemia at Temple University Hospital. The clinical efficacy of this approach was confirmed in a series of 53 patients with impending limb loss and occlusion of their runoff vessels.[13] The principle of short-duration infusion of 250,000 to 500,000 IU of urokinase into the distal limb was initially based on clinical experience and outcome observation but now is supported by the results of a prospective, randomized, placebo-controlled clinical trial.[14]

DOSING REGIMEN

Because little information was available about the regional compared to the systemic effects of intraoperative, intra-arterial thrombolysis, and because a dose–response relationship to the infused plasminogen activators was not previously evaluated, a prospective, multicenter, randomized, blinded, placebo-controlled study was performed to address a number of these basic issues regarding intraoperative delivery of UK. The purposes of this study were to evaluate (1) the regional and

systemic effects on plasma fibrinogen and the fibrinolytic system of intraoperative, intra-arterial UK infusion; (2) whether there is a dose–response relationship; (3) whether there is breakdown of cross-linked fibrin in a limb undergoing routine lower extremity revascularization (chronic limb ischemia) following a bolus infusion of UK; and (4) whether there is an increased risk of excessive bleeding, operative blood loss, or wound hematomas.

A total of 134 patients were prospectively randomized to receive one of three doses of UK or a saline placebo infusion in a blinded fashion into the distal arterial circulation during routine infrainguinal lower extremity revascularization for chronic limb ischemia. The endpoints analyzed were the degree of plasminogen activation, the regional and systemic breakdown of fibrinogen and fibrin, the degree to which a dose–response relationship could be established, and the safety of the intraoperative, intra-arterial infusion of UK. One of three doses of study drug or placebo was infused in a 30-cc volume as a bolus through the distal arteriotomy at the time of vascular reconstruction. Patient groups include (1) placebo (saline), (2) UK 125 (UK, 125,000 IU), (3) UK 250 (UK, 250,000 IU), and (4) UK 500 (UK 500,000 IU). Simultaneous blood samples were drawn from the ipsilateral femoral vein to evaluate regional effects and from an arm vein to evaluate systemic effects. Blood samples were analyzed for (1) plasminogen activity, (2) fibrinogen, (3) fibrin(ogen) degradation products (FDPs), (4) D-dimer, and (5) fibrinopeptide B-beta$_{15-42}$ breakdown products.

The patient characteristics were similar among treatment groups, except that patients in the placebo group were somewhat younger than those receiving UK (p = 0.042). There were no significant differences across treatment groups with respect to the distribution of associated risk factors, degree of ischemia at presentation, type of operative procedure, or anesthesia administered. The results of the regional and systemic blood tests are listed in Table 31–1 as maximal changes from baseline, and the patient morbidity and mortality data are listed in Table 31–2.

Compared with the placebo group, there appeared to be a dose-dependent decline in plasminogen that was significant ($p < 0.001$) only at the highest dose of UK. Even at UK 500, however, the mean values were still within the normal range. There was no significant decline in either the regional or systemic plasma fibrinogen levels following bolus UK infusion. The plasma FDP levels were elevated in the treatment group in a dose-related fashion, with increases becoming significant ($p < 0.001$) in the UK 250 and UK 500 groups regionally and in the UK 500 group systemically (p = 0.01). There were significant elevations of D-dimer regionally at each UK does level ($p < 0.001$), which increased in a dose–response fashion. Systemic levels of

Table 31–1. Maximal Changes from Baseline (Values Reported as Mean/Median)

	Placebo (n = 33)	UK 125 (n = 32)	UK 250 (n = 34)	UK 500 (n = 35)
		Regional		
Plasminogen (%)	NA	NA	NA	NA
Fibrinogen (mg/dL)	−30.72/−27.00	−28.62/−28.0	−20.35/−22.00	−38.97/−41.00
FDPs (µg/mL)	2.75/0.00	11.25/0.00	9.65/0.00	27.20/18.00 (p < 0.001)
D-Dimer (µg/mL)	−0.106/−0.003	0.035/0.008 (p < 0.001)	0.100/0.029 (p < 0.001)	0.401/0.127 (p < 0.001)
B-β_{15-42}(pmol/mL)	−0.305/−0.226	0.461/0.143	0.595/0.136 (p = 0.021)	0.952/0.296 (p = 0.017)
		Systemic		
Plasminogen (%)	−4.62/−6.50	−9.53/−10.50	−13.03/−15.00 (p = 0.052)	−27.46/−23.00 (p < 0.001)
Fibrinogen (mg/dL)	−43.78/−30.00	−30.52/−28.00	4.34/−10.00 (p = 0.018)	−50.91/−56.00
FDPs (µg/mL)	3.45/0.00	9.12/0.00	7.74/8.00 (p = 0.005)	18.00/10.00 (p < 0.001)
D-Dimer (µg/mL)	0.066/0.003	0.026/0.003	0.069/0.035 (p = 0.005)	0.288/0.111 (p < 0.001)
B-β_{15-42}(pmol/mL)	−0.249/−0.075	0.572/0.125	0.199/0.234 (p = 0.025)	0.552/0.301 (p = 0.001)

Note: p values refer to comparisons to placebo and were calculated using the Wilcoxon rank-sum analysis. p < 0.05 values are listed, but significance is assigned at $p \le 0.01$.

Table 31–2. Patient Morbidity and Mortality According to Treatment Group

	Placebo	UK 125	UK 250	UK 500	Total
Blood loss (mL)					
Mean	306.1	420.7	355.2	368.1	362.2
Median	250.0	350.0	325.0	300.0	300.0 (p = 0.12)
Blood replaced (mL)					
Mean	146.9	150.0	140.9	187.6	156.8
Median	0.0	0.0	0.0	0.0	0.0 (p = 0.89)
Excessive operative Bleeding (% of patients)	5.9	9.7	2.9	2.9	5.2 (p = 0.56)
Wound hematoma (% of patients)					
None	91.2	86.7	87.5	94.1	90.0
Mild	5.9	6.7	12.5	5.9	7.7 (p = 0.71)
Moderate-severe	2.9	6.6	0.0	0.0	2.3
Death (%)	12.1	0.0	5.9	0.0	4.5 (p = 0.034)
Length of stay (postop days)					
Mean	10.8	22.7	15.7	16.2	16.3
Median	9.5	16.0	9.0	11.0	10.0 (p = 0.06)

Significance: $p \le 0.05$.

D-dimer became significantly elevated at UK 250 and UK 500 ($p < 0.001$). Finally, fragment β-beta$_{15-42}$ levels showed a trend toward elevation at the higher doses of UK, but achieved significance only at UK 500 ($p = 0.009$).

There was no difference in blood loss, the amount of blood replaced or the assessment of operative bleeding for any patient group. There was no difference in the frequency of wound hematomas in patients receiving UK compared with those receiving placebo. There placebo group tended to have a shorter hospital stay than the treatment groups ($p = 0.06$). An unexpected finding was the higher mortality in the placebo group (12.1%) compared with 2.0% in patients receiving UK ($p = 0.033$). There were no significant differences between the maximal changes noted in the systemic and regional circulations for any of the plasma measurements.

CONTEMPORARY PRACTICE

Intraoperative, intra-arterial thrombolytic therapy is now an important part of the treatment of patients with acute limb-threatening ischemia in which distal intra-arterial thrombus is part of the pathophysiology of the patient's ongoing ischemia. Currently, several methods of intraoperative, intra-arterial thrombolysis are available to the clinician. For example, a single- or double-bolus intra-arterial infusion or a short (20- to 30-minute) infusion of 250,000 IU UK may be sufficient to lyse a small thrombus occluding the outflow from a distal tibial bypass (Fig. 31–1). On the other hand, in patients with multiple-vessel thrombosis causing critical limb ischemia, a single bolus may not be sufficient for limb salvage. If systemic thrombolysis is contraindicated, isolated limb perfusion with a high dose of plasminogen activator infused intra-arterially, with drainage of the venous effluent, can maximize clot lysis in addition to protecting the patient from any systemic lytic effect (Fig. 31–2).

Quinones-Baldrich and his colleagues have taken the isolated limb perfusion technique one step further by incorporating an extracorporeal pump to administer high-dose plasminogen activators, UK (1 to 2 million IU) or tissue plasminogen activator (125 mg) into the

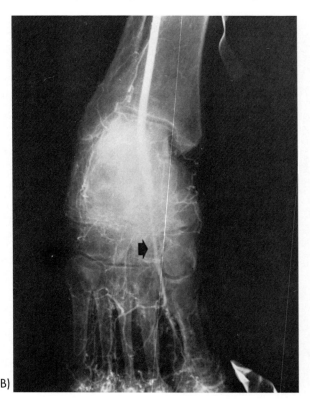

(A)   (B)

Figure 31–1. The use of intraoperative, intra-arterial thrombolysis to dissolve clots in the runoff bed before construction of a more proximal bypass. This patient presented with acute occlusion of the femoral-anterior tibial bypass graft. All named arteries below the profunda femoris artery were occluded. (A) The distal extent of the anterior tibial artery is visualized, showing progressive atherosclerotic disease in several areas. There was segmental occlusion of the dorsalis pedis artery (arrow) that appeared consistent with a thrombotic occlusion. UK (60,000 IU) was infused distally from an arteriotomy in the dorsalis pedis before thrombectomy of the femoral–anterior tibial artery bypass. Once thrombectomy was performed, the graft was extended to the dorsalis pedis with a 4-mm polytetrafluoroethylene (PTFE) graft. A completion arteriogram (B) shows complete lysis of the thrombus in the distal dorsalis pedis artery. The patient continued to receive low-dose warfarin, and the graft remained patent and the patient ambulating normally for 3.5 years.

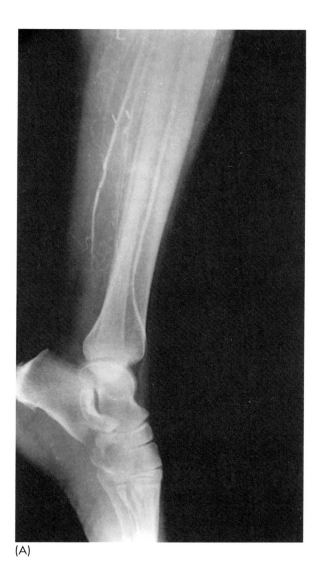

(A)

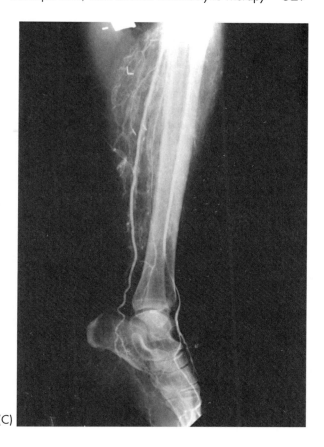

(C)

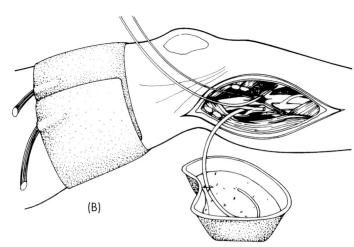

(B)

Figure 31–2. The technique of high-dose isolated limb perfusion of a thrombolytic agent in a patient who could not have any degree of systemic fibrinolysis (having had a coronary artery bypass 2 days earlier) and who had acute multivessel distal occlusion that was unlikely to resolve with a single bolus of a fibrinolytic agent. The patient had an acute embolic-thrombotic arterial occlusion after percutaneous removal of an intra-aortic balloon, which was required following her emergency coronary artery bypass. Shown is the intraopertive arteriogram after balloon catheter thrombectomy of the popliteal and tibial vessels. Additional thrombus could not be mechanically removed. Catheters were placed into the origin of the posterior tibial and anterior tibial arteries, and the arteriogram (A) was performed with this selective injection technique. There was no evidence of contrast material entering the foot. Because additional thrombus could not be retrieved, we believed the patient would require a major amputation. (B) The patient's limb was elevated and the venous blood exsanguinated with a rubber bandage. A sterile blood pressure cuff (tourniquet) was placed on the distal thigh and inflated to 250 mm Hg. The popliteal vein was cannulated with a red rubber catheter and drained into a basin. One million units of UK was infused into the lower leg in a volume of 1 L of saline (500,000 IU in each of the anterior tibial and posterior tibial arteries) over 20 minutes. Following completion of the UK infusion, the limb was flushed with a heparin-saline solution. The venotomy was closed primarily, and the arteriotomy closed with a patch. (C) A postinfusion arteriogram documented significant improvement of perfusion to the foot. The patient had a palpable dorsalis pedis pulse and a pink foot following wound closure.

Table 31–3. Applications for Intraoperative, Intra-arterial Thrombolysis

Indication	Goal of Infusion	Suggested Technique
1. Following native artery or bypass graft thromboembolectomy	Lyse residual/adherent thrombus	Bolus dose × 1–2 100–500 × 10³ IU UK 10–20 mg rt-PA
2. Open single tibial artery to provide runoff for bypass	Restore patency or dissolve residual thrombus	Bolus dose × 1–2 or short-duration infusion 100–500 × 10³ IU UK 10–20 mg rt-PA
3. Multivessel, extensive distal arterial thrombosis	Dissolve occlusive clot/thrombus	High-dose isolated limb perfusion (± extra-corporeal pump) 1000–2000 × 10³ IU UK 100–125 mg rt-PA

Abbreviation: rt-PA (recombinant tissue plasminogen activator).

distal arterial circulation. A tourniquet was placed proximal to the cannulation site and inflated above systolic pressure to maintain isolation of the circulation of the extremity. These authors noted that while perfusion pressures were maintained at a physiologic level, the volume of flow increased as lysis progressed. After patency of the distal circulation was restored, lower extremity bypass procedures could be performed. This resulted in limb salvage in 70% of these acutely ischemic patients.[15]

Although the acutely ischemic limb with suspected distal thrombi is the most frequent indication for intraoperative fibrinolytic therapy, plasminogen activators may also be of some benefit in patients with chronic lower extremity ischemia. In the prospective, randomized, placebo-controlled trial previously reported, it was evident that complexed fibrin in the distal circulation was broken down. There appeared to be a dose-related elevation of D-dimer, suggesting that lysis of fibrin in the distal circulation occurred. If this is indeed the case, small distal vessel thrombosis may be part of the pathophysiology of progressive chronic limb ischemia. Because bleeding complications were not observed with bolus doses of up to 500,000 IU, it seems reasonable to consider distal infusion of UK in patients undergoing operations for chronic but severe limb ischemia. Clearly, additional randomized trials are required to clarify this important issue.

In summary, the utility of intraoperative, intra-arterial lytic therapy is summarized in Table 31–3. Judicious use of plasminogen activators in the operating room is safe and may make an important difference in achieving limb salvage in patients with critical limb ischemia.

REFERENCES

1. Comerota AJ, Rubin R, Tyson R, et al. Intra-arterial thrombolytic therapy in peripheral vascular disease. *Surg Gynecol Obstet* 1987;165:1.
2. Chaise LS, Comerota AJ, Soulen RL, et al. Selective intra-arterial streptokinase therapy in the immediate postoperative period. *JAMA* 1982;247:2397.
3. Greep JM, Allman PJ, Janet F, et al. A combined technique for peripheral arterial embolectomy. *Arch Surg* 1972;105:869.
4. Plecha RF, Pories WJ. Intraoperative angiography in the immediate assessment of arterial reconstruction. *Arch Surg* 1972;105:902.
5. Quinones-Baldrich WJ, Ziomek S, Henderson TC, et al. Intraoperative fibrinolytic therapy: experimental evaluation. *J Vasc Surg* 1986;4:229.
6. Dunnant JR, Edwards WS. Small vessel occlusion in the extremity after periods of arterial obstruction: an experimental study. *Surgery* 1973;75:240.
7. Belkin M, Valeri R, Hobson RW. Intra-arterial urokinase increases skeletal muscle viability after acute ischemia. *J Vasc Surg* 1989;9:161.
8. Cohen LJ, Kaplan M, Bernhard VM. Intraoperative fibrinolytic therapy: an adjunct to catheter thromboembolectomy. *J Vasc Surg* 1985;2:319.
9. Quinones-Baldrich WJ, Zierler RE, Hiatt JC. Intraoperative fibrinolytic therapy: an adjunct to catheter thromboembolectomy. *J Vasc Surg* 1985;2:319.
10. Norem RF, Shrot DH, Kerstein MD. Role of intraoperative fibrinolytic therapy in acute arterial occlusion. *Surg Gynecol Obstet* 1988;167:87.
11. Garcia R, Saroyan RM, Senkowsky J, et al. Intraoperative, intra-arterial urokinase infusion as an adjunct to Fogarty catheter embolectomy in acute arterial occlusion. *Surg Gynecol Obstet* 1990:171:201.
12. Parent NE, Bernhard VM, Pabst TS, et al. Fibrinolytic treatment of residual thrombus after catheter embolectomy for severe lower limb ischemia. *J Vasc Surg* 1989;9:153.
13. Comerota AJ, White JV, Grosh JD. Intraoperative, intra-arterial thrombolytic therapy for salvage of limbs in patients with distal arterial thrombosis. *Surg Gynecol Obstet* 1989;169:283.
14. Comerota AJ, Rao AK, Throm RC, et al. A prospective, randomized, blinded and placebo-controlled trial of intraoperative, intra-arterial urokinase infusion during lower extremity revascularization: regional and systemic effects. *Ann Surg* 1993;218(4):534.
15. Quinones-Baldrich WJ, Deaton DH, Ahn SS, Nene S, Cushen C, Moore WS. Isolated fibrinolytic limb perfusion with extracorporeal pump in the management of acute limb ischemia. Presented at the Eleventh Annual Meeting of the Western Vascular Society, January 22, 1996.

Section 3
Arterial Aneurysm Disease

32

The Pathogenesis of Aortic Anerysms

Christopher K. Zarins, M.D.

INTRODUCTION

Aortic aneurysms are the most prominent and dramatic changes affecting the human aorta. Recognition that the prevalence of aortic aneurysms has increased more than threefold over the past several decades and the introduction of new endovascular methods to treat aortic aneurysms have led to a resurgence of interest in the pathogenesis of aneurysm formation. A number of theories have been proposed, including atherosclerotic aortic wall degeneration, proteolytic enzyme activation, inflammatory artery wall degradation, infectious processes, genetic predisposition, and hemodynamic influences. No single theory has been widely accepted. It is likely that aneurysm formation results from an interaction of multiple factors and influences rather than from a single process. Increased understanding of the mechanisms controlling aneurysm formation may be helpful in developing strategies to prevent and control the aneurysmal process.

ATHEROSCLEROTIC AORTIC ANEURYSMS

The relationship between atherosclerosis and aortic aneurysms has long been recognized. Most patients with abdominal aortic aneurysms have evidence of atherosclerosis in the coronary arteries, carotid arteries, or peripheral arteries, and abdominal aortic aneurysms are commonly referred to as *atherosclerotic aortic aneurysms*. Although some have suggested that no etiologic relationship exists between atherosclerosis and aneurysm formation,[1,2] increased understanding of the atherosclerotic process and its effects on the artery wall suggests a strong pathogenetic relationship.[3]

Arterial Enlargement

Atherosclerosis is a complex and dynamic process involving cellular proliferation and migration, intimal lipid deposition, inflammation, fibrosis, and necrosis with dystrophic calcification. Plaque deposition is accompanied by artery wall remodeling, which acts to counter the deleterious effects of intimal plaque deposition.[4] The primary artery wall's response to atherosclerotic plaque deposition is arterial enlargement, and this response appears to be a general characteristic of atherosclerotic arteries. Arterial enlargement can prevent or postpone the development of lumen stenosis and has been demonstrated in the coronary arteries, carotid arteries, abdominal aorta, and superficial femoral arteries in humans.[5] In the human coronary arteries, enlargement can maintain a normal or near-normal luminal caliber when the cross-sectional area of intimal plaque does not exceed approximately 40% of the area encompassed by the internal elastic lamina[6] (Fig. 32.1).

In the human aorta, enlargement is seen with increasing age and increasing atherosclerotic plaque. Both the thoracic and abdominal aorta enlarge with age, but abdominal aortic size is more prominently influenced by the amount of intimal plaque. This may

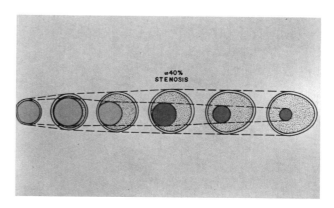

Figure 32–1. Enlargement of arteries with increasing atherosclerotic plaque. Enlargement can maintain normal or near-normal luminal caliber when plaque does not exceed 40% of the area encompassed by the internal elastic lamina. (Reprinted from Ref. 6 with permission.)

explain the particular propensity for aneurysms to develop in the infrarenal aorta, which is susceptible to plaque formation.[7] The human superficial femoral artery also enlarges with increasing atherosclerotic plaque. However, the enlargement response may be restricted in the adductor canal and thus may predispose the superficial femoral artery to the development of stenoses in this area.[8] It is not uncommon to have a twofold enlargement of atherosclerotic arteries as a result of large intimal plaques, with little or no alteration in lumen cross-sectional area. Failure of adequate dilatation, of course, will lead to stenosis. Thus, atherosclerosis characteristically causes enlargement of arteries even though a common end result is constriction of the lumen. The time-dependent enlargement of the aorta is an important consideration in therapies such as endovascular stent grafting, which depend on radial tension and friction for fixation. Enlargement of the aorta over time may result in migration of the stent graft or refill of the aneurysm.

Media Thinning

A common feature of atherosclerosis is thinning of the media beneath an atherosclerotic plaque (Fig. 32–2). The media is the major structural unit of the aorta and is composed of layers of musculoelastic fascicles. Each group of smooth muscle cells of the media is surrounded by a common collagenous basal lamina interlaced by a basketwork of type III collagen fibrils surrounded by layers of elastic fibers. Thick bundles of type I collagen fibers weave between adjacent fibromuscular layers and provide much of the tensile strength of the media. The elastic fibers distribute mural tensile stresses and provide recoil during the cardiac cycle, while the collagen network prevents overdistention, disruption, and enlargement.[9]

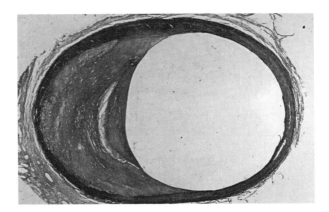

Figure 32–2. Cross section of an atherosclerotic artery with eccentric plaque, arterial enlargement, and thinning of the media beneath the plaque. Plaque erosion, ulceration, or dissolution may result in enlargement of lumen caliber and aneurysm formation.

In atherosclerosis the media frequently becomes thin and disappears under large atherosclerotic plaques. It is unclear whether this thinning is related to the mechanism of atherosclerotic enlargement or is caused by erosive effects of the plaque components on the artery wall. Cavitary excavations of the media are frequently noted in lipid-rich areas of the plaque and may be associated with regions of macrophage invasion and inflammation. Collagen and fibrous tissue in the adventitia and calcification within the plaque and media may compensate for loss of the media and provide structural support to the aortic wall. For aortic enlargement to occur in atherosclerosis, the matrix fibers of collagen and elastin of the aortic wall must be degraded and/or resynthesized in new proportions because passive distention of the aorta will not permit enlargement in excess of the diastolic dimensions without rupture. Thus, during the process of atherosclerotic artery adaptive enlargement, proteolytic enzymes must be activated for enlargement to take place. During active and rapid enlargement, which occurs during the development of aneurysms, much larger and perhaps less controlled proteolytic activities are likely to take place. Indeed, increased amounts of collagenase, elastase, and metalloproteinases have been demonstrated in aortic aneurysms, with maximal concentrations occurrng in rapidly enlarging and ruptured aneurysms.[10–13] Experimental enzymatic destruction of the medial matrix architecture results in dilatation and rupture of the aorta,[14] and experimental mechanical injury, which destroys the medial lamellar architecture, can result in aneurysm formation.[15] These observations support the importance of the media in maintenance of the integrity of the aorta.

Human atherosclerotic aneurysms, particularly those of the abdominal aorta, are characterized by extensive atrophy of the media. The normal lamellar architecture is almost totally effaced, and the aortic wall is replaced by a narrow fibrous band. Atrophic changes are also evident in the overlying atherosclerotic lesions to such an extent that plaques may be relatively thinned and contain little residual lipid. Fibrosis and calcification may predominate, depending on the region that is available for histologic study. It is rare to find human abdominal aortic aneurysms without evidence of atherosclerosis. Atherosclerotic plaques remain prominent in the neck of the aneurysm and in the iliac vessels, and frequently can be seen posteriorly along the lumbar ostia.

Aneurysm Formation

Atherosclerotic artery wall degeneration may result in aneurysm formation by the following mechanism. Intimal plaque deposition is accompanied by thinning of the media and compensatory arterial enlargement. The enlarged atherosclerotic aorta may receive structural support from the stable, fibrotic, or calcified atherosclerotic plaques, particularly in association with adventitial fibrogenesis, which is characteristic of atherosclerosis.[3]

Late in the atherosclerotic process when the aorta is enlarged, plaque senescence may occur, with reduction in plaque volume and alteration in composition, ulceration, or regression, resulting in lumen enlargement. Tensile support with an atrophic, degenerated media may be insufficient, and progressive aneurysmal enlargement may ensue.

In addition, metabolic alteration in plaque lipid composition may stimulate macrophage activity and inflammation and promote proteolytic activity in some atherosclerotic plaques. The balance between plaque formation, artery wall adaptation, and matrix protein synthesis and degradation likely plays a major role in aneurysm pathogenesis. Aneurysms appear to be a relatively late phase of plaque evolution when plaque and media atrophy predominate, rather than an earlier phase of atherosclerosis when cell proliferation, fibrogenesis, and sequestered lipid accumulation are predominant. This is consistent with the observation that patients undergoing surgery for abdominal aortic aneurysm are approximately 10 years older than those undergoing surgery for occlusive disease.[16]

PROTEOLYTIC ENZYMES

Degradation of the extracellular matrix and structural elements of the aortic wall is necessary for aneurysmal enlargement. Both collagenase and elastase activities have been shown to be elevated in aortic aneurysms, with the greatest increases occurring in rapidly enlarging or ruptured aneurysms.[10,13,17,18] While significant destruction of collagen and elastin occurs, there is also synthesis and accumulation of new collagen and elastin in the expanding aorta. This accounts for the thickening of the aortic wall observed clinically in aortic aneurysms and the maintenance of normal collagen content levels. However, the newly synthesized collagen may lack the intricate fibrillar structure and mature cross-linking necessary to maintain normal tensile strength.[19] The architecture of the aortic wall is altered by the alternation of the media and by accumulation of collagen in the adventitia and neointima. The elastin network is lost from the media, but unstructured elastin accumulates in the adventitia.[18]

Macrophages and inflammatory cells have been implicated as major sources of proteolytic enzymes involved in aneurysm formation. Macrophages are consistently found in the adventitial layer of aneurysms[20–22] as well as in association with atherosclerotic plaques. Macrophages synthesize many proteinases, including a number of important matrix metalloproteinases (MMPs) including interstitial collagenase (MMP-1), stromelysin (MMP-3), a 72-kDa gelatinase/type IV col-

lagenase (MMP-2), and a 92-kDa gelatinase/type IV collagenase (MMP-9). These have the capacity to degrade all the major connective tissue components of the aortic wall, including collagen, elastin, proteoglycans, fibronectin, and laminin. These proteinases are inhibited by tissue inhibitor of metalloproteinase (TIMP), which is also produced by macrophages. In addition, aortic smooth muscle cells,[23] mesenchymal cells,[24] monocytes,[11,25] and capillary endothelial cells[12] are sources of MMPs and/or cytokine mediators. It is likely that all these cells interact during the process of aneurysm formation. However, it is not known which cells have primary roles. Ongoing investigations will lead to a better understanding of the biochemical balance and control mechanisms regulating aortic matrix synthesis and degradation. This may lead to therapeutic interventions to modulate the excessive proteolytic activity associated with aneurysmal disease.

INFLAMMATORY CELLS

Aortic aneurysms are characterized by a chronic inflammatory infiltrate of varying degree in the outer layers of the media and adventitia. This is not present in the normal aorta, although similar inflammatory cells are seen in association with atherosclerotic plaques. Inflammatory cells are also seen in nonatherosclerotic aortic aneurysms such as those caused by various types of aortitis, including giant cell arteritis, rheumatoid arthritis, systemic lupus erythematosus, polyarteritis nodosa, syphilis, and Takayasu's, Behcet's and Kawasaki's diseases. This suggests the possibility that inflammatory cells, through the release of proteolytic enzymes, may play a primary role in either the causation or exacerbation of aneurysmal dilation.

Macrophages, along with T and B lymphocytes, are the major cellular components of chronic inflammation. Close interdependence exists among these cells during both the initial recognition of antigen and the subsequent perpetuation of inflammation. The cytokine network may play a prominent role in the bidirectional communication among inflammatory cells. Although the exact nature of the relationship between these potent polypeptides and aneurysmal disease is unclear, higher interleukin-1 release has been noted in aortic aneurysms compared to normal aorta.[26] It is clear that inflammatory cells play an important role in aneurysmal enlargement. Whether this role is primary or secondary remains to be determined.

GENETIC PREDISPOSITION

A number of investigators have reported familial clustering of aneurysms and have suggested a genetic basis for the pathogenesis of aneurysms.[27] Several specific genetic abnormalities have been identified in "nonatherosclerotic" aneurysm groups, such as fibrillin gene abnormalities in patients with Marfan syndrome and procollagen type 3 defects in patients with type 4 Ehlers-Danlos syndrome.

The search for a genetic defect in abdominal aortic aneurysm formation has centered on abnormalities of matrix proteins, particularly collagenases, elastases, metalloproteinases, and their inhibitors.[27–29] Patients with familial aneurysms have been reported to have less type 3 collagen in the aortic media, with polymorphisms on the gene for the pro-αI(III) chain of type 3 collagen.[30] A genetically determined risk has been suggested by the finding of high levels of Lp(a) in the serum of aneurysm patients with a deficiency of α-1-antitrypsin.[27]

The study of genetic abnormalities in aneurysms is complicated by the fact that aneurysms occur only late in life. Most tests of statistical association using pedigree analysis are based on analysis of first-degree relatives and sibling pairs.[31] Solid information in parents is scare, and many years will pass before substantial data on the children of probands will be available.[27]

Because 85% of patients with aortic aneurysms have no known family history of aneurysmal disease, a single primary genetic etiology is unlikely to be identified for most patients with arterial aortic atherosclerosis. Although most patients with atherosclerosis do not develop aneurysms, patients with aneurysms invariably have atherosclerotic involvement. The late onset of aneurysmal disease in affected individuals makes it highly probable that genetic factors create, at best, a predisposition and that the subsequent development of aneurysmal disease depends on environmental factors such as smoking and atherosclerotic plaque formation. Genetic factors play an important role in the development of atherosclerosis, and certain genetic predispositions may determine whether some individuals respond to atherogenic stimuli with proliferation and stenosis, while others respond primarily with dilation and aneurysmal enlargement.

MECHANISM OF ATHEROSCLEROTIC ANEURYSM FORMATION

Consideration of the atherosclerotic process of plaque formation and the compensatory arterial response suggests a possible mechanism that may account for localized aneurysm formation in the abdominal aorta.[4] Hemodynamic factors and structural vulnerabilities of the abdominal aorta may increase the propensity of the abdominal aorta to form atherosclerotic plaques.[32] Plaque deposition accompanied by compensatory arterial enlargement acts initially to maintain a normal lumen caliber. Plaque formation and enlargement are accompanied by atrophy of the underlying media, further increasing the vulnerability of the abdominal aorta. In later stages of plaque evolution, proteolytic enzymes released from the plaque or cellular inflam-

matory responses may produce localized destruction of the remaining structural matrix proteins of the aortic wall and result in progressive enlargement. Under certain circumstances, regression or absorption of plaque contents may simultaneously release proteolytic enzymes, which then act on the structural integrity of the aortic wall. Macrophages and inflammatory cells involved with repair processes and resorption or alteration of lipids during regression or evolution of atherosclerotic lesions may be important sources of the proteolytic enzymes that may play an important role in aneurysmal enlargement. Aneurysms appear to be a relatively late phase of plaque evolution, when plaque and media atrophy predominate, rather than an earlier phase of atherosclerosis, when cell proliferation and fibrogenesis, as well as lipid accumulation and sequestration, characterize plaque progression.

EXPERIMENTAL OBSERVATIONS

Experimental observations support all of these proposed theories of aneurysm pathogenesis. Genetic animal models of aneurysm formation exist, and aneurysms can be induced by exogenous cholesterol feeding in nongenetically susceptible primates. Aneurysm formation in diet-induced atherosclerosis is enhanced by regression of the atherosclerotic plaque, supporting the concept that the interaction between the plaque and the artery wall in atherosclerosis is an important pathogenic mechanism.[33] Hemodynamic models of arteriovenous fistula formation have documented enlargement in response to increased blood flow and wall shear stress,[34] and animal models utilizing proteolytic enzymes in the aorta result in focal aneurysmal dilation.[35] Enlargement of atherosclerotic arteries can be induced in hypercholesterolemic experimental animals, and such enlargement is associated with destruction of the architecture of the media.[33] This pathologic feature is particularly prominent in those primate species that are susceptible to aneurysm formation. Experimental destruction of aortic medial architecture by mechanical methods alone, or by mechanical injury along with hyperlipidemia, has also been shown to produce aneurysms.[36,37] Thus, experimental models have supported all of the hypotheses proposed in the pathogenesis of aneurysms.

CONCLUSION

The pathogenesis of aortic aneurysms is a multifactorial process involving genetic predisposition and atherosclerotic artery wall degeneration. Atherosclerotic plaque deposition, along with artery enlargement and thinning of the media, are important pathogenic processes. Inflammatory cellular and connective tissue responses and proteolytic enzyme activation are important components of the processes leading to weakening of the aortic wall and aneurysmal enlargement. Further understanding of the cellular control mechanisms and biochemical and mechanical responses of the aortic wall are needed to fully comprehend the pathogenesis of aortic aneurysms.

REFERENCES

1. Johnston KW, Rutherford RB, Tilson MD, Shah DM, Hollier L, Stanley JC. Suggested standards for reporting on arterial aneurysms. *J Vasc Surg* 1991;13:452–458.
2. Ernst CB. Abdominal aortic aneurysm. *N Engl J Med* 1993;328:1167–1172.
3. Zarins CK, Glagov S. Atherosclerotic process and aneurysm formation. In: Yao JST, Pearce WH, eds. *Aneurysms: New Findings and Treatments.* Norwalk, CT: Appleton and Lange; 1994:35–46.
4. Zarins CK, Glagov S. Artery wall pathology in atherosclerosis. In: Rutherford RB, ed. *Vascular Surgery.* 4th ed., Vol 1. Philadelphia: WB Saunders; 1995:204–221.
5. Zarins CK, Weisenberg E, Kolettis G, Stankunavicius R, Glagov S. Differential enlargement of artery segments in response to enlarging atherosclerotic plaques. *J Vasc Surg* 1988;7:386–394.
6. Glagov S, Weisenberg E, Kolettis G, Stankunavicius R, Zarins CK. Compensatory enlargement of human atherosclerotic coronary arteries. *N Engl J Med* 1987;316:1371–1375.
7. Zarins CK, Glagov S. Aneurysms and obstructive plaques: Differing local responses to atherosclerosis. In: Bergan JJ, Yao JST, eds. *Aneurysms: Diagnosis and Treatment.* New York: Grune & Stratton; 1982:61–82.
8. Blair JM, Glagov S, Zarins CK. Mechanism of superficial femoral artery adductor canal stenosis. *Surg Forum* 1990;41:359–360.
9. Clark JM, Glagov S. Transluminal organization of the arterial wall: the lamellar unit revised. *Arteriosclerosis* 1985;5:19–34.
10. Busuttil RW, Abou-Zamzam AM, Machleder HI. Collagenase activity of the human aorta: a comparison of patients with and without abdominal aortic aneurysm. *Arch Surg* 1980;116:1371–1378.
11. Cannon DJ, Read RC. Blood elastolytic activity in patients with aortic aneurysm. *Am Thorac Surg* 1982;34:10–15.
12. Herron GS. Unemori E, Wong M, et al. Connective tissue proteinases and inhibitors in abdominal aortic aneurysms. *Arterioscler Thromb* 1991;11:1667–1677.
13. Menashi S, Campa JS, Greenhalgh RM, Powell JT. Collagen in abdominal aortic aneurysm: typing, content and degradation. *J Vasc Surg* 1987;6:578–582.
14. Dobrin PB, Baker WH, Gley WC. Elastolytic and collagenolytic studies of arteries: implications for the mechanical properties of aneurysms. *Arch Surg* 1984;119:405–409.
15. Zatina MA, Zarins CK, Gewertz BL, Glagov S. Role of medial lamellar architecture in the pathogenesis of aortic aneurysms. *J Vasc Surg* 1984;1:442–448.
16. Clark ET, Gewertz BL, Bassiouny HS, Zarins CK. Current results of elective aortic reconstruction for aneurysmal and occlusive disease. *J Vasc Surg* 1990;31:438–441.
17. Campa JS, Greenhalgh RM, Powell JT. Elastin degradation in abdominal aortic aneurysms. *Atherosclerosis* 1987;65:13–21.
18. Baxter BT, McGee GS, Shively VP, et al. Elastin content, cross-links, and mRNA in normal and aneurysmal human aorta. *J Vasc Surg* 1992;16:192–200.
19. Tilson MD, Roberts MP. Molecular diversity in the abdominal aortic aneurysm phenotype. *Arch Surg* 1988;123:1202–1206.
20. Beckman EN. Plasma cell infiltrates in abdominal aortic aneurysm. *Am J Clin Pathol* 1986;85:21–24.
21. Koch AE, Haines GR, Rizzo RJ, et al. Human abdominal aortic aneurysms: immunophenotypic analysis suggesting an immune-mediated response. *Am J Pathol* 1990;137:1199–1219.
22. Brophy CM, Reilly JM, Smith GJW, Tilson MD. The role of inflammation in nonspecific abdominal aortic aneurysm disease. *Ann Vasc Surg* 1991;5:229–233.
23. Cohen JR, Sarfati I, Danna D, Wise L. Smooth muscle cell elastase, atherosclerosis and abdominal aortic aneurysms. *Ann Surg* 1992;216:327–330.
24. Evans CH, Georgescu HI, LIN CW, Mendelow D, Steed DL, Webster MW. Inducible synthesis of collagenase by cells of aortic origin. *J Surg Res* 1991;51:399–404.
25. Pearce WH, Koch A, Haines GR, Mesh C, Parikh D, Yao JST. Cellular components and immune response in abdominal aortic aneurysms. *Surg Forum* 1991;42:328–330.
26. Pearce WH, Sweis I, Yao JST, McCarthy WH, Koch AE. Interleukin-1 beta (IL-1β) and tumor necrosis factor alpha (TNF-α) release in normal and diseased human infrarenal aortas. *J Vasc Surg* 1992;16:784–789.
27. Tilson MD. A perspective on research in abdominal aortic aneurysms disease with a unifying hypothesis. In: Bergan JJ, Yao J, eds. *Aortic Surgery.* Philadelphia: WB Saunders; 1989:27.
28. Tilson MD, Roberts MP. Molecular diversity in the abdominal aortic aneurysm phenotype. *Arch Surg* 1988;123:1202–1206.
29. Tilson MD, Reilly JM, Brophy CM, Webster EL, Barnett TR. Expression and sequence of the gene for tissue inhibitor of metalloproteinases in patients with abdominal aortic aneurysms. *J Vasc Surg* 1993;18:266–270.
30. Powell J, Greenhalgh RM. Cellular, enzymatic, and genetic factors in the pathogenesis of abdominal aortic aneurysms. *J Vasc Surg* 1989;9:297–304.
31. Kulvaniemi H, Tromp G, Prockop DJ. Genetic causes of aortic aneurysms. *J Clin Invest* 1991;88:1441–1444.
32. Glagov S, Zarins CK, Giddens DP, Ku DN. Hemodynamics and atherosclerosis: insights and perspectives gained from studies of human arteries. *Arch Pathol Lab Med* 1988;112:1018–1031.
33. Zarins CK, Xu C, Glagov S. Aneurysmal enlargement of the aorta during regression of experimental atherosclerosis. *J Vasc Surg* 1992;15:90–101.
34. Zarins CK, Zatina MA, Giddens DP, Ku DN, Glagov S. Shear stress regulation of artery lumen diameter in experimental atherogenesis. *J Vasc Surg* 1987;5:413–420.
35. Anidjar S, Salzmann JL, Gentric D, et al. Elastase-induced experimental aneurysms in rats. *Circulation* 1990;82:973–981.
36. Zatina MA, Zarins CK, Gewertz BL, Glagov S. Role of medial lamellar architecture in the pathogenesis of aortic aneurysms. *J Vasc Surg* 1984;1:442–448.
37. Bomberger RA, Zarins CK, Glagov S. Medial injury and hyperlipidemia in development of aneurysm or atherosclerotic plaques. *Surg Forum* 1980;31:338–340.

33

Abdominal Aortic and Iliac Artery Aneurysms: Clinical Presentation, Natural History, and Indications for Intervention

Timothy C. Hodges, M.D.
Jack L. Cronenwett, M.D.

SIGNIFICANCE

Proper management of abdominal aortic and iliac aneurysms concerns every physician caring for the adult population. Despite the availability of effective surgical treatment, many abdominal aortic aneurysms (AAAs) go undetected until their rupture. This results in over 8500 deaths annually in the United States and represents the tenth leading cause of death for men over the age of 65.[1] Identification and treatment of life-threatening AAAs are central to reducing this high mortality. Accordingly, this chapter will address the presentation, natural history, and operative indications for aortic and iliac artery aneurysms, focusing on infrarenal AAAs as the prototype (Fig. 33–1) and then describing important special cases, such as juxtarenal aortic or isolated iliac artery aneurysms.

DEFINITIONS

An *aneurysm* is functionally defined as a focal dilation of an arterial segment to more than 1.5 times its normal diameter (Fig. 33–2). An arterial segment that is between 1 and 1.5 times its normal diameter is termed *ectatic*, while diffuse arterial enlargement is termed *arteriomegaly*. Autopsy and computed tomography (CT) studies reveal that aortic diameter is larger in men than in women and increases with age and body surface area.[2,3] Because the normal adult aortic diameter is approximately 2 cm, AAAs are often defined in the literature as aortic segments ≥ 3 cm in diameter. A *symptomatic* AAA is one that produces effects noticed by the patient, such as pain or a sense of fullness. Rupture of an AAA (disruption of the vessel wall with blood

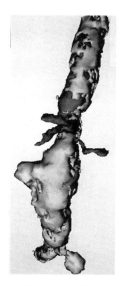

Figure 33–1. Three-dimensional reconstruction of an abdominal aortic aneurysm from spiral CT data. (Courtesy Mark F. Fillinger, M.D.)

extravasation) can be *contained*, such that the blood has escaped the vessel lumen but is localized by the surrounding perivascular tissues, or *free*, in which unrestrained blood loss into the peritoneal cavity leads rapidly to hypotension. An acutely symptomatic AAA that is not ruptured is described as *expanding*, a state believed to be the immediate precursor to frank rupture. Aneurysms can be *fusiform* (the body of the dilation is in line with the flow channel) or *saccular* (the body of the dilation is eccentric to the flow channel). AAAs are also described by location as *infrarenal* (aris-

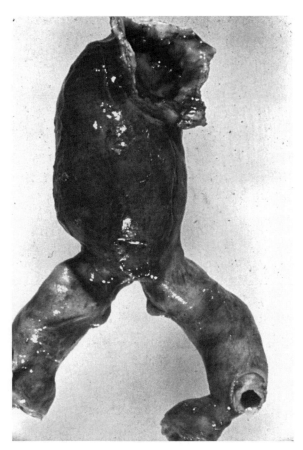

Figure 33–2. Autopsy specimen of a typical infrarenal abdominal aortic aneurysm. (Reprinted from Cronenwett JL, Sampson LN. Aneurysms of the abdominal aorta and iliac arteries. In: Dean RH, Yao JST, Brewster DC, eds. *Current Diagnosis and Treatment in Vascular Surgery.* Norwalk, CT: Appleton & Lange;1995:220–238, with permission.)

ing below the renal artery origins), *juxtarenal* (originating at the renal arteries such that repair, but not aortic control, can be accomplished below the renal arteries), or *suprarenal* (originating above the renal arteries). An aneurysm extending above the diaphragmatic hiatus is termed *thoracoabdominal*. AAAs are termed *inflammatory* when the wall is inflamed and thickened, but not infected, while aneurysms of infectious etiology are termed *mycotic*.

RISK FACTORS FOR AAA DEVELOPMENT

A number of risk factors have been identified that increase the prevalence of an AAA (Table 33–1). These have been identified in population screening studies using abdominal ultrasound.[4] Because most ruptured AAAs are not detected before rupture, many have argued that an ultrasound screening protocol should exist for older patients likely to have an AAA. This argument has been tempered by the need to contain costs by limiting screening to those patients at highest risk. If clinical risk factors are used to select high-risk

groups, it appears that AAA screening studies can be cost-effective.[5] Furthermore, it appears that AAA screening studies are not necessary if an initial ultrasound examination is normal in a patient over age 65.[6]

Demographics

AAAs increase in frequency with age, and men have a four- to sixfold higher prevalence than women. In men the onset of AAAs occurs at age 50, reaching a peak incidence at age 80. Men aged 55 to 59 have an AAA prevalence of 0.9%, but by age 80 that prevalence increases to 10.3%. Women exhibit a delay in onset, generally beginning at age 70, with a peak incidence at age 90, so that women aged 55 to 59 have an AAA prevalence of only 0.2% and by age 80 that prevalence is 2.1%.[7] Ultrasound screening studies in unselected patients aged 65 to 80 years reveal that 8% of men and 1.5% of women have aortic diameters > 3 cm.[8] Men have higher age-adjusted death rates from AAAs as well.[1] Race also affects the incidence and mortality of AAAs: Caucasian men have a 3.4-fold higher incidence of AAA and a higher mortality rate than do African-American men.[9] Advocates of screening programs recommend ultrasound examinations of white men aged 65 to 79 because this group has a relatively high prevalence of AAA and is young enough to benefit from intervention.[10]

Family History

There is considerable evidence of a familial or genetic contribution to the development of AAAs. Ultrasound screening of first-degree relatives of patients undergoing AAA repair indicates a 15 to 25% incidence of AAA compared with a 2 to 3% incidence in age-matched controls.[11,12] Because of their similar ages, it is the siblings of affected patients who are most likely to be identified with an AAA. Baird et al found that siblings of AAA patients had a greater lifetime risk of AAA development (11.7% vs 7.5%); this risk began at an earlier age and increased more rapidly than that of controls.[13] In a review of the families of 91 proband patients with AAA, Webster et al found that the relative risk for development of AAA was 10-fold higher for brothers and 23-fold for sisters of these patients.[14] Statistical analysis of this same population led Majder et al to conclude that AAA inheritance is controlled by an autosomal diallelic locus transmitted in a recessive pattern.[15]

Peripheral Arterial Disease

Peripheral arterial aneurysms are a well recognized indicator of a likely concomitant AAA. Of patients with popliteal aneurysms, approximately 40% have a concomitant AAA,[16,17] while more than 60% of patients with femoral aneurysms have an associated AAA.[18,19] The presence of peripheral arterial disease is also associated with AAA development. In a study of patients

Table 33–1.   Prevalence of ≥ 3-cm AAAs by Risk Factor, Based on Ultrasound Screening*

Risk Factor	Prevalence		Reference
	Present	Absent	
Male gender	5.6%	0.9%	7
Smoking	4.0%	1.6%	7
Peripheral arterial disease	10.8%	4.0%	4
COPD	15.5%	3.5%	4
Family history (sibling)	4.4%	1.1%	13
Giant cell arteritis	5.2%	2.1%	25
Caucasian: African-American (odds ratio)	2.4	1	9

*The prevalence in the general population age >65 is approximately 2.8%.

undergoing lower extremity vascular laboratory evaluations for suspected occlusive disease, Wolf et al screened the abdominal aorta using B-mode ultrasound. They found that the prevalence of an aortic diameter > 3.0 cm was 6.7% overall but that it increased to 15.2% in male smokers over age 65.[20] Pleumeekers et al found intermittent claudication to be more prevalent in men with AAAs.[7]

Chronic Obstructive Pulmonary Disease

Chronic obstructive pulmonary disease (COPD) is also a recognized risk factor for the development of AAAs. One theory is that both COPD and AAA formation relate to increased proteinase activity, possibly derived from circulating polymorphonuclear leukocytes or monocytes.[21] Cigarette smoking, while difficult to separate from COPD, has also been associated with an increased incidence of AAA development. In the Oxford screening program, Collin et al found that 25% of patients with AAAs were currently smoking, while only 5% had never smoked.[22] To separate the influence of cigarette smoking and the presence of COPD on AAA prevalence, more objective measurements of COPD severity have been applied to screening. Among pulmonary clinic outpatients, van Laahoven et al found an AAA prevalence of 9.9% overall and noted that those patients with more severe COPD had a higher AAA prevalence.[23]

Autoimmune Disease

Several studies have suggested that autoimmune disease increases the likelihood of AAA formation. Sato et al reported an increased incidence of AAAs in patients with autoimmune disorders receiving long-term corticosteroid therapy. In this study all the patients were female, which the authors relate to the greater incidence of autoimmune disease in women.[24] Evans et al examined patients who developed giant cell arteritis and found an AAA incidence that was double the age- and gender-matched expected incidence.[25]

CLINICAL PRESENTATION

Asymptomatic AAA

Most AAAs are asymptomatic and detected incidentally during routine physical examination or imaging studies done for other abdominal problems. Although occasionally visible to inspection in a very thin patient, the typical AAA expands without the patient's knowledge and is usually detected by a physician. To estimate aortic size more accurately by physical examination, the examiner should palpate with both hands on either side of the rectus abdominis muscle, beginning in the supraumbilical region. This technique affords a better appreciation of aortic size in the lateral dimension than direct anteroposterior palpation, in which perceived aortic size is more easily influenced by body habitus. Even for an experienced examiner, accurate measurement of aortic diameter is difficult, and only a suspicion of an aneurysm may be present. In a study of patients undergoing elective AAA repair, Chervu et al found that in only 38% was the aneurysm detected on the initial physical examination, despite the fact that its average diameter exceeded 5.5 cm. Furthermore, 23% of AAAs in this study were not palpable even when the diagnosis was known to the examiner.[26] However, because the physical examination is simple and rapid, it should not be omitted in the patient at risk for AAA development.

Symptomatic AAA

Expansion and Rupture

AAAs may cause symptoms by local compression, rupture, embolization, or thrombosis. The most common symptom is pain, which arises in one of two ways. First, an AAA may gradually enlarge and impinge on surrounding structures, causing symptoms such as back or flank pain from vertebral compression, or early satiety, nausea, or even emesis from duodenal obstruction. Some patients complain of a sense of fullness or aching in the abdomen, especially with very large aneurysms. The second mechanism for pain from an AAA is more distinctive and arises from abrupt expansion or, more often, actual rupture. This pain usually begins suddenly in the epigastrium or back, is rapidly progressive, and sometimes radiates to the flank or groin. Pain from a ruptured AAA can be confused with an acute myocardial infarction, especially in the setting of diaphoresis and hypotension, because these patients usually have risk factors for both entities. Thus, ruptured AAAs can present a challenge in diagnosis. In fact, in a review of 152 patients, Marston et al found that ruptured AAAs were misdiagnosed in 30% of cases, and the classic triad of abdominal pain, back pain, and a pulsatile abdominal mass occurred in only 26% of cases.[27]

On physical examination, the acutely expanding or ruptured AAA is tender to deep palpation. Acute expansion differs from rupture in that hemorrhage has not yet occurred but symptoms are serious enough to prompt urgent intervention. In frank rupture, the Grey-Turner sign (flank hemorrhage due to retroperitoneal dissection of blood) and scrotal or thigh ecchymosis may be present. The usual signs of shock (tachycardia, diaphoresis, skin mottling) may be present, depending on the extent of hemorrhage.

Thombosis and Embolization

Although much less frequent than rupture, AAAs can present with distal embolization or thrombosis. The presumed mechanism for these events is disruption of mural thrombus within the AAA by the motion of blood in the flow channel. This disruption can lead to local dissection and abrupt occlusion or, more likely, dislodgment of portions of the thrombus into the distal arterial tree. Depending on the size of the thrombotic debris, major proximal arterial occlusion or only very distal embolization can occur, causing digital artery occlusion ("blue toe" syndrome). In a review of 302 patients undergoing elective AAA repair, only 15 presented with embolization, but this group had a high amputation rate: 33% minor and 10% major amputations.[28] Abdominal CT findings of an irregular or fissured mural thrombus correlated with embolic symptoms, and the majority of AAAs that embolized (66%) had diameters < 5 cm. Rarely, aneurysm thrombosis results in abrupt loss of femoral pulses and severe lower extremity ischemia.[29]

NATURAL HISTORY

It is the nature of AAAs to expand in diameter, gradually increasing wall tension until the bursting strength is exceeded (tension = radius × pressure/wall thickness, after LaPlace). Thus, decision making concerning the appropriateness of elective AAA repair requires an understanding of both current rupture risk and future anticipated expansion rate.

Factors Influencing Expansion Rate

Size

Numerous studies using ultrasound or CT scans have sequentially measured the size of small AAAs. Based on these studies, there is general agreement that the AAA expansion rate is an exponential function of current size, increasing in larger AAAs. Using multivaricate analysis, Cronenwett et al determined that initial AAA diameter is an independent predictor of expansion rate, estimated at an average of 10% of the current AAA diameter per year. Thus, a 3-cm-diameter AAA would be expected to expand by 0.3 cm/year and a 6-cm-diameter AAA by 0.6 cm/year.[30] In a more sophisticated mathematical analysis, Limet et al also demonstrated that AAAs expand at an exponential rate, equivalent to an 11% diameter increase per year for small AAAs.[31] Although some studies including very small AAAs (<4 cm in diameter) identified by screening have found lower average expansion rates,[32] most AAAs being evaluated for possible repair can be anticipated to expand by approximately 10% per year.

Intuitively, hypertension would be expected to increase the AAA expansion rate as well as the rupture risk. In addition to AAA size, Cronenwett et al identified hypertension as an independent predictor of increased AAA expansion rate.[30] Specifically, this study demonstrated a positive correlation with systolic blood pressure but a negative correlation with diastolic blood pressure, suggesting that pulse pressure may be a more accurate predictor of future AAA expansion. In fact, the combination of AAA size and pulse pressure accounted for 74% of the variation observed in the expansion rate of small AAAs in this study. Conversely, Schewe et al found that both systolic and diastolic blood pressure were positively correlated with AAA expansion rate, and that diameter and diastolic blood pressure were independently predictive.[33] Not all studies have identified hypertension as having a significant influence on AAA expansion rate, which likely relates to difficulties separating treated from actual hypertension in these retrospective studies.

Thrombus Content

The amount of thrombus contained within an AAA also appears to affect the rate of expansion. Using a finite-element model, Inzoli et al demonstrated that increasing thrombus thickness raised AAA wall stress, and thereby the expansion rate and rupture risk.[34] Based on a review of CT scans, Wolf et al found that the portion of the circumference of the AAA covered by thrombus was predictive of the expansion rate.[35] If the arc of the AAA covered by thrombus (TARC) was

>120°, 34% of patients demonstrated expansion >0.5 cm/year, compared with only 7% for those with a TARC <120° ($p < 0.001$).

Smoking

MacSweeney et al analyzed the effect of cigarette smoking on expansion rate in 43 patients with small AAAs followed for a median of 2 years.[36] The median expansion rate was 0.13 cm/year in this group. It was higher for patients who continued to smoke (0.16 cm/year) than in those who no longer smoked (0.09 cm/year; $p < 0.04$).

Factors Influencing AAA Rupture Risk

Size, Hypertension, and COPD

Size, measured by diameter, is currently the best predictor of AAA rupture risk, especially for large AAAs. In an early clinical study, Szilagyi et al demonstrated that patients managed nonoperatively with AAAs >6 cm in diameter had a 5-year survival of only 6%, compared with 48% survival in patients with smaller aneurysms.[37] Autopsy studies have also demonstrated that larger AAAs are more prone to rupture. Among consecutive AAAs noted during postmortem examination, Darling et al observed that 75% of AAAs >7 cm had ruptured, compared with a 19% rupture rate in AAAs ≤7 cm in diameter.[38] In a review of patients with AAAs treated nonoperatively, Perko et al found that initial aneurysm size was the only variable with significant influence on the rate of rupture.[39] These and other studies have produced general agreement that the AAA rupture risk increases exponentially with size, even though precise size–risk estimates are difficult (Fig. 33–3).

In a series of patients with AAAs ranging from 4 to 6 cm in diameter who were followed nonoperatively, Cronenwett et al applied multivariate analysis to determine which risk factors were associated with rupture. Rupture occurred in this population at a rate of 6% per year.[40] Initial AAA size ($p < 0.01$), hypertension ($p < 0.02$), and COPD ($p < 0.001$) were independently predictive of future AAA rupture. Absolute AAA diameter was a more accurate predictor that the ratio of the AAA diameter to the more proximal aortic diameter. Similarly, diastolic blood pressure was a more accurate predictor than systolic blood pressure. COPD was the most influential risk factor, which was attributed to a possible increase in systemic proteinase activity affecting both pulmonary and aortic connective tissue.

Other studies have confirmed the influence of size, hypertension, and COPD on AAA rupture risk. Using multivariate analysis, Sterpetti et al compared patients who had died with an intact AAA versus those who had died from rupture.[41] They found that AAA size ($p < 0.001$), hypertension ($p < 0.001$), and bronchiectasis ($p < 0.025$) were independently predictive of rupture.

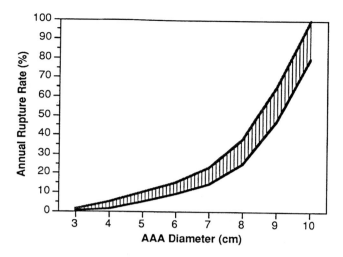

Figure 33–3. Estimated annual rupture rate basd on AAA diameter. The range shown is based on different published estimates and likely reflects other variables, such as hypertension and COPD, that also influence rupture risk (Reprinted from Sampson LN, Cronenwett JL. Abdominal aortic aneurysms. In: Zelenock GB, ed. *Problems in General Surgery in Vascular Surgery*, Vol II. Philadelphia: JB Lippincott;1994:385–417, with permission.)

These results also suggested a generalized connective tissue defect as the unifying hypothesis to explain the association between COPD and AAA rupture. Other studies have confirmed the influence of hypertension on AAA rupture risk. Among 75 patients with AAAs managed nonoperatively, Foster et al noted that death from rupture occurred in 72% of patients with diastolic hypertension but in only 29% of patients with diastolic blood pressure <100 mm Hg.[42] In a similar analysis, Szilagyi et al found that diastolic hypertension (>150/100 mm Hg) was present in 67% of patients who experienced AAA rupture but in only 23% of those without rupture.[37] Thus, diameter, hypertension, and COPD have been confirmed to be independent risk factors for AAA rupture in different studies using both clinical and autopsy data.

Family History

Although a positive family history of AAA has been demonstrated to increase the prevalence of AAAs in other first-degree relatives (FDRs), it is less clear that familial AAAs have a higher rupture risk. In one study of 86 families with 209 FDRs with AAAs, Darling et al found that the frequency of ruptured AAAs increased with the number of FDRs with AAAs: 14.8% with two FDRs, 29% with three FDRs, and 36% with four or more FDRs.[11] The incidence of rupture was particularly high for women in this series with familial AAAs. Unfortunately, this study did not consider many potentially confounding variables, such as AAA size, which might have differed in patients with familial AAAs. Thus, whether a positive family history is an independent predictor of rupture, in addition to prevalence, is not yet established.

Smoking

The potential interaction between smoking, COPD, and AAA rupture risk is not settled. Based on a large study of men in England, Strachan found that the relative risk of death from AAA rupture increased 2.4-fold for pipe/cigar smokers, 4.6-fold for cigarette smokers, and fully 14.6-fold for smokers of hand-rolled cigarettes.[43] However, it was not possible to separate the potentially confounding influence of COPD in this study because COPD was not specifically measured. Other studies that have identified COPD as a risk for rupture have not found that smoking was an independent predictor.[40,41] However, from an epidemiologic and a case management standpoint, the nearly fivefold increase in AAA rupture risk for cigarette smokers reported by Strachan should not be overlooked.[43]

Expansion Rate

Although a rapid AAA expansion rate is presumed to increase the rupture risk, it is difficult to separate this effect from the influence of expansion rate on absolute diameter, which alone could influence the rupture risk. Schewe et al found that both AAA size (7.3 vs. 6.1 cm) and expansion rate (0.47 cm/years vs 0.23 cm/year) were greater in patients with ruptured versus nonruptured AAAs.[33] Cronenwett et al found that absolute AAA size was a better predictor of rupture than expansion rate, and other studies have also demonstrated that absolute size rather than expansion rate is associated with increased rupture risk.[40,44] The question of whether expansion rate is an independent predictor of rupture may be moot, however, because more rapid AAA expansion obviously increases aneurysm size, which increases rupture risk.

Relative Size

It is generally believed that comparably sized AAAs in patients with smaller-diameter proximal aortas are at higher risk for rupture. This is difficult to prove, however, because studies that have examined this question have found that absolute size, rather than AAA/aortic ratio, is a more accurate predictor of rupture.[40,41] Ouriel et al suggested that the relative size of an AAA compared with the L-3 vertebral body may be a good predictor of rupture risk because all ruptured AAAs that they reviewed on CT scan were greater than the L-3 diameter.[45] However, many elective AAAs that had not ruptured were greater than this diameter, so this factor was only 68% accurate in discriminating the future likelihood of rupture.

AAA Shape and Thrombus Content

General clinical opinion holds that eccentric or saccular AAAs are at greater rupture risk than fusiform AAAs. By examining CT scans, however, Wolf et al were unable to confirm this suspicion.[35] Furthermore, other studies have suggested that fusiform AAAs with relative flattening of the AAA arc are associated with greater rupture, as predicted by the effectively larger radius by LaPlace's law.[46] Thus, the influence of shape on rupture risk is not clear. Similarly, the possible influence of contained thrombus within an AAA on rupture risk is unclear.

INDICATIONS FOR INTERVENTION

Decision making for elective AAA repair requires an estimate of the current AAA rupture risk and the elective operative risk in the context of a patient's life expectancy.

Rupture Risk

The rupture risk for an AAA of a specific size is not precisely known because most known AAAs undergo elective repair before rupture. However, it appears that the rupture risk increases exponentially for AAAs with diameters larger than 5 cm. Estimates for annual rupture risk of 5- to 7-cm AAAs range from 5 to 15% per year.[31,33,44,47] There is less agreement about the rupture risk of small (4- to 5-cm) AAAs, an increasingly important issue, because small aneurysms are detected more frequently with screening. In a population-based study of selective AAA management, Brown et al found that no AAAs <5 cm diameter ruptured, although a large proportion expanded to a greater diameter and required elective surgery during follow-up.[48] Nevitt et al reported that no AAAs ranging from 4 to 5 cm in diameter ruptured during follow-up, although many were electively repaired, resulting in an underestimate of the risk of rupture.[44] Glimaker et al reported a rupture risk of only 0.4% per year for patients with AAAS <5 cm in diameter but noted that all ruptures occurred in the first year, for an annual risk of 2.5%.[49] In another study of small AAAs managed nonoperatively, Limet et al found that 5.4% of AAAs 4 to 5 cm in diameter ruptured each year, even though 38% underwent elective repair during 2-year follow-up.[31] Cronenwett et al estimated the rupture risk to be 3.3% per year for AAAs 4 to 5 cm in diameter.[40,50] Thus, the estimates for rupture risk of these AAAs range from 0 to 5% per year. This relatively large range likely relates to differences in patient selection, as well as to the rate of elective repair during follow-up. More important, however, it suggests that factors other than size, such as COPD and hypertension, also have an important influence on the rupture risk of individual AAAs. Thus, for AAAs from 4 to 5 cm in diameter, we estimate the rupture risk to be 0 to 2% per year if no other risk factors for rupture are present, but as much as 5% per year if the patient has coexistent hypertension, COPD, and a positive family history. For AAAs from 5 to 7 cm in diameter, we estimate the annual rupture risk to be 5 to 15% per year, with the specific risk within this range dependent on the presence of other risk factors for rupture. For AAAs larger than 7 cm in diameter, the annual rupture risk likely exceeds 15% per year.

Operative Risk

Operative mortality after elective AAA repair is <5% in most modern series and is largely influenced by coronary artery disease (CAD), renal insufficiency and pulmonary disease.[51] In the Canadian multicenter study, these three risk factors were independently predictive of operative mortality, which was <2% when these risk factors were absent but as high as 50% if all three risk factors were severe.[51] Importantly, age does not appear to be an important risk factor for increased mortality after elective AAA repair. Multiple studies have demonstrated excellent results of elective AAA repair in appropriately selected octogenarians, indicating that physiologic, rather than chronologic age is the important determinant of the outcome. This contrasts with ruptured AAA repair, in which advanced age is an important predictor of a poor outcome. In addition to patient-specific risk factors, surgeons who seldom perform AAA surgery have a higher elective operative mortality rate.[52] Furthermore, results from statewide experience with AAA repair indicate that on average, elective operative mortality exceeds that generally reported from selected, high-volume centers. For example, in the State of Michigan elective mortality for elective AAA repair ranged from 6% to 10% during the past decade.[53] This variation indicates that each surgeon must evaluate his or her individual results to accurately estimate the elective operative risk prior to recommending AAA repair.

Because CAD is the most important cause of both early and late mortality after AAA repair, attempts to estimate operative risk more accurately have focused largely on preoperative cardiac evaluation. In this regard, clinical risk factors, such as angina, a history of myocardial infarction, (MI), Q-wave on the electrocardiogram, ventricular arrhythmia, congestive heart failure (CHF), diabetes, and age >75 years have been used to develop an algorithm to predict the risk of postoperative events (unstable angina, MI, ischemic CHF, or death).[54] A variety of algorithms have been developed (eg, by Goldman, Detsky, and Eagle) to predict perioperative morbidity/mortality, as well as the potential need for more sophisticated cardiac testing.[55] Such tests may include exercise or dipyridamole-thallium radionuclide scanning, echocardiography, or ambulatory Holter monitoring. A thorough discussion of these techniques is beyond the scope of this chapter. However, the cost effectiveness of these techniques for preoperative assessment of patients with AAAs is not established. Some reports have emphasized that an acceptably low operative mortality rate can be achieved with optimal patient selection and management based on clinical risk factors alone.[56] Others have emphasized that long-term survival, the ultimate goal of AAA repair, is improved by selective coronary revascularization prior to AAA repair.[57] Thus, it is important to individualize the preoperative assessment of patients with AAAs, depending on center-specific results and the level of clinically suspected CAD in comparison with the lkelihood of AAA rupture.

Life Expectancy

Because AAA repair is a prophylactic operation designed to prevent rupture and prolong life, it is predictably more beneficial in patients with an otherwise long life expectancy. Given that age is the best overall predictor of life expectancy, it is obvious that AAA repair in more elderly patients will yield less benefit. More difficult is the assessment of individual life expectancy for a given-age patient because individual patient-specific risk factors such as CAD influence this outcome. Identification of high-risk patients is important, however, not only to avoid perioperative complications of AAA repair but also because AAA repair is less likely to positively influence the otherwise reduced survival in this subgroup. In an analysis of survivors in the Canadian multicenter AAA study, Johnston et al found that age >75, previous MI, and creatinine ≥1.5 mg/dL were independently predictive or reduced long-term survival.[58] Thus, prior to contemplating elective AAA reapir, the life expectancy of each individual should be estimated based on these risk factors, and any other known diseases, such as malignancy, that would predictably reduce survival.

Decision Analysis and Cost Effectiveness

The interaction of AAA rupture risk, elective operative risk, and life expectancy has been formally evaluated using decision analysis techniques.[50] In addition to assisting individual decisions, such models can identify key variables that influence appropriate decision making and determine the cost effectiveness of AAA repair under different circumstances. Katz and Cronenwett have confirmed that patient age, elective operative mortality, and AAA rupture risk are the key variables that influence cost effectiveness.[59] Importantly, the influence of these key variables on cost effectiveness is an exponential rather than a linear function. For example, as patient age increases beyond 70 to 80 years, the cost effectiveness of early surgery for small

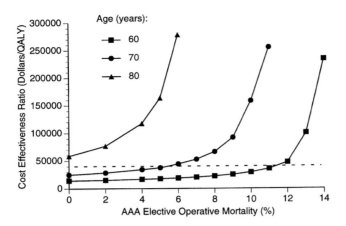

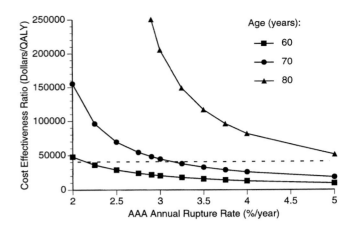

Figure 33–4. Cost effectiveness of early surgery as a function of elective operative mortality rates in three age groups. (Reprinted from Katz DA, Cronenwett JL. The cost-effectiveness of early surgery versus watchful waiting in the management of small abdominal aortic aneurysms. *J Vasc Surg* 1994;19:980–991, with permission.)

Figure 33–5. Cost effectiveness of early AAA surgery as a function of average annual rate of rupture or acute expansion in three age groups. (Reprinted from Katz DA, Cronenwett JL. The cost-effectiveness of early surgery versus watchful waiting in the management of small abdominal aortic aneurysms. *J Vasc Surg* 1994;19:980–991, with permission.)

AAAs rises exponentially. This is not surprising given the difficulty (and thus expense) of increasing life expectancy in the elderly. A conservative definition of "cost-effective" health care is that which costs $40,000 or less per quality-adjusted life year (QALY) saved. Using this criterion, if a patient has a 4 cm-diameter AAA with a rupture risk estimated to be 3.3% per year and an elective operative mortality rate of 5%, it can be seen that early repair (vs watchful waiting, with subsequent repair only if a 5-cm diameter is reached) remains cost effective for patients younger than approximately 70 years of age (Fig. 33–4). Above this age threshold, the cost of early repair increases dramatically and would not compare favorably with other health care measures competing for these same resources. In the same patient with a larger aneurysm or with other risk factors for rupture, where the estimated rupture risk is as high as 5.5% per year, early repair at 4 cm in diameter would remain cost effective until approximately age 80 (Fig. 33–5). For patients above age 80, however, AAA repair would not be cost effective unless the rupture risk were even higher, such as for an AAA >6 cm in diameter, or when many other risk factors for rupture were also present. The same nonlinear influence on cost effectiveness is observed for the other key variables of elective operative mortality and annual rupture rate. For a 70-year-old patient, early repair of a 4-cm-diameter AAA with a 3.3% annual rupture risk remains cost effective until the elective operative mortality rate exceeds 6% (Fig. 33–4). In a 60-year-old patient, however, early surgery remains cost effective even if the elective operative mortality is as high as 12% (Fig. 33–4). Finally, the effect of the most important variable on cost effectiveness, namely, AAA rupture risk, is illustrated in Figure 33–6. For a 70-year-old patient with an elective operative mortality rate of

5%, early repair remains cost effective for AAAs with a rupture risk >3% per year. This likely corresponds to any AAA ≥5 cm in diameter, as well as to AAAs from 4 to 5 cm in diameter, that are accompanied by other risk factors for rupture, such as hypertension, COPD, or a positive family history. With a lower rupture risk (<2% per year), however, such as in the patient with an AAA from 4 to 5 cm in diameter and without other factors for rupture, early AAA repair is less cost effective than watchful waiting.

Based on this decision analysis study, we recommend early AAA repair of 4- to 5-cm AAAs in patients who have risk factors that would increase their rupture risk, such as COPD, hypertension, or a positive family history. This approach applies only to young patients, particularly those under age 65, who have a long life

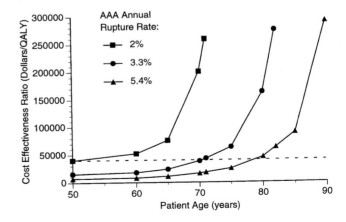

Figure 33–6. Cost-effectiveness of early AAA surgery as a function of initial age in three AAA annual rupture rate groups. (Reprinted from Katz DA, Cronenwett, JL. The cost-effectivensss of early surgery versus watchful waiting in the management of small abdominal aortic aneurysms. *J Vasc Surg* 1994;19:980–991, with permission.)

expectancy based on the absence of CAD. For patients without additional risk factors for AAA rupture, a size threshold of 5 cm is appropriate for AAA repair, but for elderly patients or those with advanced CAD, an even higher threshold may be best. These guidelines require that operative mortality for elective AAA repair be low (<5%), which usually requires a concentrated high volume of vascular surgery.

SPECIAL CONSIDERATIONS

Isolated Iliac Artery Aneurysms

Isolated iliac artery aneurysms (IAAs) are uncommon because they are usually associated with AAAs (Fig. 33–7). Due to their position in the pelvis and their relationship to nearby structures, IAAs can present in a variety of ways. Although the classic description is of a pulsatile abdominal or pelvic mass, Nachbur et al found that only a minority of patients with IAAs presented with this finding. The most common presentations for IAA in this series were a systolic murmur on physical examination, gastrointestinal or genitourinary obstruction, and acute rupture.[60] Rarely, aneurysms of the right common iliac artery can present with left lower extremity deep vein thrombosis due to compression of the left iliac vein as it crosses under the right common iliac aneurysm. The natural history of IAAs is similar to that of AAAs, and the principal complication is rupture rather than embolization on thrombosis. The precise rupture risk of IAAs is not well defined because they are infrequently detected before rupture. Most authors recommend a threshold diameter of 2.5 to 3.0 cm as the usual criterion to apply for elective repair. Other factors such as hypertension, COPD, and a positive family history should probably also influence the decision for elective repair. Internal IAAs present a technical challenge for repair due to their anatomic location deep in the pelvis. Because their size can impede control of the distal iliac artery branches prior to opening the aneurysm, it is usually safer to exclude large internal iliac aneurysms through ligation of distal branches from within the aneurysm.[61] Because of the importance of internal iliac blood flow to the pelvis and distal colon, careful assessment must be made prior to ligation, especially if both internal iliac arteries are aneurysmal. Preoperative arteriography may help delineate the adequacy of collateral flow from the inferior or superior mesenteric arteries. Intraoperative inspection of the sigmoid colon, combined with an assessment of distal internal iliac artery backbleeding, may lead to the decision that revascularization of at least one internal iliac artery is desirable in some patients.

Juxtarenal Aneurysms

Juxtarenal aortic aneurysms are uncommon, comprising 2 to 7% of all aortic AAAs. While their presentation and natural history are similar to those of infrarenal AAAs, their operative repair is more challenging. Surgical repair of juxtarenal aneurysms requires placement of the aortic clamp above the renal arteries, leading to increased cardiac afterload and transient renal ischemia. This may be associated with increased perioperative cardiac morbidity and postoperative renal insufficiency in proportion to the time required to complete the proximal anastomosis. In a study of juxtarenal aneurysm patients, Poulias et al found that a suprarenal crossclamp time exceeding 30 minutes led to a 19% incidence of postoperative renal complications, compared with 5% when the clamp time was less than 25 minutes.[62] As a result of these increased risks, many surgeons increase the size threshold for elective repair of a juxtarenal aneurysm by approximately 1 cm over the more common infrarenal AAA.

Inflammatory Aneurysms

Inflammatory AAAs are defined by noninfected but thickened inflammatory connective tissue reaction surrounding the adventitia of the artery. The inflammatory process is usually more pronounced anteriorly and may also involve the adjacent retroperitoneal tissues,

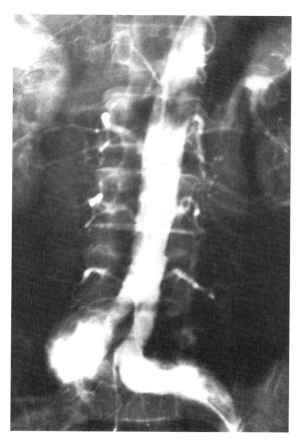

Figure 33–7. Arteriographic appearance of a large, isolated right iliac aneurysm.

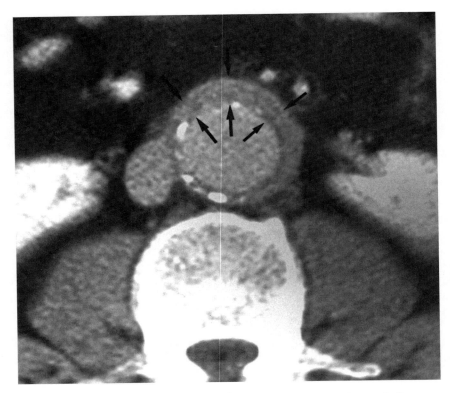

Figure 33–8. Contrast CT scan of an inflammatory aneurysm. Arrows indicate the thickness of the adventitia and retroperitoneum surrounding the anterior surface, with relative sparing of the posterior portion (Reprinted from Sampson LN, Cronenwett JL. Abdominal aortic aneurysms. In : Zelenock GB, ed. *Problems in General Surgery in Vascular Surgery*, Vol II. Philadelphia: JB Lippincott;1995:385–417, with permission.)

especially the duodenum. Preoperative diagnosis is difficult in the absence of a contrast-infusion CT scan (Fig. 33–8). The most common presentation is abdominal pain and tenderness, although as many as one-third of patients are asymptomatic.[63] Symptoms may present a management dilemma because they mimic rupture. In the absence of imaging studies, a history of chronic or progressive abdominal or back pain raises the index of suspicion that an inflammatory aneurysm is present. A history of weight loss in addition to pain, especially with evidence of medial ureteral deviation by imaging, is strongly suggestive.[63] In an acutely symptomatic but hemodynamically stable patient, expeditious CT scanning can reveal the inflammatory nature of the aneurysm, allowing better preoperative planning by the surgical and anesthetic teams. Although a markedly thickened wall of an inflammatory AAA may be regarded as less likely to rupture, the posterior portion is usually less involved and thus equally susceptible to rupture. Accordingly, detection of an inflammatory AAA in a symptomatic patient should not unduly delay intervention. Beneficial preoperative maneuvers in some patients include ureteral stenting to decompress any obstruction and to aid ureteral identification during retroperitoneal dissection.

REFERENCES

1. Gillum RF. Epidemiology of aortic aneurysm in the United States. *J Clin Epidemiol* 1995;48:1289–1298.
2. Pearce WH, Slaughter MS, LeMaire S, et al. Aortic diameter as a function of age, gender, and body surface area. *Surgery* 1993;114:691–697.
3. Sonesson B, Lanne T, Hansen F, et al. Infrarenal aortic diameter in the healthy person. *Eur J Vasc Surg* 1994; 8:89–95.
4. Simoni G, Pastorino C, Perrone R, et al. Screening for abdominal aortic aneurysms and associated risk factors in a general population. *Eur J Vasc Endovasc Surg* 1995;10:207–210.
5. Frame PS, Fryback DG, Patterson C. Screening for abdominal aortic aneurysm in men ages 60 to 80 years. A cost-effectiveness analysis. *Ann Intern Med* 1993;119:411–416.
6. Emerton ME, Shaw E, Poskitt K, et al. Screening for abdominal aortic aneurysm: a single scan is enough. *Br J Surg* 1994;81:1112–1113.
7. Pleumeekers HJ, Hoes AW, van der Does E, et al. Aneurysms of the abdominal aorta in older adults. The Rotterdam Study. *Am J Epidemiol* 1995;142:1291–1299.
8. Scott RA, Ashton HA, Kay DN. Abdominal aortic aneurysm in 4237 screened patients: prevalence, development and management over 6 years. *Br J Surg* 1991;78:1222–1225.
9. LaMorte WW, Scott TE, Menzoian JO. Racial differences in the incidence of femoral bypass and abdominal aortic

aneurysmectomy in Massachusetts: relationship to cardiovascular risk factors. *J Vasc Surg* 1995;21:422–431.

10. Norman PE, Castleden WM, and Lawrence-Brown MM. Screening for abdominal aortic aneurysms. *Aust NZ J Surg* 1992;62:333–337.

11. Darling RC, Brewster DC, Darling RC, et al. Are familial abdominal aortic aneurysms different? *J Vasc Surg* 1989;10:39–43.

12. Webster MW, Ferrell RE, St. Jean PL. Ultrasound screening of first-degree relatives of patients with abdominal aortic aneurysm. *J Vasc Surg* 1991;13:9–14.

13. Baird PA, Sadovnick AD, Yee IM, et al. Sibling risks of abdominal aortic aneurysm. *Lancet* 1995;346:601–604.

14. Webster MW, St Jean PL, Steed DL, et al. Abdominal aortic aneurysm: results of a family study. *J Vasc Surg* 1991;13:366–372.

15. Majumder PP, St Jean PL, Ferrell RE, et al. On the inheritance of abdominal aortic aneurysm. *Am J Hum Genet* 1991;48:164–170.

16. Vermilion BD, Kimmins SA, Pace WG, et al. A review of one hundred forty-seven popliteal aneurysms with long-term follow-up. *Surgery* 1981;90:1009.

17. Dawson I, Bockel HV, Brand R, et al. Popliteal artery aneurysms: long term follow-up of aneurysmal disease and results of surgical treatment. *J Vasc Surg* 1991;13:398–407.

18. Cutler BS, Darling RC. Surgical management of arteriosclerotic femoral aneurysms. *Surgery* 1973;74:764–773.

19. Graham SM, Zelenock GB, Whitehouse WM Jr, et al. Clinical significance of arteriosclerotic femoral artery aneurysms. *Arch Surg* 1981;115:502–506.

20. Wolf YG, Otis SM, Schwend RB, et al. Screening for abdominal aortic aneurysms during lower extremity arterial evaluation in the vascular laboratory. *J Vasc Surg* 1994;22:417–423.

21. MacSweeney ST, Powell JT, Greenhalgh RM. Pathogenesis of abdominal aortic aneurysm. *Br J Surg* 1994;81:935–941.

22. Collin J, Walton J, Araujo L, et al. Oxford screening programme for abdominal aortic aneurysm in men aged 65 to 74 years. *Lancet* 1988;2:613–615.

23. van Laarhoven CJH, Borstlap ACW, van Berge Henegouwen DP, et al. Chronic obstructive pulmonary disease and abdominal aortic aneurysms. *Eur J Vasc Surg* 1993;7:386–390.

24. Sato O, Takagi A, Miyata T, et al. Aortic aneurysms in patients with autoimmune disorders treated with corticosteroids. *Eur J Vasc Endovasc Surg* 1995;10:366–369.

25. Evans JM, O'Fallon WM, Hunder GG. Increased incidence of aortic aneurysm and dissection in giant cell (temporal) arteritis. A population-based study. *Ann Intern Med* 1995;122:502–507.

26. Chervu A, Clagett GP, Valentine RJ, et al. Role of physical examination in detection of abdominal aortic aneurysms. *Surgery* 1995;117:454–457.

27. Marston WA, Ahlquist R, Johnson G, et al. Misdiagnosis of ruptured abdominal aortic aneurysms. *J Vasc Surg* 1992;16:17–22.

28. Baxter BT, McGee GS, Flinn WR, et al. Distal embolization as a presenting symptom of aortic aneurysms. *Am J Surg* 1990;160:197–201.

29. Patel H, Krishnamoorthy M, Dorazio RA, et al. Thrombosis of abdominal aortic aneurysms. *Am Surg* 1994;60:801–803.

30. Cronenwett JL, Sargent SK, Wall MH, et al. Variables that affect the expansion rate and outcome of small aortic aneurysms. *J Vasc Surg* 1990;11:260–269.

31. Limet R, Sakalihassan N, Ablert A. Determination of the expansion rate and incidence of rupture of abdominal aortic aneurysms. *J Vasc Surg* 1991;14:540–548.

32. Bengtsson H, Nilsson P, Bergqvist D. Natural history of abdominal aortic aneurysm detected by screening. *Br J Surg* 1994;80:718–720.

33. Schewe CK, Schweikart HP, Hammel G, et al. Influence of selective management of the prognosis and the risk of rupture of abdominal aortic aneurysms. *Clin Invest* 1994;72:585–591.

34. Inzoli F, Boschetti F, Zappa M, et al. Biomechanical factors in abdominal aortic aneurysm rupture. *Eur J Vasc Surg* 1993;7:667–674.

35. Wolf YG, Thomas WS, Brennan FJ, et al. Computed tomography scanning findings associated with rapid expansion of abdominal aortic aneurysms. *J Vasc Surg* 1994;20:529–538.

36. MacSweeney ST, Ellis M, Worrell PC, et al. Smoking and growth rate of small abdominal aortic aneurysms. *Lancet* 1994;344:651–652.

37. Szilagyi D, Elliot J, Smith R. Clinical fate of the patient with asymptomatic abdominal aortic aneurysm and unfit for surgical treatment. *Arch Surg* 1972;104:600–606.

38. Darling PC, Messina CR, Brewster DC. Autopsy study of unoperated abdominal aortic aneurysms: the case for early resection. *Circulation* suppl II 1977;56:II-161–II-164.

39. Perko MJ, Schroeder TV, Olsen PS, et al. Natural history of abdominal aortic aneurysm: a survey of 63 patients treated nonoperatively. *Ann Vasc Surg* 1993;7:113–116.

40. Cronenwett J, Murphy T, Zelenock G, et al. Actuarial analysis of variables associated with rupture of small abdominal aortic aneurysms. *Surgery* 1985;98:472–483.

41. Sterpetti A, Cavallaro A, Cavallari N, et al. Factors influencing the rupture of abdominal aortic aneurysm. *Surg Gynecol Obstet* 1991;173:175–178.

42. Foster J, Bolasny B, Gobbel W, et al. Comparative study of elective resection and expectant treatment of abdominal aortic aneurysm. *Surg Gynecol Obstet* 1991;173:175–178.

43. Strachan DP. Predictors of death from aortic aneurysm among middle-aged men: the Whitehall study. *Br J Surg* 1991;78:401–404.

44. Nevitt MP, Ballard DJ, Hallett JW Jr. Prognosis of abdominal aortic aneurysms. *N Engl J Med* 1989;321:1009–1014.

45. Ouriel K, Green RM, Donayre C, et al. An evaluation of new methods of expressing aortic aneurysm size: relationship to rupture. *J Vasc Surg* 1992;15:12–20.

46. Veldenz HC, Schwartz TH, Endean ED, et al. Morphology predicts rapid growth of small abdominal aortic aneurysms. *Ann Vasc Surg* 1994;8:10–13.

47. Gadowski GR, Pilcher DB, Ricci MA. Abdominal aortic aneurysm expansion rate: effect of size and beta-adrenergic blockade. *J Vasc Surg* 1994;19:727–731.

48. Brown PM, Pattenden R, Gutelius JR. The selective management of small abdominal aortic aneurysms: the Kingston study. *J Vasc Surg* 1992;15:21–27.

49. Glimaker H, Holmberg L, Elvin A. Natural history of patients with abdominal aortic aneurysm. *Eur J Vasc Surg* 1991;5:125–130.

50. Katz DA, Littenberg B, Cronenwett JL. Management of small abdominal aortic aneurysms. Early surgery versus watchful waiting. *JAMA* 1992;268:2678–2686.

51. Johnston KW. Multicenter prospective study of nonruptured abdominal aortic aneurysm. Part II. Variables predicting morbidity and mortality. *J Vasc Surg* 1989;9:437–447.

52. Veith FJ, Goldsmith J, Leather RP, et al. The need for quality assurance in vascular surgery. *J Vasc Surg* 1991;13:523–526.

53. Katz DJ, Stanley JC, Zelenock GB. Operative mortality rates for intact and ruptured abdominal aortic aneurysms in Michigan: an eleven-year statewide experience. *J Vasc Surg* 1994;19:804–817.

54. Wong T, Detsky AS. Preoperative cardiac risk assessment for patients having peripheral vascular surgery. *Ann Intern Med* 1992;116:743–753.

55. Mangano DT, Goldman L. Preoperative assessment of patients with known or suspected coronary disease. *N Engl J Med* 1995;333:1750–1756.

56. Nehler MR, Taylor LM Jr, Moneta GL, et al. Indications for operation for infrarenal abdominal aortic aneurysms: current guidelines. *Semin Vasc Surg* 1994;8:108–114.

57. Bayazit M, Gol MK, Battaloglu B, et al. Routine coronary arteriography before abdominal aortic aneurysm repair. *Am J Surg* 1995;170:246–250.

58. Johnston KW. Ruptured abdominal aortic aneurysm: six-year follow-up results of a multicenter prospective study. Canadian Society for Vascular Surgery Aneurysm Study Group. *J Vasc Surg* 1994;19:888–900.

59. Katz DA, Cronenwett JL. The cost-effectiveness of early surgery versus watchful waiting in the management of small abdominal aortic aneurysms. *J Vasc Surg* 1994;19:980–991.

60. Nachbur BH, Inderbitzi RGC, Bar W. Isolated iliac aneurysms. *Eur J Vasc Surg* 1991;5:375–381.

61. Sacks NPM, Huddy SPJ, Wegner T, et al. Management of solitary iliac aneurysms. *J Cardiovasc Surg* 1992;33:679–683.

62. Poulias GE, Doundoulakis N, Skoutas B, et al. Juxtarenal abdominal aneurysmectomy. *J Cardiovasc Surg* 1992;33:324–330.

63. Curci JJ. Modes of presentation and management of inflammatory aneurysms of the abdominal aorta. *J Am Coll Surg* 1994;178:573–580.

34

Femoral and Popliteal Aneurysms: Clinical Presentation, Natural History, Indications for Intervention, and Results

James A. DeWeese, M.D.
Patrick N. Riggs, M.D.

FEMORAL ANEURYSMS

False aneurysms secondary to needle punctures for performance of angiography and cardiac catheterization, endovascular procedures, or injection of drugs are probably the most common femoral arterial aneurysms. Anastomotic aneurysms, sometimes infected, also occur. Traumatic dissections are extremely rare, and syphilitic aneurysms are of historical interest only. Femoral aneurysms secondary to arteriosclerosis are also relatively uncommon. Arteriosclerotic abdominal aortic aneurysms are approximately 40 times more common than arteriosclerotic femoral aneurysms.[1] Arteriosclerotic femoral aneurysms are generally localized to the common femoral artery but may also involve the origin of the deep and superficial femoral arteries.[2] Localized aneurysms of either the deep or superficial femoral artery are extremely rare and are still the subject of case reports.[3,4] This chapter will be limited to a discussion of arteriosclerotic aneurysms.

Clinical Presentation

Asymptomatic arteriosclerotic common femoral aneurysms may occasionally be recognized by the patient. They are more frequently diagnosed at the time of examination of patients with lower extremity occlusive or aneurysmal disease. Approximately 50% of patients with a femoral artery aneurysm will be found to have contralateral femoral aneurysms.[2,5] In a combined series of patients treated for popliteal aneurysms, 26% had femoral aneurysms.[1] On the other hand, in patients with aortic aneurysms, only 3.2% were known to have femoral aneurysms.[5]

Except in very obese patients, physical examination can identify a localized dilatation of the femoral artery. Ultrasound can provide further information.[6] Using color-flow duplex imaging, Ward found the mean diameter of the common femoral artery to be 8.68 ± 1.20 mm in 30 control subjects ranging from 52 to 85 years of age.[7] In patients with abdominal aortic aneurysms, the mean femoral artery diameter was 9.63 ± 1.86 mm. Femoral artery diameter more than twice that of the external iliac artery or greater than 2 cm is generally considered a significant aneurysm.

Natural History

The thrombus lining the wall of a femoral aneurysm may be the source of emboli, causing distal small or large vessel occlusion,[2] or may result in thrombotic occlusion of the aneurysm with distal ischemia. Compression of the femoral vein may result in venous thrombosis. Progressive enlargement may produce local pain and tenderness. Rupture occurs infrequently. Graham et al managed 105 patients with femoral aneurysms nonoperatively for an average period of 28 months.[5] Fourteen patients continued to have symptomatic ischemia unrelated to the aneurysm; six aneurysms enlarged, of which two were resected; one aneurysm ruptured, and distal embolization resulted in the amputation of the leg of one patient. Tolstedt et al reported thrombosis leading to amputation in five of nine patients followed for less than 10 years.[8] Pappas et al reported thrombosis of aneurysms in 7 of 44 patients followed for less than 13 years.[9]

Indications for Intervention

The threat of serious, untreatable complications is not as great for femoral aneurysms as it is for aortic and popliteal aneurysms. On the other hand, the operation is easier and results are better when surgery is performed electively. Therefore, an operation is recommended for any symptomatic or complicated aneurysm larger than 2 to 3 cm in size unless there are significant medical contraindications.

Interventions

Management of common femoral aneurysms has historically been surgical. More recently, endovascular therapy and lytic therapy of acute thromboses have become available. These techniques have been used for the management of popliteal aneurysms but have rarely, if ever, been used for femoral aneurysms.

Operative Methods and Results

The history of the surgical treatments of aneurysms in many respects is the history of vascular surgery. It began in the second and third century with the proximal and distal ligation and packing of a popliteal aneurysm by Antyllus.[1] Various ligature sites were subsequently advocated including proximal ligation alone, proximal ligation at a distance to avoid rupture by the ligature, and distal ligation alone to prevent embolization. Various methods for managing the sac after ligation included allowing it to thrombose with-out packing, introducing a finger into the sac for identification and ligation of branches, introducing a trocar to suck out the thrombus, incising the sac and oversewing the branches from within followed by obliteration of the sac from within, incising the sac of a saccular aneurysm and suturing closed its origin from more normal artery from within the sac, incising the sac of a fusiform aneurysm and imbricating the sac from within to construct a new channel between the proximal and distal arterial orifices, excising the sac, and partially excising the sac not adherent to the vein. Cutler and Darling and Pappas et al still reported performing aneurysmorrhaphies on femoral artery aneurysms in the 1950s.[2,9]

Beginning in the 1950s, excision of the aneurysm and replacement with a homograft, vein graft, or plastic graft became the standard operation for almost all femoral aneurysms (Fig. 34–1). If possible, the aneurysm should be excised distal to the branches of the artery at the inguinal ligament to preserve collaterals. In some patients following excision of the aneurysm, an ectatic external iliac artery can be mobilized and anastomosed end to end to the distal common femoral artery.[10] If the superficial femoral artery is thrombosed, the distal anastomosis should be made to the deep femoral artery. If the aneurysm involves one branch, the anastomosis can be made to that branch and the other branch anastomosed end to side to the graft (Fig. 34–2). If the two branches are distally normal, a new bifurcation can be constructed (Fig. 34–3). The

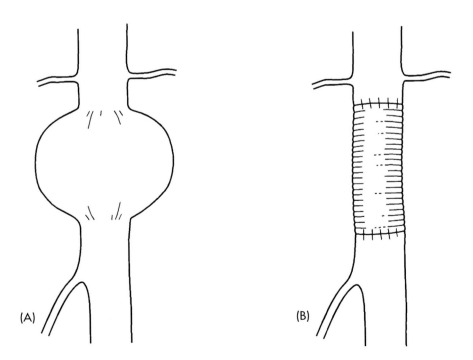

Figure 34–1. (A) Localized common femoral arterial aneurysm. (B) Common femoral aneurysm excised and replaced by interposition prosthetic graft.

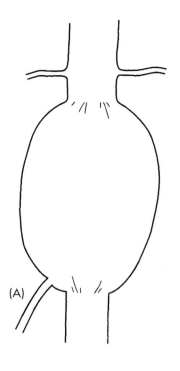

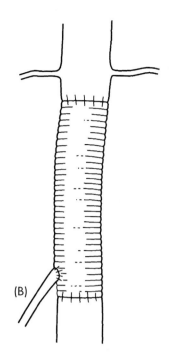

Figure 34–2. (A) Common femoral arterial aneurysm involving the proximal superficial femoral artery. (B) Aneurysm replaced by graft and profunda femorus artery anastomosed end to side to graft.

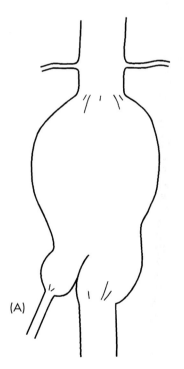

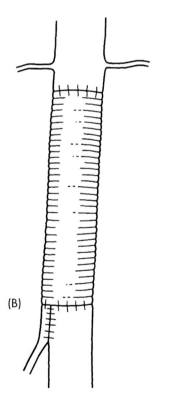

Figure 34–3. (A) Common femoral arterial aneurysm involving proximal profunda and superficial femoral arteries. (B) Aneurysm resected and replaced by graft after reconstruction of the bifurcation.

arteries are placed side to side, and a longitudinal incision is made through the ends of the arteries down the coapted walls. The cut edges of the two arteries are sutured together to reconstruct a bifurcation. An end-to-end anastomosis can be made between a graft and the resulting open end of the bifurcation. Cumulative patency rates of 83% at 5 years for autogenous vein and Dacron graft replacements of femoral aneurysms were reported by Cutler and Darling.[2] The patency rate for aneurysms without complications was 100% (18/18) compared to 75% (34/45) for patients presenting with complications. These results support the resection of asymptomatic aneurysms among patients who are medically fit.

Aneurysms of the superficial femoral artery can be excised and replaced with synthetic or vein grafts. Ligation of the superficial femoral artery and bypass with a vein graft is the preferable means of repair.[3] Aneurysms of the deep femoral artery have been successfully replaced. Vein grafts are the conduit of choice for these smaller vessels.[2,4]

POPLITEAL ANEURYSMS

Unlike femoral aneurysms, almost all popliteal aneurysms are associated with arteriosclerosis. They are more common than atherosclerotic femoral aneurysms, but aortic aneurysms are still 30 times more common than popliteal aneurysms. The aneurysms frequently occur just distal to the adductor magnus tendon or distal to the arcuate popliteal ligament, raising the possibility that they represent an accentuated poststenotic dilatation.[1,11]

Clinical Presentation

Asymptomatic, large popliteal aneurysms may occasionally be recognized by the patient. Like femoral aneurysms, they are most frequently diagnosed at the time of examination of patients with lower extremity occlusive or aneurysmal disease. Of patients presenting with a popliteal aneurysm, 48% have bilateral aneurysms.[1] Of patients with femoral aneurysms, 29% have popliteal aneurysms. On the other hand, fewer than 5% of patients with aortic aneurysms have popliteal aneurysms.

The diagnosis of popliteal aneurysms by physical examination may be quite difficult. They are frequently superior to the popliteal space. In addition, they may be confused with Baker's cysts, tumors, or an ectatic artery covered by muscle in a hypertensive patient. Duplex ultrasound can be diagnostic and can also demonstrate thrombus in the aneurysm.[12] Ward found popliteal arterial size to be 6.47 ± 0.98 mm in controls and 7.9 ± 1.74 mm in patients with abdominal aortic aneurysms.[7] Aneurysmal dilatation of more than 2.0 cm is considered significant. Arteriography is useful in demonstrating thrombus, associated occlusive disease, or abnormal anatomy in the adjacent arteries. (Fig. 34–4).

Natural History

Complications of popliteal aneurysms include thrombosis, embolization, venous compression, nerve compression, and rupture. In a collected series of 203 cases with a mean follow-up period of less than 4 years, 31% developed complications.[1] Over 68% of the complications were thromboembolic, causing gangrene in 29% and resulting in amputation in 11%.[1]

Indications for Intervention

Popliteal aneurysms that have developed complications generally require intervention. Acute thrombosis or rupture requires immediate treatment. Intervention is also recommended for asymptomatic aneurysms more than 2.0 to 2.5 cm in diameter in patients without significant medical problems. Inahara and Toledo observed nine limbs with acute ischemia secondary to thrombosed popliteal aneurysms less than 2.5 cm in diameter.[13] The mean diameter of thrombosed aneurysms seen by Vermillion et al was 1.8 cm.[14] In another

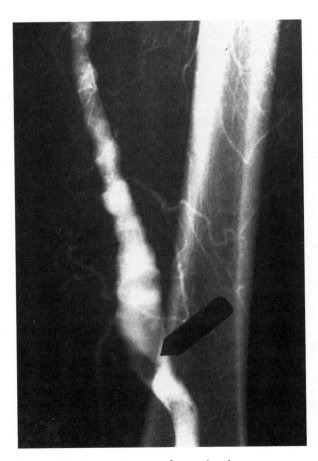

Figure 34–4. Arteriogram of a popliteal aneurysm containing a thrombus. (Reprinted from Ref. 1, Fig. 9–B, p. 126, with permission.)

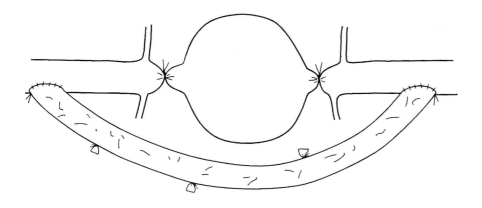

Figure 34–5. Popliteal aneurysm treated by ligation of the popliteal artery proximal and distal to the aneurysm and saphenous vein bypass.

series of patients with asymptomatic popliteal aneurysms, Lowell et al found that a diameter of more than 2 cm was one of the risk factors predictive of the development of complications.[15]

Operative Methods and Results

The historical aspects of surgery for popliteal aneurysms mimic those of surgery for femoral aneurysms. In the modern era, operations were at first performed through a posterior approach, with the patient in a prone position, through an S-shaped incision over the popliteal space. It was later found that it was possible to use a medial approach with the leg bent, which made the removal of the saphenous vein easier if it was to be used for the graft. Either approach gives adequate exposure. Originally, complete excision of the aneurysm was performed, which complicated the operation and on occasion resulted in excessive bleeding from the adherent popliteal vein. Vein or synthetic grafts are used as either transpositions with end-to-end anastomoses or ligation and bypasses with end-to-side anastomoses. The author found, as later reported by Edwards, that through the medial approach the popliteal artery could be locally exposed and ligated proximal and distal to the aneurysm and the aneurysm bypassed with a graft, usually vein[16] (Fig. 34–5). A similar procedure can be performed through the posterior approach, and for small aneurysms that can be easily excised, short transportation grafts can be inserted.

The long-term results of these operations have been quite satisfactory (Fig. 34–6). Cumulative 10-year graft patency rates have ranged from 47 to 76%, with limb salvage rates of 94 to 95%.[13,17,18] Vein graft patency rates of 84% and 94% respectively, as opposed to nonvein graft patency rates of 40% and 20%, respectively, have been reported by Dawson et al[17] and Anton et al.[19] Patency rates at 5 years for asymptomatic aneurysms were 77 to 92% compared to 39 to 54% for complicated aneurysms.[18–21] Shortell et al and Lilly et al observed 5-year patency rates of 84% and 89%, respec-

tively, for patients with good runoff compared to 65% and 24% respectively, for those with poor runoff.[18,21]

Thrombolytic Therapy

Thrombolytic therapy has been evaluated as a means of improving runoff and graft patency, particularly in patients with acute popliteal aneurysm thrombosis. Schwarz et al in 1984 successfully lysed an acutely thrombosed popliteal aneurysm.[22] Streptokinase or urokinase is infused through a catheter positioned in the aneurysm via the ipsilateral or contralateral femoral artery. During continuous infusions, arteriograms are periodically performed, usually over a 48-hour period.

In general, the results of thrombolytic therapy have been promising. Among patients treated with thrombolytic agents for acutely thrombosed popliteal aneurysms, a successful outcome was achieved in 47 (73%).[22–29] In 20 cases in which detailed information is available, complete lysis of the aneurysm was achieved in 18 cases and partial lysis in two cases.[22–24,28,29] In 14 cases, complete lysis of the runoff vessels was achieved in 12 and partial lysis in the other two.[22–24,28] Most surgeons use thrombolysis only for preoperative or intraoperative adjunctive therapy. Galland et al reported a multicenter experience with thrombolytic therapy in 866 patients with thrombosis of lower extremity arteries, grafts, or aneurysms. The lytic agents used included streptokinase, recombinant tissue-type plasminogen activator, and plasminogen–streptokinase activator complex. Acute limb deterioration occurred in 2.3% of all patients but in 6 (13%) of the 46 patients with popliteal aneurysms.[30]

Endovascular Therapy

Marin et al reported placement of an endoluminal stented graft repair in a 15 × 2.6 cm popliteal aneurysm that extended over a length of 15 cm.[31] The procedure was performed through the exposed femoral artery in the groin. A 6-mm stretch Gore-Tex graft with an attached Palmaz stent proximally was inserted. A sec-

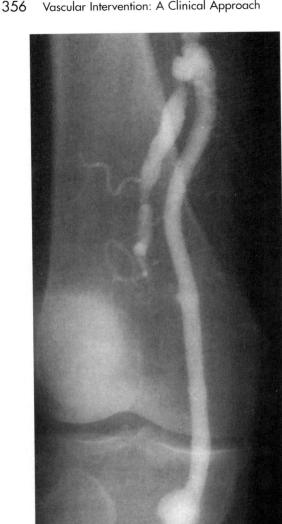

Figure 34–6. Arteriogram taken 70 months after ligation and bypass of a popliteal aneurysm using a saphenous vein graft. (Reprinted from Ref. 1, Fig. 9–3, p. 131, with permission.)

ond Palmaz stent was used to fix the distal end of the graft after it had been inserted. A postoperative arteriogram at 2 weeks and a duplex scan at 3 months demonstrated exclusion of the aneurysm and normal flow to the tibial arteries. The authors conclude that "additional experience and follow-up will be needed to assess the value of this minimally invasive procedure."

REFERENCES

1. DeWeese JA. Popliteal and femoral artery aneurysms. In: Ouriel K, ed. *Lower Extremity Vascular Disease.* Philadelphia: WB Saunders; 1995:121–139.

2. Cutler BS, Darling RC. Surgical management of arteriosclerotic femoral aneurysms. *Surgery* 1973;74:764–773.

3. Rigdon EE, Monajjem N. Aneurysms of the superficial femoral artery: a report of two cases and review of the literature. *J Vasc Surg* 1992;16:790–793.

4. Tait WF, Vohra RK, Carr HM, et al. True profunda femoris aneurysms: are they more dangerous than other atherosclerotic aneurysms of the femoropopliteal segment? *Ann Vasc Surg* 1991;5:92–95.

5. Graham LM, Zelenock GB, Whitehouse WM Jr, et al. Clinical significance of arteriosclerotic femoral artery aneurysms. *Arch Surg* 1980;115:502–507.

6. Gooding GAW, Effeney DJ. Ultrasound of femoral artery aneurysms. *AJR* 1980;134:447–483.

7. Ward AS. Aortic aneurysmal disease. A generalized dilating diathesis?. *Arch Surg* 1992;127:990–991.

8. Tolstedt GE, Radke HM, Bell JW. Late sequela of arteriosclerotic femoral aneurysms. *Angiology* 1961;12:601–602.

9. Pappas G, Janes JM, Bernatz PE, et al. Femoral aneurysms. *JAMA* 1964;190:489–493.

10. Inahara T. Aneurysms of the common femoral artery; reconstruction with the mobilized external iliac artery. *Am J Surg* 1966;111:759–763.

11. Cavallaro A, DiMarzo L, Gallo P, et al. Popliteal artery entrapment. Analysis of the literature and report of personal experience. *Vasc Surg* 1986;68:404–411.

12. Chan O, Thomas ML. Patients with arteriomegaly. *Clin Radiol* 1990;41:185–190.

13. Inahara T, Toledo AC. Complications and treatment of popliteal aneurysms. *Surgery* 1978;84:775–782.

14. Vermilion BD, Kimmins SA, Pace WG, et al. A review of one-hundred forty-seven popliteal aneurysms with long-term follow-up. *Surgery* 1981;90:1009–1014.

15. Lowell RC, Gloviczki P, Hallett JW Jr, et al. Popliteal artery aneurysms: the risk of nonoperative management. *Ann Vasc Surg* 1994;8:14–23.

16. Edwards WS. Exclusion and saphenous vein bypass of popliteal aneurysms. *Surg Gynecol Obstet* 1969;128:829–830.

17. Dawson I, van Bockel JH, Brand R, et al. Popliteal artery aneurysms. *J Vasc Surg* 1991;13:398–407.

18. Shortell CK, DeWeese JA, Ouriel K, et al. Popliteal artery aneurysms: 25-year surgical experience. *J Vasc Surg* 1991;14:771–779.

19. Anton GE, Hertzer NR, Beven ED, et al. Surgical management of popliteal aneurysms. Trends in presentation, treatment, and results from 1952 to 1984. *J Vasc Surg* 1986;3:125–134.

20. Shellack J, Smith RB III, Perdue GD. Nonoperative management of selected popliteal aneurysms. *Arch Surg* 1987;122:372–378.

21. Lilly MP, Flinn WR, McCarthy WJ III, et al. The effect of distal arterial anatomy on the success of popliteal aneurysm repair. *J Vasc Surg* 1988;7:653–660.

22. Schwarz W, Berkowitz H, Taormina V, et al. The preoperative use of intra-arterial thrombolysis for a thrombosed popliteal artery aneurysm. *J Cardiovasc Surg* 1984;25:465–468.

23. Garramore RR Jr, Gallagher JJ Jr, Drezner AD. Intraarterial thrombolytic therapy in the initial management of thrombosed popliteal artery aneurysms. *Ann Vasc Surg* 1994;8:363–366.

24. Carpenter JP, Barker CF, Roberts B, et al. Popliteal artery aneurysms: current management and outcome. *J Vasc Surg* 1994;19:65–72.

25. Varga ZA, Locke-Edmunds JC, Baird RN, et al. A multicenter study of popliteal aneurysms. *J Vasc Surg* 1994;20:171–177.

26. Ramesh S, Michaels JA, Galland RB. Popliteal aneurysm: morphology and management. *Br J Surg* 1993;80:1531–1533.

27. Hoelting T, Paetz B, Richter GM, et al. The value of preoperative lytic therapy in limb-threatening acute ischemia from popliteal artery aneurysm. *Am J Surg* 1994;168:227–231.

28. Lancashire MJR, Torrie EPH, Galland RB. Popliteal aneurysms identified by intra-arterial streptokinase: a changing pattern of presentation. *Br J Surg* 1990;77:1388–1390.

29. Bowyer RC, Cawthorn SJ, Walker WJ, et al. Conservative management of asymptomatic popliteal aneurysm. *Br J Surg* 1990;77:1132–1135.

30. Galland RB, Earnshaw JJ, Baird RN, et al. Acute limb deterioration during intra-arterial thrombolysis. *Br J Surg* 1993;80:1118–1120.

31. Marin ML, Veith FJ, Panetta TF, et al. Transfemoral endoluminal stented graft repair of a popliteal artery aneurysm. *J Vasc Surg* 1994;19:754–757.

35

The Role of Preoperative Imaging Studies in the Evaluation of Asymptomatic and Symptomatic Abdominal Aortic Aneurysms

John J. Vignati, M.D.
David C. Brewster, M.D.

Since the first repair of an abdominal aortic aneurysm (AAA) over 35 years ago, great progress has been made in the management of this potentially lethal problem. AAA repair is now quite safely accomplished in many centers and has become a common vascular surgical procedure, with approximately 40,000 operations performed annually in the United States. As the incidence of AAA increases with advancing age, the number of AAA repairs can be expected to increase as life expectancy, and hence the size of our aging population, continue to rise.

The steady improvement in the results of elective AAA repair is exemplified by several reports from the Massachusetts General Hospital detailing experience over the past 35 years. Operative mortality has decreased from approximately 10% in the 1960s to less than 2% during the most recent decade.[1-3] Much of the improvement in the outcome of AAA repair can be attributed to refinement and simplification of surgical technique, improvements in graft and suture materials, and, in particular, major advances in both intra- and postoperative care of surgical patients. However, improved results are also due in part to the evolution of technology capable of providing accurate preoperative AAA imaging that has paralleled development of surgical techniques, and that has contributed to both more accurate diagnosis of AAA and better preoperative planning, thereby allowing safer and more efficient performance of the procedure. However, in this cost-conscious era, it is clear that that the surgeon must select only those studies deemed necessary and appropriate for each patient based on the key questions and anatomic information required. The goal is to use the least expensive and least invasive imaging studies that yield the necessary information so as to allow safe, efficient, and cost-effective treatment. From a cost perspective, use of only a single imaging modality that can satisfy these needs would be ideal.

INFORMATION NEEDED BY THE SURGEON

The goals of preoperative imaging studies are to confirm the diagnosis of AAA and to provide the surgeon with sufficient information on which to base— rational management decisions. Specifically, anatomic information that influences judgments about the advisability of elective surgical repair and assessments of technical risk that may influence the decision to proceed with operation, facilitate preoperative planning, and conduct of the procedure[4] (Table 35–1).

Although the diagnosis of many asymptomatic aneurysms is currently based on an incidental finding on various radiologic studies performed for other reasons, in some patients an AAA is suspected by the finding of

Table 35–1. Preoperative Information Contributing to Successful Abdominal Aortic Aneurysm Repair

Confirmation of diagnosis
Accurate size determination
Proximal and distal extent of the aneurysm
Renal artery abnormalities
Visceral artery abnormalities
Iliofemoral occlusive disease
Associated aneurysmal disease

a pulsatile abdominal mass on physical examination. The inaccuracies of physical examination alone, however, are well recognized.[5] In obese patients, many AAAs are difficult to palpate, while in thin patients, a tortuous aorta or a prominent pulsation of a relatively normal aorta may mistakenly suggest the diagnosis. Finally, other intra-abdominal mass lesions or cysts that overlie the normal aorta may have transmitted pulsations that can confuse the examiner. Thus, it is obvious that the first need is to reliably establish the correct diagnosis.

Once the diagnosis of an AAA is verified, accurate sizing is the key to determining whether surgical correction is indicated. While controversy persists regarding operation for small (4- to 5-cm) AAAs, there is general agreement that elective repair is advisable in the low-risk patient with an AAA 5 cm in diameter or greater and even in most high-risk patients with AAAs exceeding 6 cm. Once surgical repair has been elected, a variety of anatomic issues are relevant in planning the procedure. Such anatomic data will influence both the graft configuration (tube vs bifurcated, iliac vs femoral anastomosis), the preferable operative approach (transperitoneal, retroperitoneal, medial visceral rotation, thoracoabdominal), and the site of proximal clamp control. In addition, certain anatomic data may be pivotal in deciding whether to proceed with an elective operation. For example, while a 5-cm AAA located in the infrarenal location is probably appropriate for elective surgical correction, the finding of a suprarenal extension that involves the renal and visceral arteries may suggest that watchful waiting is better, particularly in the elderly or high-risk patient. Indeed, the proximal extent of aneurysmal disease has a strong influence on operative risk and often dictates the appropriate surgical approach; therefore, this information must be accurately defined preoperatively. Similarly, knowledge of severe renal or visceral artery lesions, as well as the presence of significant accessory renal arteries and associated aneurysms, may warrant concomitant repair, and their unrecognized presence may have profound perioperative consequences. Iliofemoral occlusive disease also merits thorough evaluation prior to AAA repair, primarily by influencing the best site for the distal anastomoses.

It is often claimed that the experienced surgeon can determine virtually all such anatomic data during the course of the operation, and that information gained by various preoperative studies rarely alters the procedure or outcome and is therefore not particularly cost effective. We strongly disagree with this viewpoint. Certain features, particularly the severity and importance of stenotic lesions in major aortic branch vessels, are difficult or impossible to assess by inspection or palpation alone. In addition, even if this assessment is possible, unexpected findings may be difficult to deal with

effectively if an inappropriate surgical approach has been employed. Finally, the extra operative time and dissection required to assess the extent of pathology and reach operative decisions must be considered. At the current cost of approximately $20 per minute, the operating room is an expensive environment for a diagnostic workup. Necessary anatomic information is more safely and inexpensively obtained preoperatively by appropriate imaging evaluation.

With this perspective, it is useful to classify preoperative anatomic data into three categories: (1) those that may be crucial to a safe and successful outcome, (2) those that are quite helpful in performing the procedure but perhaps not of critical importance, and finally (3) those that are sometimes helpful but provide no essential information.[3] Crucial information includes the proximal extent of the AAA, the presence of critical renal artery abnormalities, and the presence of severe visceral or pelvic occlusive disease that makes postoperative intestinal ischemia a potential hazard. Category 2 information that may be very helpful by increasing the safety and efficiency of the planned procedure would include delineation of outflow disease in the iliofemoral and infrainguinal arterial segments and finding other unexpected features such as an inflammatory AAA, a horseshoe kidney, or other renal developmental anomalies; accessory renal arteries arising from the AAA; severe calcification of the aorta at the "neck" of the AAA; and the presence of a retroaortic renal vein or other venous anomalies. Information in the third category, which may be helpful but not essential, includes the distal extent of aneurysmal disease, other occult associated aneurysms, or the presence of other unusual findings such as dissection, arteriovenous fistulas, contained leaks, unusual lumbar arteries, and so on, all of which might influence the surgical approach or operative plan.

All imaging modalities differ considerably in the amount of information in these three categories that they may provide. It is the surgeon's task to carefully select tests that are necessary and cost effective for each particular patient. A discussion of currently utilized imaging studies follows, with emphasis on the advantages and weaknesses of each that will guide decisions for their use. Finally, our own current general practice guidelines are offered, as well as a brief consideration of what the future may bring in this field.

ULTRASOUND

Ultrasonography is perhaps the most widely employed initial imaging study for evaluation of AAAs. Its principal advantages are its wide availability, low cost, and safety due to its noninvasive nature and lack of any radiation or contrast exposure. These features have established ultrasonography as the preferred examination for establishing the diagnosis of AAA, for initial size determination, and for follow-up surveillance among patients managed conservatively. With current gray-scale sonography, longitudinal and cross-sectional sizing is usually accurate to within 3 mm of operative measurements.

However, ultrasound has widely recognized limitations. It is quite operator dependent and requires an experienced technician for reliable results. Because measurements may be taken at differing locations in serial examinations, sizing inconsistencies and inaccuracies may occur. Obesity or the presence of bowel gas may make examination difficult or impossible. Most importantly, the accurate delineation of the proximal and distal extent of the AAA and its relation to the renal, visceral, and iliac vessels is often difficult. Also, the suprarenal and thoracic aortas cannot be well visualized. Other potentially important anatomic characteristics are also not identified, such as coexistent occlusive or aneurysmal disease, the presence of an inflammatory aneurysm or retroaortic renal vein, and other features that may influence the conduct of surgery. Recent improvements in ultrasonography, including deep abdominal Doppler scanning and the addition of real-time color flow mapping, may help overcome some of these limitations, but at present, most of these areas remain a shortcoming of the technique.

Another developing role for ultrasound may be in the screening of high-risk groups for unsuspected AAAs. Wolf et al performed B-mode ultrasound examinations on 531 patients undergoing lower extremity arterial evaluations and found aortic aneurysms more than 4 cm in diameter in 3.2% of the total group and in 8.8% of male smokers over the age of 65.[6] It has been suggested that a very selective screening for occult AAAs could be both cost effective and life-saving.

Because of its low cost and risk-free performance, ultrasound continues to have an important role in diagnosis, size surveillance, and screening for AAA. However, most surgeons currently agree that additional information is important before surgical repair, and that the limitations of ultrasound examinations alone in this regard make it generally unwise to proceed with elective operation using utlrasound as the sole imaging study.

COMPUTED TOMOGRAPHY SCANNING

Conventional computed tomography (CT) scans are more expensive than ultrasound, involve ionizing radiation exposure, and, if contrast enhancement is employed, carry the potential risk of contrast-induced allergic reactions or renal dysfunction. However, in current practice, the risks and discomfort associated with this imaging modality are minimal. CT scans also provide images in only one plane (cross-sectional), and

these may be degraded by motion, metallic clips, or other metallic devices.

Despite these issues, improved CT technology has emerged as the most widely used imaging study prior to AAA repair. It is rapidly performed, available in most health care facilities, easily interpreted, and provides a wealth of information about the aneurysm and adjacent structures. Because the accuracy of CT scanning is not operator dependent, accurate size comparison of one study to a subsequent study during follow-up is also precise. In terms of operative planning, CT scanning is perhaps most valuable in its ability to define accurately the extent of the AAA in relation to the renal and iliac vessels proximally and distally. Todd et al reported a remarkable 99% accuracy rate in CT prediction of the all-important origin of the aneurysms,[7] and Papanicoleau and coworkers from our institution, determined a similar 94% accuracy rate for CT in defining the proximal extent of AAA in relation to the renal arteries.[8] In contrast to ultrasound examination, possible aneurysmal involvement of the suprarenal and thoracic aortas may also be easily evaluated. The presence of associated anomalies such as duplicated vena cava, retroaortic left renal vein, and horseshoe kidney are also clearly defined by conventional CT scanning and may help determine the advisability of further preoperative imaging studies such as angiography in the presence of a horseshoe kidney.

With the use of intravenous contrast, additional information can be obtained. Various kidney abnormalities such as hydronephrosis or nonenhancing kidneys (which may suggest unilateral renal artery occlusion) is easily visualized. The presence and pattern of intraluminal thrombus, as well as information concerning patency of the renal and visceral vessels, can be ascertained with the addition of intravenous contrast. In addition, the presence of an enhancing ring of soft tissue around the anterior and lateral aspects of the AAA is quite suggestive of an inflammatory aneurysm (Fig. 35–1). This finding may indeed influence operative management, as many authors advocate the retroperitoneal approach for known inflammatory aneurysms. Another excellent use for conventional CT is in the evaluation of *symptomatic aneurysms*, a term used to describe the AAA in a patient experiencing back or abdominal pain or other symptoms that may be related to a rapidly expanding or ruptured aneurysm. The existence of a ruptured or "leaking" AAA can be rapidly and accurately determined by the presence of fluid and asymmetry in the retroperitoneum or by disruption in the integrity of the aneurysm wall. Obviously, CT scanning is advocated only for hemodynamically stable patients under close observation. If no leak or rupture is ascertained and the patient's renal function is normal, then a contrast-enhanced CT scan should be obtained because a large

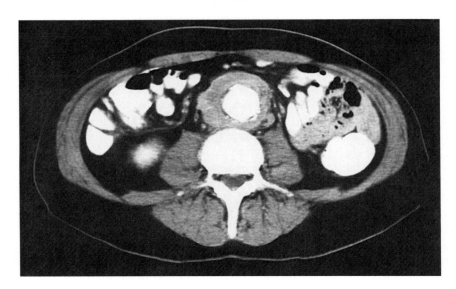

Figure 35–1. Conventional contrast CT scan demonstrating a perianeurysmal enhancing soft tissue ring suggestive of an inflammatory aneurysm.

percentage of inflammatory aneurysms present with abdominal or back pain. The ability to differentiate the ruptured AAA from the still intact but symptomatic lesion quickly and accurately is potentially very valuable in terms of immediate management decisions. Ruptured aneurysms obviously require repair as rapidly as possible. While expedient repair is also indicated for the symptomatic AAA, a better outcome can often be achieved if a brief interval is available for better preoperative preparation of the patient, as well as assembly of the best available anesthesia, surgical, and support personnel.

The major limitations of conventional CT scanning include inability to define and assess occlusive disease in the renal, visceral, and aortoiliac regions; poor visualization of accessory renal arteries; and occasional difficulty in defining the proximal neck of a large or tortuous AAA, particularly in the juxtarenal location. Because CT data are acquired in a strictly cross-sectional fashion, all surgeons have seen cases of large juxtarenal aneurysms with a tortuous neck in which conventional CT scans mistakenly suggest suprarenal extension[9] (Fig. 35–2). In cases where the proximal neck is ill-defined despite a conventional CT scan, high-resolution CT scanning has been touted by Gomes and Choyke to greatly increase the accuracy in defining the renal artery origins in relation to the proximal extent of the AAA.[10] Briefly, this technique involves taking multiple thin slices in the region of the renal arteries, which enhances resolution and decreases partial volume effects, allowing for more accurate definition of the AAA's proximal neck. If, despite high-resolution techniques, the proximal neck is still poorly defined, angiography may be warranted.

Overall, conventional CT scanning is an excellent preoperative imaging modality for AAA surgery. Because the vast majority of AAAs are infrarenal, a conventional CT scan should be used as the initial and per-

haps the only preoperative imaging study, with further imaging reserved for specific clinical or anatomic considerations.

ANGIOGRAPHY

The role of angiography prior to AAA repair has always been somewhat controversial, and current advances in other imaging modalities, as well as the current cost-conscious climate, have only intensified the debate.

Angiography is, in many ways, the ultimate preoperative imaging study to demonstrate important anatomic information such as the extent of aneurysmal disease and the anatomy of the juxtarenal aorta, as well as in the assessment of coexistent occlusive or aneurysmal disease in renal, visceral, and pelvic aortic branches (Fig. 35–3). Also, potentially important accessory renal arteries are usually displayed. Indeed, angiography often excels in areas where conventional CT scanning is admittedly weak.

Because only the true arterial lumen is opacified, angiography is relatively inaccurate in terms of diagnosis and sizing. In addition, it often fails to demonstrate other anatomic features such as venous anomalies, perianeurysmal fibrosis, contained rupture, or potentially troublesome calcification at the proximal and distal extents of the AAA. However, the major arguments against routine use of angiography are its cost, its invasiveness, and the belief that the mere demonstration of certain anatomic findings may not, in fact, alter the conduct of the operation or necessarily improve the outcome.

While all of these criticisms must be acknowledged, it is important to examine data relative to these points from the perspective of contemporary practice. Like any invasive procedure, angiography carries an inherent risk of procedure-related complications. These include local complications secondary to arterial punc-

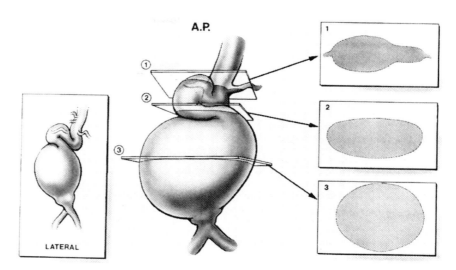

Figure 35–2. Diagrammatic representation of the inability of CT scanning to localize the aneurysm neck accurately in the presence of a tortuous juxtarenal aorta. A.P.,

ture or passage of catheters and guidewires, such as bleeding, thrombosis, embolization, dissection, or pseudoaneurysm formation, as well as systemic problems related to contrast injections, such as allergic reactions, contrast-induced renal failure, or osmotic fluid overload. However, when angiography is performed by experienced personnel with appropriate equipment and techniques, the rates of these complications are quite low. Our own experience parallels that of the literature, showing a low overall incidence of approximately 0.5% for major complications and 1 to 3% for minor complications.[5,11] The possibility of contrast-

induced renal failure is often cited as a significant danger, but with current contrast agents and widespread appreciation of the importance of periprocedural hydration and the use of limited contrast loads, clinically significant renal failure is quite infrequent in patients with normal renal function. In higher-risk patients, such as diabetics with preexisting renal insufficiency, the incidence of this problem increases to approximately 10%. However, such contrast-related renal dysfunction is almost always transient and reversible. The increased use of digital subtraction techniques and more frequent performance of outpatient studies have further reduced the potential renal risks by limiting dye loads and spacing the diagnostic and surgical procedures further apart.

Angiography is unquestionably more expensive than other imaging studies, but the differences may not be as great as suspected. Most studies are now done on an outpatient basis, eliminating the expense of an extra day of hospitalization, which formerly contributed to excess expense. In addition, it should be recognized that traditional hospital charges for the study often do not accurately reflect the true costs of the procedure. If more extensive anatomic areas need to be studied, charges for other forms of imaging may increase: for example, double charges for a patient requiring both an abdominal and a pelvic CT scan. The information gained by angiography may otherwise require use performance of several alternative imaging studies, and the potential cumulative expense of these studies may offset any cost advantages. Finally, the potential cost savings of reduced operative time and avoidance of possibly significant perioperative complications or morbidity attributable to the anatomic knowledge gleaned from angiography is difficult to quantify but needs to be considered.

Numerous studies have documented a significant incidence of ''positive'' findings on routine arteriogra-

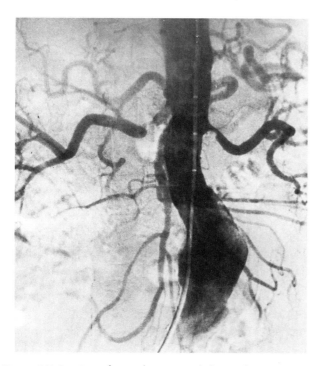

Figure 35–3. Transfemoral contrast abdominal aortagram revealing significant bilateral renal artery stenosis in addition to an infrarenal aneurysm.

Table 35–2. Selective Indications for Preoperative Angiography Prior to Aneurysm Repair

Suspicion of suprarenal extension
Suspected visceral or renal artery disease
Iliofemoral occlusive disease
Associated aneurysmal disease
Horseshoe kidney or other renal anomalies
Prior aortic or colonic surgery
Unusual aneurysms (mycotic, aortocaval fistulas, etc.)

phy performed prior to AAA repair. A cumulative review of the literature in this regard indicates that approximately 6% of AAAs extend above the renal arteries, 15 to 20% have potentially significant renal or visceral artery stenotic lesions, 10 to 15% have accessory renal arteries, and about 40% have aneurysmal or occlusive disease involving the iliofemoral segment.[4] While it is clear that not all of these findings are of great clinical importance, a review of the literature further documents that there is wide variability in the frequency with which such arteriographic findings were believed to affect or modify the operative procedure. For example, Baur et al reported a 75% incidence of procedure modification based on angiographic findings,[12] whereas Numo et al, reported procedure modification in only 6%.[13] Clearly, these figures are somewhat subjective and quite variable, but a composite mean of eight studies shows that approximately 29% of cases had a procedure modification based on angiographic findings. A prospective, randomized trial would be necessary to define this issue more accurately.

At this time, it seems appropriate to conclude that angiography may be an important preoperative imaging study in some patients, but it appears inappropriate to utilize it on a routine basis in all patients with AAAs. Hence, a policy of selective use is generally accepted by most vascular surgeons based on specific indications (Table 35–2). Most of these indications can be discerned by a careful history and physical examination as well as with clinical judgment. In other cases, the need for additional preoperative information and the use of angiography may stem from findings of other preoperative imaging studies.

MAGNETIC RESONANCE IMAGING/ MAGNETIC RESONANCE ANGIOGRAPHY

Magnetic resonance imaging (MRI) is a relatively new, noninvasive imaging modality that requires no nephrotoxic contrast agents. Images are obtained as protons are stimulated by radio waves in a magnetic field, followed by a relaxation phase. During this phase, energy is released and processed into anatomic data. Standard magnetic resonance images yield much the same data as conventional CT scanning regarding the proximal and distal extent of AAA, location of the left renal vein, and presence of other anatomic anomalies. In addition, the newer magnetic resonance angiography (MRA) sequences can now discern major renal, visceral, and aortoiliac occlusive disease, a capability conspicuously absent from conventional CT scans (Fig. 35–4). The major potential advantages of MRI/MRA are that it is a single, noninvasive study that requires no radiation or nephrotoxic contrast, is capable of yielding multipla-

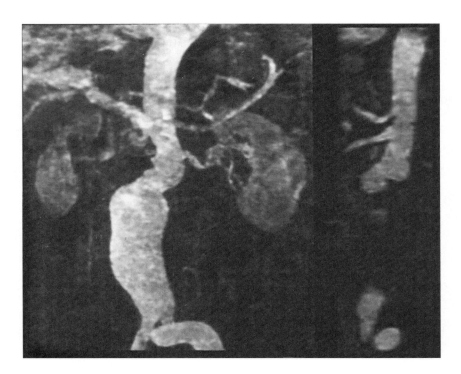

Figure 35–4. MRA scan demonstrating an adequate infrarenal proximal neck for aneurysm repair. A signal void in the right renal artery is also seen, consistent with a hemodynamically significant stenosis of the right renal artery.

nar images, and has the potential for defining renal, visceral, and iliofemoral occlusive disease. In a sense, MRI/MRA can potentially provide information similar to that produced by the combination of CT and angiography at a cost somewhere between those of CT and angiography. The addition of gadolinium, a paramagnetic contrast agent, shortens the relaxation time of blood, making it more distinct from other tissues regardless of flow rates and turbulence. This is a key advance in AAA imaging, where flow is greatly influenced by the anatomy of the AAA, often resulting in slow, turbulent flow.

The limitations of MRI/MRA include lack of general availability, inconsistent quality of studies from some facilities, and inability for use in certain patients, such as those with pacemakers or metallic hardware due to the magnetic field. In addition, patients with claustrophobia or unstable medical conditions are not optimal candidates for MRI/MRA, as the acquisition time is much longer than with CT scanning, although most claustrophobic patients can be studied successfully with supplemental benzodiazapene administration.

Petersen et al from the Massachusetts General Hospital compared the results of preoperative imaging with MRA and contrast angiography in 38 patients undergoing aneurysm repair and found the information obtained by MRA to be quite similar to that of conventional angiography.[14] In particular, the proximal extent of the AAA was correctly predicted in 87% of patients. However, MRA is still relatively insensitive in evaluating accessory renal arteries and the status of the inferior mesenteric and hypogastric arteries, as well as in defining the severity of renal and visceral vessel stenoses once they have been identified. This shortcoming is thought to be related to resolution, particularly in areas of tortuous vessels, where sharp angulations can be perceived as stenoses by this flow-based imaging technique. Prince et al also evaluated gadolinium-enhanced MRA for AAA imaging and found it to be quite accurate in sizing, predicting proximal extent, and predicting major branch vessel stenoses.[15] However, the exact severity of renal and visceral arterial stenoses was ill defined, as was the status of the inferior mesenteric and hypogastric arteries.

In summary, MRI/MRA is, a reasonable preoperative imaging technique for AAA, yielding much the same information as the combination of CT and angiography, although its present resolution regarding the exact severity of branch vessel occlusive disease remains inferior to that of angiography. While currently it may be the preoperative imaging study of choice for patients with renal insufficiency, it has the potential to become the single conventional imaging study necessary in the preoperative evaluation for elective AAA repair as the technology continues to evolve and improve.

HELICAL CT SCAN/CT ANGIOGRAPHY

Helical or spiral CT scanning is a modification of conventional CT scanning whereby a continuous volume of data is obtained rather than interrupted axial images. The X-ray tube is continuously activated and rotated while the patient is simultaneously advanced in a longitudinal direction through the scanner. Axial scans obtained in this fashion are nearly identical to conventional CT scans. However, with the addition of a properly timed bolus of IV contrast, spectacular images of the vascular anatomy can be obtained and refigured into detailed, three-dimensional images, so-called CT angiograms, which can be rotated for viewing in any projection (Fig. 35–5). This technique does require breath holding for approximately 30 seconds and a test injection to establish the optimal delay between contrast bolus and spiral scanning. Breath holding for 30 seconds can be accomplished in approximately 90% of patients with appropriate coaching and practice.[17] The total contrast load is the major drawback and is usually in the range of 120 to 150 cc. Usually with a 30-second breath hold, the abdominal aorta from the superior mesenteric artery origin to the iliac bifurcation can be imaged with a single bolus of contrast.

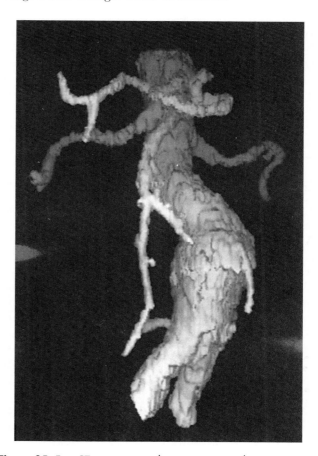

Figure 35–5. CT angiogram demonstrating a three-dimensional image of the vascular anatomy of an infrarenal aneurysm.

Gomes et al studied 32 patients with suspected AAA with helical CT scanning and found that the proximal and distal extents of the AAA, as well as the presence of renal, visceral, and aortoiliac occlusive disease, was accurately defined.[16] The presence of accessory renal arteries was also detected, a capability not possessed by MRI. It seems that helical CT provided much the same information as conventional angiography, as well as the same data as conventional CT scanning. Galanski et al described the results of spiral CT in the evaluation of renal artery stenosis in 22 patients.[18] Multiple renal arteries were correctly identified in all cases, including a total of 11 accessory renal arteries. Of the 54 arteries studied, 22 were either stenotic or occluded by spiral CT. These results correlated well with those of angiography, with complete agreement in cases with more than 50% stenosis.

In summary, helical CT/angiography is a relatively new and exciting imaging modality with tremendous potential in preoperative AAA imaging. Its major limitation is the need for a rather large volume intravenous contrast. In addition, the creation of three-dimensional CT angiograms requires a significant time investment at the computer console by the radiologist. However, the quality and detail of the images, including the presence of renal and visceral arterial stenoses and accessory renal arteries, can be quite good, certainly better than that of the images routinely obtained with MRA. The cost of spiral CT is similar to, or perhaps slightly more than, that of conventional CT scanning. Given its ability to characterize occlusive disease, as well as the extent and size of the aneurysm and periaortic structures, spiral CT may evolve into a satisfactory sole imaging modality in many patients with AAA and normal renal function.

CURRENT RECOMMENDATIONS

In the hemodynamically stable patient with a symptomatic AAA (abdominal or back pain, etc.), we recommend a rapid imaging technique to document whether rupture has occurred, define the proximal extent of the AAA, and exclude other unrelated pathology, such as diverticulitis, as the cause of the symptoms. Conventional CT, because of its universal availability, reasonable cost, and ability to acquire the necessary data, rapidly, is our imaging study of choice in these circumstances. It is critical that the patient be closely observed, with frequent blood pressure measurements during the scanning. The initial scan should be performed without contrast to minimize nephrotoxicity if emergent AAA repair is necessary. If no rupture is seen on the initial non-contrast scan and the patient has normal renal function, a contrast CT scan should then be obtained to further characterize the AAA and potentially establish the diagnosis of an inflammatory AAA, identified by a characteristic enhancing soft tissue ring around the anterior aspect of the aneurysm. The preoperative diagnosis of an inflammatory AAA, which often presents with abdominal or back pain, is important because a retroperitoneal approach may be indicated for repair.

The preferred preoperative imaging workup of asymptomatic AAA continues to evolve, and no clear consensus currently exists with respect to the optimal choice in all patients or clinical situations. The goal remains to use the fewest studies that will provide the necessary information for successful AAA repair in a safe and cost-effective manner. It seems clear that the choice of the best method will vary, depending on the desired objective of the study and the circumstances unique to each patient and clinical situation.

Ultrasound appears adequate for initial diagnosis, size assessment, and follow-up surveillance in most instances. When operation is required, conventional CT scanning, with contrast if renal function allows, seems the most logical preoperative study unless specific indications for angiography are identified. In many patients, this may suffice as the sole preoperative imaging study. If indicated by certain findings on CT scan or clinical examination (as previously outlined), however, conventional angiography should be employed in patients with reasonable baseline renal function. MRA should be performed in patients with significant renal impairment, obtaining an angiogram in this fragile patient population only if the information from MRA is inadequate.

In the future, either helical CT angiography or MRA studies may replace both CT scans and selective angiography if further technological advances improve resolution and decrease acquisition time. Also, MRI/MRA is, and will likely continue to be, the imaging modality of choice for patients with renal dysfunction in whom one wants to avoid contrast administration.

REFERENCES

1. Darling RC, Brewster DC. Elective treatment of abdominal aortic aneurysms. *World J Surg* 1980;4:661–667.
2. McCabe CJ, Coleman WS, Brewster DC. The advantage of early operation for abdominal aortic aneurysm. *Arch Surg* 1981;116:1025–1029.
3. Cambria RP, Brewster DC, Abbott WM, et al. Transperitoneal vs. retroperitoneal approach for aortic reconstruction: a randomized prospective study. *J Vasc Surg* 1990;11:314–325.
4. Petersen MJ, Brewster DC. Role of arteriography in assessment of abdominal aortic aneurysm. In: Ernst CB, Stanley JC, eds. *Current Therapy in Vascular Surgery*, 3rd ed. St Louis: Mosby Year Book; 1995:210–213.
5. Brewster DC, Retana A, Waltman AC, et al. Angiography in the management of aneurysms of the abdominal aorta, its value and safety. *N Engl J Med* 1975;292:822–825.
6. Wolf YG, Otis SM, Schwend RB, et al. Screening for abdominal aortic aneurysms during lower extremity arterial evaluation in the vascular laboratory. *J Vasc Surg* 1995;22:417–423.

7. Todd GJ, Nowygrod R, Benvenisty A, et al. The accuracy of CT scanning in the diagnosis of abdominal and thoracoabdominal aortic aneurysms. *J Vasc Surg* 1991;13:302–309.
8. Papanicolau N, Wittenberg J, Ferrucci JT, et al. Preoperative evaluation of abdominal aortic aneurysms by computed tomography. *AJR* 1986;146:711–715.
9. O'Hara PJ. Preoperative angiography vs. other imaging techniques before elective abdominal aortic aneurysm repair. In: Veith FJ, ed. *Current Critical Problems in Vascular Surgery*, Vol 6. St Louis: Quality Medical; 1994:305–312.
10. Gomes MN, Choyke P. Improved identification of renal arteries in patients with aortic aneurysms by means of high resolution computed tomography. *J Vasc Surg* 1987;6:262–268.
11. Lang EK. A survey of the complications of percutaneous retrograde arteriography: Seldinger technique: *Radiology* 1963;81:257–261.
12. Baur GM, Porter JM, Eidemiller LR, et al. The role of arteriography in abdominal aortic aneurysms. *Am J Surg* 1977;136:184–189.
13. Nuno IN, Collins GM, Bardin JA, et al. Should arteriography be used routinely in the management of abdominal aortic aneurysm? *Am J Surg* 1982;144:53–57.
14. Petersen MJ, Cambria RP, Kaufman JA, et al. Magnetic resonance angiography in the preoperative evaluation of abdominal aortic aneurysms. *J Vasc Surg* 1995;21:891–898.
15. Prince MR, Narasimhan DL, Stanley JC. Gadolinium-enhanced magnetic resonance angiography of abdominal aortic aneurysms. *J Vasc Surg* 1995;21:656–669.
16. Gomes MN, Davros WJ, Zeman RK. Preoperative assessment of abdominal aortic aneurysm: the value of helical and three-dimensional computed tomography. *J Vasc Surg* 1994;20:367–376.
17. Rubin G. Three dimensional angiography using spiral CT. In: Veith FJ, ed. *Current Critical Problems in Vascular Surgery*, Vol 6. St. Louis: Quality Medical; 1994;305–312.
18. Galanski M, Prokop M, Chavan A, et al. Renal arterial stenoses: spiral CT angiography. *Radiology* 1993;189:185–192.

36

Results of the Surgical Treatment of Intact and Ruptured Abdominal Aortic Aneurysms: Factors Influencing Outcome

David A. Lipski, M.D.
Calvin B. Ernst, M.D.

Since the first successful repair of an abdominal aortic aneurysm (AAA) by Dubost in 1951, repair by prosthetic graft replacement has become standard treatment. Indeed, until recently, open aneurysmorrhaphy was the only definitive treatment available. Pivotal in the case supporting elective aneurysm repair have been data documenting a marked survival advantage for patients undergoing AAA repair compared to that of patients treated nonoperatively, first reported in a classic study by Szilagyi and others in 1966.[1] Although nearly all aspects of AAA genesis, evaluation, treatment, and results have been extensively investigated, different methods of data collection and presentation have made study findings difficult to validate.

To standardize the interpretation and comparability of results reported by different investigators, guidelines for reporting the results of the management of arterial aneurysms were suggested by a joint subcommittee of the Society for Vascular Surgery (SVS) and the North American Chapter of the International Society for Cardiovascular Surgery (ISCVS-NA).[2] Since the time of this publication in 1991, many authors have adopted these guidelines. The subcommittee further promoted uniformity by recommending the presentation of survival data in life-table form and the evaluation of statistical significance of outcome differences based on a Cox proportional hazards model. This latter statistical technique eliminates the influence of factors other than the one under consideration.

EARLY MORTALITY

Operative repair of an AAA improves survival (Table 36–1). Two early studies examined the survival of

Table 36–1. Factors Adversely Affecting the Outcome of AAA Repair

Operative repair

Rupture

Preoperative (elective)
  Age >90 years
  Significant coronary artery disease
  Chronic lung disease requiring home oxygen use
  Significant renal insufficiency

Preoperative (ruptured)
  Hemodynamic instability
  Advanced coronary artery disease
  Renal insufficiency

Technical factors (elective and ruptured)
  Inflammatory aneurysm
  Renal vessel anomalies
  Pararenal aneurysm
  Primary aortocaval fistula
  Primary aortoenteric fistula
  Meandering mesenteric artery

Operative (ruptured)
  Large transfusion requirements
  Free, intraperitoneal rupture
  Suprarenal cross-clamp placement
  Prolonged cross-clamp time

Postoperative (elective and ruptured)
  Myocardial infarction
  Congestive heart failure
  Prolonged mechanical ventilation
  Acute renal failure
  Intestinal ischemia
  Stroke
  Bleeding
  Limb ischemia
  Distal embolism
  Multisystem organ failure

patients with aneurysms who did not undergo repair. Estes reported 81% patient mortality after 5 years, and 63% of deaths resulted from aneurysm rupture.[3] Szilagyi and colleagues noted 83% 5-year mortality of patients managed nonoperatively, and 35% of deaths followed aneurysm rupture.[1] In both studies, the reported mortality rate far exceeded the expected age-adjusted mortality rate. In a contemporary study, Perko and associates reported an 85% 5-year mortality rate for patients not undergoing repair and a 30% death rate from rupture.[4] Median survival was only 18 months. Because most surgeons agree that the behavior of an AAA cannot be predicted for any individual patient, elective repair is recommended for nearly all patients with sizable AAAs who do not have a limited life expectancy. (See Chapter 33).

Furthermore, reported data demonstrate a marked reduction in perioperative morbidity and mortality when repair is undertaken before rupture.[5] Operative mortality rates following repair of intact and ruptured AAAs reported since 1990 are tabulated in Tables 36–2 and 36–3. The mean 30-day mortality for repair of intact AAAs is 6%, contrasting sharply to the 48% mortality rate for repair of ruptured AAAs. These data are even more persuasive when the total mortality of AAA rupture is considered. Fully 60% of patients with ruptured AAA die before reaching the operating room, and the frequently reported mortality rates apply only to the remaining 40% who survive long enough to undergo attempted repair. Consequently up to 90% of patients die following AAA rupture. These data emphasize the advantage of operative repair of intact AAAs.

In addition, operative mortality rates for patients with intact AAAs have been declining, especially among reports from major vascular centers. The operative mortality rates reported during the 1970s and 1980s were generally higher than those reported during the 1990s. Reports including data accumulated over several decades also document lower contemporary mortality rates. Recent mortality rates cluster between 3% and 5%. This decline in operative mortality has occurred despite the fact that AAA repair is being offered to an older and more infirm patient population. Improvements in perioperative care and anesthesia, as well as refinements in operative techniques, have contributed to the lower operative mortality rates.

There has not been a similar trend toward lower operative mortality following repair of ruptured AAAs. The reasons for this are not clear but may include the aging of the general population and the greater prevalence of underlying medical problems in patients who develop ruptured AAA; prompt transport of living but unresuscitatable patients to hospitals; and improved operative techniques without parallel improvements in the ability to prevent and treat multisystem organ failure.

In 1992, a subcommittee of the SVS and ISCVS-NA ranked several risk factors predictive of operative morbidity and mortality following AAA repair.[6] Factors believed to confer a moderate to major (3 to 7%) increase in operative mortality rate included the following:

1. Age above 90 years.
2. Significant coronary artery disease (CAD), characterized by class II or III angina, cardiac catheterization or thallium scintiscan data documenting significant myocardium at risk, recent congestive heart failure (CHF), or a left ventricular ejection fraction of <20%.
3. Chronic obstructive pulmonary disease requiring home oxygen use.
4. Baseline serum creatinine level of >3.5 mg/dL.

Lesser degrees of impairment in these categories were associated with a mild (1 to 3%) increase in risk. However, in light of the dramatically higher mortality rates associated with aneurysm rupture, AAA repair should not be denied based solely on the presence of these factors when repair is otherwise indicated. Coexisting conditions, particularly CAD, must be identified and treated for optimal results. Hertzer's comprehensive analysis of AAA treatment documented that untreatable cardiac disease caused 37% of early portoperative deaths.[7] In addition, 39% of deaths within 5 years resulted from CAD. Although CAD is prevalent among patients with AAA and is responsible for many early and late deaths, the correlation between preoperative correction of CAD and outcome has been variable. Preoperative screening of asymptomatic individuals followed by ''prophylactic'' coronary artery bypass grafting (CABG) before elective AAA repair has not produced a significant reduction in cardiac morbidity and mortality following CABG and AAA repair.[8–11] Mason and colleagues asserted that as overall mortality from elective AAA repair continues to decrease, a benefit from preoperative coronary revascularization will be progressively more difficult to demonstrate.[10]

Several variables predictive of outcome following repair of ruptured AAA have been identified, although the findings vary from series to series. Hemodynamic instability, evidenced by hypotension, hypovolemic shock, and frank cardiac arrest, correlates with a poor outcome. Preoperative renal insufficiency is also associated with early death. Advanced age, preexisting CAD, the presence and number of comorbid conditions, low or high admission hematocrit, large transfusion requirements, free intraperitoneal rupture, suprarenal clamp placement, prolonged aortic cross-clamp time, and female gender are also associated with high perioperative mortality rates. Significant increases in operative mortality follow the development of cardiopulmonary, renal, and neurologic complications.[12–16]

Table 36–2.   Operative Mortality Rates for Repair of Intact AAA

Author	Year	Dates	n	Died	Mortality Rate, %
Golden[8]	1990	1973–89	500	8	1.6
AbuRahma[24]	1991	1983–87	332	12	3.6
Olsen[25]	1991	1979–88	287	14	4.8
Hannan[26]	1992	1982–86	1397	100	7.2
Magee[27]	1992	1988–89	134	11	8.2
Calligaro[28]	1993	1986–92	181	3	1.7
Ernst[5]	1993	1980–89	710	25	3.5
Hallett[29]	1993	1971–87	130	6	4.6
Stonebridge[30]	1993	1980–89	311	12	3.8
Akkersdijk[21]	1994	1990	1289	88	6.8
Johnston[31]	1994	1986	680	37	5.4
Katz, DJ[13]	1994	1980–90	8185	614	7.5
Feinglass[32]	1995	1985–87	280	8	2.9
DAV PTF*[32]	1995	1990–93	5799	302	5.2
O'Hara[22]	1995	1984–93	731	22	3.0
Totals			20,946	1262	6.0

* Department of Veterans Affairs Patient Treatment File.

Table 36–3.   Operative Mortality Rates for Repair of Ruptured AAA

Author	Year	Dates	n	Died	Mortality Rate, %
Chang[33]	1990	1983–89	63	16	25
Ouriel[34]	1990	1979–88	243	133	55
Sullivan[35]	1990	1978–89	69	24	35
AbuRahma[24]	1991	1983–87	73	45	62
Harris[12]	1991	1980–89	113	72	64
Johansen[36]	1991	1980–89	180	124	69
Gloviczki[37]	1992	1980–89	214	97	45
Hannan[26]	1992	1982–86	372	223	60
Magee[27]	1992	1988–89	77	27	35
Bauer[14]	1993	1979–91	340	92	29
Bengtsson[38]	1993	1971–86	61	35	57
D'Angelo[39]	1993	1966–78	170	91	54
Ernst[5]	1993	1980–89	91	41	45
McCready[40]	1993	1980–89	208	103	50
Stonebridge[20]	1993	1980–89	227	61	27
Akkersdijk[21]	1994	1990	709	309	44
Johnston[16]	1994	1986	147	74	50
Katz[13]	1994	1980–90	1829	911	50
Katz[18]	1994	1984–92	99	57	57
Tromp Meesters[23]	1994	1985–92	110	60	55
Browning[15]	1995	NS	49	22	45
O'Hara[22]	1995	1984–93	47	13	28
Totals			5491	2630	48

Abbreviation: NS, not stated.

A number of technical factors may also affect the outcome of AAA repair. An inflammatory aneurysm is more difficult to expose and control, and injury to nearby structures (eg, duodenum, renal vessels, ureter) may occur. Such injuries are associated with a poorer outcome, but better results have been reported when a retroperitoneal approach was utilized. Accessory renal arteries originating from or near the aneurysm that require reimplantation prolong the procedure and may increase morbidity and mortality. This is also true when a horseshoe kidney is present. Similarly, complexity and risk increase when coexistent renal or mesenteric artery stenoses are treated at the time of aortic reconstruction.

Injuries to unsuspected circum- or retroaortic left renal veins, double or left-sided inferior vena cavae, and other venous anomalies cause troublesome bleeding that may be very difficult to control. Such variants may be undetectable if a retroperitoneal hematoma from a ruptured AAA obscures anatomic landmarks.

The results of reconstruction for pararenal AAAs tend to be slightly worse than those for aneurysms confined to the infrarenal aorta.[17] Two additional problems, spontaneous aortoenteric fistula and aortocaval fistula, are difficult to treat, and patients who survive the initial operation face high morbidity and mortality rates.

Katz and Kohl noted that little can be done to change the acute and chronic medical conditions of patients once they present with ruptured AAA (*patient-determined* factors), but that factors such as technical errors (inadvertent arterial and venous injuries and anastomotic failures) associated with higher operative morbidity and mortality rates were *surgeon determined* and may be preventable.[18] Others have also noted poorer survival rates among patients treated in hospitals caring for fewer than five ruptured AAAs annually and among patients treated by inexperienced surgeons.[19-21] The negative correlation of low hospital volume and surgeon inexperience with outcome suggests that management of AAA may be improved by the regionalization of care to those most experienced in treating patients with vascular diseases.

In addition to prolonging the length of the hospital stay and increasing costs, postoperative complications are associated with early death. Postoperative renal failure, CHF or myocardial infarction, respiratory failure requiring prolonged mechanical ventilation, and colonic ischemia are ominous. This is especially true following repair of ruptured AAA because sepsis and multisystem organ failure are commonly lethal.

LATE MORTALITY

Late survival data are summarized in Table 36–4. One- and 5-year survival rates of 90% and 70%, respectively, have been reported following elective AAA repair. The 5-year survival rate after ruptured AAA repair approximates 50%. There is controversy regarding whether patients undergoing successful AAA repair experience the same life expectancy as an age-matched patient population without AAAs. No author has reported longer survival following repair, and the majority of reports suggest shorter survival.

Advanced age is negatively associated with late survival following AAA repair. Electrocardiographic evidence of left ventricular hypertrophy or of an old myocardial infarction also predict lower late survival, as do chronic obstructive pulmonary disease, cerebrovascular disease, and renal insufficiency.

Johnston and O'Hara and their colleagues have reported late survival data.[16,22] Death from cardiovascular disease, specifically from myocardial infarction, was most common, and cardiovascular disease and cancer together accounted for more than 60% of all late deaths. Pulmonary and renal diseases and rupture of thoracic aortic aneurysms were less common but notable causes of late mortality. In summary, following AAA repair, mean survival rates approximating 90% at 1 year and 60% at 5 years may be anticipated following hospital discharge.

MORBIDITY

Systemic, nonvascular complications of AAA repair predominate over vascular complications, and cardiopulmonary complications are the most frequent. However, late vascular complications contribute to the cumulative mortality related to the surgical management of AAA.[5] Late graft infection, aortoenteric fistula, graft occlusion, and anastomotic pseudoaneurysms typically develop 3 to 5 years after aortic reconstruction, and their presence and treatment are associated with increased morbidity and mortality. Aortoenteric fistula and late graft infection occur in about 1% and 2% of patients, respectively. Anastomotic pseudoaneurysms are more common, being observed in 3 to 6% of AAA repairs requiring aortofemoral reconstructions. The collective late mortality rate from these factors approximates 2% and, when added to an early mortality rate of 4 to 6%, results in a cumulative mortality rate of elective AAA repair of about 6 to 8%.

Cardiac complications follow 10 to 20% of operations, depending on the patient population and on how complications are defined and reported. Perioperative myocardial infarction may be identified in 3 to 6%, and CHF in up to 10% of patients. Approximately 10% of patients develop new arrhythmias or arrhythmias requiring treatment.

Mild pulmonary insufficiency frequently develops after major abdominal operations, but respiratory failure requiring reintubation or prolonged mechanical ventilation may be anticipated in 5 to 8% of patients following aortic reconstruction. Marginal pulmonary

Table 36–4.   Late Survival After AAA repair

Author	Year	Dates	n	1 Year	5 Year
		Intact Aneurysms			
Reigel[41]	1987	1980–85	485	95	74
Vohra[42]	1990	1981–86	235	NS	69
Olsen[25]	1991	1979–88	287	NS	80
Hallett[29]	1993	1971–87	130	NS	61
Stonebridge*[20]	1993	1980–89	311	97	75
Johnston[31]	1994	1986	680	91	68
Feinglass[32]	1995	1985–87	280	89	64
		Ruptured Aneurysms			
Olsen[25]	1991	1979–88	218	NS	48
Stonebridge*[20]	1993	1980–89	227	95	68
Johnston[16]	1994	1986	147	42	26
		Rupture Not Indicated/Combined			
Crawford[43]	1981	1955–80	860	90	63
Hollier[44]	1984	1970–75	1066	91	68
Johanson[36]	1990	1981–85	134	90	65
Ernst[5]	1993	1980–89	801	87	64
O'Hara[22]	1995	1984–93	114	NS	41

*Includes only patients who survived initial hospitalization.
Abbreviation: NS, not stated.
Source: Reprinted by permission of *The New England Journal of Medicine*, Ernst CB, Volume 328, page 1171, 1993.
Copyright 1993. Massachesetts Medical Society. All rights reserved.

function, with forced vital capacity (FVC) and forced expiratory volume in 1 second (FEV_1) of less than 50% of the predicted value, are harbingers of postoperative pulmonary complications. Renal dysfunction marked by an increase in blood urea nitrogen or serum creatinine occurs in about 5% of patients, but frank acute renal failure requiring hemodialysis is rare. The most important clinical marker predicting perioperative renal dysfunction (serum creatinine increase 50% above the baseline value) is preexisting parenchymal disease. Prolonged intestinal ileus is observed among approximately 10% of patients, but clinically significant ischemic colitis is much less frequent, developing in 2% of patients. Ischemic central nervous system events occur in less than 1% of patients. Penile erectile dysfunction and retrograde ejaculation may affect one-third or more of men, although this is difficult to document. The cumulative incidence of complications following elective aortic reconstruction for AAA may be 25 to 45%. Unfortunately, many of the complication predictors cannot be modified (eg, gender, preoperative hemodynamic instability, preoperative creatinine level) or anticipated (eg, technical errors, intraoperative fluid requirements, prolonged aortic clamp time). Contemporary data regarding the incidence of both vascular and nonvascular complications after repair of ruptured AAA indicate at least a twofold increase compared to elective AAA repair; for some factors the increase approaches fivefold. As noted above, operative mortality is 8- to 10-fold greater than associated with elective aneurysm repair. Postoperative bleeding is seen following approximately 15% of operations. Limb ischemia and distal embolization are observed in about 10% of patients. Single-system and multisystem organ dysfunction often complicate ruptured AAA operations, and multisystem organ failure strongly correlates with mortality.[23]

As with intact aneurysms, cardiac morbidity following repair of ruptured AAA is frequent, occurring in nearly half of patients. Prolonged mechanical ventilation is required in about 25% of patients. Renal dysfunction is frequent, and hemodialysis is neded in 10 to 15% of survivors. Varying degrees of ischemic colitis may be identified in up to 50% of patients, and associated mortality exceeds 50% in the severest cases. Stroke and paraplegia are distinctly rare complications following elective AAA repair but develop in nearly 5% of patients with ruptured AAA.

SUMMARY

Morbidity and mortality rates following elective repair of intact abdominal aortic aneurysms are decreasing, but the frequency of death and complications after ruptured AAA remains high. Although certain factors are known to increase the operative risk, only patients known to have short life expectancies for other reasons should be denied elective repair because acceptable 1- and 5-year survival rates may be anticipated following successful aortic reconstruction. Cardiac disease continues to be the most common source of morbidity, as well as early and late mortality. Advanced age, as well as underlying renal and pulmonary diseases, are also important factors.

REFERENCES

1. Szilagyi DE, Smith RF, DeRusso FJ, Elliott JP, Sherrin FW. Contribution of abdominal aortic aneurysmectomy to prolongation of life. *Ann Surg* 1966;164:678–699.
2. Johnston KW, Rutherford RB, Tilson MD, Shah DM, Hollier LH, Stanley JC. Suggested standards for reporting on arterial aneurysms. *J Vasc Surg* 1991;13:444–450.
3. Estes JE Jr. Abdominal aortic aneurysm: a study of one hundred and two cases. *Circulation* 1950;2:258–264.
4. Perko MJ, Schroeder TV, Olsen PS, Jensen LP, Lorentzen JE. Natural history of abdominal aortic aneurysm: a survey of 63 patients treated nonoperatively. *Ann Vasc Surg* 1993;7:113–116.
5. Ernst CB. Abdominal aortic aneurysm. *N Engl J Med* 1993;328:1167–1172.
6. Hollier LH, Taylor LM, Ochsner J. Recommended indications for operative treatment of abdominal aortic aneurysms. *J Vasc Surg* 1992;15:1046–1056.
7. Hertzer NR. Fatal myocardial infarction following abdominal aortic aneurysm resection. *Ann Surg* 1980;192:667–673.
8. Golden MA, Whittemore AD, Donaldson MC, Mannick JA. Selective evaluation and management of coronary artery disease in patients undergoing repair of abdominal aortic aneurysms: a 16-year experience. *Ann Surg* 1990;212:415–419.
9. Hertzer NR, Beven EG, Young JR, et al. Coronary artery disease in peripheral vascular patients: a classification of 1,000 coronary angiograms and results of surgical management. *Ann Surg* 1984;199:223–233.
10. Mason JJ, Owens DK, Harris RA, Cooke JP, Hlatky MA. The role of coronary angiography and coronary revascularization before noncardiac vascular surgery. *JAMA* 1995;273:1919–1925.
11. Seegar JM, Rosenthal GR, Self SB, Flynn TC, Limacher MC, Harward TRS. Does routine stress-thallium cardiac scanning reduce postoperative cardiac complications? *Ann Surg* 1994;219:654–663.
12. Harris LM, Faggioli GL, Fiedler R, Curl GR, Ricotta JJ. Ruptured abdominal aortic aneurysm: factors affecting mortality rates. *J Vasc Surg* 1991;14:812–820.
13. Katz DJ, Stanley JC, Zelenock GB. Operative mortality rates for intact and ruptured abdominal aortic aneurysms in Michigan: an eleven-year statewide experience. *J Vasc Surg* 1994;19:804–817.
14. Bauer EP, Redaelli C, von Segesser LK, Turina MI. Ruptured abdominal aortic aneurysms: predictors for early complications and death. *Surgery* 1993;114:31–35.
15. Browning NG, Long MA, Barry R, Nel CJC, Schall R, Monk E. Ruptured abdominal aortic aneurysms—prognostic indicators and complications affecting mortality. *South Afr J Surg* 1995;33:21–25.
16. Johnston KW and the Canadian Society for Vascular Surgery Aneurysm Study Group. Ruptured abdominal aortic aneurysm: six-year follow-up results of a multicenter prospective study. *J Vasc Surg* 1994;19:888–900.
17. Nypaver TJ, Shepard AD, Reddy DJ, Elliott JP, Smith RF, Ernst CB. Repair of pararenal abdominal aortic aneurysms: an analysis of operative management. *Arch Surg* 1993;128:803–813.
18. Katz SG, Kohl RD. Ruptured abdominal aortic aneurysms: A community experience. *Arch Surg* 1994;129:285–290.
19. Veith FJ, Goldsmith J, Leather RP, Hannen EL. The need for quality assurance in vascular surgery. *J Vasc Surg* 1991;13:523–526.
20. Stonebridge PA, Callam MJ, Bradley AW, Murie JA, Jenkins AML, Ruckley CV. Comparison of long-term survival after successful repair of ruptured and non-ruptured abdominal aortic aneurysm. *Br J Surg* 1993;80:525–586.
21. Akkersdijk GJM, van der Graaf Y, van Bockel JH, de Vries AC, Eikelboom BC. Mortality rates associated with operative treatment of infrarenal abdominal aortic aneurysm in The Netherlands. *Br J Surg* 1994;81:706–709.
22. O'Hara PJ, Hertzer NR, Krajewski LP, Tan M, Xiong X, Beven EG. Ten-year experience with abdominal aortic aneurysm repair in octogenarians: early results and late outcome. *J Vasc Surg* 1995;21:830–838.
23. Tromp Meesters RC, van der Graaf Y, Vos A, Eikelboom BC. Ruptured aortic aneurysm: early postoperative prediction of mortality using an organ failure score. *Br J Surg* 1994;81:512–516.
24. AbuRahma AF, Robinson PA, Boland JP, et al. Elective resection of 332 abdominal aortic aneurysms in a southern West Virginia community during a recent 5-year period. *Surgery* 1991;102:244–251.
25. Olsen PS, Schroeder T, Agerskov K, et al. Surgery for abdominal aortic aneurysms: a survey of 656 patients. *J Cardiovasc Surg* 1991;32:636–642.
26. Hannan EL, Kilburn H, O'Donnell JF, et al. A longitudinal analysis of the relationship between in-hospital mortality in New York State and the volume of abdominal aortic aneurysm surgeries performed. *Health Serv Res* 1992;27:517–542.
27. Magee TR, Scott DJ, Dunkley A, et al. Quality of life following surgery for abdominal aortic aneurysm. *Br J Surg* 1992;79:1014–1016.
28. Calligaro KD, Azuring DJ, Dougherty MJ, et al. Pulmonary risk factors of elective abdominal aortic surgery. *J Vasc Surg* 1993;18:914–921.
29. Hallett JW, Naessens JM, Ballard DJ. Early and late outcome of surgical repair for small abdominal aortic aneurysms: a population-based analysis. *J Vasc Surg* 1993;18:684–691.
30. Stonebridge PA, Callam, MJ, Bradley AW, Murie JA, Jenkins AML, Ruckley CV. Comparison of long-term survival after successful repair of ruptured and nonruptured abdominal aortic aneurysm. *Br J Surg* 1993;80:585–586.
31. Johnston KW and the Canadian Society for Vascular Surgery Aneurysm Study Group. Nonruptured abdominal aortic aneurysm: six-year follow-up from the multicenter prospective Canadian aneurysm study. *J Vasc Surg* 1994;20:163–170.
32. Feinglass J, Cowper D, Dunlop D, Slavensky R, Martin GJ, Pearce WH. Late survival risk factors for abdominal aortic aneurysm repair: experience from fourteen Department of Veterans Affairs hospitals. *Surgery* 1995;118:16–24.
33. Chang BB, Shah DM, Pary PSK, Kaufman JL, Leather RP. Can the retroperitoneal approach be used for ruptured abdominal aortic aneurysm? *J Vasc Surg* 1990;11:326–330.

34. Ouriel K, Geary K, Green RM, Fiore W, Geary JE, De-Weese JA. Factors determining survival after ruptured abdominal aortic aneurysm: the hospital, the surgeon, and the patient. *J Vasc Surg* 1990;11:493–496.

35. Sullivan CA, Roher MJ, Cutler BS. Clinical management of the symptomatic but unruptured abdominal aortic aneurysm. *J Vasc Surg* 1990;11:799–803.

36. Johansen K, Kohler TR, Nicholls SC, Zieler RE, Clowes AW, Kazmers A. Ruptured abdominal aortic aneurysm: the Harborview experience. *J Vasc Surg* 1991;13:240–247.

37. Gloviczki P, Pairolero PC, Mucha P Jr, et al. Ruptured abdominal aortic aneurysms: repair should not be denied. *J Vasc Surg* 1992;15:851–859.

38. Benggtsson H, Berqvist D. Ruptured abdominal aortic aneurysm: a population-based study. *J Vasc Surg* 1993;18:74–80.

39. D'Angelo MD, Vaghi M, Mattassi R, Bisetti P, Tacconi A. Changing trends in the outcome of urgent aneurysms surgery. *J Cardiovasc Surg* 1993;34:237–239.

40. McCready RA, Siderys H, Pittman JN, et al. Ruptured abdominal aortic aneurysm in a private hospital: a decade's experience (1980–1989). *Ann Vasc Surg* 1993;7:225–228.

41. Reigel MM, Hollier LH, Kazmier FJ, et al. Late survival in abdominal aortic aneurysm patients: the role of selective myocardial revascularization on the basis of clinical symptoms. *J Vasc Surg* 1987;5:222–527.

42. Vohra R, Reid D, Groome J, Abdool-Carrim AT, Pollock JG. Long-term survival in patients undergoing resection of abdominal aortic aneurysm. *Ann Surg* 1990;4:460–465.

43. Crawford ES, Saleh SA, Babb JW III, Glaeser DH, Vaccaro PS, Silvers A. Infrarenal abdominal oartic aneurysm: factors influencing survival after operation performed over a 25-year period. *Ann Surg* 1981;193:699–709.

44. Hollier LH, Plate G, O'Brien PC, et al. Late survival after abdominal aortic aneurysm repair: influence of coronary artery disease. *J Vasc Surg* 1984;1:290–299.

37

Aortic Dissection: Clinical Presentation, Medical Management, and Indications for Surgical Intervention

G. Melville Williams, M.D.

Aortic dissection is caused by multiple factors, some known and some still unknown. Its treatment varies according to location and urgency. It may result in either aneurysmal expansion and rupture or aortic occlusion. These variations, combined with the potential for sudden demise, render patients with this condition some of the most interesting and challenging in all of medicine and surgery. The author hopes to be forgiven for expressing many of his personal observations in methods for establishing the diagnosis and management of these patients.

CLASSIFICATION OF DISSECTING ANEURYSMS

There are currently two schemes for classifying dissecting aneurysms, the DeBakey and the Stanford (Table 37–1). DeBakey divided dissecting aneurysms into three types. Type I begins in the ascending aorta and extends through the arch, thoracic, and abdominal aortas. Type II begins in the ascending aorta and is limited to it. Type III begins in the descending thoracic aorta and either stops there (IIIa) or extends into the abdominal aorta (IIIb).

When more experience was gained in the management of dissecting aneurysms, it became apparent that patients with type I or type II aneurysms were at severe risk of extension of the dissection into the coronary ves-

sels, of disruption of the aortic valve, or of rupture into the pericardium. Therefore, these two types were classified as type A by the group at Stanford because they were treated with emergency surgery. By contrast, aneurysms originating in the descending thoracic aorta or abdominal aorta proved to be more benign, frequently stabilizing in patients whose blood pressure was controlled. The distinctions between types A and B are so obvious that they are used by many surgeons and cardiologists. Of course, this is confusing because others might interpret A and B as subdivision types of DeBakey type III aneurysms. While each classification has its own merits, the author prefers the more comprehensive classification proposed by DeBakey.

ETIOLOGY

Having sent multiple specimens of aorta to pathologists for their review, I have become convinced that there is no uniform histopathology associated with aortic dissection. I have rarely, if ever, received a pathology report stating that the patient has classical medial cystic necrosis.[1] In my experience, dissections of the aorta appear to be caused by one of two processes: an inherited connective tissue deficit or hypertension associated with atherosclerosis.

In patients with Marfan syndrome and Ehlers-Danlos syndrome type IV with dissections, dissection occurs in the context of aneurysmal dilatation of the involved artery. In Marfan syndrome, sufficient information has accumulated to suggest that dilation of the aortic root to a diameter of 5 cm creates the risk of dissection, and one measuring 6 cm should be repaired. My experience with Ehlers-Danlos syndrome involves one patient who had large arteries throughout her body that devel-

Table 37–1. Classification of Dissecting Aneurysms

Stanford	A	B
DeBakey	I, II	IIIa
		IIIb

DIAMETER AND COMPLICATIONS

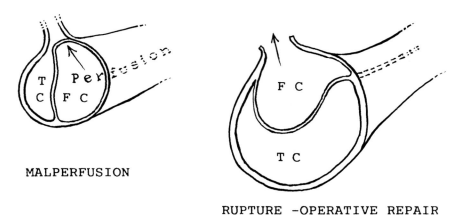

MALPERFUSION

RUPTURE –OPERATIVE REPAIR

Figure 37–1. Diagrammatic illustration demonstrating that dissections occurring in normal-sized aortas generally crowd branches with the dissecting membrane, while those occurring in dilated aortas tend to rupture. It is important to consider visceral, renal, or limb ischemia when dissections occur in a normal-sized aorta.

oped both fusiform and dissecting aneurysms. Two other patients with this condition simply had multiple ruptures from fusiform aneurysms.

We now know that Marfan syndrome is caused by defects in the gene coding for fibrillin, a protein that acts as a glue holding together the various layers of the aorta.[2] There are many varieties of gene defects that are probably responsible for the varying presentation of individuals with Marfan syndrome. For example, some of these patients have minimal aortic disease. Others may have simple fusiform infrarenal abdominal aortic aneurysms at the age of 60 or older, and still others develop acute dilatation and dissection of the entire aorta in childhood.

Among patients, who have a hypertensive atherosclerotic etiology, dissections occur in aortas of relatively normal diameter and develop in a natural endarterectomy plane. In the event of a reentry of considerable size, the condition may well stabilize. However, others may develop malperfusion caused by dissection in important vessels of the arch, viscera, kidneys, or lower extremities. The aorta may expand over time, principally in the superior descending thoracic aorta.

The lesson I have learned is that when dissection begins in an enlarged artery, watch for rupture; when it begins in a normal-sized or minimally enlarged aorta, watch for malperfusion (Fig. 37–1).

CLINICAL PRESENTATION

Type I and Type II Dissections

There is no set of clinical symptoms or physical findings absolutely diagnostic of aortic dissection (Table 37–2). Patients presenting with acute type I or type II

Table 37–2. Symptoms of Aortic Dissection

	Types I and II	Type III
Location	Substernal, neck, intrascapular	Interscapular, left upper quadrant, epigastrium
Intensity	Mild → Severe, tearing	Mild → severe, constant

dissections usually have severe pain that mimics myocardial infarction. The pain is retrosternal and may radiate to the neck or back. A normal electrocardiogram and cardiac enzymes are an indication to proceed to an emergent computed tomography (CT) scan. If transesophageal echocardiography (TEE) is available, it is also diagnostic. The magnetic resonance imaging (MRI) scan may provides more information regarding the extent of the dissection in the aortic arch but takes more time. A "spiral" CT scan taken after infusion of a contrast bolus can be done in 15 minutes and is the procedure of choice in the unstable or severely symptomatic patient.

At the other end of the spectrum are individuals who complain initially of mild to moderate substernal or upper chest discomfort followed hours later by severe substernal pain and prostration. This type of presentation is very upsetting to the patient and the family, for they believe that somehow the physician should have recognized impending doom at the initial presentation. Inasmuch as the only diagnostic procedures are cumbersome and expensive, I find it very easy to forgive the primary care physician under these circumstances. However, any type of chest discomfort in a patient with the features of Marfan syndrome should be taken very seriously (Table 37–3).

Table 37–3. Symptoms of Marfan Syndrome

Eyes:	dislocation of lens
Back:	scoliosis
Extremities:	long fingers
	long narrow foot
Heart:	aortic regurgitation
	mitral prolapse
	mitral regurgitation
Family history	

Table 37–4. Diagnosis of Aortic Dissection

ECG	If normal, think dissection
X-ray	Chest, kidney, ureters, bladder a waste of time
	CT scan with IV contrast
	Tee only to localize origin of tear
	MRI when in doubt

Table 37–5. Treatment of Aortic Dissection

Medical	Labetalol, lorazepam, nitroprusside
Type I, II	Postoperative monitoring
Type III	ICU monitoring

Type III Dissections

Patients with dissections of the descending thoracic aorta also have varying symptoms. The majority of them complain of severe interscapular back pain described as constant and unrelieved by changes in position. Others may present with left upper quadrant and even epigastric pain. Malperfusion may cause lower extremity pain. However, a minority of patients experience so few symptoms that their type III dissection is found incidentally. Acute pain different from any ever experienced by the patient should raise the suspicion of aortic dissection.

As with proximal dissections, pain may ease and the second episode of pain, occurring hours to days later, brings the patient to medical attention. It is likely that the second episode represents extension of the dissection. Pain is a valuable means of assessing the stability of the dissection, and it should cease with blood pressure control. Continued episodes of pain with systemic pressures less than 130 mm Hg are just as serious as a decline in the hematocrit.

In summary, the definitive diagnosis of aortic dissection is established by means of CT or MRI scans and/or TEE (Table 37–4). Aortography, the former gold standard should be avoided in the acute phase to spare the kidneys the large dose of contrast.

THERAPY (Table V)

Patients with types I and II dissections deserve emergency operation (Table 37–5). At operation, it is essential to determine whether the aortic valve can be preserved and made competent by suspending the aortic intima and the valve annulus or whether a composite Dacron graft mechanical valve with coronary implantation should be carried out. In the young patient, a biological valve should also be considered. Judgment is also needed to repair the distal aspect of the dissection. An inadequate repair of the distal aorta almost invariably leads to expansion in the arch, requiring a very difficult repeat operation. In the long run, it is probably better to open the aorta along the arch inferiorly, employing cold circulatory arrest. This enables the surgeon to deal with the dissection membrane,

removing or tacking it down in the arch. European cardiac surgeons have employed "glue" to facilitate membrane attachment and suture retention, and this appears to have distinct advantages.[3] Opening the arch inferiorly also allows the surgeon to determine whether to employ the "elephant trunk" technique, which basically replaces the arch and provides a conduit through a large or normal-sized descending thoracic aorta for a staged repair in individuals with type I aortic dissections.

Treatment of patients with dissections of the descending thoracic aorta remains somewhat controversial. Miller and his associates at Stanford still believe in the role of urgent surgical repair and have pointed out that operative survival of 87% is possible.[4] Svensson et al reported a 95% survival rate in patients operated on after 1984.[5] Older age, rupture, renal visceral ischemia and/or infarction, and the intensity of pain were the only independent determinants of mortality in these studies.

Wheat deserves much credit for advocating medical management with antihypertensive medications, including beta-adrenergic blocking agents.[6] In 1980, he reported on the outcome of 17 patients designated to be treated by antihypertensive medications. In this group, three patients required surgery for uncontrollable symptoms, hemorrhage, or expansion, and two of them died. Thirteen of the remaining 14 treated medically survived, and on follow-up their dissections remain stable.

Glower et al[7] attempted to assess the role of medical versus surgical therapy, combining the experience at Duke with that at Stanford. Their results in managing 136 patients illustrate vividly the complexity of the patient population and therapy for patients with dissections of the descending thoracic aorta. Among 89 patients with *acute* dissections, the 30-day mortality was 18% for those managed medically and 33% for those managed surgically. However, it is evident that patients with rupture and those with significant malperfusion problems undergo surgery urgently, thereby biasing the outcome. In fact, 30 of the 136 patients presented with operative indications, and only 22 patients were judged to be operative candidates. Of these, 14 survived for 30 days. However, two of the survivors died of rupture at 5 and 14 months, and four were subjected to reoperation, leaving eight alive and well long-term. Among the 106 remaining patients, 50 were judged to have medical problems, making them high-risk candidates for surgery. Medical therapy failed in 10 of these patients, mandating desperate surgery. An additional 12 of the 40 medically treated patients died. Thus, in the mixed group of patients with acute and chronic type III dissections, the intention to treat medically because of heart, lung, or kidney disease failed in 22 of 50 patients (44%). The remaining core group of 56 patients could be treated either way, having contraindications for neither medical nor surgical therapy. Only 30 of these patients had acute dissections, leaving very few patients for statistical analysis. Three of 19 patients died after receiving medical therapy, whereas 1 of 11 patients died following surgery. In our experience, two-thirds of the patients are at high risk and have no specific indications for surgery. The remainder are split between those requiring surgery to save life or limb and younger patients with neither immediate indications nor contraindications to surgery (Fig. 37–2). Because there is no clear-cut survival advantage with surgery and because the hospital stay is nearly twice as long for surgical as for medical patients, we also advocate initial medical management.

In addition to a longer hospital stay, the repair of acute extensive dissections with aneurysms runs the risk of paraplegia secondary to spinal cord ischemia. The frequency was reported to be 5% in the Duke/Stanford experience, which basically limited repairs to the descending thoracic aorta. Crawford's group, operating on more extensive dissections, showed clearly that the frequency of paraplegia varied from 5 to 36%, depending on the extent of the thoracoabdominal aorta replaced.[5] Severe symptoms of aneurysm often secondary to malperfusion problems, preoperative hypertension, aneurysm extent, and aortic cross-clamp time were all independent determinants of the risk of paraplegia.

Thus, the surgeon managing patients with acute dissections of the descending thoracic aorta is forced to exercise judgment in the care of these patients. We, as well as most others, now treat patients with acute type III dissections with antihypertensive medication, reserving surgery for complications. It is my impression that with better antihypertensive agents, the proportion of patients requiring surgery for expansion is diminishing and intervention is reserved mainly for those with malperfusion of an extremity or a visceral or renal artery.

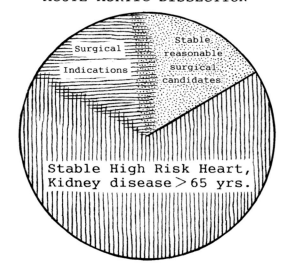

CONDITION AT PRESENTATION TYPE III
ACUTE AORTIC DISSECTION

Surgical Indications

Stable reasonable surgical candidates

Stable High Risk Heart, Kidney disease > 65 yrs.

Figure 37–2. Schematic diagram illustrating the mix of patients presenting with acute aortic dissection. The majority of patients are referred to our institution with a known dissection and are poor candidates for operative intervention because of significant heart, kidney, or pulmonary disease or because of advanced age. We hope that all of these patients can be satisfactorily managed medically, but some of them present with or develop clear-cut indications for surgery. The surgical outcome depends entirely on whether the surgeons are willing to assume the risk of operating on desperately ill patients. A relatively small proportion of patients are young and have neither indications nor contraindications for medical or surgical management. We still advocate medical management, reserving surgery for specific indications.

MALPERFUSION SYNDROMES

Dissections progress down the descending thoracic aorta, causing ischemic symptoms by two mechanisms (Fig. 37–3): (1) when there are inadequate reentry sites in the abdominal aorta and the true lumen becomes compressed and (2) when the dissection extends into the lumen of a vessel, creating an obstructing intimal flap. In general, the dissection membrane splits the abdominal aorta so that the left kidney is most often supplied by the false or thinner channel and the celiac axis, superior mesenteric artery, and right renal artery continue to originate from the true lumen. At times, the dissection membrane crosses the origins of the celiac axis and superior mesenteric artery, creating a partial occlusion. In reality, these occlusions can be thought of as incomplete endarterectomies. If the dissection has extended to the aortic bifurcation, a similar problem may exist in either common iliac or at the common iliac bifurcation, resulting in lower limb ischemia. Patients may present with distal aortic occlusion as the hematoma in the dissection channel obliterates the true lumen.

MECHANISM OF MALPERFUSION

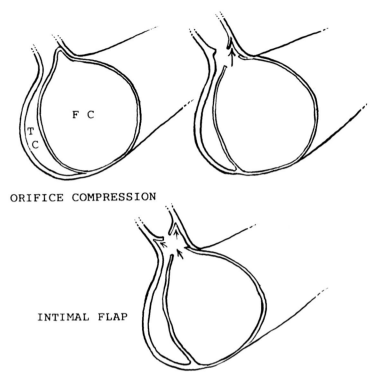

ORIFICE COMPRESSION

INTIMAL FLAP

Figure 37–3. Illustrated here are the two mechanisms producing malperfusion in patients with aortic dissections. In some patients, the lumen of an important aortic branch is compressed by the expanded intima. Decompression of the false channel will restore an important blood supply. This problem occurs frequently at the celiac axis, where on can frequently see the intimal membrane straddling the orifice on CT scan. Commonly, the intima is disrupted, resulting in a dissection of the intima of the branch itself. This may result in either acute or chronic stenosis/occlusion.

Proximal aortic surgery to repair the tear in type IIIA dissections may reduce the frequency of malperfusion problems. Theoretically, an operation designed to provide an anastomosis proximal to the tear in the intima and an anastomosis distal to the dissection, that is, to a single lumen, provides ideal management. While the proximal anastomosis can most often be carried out to a single lumen, the distal anastomosis is problematic in many patients. Teflon felt and/or tissue glue has been used to reapproximate the dissected intima to the outer wall of the aorta, enabling an end-to-end anastomosis without leakage into the false channel. However, despite the use of these adjunctive measures, leaks are very common because the dissected intima fails to retain sutures or is much smaller than the whole aorta, so that flow continues down the false channel into the renal/visceral artery segment.

There are other problems with the repair of the tear technique. In patients with type IIIb dissections, there is frequently a loss of continuity between the left renal artery and the main channel. Consequently, if flow is directed only through the main channel, the left kidney is lost. A final problem exists if there is an established reentry site lower down in the abdomen. With the proximal tear repaired, the reentry may distend and serve as the point of additional dissection. Thus this straightforward remove-the-tear approach is best restricted to the therapy of patients with type IIIa dissections.

FLOW SHEET FOR THE MANAGEMENT OF PATIENTS WITH DISTAL ACUTE AORTIC DISSECTIONS

In type I dissections, only a proportion of patients will have the false channel obliterated with the primary operation. Therefore, they should be monitored postoperatively as if they had type III dissections.

Our experience, and that of others using the selective approach, suggests that only 1 of 10 patients with type III dissections managed medically has indications for endovascular or open surgery. The goal of medical management is to reduce and sustain the blood pressure below 130/80 and to decrease the force of left ventricular ejection. To do so, all patients should be admitted to an intensive care unit where they can be monitored from minute to minute (Tables 37–5, 37–6). A large intravenous catheter should be placed together with an intra-arterial cannula to monitor blood pressure instantaneously. A catheter should also be inserted into the bladder to provide an accurate, moment-to-moment index of urine volume.

Blood pressure must be controlled immediately, and labatalol is a very effective agent. A bolus of 0.25 mg/kg is given IV, followed by a constant IV infusion of 40 to 50 mg/hr. Labetalol has some alpha-1 blocking action together with widespread beta blockade. Esmolol is indicated for immediate blood pressure control in the presence of sinus tachycardia. An infusion of nitroprus-

Table 37–6. Medical Management of Aortic Dissection

Monitoring
  Arterial catheter, Foley catheter
  Pain, pulses, urine output
  Sodium, potassium, blood urea nitrogen, creatinine, bilirubin twice daily
  ECG, chest X-ray daily, echocardiography
  CT scan at 48°, abdominal duplex scan
Medications
  Goal: blood pressure <130/80 and freedom from pain
  Beta blockers
  Nitrates → calcium channel blockers

Table 37–7. Outcomes of Therapy

1. Stable, Pain Free
   Repeat CT scan on day 7
   Discharge
2. Moderate pain, increased or decreased blood pressure
   Sustain ICU therapy
   Repeat CT scan on day 7
   Discharge
3. Decreased hemoglobin, increased pain, increased size of dissection by CT or TEE
                        or
4. Pain, decreased to 0 pulse, decreased urinary output
   Stable CT scan
   Duplex abdomen scan
   Angiography suite for repair or surgery

side should also be started and titrated down as a calcium channel blocker is added. Nicardipine or diltiazin offers good vasodilation by IV infusion. The aim is to eliminate nitroprusside and rely on longer-acting agents offering beta and calcium channel blockade. I would not use an ACE inhibitor initially because of the possibility of interfering with glomerular filtration. The patient should be sedated and kept on bed rest.

Monitoring consists of observing the patient from moment to moment, as well as hourly and daily. The existence of pain and its location should be queried at least hourly together with the presence or absence of pulses. Pulses that cannot be palpated should be judged by extremity pressures taken by Doppler. Hypotension or hypertension, the recurrence of pain, the absence of pulses, and a decline in urine volume to less than 30 mL/hr are causes for concern. Daily chest X-rays should be obtained. A CT scan should be obtained at 48 hours and compared to the admission CT scan. Cardiac function should be tested with two-dimensional echocardiography or in the cooperative patient, with transesophageal echocardiography.

There are four possible outcomes (Table 37–7). These will now be described.

The Stable Group

About half of the patients become pain free during this first 48 hours and can be discharged from the intensive care unit on oral medication. Seven days after admission reassessment is carried out, measuring parameters of liver and renal function, thoroughly evaluating the peripheral circulation, and determining the aortic diameter and perfusion by spiral CT scan. If all is well, the patient can be returned to his or her own physician with the advice of sustaining the medication and repeating the CT scan in 3 months and, if stable, at 6-month intervals for the rest of his or her life.

The Semistable Group

Another group of patients have some disquieting problem. Some residue of pain may persist. There may be a decline in hemoglobin perhaps secondary to hydration. Blood pressure may be erratic and uncontrolled, so a

switch to oral agents is not feasible. These patients should remain in the intensive care unit for another 48 hours. During this time, the goal is to stabilize them on antihypertensive medications, relying on a longer-acting beta blocker (propranolol, atenolol) and a calcium channel blocker (Procardia XL Calan SR).

The Group Experiencing Expansion

Expansion is the least likely outcome. Patients who continue to have moderate to severe pain, diminution in hemoglobin sufficient to require blood transfusions, pleural effusion, and expansion by CT scan should be operated on urgently. I would do so without an aortogram, relying on previous CT scans to localize the tear. A portable duplex scan is valuable to assess the possibility of simultaneous occlusion of major aortic branches.

The Group Experiencing Malperfusion

The loss of circulation to the kidneys, viscera, or legs prompts an urgent visit to the angiography suite. It is possible, even likely, that definitive therapy can be carried out there; if not, angiography will provide a road map for surgery.

A recent publication from Stanford reports the outcome of 22 patients treated by endovascular techniques.[8] In the case of encroachment of the main lumen, decompression of the other lumen can be carried out by fenestration. Initially, this sounded to me like radiology gymnastics, as each channel had to be catheterized and a puncture made between the two that was subsequently expanded by balloon dilatation. I could imagine an error in puncture leading to exsanguination. However, with good imaging techniques, a contrast-filled balloon placed in one of the two channels serves as a good target for a puncture and window (Fig. 37–4). Additionally, I was fearful that fresh clot might be present in the high-pressure, slow-flow lumen that could embolize distally as flow was reestablished. However, this complication did not occur in the 15 patients treated acutely.

FENESTRATION

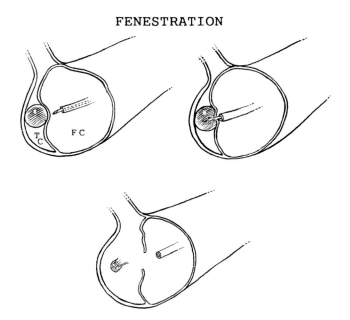

Figure 37–4.   Schematic representation of the ingenious method for producing a reliable communication between the distended false channel (FC) and the true lumen (TC) using a contrast-filled balloon.[8] Interaortic ultrasound has also been advocated by the group at Stanford to determine where the window should be made, reducing the load of contrast.

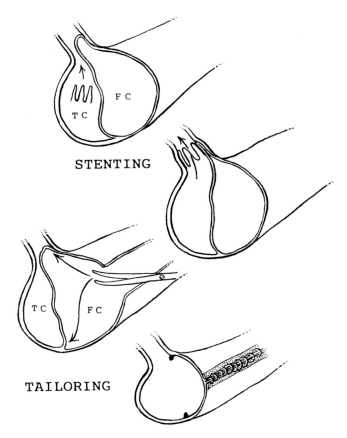

Figure 37–5.   Schematic representation of methods of restoring perfusion to important aortic branches. Stents can clearly be placed within the aortic lumen itself to compress the false channel, opening up the true channel, or to tack down the intima and sustain the patency of aortic branches. This would seem to be an ideal method for the treatment of malperfusion in patients presenting with chronic aortic dissection. In our experience, surgical removal of the dissected membrane (tailoring) has proved to be definitive treatment for significant malperfusion problems in the acute, unstable patient. The operation basically consists of completing the aortic endarterectomy.

Stent angioplasty is the logical way to treat partial occlusions caused by disrupted intima, and the authors were able to restore circulation in all vessels treated. Three patients required additional stenting. There were two deaths in this series, both in patients with visceral malperfusion. In one patient, the process had progressed too far and was irreversible. In the second patient reported in the discussion of this article, more expeditious reintervention may have avoided sigmoid colon necrosis, which ultimately led to the patient's demise several months later.

This new technique relies on the principle of creating a reentry point or window, a procedure that many surgeons previously tried and abandoned. However, the concept has been revitalized. The group at Yale have performed 14 procedures, using the retroperitoneal approach to the aorta to create a membranectomy.[9] The aorta is transected. The distal intima is reattached to the outer wall with glue or felt, and an end-to-end anastomosis is constructed to the *outer* wall of the proximal aorta. This was successful in 13 of 14 instances, and it proved durable on chronic follow-up.

I have taken an even more aggressive approach in five patients, removing all of the obstructing dissected aorta intima through a longitudinal aortotomy. In two patients using the posterior retroperitoneal approach, the aorta was "tailored" from the renal arteries to its bifurcation (Fig. 37–5). The intimal membranes causing bilateral leg ischemia were excised, and the longitudinal aortotomy was closed. Three other patients

were treated by total abdominal membranectomy, removing all of the dissected intima from diaphragm to iliacs. The long aortotomy was closed to a normal diameter. All patients survived. Three anuric patients recovered renal function, and all limbs were salvaged.

Thus, it appears that there are several good ways to address the problem of malperfusion, which vary in the degree of invasiveness. In the absence of renal failure or mesenteric ischemia, my first choice would be to restore the circulation by fenestration and stenting using endovascular techniques. This is far less traumatic than either operation. However, in the presence of oliguria, acidosis, and high lactate levels, particularly when there is considerable thrombus in the lumen with poor blood flow, it may be safer to inspect the aorta directly by operative techniques (Fig. 37–6). Additionally, in some patients it is difficult to determine the dis-

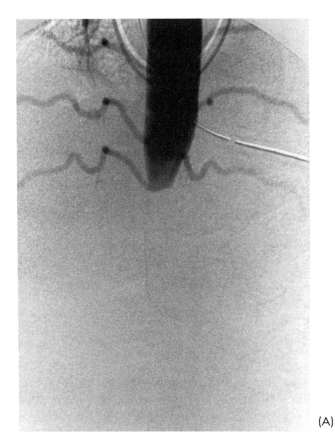

(A)

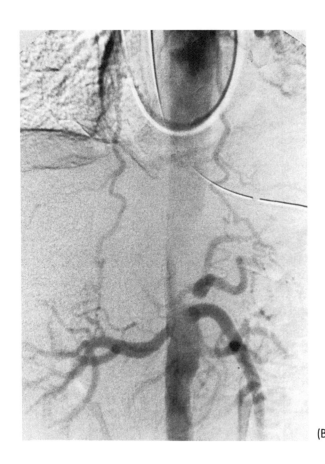

(B)

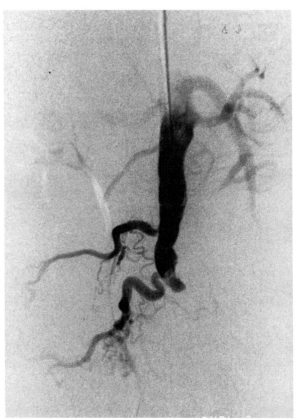

(C)

Figure 37–6. Aortogram in a patient presenting with congestive heart failure and absent femoral pulses. The aortogram was performed through the left brachial artery. (A) This illustrates a contrast-filled false channel that ends at the level of the renal arteries. The false channel supplies all of the large intercostal arteries. If this is ablated successfully with a proximal operation, paraplegia is a likely outcome. (B) Injection into a second lumen that supplies the kidney and the gut. Contrast appeared in the right renal artery after considerable delay, suggesting that this artery was supplied from a third channel. (C) The channel supplying the visceral and renal arteries also ended abruptly, as illustrated. Because the patients was gravely ill and respirator dependent at this time, and because the dissection was so complex, he was taken to the operating room for membranectomy of the renal/visceral artery segment, terminating this in an aortobifemoral bypass. His recovery was uneventful.

section. Coexisting occlusive disease may prevent retrograde access. A kidney may excrete contrast without visualizing any artery. When the questions of visceral ischemia exists, I believe that the operative approach, removing the entire dissected membrane and leaving the patient with a single lumen, is the most certain and definitive treatment. However, this procedure necessitates additional renal ischemia, places greater strain on the heart from the high position of the aortic cross-clamp, and is associated with significant blood loss. Thus, it should be reserved for the younger patient free of serious heart disease.

Aortic dissection is a complex problem that sets in motion a concatenation of often dramatic and lethal circulatory disturbances. Earlier operation in patients with Marfan syndrome and better education in blood pressure control may prevent later complications. When these occur, optimal management involves application of the best medical, radiologic, and surgical techniques, sometimes directed to aortic repair and sometimes to specific complications.

REFERENCES

1. Hirst AE, Gore I. Is cystic medionecrosis the cause of dissecting aortic aneurysm? *Am Heart J* 1976;53:915–916.

2. Dietz HC, Cutting GR, Pyeritz RE, et al. Marfan syndrome caused by a recurrent de novo missense mutation in the fibrillin gene. *Nature* 1991;352:337–339.

3. Carpentier AF. Discussion of Bachet J, Gigou F, Laurian C, et al. Four-year clinical experience with the gelatin-resorcine-formol biological glue in acute aortic dissection. *J Thorac Cardiovasc Surg* 1982;83:212–217.

4. Miller DC, Mitchell RS, Oyer PE, et al. Independent determinants of operative mortality for patients with aortic dissections. *Circulation* 1984;70(suppl 1):153.

5. Svensson LG, Crawford ES, Hess, KR, et al. Dissection of the aorta and dissecting aortic aneurysms: improving early and long-term surgical results. *Circulation* 1990;82(suppl 4):24–38.

6. Wheat MW Jr, Harris PD, Malm JR, et al. Acute dissecting aneurysms of the aorta: treatment of results in 64 patients. *J Thorac Cardiovasc Surg* 1969;58:344–351.

7. Glower DD, Fann JI, Speier RH, et al. Comparison of medical and surgical therapy for uncomplicated descending aortic dissection. *Circulation* 1990;82(suppl 4):39–46.

8. Slonim SM, Nyman U, Semba CP, et al. Aortic dissection: percutaneous management of ischemic complications with endovascular stents and balloon fenestration. *J Vasc Surg* 1996;23:241–253.

9. Elefteriades JA, Hartleroad J, Gusberg RJ, et al. Long-term experience with descending aortic dissection: the complication-specific approach. *Ann Thorac Surg* 1992;53:11–21.

38

The Role of Spinal Arteriography in the Evaluation of the Patient with a Thoracoabdominal Aortic Aneurysm

Scott J. Savader, M.D.

An anatomic description of the blood supply to the spinal cord was first recorded in the late nineteenth century by Adamkiewicz[1] and Kadyi.[2] Angiographic evaluation was not to follow until 65 years later, with numerous articles from Doppman and Di Chiro[3–5] and Lazorthes et al.[6] Although the main focus during the infancy of this technique was on diagnostic angiography and percutaneous embolization of spinal cord arteriovenous malformations, the concept of angiographically road-mapping the blood supply of the spinal cord prior to aortic surgery had also come of age.[5]

Almost 30 years later, one can still ask, "What is the role of spinal angiography in patients requiring surgery for thoracoabdominal aneurysms?" and receive a variety of answers. If one were to search the literature for an article that, by content, clarity, and scientific means, unequivocally demonstrated the value of spinal arteriography, one would very likely complete this task somewhat disappointed. That literature search would, however, clearly show that there are both proponents and opponents of presurgical spinal artery road-mapping,[7–12] in addition to those still searching for an answer to the perplexing question initially presented.

The elusiveness of the answer lies in the ethics of a randomized, double-blind study designed to address the question. Could one possibly implement a study in which patients were randomized into two groups, both of which would undergo diagnostic spinal angiography, only one of which, however, would undergo spinal cord revascularization? The stakes of such a study, namely, postoperative paraplegia or anterior spinal artery syndrome, are rather high. How many participants would have to demonstrate a neurologic deficit before the answer to the question was believed to have been found? One can surely appreciate the ethical issues that would abound in regard to such a study. Thus, this author will attempt to present the pros and cons of the issue rather than to specifically answer the question. The reader can then weigh this information and make his or her own decision.

ANATOMY

At the level of the foramen magnum, each vertebral artery gives rise to an anterior spinal ramus; these rami join in the midline to form the origin of the anterior spinal artery (ASA) (Fig. 38–1). The blood supply to the anterior two-thirds of the spinal cord is derived primarily from the ASA, which runs along the anterior median fissure of the spinal cord inferiorly to the level of the conus medullaris. The posterior one-third of the spinal cord is supplied by paired posterior spinal arteries that originate from the vertebral arteries proximal to the takeoff of the anterior spinal rami. The posterior spinal arteries, interconnected by a mesh-like network of small vessels, are fed at each intervertebral level by the posterior radiculomedullary artery arising from the radiculomedullary trunk.

Inferior to its origin, the ASA is further supplied by multiple small vessels arising directly or indirectly from the aorta. Radiculomedullary branches from the cervical portion of the vertebral arteries traverse horizontally to unite with the descending ASA. At the lower cervical level, either costocervical trunk may give rise to a relatively large radiculomedullary branch. The thyrocervical trunk very rarely contributes to the arterial supply of the cord. At the level of T-4 to T-6, the thoracic (lesser) radicular artery (TRA) arises from the corresponding intercostal artery to infuse the upper thoracic

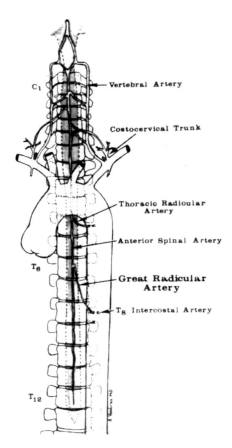

Figure 38–1. Classic arterial supply to the spinal cord. (Reprinted from Ref. 7 with permission.)

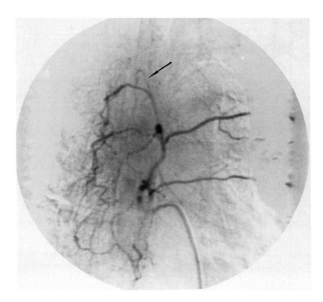

Figure 38–2. Digital subtraction angiogram obtained following injection of the left T-5 intercostal artery that demonstrates filling of the thoracic radicular artery (arrow). The vessel originates from the left T-4 intercostal artery. Note the similar appearance to the GRA. (Reprinted from Ref. 7 with permission.)

portion of the ASA (Fig. 38–1). Though not as large as the great radicular artery (GRA) or the artery of Adamkiewicz, this vessel can provide a critical collateral pathway in cases of occlusion of its lower thoracic counterpart. It can often be demonstrated angiographically if a dedicated search of the upper thoracic intercostal vessels is performed (Fig. 38–2). The lower thoracic and lumbar portions of the cord are fed by the GRA. Typically arising from the proximal 1 to 2 cm of the T-8 to L-1 intercostal vessel (left side in 80% and T-9 level most commonly), this relatively large supplying vessel has a characteristic upward course as it angles toward the midline.[7] The "downward" component that completes the classic hairpin appearance of this vessel is the ASA itself (Fig. 38–3).

At the level of lower lumbar and pelvic vessels, the internal iliac artery's posterior division gives rise to the iliolumbar artery. This vessel subsequently divides, yielding a spinal branch that anastomoses with the terminal branches of the ASA.[13,14] In addition, at each thoracic and lumbar level, the intercostal artery bifurcates into an anterior and a posterior division (Fig. 38–4). The posterior division gives rise to the radiculomedullary arteries, which subsequently divide into the anterior and posterior radiculomedullary arteries

that supply the ASA and the posterior spinal arteries, respectively. Only a few of the anterior radiculomedullary arteries actually continue to supply the cord, and these are in fact predominantly the GRA and TRA.[13,15]

TECHNIQUE

Patients requiring spinal angiography prior to resection of a thoracoabdominal aortic (TAA) aneurysm have usually had noninvasive imaging studies such as computed tomography and magnetic resonance imaging performed prior to the scheduled angiogram. Thus, a detailed multiview arteriogram of the thoracolumbar aorta is rarely needed to define the extent and size of the aneurysm. However, many surgeons still like to see the aorta in its entirety, as demonstrated angiographically. More important, this study can aid the interventionalist by road-mapping the regions from which the intercostal artery supplying the GRA might arise.

This author initially begins by placing a vascular sheath to reduce trauma during the multiple catheter changes common to this procedure. A standard digital subtraction angiogram (DSA) of the arch at a 35 to 40° left anterior oblique angle is initially performed. Filming is at three to four frames per second with a 25-cc injection for a total of 40 to 60 cc (depending on the size of the aneurysm) utilizing half-strength contrast. An anteroposterior view of the remaining thoracic and abdominal aorta including the common iliac arteries at a similar injection rate map out the entire thoracoabdominal aneurysm using less than 90 cc of contrast

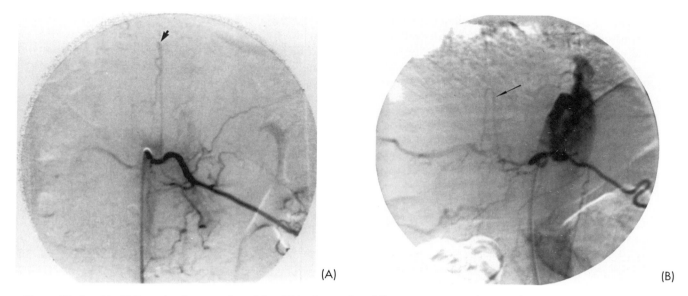

Figure 38–3. (A, B) Two classic examples of the GRA obtained in different patients. Both examples demonstrate the classic hairpin appearance of the GRA (arrow) as it unites with the anterior spinal artery.

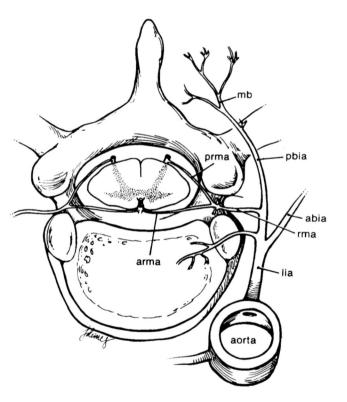

Figure 38–4. Illustration demonstrating the segmental blood supply anatomy to the spinal cord lia, left intercostal artery; abia and pbia, anterior and posterior branches of the intercostal artery, respectively; rma, radiculomedullary artery; arma and prma, anterior and posterior radiculomedullary arteries, respectively; mb, muscular branches. (Reprinted from Kadir S. *Diagnostic Angiography.* Philadelphia: WB Saunders; 1986:497, with permission.)

material. In patients with normal renal function, this leaves about 170 to 210 cc of nondiluted, nonionic contrast such as Omnipaque, 350 to 300, respectively, to search for and identify the GRA before one reaches the average patient's contrast limit.[16] Dilution of the contrast material easily yields about 300 cc of contrast material to search for the spinal artery. Patients with compromised renal function should have the total con-

trast dose limited according to the equation by Cigarroa for high-osmolality contrast media[17]:

Contrast media (mL) limit =
$$5 \text{ mL} \times \text{pt wt (kg)/serum CR (mg/100/mL)}.$$

Choosing a catheter to select the intercostals is, for the most part, a personal decision of the interventionalist. However, the anatomy of the aneurysm often dictates which catheter will ultimately prove most useful.

For example, a standard No. 5 French shepherd's crook catheter does not ordinarily work well with a large aneurysm because the angle of the limb is too acute to reach the wall of the aorta. A Sidewinder II (Cook, Bloomington, IN) might function far better in this case, but in a small aneurysm, this catheter may prove to be too clumsy. Spinal artery (Cook), Judkins JR1 (Cordis, Miami, FL), or Headhunter (Cook) catheters are also commonly employed. Selection of aortic branches other than the intercostals that might supply the ASA, such as the costocervical trunk, requires standard catheterization techniques. A radiopaque ruler taped underneath the table of the angiographic unit serves as an excellent marker of the intervertebral level during the selective catheterization portion of the procedure. This avoids the need for continuous magnification and demagnification to count vertebral bodies to orient oneself to the level of the intercostal being catheterized. Extreme care should be used to avoid burying the catheter tip in clot or atheroma lining the aortic wall.

As the catheter is manipulated, small puffs of dilute contrast material should be used to help identify the origins of the intercostal vessels. Any vessel initially seen on the road-mapping aortogram should be catheterized initially, keeping in mind that the GRA arises from the left intercostal vessel in up to 80% of cases and most commonly at the level of T-9 to T-11.[7] If intercostal vessels are not seen on the road map or cannot be selected, the posterior aortic flush method can be used. The catheter is positioned facing posteriorly, and 7 to 10 mL of nondilute contrast material is rapidly injected manually during digital subtraction imaging. The aortic contrast material is flushed away, while patent intercostal vessels opacify.

The most significant complication associated with spinal angiography is permanent neurologic injury. The majority of reports indicate that these injuries occur during inadvertent catheterization of the intercostal arteries supplying the GRA or TRA during aortography or bronchial angiography rather than during selective spinal arteriography.[18–20] Direct neurotoxicity from hyperosmolar ionic contrast media has also been implicated. The risk of a permanent cord injury following spinal angiography is about 0.2 to 1.0%.[21,22] The use of nonionic contrast media and low-volume injections, with removal of the catheter from the intercostal vessel ostia after the injection to restore normal blood flow, could help to reduce the possibility of permanent neurologic injury.

THE ARGUMENT FOR DEDICATED SPINAL ARTERY REVASCULARIZATION

This portion of the debate should begin with the understanding that few, if any, investigators would repudiate the statement that spinal cord ischemia occurring during TAA aneurysm repair is responsible for the neurologic injury that can complicate this procedure. Rather, the debate centers on whether dedicated spinal cord revascularization can result in a lower overall neurologic injury rate.

In studies in which TAA aneurysmectomy was performed in conjunction with spinal cord revascularization, the reported occurrence of a neurologic injury has ranged from 5 to 28%.[7–9] Studies have also shown that in patients undergoing TAA aneurysm repair, the incidence of spinal cord injury was 0% when the GRA, preoperatively identified on spinal angiography, was not included in the surgical field.[7,9] When the GRA was included in the surgical field and revascularized, the neurologic injury rate was 50%. However, when both the GRA and the TRA were included in the revascularization procedure, or when the GRA alone was shown on preoperative angiography to supply the thoracic portion of the spinal cord adequately, the neurologic injury rate was reduced to 5%.[9] Anatomic studies of the ASA in normal human subjects have shown that this vessel may not be continuous, but rather segmental. When continuous, this vessel may demonstrate a variable caliber at different levels.[23] Thus, the more standard surgical procedure utilizing revascularization of the GRA alone may not be adequate to reperfuse the entire spinal cord. Complete revascularization of the spinal cord with reimplantation of both the GRA and TRA might further reduce the neurologic injury rate below that seen with isolated GRA revascularization alone.

Multiple studies have clearly demonstrated that the neurologic injury rate can be reduced to 0% if the GRA and/or the TRA can be excluded from the surgical resection.[7,9] While this may seem to be an obvious declaration, the implications are important. The demonstration of the GRA or TRA arising from the margin of an aneurysm could influence the surgeon to exclude those vessels from the resection, thus reducing the morbidity and mortality rates from up to 50% to 0%.[7] In addition, in patients with smaller aneurysms, marginal indications for surgery, or high-risk spinal artery anatomy, surgery might be delayed if the overall risk of a permanent neurologic injury was believed to be significantly greater than the possibility of aneurysm rupture. Spinal cord angiography can also help to decrease the overall operative time. In patients in whom no spinal artery is identified, or in whom the GRA or TRA is not arising from the critical aortic segment, revascularization of the intercostal or lumbar arteries is unnecessary. In such cases, valuable aortic cross-clamping time is not lost by random and unnecessary intercostal revascularization, which has been shown not to decrease spinal cord complications.[11]

Williams et al originally reported that patients with a patent spinal artery (ie, GRA identified on spinal angiography) who undergo spinal cord revascularization have a greater incidence of neurologic injury (38%) than those in whom the GRA was not identified (16%) on spinal angiography.[18] This latter group was presumed to have already established adequate collateralization of the spinal cord blood supply. Thus, further support is lent to the notion that the demanding and time-consuming exercise of dedicated spinal cord revascularization may not in itself be adequate to prevent neurologic injury if the primary cord blood supply is not addressed.

THE ARGUMENT AGAINST DEDICATED SPINAL CORD REVASCULARIZATION

The overall reported incidence of paraplegia in patients undergoing TAA aneurysm repair ranges from 6.5 to 60%.[9–12,24] These statistics incorporate the range reported previously for those patients in whom dedicated spinal cord revascularization is performed, as well as present evidence of very comparable results at the lower end of the range. In light of the data on the incidence of spinal cord injury in patients who undergo preoperative spinal angiography, one would need to compare the data (nonrandomized study) to data on a similar group of patients not undergoing spinal angiography prior to TAA aneurysm repair to determine if the former group benefited significantly from dedicated spinal cord revascularization.

In a report by DeBakey et al, 527 patients with dissecting thoracic and TAA aneurysms treated surgically without dedicated spinal cord revascularization experienced an overall neurologic injury rate of 18%.[10] This figure, however, was increased to 34% when the dissection involved the descending thoracic aorta. Attempts to maintain aortic and spinal cord perfusion during the operation using various shunts and bypasses did not decrease the neurologic injury rate. Other studies have supported these statistics. In two similar studies incorporating a total of 433 patients undergoing repair of a TAA aneurysm without preoperative spinal angiography or dedicated cord revascularization, only 3.6% incurred a spinal cord injury.[12,25] In both of these studies, backbleeding intercostals in the critical aortic segment were simply ligated.

Crawford et al later reported on 605 patients, 169 of whom underwent intercostal artery revascularization without preoperative angiography to identify the actual supply to the ASA. This study failed to demonstrate a significant difference in the neurologic injury rate between patients in whom revascularization was performed versus those in whom it was not (11% overall).[11] Although it is true that preoperative spinal angiography was not performed in the revascularization group, the fact that the neurologic injury rate was also not reduced in this group lends further support to the notion that nondedicated revascularization alone does not significantly decrease the spinal cord injury rate.

ADJUNCTS TO SPINAL CORD REVASCULARIZATION

As noted, spinal cord injury in this group of patients is a complex, multifactorial issue, extending beyond the boundaries of mechanical spinal artery revascularization. There are certainly data to support spinal artery revascularization, with the most convincing arguments presented by Kieffer et al. Dedicated spinal cord revascularization with particular attention to both the GRA and the TRA may result in a spinal cord injury rate as low as 5%.[9] Opponents would probably argue that this study was relatively small compared with those by DeBakey et al and Crawford et al, which both indicated that TAA aneurysmectomy can be safely accomplished without the need for preoperative spinal angiography and time-consuming revascularization of small intercostal vessels.[10,11,25]

Because of the multifactorial nature of this most unfortunate complication, one single adjunct most likely will not significantly decrease the incidence of spinal cord injury further than the reported rates at the lower end of the range, that is, 3.6 to 5%.[7,9,12,24,25] Successful revascularization would seem to be the obvious solution. However, the complexity of the spinal cord blood supply, technical difficulties associated with the complete vascular mapping of the spinal cord, and the labor-intensive nature and technical difficulties of surgical revascularization may be such that alternative and/or multiple techniques will be required to further minimize the incidence of intraoperative spinal cord ischemia. In an attempt to further decrease the incidence of postoperative paraplegia, investigators have evaluated numerous other surgical adjuncts. The first technique is intraoperative cerebrospinal fluid (CSF) drainage to increase spinal cord perfusion by decreasing the extrinsic pressure on the cord imparted by the surrounding CSF. This technique has shown promising results in both animal and human studies.[26,27] The second technique is monitoring of spinal cord evoked potentials to evaluate the intensity of the signal sent to the lower extremities from the spinal cord during surgery. Baseline evoked potentials are obtained and then continuously monitored during the procedure. A decrease in the intensity or a change in waveforms of the evoked potentials may indicate spinal cord ischemia.[28,29] The third technique is cardiac and distal shunts to increase the perfusion pressure in the aorta below the inferior aortic cross-clamp so that cord perfusion pressure through lower collaterals is maintained above a critical level.[10,30,31]

SUMMARY

The issue of spinal cord revascularization during TAA aneurysmectomy remains controversial. The decision to perform this challenging procedure is generally based on the surgeon's training. While there are large series that suggest that TAA aneurysmectomy can be performed safely without dedicated spinal cord revascularization, there are other studies that show that this surgical adjunct is paramount in decreasing the neurologic injury rate to an even more acceptable level. For the interventionalist, the technically challenging procedure of selective spinal arteriography can be safely and effectively performed with an acceptable complication rate. Finally, regarding its value, further investigations specifically designed to evaluate the benefit-risk ratio of spinal angiography and dedicated spinal cord revascularization will surely be required to put this issue at rest.

REFERENCES

1. Adamkiewicz A II. Theil. Die Gefässe der Rucken marks oberfläche. Sitzungberiche der Kaiserlichen Akademie der Wissenchaften. *Mathematisch-Natur Wissenchaftliche classe* 1882;85:101.
2. Brody P, Doppman JL, Bisaccia LJ. An unusual complication of aortography with the pigtail catheter. *Radiology* 1974;110:711.
3. Di Chiro G, Doppman JL, Ommaya AK. Selective arteriography of arteriovenous aneurysms of the spinal cord. *Radiology* 1967;88:1065–1077.
4. Doppman JL, Di Chiro G. The arteria radicularis magna: radiographic anatomy in the adult. *Br J Radiol* 1968; 41:40–45.
5. Doppman JL, Di Chiro G, Morton DL. Angiographic identification of thoracolumbar spinal cord blood supply prior to aortic surgery. *JAMA* 1968;204:174–175.
6. Lazorthes G, Gouaze A, Zaden JO, Santini JJ, Lazorthes Y, Burdin P. Arterial vascularization of the spinal cord: recent studies of the anastomotic substitution pathways. *J Neurosurg* 1971;35:253–269.
7. Savader SJ, Williams GM, Trerotola SO, et al. Preoperative spinal artery localization and its relationship to postoperative neurologic complications. *Radiology* 1993;189:165–171.
8. Williams GM, Perler BA, Burdick JF, et al. Angiographic localization of spinal cord blood supply and its relationship to postoperative paraplegia. *J Vasc Surg* 1991;13(1):23–35.
9. Kieffer E, Thierry R, Chiras J, Godet G, Cormier E. Preoperative spinal cord arteriography in aneurysmal disease of the descending thoracic and thoracoabdominal aorta: preliminary results in 45 patients. *Ann Vasc Surg* 1989;3(1):34–46.
10. DeBakey ME, McCollum CH, Crawford ES, et al. Dissection and dissecting aneurysms of the aorta: twenty-year follow-up of five hundred twenty-seven patients treated surgically. *Surgery* 1982;92(6):1118–1134.
11. Crawford ES, Crawford JL, Hazim JS, et al. Thoracoabdominal aortic aneurysms: preoperative and intraoperative factors determining immediate and long-term results of operations in 605 patients. *J Vasc Surg* 1986;3:389–404.
12. Livesay JJ, Cooley DA, Ventemiglia RA, et al. Surgical experience in descending thoracic aneurysmectomy with and without adjuncts to avoid ischemia. *Am Thoracic Surg* 1985;39(1):37–46.
13. Doppman JL. Spinal angiography. In: Abrahms HL, ed. *Angiography. Vascular and Interventional Radiology.* 3rd ed. Boston: Little, Brown; 1983:315–335.
14. Djinjian R. Arteriography of the spinal cord. *Am J Roentgenol Rad Ther Nucl Med* 1969;107(3):461–478.
15. Hollingshead WH. The pelvis. In: Hollingshead WH, ed. *Textbook of Anatomy,* 3rd ed. New York: Harper & Row; 1974:677–747.
16. Omnipaque (Iohexal) Package Insert. New York: Nycomed, Inc. 1992;8.
17. Mohamed MA, Cohan RH, Dunnick NR. Ionic and nonionic contrast media: current status and controversies. *Appl Radiol* 1993;41–55.
18. Di Chiro G. Unintentional spinal cord arteriography: a warning. *Radiology* 1974;112:231–233.
19. Ederli A, Sassaroli S, Spaccarelli G. Vertebral angiography as a cause of necrosis of the spinal cord. *Br J Radiol* 1962;35:261–264.
20. Kardjiev V, Symeonov, Chankov I. Etiology, pathogenesis, and prevention of spinal cord lesions in selective angiography of the bronchial and intercostal arteries. *Radiology* 1974;112:81–83.
21. Djindjian R. *Angiography of the Spinal Cord.* Baltimore: University Park Press; 1970.
22. Djindjian R. Arteriography of the spinal cord. *AJR* 1969;107:461–478.
23. Taveras JM, Wood EH. Diseases of spinal cord. In: *Diagnostic Neuroradiology, Vol II,* 2nd ed. Baltimore: Williams & Wilkins; 1976;1180–1192.
24. McCullough JL, Hollier LH, Nugent M. Paraplegia after thoracic aortic occlusion: influence of cerebrospinal fluid drainage—experimental and early clinical results. *J Vasc Surg* 1988;7:153–160.
25. Crawford ES, Rubio PA. Reappraisal of adjuncts to avoid ischemia in the treatment of aneurysms of descending thoracic aorta. *J Thorac Cardiovasc Surg* 1973;66(5):693–704.
26. Miyamoto K, Ueno A, Wada T, Kimoto S. A new and simple method of preventing spinal cord damage following temporary occlusion of the thoracic aorta by draining the cerebrospinal fluid. *J Cardiovasc Surg* 1960;1:188–197.
27. Blaisdell FW, Cooley DA. The mechanism of paraplegia after temporary thoracic aortic occlusion and its relationship to spinal fluid pressure. *Surgery* 1963:51:351–355.
28. North RB, Drenger B, Beattie C, et al. Monitoring of spinal cord stimulation evoked potentials during thoracoabdominal aneurysm surgery. *Neurosurgery* 1991;28:325–330.
29. Swensson LG, Vasishta P, Robinson MF, Toshihiko U, Roehm OF Jr, Crawford ES. Influence of preservation or perfusion of intraoperatively identified spinal cord blood supply on spinal motor evoked potentials and paraplegia after aortic surgery. *J Vasc Surg* 1991;13:355–365.
30. Katz NM, Blackstone EH, Kirklin JW, Karp RB. Incremental risk factors for spinal cord injury following operation for acute traumatic aortic transection. *J Thorac Cardiovasc Surg* 1991;81:669–674.
31. Jex RK, Schaff HV, Piehler JM, et al. Early and late results following reapir of dissection of the descending thoracic aorta. *J Vasc Surg* 1986;3:226–237.

39

Endovascular Suite for Endograft Placement and Other Combined Interventional-Surgical Procedures

Gary J. Becker, M.D.
Barry T. Katzen, M.D.
James F. Benenati, M.D.
Gerald Zemel, M.D.

By 1997, it had become clear that transluminal endovascular graft placement for thoracic and abdominal aortic aneurysms is not a fad but rather a therapy that is here to stay.[1-8] Improved devices and methods are still to come, and with these refinements, procedures will evolve from their current form. Although this field is in its infancy, a variety of devices are under investigation, including covered stents (stents covered with graft material), conventional bypass materials with stents or stent-like devices for endovascular attachment, and devices that combine integrated weaves of metal and fabric.

Most iliac aneurysms, arteriovenous (AV) fistulae, and aneurysms involving smaller vessels can be treated with covered stents utilizing percutaneous access (10F sheath). However, because of the large size of the delivery catheters/sheaths involved in the treatment of aortic aneurysms (18F to 27F), surgical access utilizing open arteriotomy is required.

At the Miami Cardiac and Vascular Institute, a multidisciplinary team was organized to determine the optimal environment for performing combined surgical and interventional procedures. This chapter reviews the factors considered, the process itself, and the ultimate establishment of and experience with a modified interventional suite for procedures that require surgical access and others with significant potential for conversion to open conventional (nontransluminal) surgery.

DEVELOPMENT OF THE ENDOVASCULAR SUITE

In the initial discussions, representatives of the vascular surgery and interventional radiology departments examined the imaging equipment in our operating room and in our angiographic-interventional suite, as well as the optimal imaging and operative requirements for endografting. Optimal requirements were determined based on previous work and on visits to other investigational centers in the field of clinical and laboratory endograft research. The most obvious common thread in all of these endeavors was that endograft procedures are heavily dependent on high-quality imaging and on interventional skills, techniques, and tools. It was also clear that interventional angiographic suites lack several elements necessary for optimal patient care.

In several institutions, radiographic and angiographic equipment had been placed in operating room environments, and its use was being advocated by some for political purposes. On review, it became evident that many of the latter facilities consisted of surgical tables with a C-arm and associated digital imaging. These facilities are useful in providing imaging that can be used as an adjunct to a wide variety of surgical procedures. However, they are clearly are not *optimal* for endograft deployments, a range of procedures in which the primary operation being performed is guided by imaging and in which surgical access is a necessary but secondary consideration. The most common problems with intraoperative angiography are a small field of view, narrow apertures, slower frame rates, limitations in hard copy format, and, in some cases, lack of sophisticated road mapping techniques.

At our institution, because of low ceilings and lighting limitations precluding installation of the necessary ceiling rails, placement of a new, complete angiography suite in an operating room would involve major reconstruction. Additionally, it was agreed that placing a new, complete angiography stand and imaging equipment in the operating room (OR) would not be justifiable financially because utilization of the equipment would be limited. Such has been the experience in many operating rooms that have been modified with high-tech angiographic equipment.

Our interdisciplinary task force considering this issue comprised representatives from interventional radiology, vascular surgery, anesthesia, critical care, infection control, surgical services, interventional services, nursing, quality assurance, and risk management.

The following were the goals of the task force:

- Assess the feasibility of modifying one angiographic/interventional suite to accommodate procedures requiring surgical access, including emergency open surgery if necessary
- Identify deficiencies in personnel, procedures, and facilities existing in the interventional radiology department and in the operating room environment
- Identify regulatory requirements for the performance of these combined procedures
- Take the steps necessary to establish an optimal environment for transluminal endografting and for combined interventional-surgical procedures
- Develop an ongoing quality assurance process to monitor the safety of procedures performed in the new environment

Florida State statutes and published guidelines derived from several major professional groups were reviewed to establish the specific requirements of the new endovascular suite. The groups included the Committee on Operating Room Environment (CORE) of the American College of Surgeons, the Association of Operating Room Nurses, the Centers for Disease Control, the American Hospital Association, the Joint Commission on the Accreditation of Health Care Organizations, the National Fire Protection Association, the U.S. Public Health Service, and the Medical Research Council of Great Britain.

Our goal was to create an environment for optimal imaging and interventional capabilities, optimal working capacity for surgery, optimal conditions for anesthesia, and optimal patient care. Additional considerations were the inventory requirements of both surgery

and interventional radiology. The task force identified the critical elements in operations and physical setting required to ensure patient safety. It recognized a long history of surgical access outside of the traditional operating room environment for brachial artery exposure, venography, and lymphography, as well as other institutional precedents for combined procedures, such as intraoperative radiation therapy.

The critical elements that were identified will now be identified.

General Measures

- Minimum of 600 ft^2 of space[9]
- Adequate lighting (overhead surgical lamp required in addition to 100 foot-candles from overhead fluorescent lights)
- Full complement of OR personnel as needed (case-by-case basis)
- Full complement of interventional radiology personnel as needed (case-by-case basis)
- Full complement of anesthesia personnel and equipment as needed (case-by-case basis)
- Immediate access to all surgical trays, equipment, and support devices, including the cell saver
- Immediate access to all angiographic and interventional catheters, wires, and equipment
- Integrated scheduling (interventional radiology/OR/anesthesia)

Measures to Reduce the Likelihood of Infection

- Twenty to 25 air exchanges per hour, at least 20% of which involve fresh air[10–12]
- Positive air pressure in the procedure room relative to surrounding corridors[10–12]
- Temperature of 65°F to 75°F (18°C to 24°C)[10–12]
- Humidity of 50 to 55%[10–12]
- Washable ceilings to avoid contamination with bacteria-harboring dust particles[13]
- Seamless floors with integral wall bases to avoid areas that can harbor bacteria[13]
- Preprocedure disinfection and environmental preparation of the procedure suite[10,14,15]
- Adequate traffic control procedures and barriers during combined interventional-surgical operations; the likelihood of procedure-related infection is proportional to the number of people in the room[10,12]
- Surgical scrubbing by all physicians and assistants in all cases
- Maintenance of maximum aseptic technique

The task force took the following actions:

1. Recommended reconfiguring an angiographic-interventional suite as an endovascular suite with unique specifications for endografting and other combined interventional-surgical procedures

2. Identified modifications to the interventional suite that, if made, would meet regulatory requirements and ensure an optimal environment for patient care

The recommendations of the task force resulted in the following actions:

1. Development of an endovascular suite for performing interventional procedures in conjunction with surgical access. One of the interventional suites in the institute with a Philips Integris V-3000 (Best, the Netherlands) angiography stand was identified for this purpose. It is located in a mixed cardiac-vascular interventional environment (alternating cardiac and peripheral vascular suites). (*Note:* This equipment is completely washable and is regularly disinfected with a bleach-containing compound before endograft procedures and between all procedures.)

2. Installation of a surgical light with ceiling suspension

3. Minor modifications to ensure adequate air flow (*Note:* In some institutions, this important step may require installation of a new air handler, which can be quite expensive; engineering and/or architectural expertise may be required to determine specific needs)

4. Replacement of old ceiling tiles with washable ceiling tiles

5. Minor modifications to render the floor seamless

6. Additional training of the interventional technical and nursing personnel in surgical sterile technique, including surgical scrubbing and traffic flow

7. Additional training of the surgical staff in radiation protection and working in a fluoroscopic environment

8. Combined training of staff in the purpose and scope of combined endovascular procedures

9. Identification of procedures to deal with adverse events, including conversion to open surgical procedures

10. Formation of operations group to monitor activities and provide case-by-case quality assurance

Once these actions were implemented, it was agreed that this suite would be suitable for providing surgical access. In the event that conversion to open surgery becomes necessary, this could be accomplished in the endovascular suite. If this approach proved inadequate, transportation to the operating room (immediately below via elevator) could be accomplished in less than 10 minutes. Because many of the initial procedures performed in this suite would be investigational, it was agreed that the suite itself would be viewed as investigational and closely monitored.

Experience in the Endovascular Suite

Since the establishment of the endovascular suite, more than 100 procedures have been performed, including endografts and other combined procedures for a diverse group of indications. In addition to aortic and nonaortic endografting, other combined procedures have included iliac stenting in combination with common femoral endarterectomy and patch grafting, femoropopliteal bypass in combination with tibial angioplasty, carotid endarterectomy in combination with common carotid stenting, and others. Experience has now extended beyond vascular cases. One of the more interesting and gratifying procedures has been fluoroscopically guided transhepatic hepaticogastrostomy in combination with laparoscopically guided gastrojejunostomy for patients with combined biliary and gastric outlet obstruction due to periampullary carcinoma.

Preprocedure evaluations have been thorough. Most often they have involved an outpatient consultation with both the interventional radiologist and the vascular surgeon, as well as imaging studies and other studies as needed on an individual basis. As with all preplanned procedures, the anesthesiologists have evaluated the patients after admission, but before the procedure, so that they are able to implement the best management plan. All of the aortic aneurysm cases and a few of the other cases have also involved a preoperative cardiology consultation or referral directly from a cardiologist, and almost all of our patients have had a cardiologist on the team caring for them during hospitalization.

Endograft patients each receive 1 g of cefazolin sodium at the beginning of the procedure. Allergic patients receive vancomycin hydrochloride, 500 mg, at the time of the procedure followed by 500 mg 12 hours after the first dose. In all cases, all physicians and assistants directly participating in the procedure perform a complete surgical scrub. In each case, initial preparation of the sterile field is carefully contingency planned for emergency conversion to an open conventional operative approach. Therefore, in those cases that require emergency conversion, the transition has, to date, been accomplished within 5 minutes. Conversion involves moving the C-arm to an unobtrusive position, bringing the operating room nurses and trays into a central position, and making the incision.

In each endograft case, from start to finish, a sterile plastic cover with an elastic band (Pulse Medical, Inc., Davie, FL) fitted snugly over the image intensifier serves as a sterile barrier, as depicted during an endograft implantation (Fig. 39–1a). Fig. 39–1b provides a view of the endovascular suite configuration. In aortic aneurysm cases, the potential for significant blood loss is a concern. Therefore, preprocedural and

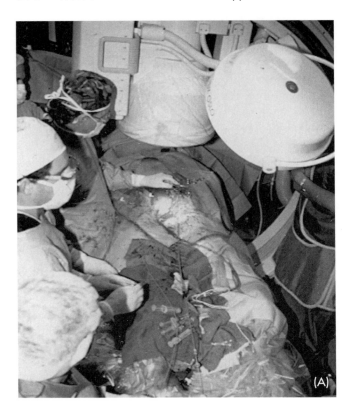

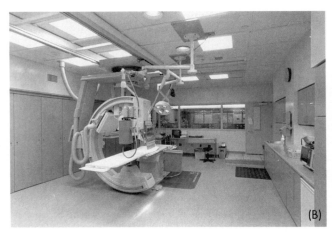

Figure 39–1. The endovascular suite. (A) View over the operative field during endograft deployment. Note the plastic barrier over the image intensifier. (B) Overview of the room configuration. Note the spacious room size, the ceiling-suspended C-arm of the Philips Integris angiographic stand, and the surgical lamp. The windows at the far end provide a view into the control room, so that visitors and onlookers can see the procedures.

procedural measures are taken. First, patients are asked to bank 1 unit of their own blood prior to the procedure, and are provided with directions to and an appointment with the nearest Red Cross center. In some instances, patients are able to bank 2 units prior to surgery. On the day of the procedure, in preparation, a urologic barrier drape with a U-pouch (No. 1067 U-Pouch, Medical-Surgical Division, 3M Health Care, St. Paul, MN, assembled in Mexico) is adapted to the tabletop's sterile field and used in conjunction with a Compact-A cell saver (DIDECO, Italy) to preserve the patient's own blood and minimize the necessity for transfusion.

Fig. 39–2 depicts a procedure that was performed in the endovascular suite.

Four of the abdominopelvic operations performed in the endovascular suite to date were not planned at the outset, including two emergency conversions, each of which occurred within 5 minutes of the decision to convert. One was required for emergency conventional aortobifemoral grafting after a bifurcated endograft failed to deploy from a right femoral cutdown approach. The other was required for emergency iliofemoral grafting when a thoracic endograft deployment sheath too large for the right iliac artery transected the artery on withdrawal.

No instances of inadequate access to surgical instruments or lack of inventory in the department have occurred. Even under the adverse conditions requiring conversion to open surgical procedures, there have

been no delays. No occurrences have necessitated moving the patient to an operating room to handle a surgical emergency. No conflicts in room scheduling or utilization have occurred. This topic is discussed further below. Acceptance of the endovascular suite by the surgeons, interventionalists, and anesthesiologists has been unanimous.

So far in our experience, there has been one major (endograft) infection in 75 endograft procedures. This infection required surgical excision and extra- anatomic bypass grafting. There have also been a few cases of minor wound infection involving the inguinal incision site for endovascular therapy; these have resolved with antibiotic administration.

DISCUSSION

As the field of vascular intervention rapidly evolves, it is more important than ever for interventional radiologists to assume a significant clinical role in the management of patients with vascular disease. Patients will clearly benefit from the combined skills of interventionalists and vascular surgeons, and close collaboration will benefit all parties involved. Our approach regarding combined interventional-surgical procedures has been to begin with the optimal imaging environment and to make modifications that provide safe conditions for the performance of these procedures. This helps to take maximum advantage of the complementary skills that interventionalists and surgeons have to offer.

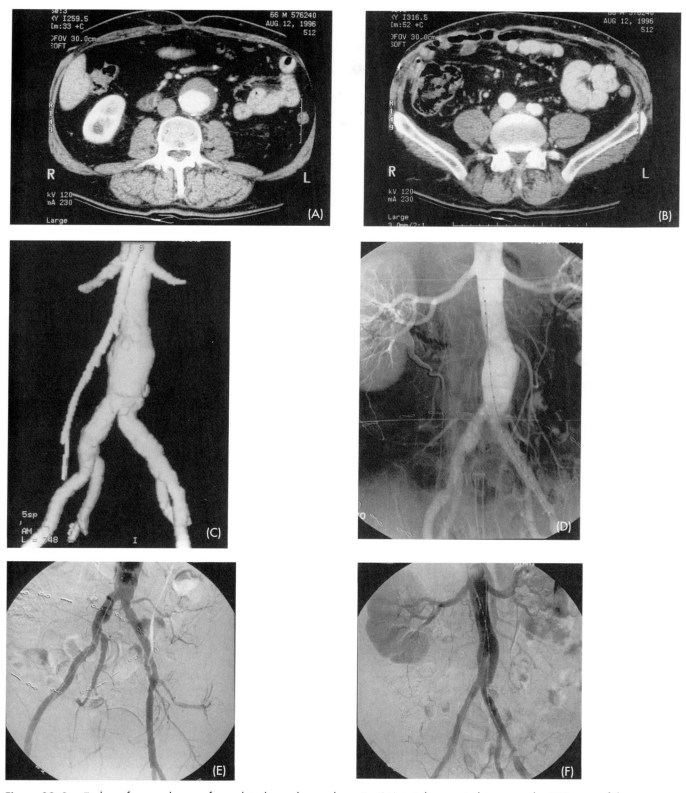

Figure 39–2. Endograft procedure performed in the endovascular suite. (A) Axial computed tomography (CT) scan of the abdomen demonstating an infrarenal abdominal aortic aneurysm. (B) Three-dimensional shaded surface displays a reconstructed CT image of the abdominal aortic aneurysm. (C) Aortogram with calibrated marker catheter demonstrating an infrarenal abdominal aortic aneurysm. (D) Fluroscopic spot film image taken during deployment of a bifurcated Endovascular Technologies (EVT) endograft. Note that the distal anchor mechanism in each iliac has already been deployed. (E) Intravascular ultrasound image of the right iliac limb of the graft after deployment. Note the infolding of the graft. (F) Kissing balloon technique is used at the bifurcation of the graft to "iron" the folds.

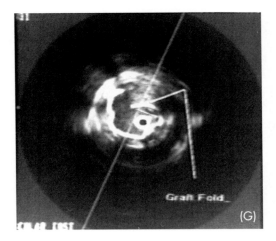

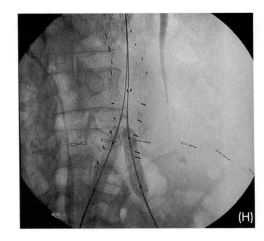

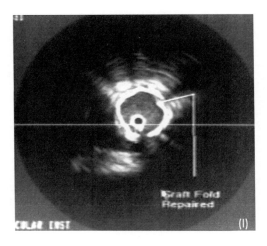

Figure 39–2 *(cont'd)* (G) Intravascular ultrasond image after ironing of the graft shows improvement in the appearance of the graft material and the lumen. (H) Final aortogram shows excellent appearance of the bifurcated aortic endograft. (I) copy to come.

We acknowledge, however, that in the long run, having both an interventionalist and a vascular surgeon on every case may not be a practical solution in many (particularly smaller) institutions. Ultimately, the long-term solution should be the training of solo practitioners with expertise in both interventional and vascular surgical methods. This group of new hybrids would likely be heterogeneous, comprising some who have similar backgrounds but whose training, interests, and experience lead them to practice predominantly vascular surgical techniques (eg, thoracoabdominal aneurysm surgery or femoral-tibial bypass) and some who have similar skills but whose training, interests, and experience lead them to practice predominantly intervention (eg, peripheral and renal angioplasty, thrombolytic therapy).

No immediate adverse consequences owing to the use of an endovascular suite have occurred in our relatively small series. The one major endograft infection occurred in a patient who had had an aortobiiliac graft 15 years earlier and who now had a large pseudoaneurysm of the left distal anastomosis that occupied approximately half of the pelvis. In retrospect, this pseudoaneurysm probably represented a graft infection even before the endografting took place. Regardless,

the major infection rate is small; however, we continue to maintain a vigilant attitude as we continue to expand our experience in the endovascular suite.

Thus far, a review of our hospital billing for combined procedures gives the impression of cost inefficiency. This is because there are hospital charges for the endovascular suite and materials, as well as charges for the backup operating room, personnel, and equipment. We anticipate that this process will be streamlined in the future. More important, the overall hospitalization in the combined cases turns out to be very cost efficient relative to conventional operation, primarily because of differences in length of stay.

At our institution, we are fortunate to have enough angiography suites, so that creation of the endovascular suite described herein has not impacted the work schedule to the degree it might in a department with only one or two suites. Still, more recently, the schedule of combined procedures in the endovascular suite has affected room availability and the remainder of our interventional case schedule. For departments with only one or two angiography suites or with one fully operational suite and one backup room, a modified approach may be required. Under such circumstances, an environment like that of our endovascular suite could be created in the angiography suite, but to optimize room utilization, the plan could entail moving patients who require conversion to a conventional operation into the operating room. This plan should work particularly well for angiography suites in close proximity to the operating room. For departments planning to keep their endovascular suite busy as a combined facility and an angiography suite each day, it is important to know that the room can be scrubbed down and prepared and the surrounding corridors appropriately cordoned off for a room turnover time of about 30 to 45 minutes.

In some environments, it may be difficult to achieve the recommended number of air exchanges per hour. If the existing number of air exchanges per hour is far too low in the angiography area, installation of a new, separate air handler may be required. This can be an expensive endeavor, albeit less expensive than purchasing and installing high-quality angiographic imaging equipment for the operating room.

Because of space limitations, other physical limitations, and lack of resources, in some hospitals it will not be possible to reconfigure an angiographic-interventional suite to function as an endovascular suite. In this situation, it may be appropriate to consider establishing a plan for performing combined procedures in the operating room with the use of portable digital angiographic imaging equipment with expanded memory and good-quality hard copy imaging. Whatever the ultimate solution, to maintain the optimum standard of care, every imaging-guided procedure performed in the hospital should be accompanied by a dictated report.

Finally, for all those in the process of developing or finalizing plans for a new angiographic-interventional suite, the guidelines provided herein should serve to help plan the new room as an endovascular suite.

REFERENCES

1. Parodi JC, Palmaz JC, Barone HD. Transfemoral intraluminal graft implantation for abdominal aortic aneurysms. *Ann Vasc Surg* 1991;5:491–499.

2. Parodi JC. Endovascular repair of abdominal aortic aneurysms and other arterial lesions. *J Vasc Surg* 1995;21:549–557.

3. Yusuf SW, Baker DM, Chuter TAM, et al. Transfemoral endoluminal repair of abdominal aortic aneurysm with bifurcated graft. *Lancet* 1994;344:650–651.

4. Chuter TAM, Donayre C, Wendt G. Bifurcated stent-grafts for endovascular repair of abdominal aortic aneurysm. *Surg Endosc* 1994;8:800–802.

5. Moore WS, Rutherford RB for the EVT Investigators. Transfemoral endovascular repair of abdominal aortic aneurysm: results of the North American EVT phase 1 trial. *J Vasc Surg* 1996;23:543–553.

6. Blum U, Langer M, Spillner G, et al. Abdominal aortic aneurysms: preliminary technical and clinical results with transfemoral placement of endovascular self-expanding stent-grafts. *Radiology* 1996;198:25–31.

7. White GH, Yu W, May J, et al. A new nonstented balloon-expandable graft for straight or bifurcated endoluminal bypass. *J Endovasc Surg* 1994;1:16–24.

8. Dake MD, Miller DC, Semba CP, et al. Transluminal placement of endovascular stent-grafts for the treatment of descending thoracic aortic aneurysms. *N Engl J Med* 1994;331:1729–1734.

9. Altemeier WA, Burke JF, Clowes GHA Jr, et al. Hospital design requirements for safe surgery. In: Altemeier WA, Burke JF, Pruitt BA Jr, et al, eds. *Manual on Control of Infection in Surgical Patients* (2nd ed.). Philadelphia: JB Lippincott, 1984;269–270.

10. Altemeier WA, Burke JF, Clowes GHA Jr, et al. Preparation and maintenance of a safe operating room environment. In: Altemeier WA, Burke JF, Pruitt BA Jr, et al, eds. *Manual on Control of Infection in Surgical Patients* (2nd ed.). Philadelphia: JB Lippincott, 1984;111–120.

11. Nichols RL. The operating room. In: Bennett JV, Brachman PS, Sanford JP, eds. *Hospital Infections* (3rd ed.). Boston: Little, Brown, 1992;461–467.

12. Soule BM. *The APIC Curriculum for Infection Control Practice*, Dubuque: 1983;850–851.

13. Florida Statutes on Hospital Licensure. Specific Authority 395.005 FS. Law implemented 395.001, 395.005 FS. History — New 1-1-77, formerly 10D-28-82, amended 1-16-87, formerly 10D-28.082, Amended 9-3-92; 59A-3.082;16:81–82.

14. Rutala WA. APIC guideline for selection and use of disinfectants. In: *APIC Guidelines for Infection Control Practice.* 1990;18(2):100–117.

15. Recommended practices for sanitation in the surgical practice setting. *AORN J* 1975; revised 1978, 1982, 1984, 1988, and 1992;251–254.

40

Endovascular Grafts for the Treatment of Arterial Aneurysms, Pseudoaneurysms, and Arteriovenous Fistulas

Michael L. Marin, M.D.
Frank J. Veith, M.D.

Over the past 5 years, intravascular stents have gradually achieved acceptance for treating arterial occlusive disease. Unfortunately, currently available stents are extremely porous, and thus unsuitable for treating other forms of arterial pathology. Aortic and peripheral aneurysms, traumatic pseudoaneurysms, and arteriovenous fistulas require devices with the capacity to form a blood-tight seal to treat the pathology. To address these problems, an alternative approach has been developed that combines intravascular stent and prosthetic graft technologies, thereby using the efficient "anchoring" qualities of stents and the flexible hemostatic sealing properties of vascular grafts. Such "stent graft" devices can be used to treat arterial aneurysms, occlusions, and traumatic vascular injuries.[1–5]

STENT GRAFTS FOR ARTERIAL ANEURYSMS

The clinical significance of arterial aneurysms was recognized over 2000 years ago. However, the modern therapy of aortic and peripheral artery aneurysms began in the 1950s. The seminal contributions of Dubost et al,[6] who advocated the use of aortic homografts to bridge the defect of aortic aneurysms, followed by the discovery of Voorhees et al[7] of the utility of prosthetic vascular grafts, marked the beginning of modern aortic surgery. Similar techniques for aneu-

rysm exclusion and endoaneurysmorrhaphy evolved for treating peripheral arterial aneurysms.

Improvements in surgical technique and pre- and postoperative care of patients with aortic aneurysms were primarily responsible for a marked reduction in the morbidity and mortality from this disease. However, problems in treating patients with large aortic aneurysms and significant comorbid medical illnesses persist. The reintroduction of older techniques such as aneurysmal thrombosis, and new approaches to external aortic wrapping, have been pursued, but it is generally believed that they do not provide significant protection against the complication of aortic rupture.[8–10]

An important potential advance in the management of aneurysmal disease was the first clinical application of endovascular stent grafting to treat aortic aneurysms, reported by Parodi et al in 1991.[1] The idea of endovascular grafting was actually first conceptualized by Charles Dotter in the late 1960s.[11] Following Dotter's suggestion that such stent grafts could be used to repair aneurysms and arteriovenous fistulas, a number of experimental studies were performed to evaluate the feasibility of these techniques.[12–14] Clinical experience with endovascular grafts for aneurysms continues to grow.[15–22]

The endovascular graft is commonly composed of a prosthetic graft that is inserted through a remote site in the vasculature and fixed to the arterial wall by means of an attachment device such as an intravascular stent (Fig. 40–1). Several different graft and stent combinations have been tested in experimental settings; how-

Supported by grants from the U.S. Public Health Service (HL 02990-02), the James Hilton Manning and Emma Austin Manning Foundation, The Anna S. Brown Trust and the New York Institute for Vascular Studies

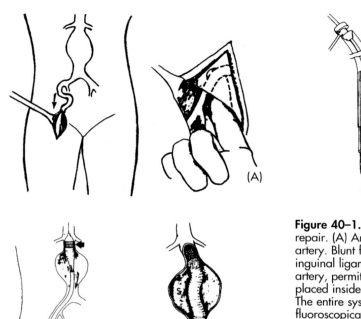

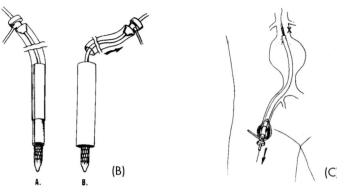

Figure 40–1. Transfemoral endovascular stented graft aortic aneurysm repair. (A) An incision is made in the groin to expose the common femoral artery. Blunt finger dissection is used to mobilize the vessel from beneath the inguinal ligament (L). This allows downward traction on the external iliac artery, permitting vessel straightening. (B) A stented graft (A) is folded and placed inside a delivery catheter (B) equipped with a hemostatic valve. (C) The entire system is inserted through an arteriotomy over a wire to a fluoroscopically confirmed proximal attachment site (X). (D) After manual withdrawal of the sheath (arrows), a balloon is inflated, sealing the stent to the arterial wall (large arrow). (E) A second stent is deployed to seal the lower end of the graft, excluding the aneurysm sac (S). (Reprinted from Marin ML, Veith FJ. Endovascular stents and stented grafts for the treatment of aneurysms and other arterial lesions. In: Cameron JL, ed. *Advances in Surgery*, Vol 29. St. Louis, MO; Mosby: 1995:93–109, with permission.)

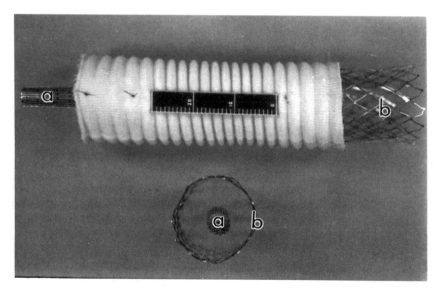

Figure 40–2. A Parodi-type stented graft composed of two balloon-expandable Palmaz stents sutured to the end of a crimped Dacron vascular graft. The stainless steel tubular stent expands from a relatively compact outer diameter (a) to an expanded form (b) after deployment. (Reprinted from Marin ML, Veith FJ. Endovascular stents and stented grafts for the treatment of aneurysms and other arterial lesions. In: Cameron JL, ed. *Advances in Surgery*, Vol 29. St. Louis, MO; Mosby: 1995:93–109, with permission.)

ever, one of the first such devices to be used employed a modified Palmaz stent and a Dacron knitted graft[1] (Fig. 40–2). The stent graft device is packaged inside an introducer sheath ranging from No. 18 to 28 French and equipped with a hemostatic valve. For repair of abdominal aortic aneurysms, the entire device is inserted through a remote arteriotomy in the femoral artery and advanced in a retrograde fashion to the infrarenal aorta. The locations for the proximal and distal portions of the stent graft device are identified by fluoroscopy. After fixation of the proximal and distal

portions of the prosthetic graft with its respective stents, a completion arteriogram and follow-up computed tomography (CT) scan are performed to confirm proper placement and adequate exclusion of the aortic aneurysm. The complication of an inadequate seal at either the proximal or distal fixation sites may occur in up to 30% of procedures with currently available devices.

Using these techniques, initial experiences with a number of devices have recently been reported.[15–23] Parodi reported the treatment of 50 patients with

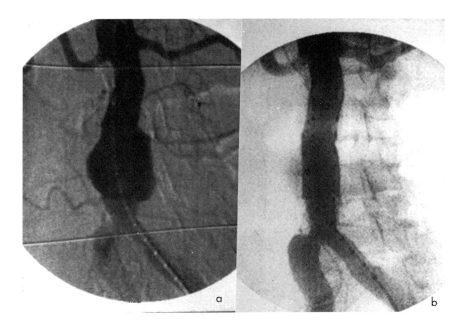

Figure 40–3. Transfemoral, endoluminal repair of an abdominal aortic aneurysm using the Endovascular Technologies' Endograft. (A) Preoperative arteriogram demonstrates a suitable proximal and distal segment of normal aorta above and below the aneurysm. (B) Following transfemoral insertion of the Endograft, the aneurysm is excluded from the circulation. (Reprinted from Ref. 22 with permission.)

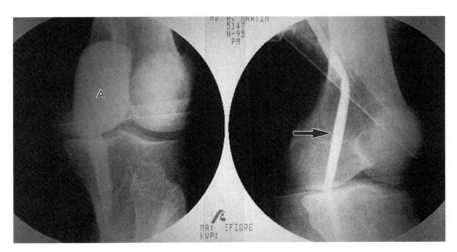

Figure 40–4. Transluminal repair of a popliteal artery aneurysm. (A) A transfemoral digital arteriogram demonstrates a large popliteal artery aneurysm (A). (B) Following insertion of an endovascular graft (arrow) that is fixed to the below-knee popliteal artery with a 1-cm Palmaz stent, the popliteal artery aneurysm is excluded. (Reprinted from Ref. 22 with permission.)

abdominal aortic aneurysms, with a technical success rate of 80%.[19] Several of these patients have required supplemental procedures, however. In addition, a 10% mortality rate was reported among this group of patients with large aneurysms and significant medical comorbidities.[19] Our experience with this technique at the Montefiore Medical Center in New York has paralleled that of Parodi[22] (Fig. 40–3). Moore and Vescera reported their experience using Endovascular Technologies' Endograft to treat abdominal aortic aneurysms in low-risk patients.[20] There were no deaths or perioperative complications in their group.

These stent graft devices are not limited to the treatment of aneurysms within the aorta. A similar approach can be used to repair aneurysms in the popliteal and iliac arteries. Successful exclusion of aneurysms in these locations has been demonstrated at the Montefiore Medical Center in New York using polytetrafluoroethylene (PTFE) and Dacron grafts. In one patient, a large, clot-filled popliteal artery aneurysm was successfully excluded using a 6-mm PTFE graft and two Palmaz stents[2] (Fig. 40–4). Experience with aneurysms in the common and internal iliac arteries has also been favorable[23] (Fig. 40–5). The long-term results of endovascular grafting for aortic and peripheral artery aneurysms are still unclear. Potential changes in the arterial tissue above and below the aneurysm in which the fixation device has been embedded remain uncertain. For

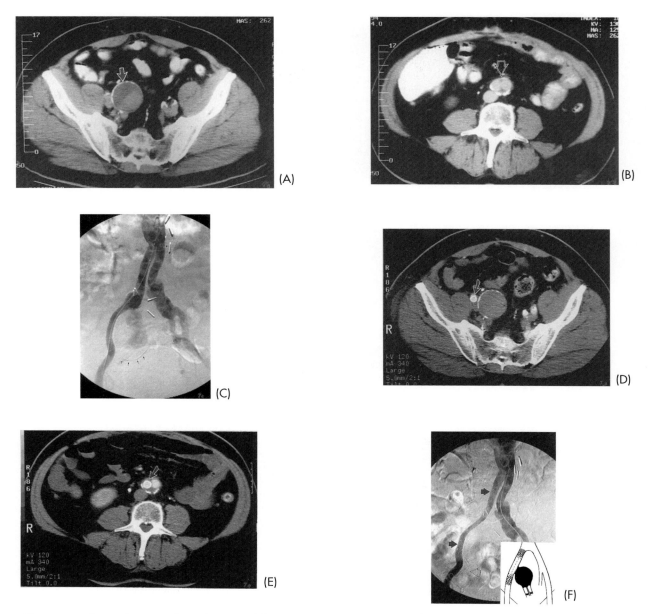

Figure 40–5. Transfemoral repair of a right internal iliac artery aneurysm 5 years after a bifurcated graft repair of aortic and common iliac artery aneurysms. (A) CT scan documents the presence of the right internal iliac artery aneurysm (arrow). (B) The two limbs of the bifurcated graft can be identified (arrow). (C) Transfemoral arteriography documents filling of the aneurysm prior to coil embolization of the anterior and posterior divisions of the vessel. (Note the aneurysmal wall calcification [small arrows].) (D) Following endovascular graft repair, the aneurysm has thrombosed. Contrast material can be identified within the endovascular graft (arrow). (E) This CT scan documents fixation of the Palmaz stent (arrow) within the old bifurcated graft. (F) Postoperative digital arteriogram shows the anchoring stents (arrows) and coils in the posterior and anterior divisions of the vessel to prevent retrograde flow (open arrow). Inset: Drawing of the completed repair. (Reprinted from Ref. 22 with permission.)

example, dilatation of these portions of the artery could result in dislodgment of the stent graft device, with prosthesis migration. In addition, whether endovascular grafting for the treatment of aortic aneurysms will truly eliminate the risk of aneurysmal rupture will require a longer follow-up period in more patients with aneurysms of varying sizes.

ENDOVASCULAR STENT GRAFTS FOR ARTERIAL TRAUMA

Techniques and Devices

Transluminally placed stented grafts for treating traumatic arterial lesions were first conceptualized by Dotter in 1969,[11] and one of the first clinical applications

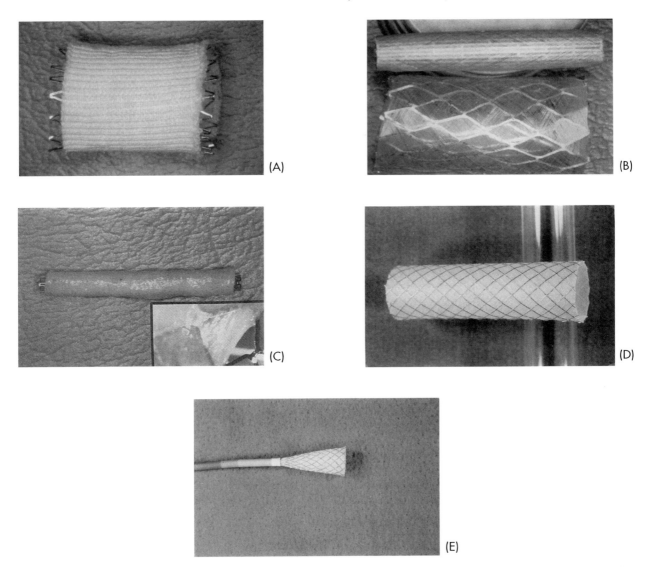

Figure 40–6. Endovascular covered stents. (A) Dacron graft material may be used to cover the balloon-expandable stents. These devices have been used by Parodi et al[19] to treat traumatic lesions. (B) Polyurethane can be attached directly onto a stent. This material has "elastic" properties, permitting a closed stent (top) to remain well covered following deployment (bottom). (C) Autogenous vein can be used to cover stents, creating biological stented grafts. The collapsed stent graft assumes a small profile that effectively covers the struts of the stent following deployment (inset). (D) Corvita graft for arterial trauma. This device is currently being used in clinical trials in the United States. (E) A specialized introducer catheter is supplied with each device. After the Corvita stent graft is custom cut to the desired length, it is inserted into this delivery sheath equipped with a central pusher catheter.

of this technology was used by Volodos et al, employing a Dacron graft and a self-expanding stent.[24] Experimental and clinical experience to date has demonstrated success with several different devices for treating traumatic arterial lesions[19,25,26] (Fig. 40–6). The ideal composition of the external covering on the stent, as well as the structure of the stent itself, has not yet been determined.

At Montefiore Medical Center, we have used the Palmaz balloon-expandable stent in conjunction with thin-walled PTFE graft material, as well as the Corvita graft, to perform arterial repairs of pseudoaneurysms and arteriovenous fistulas from remote access sites (Fig. 40–7).

The Palmaz stent grafts varied between 2 and 3 cm in length, with the stents fixed inside 6-mm Gore-Tex grafts (W.L. Gore and Associates, Flagstaff, AZ) by two "U" stitches. The balloon-expandable stented graft was mounted on a balloon angioplasty catheter that had a tapered dilator tip. The entire device was loaded into a No. 12 French delivery catheter for over-the-wire insertion either percutaneously or through an arterial cutdown. The Corvita device is supplied by the manufacturer (Corvita, Inc., Miami Beach, FL) ready to be cut to a desired length in the operating room. A custom introducer catheter complete with a "pusher" stylet is also supplied with the device (Fig. 40–6D and E).

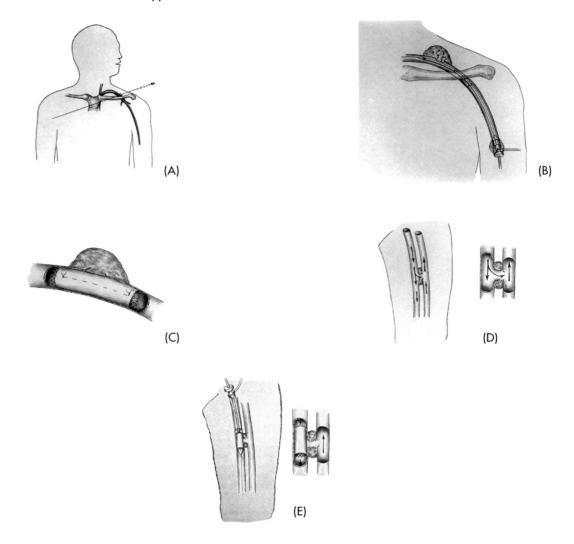

Figure 40–7.   Schematic drawing of stented graft repair of an arterial injury. (A) A bullet wound partially disrupts the wall of the vessel. (B) The stent graft device is delivered to the site of injury via a remote arteriotomy. (C) Once deployed, the stented graft covers the hole in the vessel. (D) When an arteriovenous fistula forms following a vascular injury, the same principles apply for stented graft repair. In this example, the stent graft device is inserted in the superficial femoral artery at a site remote from the arterial injury. (E) Following deployment, the stented graft occludes the arteriovenous fistula. (Reprinted from Ref. 25 with permission.)

Results

As shown in Table 40–1, 11 patients, ranging in age from 18 to 85 years, received 11 stented grafts to treat traumatic arterial lesions. Seven injuries occurred as a result of gunshot wounds (Fig. 40–8). In addition, there was one knife wound and three iatrogenic (needle catheterization or surgical) injuries. All injuries were associated with an arterial pseudoaneurysm. In three instances, the arterial injury formed a fistula to an injured adjacent vein. Associated injuries were present in eight patients (Table 40–1). The hospital length of stay averaged 5 days (excluding case number 6), and stented graft patency was 100%. Mean follow-up time was 24 months (range, 3 to 38 months). One

patient with a left axillary-subclavian stent graft developed compression of the stent at 12 months, which was successfully treated with balloon angioplasty. This problem recurred 3 months later. The device did not thrombose, and it is currently being observed without further intervention. One patient who had an axillary pseudoaneurysm repaired with a stented graft required a vein patch of a small brachial artery at the catheter insertion site. There have been no occlusions.

SUMMARY

The blending of prosthetic graft and intravascular stent technologies may rapidly become an important part of therapy for aneurysmal and traumatic vascular injuries.

Table 40–1. Stented Grafts for Arterial Trauma

Sex/Age	Mechanism of Injury	Vessel(s) Involved	Pseudo-aneurysm	Arterio-venous Fistula	Anes-thesia	Associated Injuries	Time Interval from Injury to Repair	Stent Graft Length (cm)	Access	Hospital Stay (days)	Patency (mo)	Complications
M 20	Bullet	LSFA LSFV	Yes	Yes	General	Soft tissue buttock	36 hr	3	LSFA percutaneous	5	38	—
M 28	Bullet	RSFA	Yes	No	Local	Left open femur fracture	12 hr	3	RSFA arteriotomy	9	36	—
M 22	Bullet	LSFA	Yes	No	Local	Soft tissue right thigh; left deep venous thrombosis	12 hr	3	LSFA arteriotomy	6	2*	—
M 24	Knife	LASA	Yes	No	General	Pneumothorax; hemothorax	4 hr	3	Left brachial arteriotomy	7	33	Stent compression
M 35	Bullet	RASA	Yes	No	Local	Brachial plexus	3 wk	3	Right brachial arteriotomy	4	29	—
F 78	Catheterization	RSA	Yes	No	Local	Hemothorax	24 hr	3	Right brachial arteriotomy	8 wk†	28	—
M 78	Catheterization	LCIA	Yes	No	Epidural	None	4 mo	2	LCFA arteriotomy	2	28	—
M 18	Bullet	RSA	Yes	Yes	Local	Hemothorax	48 hr	3	Right brachial artery	4	21	—
M 18	Bullet	RASA	Yes	No	Local	None	6 hr	3	Right brachial artery	3	12	—
M 22	Bullet	RASA	Yes	No	Local	Hemothorax	3 hr	3	Right brachial artery	6	12	—
F 85	Surgical trauma	RCIA	Yes	Yes	Local	None	8 yr	5cm‡	LCFA Percutaneous	4	3	Distal emboli (treated with catheter suction thrombectomy)

*Died 2 months postprocedure (homicide).
†Hospitalized for multiple medical problems.
‡Corvita stent graft.

Abbreviations: LSFV, left superficial femoral vein; LSFA, left superficial femoral artery; RSFA, right superficial femoral artery; RSA, right subclavian artery; LCIA, left common iliac artery; RCIA, right common iliac artery; RASA, right axillary subclavian artery; LASA, left axillary subclavian artery; LCFA, left common femoral artery.

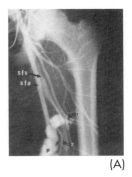
(A)

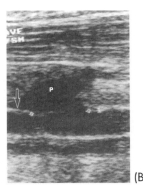
(B)

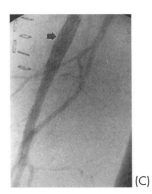
(C)

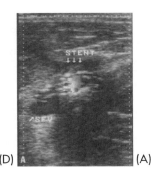
(D) (A)

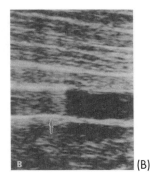
(B)

Figure 40–8.   (A) Femoral arteriogram after a gunshot wound to the left thigh. An arteriovenous fistula associated with a large pseudoaneurysm is seen between the left superficial femoral artery (SFA) and the superficial femoral vein (SFV). Selective catheterization of the deep femoral artery (1) and the SFA branch (2) showed that these vessels were not injured. (p, pseudoaneurysm.) (B) Duplex ultrasonographic image of the SFA depicted in (A). Loss of the intimal stripe (arrow) and associated pseudoaneurysm (p) is seen. The arterial defect measures approximately 13 mm (distance between the stars). (C) Completion arteriogram demonstrates patency of the SFA, proper positioning of the stented graft (arrow), and no evidence of the arteriovenous fistula or extravasation. Metal clips were placed in the skin before the procedure to facilitate fluoroscopic localization of the arteriovenous fistula and proper placement of the stented graft. (D) Transverse and longitudinal duplex ultrasonographic images of stented graft repair of the SFA after 3 months. A: Transverse image of the artery and vein at the level of the stent can be identified, with evidence of normal flow in arteries. B: Longitudinal duplex ultrasonogram identifies the stented graft within the artery (arrow). Minimal changes in peak systolic velocities are appreciated between the native SFA and the portion of the vessel that is covered by the stented graft. (Reprinted from Ref. 5 with permission.)

It is conceivable that the use of this technology may result in reduced operative morbidity and mortality, as well as decreased operative blood loss, hospital stay, and cost. Once additional experience with this important new technique has been obtained, controlled clinical trials comparing standard therapy to endovascular grafting techniques will be needed to substantiate using this approach for the more widespread treatment of arterial disease.

REFERENCES

1. Parodi JC, Palmaz JC, Barone HD. Transfemoral intraluminal graft implantation for abdominal aortic aneurysms. *Ann Vasc Surg* 1991;5:491–499.
2. Marin ML, Veith FJ, Panetta TF, et al. Transfemoral endoluminal stented graft repair of a popliteal artery aneurysm. *J Vasc Surg* 1994;19:754–757.
3. Cragg AH, Dake MD. Percutaneous femoropopliteal grafting: report of a new technique. *J Vasc Intervent Radiol* 1993;4:64–65.
4. Marin ML, Veith FJ, Cynamon J, et al. Transfemoral endovascular stented graft treatment of aorto-iliac and femoropopliteal occlusive disease for limb salvage. *Am J Surg* 1994;168:156–162.
5. Marin ML, Veith FJ, Panetta TF, et al. Transfemoral endolumisal stented graft repair of a traumatic femoral arteriovenous fistula. *J Vasc Surg* 1993;18:298–301.
6. Dubost C, Allary M, Oeconomos N. Resection of aneurysm of abdominal aorta: reestablishment of continuity by preserved human arterial graft, with result after five months. *Arch Surg* 1952;64:405–408.
7. Voorhees AB Jr, Jaretzki A III, Blakemore AH. The use of tubes constructed from vinyon "N" cloth in bridging arterial defects; preliminary report. *Ann Surg* 1952;135:332–338.
8. Blakemore AH. Progressive constrictive occlusion of abdominal aorta with wiring and electrothermic coagulation: one-stage operation for arteriosclerotic aneurysms of abdominal aorta. *Ann Surg* 1951;133:447–462.
9. Robicsek F, Daugherty HK, Mullen DC. External grafting of aortic aneurysms. *J Thorac Cardiovasc Surg* 1971;61:131–134.

10. Berguer R, Schneider J, Wilner HL. Induced thrombosis of inoperable abdominal aortic aneurysm. *Surgery* 1978;84:425–429.
11. Dotter CT. Transluminally-placed coilspring endarterial tube grafts. Long-term patency in canine popliteal rtery. *Invest Radiol* 1969;4:329–332.
12. Balko A, Piasecki GJ, Shah DM, et al. Transfemoral placement of intraluminal polyurethane prosthesis for abdominal aortic aneurysm. *J Surg Res* 1986;40:305–309.
13. Mirich D, Wright KC, Wallace S, et al. Percutaneously placed endovascular grafts for aortic aneurysms: feasibility study. *Radiology* 1989;170:1033–1037.
14. Laborde JC, Parodi JC, Clem MF, et al. Intraluminal bypass of abdominal aortic aneurysm: feasibility study. *Radiology* 1992;184:185–190.
15. Blum U, Langer M, Spillner G, Mialhe C, et al. Abdominal aortic aneurysm: preliminary technical and clinical results with transfemoral placement of endovascular self-expanding stent-grafts. *Radiology* 1996;198:25–31.
16. May J, White G, Yu W, et al. Treatment of complex abdominal aneurysms by a combination of endoluminal and extraluminal aortofemoral grafts. *J Vasc Surg* 1994;19:924–933.
17. Dake M, Miller C, Semba CP, et al. Transluminal placement of endovascular stent-grafts for the treatment of descending thoracic aortic aneurysms. *N Engl J Med* 1994;331:1729–1734.
18. Yusef SW, Baker DM, Chuter TA, et al. Transfemoral endoluminal repair of abdominal aortic aneurysms with bifurcated graft. *Lancet* 1994;334:650–651.
19. Parodi JC. Endovascular repair of abdominal aoric aneurysms and other arterial lesions. *J Vasc Surg* 1995;21:549–557.
20. Moore WS, Vescera CL. Repair of abdominal aortic aneurysm by transfemoral endovascular graft placement. *Ann Surg* 1994;220:331–341.
21. May J, White GH, Yu W, et al. Endoluminal grafting of abdominal aortic aneurysms: causes of failure and their prevention. *J Endovasc Surg* 1994;1:44–52.
22. Marin ML, Veith FJ, Cynamon J, et al. Initial experience with transluminally placed endovascular grafts for the treatment of complex vascular lesions. *Ann Surg* 1995;222:449–469.
23. Marin ML, Veith FJ, Lyon RT, Cynamon J, Sanchez LA. Transfemoral, endovascular repair of iliac artery aneurysms. *Am J Surg* 1995;170:179–182.
24. Volodos NL, Karpovich IP, Troyan VI, et al. Clinical experience of the use of self-fixing synthetic prostheses for remote endoprosthetics of the thoracic and the abdominal aorta and iliac arteries through the femoral artery and as intraoperative endoprosthesis for aorta reconstruction. *Vasa* suppl 1991;33:93–95.
25. Marin ML, Veith FJ, Panetta TF, et al. Transluminally placed endovascular stented graft repair for arterial trauma. *J Vasc Surg* 1994;20:466–473.
26. Rivera FJ, Palmaz JC, Encarnacion CE, et al. Aneurysm and pseudoaneurysm balloon expandable stent/graft bypass: clinical experience. *J Vasc Intervent Radiol* 1994;5:19. Abstract.

41

Endoluminal Repair of Thoracic Aortic Dissections

Kenneth S. Ostrow, M.D.
Charles P. Semba, M.D.
Michael D. Dake, M.D.

Aneurysm of the thoracic aorta is an uncommon though life-threatening condition. The vast majority of thoracic aneurysms are arteriosclerotic in origin and are often asymptomatic, presenting as an unsuspected mass on chest radiographs.[1,2] Clinical manifestations are related to aneurysm expansion, with compression or erosion of adjacent structures, associated aortic dissection, or rupture.[3,4] The natural history of thoracic aneurysm is progressive dilatation and rupture, with almost uniform mortality.[5,6] Survival is further compromised by a strong association with comorbid conditions including cardiovascular disease and hypertension.[2,6] Twenty-five percent of patients with thoracic aortic aneurysms have additional aneurysms, usually of the abdominal aorta.[6] Without intervention, 1- and 3-year survival rates of non-dissecting thoracic aneurysms have been reported to be 58.2% and 25.7%, respectively.[6]

Given its high mortality rate and associated comorbid factors, thoracic aneurysm presents a significant therapeutic challenge. Standard treatment consists of surgical resection and replacement of the aneurysm with a segment of synthetic graft material.[1,4,7–9] Though extracorporeal circulation can be avoided in lesions distal to the left subclavian origin, the procedure is not without risk, with a mortality rate of 12% increasing to 50% in emergent conditions.[10] Morbidity is also significant, with paraplegia seen in 2 to 10%.[9,10]

Transluminal endovascular stent grafting provides a therapeutic alternative for these clinically challenging patients. The idea of transluminal placement of stented grafts was first proposed by Dotter in 1969.[11] Subse-

quently, the feasibility of graft placement was established in both animal models[12–17] and early clinical trials.[16] Transluminal graft placement has been described in the treatment of femoral arteriovenous fistula,[18] subclavian aneurysm,[19] and femoro-popliteal atherosclerotic disease.[20] Reports of several series have also described placement of stented grafts for the treatment of abdominal aortic aneurysms.[16,21]

Our initial experience with transluminally placed endovascular stent-grafts for the treatment of descending thoracic aortic aneurysm at Stanford University Hospital in 44 patients demonstrated the potential of this procedure as a safe and efficacious alternative to traditional surgical correction.[22–24] Since the time of these reports, we have treated a total of 84 patients, with continued promising results. In the following sections, the clinical and technical considerations involved in the endovascular treatment of thoracic aortic aneurysms will be discussed, as well as results of the ongoing trial at Stanford.

ANATOMIC CONSIDERATIONS

Each patient undergoes pre-operative spiral computed tomography (CT) and thoracic aortography to determine the dimensions of the aneurysm for stent construction and to ensure that the patient is anatomically suitable for stent-graft placement. The primary anatomic consideration during the initial evaluation for stent-graft placement is the presence of an adequate proximal and distal aneurysm neck. A neck measuring at least 1.5 cm is necessary to ensure adequate anchoring of the stent across the aneurysm. In addition, the proximal aneurysm neck should be at least 1.5 to 2.0 cm distal to the origin of the left subclavian artery to avoid inadvertent extension of the graft over the subclavian artery origin. Similarly, a 1.5 to 2-cm margin must exist between the distal aneurysm neck and the ostium of the celiac axis. The stent-graft is made as short as possible to minimize the number of intercostal arteries covered by the prosthesis.

Measurements are also made of the iliac vessels to ensure that they can accommodate the No. 24 Fr. stent-graft delivery sheath introduced via a transfemoral approach. If the iliac vessels are of insufficient caliber (<9 mm), a retroperitoneal infrarenal aortic approach is used. Procedures that combine endovascular stent-graft placement for treatment of a thoracic aneurysm with surgical graft placement for treatment of a coexisting abdominal aortic aneurysm provide the opportunity to access the thoracic aorta via a side limb attached to the surgical graft.

STENTS

The stent is the metallic framework onto which the graft material is sutured. Stents are manufactured from stainless steel, nitinol, or tantalum and may be self-expanding or balloon-expandable. Self-expanding stents, such as the Wallstent (Schneider, Inc., Plymouth, MN) and the modified Z-stent (Cook, Inc., Bloomington, IN) return to a preformed shape when released from a protective sheath. Balloon-expandable stents such as the Palmaz stent (Johnson and Johnson Interventional Systems, Inc., Warren, NJ) are mounted on an angioplasty balloon catheter and expanded by balloon dilatation.

Techniques for stent-grafts using both balloon-expandable and self-expanding stents have been described.[16,22] However, the unique anatomic and physiologic factors associated with the endovascular treatment of thoracic aneurysms confer a significant advantage on a self-expanding stent. In our experience, the mean diameter of the proximal aneurysm neck is 35 mm, significantly larger than the largest commercially marketed angioplasty balloon (25 mm). Further, as the balloon inflates to partially occlude the aortic lumen, the force of aortic blood flow may cause distal migration of the balloon, resulting in sub-optimal stent graft placement. The self-expanding stents offer less resistance to aortic blood flow during deployment than balloon-expandable devices.

Our stents are constructed from 0.02-inch surgical-grade stainless steel wire formed into Z-shaped elements. Individual stent bodies are 2.5 cm in length, with combinations sewn together using 2-0 polypropylene suture.

GRAFTS

The graft material used for our device is woven polyethylene terephthate (Cooley Veri-Soft; Meadox Medicals, Inc., Oakland, NJ). The crimps are ironed out using a standard laundry iron. A single piece of graft material is secured to the stent at each end with interrupted 5-0 polypropylene sutures (Fig. 41–1). The completed device is gas sterilized with ethylene oxide prior to use.

DELIVERY SYSTEM

The delivery system consists of four components: (1) a No. 24 Fr. introducer sheath with a hemostatic valve; (2) a tapered dilator that allows the sheath to be advanced over a 0.035-inch guidewire; (3) a No. 24 Fr. loading cartridge in which the stent-graft is placed to facilitate introduction into the sheath via the hemostatic valve; and (4) a No. 24 Fr. Teflon pusher to advance the loaded stent-graft through the delivery sheath (Figs. 41–1 and 41–2).

PATIENT PREPARATION

At Stanford University Hospital, all thoracic stent-grafts are placed in the operating room under general anesthesia. Both radiologists and surgeons participate in the procedure, acting as a team. The patient is placed on the operating table in a shallow right lateral decubitus position, with the thorax prepared for a left thoracotomy in case conversion to an open surgical procedure becomes necessary. The groin (selection of the left or right side is based on the preoperative angiogram) is prepared for a femoral cutdown when using a femoral approach. Alternatively, if a retroperitoneal approach is necessary due to inadequate iliac artery diameters or extreme tortuosity, the left lower abdomen is prepared for a retroperitoneal approach.

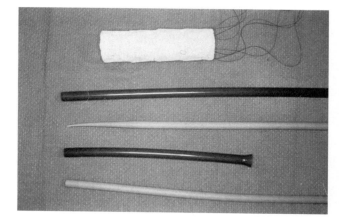

Figure 41–1. Delivery system for stent-graft deployment. Top to bottom: self-expanding endovascular stent-graft, introducer sheath, tapered dilator, loading cartridge, Teflon pusher.

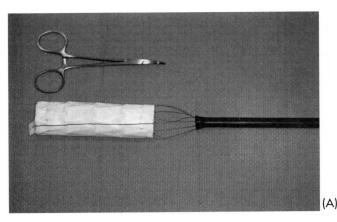
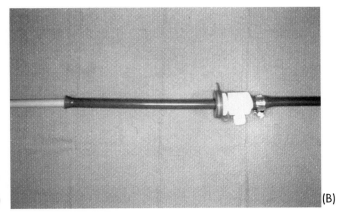

Figure 41–2 (A) Loading stent-graft. The stent-graft is pulled into the loading cartridge by sutures that are cut after the device has been loaded. (B) Stent-graft with loading cartridge is advanced into the introducer sheath by the Teflon pusher.

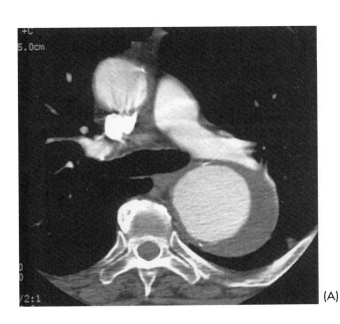
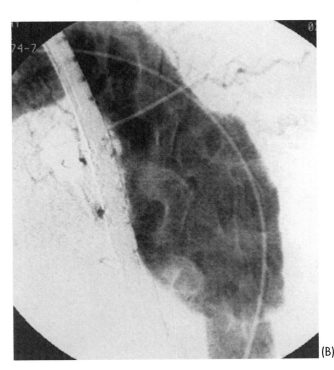

Figure 41–3 (A) Contrast-enhanced CT scan of a 69-year-old man with a large aneurysm of the descending thoracic aorta. (B) Corresponding intraoperative angiogram during stent-graft deployment demonstrates fusiform thoracic aortic aneurysm.

A C-arm fluoroscopic unit with digital subtraction capability is centered over the thorax at the beginning of the procedure.

PROCEDURE

A surgical cutdown is performed on the chosen femoral artery access site. An 18-gauge needle is used to puncture the artery, and a soft-tipped, 0.035-inch guidewire is advanced into the thoracic aorta, across the aneurysm, under fluoroscopic guidance. A pigtail angiographic catheter is advanced over the wire, and the wire is withdrawn. An initial aortogram is performed in the optimal obliquity, as determined by the preoperative arteriogram (Fig. 41–3). Both proximal and distal aneurysm necks are identified and localized in relation to body landmarks and/or radioopaque markers. An exchange length (260-cm) 0.035-inch extra stiff guidewire is advanced through the pigtail catheter, and the catheter is withdrawn. The patient is anticoagulated with intravenous heparin (300 IU/kg), a transverse femoral arteriotomy is performed, and the No. 24 Fr. dilator/sheath assembly is advanced over the wire under fluoroscopic guidance until the sheath tip is proximal to the proximal aneurysm neck. Both the dilator and the guidewire are removed, and the stent-graft is introduced into the sheath from its loading cartridge

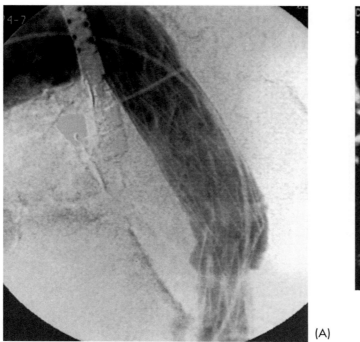

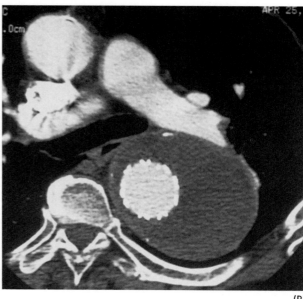

Figure 41–4 (A) Intraoperative arteriogram following placement of a stent-graft demonstrates interval exclusion of flow to the thoracic aortic aneurysm. (B) Contrast-enhanced CT scan following placement of a stent-graft, with interval thrombosis of the excluded aneurysm.

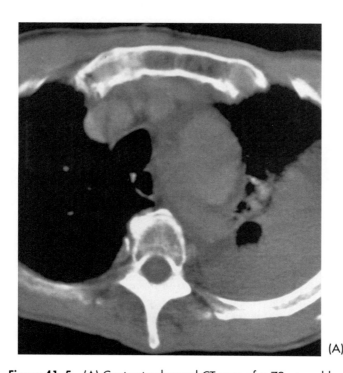

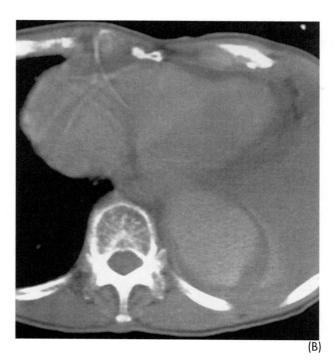

Figure 41–5 (A) Contrast-enhanced CT scan of a 72-year-old man with a large aneurysm extending from the aortic arch. An aneurysm leak was suspected. Note the large left pleural effusion. (B) Contrast-enhanced CT scan in the same patient demonstrates an additional aneurysm of the descending thoracic aorta. Note the luminal countour abnormality within the posterior aspect of the aneurysm, which may represent the leak site.

using the Teflon mandrel as a "pusher." The device is pushed to the sheath tip and, if necessary, the components are partially withdrawn as a unit to the level of the desired deployment site.

Prior to deployment, the arterial blood pressure is lowered to a mean of 50 to 60 mm Hg using an intravenous infusion of sodium nitroprusside to decrease the risk of inadvertent deployment of the graft downstream of the target due to the force of aortic blood flow. With the Teflon pusher held firmly in place, the sheath is rapidly withdrawn and the stent-graft expands into position. Blood pressure is allowed to normalize immediately following deployment.

Following deployment, a soft-tipped 0.035-inch is advanced across the graft through the delivery sheath, followed by a pigtail angiographic catheter. A postdeployment angiogram is performed (Fig. 41–4A), the delivery sheath is removed, protamine sulfate is administered to reverse the anticoagulant effects of heparin, and surgical closure of the arteriotomy site is performed.

POSTPROCEDURE ROUTINE

Typically, patients are observed in the intensive care unit for 24 hours following the procedure. They are then transferred to a ward for 1 to 2 days and subsequently discharged. All patients undergo a postprocedure spiral CT scan (Fig. 41–4B) and a thoracic aortogram before discharge to evaluate the graft position and detect persistent aneurysm filling via perigraft leakage. Patients do not receive anticoagulant therapy after the procedure. Our current protocol requires a follow-up CT scan 6 months after placement of the stent-graft and yearly thereafter.

PROBLEM SOLVING

Though the procedure is conceptually elementary, complexities in patient anatomy and graft deployment often require percutaneous manipulation of the stent-graft, either intraoperatively or postoperatively, to ensure complete exclusion of flow to the aneurysm.

In cases where there is an insufficient margin between the origin of the left subclavian artery and the aneurysm, surgical transposition of the left subclavian to the left common carotid artery allows more proximal placement of the graft, and thereby creates a more favorable situation for anchoring of the graft and exclusion of the aneurysm. If a sufficient but suboptimal proximal neck is present, access across the left subclavian artery is maintained during graft deployment using a 0.035-inch, soft-tipped guidewire placed from the left arm into the ascending aorta. The origin of the left subclavian can then be stented to ensure patency if there is encroachment by the stent-graft.

Faint filling of the aneurysm on the intra-operative postdeployment arteriogram is often seen and frequently represents leak of contrast medium through the semiporous graft material. This typically ceases following normalization of the patient's coagulation parameters, and no further intervention is necessary.

Persistent perigraft leakage due to inadequate stent-graft size or suboptimal orientation of the stent-graft within the aneurysm neck may require placement of an additional covered stent during the initial procedure. This extension of the stented area can create a tight seal by obtaining ideal apposition of the graft to the aortic wall. However, persistent filling of the aneurysm may occur even in optimally placed stent-grafts due to an incomplete seal of the stent-graft at the proximal or distal aneurysm neck (Figs. 41–5 to 41–9). These leaks can be eliminated by additional stent-grafts or selective catheter-directed coil embolization of the leaking tract in the angiography suite (Fig. 41–10).

RESULTS

To date, we have treated 84 patients with thoracic aortic aneurysms using covered stent-grafts at Stanford University Hospital. The majority of patients were judged to have a high surgical risk due to coexisting cardiovascular or pulmonary disease or prior surgeries. Complete thrombosis of the aneurysm is documented in 79 patients. Additional stents or coils were required to completely exclude the aneurysm from aortic flow in five cases. Five (6.0%) periprocedural deaths (less than 30 days after the procedure) and six deaths that occured more than 30 days following the procedure were documented. Paraplegia occured in three patients (3.6%), two of whom underwent combined surgical correction of an abdominal aortic aneurysm and thoracic aortic stent-graft placement. The third case of paraplegia occurred following stent-grafting of a long-segment thoracic aortic aneurysm in a patient who had previously undergone operative placement of an aorto-bifemoral bypass graft. Four patients in the series (4.8%) suffered a stroke. The mean follow-up time has been 14.1 months, ranging from 1 month to 45 months. There have been no episodes of distal embolization or infection, and conversion to a surgical aneurysm repair has not been necessary.

CONCLUSION

The morbidity and mortality of our series compare favorably to the best results from surgical trials. Furthermore, transluminal endovascular stent-grafting possesses the additional advantages of a minimally invasive procedure, with the attendant decrease in hospital stay and cost. To date, all stent-grafts are custom-made to the specifications of each patient's anatomy. Ultimately, the ease and availability of the procedure will improve

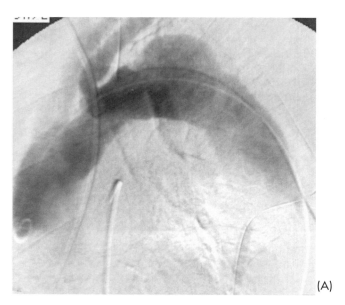

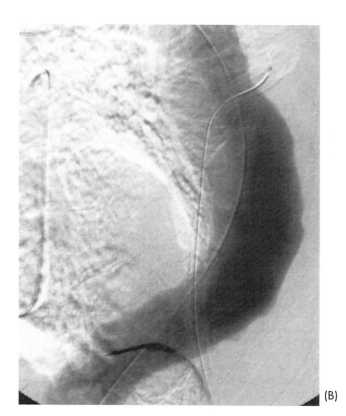

Figure 41–6   (A) Corresponding thoracic arteriogram demonstrates a saccular aneurysm of the aortic arch. (B) Thoracic arteriogram demonstrates a fusiform aneurysm of the descending thoracic aorta.

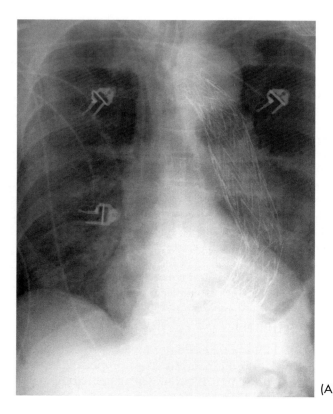

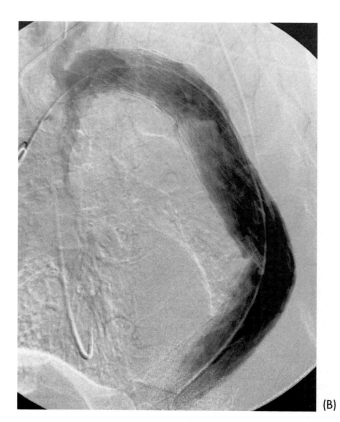

Figure 41–7   (A) Chest radiograph in the same patient after deployment of overlapping stent-grafts to exclude both aneurysms. (B) Intraoperative arteriogram following stent-graft deployment, with complete exclusion of both the saccular aortic arch aneurysm and the fusiform aneurysm of the descending thoracic aorta.

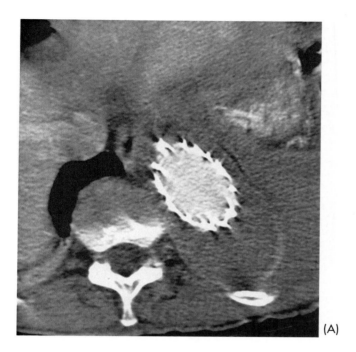

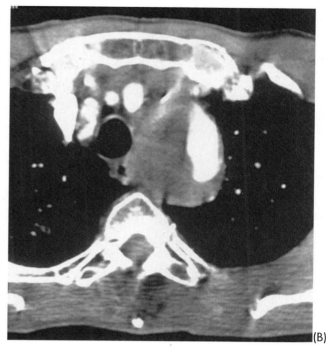

Figure 41–8 (A) Postoperative contrast-enhanced CT scan in the same patient demonstrates complete exclusion of the descending thoracic aortic aneurysm. (B) Portoperative contrast-enhanced CT scan showing persistent flow within the saccular aortic arch aneurysm consistent with proximal stent-graft leakage.

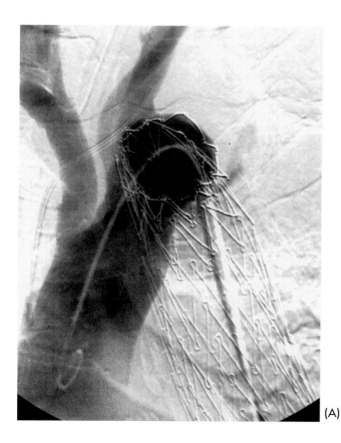

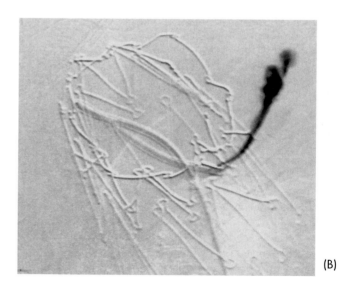

Figure 41–9 (A) Thoracic arteriogram of the same patient, with a faint leak seen filling the aneurysm from the inferolateral aspect of the stent-graft. (B) Selective injection within the leaking tract filling the aneurysm.

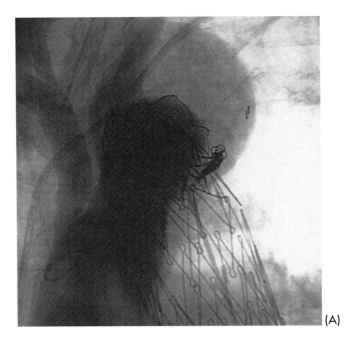

(A)

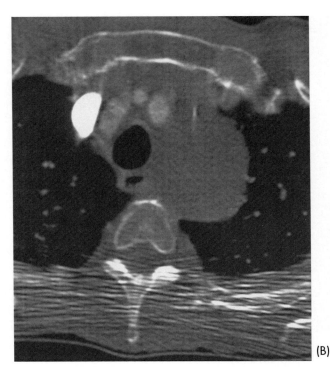

(B)

Figure 41-10   (A) Thoracic arteriogram following coil embolization of the leak tract, with successful exclusion of flow to the aneurysm. A single coil is also seen within the thrombosed aneurysm. (B) Contrast-enhanced CT scan demonstrates complete thrombosis of the aortic arch aneurysm after coil embolization of the leaking tract.

as commercially produced covered stent-grafts and deployment systems for treatment of aortic aneurysms are introduced.

The procedure itself demands both surgical and interventional skills. As stated above, many of our stent-grafts have required extensive endovascular manipulations. These procedures should be undertaken only by individuals with considerable experience in catheter manipulation techniques. At Stanford, interventional radiologists and vascular surgeons act as a team. We have found that this combined approach maximizes the chances of a successful procedure.

Though the ultimate safety and efficacy of this alternative therapy can be determined only by further long-term follow-up, our initial results suggest that endovascular stent-graft treatment of thoracic aortic aneurysm is a promising therapeutic alternative to extensive surgery in clinically challenging patients.

REFERENCES

1. Najafi H, Javid H, Hunter J, et al. An update of treatment of the descending thoracic aorta. *World J Surg* 1980;4:553–561.
2. Pressler V, McNamara J. Thoracic aortic aneurysm: natural history and treatment. *J Thoracic Cardiovasc Surg* 1980;79:489–498.
3. Joyce J, Fairbairn JI, Kincaid O, et al. Aneurysms of the thoracic aorta: a clinical study with special reference to prognosis. *Circulation* 1964;29:176–181.
4. DeBakey M, McCollum C, Graham J. Surgical treatment of aneurysms of the descending thoracic aorta: long term results in five hundred patients. *J Cardiovasc Surg* 1978;19:571–576.
5. McNamara J, Pressler V. Natural history of arteriosclerotic thoracic aortic aneurysms. *Ann Thorac Surg* 1978;26:468–472.
6. Bickerstaff L, Pairolero P, Hollier L, et al., Thoracic aortic aneurysms: a population-based study. *Surgery* 1982; 92:1103–1108.
7. Connolly J, Wakabayashi A, German J, et al. Clinical experience with pusatile left heart bypass without anticoagulation for thoracic aneurysms. *J Thorac Cardiovasc Surg* 1971;62:568–576.
8. Crawford E, Rubio P. Reappraisal of adjuncts to avoid ischemia in the treatment of aneurysms of the descending thoracic aorta. *J Thorac Cardiovasc Surg* 1973;66:693–704.
9. Carlson D, Karp R, Kouchoukos N. Surgical treatment of aneurysms of the descending thoracic aorta: an analysis of 85 patients. *Ann Thorac Surg* 1983;35:58–69.
10. Moreno-Cabral C, Miller D, Mitchell R, et al. Degenerative and atherosclerotic aneurysms of the thoracic aorta: determinants of early and late surgical outcome. *J Thorac Cardiovasc Surg* 1984;88:1020–1032.
11. Dotter C. Transluminally placed coilspring endarterial tube grafts: long-term patency in canine popliteal artery. *Invest Radiol* 1969;4:329–332.
12. Blako A, Piasecki G, Shah D, et al. Transfemoral placement of intraluminal polyurethane prosthesis for abdominal aortic aneurysm. *J Surg Res* 1986;40:305–309.
13. Lawrence DJ, Chansangavej C, Wright K, et al. Percutaneous endovascular graft: experimental evaluation. *Radiology* 1987;163:357–360.

14. Yoshioka T, Wright K, Wallace S, et al. self-expanding endovascular graft: an experimental study in dogs. *AJR* 1988;151:673–676.
15. Mirich D, Wright K, Wallace S, et al. Percutaneously placed endovascular grafts for aortic aneurysms: feasibility study. *Radiology* 1989;170:1033–1037.
16. Parodi J, Palmaz J, Barone H. Transfemoral intraluminal graft implantation for abdominal aortic aneurysms. *Ann Vasc Surg* 1991;5:491–499.
17. Laborde J, Parodi J, Clem M, et al. Intraluminal bypass of abdominal aortic aneurysm: feasibility study. *Radiology* 1992;184:185–190.
18. Marin M, Veith F, Panetta T, et al. Percutaneous transfemoral insertion of a stented graft to repair a traumatic femoral arteriovenous fistula. *J Vasc Surg* 1993;18:299–302.
19. May J, White G, Waugh R, et al. Transluminal placement of a prosthetic graft-stent device for treatment of subclavian artery aneurysms. *J Vasc Surg* 1993;18:1056–1059.
20. Cragg A, Dake M. Percutaneous femoropopliteal graft placement. *Radiology* 1993;187:643–648.
21. Chuter T, Green R, Ouriel K, et al. Transfemoral endovascular aortic graft placement. *J Vasc Surg* 1993;18:185–197.
22. Dake M, Miller D, Semba C, et al. Transluminal placement of endovascular stent-grafts for the treatment of descending thoracic aortic aneurysms. *N Engl J Med* 1994;331:1729–1734.
23. Fann J, Dake M, Semba C, et al. Endovascular stent-grafting after arch aneurysm repair using the "Elephant Trunk." *Ann Thorac Surg* 1995;60:1102–1105.
24. Mitchell RS, Dake MD, Semba CP, et al. Emdovascular stent-graft repair of thoracic aortic aneurysms. *J Thorac Cardiovasc Surg* 1996;III:1054–1062.

42

Thrombolytic Therapy for Iliofemoral Deep Vein Thrombosis: Catheter-Directed Techniques

Charles P. Semba, M.D.
Michael D. Dake, M.D.

In recent years, significant advances have been achieved in the approach to the patient with extensive lower extremity deep venous thrombosis (DVT). Noninvasive diagnosis using color flow Doppler or magnetic resonance angiography has replaced conventional ascending venography, and new treatment algorithms using low molecular weight heparin have been introduced that may eliminate the need for hospitalization during the initial period of anticoagulation.[1–3] Despite these achievements, patients with iliofemoral DVT remain challenging for the clinician. Though anticoagulation is the primary treatment for DVT, aggressive therapy using endovascular techniques is rapidly emerging as an alternative method for patients with extensive, high-risk iliofemoral DVT in which anticoagulation therapy alone is insufficient. The purpose of this chapter is to outline the role of catheter-directed thrombolytic therapy in patients with iliofemoral DVT.

ILIOFEMORAL DVT: DEFINING THE PROBLEM

Many physicians view the workup of DVT as an all-or-nothing phenomenon. The diagnostic emphasis is on determining the presence or absence of DVT, with generally little regard for the location, length, and extent of the venous obstruction. The patient with a short-segment popliteal DVT is treated similarly to the patient with massive iliofemoral DVT—anticoagulation with heparin followed by oral warfarin. Because the long-term disability due to postphlebitic syndrome takes years to develop, the clinical management of DVT is strongly biased toward prevention of pulmonary emboli. DVT has a spectrum of severity and risk. The patients at highest risk for developing long-term sequelae from postphlebitic syndrome have iliofemoral DVT.[4,5]

Postphlebitic syndrome is due to chronic ambulatory venous hypertension. It consists of chronic leg edema, hyperpigmentation, venous claudication, and, in advanced cases, venous stasis ulcers.[6,7] Ambulatory venous hypertension is caused by venous obstruction, valvular incompetence, or both.[8] The natural history of iliofemoral DVT treated with adequate long-term anticoagulation is striking, with significant socioeconomic consequences. O'Donnell et al followed a group of 24 patients with iliofemoral DVT treated with anticoagulation therapy over a 10-year period. Fifty percent of these patients developed venous claudication and job disability, 86% developed venous stasis ulcers, 95% lost valvular competency, and all of them had chronic leg edema.[4,9] Furthermore, these patients had an increased need for health care services. They averaged eight clinic visits per year and five hospitalizations over the 10-year period due to problems related to the care of their chronic venous disease.

Another major misconception among treating physicians is that "thinning the blood" helps to dissolve thrombus. Anticoagulation does not promote thrombolysis. Anticoagulation is merely prophylactic, preventing further thrombus propagation. In patients who are anticoagulated appropriately, less than 10% resolve their DVT within 10 days of therapy and up to 40% continue to propagate the thrombus despite adequate heparinization.[10,11]

The benefits and superiority of thrombolytic agents over heparin have been known for the past 25 years.[12,13] A retrospective meta-analysis of 13 major clinical trials involving over 600 patients, comparing systemic streptokinase with heparin, have clearly demonstrated the clinical benefits of lytic therapy.[14] The heparin group had a complete thrombolysis rate of only 4% versus 45% for the streptokinase group. However, in the setting of long-segment iliofemoral DVT, systemic infusion of lytic agents is ineffective in dissolving thrombus.[15]

RATIONALE FOR CATHETER-DIRECTED THROMBOLYSIS

While anticoagulation therapy has been the standard of care for the past 40 years in managing DVT, it is our opinion that high-risk iliofemoral DVT should be treated more aggressively, using endovascular techniques to reduce or eliminate the potential for developing irreversible chronic venous disease. Though systemic thrombolysis is better than heparin in restoring vessel patency, it is relatively inefficient because the majority of the infused dose is drained through venous collaterals instead of within the obstructing thrombus. Streptokinase is not the optimal lytic agent because of its immunogenicity, which leads to drug fevers, an antibody response that reduces its effectiveness over time, and significant hemorrrhagic complications.[16,17] Catheter-directed techniques involving urokinase have been used extensively for the treatment of upper-extremity DVT and for arterial thrombus for decades, with excellent records of safety and efficacy.[18–20]

The goals of catheter-directed therapy are to improve the efficiency of drug delivery to the thrombus, reduce the potential for secondary bleeding complications by minimizing systemic fibrinolysis, and allow for adjunctive endovascular therapies such as angioplasty and stent placement.[21–23] For iliofemoral DVT, the long-term sequelae can be eliminated if the obstructing thrombus is removed and valve integrity ir preserved by avoiding ambulatory venous hypertension.

CATHETER-DIRECTED THROMBOLYSIS: PATIENT SELECTION AND TECHNIQUE

Because the goal of therapy is to reduce the risk of chronic venous hypertension, we prefer to treat active, ambulatory patients who have documented iliofemoral DVT and are acutely (≤10 days) symptomatic, with leg edema and pain. Therapy is contraindicated if patients have one or more of the following: contraindications for anticoagulation, a recent history of hemorrhagic stroke (≤1 year), generalized metastatic disease with central nervous system involvement, pregnancy, coagulopathic disorders, or septic thrombophlebitis. Thrombolytic therapy in the postoperative period is a relative

contraindication, depending on the nature and type of the surgical intervention. In general, we do not recommend catheter-directed therapy within 10 days of surgery. In addition, the patient's quality of life must be considered. We do not recommend therapy for patients who have limited ambulation and thus are at low risk of developing ambulatory venous hypertension (eg, paraplegic patients who are wheelchair bound) unless the limb is threatened due to phlegmasia.[24]

The entire procedure is performed in the angiographic suite (Fig. 42–1). Initially, a Foley urinary catheter is placed and the patient is then positioned prone. The popliteal fossa of the affected extremity is prepared and draped in a sterile manner and the popliteal vein is localized using ultrasound. A small, portable ultrasound unit (Site-Rite; Dymax Inc., Pittsburgh, PA) equipped with a 5- to 7-MHz probe is used. A micropuncture needle set is used (Cook, Inc., Bloomington, IN), which contains a 21-gauge needle, a 0.018-inch guidewire, and a No. 5 Fr. dilator, and meticulous technique must be applied to avoid errant puncture of the popliteal artery. If the vein is thrombosed, attention must be paid to the needle tip within the lumen of the hypoechoic vein. A small amount of iodinated contrast material is injected to confirm the needle position prior to probing the clot with the 0.018-inch wire. Following placement of the No. 5 Fr. dilator, an ascending venogram is performed. The thrombus is then probed with 0.035-inch hydrophilic guidewire (Terumo; Boston Scientific, Inc., Watertown, MA) and a No. 6 Fr. sheath is inserted. Occasionally, a hydrophilic catheter (Glidecath; Boston Scientific, Inc.) is needed to navigate the thrombus.

Similar to endovascular thrombolytic techniques in the arterial circulation, coaxial thrombolysis systems or multi-side-hole catheters can be used to infuse the thrombus. We generally prefer to use a valve-tipped, multi-side-hole catheter (Cragg-McNamara infusion catheter; Microtherapeutics, Inc., Ventura, CA) and embed the catheter approximately two-thirds of the way into the thrombus. The popliteal access sheath is usually embedded in the caudal portion of the thrombus, and we often create multiple side holes in the venous portion of the sheath and infuse urokinase through both the sheath and the multi-side-hole catheter.

Urokinase (Abbokinase; Abbott Laboratories, Abbott Park, IL) is manufactured in 250,000-IU vials and is reconstituted using 10 mL of sterile water. Reconstituted urokinase is added to a 250-mL IV bag of normal saline (NS) (500,000 IU urokinase/250 mL NS). Most cases involve two IV bags of urokinase (2000 IU urokinase/mL) and three automated IV pumps (Valley Lab, Boulder, CO). One urokinase pump is connected to the multi-side-hole catheter, and the other urokinase pump is connected to the sheath. The third pump is used for systemic anticoagulation therapy

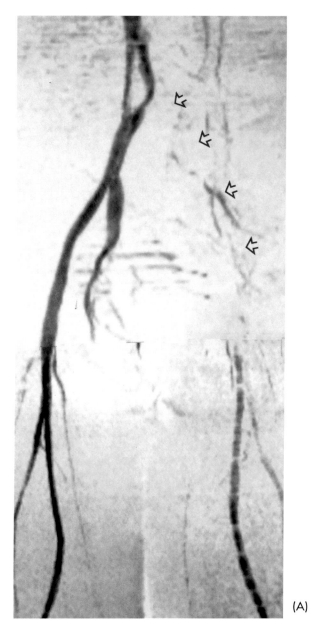

(A)

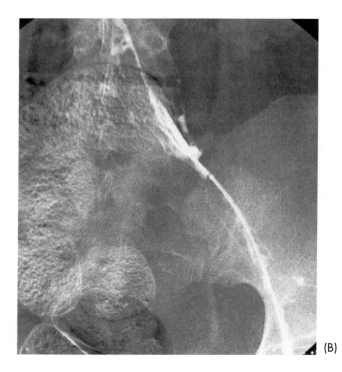

(B)

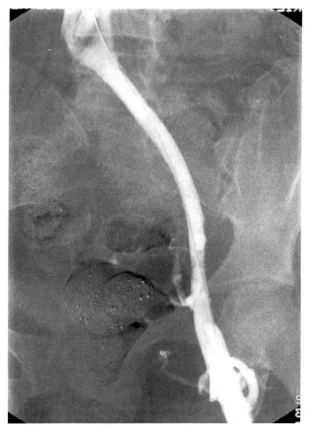

(C)

Figure 42–1. A 28-year-old woman with acute left leg swelling and pain underwent (A) a magnetic resonance venography, which demonstrated a patent left femoral-popliteal vein and thrombosis of the left iliac vein (open arrow). The right leg is clinically normal, however, a non-occlusive thrombus is present at the caval bifurcation (dark arrow). Through a popliteal approach (B) a multi-side-hole catheter was placed in the iliac vein; contrast venography confirms the presence of occlusive thrombus. Following 72 hours of continuous infusion thrombolysis with urokinase (C), patency of the vein was fully restored after adjunctive angioplasty and deployment of a self-expanding Wallstent in the common iliac vein. The patient's leg thigh edema and pain resolved. (Courtesy of Richard Hoffman, M.D., Torrance, CA)

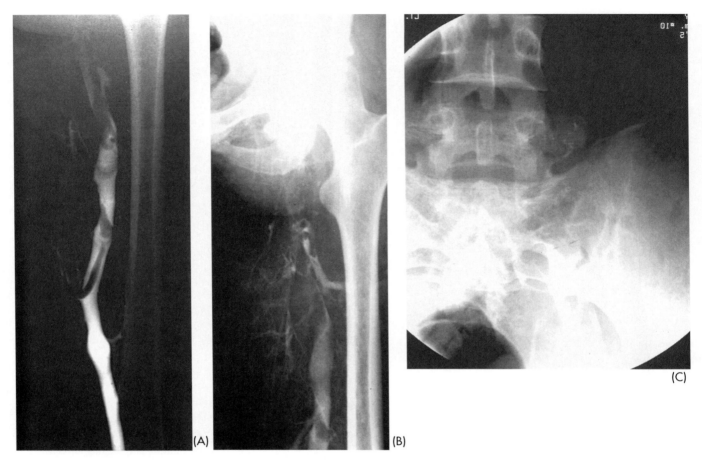

Figure 42–2. A 24-year-old woman with a two-day history of progressive left leg edema and pain. (A) Popliteal venography revealed acute thrombus in the distal and midsuperficial femoral vein, which led to (B) complete occlusion of the common femoral and (C), iliac veins.

through a peripheral IV following an intravenous bolus of 5000 units of unfractionated heparin. Typical urokinase infusions are between 100,000 and 200,000 IU/hr (eg, 80,000 IU through the sheath and 80,000 IU through the catheter, for a total infused dose of 160,000 IU urokinase/per hour). We have found the popliteal approach to be much simpler to perform because shorter catheter lengths are involved (compared to the transjugular approach). There is also less potential for causing damage to the venous valves. Patients are more comfortable, and can sit upright in bed and have limited ambulation.

The popliteal lines and sheath are secured in place, and the patient is transferred to a cardiac step-down unit rather than the intensive care unit. The partial thromboplastin time (PTT) and fibrinogen level are monitored every 8 hours and maintained between 60 and 90 seconds and >100mg/dL, respectively. Whenever possible, the patient also receives the first oral dose of warfarin (10 mg PO) on the evening of the first day of intervention (target (INR) international normalized ratio = 2.0 and 3.0).

The patient is brought back to the angiography suite the following day for repeat venography. If there is complete lysis and no underlying venous stenosis, the procedure is terminated (Fig. 42–2). Intravenous heparin is maintained through the popliteal sheath to bathe the treated venous segment until the INR is therapeutic on oral warfarin. The sheath can be safely removed, with minimal risk of a hematoma, due to the low pressure of the popliteal venous flow.

If the venogram demonstrates complete lysis and an underlying venous stenosis of the iliac vein, the lesion is treated using angioplasty and stents. Rarely is angioplasty a stand-alone technique. For iliac vein stenoses, we favor using longitudinally flexible Wallstents (Schneider, Inc., Plymouth, MN) using diameters of at least 10 mm (range, 10 to 20 mm). Venous stenting below the inguinal ligament is not recommended due to premature occlusion from intimal hyperplasia.

If there is no appreciable lysis on the follow-up venogram, we then proceed directly to endovascular reconstruction of the chronically occluded iliac vein only if there is sufficient inflow from the superficial femoral,

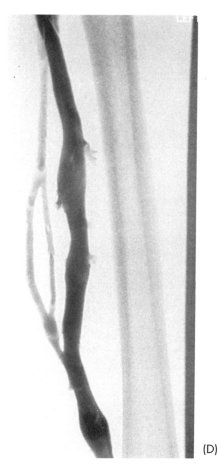
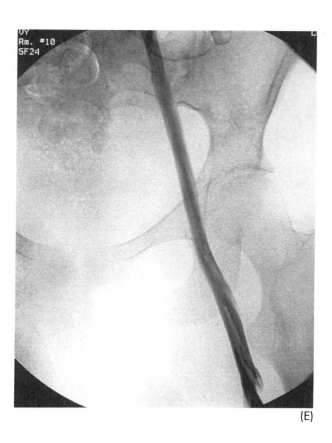

Figure 42–2 *(cont)*   Following overnight catheter-directed infusion of the thrombus with urokinase (D), there was complete restoration of patency of the superficial femoral and (E) iliofemoral outflow. At 1 year of follow-up she remained asymptomatic, with preservation of valve function and venous patency.

profunda, and saphenous veins. In our experience, stenting of the iliac vein in the presence of chronic occlusion of the inflow veins is not recommended due to a high rate of immediate rethrombosis of the iliac vein stents.

After completion of thrombolytic therapy, the patient undergoes regular surveillance using Doppler at 3, 6, and 12 months and annually thereafter. We document the patency of the vein and evaluate for the presence of valvular insufficiency. Patients also remain on warfarin therapy for a minimum of 6 months.

Prophylactic placement of inferior vena cava filters is not recommended unless the patient meets the traditional criterion for filter placement or a free-floating thrombus is identified in the iliac vein.

RESULTS

For treatment of acute iliofemoral DVT, we have achieved a complete or partial thrombolysis rate of 85% (Tables 42–1 and 42–2).[25] Many patients have an underlying iliac lesion that may require further intervention. Long-term patency rates are excellent in patients with

nonmalignant iliofemoral DVT (>90% at 1 year). Patients with iliac vein compression syndrome (May-Thurner syndrome) also have an excellent prognosis following angioplasty and stent placement provided that the infrainguinal venous inflow is normal.[26,27]

COMPLICATIONS

In our small series, there have been no cases of pulmonary emboli, hemorrhagic stroke, or death. Minor complications include access site hematomas and stent migration during deployment.

CONCLUSION

Because patients with iliofemoral DVT have a high long-term risk of postphlebitic syndrome despite adequate anticoagulation therapy, in our opinion catheter-directed thrombolysis is the treatment of choice. The experiential database gathered through the National Venous Thrombolysis Registry is compelling, showing initial complete and partial lysis rates of over 90%.[28] With the recent enthusiasm for low molecular weight heparin compounds, the long-term

Table 42–1. Presenting Symptoms, Location, and Cause of DVT in 41 Limbs (32 Patients)

	No. of Limbs	
Initial symptoms		
Lower extremity edema	40	(98)
Lower extremity pain	41	(100)
Phlegmasia	4	(10)
Type of symptoms		
Acute*	25	(61)
Chronic†	16	(39)
Location of thrombus		
Left lower extremity	28	(68)
Right lower extremity	13	(32)
IVC, iliac vein	5	(12)
IVC, iliac, femoral veins	11	(27)
Iliac vein	7	(17)
Iliac and femoral veins	18	(44)
Cause		
Retroperitoneal fibrosis	2	(5)
May-Thurner syndrome	2	(5)
Recurrent DVT	3	(7)
Oral contraceptives	3	(7)
Femoral vein catheter	3	(7)
Radiation injury	6	(15)
Postoperative DVT	8	(20)
Unknown	14	(34)

Note: Numbers in parentheses are percentages.
Abbreviation: IVC, inferior vena cava.
*Average duration of acute symptoms was 10.5 days (range, 7–28 days).
†Median duration of chronic symptoms was 270 days (range, 35–5475 days).

Table 42–2. Treatment Outcomes in 41 Limbs (32 Patients) Treated for Iliofemoral DVT

Treatment Outcome	No. of Limbs	
No thrombolysis		
Angioplasty, stent replacement	5	(12)
Thrombolysis		
Complete	21	(12)
No further intervention	8	
Angioplasty	2	
Angioplasty, stent replacement	11	
Partial	9	(22)
No further intervention	1	
Angioplasty, stent replacement	8	
None	2	(5)
No further intervention	1	
Angioplasty, stent replacement	1	
Technical failure		
Occluded vein unable to be crossed with guidewire	4	(10)
No thrombolysis achieved, no further intervention	1	
Partial thrombolysis, no further intervention	1	
Resolution of leg edema and pain		
Complete	33	(80)
Partial	2	(5)
None	6	(15)
Technical success	35	(85)
Clinical success	35	(85)

Note: Numbers in parentheses are percentages.

risk of limb complication of DVT has been virtually ignored. Through a planned future randomized, prospective trial comparing the treatment of iliofemoral DVT with catheter-directed thrombolysis versus anticoagulation, we are optimistic that thrombolytic therapy will prove to be extremely beneficial for the immediate and long-term well-being of the patient.

REFERENCES

1. Geerts WH, Jay RM, Code KI, et al. A comparison of low-dose heparin with low molecular weight heparin as prophylaxis against venous thromboembolism after major trauma. *N Engl J Med* 1996;335:701–707.
2. Bergovist D, Benoni G, Bjorgell O, et al. Low molecular weight heparin (enoxaparin) as prophylaxis against venous thromboembolism after total hip replacement. *N Engl J Med* 1996;335:696–700.
3. Hull R, Raskob G, Pineo G, et al. A comparison of subcutaneous low molecular weight heparin with warfarin sodium for prophylaxis against deep-vein thrombosis after hip or knee implantation. *N Engl J Med* 1993; 329:1370–1376.
4. O'Donnell TF, Browse WL, Burnand KE, Thomas ML. Socioeconomic effects of an iliofemoral deep venous thrombosis. *J Surg Res* 1977;22:483–488.
5. Strandness DE, Langlois YE, Cramer M, et al. Long-term sequelae of acute venous thrombosis. *JAMA* 1983; 250:1289–1292.
6. Shull KC, Nicolaides AN, Fernandes E, et al. Significance of popliteal reflux in relation to ambulatory venous pressure and ulceration. *Arch Surg* 1979;114:1304–1306.
7. Johnson DF, Manzo RA, Bergelin RO, Strandness DE. Relationship between changes in the deep venous system and the development of the postthrombotic syndrome after an acute episode of lower limb deep vein thrombosis: a one to six year follow-up. *J Vasc Surg* 1995;21:307–312.
8. Welkie JF, Comerota AJ, Katz ML, Aldridge SC, Kerr RP, White JV. Hemodynamic deterioration in chronic venous disease. *J Vasc Surg* 1992;16:733–740.
9. Akesson H, Brudin L, Dahlstrom JD, et al. Venous function assessed during a five year period after acute iliofemoral venous thrombosis treated with anticoagulation. *Eur J Vasc Surg* 1990;4:43–48.
10. Sherry S. Thrombolytic therapy for deep venous thrombosis. *Semin Intervent Radiol* 1985;4:331–337.
11. Krupski WC, Bass A, Dilley RB, et al. Propagation of deep venous thrombosis identified by duplex ultrasonography. *J Vasc Surg* 1990;12:467–475.
12. Arnesen H, Hoiseth A, Ly B. Streptokinase or heparin in the treatment of deep vein thrombosis: follow-up results of a prospective study. *Acta Med Scand* 1982;211:65–68.
13. Elliot MS, Immelsman EJ, Jeffrey L, et al. A comparative randomized trial of heparin versus streptokinase in the treatment of acute proximal venous thrombosis: an interim report of a prospective trial. *Br J Surg* 1979; 66:838–843.

14. Comerota AJ, Aldridge S. Thrombolytic therapy for acute deep vein thrombosis. *Semin Vasc Surg* 1992;5:76–81.
15. Hill SL, Martin D, Evans P. Massive vein thrombosis of the extremities. *Am J Surg* 1989;158:131–136.
16. van Breda A, Graor RA, Katzen BT, et al. Relative cost-effectiveness of urokinase versus streptokinase in the treatment of peripheral vascular disease. *J Vasc Intervent Radiol* 1991;2:77–89.
17. Hirsh J. Coronary thrombolysis: hemorrhagic complications. *Can J Cardiol* 1993;9:505–511.
18. McNamara TO, Gardner KR, Bomberger RA, Greaser LE. Clinical and angiographic selection factors for thrombolysis as initial therapy for acute lower limb ischemia. *J Vasc Intervent Radiol* 1995;6:36S–47S.
19. Kandarpa K. Technical determinants of success in catheter-directed thrombolysis for peripheral arterial occlusions. *J Vasc Intervent Radiol* 1995;55S–61S.
20. Crowe MT, Davies CH, Gaines PA. Percutaneous management of superior vena cava occlusions. *Cardiovasc Intervent Radiol* 1995;18:367–372.
21. Semba CP, Dake ML. Iliofemoral deep venous thrombosis: aggressive therapy using catheter-directed thrombolysis. *Radiology* 1994;191:487–494.
22. Okrent D, Messersmith R, Buckman J. Transcatheter fibrinolytic therapy and angioplasty for left iliofemoral venous thrombosis. *J Vasc Intervent Radiol* 1991;2:195–197.
23. Molina JE, Hunter DW, Yedlcika JW. Thrombolytic therapy for iliofemoral venous thrombosis. *Vasc Surg* 1992;26:630–637.
24. Robinson DL, Teitelbaum GP. Phlegmasia cerulea dolens: treatment with pulse-spray and infusion thrombolysis. *AJR* 1993;160:1288–1290.
25. Semba CP, Dake MD. Catheter-directed thrombolysis for iliofemoral venous thrombosis. *Semin Vasc Surg* 1996;9:26–33.
26. Berger A, Jaffe JW, York TN. Iliac compression syndrome treated with stent placement. *J Vasc Surg* 1995;21:510–514.
27. Michel C, Laffy PY, Leblanc G, Bonnet D. Treatment of Cockett syndrome by percutaneous insertion of a vascular endoprosthesis (Gianturco). *J Radiol* 1994;75:327–330. In French.
28. Mewissen M. Report of the National Venous Thrombosis Registry, Monterey, CA, October 12, 1996.

43

Ultrasound-Guided Compression of Iatrogenic Femoral Pseudoaneurysms: Indications and Results

Anne C. Roberts, M.D.

A pseudoaneurysm is an extraluminal cavity that occurs after injury to all the layers of the arterial wall. Unlike a true aneurysm, a pseudoaneurysm has no arterial wall lining. Unlike a hematoma, the pseudoaneurysm has a communication with the arterial circulation, with pulsatile flow between the cavity and the artery. Diagnosis of pseudoaneurysms has been difficult because of problems in differentiating between a hematoma that pulsates due to transmitted pulsation from the adjacent artery and a pseudoaneurysm. Pseudoaneurysms have been called "pulsatile hematomas," which indicates the diagnostic difficulty. Accurate diagnosis of these injuries can now be made noninvasively with duplex sonography and color flow imaging.[1,2] The color flow ultrasound image shows a very characteristic image of to-and-fro flow within the cavity. (Fig. 43–1).

Pseudoaneurysms have a number of causes, including penetrating and blunt trauma, iatrogenic injury, complications of arterial reconstruction, and infection. When discussing ultrasound-guided compression repair of pseudoaneurysms, one should understand that the pseudoaneurysms are due to iatrogenic injury, usually resulting from a catheterization procedure.

Until recently, postcatheterization femoral artery pseudoaneurysms or arteriovenous fistulas were rare, with a reported incidence of about 0.02%.[3] With the increasing sizes of percutaneous catheters and sheaths and the increasing use of periprocedural heparin, urokinase, tissue plasminogen activator (tPA), and other anticoagulation measures, there appears to be an increase in the frequency of such complications. One recent study found that over a 33-month period with almost 9500 femoral artery catheterizations, there were 89 femoral artery injuries (0.9%).[4] A study of cardiac catheterization procedures with 5042 patients found an incidence of groin complications of 6.1%; of these, 3.8% required vascular repair.[5] Many of these patients had undergone procedures with newer devices such as atherectomy, laser angioplasty, and stenting. Among the patients undergoing procedures with new devices, there was significant increase in the rate of vascular complications (10.0%) and vascular repair (6.0%) compared with balloon angioplasty (5.3% and 1.6%, respectively).[5] Coronary stent procedures have the greatest number of vascular complications, 16% in one study.[6] Another study looked prospectively at the incidence of pseudoaneurysm complicating percutaneous transluminal angioplasty (PTA), PTA with local lysis, or diagnostic angiography.[7] This study included 565 patients with 581 procedures. The incidence of pseudoaneurysm formation was 7.7%, and the size of the pseudoaneurysms ranged from $5 \times 5 \times 5$ mm to $40 \times 30 \times 25$ mm (mean, $15 \times 12 \times 10$ mm). Interestingly, only two patients were clinically symptomatic.[7] This study found that obesity and anticoagulation were associated with a significantly higher ($p < 0.05$) rate of pseudoaneurysm formation. Other ultrasound studies of suspected pseudoaneurysms have found an incidence of 1 to 6%.[7] Some of the increased prevalence may be attributed to the more common use of ultrasound examinations, which lead to earlier evaluation of patients with groin hematomas following catheterization.[8] Studies have reported risk factors for the development of pseudoaneurysms including increasing age, female gender, hypertension, obesity, thrombolytic therapy, postprocedure anticoagulation, catheter size larger than No. 8 French, and intracoronary stenting.[4,7,9–11]

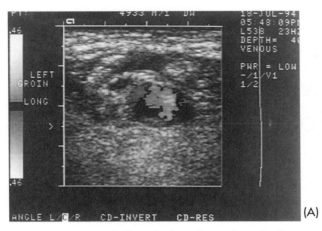
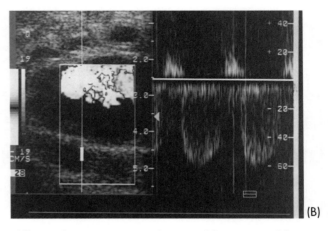

Figure 43–1. (A) Black-and-white photo of a color flow image. The different densities represent the to-and-fro pattern of the turbulent flow within the pseudoaneurysm. (B) Duplex scan of the pseudoaneurysm, with the Doppler waveforms demonstrating graphically the turbulent to-and-fro blood flow.

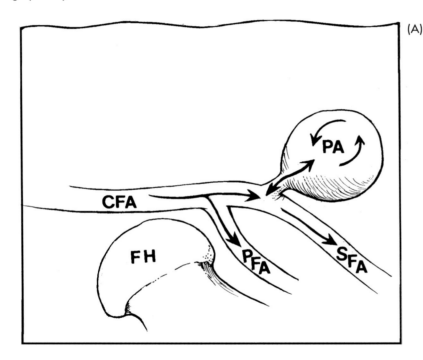

Figure 43–2. (A) Pseudoaneurysm arising from the superficial femoral artery. This is a common site of pseudoaneurysms, probably due to the difficulty in obtaining good compression during the initial puncture compression. This is unlike the common femoral artery, which allows compression to be applied against the femoral head.

Long-term sequelae of pseudoaneurysms include pain, infection, progressive enlargement, arterial thrombosis, peripheral embolization, venous and neurologic compression, and rupture. Once the diagnosis is established, the standard treatment is open surgical repair of the arterial defect. Surgical repair is very effective in repairing pseudoaneurysms, but surgical procedures have a varied incidence of complications (1.4 to 30%),[12] including wound infections, seromas, leg edema, venous and arterial thrombosis, femoral neuralgia, and, rarely, myocardial infarction and death.[5,11,13] In addition, the surgical repair usually requires several days of postoperative inpatient recovery.[13]

After observing the color flow features of several pseudoaneurysms with ultrasound, radiologists realized that applying pressure over the extraluminal track until blood flow was eliminated might seal the track.[14] This is identical to the blind manual compression routinely employed to close the arterial puncture after angiography, except that real-time color flow sonography is used to determine the location and the intensity of compression.

TECHNIQUE

All patients with sonographically demonstrated pseudoaneurysms are considered candidates for ultrasound-guided compression repair (UGCR). Contraindications to UGCR include suspected infection, coexisting very large hematomas with impending com-

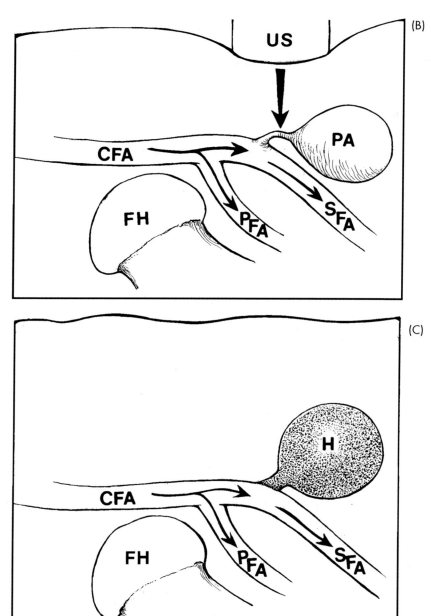

Figure 43–2 *(cont.)*   (B) Compression applied by the ultrasound transducer, with decreased caliber of the track and elimination of flow into the pseudoaneurysm. There is continued blood flow through the arteries. (C) With successful compression, the track and pseudoaneurysm are thrombosed. The pseudoaneurysm now appears as a hematoma. There continues to be normal flow in the arteries. CFA, common femoral artery; SFA, superficial femoral artery; PFA, profunda femoral artery; PA, pseudoaneurysm; FH, femoral head; US, ultrasound transducer; H, hematoma.

partment syndrome or overlying skin ischemia, high injuries above or near the inguinal ligament where delayed rupture could be catastrophic, and severe groin tenderness precluding adequate compression.

Informed consent is obtained before treatment. The most important complications the patient should be aware of are possible thrombosis of the femoral artery and/or distal embolization; both eventualities may require surgical therapy. The possibility that the procedure may not be successful, which would then mandate a surgical repair, should also be discussed with the patient.

The groin is scanned, keeping the transducer perfectly vertical. A longitudinal, cross-sectional, or oblique projection is selected, depending on which best visualizes the narrow track of flow that connects the arterial lumen to the pseudoaneurysm of the arteriovenous fistula. The transducer is then positioned so the track is centered in the color flow image, and straight downward force is applied with the transducer until flow through the track is eliminated (Fig. 43–2). This position is maintained for 20 minutes (30 minutes in anticoagulated patients), after which compression is slowly released. If sonography demonstrates persistent extralu-

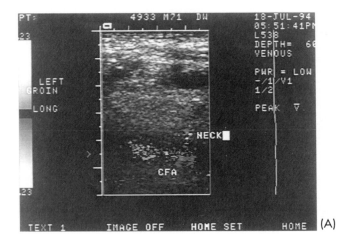 (A)

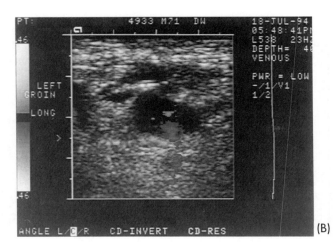 (B)

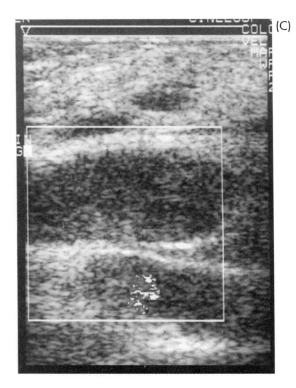 (C)

Figure 43–3. (A) The ultrasound image shows the flow within the common femoral artery (CFA) and the flow within the neck or track of the pseudoaneurysm. The flow in the pseudoaneurysm is not seen because of the transducer's position. (B) The transducer has been moved slightly, and now the flow is demonstrated entering the pseudoaneurysm, with a small portion of the track seen just below the pseudoaneurysm. In performing compression, the most important area to compress is the track of the pseudoaneurysm. If the track is thrombosed, the pseudoaneurysm will also become thrombosed. (C) Image of the pseudoaneurysm following successful compression. Flow remains in the common femoral artery below the pseudoaneurysm. No flow is demonstrated in the pseudoaneurysm, which now appears as a echogenic area, or hematoma.

minal color flow on gradual release, compression is immediately reapplied and held for an additional 20 minutes. Commonly, as the compression is released, echogenic material appears within the pseudoaneurysm. This is a very positive sign and portends success; compression should immediately be reapplied and held for 10 to 15 minutes. Usually at the end of this compression cycle, complete thrombosis is achieved. The echogenic material undoubtedly represents some intracavitary thrombus within the pseudoaneurysm, and with continued compression this thrombus acts as a nidus for continued thrombosis. Compression cycles are continued until all abnormal flow ceases or operator (or patient) fatique mandates termination. The minimum pressure required to stop the abnormal flow

is used, and patent color flow through the artery beneath is maintained and monitored during UGCR (Fig. 43–3).

Tenderness at the compression site is common. For some patients, once the compression is started and the pressure needed to close the track is achieved, the discomfort is much less intense and is bearable, if not comfortable. For other patients, the pain of the compression is very uncomfortable; these patients benefit from some sedation. Versed and fentanyl given intravenously with appropriate monitoring are very helpful. Other analgesics, such as Demerol and morphine, are alternative medications. Infiltration of local anesthestic is also helpful in decreasing pain at the site.

After successful closure, the patient is placed at bed rest, with the affected leg straight for 6 hours. Anticoagulation is withheld if clinically feasible. A follow-up scan should be performed in 24 to 72 hours to confirm closure, after which the patient is followed clinically.

Although most of the compressions performed in our institution are done with manual compression of the pseudoaneurysm track, there have been several reports of UGCR with a variety of devices to maintain pressure, thus conserving the operator's strength. These devices include a C-clamp[15,16] and a commercially market device, the Femostop (Bard, Billerica, MA).[17,18] The Femostop is quite appealing for this application. The device consists of a plastic "pressure arch" that is positioned over the groin and held in place by a belt that passes around the patient. The arch contains a "pressure bubble" that can be filled with saline. As the saline fills the bubble, the bubble expands and exerts pressure on the neck of the pseudoaneurysm. The amount of pressure and its effect on the artery can be evaluated by placing the ultrasound probe directly over the water-filled compression device for direct visualization of the arterial flow.

RESULTS

The overall success rate of UGCR was 74% in our initial study. If only the cases in which compression was technically feasible are considered, the success rate was 90%.[14]

In a later and larger study, there were 133 patients with pseudoaneurysms.[3] Of those, seven were not candidates for compression because of skin ischemia, infection, or spontaneous thrombosis. Other cases that were technically not feasible involved patients with severe pain precluding adequate compression, marked obesity, very large hematomas precluding adequate compression, and those in whom the force of adequate compression caused occlusion of the underlying femoral artery. There were 117 patients in whom compression was successfully attempted. The initial success rate was 86%. Of the 18 initial patients who failed, 14 were brought back for an additional attempt at UGCR; only 1 of these required subsequent surgery. In 3 patients the pseudoaneurysm spontaneously thrombosed, and the other 10 were successfully treated. Eight of these patients had been taken off anticoagulation. Thus among the patients who could be compressed, 86% were successful, and among the patients who were candidates for therapy, the success rate was 82%.

Compression times ranged from 10 to 300 minutes, with a majority of the compressions requiring less than 40 minutes. In a few patients an experimental compression device was used; some of the exceptionally long compressions involved this device.

Anticoagulation does affect the success of this therapy. Anticoagulation data were available on 112 patients. Of these, 37 (33%) were anticoagulated at the time of compression. Of the 18 patients in whom UGCR initially failed, 14 were receiving anticoagulation. The initial failure rate in patients on anticoagulants was 38%. However, 62% of the anticoagulated patients were treated successfully. Another study, by Dean et al,[19] was even more successful, with 73% of the patients who were anticoagulated at the time of compression being successful treated.

Other characteristics of the pseudoaneurysm that seem to be important are the size and nature of the pseudoaneurysm. There was a relationship, although not a statistically significant one, between pseudoaneurysm size and the success of UGCR. Compression of pseudoaneurysms smaller than 4 cm was more successful than compression of larger pseudoaneurysms. The nature of the pseudoaneurysm, that is, whether it was unilocular or multiloculated, was not significantly different in terms of success but was important in terms of the time required for compression. As might be expected, multiloculated pseudoaneurysms required a longer compression time.

These results have been duplicated in other reports,[7,19,20] with some 400 cases in the literature and a consensus that more than 90% of pseudoaneurysms can be successfully thrombosed with negligible complications.[21] Ultrasound-guided compression repair has become an accepted first-line therapy for catheter-related pseudoaneurysms.

COMPLICATIONS

There was one major complication in our series. One patient had a combination of an arteriovenous fistula and a pseudoaneurysm that was present for 3 months following the removal of a large-gauge, double-lumen femoral venous dialysis catheter. Despite the concern that the involved track would be lined with nonthrombogenic endothelium, UGCR was attempted. Very high transducer pressure was needed to close the track, and although femoral artery patency could not be maintained, UGCR was applied for 50 minutes. The pseudoaneurysm was successfully closed, but the fistula persisted. Twenty minutes after the procedure, coolness and paresthesia of the calf occurred. Angiography revealed thrombus in the distal femoral artery, which was successfully lysed with transcatheter urokinase. The fistula was then surgically repaired. This thrombus likely formed because of stagnation from excessive compression of the femoral artery. After experiencing the above complication, we believe that the inability to maintain patent femoral artery flow during UGCR is a contraindication to this procedure. Other groups do not believe as strongly that the maintenance of femoral artery blood flow is an absolute requirement.[12,22] It may be that a short period of complete compression does not lead to thrombosis. This is particularly true in patients who are anticoagulated. Other complications that have been reported are pseudoaneurysm rupture and femoral vein thrombosis.

The success of this procedure depends on the thrombogenicity of the wall of the track from the artery through the tissues. Compression temporarily eliminates the blood flow that inhibits thrombosis, facilitating formation of a hemostatic plug and thus converting the injury into a simple hematoma. We assumed that long-standing injuries would be more resistant to UGCR due to the development of endothelium and decreased thrombogenicity of the track walls. However, in our study, the success rate was the same whether the pseudoaneurysms existed for 21 days or more or for 5 or fewer days (89% vs 88%, respectively).

Recurrences were rare. Pseudoaneurysm recurred in four patients (3.7%), in three within 24 hours and in one within 72 hours. Three were recompressed successfully. The fourth patient had undergone repeat cardiac catheterization the day following the compression. This patient was treated with urokinase, heparin, Dextran, and continued anticoagulation. Repeat UGCR was attempted with the patient anticoagulated, but without success. There were no late recurrences.

This rate of complications compares favorably to the rate given in surgical reports. In one report, minor complications included wound infections treated with antibiotics in 13% of patients, mild ankle edema in 13%, and femoral neuralgia in 6%. One major complication of a postoperative myocardial infarction (3%) was reported.[13]

CONCLUSION

Our experience leads us to believe that UGCR should be the first-line therapy for patients with catheter-associated pseudoaneurysms. Unsuccessful UGCR in no way hinders subsequent surgical repair if necessary. Because an ultrasound study is the best way to confirm the diagnosis of pseudoaneurysm, an on-the-spot repair is extremely cost effective. Morbidity is limited the discomfort of compression of a tender groin and the very low likelihood of thrombosis of the femoral artery.

Small pseudoaneurysms may and do close spontaneously, as occurred in some of our cases.[7,23–25] However, pseudoaneurysms may also increase in size,[16] requiring emergency surgery, and occasionally rupture. An attempt has been made to develop color Doppler ultrasound criteria to determine which pseudoaneurysms are likely to thrombose spontaneously. The only criterion that appeared to reach statistical significance was the volume of flow in the pseudoaneurysm. The volume of flow in pseudoaneurysms that thrombosed spontaneously was smaller than the volume of flow of those treated surgically. No other criteria, such as volume, length of the pseudoaneurysm neck, or percentage of flow, were predictive of spontaneous thrombosis.[24] Because of this uncertainty, we believe that an attempt at UGCR is justified in all patients who do not have contraindications to the procedure. Clinical follow-up of such patients may result in continued hospitalization, multiple office visits, and repeated ultrasound evaluations to assess the status of the pseudoaneurysm. UGCR may very well be quite cost effective compared to continued follow-up.

If possible, anticoagulation should be withheld prior to UGCR. Our experience,[3] as well as other reports,[12,22,26] suggests that compression is more effective when the patient is not anticoagulated. However, if anticoagulation cannot be discontinued, then our experience, along with others,[19] indicates that successful thrombosis can be achieved even with patients who are fully anticoagulated at the time of compression.

Other percutaneous methods have been used to close pseudoaneurysms. Direct intracavitary injection of thrombin,[27] injection of bucrylate,[28] and transcatheter embolization of pseudoaneurysms have been reported.[29]

UGCR of pseudoaneurysms in arteries other than the femoral artery has been performed both by ourselves and by others. Brachial artery pseudoaneurysms have been repaired utilizing UGCR.[19,30] These injuries should be carefully assessed so that the ones treated by this method are appropriate for such therapy.

We continue to advocate surgical treatment in patients who have extreme tenderness precluding compression or associated clinical findings that mandate surgery anyway, such as infection, a very large or tense hematoma, or critical leg ischemia that requires surgical reconstruction. A rapidly enlarging mass could be a pseudoaneurysm that is prone to rupture or may be due to infection. Pseudoaneurysms can become infected secondarily, but pseudoaneurysms developing in response to infection may occur following surgery or injection of illicit medications.[31,32] Infected pseudoaneurysms should not be treated with UGCR. Patients with hematomas causing neurologic compromise should be treated with surgical repair and drainage of the hematoma. Defects high in the common femoral artery should also be considered a contraindication because of the risk of an uncontrolled rupture into the retroperitoneum demanding a prompt, definitive surgical repair. Injuries that cannot be compressed without also occluding the underlying artery are contraindicated because of the risk of thrombus forming in the arterial lumen.

In the future, the incidence of pseudoaneurysms may decrease with the development of the various mechanical plugs that have been created. These devices have been touted as a way of both shortening the compression times required to achieve hemostasis and reducing arterial complications such as pseudoaneurysms.[33,34] Although such devices have been approved for marketing in the United States, they are not in widespread use at this time.

As more invasive endovascular procedures are performed, with concomitant use of anticoagulation and thrombolytic medications, a significant number of iatrogenic injuries will occur. A majority of these injuries will be pseudoaneurysms. UGCR offers a minimally invasive method of treating these pseudoaneurysms. The technique is safe and effective, has no long-term complications, and appears to be cost effective. It is the first choice for the treatment of iatrogenic femoral artery pseudoaneurysms.

REFERENCES

1. Fitzgerald E, Bowsher W, Ruttley M. False aneurysm of the femoral artery: computed tomographic and ultrasound appearances. *Clin Radiol* 1986;37:585–588.

2. Sacks D, Robinson M, Perlmutter G. Femoral artery injury following catheterization. *J Ultrasound Med* 1989;8:241–246.

3. Coley BD, Roberts AC, Fellmeth BD, et al. Postangiographic femoral artery pseudoaneurysms: further experience with US-guided compression repair. *Radiology* 1995;194(2):307–311.

4. Waksman R, King SBR, Douglas JS, et al. Predictors of groin complications after balloon and new-device coronary intervention. *Am J Cardiol* 1995;75(14):886–889.

5. Lumsden AB, Miller JM, Kosinski AS, et al. A prospective evaluation of surgically treated groin complications following percutaneous cardiac procedures. *Am Surg* 1994;60(2):132–137.

6. Katzenschlager R, Ugurluoglu A, Ahmadi A, et al. Incidence of pseudoaneurysm after diagnostic and therapeutic angiography. *Radiology* 1995;195(2):463–464.

7. Kresowik T, Khoury M, Miller B, et al. A prospective study of the incidence and natural history of femoral vascular complications. *J Vasc Surg* 1991;13:328–336.

8. DiPrete DA, Cronan JJ. Compression ultrasonography. Treatment for acute femoral artery pseudoaneurysms in selected cases. *J Ultrasound Med* 1992;11(9):489–492.

9. Messina L, Brothers T, Wakefield T. Clinical characteristics and surgical management of vascular complications in patients undergoing cardiac catheterization: intervention versus diagnostic procedures. *J Vasc Surg* 1991;13:593–600.

10. Karfonta T, Mielcarek F. Pseudoaneurysm of the femoral artery following cardiac intervention: identification and management. *Prog Cardiovasc Nurs* 1994;9(4):13–17.

11. Ricci MA, Trevisani GT, Pilcher DB. Vascular complications of cardiac catheterization. *Am J Surg* 1994;167(4):375–378.

12. Hajarizadeh H, LaRosa CR, Cardullo P, et al. Ultrasound-guided compression of iatrogenic femoral pseudoaneurysm: failure, recurrence, and long-term results. *J Vasc Surg* 1995;22(4):425–430; discussion 430–433.

13. Perler BA. Surgical treatment of femoral pseudoaneurysm following cardiac catheterization. *Cardiovasc Surg* 1993;1(2):118–121.

14. Fellmeth B, Roberts A, Bookstein J. Postangiographic femoral artery injuries: nonsurgical repair with US-guided compression. *Radiology* 1991;178:671–675.

15. Fellmeth D, Buckner N, Ferreira J, et al. Postcatheterization femoral artery injuries: repair with color flow US guidance and c-clamp assistance. *Radiology* 1992;182:570–572.

16. Agrawal SK, Pinheiro L, Roubin GS, et al. Nonsurgical closure of femoral pseudoaneurysms complicating cardiac catheterization and percutaneous transluminal coronary angioplasty. *J Am Coll Cardiol* 1992;20(3):610–615.

17. Trertola SO, Savader SJ, Prescott CA, Osterman FA Jr. US-guided pseudoaneurysm repair with a compression device. *Radiology* 1993;189(1):285–286.

18. Sabri N, Eddy P, Traverso R, Khania S. Closure of a persistent femoral artery pseudoaneurysm complicating coronary angioplasty using the Femostop compression device and direct ultrasound visualization. *Int J Card Imag* 1995;11(4):273–275.

19. Dean S, Olin J, Piedmonte M, et al. Ultrasound-guided compression closure of postcatheterization pseudoaneurysms during concurrent anticoagulation: a review of seventy-seven patients. *J Vasc Surg* 1996;23:28–35.

20. Currie P, Turnbull CM, Shaw TR. Pseudoaneurysm of the femoral artery after cardiac catheterisation: diagnosis and treatment by manual compression guided by Doppler colour flow imaging. *Br Heart J* 1994;72(1):80–84.

21. Cutler B. Discussion of paper: ultrasound-guided compression closure of postcatheterization pseudoaneurysms during concurrent anticoagulation: a review of seventy-seven patients. *J Vasc Surg* 1996;23:34.

22. Schaub F, Theiss W, Heinz M, et al. New aspects in ultrasound-guided compression repair of postcatheterization femoral artery injuries. *Circulation* 1994;90(4):1861–1865.

23. Johns J, Pupa LJ, Bailey S. Spontaneous thrombosis of iatrogenic femoral artery pseudoaneurysms: documentation with color Doppler and two-dimensional ultrasonography. *J Vasc Surg* 1991;14:24–29.

24. Paulson EK, Hertzberg BS, Paine SS, Carroll BA. Femoral artery pseudoaneurysms: value of color Doppler sonography in predicting which ones will thrombose without treatment. *AJR* 1992;159(5):1077–1081.

25. Kent K, McArdle C, Kennedy B, et al. A prospective study of the clinical outcome of femoral pseudoaneurysm and arteriovenous fistulas induced by arterial puncture. *J Vasc Surg* 1993;17:125–131.

26. Cox GS, Young JR, Gray BR, et al. Ultrasound-guided compression repair of postcatheterization pseudoaneurysms: results of treatment in one hundred cases. *J Vasc Surg* 1994;19(4):683–686.

27. Cope C, Zeit R. Coagulation of aneurysms by direct percutaneous thrombin injection. *AJR* 1986;147:383–387.

28. Jenas W, Leven H. A new technique for nonsurgical repair of peripheral pseudoaneurysm. *Acta Radiol* 1995;36:100–101.

29. Sclafani S, Cooper R, Shaftan G, et al. Arterial trauma: diagnostic and therapeutic angiography. *Radiology* 1986;161:165–172.

30. Schwend RB, Hambsch KP, Kwan KY, et al. Color duplex sonographically guided obliteration of pseudoaneurysm. *J Ultrasound Med* 1993;12(10):609–613.

31. Cheng SW, Fok M, Wong J. Infected femoral pseudoaneurysm in intravenous drug abusers. *Br J Surg* 1992;79(6):510–512.

32. Padberg F Jr, Hobson RD, Lee B, et al. Femoral pseudoaneurysm from durgs of abuse: ligation or reconstruction?
J Vasc Surg 1992;15(4):642–648.
33. Ernst SM, Tjonjoegin RM, Schräder R, et al. Immediate
sealing of arterial puncture sites after cardiac catheterization and coronary angioplasty using a biodegradable collagen plug: results of an international registry. *J Am Coll
Cardiol* 1993;21(4):851–855.

34. Kussmaul WGR, Buchbinder M, Whitlow PL, et al. Rapid
arterial hemostasis and decreased access site complications after cardiac catheterization and angioplasty: results
of a randomized trial of a novel hemostatic device. *J Am
Coll Cardiol* 1995;25(7):1685–1692.

Section 4

Cerebrovascular Disease

44

The Clinical Presentation, Natural History, and Medical Management of Patients with Cerebrovascular Disease

Stephen Oppenheimer, M.D.

Approximately 350,000 patients suffer from acute cerebral infarction or hemorrhage each year in the United States. It is the most prevalent cause of neurologic disease in the community and the third most common cause of death. Over the past 5 years or so, there have been considerable advances in our understanding of the pathophysiology of this condition. New advances in imaging, in basic science research, and in therapeutics have made this a most exciting time for those involved in the management of such patients. It is no longer tenable to suggest that nothing can be done for the stroke patient. Over the next few years, it is likely that considerable advances will be made in the therapeutics of stroke and its prophylaxis, based on an increased understanding of the metabolic changes unleashed in this form of acute cerebral trauma. Future advances will continue at great speed in the fields of interventional radiology, surgical procedures, and medical therapy for stroke prevention and therapy. This chapter will provide an overview of the pathophysiology of this condition, its clinical presentation, and its treatment. Many of the recent advances concern actue ischemic stroke and its prophylaxis. It is on this condition that this chapter focusses.

CAUSES OF STROKE

By far the most common cause of stroke is embolism from an atheromatous source within the great vessels of the neck. The origin of emboli from the extracranial vasculature was first emphasized by Thomas Willis in his 1679 treatise.[1] Although Willis' genius was well recognized in his day, he was an unpopular figure and many of his seminal thoughts were ignored. Using the same approach of correlating clinical presentation with autopsy findings, C. Miller Fisher came to the same conclusions about the origins of acute ischemic stroke in the late 1950s.

A variety of factors, including hypertension, cigarette smoking, and hemorrheologic abnormalities, alone or in concert, result in significant damage to the endothelial lining of an artery and predispose to the development of an atheromatous plaque (Fig. 44–1). This is likely to occur at major arterial branch points or sites where hemorrheologic forces result in relentless impacting of jets of blood on the vascular wall. In the anterior extracranial circulation, such sites include the bifurcation of the common carotid artery and the carotid sinus; in the posterior cerebral circulation, the origins of the vertebral arteries are most frequently involved. However, more distal disease is not uncommon. This may involve the basilar artery and its tributaries or the distal internal carotid artery and branches of the middle cerebral artery. Such distal involvement, as in the case of the coronary circulation, is most common in diabetics, severely hypertensive patients, and/or those with serious abnormalities of lipid metabolism.

Distal embolization to the intracranial vasculature from extracranial vessels is the cause of stroke in up to 80% of all cases.[2] The atheromatous plaque occurs as cholesterol and its esters are deposited in and around proliferating myointimal cells in the subintimal region beneath the vascular endothelium. In response to trauma to the endothelium and to proliferative factors released by the platelets and leukocytes that congregate at the surface of damaged vascular tissue, these myointimal cells divide and accumulate cholesterol esters. In addition, fibroblasts in the vicinity proliferate and form

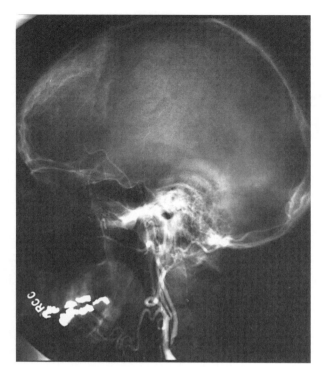

Figure 44–1. Right common carotid arteriogram showing 90% stenosis at the origin of the internal carotid artery.

a fibrous stroma.[3] Calcification may occur. Hemorrhage may be associated with plaque rupture and dislodgment of part of the fibrocalcific plaque distally, where it may block a smaller branch of the anterior or posterior circulation. On the other hand, such maturation changes in the plaque may be associated with intermittent denuding of the overlying endothelium, exposing underlying matrix material, which can encourage the formation of platelet fibrin clots and which ultimately may result in the formation of a thrombus that itself can occlude the vessel or embolize distally. Plaque hemorrhage, progression of the atherothrombotic subintimal plaque, or fibrocalcific maturation may also result in progression of stenosis to the point of complete vascular occlusion. The process of clot formation, plaque extension, and platelet and white cell accretion to the abnormal regions of the vasculature is balanced by protective mechanisms leading to dissolution of the same. Thus the probabilty of stroke after either a transient ischemic attack or a cerebral infarction varies with time and can be considered to wax and wane.

The significance of plaque ulceration is controversial (Fig. 44–2). Theoretically, by denuding the vascular endothelium and providing a nidus for the deposition of platelet fibrin clots, this phenomenon should increase the risk of distal embolization. The recent results of the North American Symptomatic Carotid Endarterectomy Study confirm this. Specifically, this study demonstrated that ulceration signifi-

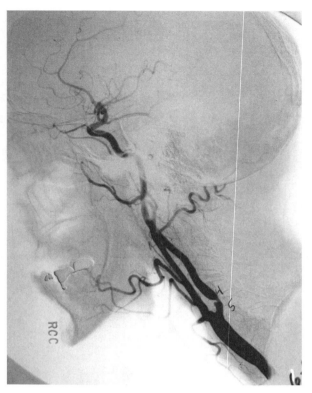

Figure 44–2. Right common carotid arteriogram showing an ulcerated plaque at the origin of the right internal carotid artery.

cantly increases the risk of stroke at each level of carotid stenosis, above the risk of that stenosis alone. The relative risk compared to that of stenosis without ulceration increases from 1.2 at 75% stenosis to 3.4 at 96% stenosis.[4]

Lacunar strokes occur in approximately 20% of stroke cases.[5] These are small strokes, less than 1 cm in diameter, usually associated with a discrete neurologic syndrome such as pure motor hemiparesis involving the face, arm, and leg, and typically result from thrombosis of a distal cerebral penetrating vessel.

Other etiologies of cerebral ischemia are less common. These include cardioembolic causes, which may be responsible for 10 to 20% of all ischemic strokes; hematologic disorders (eg, protein S, protein C, and anticardiolipin antibody disorders), which occur in 1 to 4% of all stroke cases; and abnormalities of the cranial vasculature including fibromuscular dysplasia in 1 to 5% of all strokes. In general, these unusual causes of stroke are more common in younger patients (ie, those less than 40 years of age). Dissections of the extracranial or intracranial vasculature are probably among the most common causes of stroke among younger individuals (Fig. 44–3). They may be associated with head trauma, but most often a precipitating cause is not identified. A tear occurs in the intimal lining, followed by intravasation of blood. This may be suffieient to

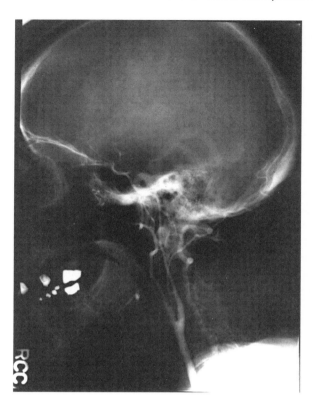

Figure 44–3. Right common carotid arteriogram showing a significant tapering of the internal carotid artery above the carotid bulb, which is characteristic of a carotid dissection and in this case is associated with fibromuscular dysplasia. The dissection extends superiorly to involve the intracranial carotid artery. Dissection is one of several etiologies of this carotid "string sign."

occlude the artery completely and result in stroke. Alternatively, any stenosis caused by a dissection may serve as a nidus for clot formation and subsequent distal embolization. In the posterior circulation, this often occurs more distally within the brain and is associated with hemorrhage, as the friable arterial lumen ruptures into the surrounding tissue.

One of the more common causes of cerebral infarction or hemorrhage recently relates to the use of sympathomimetic drugs. For example, cocaine can cause stroke in a variety of ways.[6] Cardiogenic emboli may result from myocardial damage, with resultant reduction in the ejection fraction and deposition of platelet-fibrin thrombus onto a damaged endocardium. Cardiac arrhythmias are also commonly induced by cocaine. This also may encourage the formation of emboligenic material. Vasculitis may occur as a result of the use of these agents, and when this occurs within the brain, it may reuslt in local infarction. Such agents may also elevate the blood pressure to levels beyond the autoregulatory ability of the cerebral vasculature, so that severe damage may occur to these vessels, leading to rupture and intracerebral hemorrhage.

CLINICAL PRESENTATION

In general, cerebral ischemia can present in one of three ways, depending on the duration of symptoms: these may last for less than 24 hours (a transient ischemic attack or TIA); the symptoms may resolve over a period of a few days to a week (reversible ischemic neurologic deficit or RIND, or minor stroke); or the symptoms may last for a longer period of time and resolve gradually or remain without amelioration, indicating a completed stroke. It is not clear what pathophysiology underlies these various manifestations. For example, in the case of a TIA in the simplest conceptual terms, the embolus may break down quickly and/or the collateral circulation may be sufficient so that vascular occlusion does not cause prolonged ischemia. Alternatively, a TIA may occur when the intracerebral clot persists, but the brain tissue supplied by the involved vessel recovers from the initial ischemia, although the artery remains occluded. Finally, recovery may occur when other areas of the brain assume the function of the involved tissue. If the temporal course of the vascular occlusion is prolonged or if any of the briefly discussed mechanisms fail, a stroke with persistent neurologic deficit occurs rather than a transient deficit.

Initially, a TIA may be difficult to differentiate from a completed stroke. In fact, most TIAs resolve within 5 to 10 minutes. If the symptoms persist for longer than an hour, the likelihood of a radiographically demonstrable abnormality is high even if the symptoms resolve completely.[7]

The clinical presentation also depends on the vascular territory involved. It is often difficult to differentiate between stroke involving the anterior or posterior circulations. In general, posterior circulation strokes are more likely to involve a larger area of the body, and this may be bilateral. In addition, there may be a hemianopsia and ataxia. Lower motor neuron cranial nerve involvement may also indicate that the stroke has involved the posterior circulation. Conversely, aphasia, apraxia, seizure abnormalities, and a more circumscribed involvement of the limbs and face may indicate anterior circulation involvement.[8]

Amaurosis fugax is another manifestation of acute ischemia. There is sudden loss of vision, either within the entire visual field of one eye or a part thereof. The symptom is often described as being like a shutter coming down and obscuring sight. While usually due to an embolus lodging in the ophthalmic artery or a branch thereof and originating from a plaque within the ipsilateral carotid artery, amaurosis fugax is less ominous in terms of the risk of subsequent stroke.[9] Specifically, the risk of stroke after a hemisphere TIA may be as much as three times that of amaurosis fugax.

Other symptoms are uncommonly associated with stroke, although they may initially be diagnosed as such, including loss of consciousness in the absence of focal neurologic symptoms or signs and vertigo without concomitant light-headedness or dizziness. While occasionally these symptoms may be due to focal brain ischemia, in general they are more often associated with a more peripheral disturbance either involving the inner ear (vertigo) or the systemic circulation (loss of consciousness) or due to seizure (loss of consciousness).

PATHOPHYSIOLOGY OF ACUTE STROKE

Although an occluded artery may result in the death of brain cells, this dead zone may be surrounded by a rim of surviving, salvageable tissue. This region is termed the *penumbra*. Furthermore, not all cerebral tissue has the same susceptibility to ischemia. Some regions of the brain appear to be more resistant than others and infarct late, if at all. Astrup et al demonstrated in monkeys that if the middle cerebral artery is occluded, blood flow within the center of the tissue is reduced to very low levels,[10] and this central area will infarct within a few minutes. The cells within the penumbra, however, do not function normally and contribute to the clinical expression of ischemia. If cerebral blood flow is not reestablished, the infarction may extend into the penumbra.

Whether a penumbra exists in human clinical stroke has been debated. Recent positron emission tomography (PET) studies have indicated the existence of a region of reduced blood flow and abnormal metabolism surrounding infarcted tissue.[11] It has been argued, however, that because of the relatively low resolution of this technique, the findings result from partial volume averaging whereby normal tissue, juxtaposed to inviable tissue, is included in overlapping areas of imaging averaging the two regions. Recently we have used magnetic resonance imaging (MRI) techniques to attempt to ascertain whether penumbratous areas exist in human infarction. In a study of 12 patients, we have applied spectroscopy that uses the information obtained in the MRI scan not to provide a picture of the cerebral structure, but to investigate cerebral metabolism.[12] N-acetyl aspartate (NAA) is a compound that is virtually unique to neurons. At the center of the infarction imaged on average 13 hours after symptom onset, we have shown that this neuronal marker is absent. This probably represents the core of the infarct. Surrounding this region, however, is an area of intermediate NAA levels representing partial cellular death. In this latter area, but not in the infarct core, we find markedly increased lactate levels, which, using our imaging techniques, are not found in normal cerebral tissue. We suggest that this represents the surrounding penumbra. Interestingly, on follow-up MRI scanning, the infarcted area may be seen to extend into this metabolically compromised region in some patients, whereas in others the area

appears to recover. The data imply that the penumbra exists and that efforts to protect this region might translate into significant clinical benefit.

A further point of practical interest in the management of patients with acute ischemic stroke relates to the period of time during which this tissue remains viable. Studies in rats and gerbils, as well as early PET studies in humans,[13,14] suggest that cytoprotective therapy may be of benefit for at least 3 to 4 hours after reversible ischemia. These studies also suggest that survival of viable tissue is a function of the degree of blood flow reduction and the length of time this reduction persists[15] (Fig. 44–4). In other words, the viability of the penumbra may well depend on the overall condition of intracranial and extracranial vessels, in addition to that specifically involved in the cause of the infarct. Persons having high-grade stenoses in multiple extracranial vessels consequently might only be able to sustain a small penumbra, if any at all. In addition, viability would be greater in regions of the cerebral circulation where considerable anastomoses with collateral vessels occur, such as the posterior circulation. The data are less clear

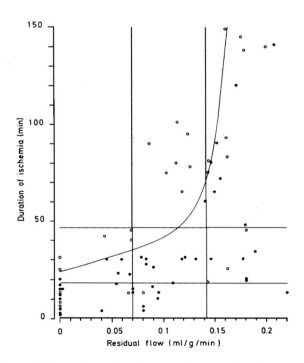

Figure 44–4. Relationship between duration of ischemia and incidence of cell death (see Ref. 15). Cats were subjected to reversible occlusion of the middle cerebral artery; blood flow was measured in the middle cerebral artery territory using a hydrogen clearance technique. Neuronal extracellular recordings were made within this region, and the probability of recovery of function was ascertained according to residual cerebral blood flow and the length of time during which this was reduced. Filled circles show cells that recovered function; open circles show cells with no functional recovery. The transition between cell recovery and cell death is demonstrated by the fitted curve.

in humans. Recently, for example, the results of acute interventional trials involving reperfusion, as with recombinant tissue plasminogen activator, suggest that intervention, if it is to be of benefit, should be applied within 3 hours of infarct onset.[16]

In animal studies, there is also evidence that different brain regions are variably susceptible to ischemia. In the rat subjected to global ischemia and then reperfusion, different regions of the hippocampus, although possessing the same blood supply, showed histologic evidence of infarction at different rates. Some regions remained viable for several days.[17] Petito et al have produced some evidence suggesting that this occurs in humans.[18] Various agents, including glutamate, nitric oxide, and a variety of free radicals, may be generated at different times during ischemia, and cells may have different abilities to withstand the metabolic effects of these agents, thus explaining the differential tissue susceptibility to ischemia.

Another phenomenon may also be important in the recovery from stroke, or may add to its burden of deficit. *Diaschisis* is the term given to dysfunction of a cerebral region not principally involved in the infarct. PET and single photon emission computed tomography (SPECT) studies have shown that such a region might well exist, although this is still a matter of some controversy.[19,20] It is believed that the abnormal area involved in diaschisis results from a sudden interruption in connectivity. Pathways normally synapsing in these areas are destroyed by the stroke, resulting in hypometabolism and a reduction in blood flow. By definition, this area is not directly involved in the vascular infarct. If this pathophysiologic mechanism is further delineated, therapeutic interventions aimed at the protection of such tissue may be clinically beneficial.

NATURAL HISTORY OF TRANSIENT AND PERSISTENT CEREBRAL ISCHEMIA

The incidence of stroke is 1.6 to 2.0 per 1000 and increases dramatically with age.[21] The odds of a male suffering a stroke are 26% higher than those of a female. The overall 30-day case fatality for ischemic stroke is 10% compared to 50% for intracerebral and subarachnoid hemorrhage. By 1 year of follow-up, 23% of all ischemic stroke patients die; 65% are functionally independent. Lacunar strokes occur at a rate of 0.33 per 1000 but without a male preponderance. The case fatality rate is 1% at 30 days and 10% at 1 year.[5] Sixty-six percent of patients are functionally independent after 1 year.

Primary prevention of stroke involves, among other things, attention to the risk factors for this condition (including hypertension, smoking, hypercholesterolemia, control of diabetes), which are directly implicated in the production of extracranial and intracranial

atheroma. The single most important preventive measure is effective treatment of hypertension.

The frequency of anterior circulation ischemic stroke after the warning of TIA, amaurosis fugax, or minor, nondisabling stroke may be ascertained by reference to the medical treatment group of patients included in the North American Symptomatic Carotid Endarterectomy Trial (NASCET).[22] The risk of reinfarction was dependent on the presence or absence of ulceration within the symptomatic carotid artery. In the absence of ulceration, the stroke rate after 24 months was 21% in patients treated solely with aspirin. In the medical arm of the trial, the presence of an ulcer not only increased the rate of reinfarction but also exposed a stenosis-dependent risk. At 75% stenosis with ulceration, the reinfarction rate was 26%, rising to 73% with 95% stenosis over the 24-month period. In general, the likelihood of a new or second stroke is greatest within the first 3 months after TIA or stroke, when it may be as high as 15%, and then falls somewhat during the first year. It then plateaus to an annual rate of 4 to 10% thereafter. In the case of lacunar infarction, the reinfarction rate is on the order of 12%.

Complete occlusion of the internal carotid artery may occur without symptoms (Fig. 44–5). Alternatively, it may be associated with stroke. Often the symptoms are suggestive of extensive middle cerebral artery occlusion. Once the internal carotid artery has occluded,

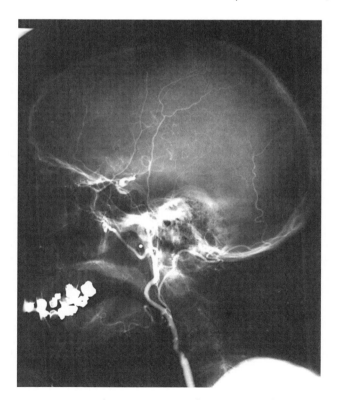

Figure 44–5. Right common carotid arteriogram showing complete occlusion of the right internal carotid artery at its origin.

surgical intervention is not possible due to fibrosis and superimposed clot extension far into the intracranial portion of this vessel. On the other hand, carotid occlusion does not protect the brain from further embolization from the vessel. The mechanism may involve stagnation and retrograde flow into the artery from more distal vessels, causing the buildup of friable fibrin-platelet clots above the region of occlusion. These may dislodge and embolize into the cerebral vasculature. The frequency of infarction following carotid occlusion may be as high as 5% per annum.[24] Following cerebral infarction or TIA, if a thrombus is found within a carotid artery with more than 70% stenosis, anticoagulation can be effective in promoting dissolution of the clot, although surgical thrombectomy should be considered seriously.[25] The timing of surgery will depend on the specific angiographic findings and the extent of the infarction.

Reinfarction within the posterior circulation has been less well studied. Bamford and colleagues showed that patients with posterior circulation strokes were more likely to suffer reinfarction than those with anterior circulation strokes, although such patients had a better functional outcome.[26] Spontaneous reperfusion can occur when an artery occludes. In investigations where arteriography was performed within 6 hours of stroke onset, the absence of an arterial occlusion appropriate to the symptoms was demonstrated in 17 to 25% of patients, and it was assumed that complete recanalization had occurred by this time in these patients.[27,28]

DIAGNOSTIC TESTS

In view of the availability of reperfusion therapy (vida infra), it is clearly of paramount importance to distinguish ischemic infarction from hemorrhage as early as possible because hemorrhage is an absolute contraindication to thrombolytic therapy. The computed tomography (CT) scan has excellent resolution for the demonstration of blood. On the other hand, ischemic infarction may become visible on the CT scan only after 16 to 24 hours later. MRI, while often not available on an emergency basis, tends to demonstrate the infarct earlier (within 8 to 12 hours). Newer techniques such as diffusion weighted imaging and MR spectroscopy may show changes within minutes to a few hours after the stroke.[12]

In the subsequent evaluation of a patient in the subacute or more chronic phase, when surgical intervention might be considered, investigation of the extracranial circulation can proceed with carotid duplex ultrasound scanning. The noninvasive procedure will detect the presence of stenosis, determine their severity, and characterize plaque morphology such as ulceration. The accuracy of the scan is highly dependent on the skill of the examiner, and in some

centers has been associated with a specificity of 99% and a sensitivity of 89% compared to angiography.[29] In general, I consider the technique a useful screening tool but never use it alone. A second noninvasive technique that may be usefully combined with ultrasonography is MR angiography (MRA). The anterior circulation is usually well visualized, often including the M2 branches of the middle cerebral artery. Although MRA tends to overestimate the degree of stenosis, when combined with ultrasonography a good approximation to arteriography is possible. If a high-grade stenosis is demonstrable by these techniques, and if either endarterectomy or angioplasty is contemplated, it is my practice to proceed to arteriography. This procedure is not without risks; Major stroke or death has been reported in approximately 1% of patients, and less severe complications in 3 to 5%.[30] The rationale for performing this test is severalfold. First, noninvasive investigations may yield false-positive results. Second, an operable high-grade stenosis may appear as an inoperable occlusion on the MRA scan, thirdly, conditions that may resemble atherosclerotic disease, such as fibromuscular dysplasia, may not be amenable to surgical intervention. Fourth, the more distal vessels are not well visualized with duplex ultrasonography or very precisely delineated with MRA. If a carotid stenosis occurs in tandem with a complete occlusion of the symptomatic middle cerebral artery, many stroke neurologists would argue against the performance of endarterectomy. Finally, there are some inflammatory conditions that, although rare, may involve both the extracranial and intracranial vessels, resulting in stroke. Imaging of the smaller arteries may yield the telltale beaded appearance of vasculitis, which is not amenable to surgical intervention.

MRI should be performed in the patient with a high-grade stenosis who has no symptoms or signs of stroke and who is being considered for endarterectomy for asymptomatic carotid disease because silent infarction is not infrequently demonstrated in a neurologically noneloquent area. Using CT scanning, the likelihood of finding an asymptomatic infarct increases with the degree of stenosis; with less than 50% stenosis, 10% of scans may show an ipsilateral infarct. With more than 75% stenosis, this figure reaches 30%.[31] In my opinion, this converts the disease into a symptomatic form in that a radiographic lesion has occurred. It should be noted that whether the prognosis is different for patients with asymptomatic stroke and high-grade stenosis compared with those with clinically silent but radiographic infarction is unclear.

Information about the status of the intracranial vasculature may be obtained indirectly using transcranial doppler insonation (TCD). This technique is also highly operator dependent. In one report, the sensitivity was 87% and the specificity was 80% when used in the posterior circulation compared with the results of intra-arterial digital subtraction angiography.[32] The technology relies on applying pulsed waves to the intracranial vessels and determining Doppler shifts in the reflected waveforms from moving blood. It requires the presence of a temporal window (an area of thinning of the temporal bone) through which insonation of the middle cerebral arteries and anterior cerebral arteries may occur. This is lacking in as many as 25% of all patients. It may also be used to investigate the posterior circulation (vertebral and basilar arteries). On the other hand, the technique does not produce images of the cerebral circulation or a direct measure of blood flow. It measures cerebral blood flow velocity, which is nonlinearly related to cerebral blood flow and depends on a variety of factors, including blood volume and vascular patency. It may, however, be useful in screening for subclavian steal syndrome, in which case turning of the head or repetitive hand clenching may result in retrograde flow down the vertebral artery. In addition, it is a very sensitive indicator of retrograde flow in the ophthalmic arteries, which may occur with occlusion of the ipsilateral carotid. It therefore accurately indicates certain types of collateral flow through the anterior circulation.

The newest technique of noninvasive imaging is spiral CT.[33] This technique images the extracranial circulation and circle of Willis. It may be of great benefit as a screening test in patients with pacemakers in or those who are claustrophobic and unable to undergo MRA. The technique involves a continuous sequential acquisition of images as the patient is moved rapidly through the scanner. Instead of stopping after each tomographic slice, the gantry moves helically to the next plane to obtain data. This allows for very fast imaging, which is prevented by routine CT scanning. The scan commences after injection of contrast material into the peripheral circulation, and the timing of the acquisition in relation to this injection is crucial. In the case of a carotid stenosis, nearly 90% correlation has been obtained between this technique and conventional arteriography. It has also been found to be accurate in differentiating between complete occlusion and a high-grade stenosis, a failing of MRA. Imaging of the circle of Willis achieves a level of accuracy similar to that of MRA.

TREATMENT (ACUTE AND PROPHYLACTIC)

There have been startling developments in the treatment of acute stroke and its prophylaxis over the past few years, and preservation of the penumbratous tissue is the key. In this respect, control of blood sugar, blood pressure, and temperature is of paramount importance.[34] Most attention has been paid to reperfusion therapy, which has well-defined risks. First, vascular tissue distal to the site of the arterial blockage is ischemic.

The acute restoration of blood flow under normal or high arterial pressure could have several consequences, including the disruption of damaged endothelium resulting in hemorrhage, and the extravasation of plasma through the damaged tight junctions that normally comprise the intact blood-brain barrier. This results in severe cerebral edema. Second, the restoration of oxygen to a previously ischemic region may result in profound and potentially deleterious metabolic changes. Free radicals are often generated under these circumstances. These highly reactive species damage the plasma membrane, causing an inability to maintain appropriate ionic currents, particularly of calcium. The consequent changes in osmotic gradients and changes in secondary messenger systems result in cellular necrosis. In view of this, I believe the future optimal care of the acute stroke patient will include cytoprotective therapy, which protects viable but unstable cells in the penumbra, coupled with acute reperfusion methods. Selection of patients for these treatments will be based on noninvasive (probably MR) methods of evaluating the extent of damaged but viable tissue (the penumbra) and the blood flow in this region.

Recently there has been considerable interest in the use of tissue plasminogen activator (t-PA) in the treatment of acute stroke patients.[16] Unlike other thrombolytic agents, this agent has the advantage of being activated mainly in the principal region of thrombus formation. When such therapy was instituted intravenously within 3 hours of stroke onset, a statistically significant improvement was seen in Barthel, Rankin, National Institutes of Health, and Glasgow outcome scores at 3 months. Interestingly, no improvement was seen within 24 hours of therapy. All the gains occurred later. The absolute degree of improvement was 10 to 12% (depending on the scoring system). Thus, for the Barthel index, 38% of patients treated with placebo were in the highest functional category after 3 months, whereas for the t-PA-treated patients, this figure was 50%. However, 6% of patients treated with t-PA suffered a hemorrhage compared with 0.6% of patients treated with placebo ($p < 0.001$). The import of this result was that those patients who sustained a hemorrhage often deteriorated significantly or died. It is unclear which patients might become so afflicted. The results of this and a similar European study suggest that patients whose CT scan demonstrates a lesion at the time of therapy with t-PA, who receive treatment after 3 hours, and who may have suffered a cardioembolic infarction are most vulnerable to hemorrhage and an adverse outcome.

A recent study performed in Hong Kong suggests that the subcutaneous treatment of acute stroke patients with low molecular weight heparinoids significantly improves functional recovery at 6 months.[35] This treatment uses anticoagulant agents that do not alter the prothrombin time or the partial thromboplastin time, so that there is little risk of systemic hemorrhage. There was no significant difference in the incidence of intracerebral hemorrhage in patients treated with heparinoids and those treated with placebo.

The NASCET demonstrated a significant benefit associated with carotid endarterectomy among patients with more than 70% carotid stenosis who had experienced either an anterior circulation TIA or a minor, nondisabling stroke within 3 months of randomization.[22] The efficacy of this procedure was demonstrated by a significant reduction in ipsilateral stroke over 2 years of follow-up. The effect of treatment was directly proportional to the degree of stenosis. For patients with the highest degree of stenosis (90 to 99%), the absolute stroke risk reduction was 26 ± 8%; for those with 70 to 79% stenosis, the corresponding figure was 12 ± 5%. This intervention was assessed with reference to what was considered by the investigators to be the best available medical therapy (usually 1300 mg aspirin daily). The study assigned treatment to centers with a low incidence of severe side effects of surgery (significant stroke or death); in addition, the significant complication rate of carotid angiography was 1% or less. The evidence is therefore strongly in favor of carotid endarterectomy for stroke prophylaxis in patients with symptomatic carotid stenoses greater than 70%. It is a subject of conjecture only in patients without this degree of stenosis, whose symptomatic event occurred more than 3 months previously or whose general medical condition indicates that surgery might be contraindicated.

With respect to the treatment of patients with asymptomatic carotid arterial disease, the studies are somewhat more controversial. It is not clear exactly what the natural history of such patients may be. Bornstein and Norris performed carotid duplex ultrasound in 500 patients with cervical bruits and followed them for 4 years.[36] The incidence of stroke in this group was 1.7% at 1 year, and 80% of strokes were ipsilateral to the asymptomatic stenosis. Among patients with the highest degree of stenosis (>75%), the infarction rate was 5.5% at 1 year; however, only 50% of these strokes were ipsilateral. On the other hand the results of the recent ACAS have suggested a beneficial effect for endarterectomy in patients with carotid stenoses greater than 60%.[37] The incidence of stroke was reduced from 11% to 5% over 5 years of follow-up (an absolute risk reduction of 53% over 5 years). The benefit in women was not statistically significant.[37] Further, some would argue that this absolute reduction in the incidence of stroke is too small to merit surgical intervention. In general, the American Heart Association has determined that carotid endarterectomy in asymptomatic patients may result in a modest reduction in stroke risk. A screening and intervention program for asymptomatic disease is not recommended at this stage.

Medical treatment alone may be considered in symptomatic patients unsuitable for surgery or in those who have an asymptomatic stenosis. Two therapeutic interventions have been of benefit in such cases. An early study showed a significant benefit of aspirin in preventing cerebral infarction.[38] The dosage used was 1300 mg daily if tolerated, although such high doses were associated with a greater likelihood of gastrointestinal and hematologic side effects. Other studies have suggested comparable stroke prevention using lower aspirin dosages (eg, 325 or even 81 mg).[39] However, several points must be considered. First, aspirin causes irreversible blockade of cyclooxygenase. This enzyme is present within platelets, where it mediates the formation of procoagulant and vasoconstrictive prostanoids. In the endothelium, aspirin blocks the same enzyme that produces a vasodilator substance, prostacyclin. It is unclear what dosage of the medication achieves the best balance between prostanoid product inhibition and prostacyclin inhibition. Also, patients metabolize aspirin at different rates. There have been reports suggesting that even with high doses, a small number of patients may not achieve appropriate platelet inhibition. Consequently, it is my practice to prescribe the maximally tolerable dose, keeping in mind the age of the patient. Older individuals (70 or above) may tolerate only 350 mg of the enteric-coated preparation with meals twice a day. Higher doses may cause indigestion and gastrointestinal hemorrhage. Younger patients may tolerate 650 mg of the enteric-coated preparation twice daily. It should be noted that aspirin was not shown to be of benefit in women in this and in other studies where gender relationships were investigated. As fewer strokes occur in women, a larger number might need to be recruited before beneficial effects can be demonstrated.

Ticlopidine hydrochloride is a new antiplatelet agent, and within the first year of symptom onset (TIA or nondisabling stroke) it has been associated with a 50% greater relative efficacy than aspirin in the prevention of stroke.[40] This effect was dissipated during the next 4 years of follow-up when the effects were similar. On the other hand, ticlopidine produces less gastrointestinal hemorrhage, and subgroup analysis suggested that it was of greater benefit in women, in patients with posterior circulation events, and in those who have failed treatment with aspirin. The most important side effect of this medication is the induction of neutropenia, which occurs in about 2 to 4% of treated patients and is reversible if the medication is stopped. Patients are advised to have a complete blood count every 2 weeks for 3 months after institution of this therapy. Thereafter, the incidence of neutropenia is low. I suggest the use of this agent in patients who are unable to tolerate aspirin, and those who have failed aspirin therapy and whose lesions are not amenable to any other form of intervention.

The most recent form of therapeutic intervention is carotid angioplasty.[41] This investigational endovascular approach requires advancing a guidewire across the region of stenosis, and a balloon catheter is threaded over it. The balloon is inflated within the region of stenosis, cracking the plaque and enlarging the artery. Remodeling of the artery and plaque then occurs over subsequent weeks and months. Theoretical concerns include the production of embolic material during the procedure, which could result in distal embolization and stroke, dissection of the artery, and aneurysm formation. The restenosis rate is unclear. In general, preliminary data suggest a low complication rate when the procedure is performed by specialists with appropriate experience. Most patients are anticoagulated briefly following the procedure. The indication for stenting is also unclear. The potential of this procedure will depend on the complication and restenosis rates associated with it, and on whether it can be shown to reduce the recurrence of cerebral infarction with comparable efficacy to that achieved with surgery. Angioplasty could be of benefit in patients too debilitated to undergo surgery. It could be applied to the posterior circulation and used in the treatment of more distal intracerebral disease that has hitherto proven inaccessible to surgical intervention.

CONCLUSIONS

The past few years have seen striking changes in our understanding of the pathophysiology of stroke. Significant research is being devoted to the development of cytoprotective therapy that could prevent destruction of ischemic tissue, at risk of total infarction. Reperfusion therapy in the acute phase, while promising, is not without hazards. The incidence of hemorrhage is high with systemic administration of these agents, but might be less when these agents are delivered directly into the involved artery. This, however, requires the immediate availability of expert interventionalists. In the future, I suspect that a mixture of cytoprotective agents, reperfusion, and optimized medical management in specialized units will be the most productive approach. At present, among patients who have more than 70% carotid stenoses and who are within 3 months of stroke or TIA onset, endarterectomy is the treatment of choice. For those with asymptomatic disease, medical therapy is warranted, and endarterectomy should be reserved for those with the highest grade of stenosis (>90%) who are otherwise in good health. This latter is a personal view.

ACKNOWLEDGMENTS

Supported by the EL Wiegand Foundation and the NIH (1RO1-NS 33770)

REFERENCES

1. Willis T. Instructions and prescripts for curing the apoplexy. In: *The London Practice of Physick.* 1679.
2. Bamford J, Sandercock P, Dennis M, Burn J, Warlow C. A prospective study of acute cerebrovascular disease in the community: the Oxfordshire community stroke project—1981–6. 2. Incidence, case fatality rates and overall outcome at one year of cerebral infarction, primary intracerebral and subarachnoid haemorrhage. *J Neurol, Neurosurg Psychiatry* 1990;53:16–22.
3. Ross R. The pathogenesis of atherosclerosis: a perspective for the 1990s. *Nature* 1993;362:801–809.
4. Eliaziw M, Streiffler J, Fox A, Hachinski V, Ferguson G, Barnett H. Significance of plaque ulceration in symptomatic patients with high-grade carotid stenosis. *Stroke* 1994;25:304–308.
5. Bamford J, Sandercock P, Jones L, Warlow C. The natural history of lacunar infarction: the Oxfordshire community stroke project. *Stroke* 1987;18:545–551.
6. Daras M, Tuchman A, Marks S. Central nervous system infarction related to cocaine abuse. *Stroke* 1991;22:1320–1325.
7. Giroud M, Gras P, Milan C, Vion P, Essayagh E, Dumas R. Prognostic des accidents ischemiques transitoires revelant un infarctus. *Rev Neurol* 1992;148:576–579.
8. Victor M, Adams R. *Principles of Neurology* 3rd ed. New York: McGraw-Hill; 1985.
9. Streiffler J, Eliasziw M, Benavente O, et al. The risk of stroke in patients with first ever retinal vs hemispheric transient ischemic attacks and high grade carotid stenosis. *Arch Neurol* 1995;52:246–249.
10. Astrup J, Siesjo B, Symon L. Thresholds in cerebral ischemia—the ischemic penumbra. *Stroke* 1981;12:723–725.
11. Heiss WD, Graf R. The ischemic penumbra. *Curr Opin Neurol* 1994;7:11–19.
12. Gillard JH, Barker PB, van Zijl P, et al. Identification of the metabolic penumbra in acute ischemic middle cerebral artery stroke using proton MR spectroscopic imaging. *Am J Neuroradiol* 1996;17:873–886.
13. Toulmond S, Serrano A, Benavides J, Scatton B. Prevention by eliprodil of traumatic brain damage in the rat. Existence of a large therapeutic window. *Brain Res* 1993;620:32–41.
14. Xue D, Huang Z, Barnes K, Lesiuk H, Smith K, Buchan A. Delayed treatment with AMPA but not NMDA antagonists reduces neocortical infarction. *J Cereb Blood Flow Metab* 1994;14:251–261.
15. Heiss W-D, Rosner G. Functional recovery of cortical neurons as related to degree and duration of ischemia. *Ann Neurol* 1983;14:294–301.
16. National Institute of Neurological Disorders and Stroke rt-PA Stroke Study Group: Tissue plasminogen activator for acute ischemic stroke. *N Engl J Med* 1995;33:1581–1587.
17. Pulsinelli W, Brierley J, Plum F. Temporal profile of neuronal damage in a model of transient forebrain ischemia. *Ann Neurol* 1982;11:491–498.
18. Petito C, Feldmann E, Pulsinelli W, Plum F. Delayed hippocampal damage in humans following cardiorespiratory arrest. *Neurology* 1987;37:1281–1286.

19. Giroud M, Creisson E, Fayolle H, et al. Homolateral ataxia and crural paresis: a crossed cerebral-cerebellar diaschisis. *J Neurol Neurosurg Psych* 1994;57:221–222.

20. Tanaka M, Kondo S, Hirai S. Crossed cerebellar diaschisis accompanied by hemiataxia: a PET study. *J Neurol Psych* 1992;55:121–125.

21. Bamford J, Sandercock P, Dennis M, et al. A prospective study of acute cerebrovascular disease in the community: the Oxfordshire community project 1981–86.1 Methodology, demography and incident cases of first ever stroke. *J Neurol Neurosurg Psychiatry* 1988;51:1373–1380.

22. North American Symptomatic Carotid Endarterectomy Trial Collaborators. Beneficial effect of carotid endarterectomy in symptomatic patients with high-grade stenosis. *N Engl J Med* 1991;325:445–453.

23. Bogousslavsky J, Despland P, Regli F. Prognosis of high risk patients with nonoperated symptomatic extracranial carotid tight stenosis. *Stroke* 1988;19:108–111.

24. Barnett H, Peerless S, Sutherland G. The stump syndrome. In: Smith RR, ed. *Stroke and the Extracranial Vessels.* New York: Raven Press; 1984:295–306.

25. Buchan A, Gates P, Pelz D, Barnett H. Intraluminal thrombus in the cerebral circulation. Implications for surgical management. *Stroke* 1988;19:681–687.

26. Bamford J, Sandercock P, Dennis M, Burn J, Warlow C. Classification and natural history of clinically identifiable subtypes of cerebral infarction. *Lancet* 1991;337:1521–1526.

27. Mori E, Yoneda Y, Tabuchi M, Yoshida T, et al. Intravenous recombinant tissue plasminogen activator in acute carotid artery territory stroke. *Neurology* 1992;42:976–982.

28. Fieschi C, Argentino C, Lenzi G, et al. Clinical and instrumental evaluation of patients with ischemic stroke within the first six hours. *J Neurol Sci* 1989;91:311–321.

29. Ratliffe D, Hames T, Humphries K, Birch S, Chant A. The reliability of Doppler ultrasound techniques in the assessment of carotid disease. *Angiology* 1985;36:333–340.

30. Hankey GJ, Warlow CP, Sellar RJ. Cerebral angiographic risk in mild cerebrovascular disease. *Stroke* 1990;21:209–222.

31. Norris J, Zhu C. Silent stroke and carotid stenosis. *Stroke* 1992;23:483–485.

32. Cher LM, Chambers BR, Smidt V. Comparison of transcranial Doppler with DSA in vertebrobasilar ischemia. *Clin Exp Neurol* 1992;29:143–148.

33. Beauchamp NJ. Spiral CT angiography: a new technique for evaluating the neurovasculature. *App Radiol* 1995;(suppl 14):15–20.

34. Oppenheimer SM, Hachinski VC. The complications of acute stroke. *Lancet* 1992;329:721–724.

35. Kay R, Wong K, Yu Y, et al. Low molecular weight heparin for the treatment of acute ischemic stroke. *N Engl J Med* 1995;333:1588–1593.

36. Bornstein N, Norris J. Management of patients with asymptomatic neck bruits and carotid stenosis. *Neurol Clin North Am* 1992;10:269–280.

37. Executive Committee for the Asymptomatic Carotid Atherosclerosis Study. Endarterectomy for asymptomatic carotid artery stenosis. *JAMA* 1995;273:1421–1428.

38. Canadian Co-operative Study Group. A randomised trial of aspirin and sulfinpyrazone in threatened stroke. *N Engl J Med* 1978;299:53–59.

39. Van Gijn J. Aspirin—dose and indications in modern stroke prevention. *Neurol Clin North Am* 1992;10:193–208.

40. Hass W, Easton J, Adams H, et al. A randomised trial of ticlopidine hydrochloride with aspirin for the prevention of stroke in high risk patients. *N Engl J Med* 1989;321:501–507.

41. Brown M. Angioplasty for stroke prevention. In: Ginsburg M, Bogousslavsky J, eds. *Cerebrovascular Disease.* Cambridge: Blackwell.

45

The Role of Duplex, MRA, and Angiography in the Evaluation of Carotid Artery Disease

Michael D. Colburn, M.D.
Wesley S. Moore, M.D.

Despite the recent development of sophisticated diagnostic techniques, the backbone of any thorough evaluation of patients suffering from the manifestations of cerebrovascular disease remains an accurate history and physical examination. However, because recent randomized prospective studies have established the efficacy of carotid endarterectomy in preventing subsequent ischemic strokes in both symptomatic and asymptomatic patients, developing cost-effective and safe methods of assessing carotid bifurcation lesions has taken on new importance. In addition, because these trials categorize and compare patients with very specific degrees of carotid stenoses, accurate methods of measuring these lesions have become essential.

In the last decade, duplex scanning has emerged as the preferred noninvasive method of evaluating patients with extracranial cerebrovascular disease. This new technology has research and clinical as well as economical implications. The availability of a noninvasive method for imaging atherosclerotic plaques in the carotid bifurcation has led to important information regarding the nature and progression of these lesions. The cost of this test is only a few hundred dollars compared to several thousand dollars for an angiographic procedure. Apart from these advantages, the real debate as to the proper role of duplex scanning involves clinical management issues. There is no argument that routine angiography significantly increases the risk of surgical treatment of cerebrovascular disease. This morbidity must be added to the overall risk associated with surgical intervention. The question is whether duplex scanning alone, or in combination with other noninvasive methods of carotid imaging, is a reliable and safe method of evaluating these lesions; and if

they are capable of accurately selecting patients for whom surgical intervention is appropriate.

In this chapter we will review the role of duplex scanning, magnetic resonance angiography (MRA), and contrast angiography in the preoperative evaluation of patients with cerebrovascular disease. In addition, to determine whether noninvasive testing is a sufficient workup for patients with cerebrovascular disease, we will review the combined experience with carotid endarterectomy without the preoperative use of contrast angiography.

DUPLEX ULTRASONOGRAPHY

Duplex scanning is a very accurate, noninvasive method of imaging the carotid bifurcation, and it has many advantages over angiography. Compared to the multiple puncture site and contrast-related problems associated with angiography, duplex scanning is essentially without risk. The examination involves little or no patient discomfort, and it is entirely noninvasive. The anatomic detail, while not as good as with angiography, is satisfactory. In fact, some information, such as plaque composition, is better demonstrated by duplex ultrasonography. In addition, the duplex study can provide additional important physiologic information such as hemodynamic measurements. The ability to characterize the relative proportions of fatty, fibrous, and calcific material within a lesion is a major advantage of duplex technology. Soft, irregular, fatty plaques that are not calcified are high-risk lesions. On the other hand, smooth, fibrous, and calcified lesions are more stable and represent a lower embolic risk. Finally, a four-vessel cerebral angiogram in most hospitals can cost several thousand dollars compared to only a few hundred for a complete duplex study.

The announcement of significant benefit from surgical endarterectomy of carotid stenoses in both symptomatic and asymptomatic patients has led to a large number of publications aimed at determining the ultrasonographic efficacy and criteria for identifying hemodynamically significant carotid artery stenoses.[1-5] In general, there appears to be a clear, positive correlation between ultrasonographic and angiographic measurement. There is, however, some well-established variability, and the amount of variation increases as the severity of the imaged stenosis increases.

The major limitation of duplex scanning is its inability to image clearly other areas within the cerebrovascular circulation. Proximal lesions are poorly visualized, and significant intracranial disease (arteriovenous malformations, aneurysms, tumors, and siphon lesions) also go unrecognized. Also, even though the vertebral vessels can be studied, the results can often be unreliable. Occasionally, in patients with short, broad necks, even the evaluation of the anterior circulation can be difficult. Furthermore, even though the ability to measure hemodynamic data was cited as an advantage of duplex technology, its reliance on flow characteristics can at times be a disadvantage. Because duplex scans depend on flow velocities for the determination of lesion severity, hyperdynamic states caused by sepsis, inotropic agents, or a contralateral carotid occlusion can lead to an inaccurate estimation of the degree of stenosis. Ultrasonography may also not identify the presence of intraluminal thrombus or dissection, and it is unreliable for the detection and quantification of plaque ulceration. Another important limitation of duplex scanning is that it is inaccurate in differentiating a totally occluded from a nearly occluded internal carotid.[6] Thus, cerebral angiography is strongly recommended in a symptomatic patient when the duplex scan suggests a total occlusion of the affected side. Finally, and perhaps most importantly, the reliability of duplex scanning depends on the individual performing the examination, and results from different laboratories vary greatly.

Clearly, none of these conditions occur in large numbers but, taken together, the aggregate has deterred many clinicians from relying solely on duplex ultrasonography for the screening and evaluation of patients with cerebrovascular disease.

MAGNETIC RESONANCE ANGIOGRAPHY

Magnetic resonance angiography (MRA) is a recently developed variation of magnetic resonance imaging that has increasingly been applied to the evaluation of patients with cerebrovascular occlusive disease. In general, an MR image is created by the application of pulses of radiofrequency energy to a selected anatomic area that has been oriented within a magnetic field. Depending on the composition of the selected anatomic structure, the imaged tissue emits radio signals in response to these energy pulses. At appropriate intervals, the imaging machine and its computer software receive the tissue signals and use them to generate an image.

Since the inception of MRA, many different MRA techniques have been developed. Currently, the most frequently used methods for studying the carotid bifurcation are the techniques such as two-dimensional (2D) and three-dimensional (3D) time-of-flight (TOF) sequences. These methods are based on an imaging technique referred to as *flow-related enhancement*. To briefly summarize, these techniques are based on the fact that, within a given imaging volume, the *spin* characteristics of hydrogen ions in flowing blood are different from the spin characteristics of these ions in fixed tissue. Because the blood is moving, by the time the MR equipment receives the returned radio pulses emitted by the imaged tissue, the blood appears to be relatively unsaturated with signal compared to the stationary surrounding tissue. As a result, the correct imaging software is able to produce an intense or "bright" image representing the blood vessel being studied.

Two-dimensional TOF methods scan a tissue volume by obtaining multiple-sequential 2D images. The computer software then stacks these data to generate the angiogram-like pictures produced on the film. The technique of 3D TOF imaging scans and reproduces an entire tissue volume all at once. Both of these techniques have advantages and disadvantages. Two-dimensional TOF imaging is much faster and is therefore less affected by slow-flowing blood. Also, because of its greater speed, it is better suited for scanning larger body tissue areas. Three-dimensional TOF imaging is slower and is therefore less sensitive to areas of slow flow where signal is lost when blood flows across the volume being studied. However, although the anatomic detail still does not approach that which can be achieved with conventional angiography, 3D TOF does allows for better detail than 2D TOF and can identify some vessel wall irregularities and ulcerations.

Overall, MRA is an exciting new technique that, when used correctly, can be an important addition to the evaluation of selected patients with cerebrovascular disease. However, as a precise method of evaluating the degree of carotid artery stenosis to determine the appropriateness of carotid endarterectomy, MRA has unfortunately proven to be inadequate. The correlation of MRA with contrast angiography in the assessment of carotid artery stenosis has been studied by a number of investigators (Table 45–1). In general, even in recent series, the accuracy of MRA compared to angiography is reported to be between 50 and 95%, with an average accuracy of approximately 75%. As expected, the vast

Table 45–1. Accuracy of MRA Compared with Contrast Angiography in the Evaluation of Carotid Artery Stenosis

Author	Yr	MRA Technique	No. of Observations	% Accurate	% Overcalls	% Undercalls
Masaryk[41]	1989	3D TOF	22	95%	0%	5%
Wilkerson[42]	1991	3D TOF	25	80%	20%	0%
Anderson[43]	1992	2D & 3D	61	64%	29%	7%
Heiserman[7]	1992	2D TOF	292	79%	12%	9%
Riles[10]	1992	2D TOF	75	52%	44%	4%
Wesbey[44]	1992	3D TOF	37	86%	9%	5%
Huston[8]	1993	2D TOF	93	59%	39%	2%
Mittl[9]	1994	2D TOF	219	75%	20%	5%

Observations = (No. of Observers) × (No. of Arteries).

majority of inaccurate MRA readings represent overcalls. This is not surprising because MRA is most accurate in areas of laminar blood flow that are perpendicular to the imaging plane. When flow is slow or turbulent, such as in a carotid bulb or stenosis, bright blood MRA techniques are subject to areas of *flow void* or *signal dropout* where no signal is generated from the flowing blood because it is moving too slowly or in a different direction. Because such an area appears dark on the processed image, the MRA scan tends to overestimate the narrowing in these areas of moderate or severe stenoses where flow is typically highly turbulent.

One area where MRA does seem to be extremely accurate, and perhaps one of its most important benefits, is in the detection of a complete carotid artery occlusion. As mentioned previously, this is also one clinical situation in which the accuracy of duplex ultrasonography has been questioned. The ability of MRA to detect very slow laminar flow, as occurs in the internal carotid artery distal to a very high grade stenosis, has made this technique highly accurate in identifying total carotid occlusions. Many reports in the literature have claimed 100% sensitivity and specificity for MRA in the detection of complete carotid occlusions,[7–9] and only a very rare series has not reported complete accuracy in this regard.[10] In addition, many investigators have been impressed by the ability of MRA to image the intracranial circulation easily. Unfortunately, data to determine the accuracy of these intracranial views are lacking at this time.

One noninvasive imaging strategy that has been suggested for the evaluation of patients with cerebrovascular disease is the combination of duplex ultrasonography and MRA. The logic and benefits of combining these two techniques are readily apparent. The duplex scan provides accurate assessment of the degree of stenosis and plaque characterization that MRA lacks. Likewise, the addition of MRA provides both proximal and intracranial anatomic information and increases the ability to differentiate between high-grade carotid stenoses and total occlusions. Although both duplex ultrasonography and MRA have been studied as potential substitutes for conventional angiography, the concept of combining the two tests has not been thoroughly investigated. One recent study evaluated whether concordant data from 3D TOF MRA and duplex ultrasonography could provide sufficient diagnostic accuracy to obviate the need for contrast angiography.[11] A total of 148 arteries were imaged with both noninvasive tests, and in 124 of these arteries, the studies were in agreement. For these 124 lesions, the accuracy of the combined concordant data from both noninvasive studies was 94%. Imaging of the other 24 lesions resulted in divergent data, and accurate assessment of these arteries would have required contrast angiography. In summary, combining data from both noninvasive tests markedly increased the overall accuracy (94%) compared with either 3D TOF MRA (88%) or duplex ultrasonography (86%) alone. Importantly, in this study, contrast angiography identified 17 total occlusions, and MRA was able to differentiate between high-grade stenoses and occlusions in all cases. By comparison, two occluded arteries were identified as patent by duplex ultrasonography.

There are a number of other problems with MRA. For instance, MRA can have difficulty imaging highly tortuous vessels that do not maintain a constant orientation with respect to the imaging plane. Also, despite recent advances in software, up to 20% of MRA evaluations of the carotid arteries are technically inadequate because of motion artifact. In addition, some patients cannot be studied because of claustrophobia or the presence of an implanted metallic device.

CONTRAST ANGIOGRAPHY

Cerebral angiography has traditionally been the gold standard for the evaluation of patients with cerebrovascular disease. The unmatched demonstration of anatomic detail, in a familiar format that is easily interpreted by most clinicians, is frequently cited as the main advantage of this procedure. By imaging the lumen of the carotid vessels, this technique provides a clear assessment of occlusive lesions, plaque ulcerations, and the presence of any unsuspected anatomic variations. Information regarding the degree of stenosis and the size of an ulceration is easily and reliably gathered. Also, additional anatomic information, such as the presence of kinks, coils, carotid body tumors, and aneurysms, can readily be provided with this technique and is useful for operative planning.

Perhaps the most important advantage of angiography is its ability to evaluate the entire cerebrovascular system. This includes the origin of the brachiocephalic vessels as they arise from the aortic arch, as well as the intracranial portion of the branch vessels. Many neurologists and surgeons maintain that a complet evaluation of patients with cerebrovascular symptoms must include an accurate anatomic delineation of the aortic arch, carotid bifurcation, and intracranial vasculature. Significant proximal pathology can cause identical neurologic symptoms, and if they are not specifically looked for, their presence may be easily missed. Arteriovenous malformations, cerebral aneurysms, and significant siphon stenoses are among the many intracranial lesions that can be identified and may influence management decisions.

The risks associated with cerebral angiography are numerous. First, because this is an invasive procedure requiring arterial access, puncture site complications are not infrequent. Hematoma formation, acute arterial dissection or thrombosis, false aneurysms, and distal embolization have all been reported. The exact incidence of these complications has unfortunately not been consistently reported. However, they probably occur in 1 to 2% of cases.[12,13] Second, catheter manipulation within the carotid artery can lead to serious complications such as dissection or embolization. In one review of over 5000 cerebral angiographic procedures, the overall risk of neurologic sequelae was 0.9%, with 0.06% of patients suffering a permanent stroke.[14] Others have placed the risk of neurologic events and stroke at 2.6% and 0.6%, respectively.[15] In a 1990 review of eight prospective studies, the risk of stroke following angiography was 1.0% and the overall mortality rate was 0.06%.[16] Finally, although exact results are still unpublished, it appears that the stroke rate in patients entered into the North American Symptomatic Carotid Endarterectomy Trial (NASCET) trial is approximately 0.78%.[5] The risk of stroke does seem to vary based on the clinical presentation. In general, asymptomatic patients have a lower risk, whereas angiography in the setting of transient ischemic episodes is associated with a slightly higher complication rate.[15,17,18] Two groups of patients that deserve special mention are those who undergo angiography to evaluate a stroke in evolution and those with bilateral severe carotid stenoses. The former group has been associated with a neurologic complication rate of 7.7%, and a rate of 12.5% has been reported for the latter.[18] Finally, the contrast material injected during angiography can induce allergic reactions and renal failure, as well as alterations in the coagulation system. Allergic reactions range from mild rashes and gastrointestinal upset to life-threatening hypotension, bronchospasm, pulmonary edema, and cardiac arrhythmias. The risk of contrast reactions in all types of angiographic studies varies between 2 and 8%.[13] For cerebral examinations it is at the lower end of the range, with a rate of approximately 2%.[13] In high-risk patients with antecedent renal disease, the risk of acute renal failure following the administration of contrast material can be as high as 40%, with over 8% of patients requiring permanent dialysis.[19] The same center has reported an overall rate of acute renal dysfunction following angiography of 11.3%, with 1.5% of patients requiring permanent dialysis.[19] An increased thrombotic tendency has been observed in association with injection of radiocontrast material and may be related to a transient decrease in endothelial prostacyclin production.[20]

In addition to these well-known complications, there are other drawbacks to angiography that should be mentioned. First, angiography does not provide information regarding plaque composition. Although the degree of stenosis is easily quantified, the character of the lesion in question remains unknown. This is an important limitation because, as mentioned above, the content of a given plaque (soft, calcified, or mixed) has implications in predicting the natural history of the lesion. Finally, depending on the institution, the cost of angiography is as high as several thousand dollars per procedure. If one estimates that 100,000 carotid endarterectomies are performed in the United States each year,[21] then the cost of obtaining a routine angiogram on every patient would be millions of dollars annually.

CAROTID ENDARTERECTOMY WITHOUT ANGIOGRAPHY

Background

Although many surgeons consider angiography mandatory prior to performing a carotid endarterectomy,[22] with the emergence of newer noninvasive imaging technologies, others have questioned whether this study is necessary in all cases. In 1982, Blackshear and Connar were the first to demonstrate that carotid endarterectomy could be performed on the basis of the analysis of carotid Doppler signals without the use of angiography.[23] Since then, several forces have motivated clinicians to evaluate this policy. First, in this era of cost containment, the prospect of reducing the cost of evaluating patients is very attractive. Second, the morbidity associated with angiography is significant and has remained relatively unchanged because these patients are often afflicted by concurrent cardiac and renal dysfunction. Finally, because the morbidity of any preoperative examination must be added to the overall risk associated with the surgical intervention, methods of treating these patients safely without routine angiography are even more desirable. These forces have led several investigators to review their own experience in managing carotid lesions in an attempt to determine the relative value of angiographic data.

Ricotta and associates were the first to present a retrospective analysis comparing the value of angiography versus duplex scanning in the preoperative evaluation of patients being considered for carotid endarterectomy.[24] These authors reviewed the hospital records of 111 patients who had undergone both examinations prior to surgery. The results suggested that at least two-thirds of their patients, with either asymptomatic lesions or hemispheric symptoms, derived no benefit from carotid angiography. Two years later, Walsh and colleagues reported on their experience in treating 28 patients who presented with amaurosis fugax.[25] In no instance did they find that preoperative angiography added important information to the workup. In fact, angiography correctly characterized only 17 of the 28 recorded pathologic specimens. By comparison, the combination of duplex scanning and routine cerebral computed tomography (CT) accurately predicted the operative findings in every case. The authors concluded that routine angiography was not necessary in patients with amaurosis fugax and no other complications. The same conclusion was reached by Goodson et al after a review of 78 carotid endarterectomies performed in patients with focal anterior circulation symptoms.[26] By comparing the results of both angiography and duplex scanning, they determined that the sensitivity of the duplex data was superior to that of angiography (99% vs 91%). This was particularly true for the detection of luminal surface abnormalities, where the sensitivity of duplex scanning was 92% compared to 64% for angiography. The authors suggested that selected patients with positive duplex studies, associated with focal symptoms in the appropriate distribution, could undergo carotid endarterectomy without angiography.

With these retrospective reviews as a background, Moore et al designed a prospective study in which physicians were asked to predict anatomic findings from a group of 85 patients.[27] The clinicians were provided with complete histories and physical exam reports, as well as the results of duplex studies. After comparison with angiographic findings, 93.5% of the recorded predictions were noted to be correct. Based on this diagnosis rate, the authors performed 32 carotid endarterectomies without angiography. There were no complications, and the predicted lesion was confirmed at operation in every patient. Furthermore, intraopera-

tive angiography, which was obtained after every procedure, failed to identify any abnormalities that would have altered a single patient's management. A similar simulated treatment technique was later employed by Farmilo and associates.[28] In this study, the records of 63 patients who had undergone both carotid duplex scanning and angiography were reviewed. It was found that in patients with angiographic evidence of a stenosis of 50% or greater, duplex scanning achieved a sensitivity and specificity of 96% and 95%, respectively. In patients later documented to have a totally occluded vessel, however, the sensitivity of duplex scanning was only 50%. These authors also concluded that routine angiography was unnecessary in selected patients.

It should be noted that not all investigators performing similar reviews have arrived at the same conclusion. Geuder and colleagues compared the results of preoperative angiography and duplex scanning in 100 patients.[22] They surmised that eight of these patients would have been treated incorrectly on the basis of duplex data alone. For this reason, the authors concluded that routine preoperative angiography should be performed in all patients being considered for carotid endarterectomy. Despite these recommendations, on careful review of this series it is apparent that angiography would not have altered the management in over 90% of these patients. Furthermore, most of the patients in whom angiography uncovered unsuspected information had intracranial or posterior circulation lesions and would have undergone a bifurcation endarterectomy anyway.

To summarize the experience gained from these retrospective reviews, it is clear that carotid endarterectomy can be performed safely in selected patients based on carotid duplex scanning alone without preoperative angiography.

Published Results of Carotid Endarterectomy without Angiography

To date, hundreds of carotid endarterectomies performed without preoperative angiography have been reported in the English literature. This experience is summarized in Table 45–2. The first report, which appeared in 1982, was by Blackshear and Connar.[23] These authors performed carotid endarterectomy without angiography in four patients using only duplex scanning for diagnostic data. There were no perioperative neurologic events. The following year, Sandmann et al[45] published a series of 91 carotid endarterectomies done without angiography. Again, there were no postoperative strokes, and the authors suggested that preoperative angiography was unnecessary in the majority of patients. Following these early reports, several additional investigators have submitted for review their experience in performing carotid endarterectomy without angiography. The combined number of cases

Table 45–2. Early Results of Carotid Endarterectomy Performed without Preoperative Angiography

Author	Year	No. of Cases	Perioperative		
			Stroke	TIA	Event
Blackshear[23]	1982	4	0 (0.0%)	0 (0.0%)	0 (0.0%)
Sandmann[45]	1983	91	0 (0.0%)	0 (0.0%)	0 (0.0%)
Gonzalez[46]	1984	5	0 (0.0%)	0 (0.0%)	0 (0.0%)
Crew[47]	1984	65	1 (1.5%)	1 (1.5%)	2 (3.0%)
Thomas[48]	1986	32	0 (0.0%)	0 (0.0%)	0 (0.0%)
Marshall[49]	1988	26	1 (3.8%)	1 (3.8%)	2 (7.6%)
Moore[27]	1988	32	0 (0.0%)	0 (0.0%)	0 (0.0%)
Hill[50]	1990	130	1 (0.7%)	2 (1.4%)	3 (2.1%)
Wagner[51]	1991	255	6 (2.4%)	0 (0.0%)	6 (2.4%)
Cartier[52]	1993	130	3 (2.3%)	2 (1.5%)	5 (3.8%)
Total		770	12 (1.6%)	6 (0.8%)	18 (2.4%)

Abbreviation: TIA, transient ischemic attack.

reaches several hundred, and the overall incidence of perioperative neurologic events, at least in this review, can be expected to be approximately 2.4%. It is important to note that in the majority of these reports, the anatomic location of these strokes relative to the operative side was not specified. Regardless, the combined incidence of stroke in these series compares favorably with the expected rates of perioperative stroke following carotid endarterectomy for asymptomatic (1 to 2%) as well as symptomatic (3 to 5%) patients.[29–32]

Selection of Patients for Carotid Endarterectomy without Angiography

The most important criterion that must be satisfied prior to subjecting a patient to carotid endarterectomy on the basis of duplex scan data alone is that the duplex scan be a reliable study from a laboratory that has validated its results by sequential comparison of previous duplex and angiographic data. This point is essential and cannot be overemphasized. Results of duplex scanning can vary greatly, depending on the operator, and it is therefore very important to have well-trained and experienced personnel performing the examination.

In general, the more suitable patients for carotid endarterectomy without angiography are symptomatic or asymptomatic patients with hemodynamically significant carotid bifurcation lesions. Even in this setting, however, certain criteria must be met. First the history and physical examination should be consistent and should correlate accurately with the duplex scan findings. Second, a head CT scan should be obtained to rule out any intracranial explanation for the patient's complaints. Vertebrobasilar symptoms, abnormal flow patterns in the common carotid, unequal upper extremity blood pressures, or any other signs that

proximal disease may be present are an indication for preoperative angiography. Likewise, any discrepancy among the history, physical examination, and duplex data should suggest the need for a contrast study. Lastly, patients with focal cerebral symptoms and either a stenosis below 50% or duplex findings suggestive of total carotid occlusion should undergo further carotid imaging. The former will rule out an ulcerative plaque or significant disease in another location, and the latter is important because duplex scanning has proven less accurate in distinguishing a "string sign" from a total carotid occlusion.

Several types of patients are well suited to carotid endarterectomy without angiography. These include patients with severe contrast allergies associated in the past with an episode of anaphylactic shock, patients with severe peripheral vascular disease in whom no adequate arterial access site is available, and patients requiring urgent intervention such as those with crescendo ischemic attacks or a stroke in evolution.

As mentioned earlier, the main disadvantage of duplex imaging is its inability to evaluate both proximal and intracranial disease. Opponents of the policy of operating on suspected bifurcation lesions without the benefit of angiography traditionally point to these deficiencies when arguing in favor of angiography in all cases. However, careful analysis of these objections fails to provide sufficiently strong evidence to discourage the selective use of angiography. Significant proximal stenoses will often be associated with innominate or subclavian arterial disease that can easily be identified on physical examination. Even in the absence of associated arch vessel disease, duplex scanning is capable of suggesting the presence of an isolated proximal carotid lesion by the finding of turbulent flow and spectral broadening in the carotid artery at the base of the neck. Abnormal turbulence and low flow velocities in the distal internal carotid can also be used to detect carotid siphon disease and should prompt the clinician to obtain additional studies.

The presence of most other types of intracranial disease can be detected by the use of routine head CT scans. This examination is capable of identifying arteriovenous malformations, tumors, and aneurysms 1 cm or more in size. In addition, it should be recognized that most experienced surgeons recommend correcting significant carotid bifurcation disease even in the presence of many intracranial lesions.[33–39] The incidence of intracranial aneurysms that are too small to be detected by routine CT scans is quite low. After reviewing cerebral angiograms in 3684 patients, Winn found berry aneurysms in only 0.65% of cases.[40] In addition, it is unlikely that the incidental finding of an asymptomatic intracranial aneurysm has any clinical significance in the management of a patient presenting for repair of an extracranial carotid stenosis. Orrechia et al safely performed carotid endarterectomies in 10 patients with associated berry aneurysms despite the presence of significant hypertension in 70% of this group.[39] Similarly, Ladowski et al reported no postoperative complications after carotid endarterectomy in 19 patients with asymptomatic intracranial aneurysms.[38] Both Schuler et al[33] and Borozan et al[35] found no difference in the incidence of late cerebrovascular symptoms following carotid endarterectomy in patients with or without carotid siphon disease. Roederer and associates reported that only 9% of identified siphon lesions had a stenosis of 50% or greater and that the degree of siphon stenosis did not predict the recurrence of focal symptoms in patients operated on for bifurcation lesions.[34] Finally, Akers et al demonstrated that patients undergoing carotid endarterectomy in the presence of a siphon stenosis are relieved of their symptoms, and in their series no patient suffered any perioperative complications as a result of the untreated distal disease.[37]

SUMMARY

The recent publication of prospective randomized trials establishing the benefit of carotid endarterectomy in selected symptomatic and asymptomatic patients with carotid artery stenoses clearly highlights the importance of accurate, safe, and cost-effective ways to assess the cerebrovascular circulation. An accurate history and physical examination remains the mainstay of this evaluation. Following this, we believe that patients with well-defined symptoms, appropriate physical findings, and concurring CT and duplex scans can safely undergo carotid endarterectomy without preoperative arteriography. It is extremely important, however, that the duplex scan be a reliable study from a laboratory that has validated its results by sequential comparison of previous duplex and angiographic data.

Contrast angiography remains appropriate in patients with atypical symptoms; with conflicting findings among the history, physical exam, and duplex data; or when there is evidence of proximal disease. Also, in a symptomatic patient, when the duplex scan suggests a total occlusion, angiography is still indicated because duplex data cannot accurately differentiate between a tight lesion and total occlusion. Of course, patients suspected of having carotid pathology other than atherosclerotic occlusive disease such as aneurysms, fibromuscular dysplasia, tortuosities, or tumors are all currently considered candidates for angiography. Alternatively, 2D and 3D TOF magnetic resonance imaging is a promising new technique that may be able to replace conventional angiography in some clinical situations. The major advantages of MRA are its ability to display the bifurcation in a format similar to that of contrast angiography, its ability to distinguish high-grade from total carotid occlusions, and its impressive demonstration of the intracranial vascular anatomy. Unfortunately, signal void related to turbulence remains a serious problem, and even the latest MR imaging technology tends to overestimate the degree of bifurcation stenoses.

REFERENCES

1. Hunink MGM, Polak JF, Barlan MM, et al. Detection and quantification of carotid artery stenosis: efficacy of various Doppler velocity parameters. *AJR* 1993;160:619–625.
2. Moneta GL, Edwards JM, Chitwood RW, et al. Correlation of North American Symptomatic Carotid Endarterectomy Trial (NASCET) angiographic definition of 70% to 99% internal carotid artery stenosis with duplex scanning. *J Vasc Surg* 1993;17:152–159.
3. Faught WE, Mattos MA, van Bemmelen PS, et al. Color-flow duplex scanning of carotid arteries: new velocity criteria based on receiver operator characteristic analysis for threshold stenoses used in the symptomatic and asymptomatic carotid trials. *J Vasc Surg* 1994;19:818–828.
4. Neale ML, Chambers JL, Kelly AT, et al. Reappraisal of duplex criteria to assess significant carotid stenosis with special reference to reports from the North American Symptomatic Carotid Endarterectomy Trial and the European Carotid Surgery Trial. *J Vasc Surg* 1994;20:642–649.
5. Eliasziw M, Rankin RN, Fox AJ, et al. Accuracy and prognostic consequences of ultrasonography in identifying severe carotid artery stenosis. *Stroke* 1995;26:1747–1752.
6. Bornstein NM, Beloev ZG, Norris JW. The limitations of diagnosis of carotid occlusion by Doppler ultrasound. *Ann Surg* 1988;207:315–317.
7. Heiserman JE, Drayer BP, Fram EK, et al. Carotid artery stenosis: clinical efficacy of two-dimensional time-of-flight MR angiography. *Radiology* 1992;182:761–768.
8. Huston J, Lewis BD, Wiebers DO, et al. Carotid artery: prospective blinded comparison of two-dimensional time-of-flight MR angiography with conventional angiography and duplex US. *Radiology* 1993;186:339–344.
9. Mittl RL Jr, Broderick M, Carpenter JP, et al. Blinded-reader comparison of magnetic resonance angiography

and duplex ultrasonography for carotid artery bifurcation stenosis. *Stroke* 1994;25:4–10.

10. Riles TS, Eidelman EM, Litt AW, et al. Comparison of magnetic resonance angiography, conventional angiography, and duplex scanning. *Stroke* 1992;23:341–346.

11. Patel MR, Kuntz KM, Klufas RA, et al. Preoperative assessment of the carotid bifurcation. Can magnetic resonance angiography and duplex ultrasonography replace contrast arteriography? *Stroke* 1995;26:1753–1758.

12. Hessel SJ, Adams DF, Abrams HL. Complications of angiography. *Radiology* 1981;138:273–281.

13. Rose JS. Contrast media, complications, and preparation of the patient. In: Rutherford RB, ed. *Vascular Surgery*. 2nd ed. Philadelphia: WB Saunders; 1984:244–252.

14. Mani RL, Eisenberg RL, McDonald EJ, et al. Complications of catheter cerebral angiography: analysis of 5,000 procedures. I. Criteria and incidence. *Am J Roentgenol* 1978;131:861–865.

15. Earnest F, Forbes G, Sandok BA, et al. Complications of cerebral angiography: prospective assessment of risk. *Am J Radiol* 1984;142:247–253.

16. Hankey GJ, Warlow CP, Sellar RJ. Cerebral angiographic risk in mild cerebrovascular disease. *Stroke* 1990;21:209–222.

17. Dion JE, Gates PC, Fox AJ, et al. Clinical events following neuroangiography: a prospective study. *Stroke* 1987;18:997–1004.

18. Theodotou BC, Whaley R, Mahaley MS. Complications following transfemoral cerebral angiography for cerebral ischemia: report of 159 angiograms and correlation with surgical risk. *Surg Neurol* 1987;28:90–92.

19. Martin-Paredero V, Dixon SM, Baker JD, et al. Risk of renal failure after major angiography. *Arch Surg* 1983;118:1417–1420.

20. Osborne RW, Malone JM, Hunter GC, et al. Endothelial fibrinolytic activity: the key to postangiographic thrombosis? *Surg Forum* 1981;32:328–330.

21. Pokras R, Dyken ML. Dramatic changes in the performance of endarterectomy for diseases of the extracranial arteries of the head. *Stroke* 1988;19:1289–1290.

22. Geuder JW, Lamparello PJ, Riles TS, et al. Is duplex scanning sufficient evaluation before carotid endarterectomy? *J Vasc Surg* 1989;9:193–201.

23. Blackshear WM, Connar RG. Carotid endarterectomy without angiography. *J Cardiovasc Surg* 1982;23:477–482.

24. Ricotta JJ, Holen J, Schenk E, et al. Is routine angiography necessary prior to carotid endarterectomy? *J Vasc Surg* 1984;1:96–102.

25. Walsh J, Markowitz I, Kerstein MD. Carotid endarterectomy for amaurosis fugax without angiography. *Am J Surg* 1986;152:172–174.

26. Goodson SF, Flanigan DP, Bishara RA, et al. Can carotid duplex scanning supplant arteriography in patients with focal carotid territory symptoms? *J Vasc Surg* 1987;5:551–557.

27. Moore WS, Ziomek S, Quiñones-Baldrish WJ, et al. Can clinical evaluation and noninvasive testing substitute for arteriography in the evaluation of carotid artery disease? *Ann Surg* 1988;298:91–94.

28. Farmilo RW, Scott DJA, Cole SEA, et al. Role of duplex scanning in the selection of patients for carotid endarterectomy. *Br J Surg* 1990;77:388–390.

29. Thompson JE. Carotid endarterectomy for asymptomatic carotid stenosis: An update. *J Vasc Surg* 1991;13:669–676.

30. North American Symptomatic Carotid Endarterectomy Trial Collaborators. Beneficial effect of carotid endarterectomy in symptomatic patients with high-grade carotid stenosis. *N Engl J Med* 1991;325(7):445–453.

31. European Carotid Surgery Trialists' Collaborative Group. MRC European Carotid Surgery Trial: interim results for symptomatic patients with severe (70–99%) or with mild (0–29%) carotid stenosis. *Lancet* 1991;337:1235–1243.

32. Mayberg MR, Wilson SE, Yatsu F, et al. Carotid endarterectomy and prevention of cerebral ischemia in symptomatic carotid stenosis. *JAMA* 1991;266:3289–3294.

33. Schuler JJ, Flanigan DP, Lim LT, et al. The effect of carotid siphon stenosis on stroke rate, death, and relief of symptoms following elective carotid endarterectomy. *Surgery* 1982;92:1058–1067.

34. Roederer GO, Langois YE, Chan ARW, et al. Is siphon disease important in predicting outcome of carotid endarterectomy? *Arch Surg* 1983;118:1177–1181.

35. Borozan PG, Schuler JJ, LaRosa MP, et al. The natural history of isolated carotid siphon stenosis. *J Vasc Surg* 1984;1:744–749.

36. Moore WS. Does tandem lesion mean tandem risk in patients with carotid artery disease? *J Vasc Surg* 1988;7:454–455.

37. Akers DL, Bell WH, Kerstein MD. Does intracranial dye study contribute to evaluation of carotid artery disease? *Am J Surg* 1988;156:87–90.

38. Ladowski JS, Webster MW, Yonas HO, et al. Carotid endarterectomy in patients with asymptomatic intracranial aneurysm. *Ann Surg* 1984;200:70–73.

39. Orrechia PM, Clagett GP, Youkey JR, et al. Management of patients with symptomatic extracranial carotid artery disease and incidental intracranial berry aneurysm. *J Vasc Surg* 1985;2:158–164.

40. Winn HW. What's new in neurosurgery: aneurysm. *Bull Am Coll Surg* 1984;70:17–21.

41. Masaryk TJ, Modic MT, Ruggieri PM, et al. Three-dimentional (volume) gradient-echo imaging of the carotid bifurcation: preliminary clinical experience. *Radiology* 1989;171:801–806.

42. Wilkerson DK, Keller I, Mezrich R, et al. The comparative evaluation of three-dimentional magnetic resonance for carotid artery disease. *J Vasc Surg* 1991;14:803–811.

43. Anderson CM, Saloner D, Lee RE, et al. Assessment of carotid artery stenosis by MR angiography: comparison with x-ray angiography and color-coded doppler ultrasound. *Am J Neuroradiol* 1992;13:989–1003.

44. Wesbey GE, Bergan JJ, Moreland SI, et al. Cerebrovascular magnetic resonance angiography: a critical verification. *J Vasc Surg* 1992;16:619–632.

45. Sandmann W, Hennerici M, Nullen H, et al. Carotid artery surgery without angiography: risk or progress. In: Greenhalgh RM, Rose FC, eds. *Progress in Stroke Research* II. London: Pittman; 1983:447–461.

46. Gonzalez LL, Partusch L, Wirth P. Noninvasive carotid artery evaluation following endarterectomy. *J Vasc Surg* 1984;1:403–408.

47. Crew JR, Dean M, Johnson JM, et al. Carotid surgery without angiography. *Am J Surg* 1984;148:217–220.

48. Thomas GI, Jones TW, Stavney LS, et al. Carotid endarterectomy after Doppler ultrasonographic examination without angiography. *Am J Surg* 1986;151:616–619.

49. Marshall WG, Kouchoukos NT, Murphy SF, et al. Carotid endarterectomy based on duplex scanning without preoperative arteriography. *Circulation* 1988;78(suppl I):I1–I5.

50. Hill JC, Carbonneau K, Baliga PK, et al. Safe extracranial vascular evaluation and surgery without preoperative arteriography. *Ann Vasc Surg* 1990;4:34–38.

51. Wagner WH, Treiman RL, Cossman DV, et al. The diminishing role of diagnostic arteriography in carotid artery disease: duplex scanning as definitive preoperative study. *Ann Vasc Surg* 1991;5:105–110.

52. Cartier R, Cartier P, Fontaine A. Carotid endarterectomy without angiography. The reliability of Doppler ultrasonography and duplex scanning in preoperative assessment. *Can J Surg* 1993;36:411–416.

46

The Current Status of Carotid Endarterectomy: Indications and Results

Peter N. Purcell, M.D.
Richard P. Cambria, M.D.

BACKGROUND

In 1951, C. Miller Fisher, in two sentinel reports, emphasized the relationship between disease of the extracranial carotid artery and ipsilateral hemispheric stroke.[1,2] He realized that the disease process was atherosclerotic in origin and could cause neurologic symtoms prior to causing a stroke. He cogently stated that "it is even conceivable that some day vascular surgery will find a way to bypass the occluded portion of the artery during a period of ominous fleeting symptoms."[1] This prediction was rapidly followed by the first description of a surgical carotid reconstruction in 1952 by Eastcott et al.[3]

After the first successful carotid endarterectomy (CEA), performed by DeBakey in 1953, the operation became an accepted treatment for symptomatic carotid disease.[4] However, the lack of prospective data demonstrating the efficacy of CEA compared to medical treatment in preventing stroke and a lack of valid natural history data in general, particularly in patients with asymptomatic disease, led to decades of controversy about the operation. For example, the Framingham Study identified an asymptomatic carotid bruit in 66 men and 105 women. Stroke appeared in 21 patients, a rate more than twice that in sex- and age-matched controls, yet more often than not, cerebral infarction occurred in a vascular territory different from that of the carotid bruit. Therefore, the carotid bruit was believed to be an indicator of increased stroke risk but not predictive of a specific anatomic cause of stroke.[5]

The surgical treatment of asymptomatic carotid disease continued to generate controversy. Natural history studies began to appear in the 1980s, suggesting that while asymptomatic carotid disease was not benign, the onset of symptoms often preceded stroke. Furthermore, the incidence of cardiac ischemic events in this population tended to negate the potential benefits of prophylactic carotid surgery. For example, Norris and colleagues followed 696 patients with asymptomatic carotid stenoses with duplex scans for a mean period of 41 months. The annual stroke rate was 1.3% among patients with a carotid stenosis less than 75% and 3.3% (2.5% ipsilateral) among those with stenoses greater than 75%. In contrast, the annual cardiac event rate was 8.3%[6] In another study, Chambers and Norris followed 500 asymptomatic patients with cervical bruits for a mean period of 23.2 months. The overall incidence of stroke at 1 year was 1.7% but increased to 5.5% in patients with carotid stenoses greater than 75%. The incidence of cardiac ischemic events at 1 year was 6%. Furthermore, most patients did not have strokes without first developing transient ischemic attacks (TIAs).[7] These data, and the risk of significant surgical morbidity, further reinforced a conservative management posture among many clinicians. For example, in one study, 228 consecutive CEAs performed in two hospitals were examined retrospectively.[8] The combined stroke-mortality rate was 21.1%, with an operative stroke rate for the series of 14.5% Although an interim update from the same group showed significant improvement in stroke and mortality rates,[9] these alarmingly high morbidity and mortality rates convinced many clinicians that CEA should not be performed for asymptomatic disease, and perhaps only in selected symptomatic cases.

Further natural history data were reported from the University of Washington. Roderer and colleagues followed 167 patients with asymptomatic cervical bruits with annual duplex exams and noted a close relationship between disease progression and the appearance of ischemic neurologic symptoms or subsequent carotid artery occlusion. The annual rate of symptom occurrence was 4%. The mean annual rate of disease progression to a stenosis greater than 50% was 8%. Progression of a lesion to a stenosis greater than 80% was found to carry a 35% risk of ischemic symptoms or ipsilateral occlusion within 6 months and a 46% risk at 12 months. The authors believed that surgical treatment could safely be delayed until the appearance of TIAs or progression of disease to a stenosis greater than 80% in diameter.[10] In a follow-up study, Moneta et al. documented 129 asymptomatic, high-grade (80 to 99%) lesions in 115 patients. Fifty-six CEAs were performed, and 73 patients were followed without surgery. Life table analysis at 24 months revealed a 19% incidence of stroke and a 28% incidence of TIAs for the nonoperative group versus 4% and 5%, respectively, for the operative group. Furthermore, none of the strokes in the nonoperative group were preceded by a TIA.[11] This study, though not randomized, was one of the first of the "modern" studies to demonstrate the efficacy of surgery for patients with asymptomatic lesions.

The current indications for CEA have been clarified through several large, prospective studies of symptomatic and asymptomatic patients. In addition, two clinical scenarios for which no conclusive data exist, that is, for patients with evolving or recent stroke and patients with symptomatic noncritical stenosis, are reviewed. Because these two clinical presentations are uncommon, definitive data in the form of large clinical trials may not be forthcoming.

INDICATIONS FOR SURGERY

Symptomatic Carotid Artery Stenosis

The two largest studies to address the role of CEA in symptomatic patients were the European Carotid Surgery Trial (ECST) and the North American Symptomatic Carotid Endarterectomy Trial (NASCET). In the ECST, 2518 patients with a carotid stenosis and a nondisabling carotid territory ischemic stroke, TIA, or amaurosis fugax were randomized to CEA or aspirin. The mean follow-up period for the cohort was 3 years. Carotid stenoses were categorized angiographically as "mild" (0 to 29% stenosis) "moderate" (30 to 68% stenosis), "severe" (70 to 99% stenosis). The recruitment criteria for the ECST deserve comment. Patients who had suffered a stroke or the above symptoms within 6 months underwent carotid arteriography. They were then offered participation in the study only if the local surgeon and neurologist were "substantially uncertain" whether to recommend CEA. Patients randomized to surgery underwent an operation within 6 weeks. Both groups received similar medical therapy—aspirin, treatment of hypertension, and advice to stop

smoking. Patients underwent surgery at multiple institutions in 14 countries. For patients with mild stenosis a minimal risk of ischemic stroke at 3 years was found, and the risks of surgery in this group outweighed the benefits. Randomization continues for patients with moderate stenoses. However, among patients with severe stenoses ($n = 778$), the benefit of surgery was clear despite a substantial (and, by current standards, unacceptable) stroke-mortality rate of 7.5% after CEA. The 3 year stroke risk was 2.8% for the surgical group and 16.8% for the medical group ($p < 0.001$, a sixfold risk reduction). The investigators concluded that while CEA clearly was associated with a 30-day risk of stroke or mortality, patients with severe stenosis undergoing surgery may be expected to benefit from the stroke-reducing effect of CEA within 1 to 2 years.[12]

In the NASCET, 659 patients less than 80 years of age with carotid stenoses of 70 to 99% who had experienced TIAs, amaurosis fugax, or nondisabling stroke within 120 days prior to entry into the study were randomized to medical versus surgical treatment in 50 centers in the United States and Canada. Approximately two-thirds of both groups were male. All patients received aspirin and, as indicated, antihypertensive and antilipid therapy. The perioperative stroke rate was 5.5% (18 patients); of these, 12 had minor strokes, 5 major, and 1 fatal. In addition, one patient died suddenly after surgery, for a combined perioperative stroke-death rate of 5.8%. In a comparable time period, the stroke rate in the medical group was 3.3%. Life-table estimates demonstrated that the cumulative risk of ipsilateral stroke at 2 years was 26% in the medical group and 9% in the surgical group. These data, which included perioperative stroke in the surgical group, demonstrated that for every 100 patients treated surgically, 17 were spared an ipsilateral stroke over the next 2 years, or that 6 patients would need surgery to prevent one stroke every 24 months. Further, the early disadvantage of perioperative stroke or death was overcome at 3 months. There was no evidence of the advantage of CEA declining for as long as 30 months postoperatively. Thus, CEA was found to be highly beneficial in symptomatic patients with high-grade carotid artery stenoses. As in the ECST, results have not been reported for patients with lesser degrees of stenosis (30 to 69%).[13]

The NASCET also demonstrated a correlation between the degree of stenosis and the magnitude of risk reduction. Absolute risk reduction for ipsilateral stroke at 2 years in the surgical group was 26% for 90 to 99% stenosis, 18% for 80 to 89% stenosis, and 12% for 70 to 79% stenosis. The NASCET was terminated early due to evidence of treatment efficacy in the high-grade stenosis group. This study emphasized the need for low complication rates to confer benefit from CEA. The data analysis predicted that if perioperative complications approached 10%, the stroke-reducing benefit of CEA would vanish entirely.[13,14]

Carotid Artery Stenosis and Acute Stroke

Two subsets of symptomatic CEA candidates deserve separate consideration: those with acute, unstable neurologic symptoms, and those with acute stroke. Historically, CEA for evolving stroke has been discouraged due to the poor neurologic outcome and high operative mortality. In Thompson's landmark 1970 review of 748 CEAs, 262 were performed for acute stroke and the mortality for this group was 7.4%; only 64% of patients improved neurologically after operation. The high mortality was presumed to be due, in part, to reperfusion hemorrhage. Thompson recommended that patients with acute profound and rapidly progressing strokes should not be treated with emergent surgery, but rather should be allowed to stabilize for several weeks before considering an operation.[14] More recently, Gertler et al examined the outcomes of 55 patients undergoing CEA who had neurologically unstable conditions, such as crescendo TIAs despite anticoagulation, stroke in evolution, or a radiographic "string sign." Overall morbidity was 3.5%, and there was no mortality. The survival rate was equivalent to that of a matched control population at 5 years, and the cumulative TIA/stroke-free survival rate was 75% at 5 years, suggesting that early intervention in these patients is warranted.[15]

A related issue involves the timing of CEA after a completed stroke. Historically, it had been suggested that patients with a completed stroke should undergo CEA only after a 6-week waiting period.[16] This conclusion was challenged in a prospective trial by Piotrowski et al at the University of Arizona in which 129 patients underwent CEA after stroke. In 82 patients CEA was performed after the evolving stroke "plateaued," based on symptoms, and in all cases within 6 weeks. In the remainder, operation was not performed until recovery from stroke was documented, and no patients underwent surgery for at least 6 weeks. No significant difference in morbidity or mortality was noted between the two groups, and no significant difference was found between patients operated on at 2, 4, 6, or more than 6 weeks after a stroke. The authors concluded that a delay of 6 weeks was not necessary as long as neurologic symptoms had plateaued.[17] Other studies agree with the conclusion that CEA after a stroke may be safely undertaken once symptoms have stabilized.[18]

Our experience confirms that the truly emergency CEA is quite rare. Circumstances of compelling radiographic anatomy (string sign, intraluminal thrombus) are the more common dictators of truly urgent operation. CEA for patients with acute or recent stroke depends on the anatomy of the lesion, the extent of the cerebral injury, and the clinical status of the patient.

Refinement of catheter-based thrombolytic therapy has made this technique the inital choice of many clinicians in patients with acute carotid thrombosis, but surgical intervention may still be indicated as a primary or secondary therapy in some cases.[19]

Symptomatic Noncritical Carotid Artery Stenosis

The management of symptomatic patients with noncritical carotid artery stenoses remains unsettled. These patients are uncommon, and studies such as the NASCET have had considerable difficulty with patient recruitment. We believe that neurologic events related to lesser degrees of carotid stenosis represent dynamic events in the carotid bifurcation plaque, such as intraplaque hemorrhage and/or communication of the necrotic plaque core (ie, a source of emboli) with the vascular lumen. The angiographic correlate of this condition (plaque ulceration) may be present.

The significance of plaque ulceration as an independent risk factor for stroke has been recognized for some time. Tow earlier studies examined the stroke risk among 153 asymptomatic patients with nonstenotic carotid ulcerative lesions classified as small (grade A), large (grade B), or compound (multiple cavities; grade C). The interval annual stroke rates were 0.9%, 4.5%, and 7.5%, respectively, suggesting that an aggressive surgical approach is indicated in patients with grade B and C ulcers.[20,21] The relationship between plaque ulceration and stroke risk in symptomatic patients was examined by Eliasziw et al in a study of 659 patients from the NASCET with severe carotid stenoses. Among medically treated patients with plaque ulceration, the risk of stroke at 24 months increased incrementally from 26% to 73% as stenosis increased from 75% to 95%, whereas the risk of stroke remained constant at 21% in the absence of ulceration.[22] These data suggest that plaque ulceration in symptomatic patients is an independent risk factor for stroke, and CEA should be considered in these patients even if the degree of stenosis is less than 70%. It is our practice to recommend CEA in patients with complex/ulcerated bifurcation plaques, irrespective of the degree of stenosis, when the clinical and angiographic data implicate the carotid disease as the source of hemispheric or retinal symptoms.

A related problem among patients with noncritical stenoses is the significance of retinal findings such as ischemic retinopathy and Hollenhorst plaques, which may result from thromboemboli secondary to carotid artery atherosclerosis. While amaurosis fugax is known to correlate strongly with the presence of hemodynamically significant disease,[23,24] several studies suggest that patients with clinical evidence of retinal embolic events carry an increased risk of significant carotid disease and subsequent stroke. One study found that patients with retinal plaques were significantly more likely to have ipsilateral ulcerated carotid artery plaques,[25] and another study reported that patients with Hollenhorst plaques were more likely to develop subsequent TIAs than those without retinal pathology.[26] Although the presence of asymptomatic retinal lesions may not be a specific indication for CEA, it warrants noninvasive carotid artery examination, and if symptoms develop even in the presence of noncritical carotid disease, CEA may be indicated (Fig. 46–1).

Asymptomatic Carotid Artery Stenosis

Two recent randomized trials have clarified the role of CEA in asymptomatic carotid disease. In the multi-center Veterans Affairs (VA) Cooperative Studies Pro-

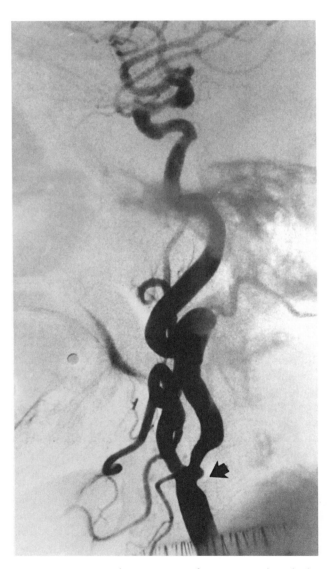

Figure 46–1. Carotid arteriogram of a patient with multiple episodes of retinal cholesterol emboli documented by fundoscopic examination and complicated by a partial retinal infarct. Arch vessels were normal. Note the significant ulceration (arrow) in plaque and the modest degree of stenosis.

gram Asymptomatic Stenosis Trial, 444 men with asymptomatic carotid stenoses shown by arteriography to be at least 50% diameter-reducing were randomly assigned to medical therapy alone or in conjunction with CEA. After a mean follow-up period of 48 months, the combined incidence of ipsilateral neurologic events (TIA, retinal symptoms, and stroke) was 8% in the surgical group and 20.6% in the medical group ($p < 0.001$). The incidence of ipsilateral stroke was 4.7% in the surgical and 9.4% in the medical group, a difference that did not reach statistical significance due to the relatively small sample size of the study.[27] While providing important evidence of the efficacy of CEA in selected patients with asymptomatic carotid disease, this study suffered from several problems. The study population was considerably smaller than the 500-patient target established by power calculations at the beginning of the study.[28] An alpha power calculation indicates that with the addition of another 150 patients to each group, the difference in the ipsilateral stroke rate alone would have reached statistical significance.[29] The study also was criticized for the inclusion of TIA/retinal events as endpoints. This was done because some patients in the medical group who experienced these symptoms were allowed to cross from medical to surgical treatment, thus possibly preventing an impending stroke. Finally, the study can be criticized for examining all patients with stenoses greater than 50% as a single group.[30] The VA study confirmed that significant numbers of asymptomatic patients with carotid stenoses will experience stroke without antecedent symptoms because half of the neurologic outcome events were strokes that were not preceded by TIAs. Surgical complications included an operative mortality of 1.9%, a permanent stroke rate of 2.4%, and an angiography-related stroke incidence of 0.4%. This study provided the first randomized, multi-institutional data showing the benefit of CEA in asymptomatic patients. The authors also noted a 20% incidence of late cardiac death in both groups and suggested that because most of these patients would succumb to coronary artery disease, the recommendation for CEA in the presence of asymptomatic carotid disease should always be considered in terms of the patient's longevity from a cardiac standpoint.

The second of the two major asymptomatic trials, the Asymptomatic Carotid Atherosclerosis Study (ACAS), provided the most comprehensive data to date on the role of CEA for asymptomatic stenoses and was the first study to address the question of whether CEA prevents unhearalded stroke. Patients between 40 and 79 years of age with asymptomatic, surgically accessible carotid stenosis of 60% or greater were eligible. The degree of carotid stenosis was determined by two of three methods: ocular pneumoplethysmography, carotid duplex exam, or contrast arteriography.[31] Many patients in the medical cohort did not undergo arteriography. End-points were cerebral infarction occurring in the distribution of the study artery or any stroke or death occurring in the perioperative period.[32] Of 42,000 patients screened, 1662 were randomized from 39 clinical sites across the United States and Canada. Two-thirds of the patients were men, and 95% were white. The study reached statistical significance at a median follow-up time of 2.7 years, though the benefit of surgery was apparent by 10 months. The estimated 5-year risk of ipsilateral stroke and any perioperative stroke or death was 5.1% for surgical patients and 11.0% for medical patients, an aggregate risk reduction of 53% ($p = 0.004$). Perioperative stroke or death occurred in 2.3% of surgical patients and included an arteriographic stroke rate of 1.2%. These results again emphasized the need for low surgical morbidity and mortality rates to realize the benefits of CEA.

The ACAS trial has been criticized for a number of perceived flaws. Siome critics believed that all patients should have undergone arteriography prior to entering the study to ensure that only patients with arteriographically proven stenoses of 60% or greater were allowed to participate. However, duplex ultrasonography in this study had a positive predictive value of 93%, indicating that fewer than 5% of patients had stenoses of less than 60%. The results have also been criticized as perhaps not applicable to women because the 5-year stroke risk reduction was 66% for men but only 17% for women. This discrepancy was due, at least in part, to a higher perioperative complication rate in women (excluding arteriographic and perioperative complications, the risk reduction was 79% in men and 56% in women). The reasons for the higher perioperative complication rate among women are not clear.

It should be mentioned that the major randomized trials have utilized different methods of calculating arteriographic percent stenosis, which has resulted in some confusion. For example, the ECST used as its measurement of maximal diameter a visual estimate of the "normal" inner diameter of the carotid bulb at the site of maximal lumen narrowing.[12] The NASCET (and the ACAS) used the diameter of the distal internal carotid artery beyond the stenosis at the point at which the artery walls became parallel.[13] To add to the confusion, the widely used University of Washington duplex criteria utilize the ECST method when correlating ranges of stenosis.[33] As Hertzer points out, unless an allowance is made for this, patients in the NASCET and ACAS will appear to have had lesser degrees of stenosis by traditional standards than is the case. He believes that surgeons who perform CEA for patients who have a stenosis of at least 75% on the basis of conventional duplex or arteriographic measurements do not need to change their recommendations based on the ACAS.[34] In fact, many surgeons have recently adapted a policy of selectively performing preoperative arteriography in patients undergoing CEA (see Chapter 46). For example, among the 110 CEAs performed by the senior author in 1995, only 28 patients underwent preoperative carotid arteriography due to the availability of an accredited vascular diagnostic laboratory where duplex results have been repetitively validated against both contrast arteriography and actual measurements of intact CEA specimens.[35]

Finally, the VA Study and the ACAS demonstrated that patients with significant carotid disease suffered a high late cardiac event rate, whether or not they underwent CEA. Mackey et al also found myocardial infarction (MI) to be the most frequent cause of death in patients undergoing CEA.[36] In light of the very significant late cardiac morbidity and mortality of this population, we believe that patient selection for CEA based on cardiac risk evaluation is particularly important. In treating patients with asymptomatic carotid disease, good surgical judgment requires consideration not only of the patient's age and general health, but also of the short- and long-term cardiac prognosis.[37]

PATIENT SELECTION FOR SURGERY

The difference between having a surgical indication and being an appropriate candidate for surgery is the essence of surgical judgment. As noted above, the indicence of coexistent coronary artery disease (CAD) in patients with carotid disease is quite high. For example, in a prospective study of 1000 patients with vascular disease, all of whom underwent coronary arteriography, severe CAD was present in one-third of the patients presenting for CEA.[38] The high incidence of CAD in this population affects not only the perioperative cardiac event rate but also late servival. In a recent study by L'Italien et al, late cardiac events were examined re

hptrospectively among 914 patients undergoing vascular surgery. Patients undergoing CEA had the highest annual incidence of cardiac events, 11%, versus 10% for infrainguinal procedures and 4% for aortic procedures.[37] Furthermore, the high late cardiac morbidity and mortality were noted even among patients without overt coronary disease. Mackey et al studied the course of patients with and without overt CAD (prior MI, angina, significant electrocardiographic [ECG] abnormalities) who underwent CEA and reported a 15-year life-table survival of 36.4% for those with overt coronary disease and 54.3% for those free of overt disease. MI was the most frequent cause of death in both groups.[36] Therefore, one of the most important determinations the clinician should make is the potential surgical candidate's cardiac risk, not only perioperative but also late. In our unit, patients who are elective CEA candidates undergo cardiac risk stratification (CRS) to define that risk.

The rationale for CRS is that it allows one to select individuals in whom appropriate coronary interventions (ie, cardiac artery bypass graft [CABG] or coronary angioplasty) will decrease the perioperative and long-term cardiac risks. Alternatively, patients whose cardiac risk is prohibitive and who are not candidates for coronary intervention may not be appropriate candidates for CEA, even if their carotid anatomy suggests otherwise. Finally, appropriate CRS and selected intervention may prolong the life and enhance the quality of life of selected patients, independent of intervention for their carotid disease.

The clinical presentation of the patient's carotid disease is the most important factor in deciding which patients to test. Patients with a truly urgent need for CEA, namely, those with evolving stroke, crescendo or multiple TIAs, or truly compelling anatomy (such as a 95% stenosis with an occluded contralateral carotid artery) should not undergo cardiac testing; they should proceed directly to surgery after optimization of their medical therapy, not only because of the urgent nature of their carotid disease, but also because of the possibility that stress testing and/or coronary arteriography may precipitate complications referable to the severe carotid disease. Asymptomatic patients or those with lesser degrees of stenosis may be candidates for CRS.

Which patients with asymptomatic carotid stenosis should undergo preoperative CRS? Some advocate preoperative testing for all elective CEA candidates based on the high incidence of CAD in this patient population and the incidence of late cardiac mortality after successful CEA.[39,40] There seems little doubt that the ready availability of noninvasive testing has resulted in the indiscriminate use of CRS and the corresponding overuse of coronary arteriography in preoperative patients. For example, a prospective study of 457 vascular surgery patients undergoing dipyridamole-thallium(D-THAL) scanning illustrated that routine testing of all patients without regard to clinical profiling results in low specificity and a poor predictive value for perioperative cardiac events.[41] Therefore, many patients who do not require intervention will be referred for coronary arteriography, which is expensive and exposes the patient to further risks. These results are not surprising because it is clear that many patients with significant CAD can safely undergo vascular surgery. A decade of experience with CRS has convinced us that a selective approach to CRS based on clinical profiling is the best strategy for identifying those patients at risk of having significant CAD that would impact on the subsequent management.

The clinical scoring system we utilize is detailed in a series of reports from Eagle and colleagues.[42,43] Five clinical markers of CAD—Q waves on the preoperative ECG, history of angina, history of ventricular arrhythmias, diabetes, and age older than 70 years—were found to be independent predictors of postoperative ischemic events.[43] Thallium redistribution and ischemic ECG changes after thallium injection on D-THAL scans were also predictive of postoperative ischemia. However, greater specificity (81%) with equal sensitivity for the prediction of postoperative cardiac ischemic changes was obtained using a model combining clinical and D-THAL features rather than using either alone. In addition to these occult clinical markers of CAD, some patients will present with major markers of CAD, such as a history of recent MI, the presence of unstable or new-onset angina, and recent or poorly controlled left ventricular dysfunction (Table 46–1), and are best served by eliminating the preliminary step of performing D-THAL. If believed to be potential candidates for CABG or angioplasty prior to CEA, they should proceed directly to coronary arteriography, presuming CEA is elective,

Clinical factors alone can distinguish patients with a very low risk, that is, those with none of the five clinical markers, and those at high risk, that is, with three or more of the clinical markers. These high- and low-risk groups are not further distinguished by the presence or absence of thallium redistribution. Patients in the intermediate-risk group (those with one or two clinical markers) benefit most from D-THAL. Therefore, those at low risk could undergo CEA without further noninvasive testing, and those at high risk could proceed directly to coronary arteriography if further knowledge of their coronary anatomy would influence their management. Those at intermediate risk would undergo D-THAL. Paul et al applied this clinical risk index to arteriographic data from Hertzer's original database of 1,000 coronary angiograms[44] and found that a gradient of risk for severe CAD was seen with the presence of an increasing number of clinical markers. The clinical risk index alone accurately predicted the severity of CAD. If a "positive" coronary angiogram were defined as either (1) three-vessel CAD with at least 50% stenosis in each vessel, (2) two-vessel CAD with at least 70% stenosis of the left anterior descending artery, or (3) left main CAD with at least 50% stenosis, then the clinical index alone was accurate in predicting negative angiograms in 83% of patients clinically classified as

Table 46–1. Major Versus Occult Markers of Coronary Artery Disease

Occult Markers	Major Markers
Diabetes mellitus	Recent MI
Age >70 years	Unstable/new-onset angina
History of angina	New/poorly controlled LV dysfunction
Prior MI/Q waves on ECG	
History of CHF/ventricular arrhythmias	

Abbreviations: CHF, congestive hearts failure; LV, left ventricle.

low risk. Similarly, 77% of patients classified as high risk based on the clinical index profiling had positive coronary angiograms. Finally, the anatomic discrimination for those whose clinical profile was classified as intermediate was poor, and, as noted above, it is these patients in whom D-THAL imaging is most useful.[45] Based on these observations, an algorithm has been developed at our institution that can be applied to CEA candidates (see Fig. 46–2).

Patients with severe CAD and an urgent need for CEA may benefit from simultaneous CEA/CABG. Though many institutions have adopted a conservative policy toward this option, invoking unacceptable operative risks, we believe that selected patients may benefit from a combined approach. A detailed classification of which patients should undergo simultaneous CEA/CABG is beyond the scope of this chapter, but patients with symptomatic and/or severe carotid stenosis and the need for coronary revascularization may be best served by simultaneous repair. The senior author reviewed 71 patients receiving CEA/CABG and contrasted the results with those of both CEA and CABG performed as separate procedures.[46] Most complications in CEA/CABG patients occurred in the early years of the 9-year study. In the last 4 years of the study, there was no significant difference in either operative mortality or perioperative stroke between the two groups. More recently, Akins and colleagues extended this review to include 200 patients who had CEA/CABG from 1979 to 1993. Hospital death occurred in 3.5% of these patients, MI in 2.5%, and stroke in 3%.[47] While this approach is not necessary for all patients with carotid and coronary disease, in cases of critical carotid stenosis and an urgent need for coronary revascularization it may be performed with reasonable safety.

RESULTS OF CEA

Long-term stroke prevention and surgical morbidity are the principal endpoints of CEA. A consistent message of the prospective trials is that CEA must be performed with low perioperative morbidity and mortality to confer the stroke-reducing benefit of the procedure. The incidence of late complications of CEA is also an important parameter and will be examined separately.

Surgical Morbidity and Mortality

While our own data are consistent with others demonstrating that cardiac, not neurologic, events are the more common source of morbidity after CEA,[36] most patients and referring physicians focus on the potential stroke morbidity of CEA. As shown by the NASCET and ACAS trials, perioperative morbidity and mortality rates of 3% or less are necessary if patients are to realize the full protective benefits of CEA, and multiple contemporary series have demonstrated that this goal is realistic. In a large retrospective study from New York University Medical Center, including more than 3000 CEAs performed over a 26-year period, it was noted that the cause of most perioperative strokes could be identified, and most were technical in nature. The overall stroke rate was 2.2%.[48] Identifiable causes of stroke included cerebral ischemia during surgery (10 cases) related to difficulty placing the shunt, hypotension with the shunt in place, or contralateral stroke; postoperative thrombosis/embolism (25 cases); intracranial hemorrhage (12 cases); strokes from other surgical mechanisms (8 cases)—intraoperative embolism during carotid dissection or unclamping, thrombosis, or reperfusion injury; and strokes unrelated to the operated artery (8 cases). When examined with univariate analysis, patients who had a stroke were found to have a significantly higher incidence of hypertension, contralateral carotid artery occlusion, preoperative stroke, use of an intra-arterial shunt, and use of general anesthetic. In short, while the stroke rate was higher among symptomatic patients, mechanisms attributable to technical factors accounted for most perioperative strokes, regardless of the preoperative neurologic status.

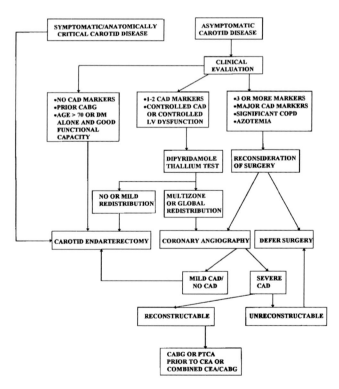

Figure 46–2. Suggested algorithm for management of patients with carotid disease. Clinical markers of CAD are age older than 70 years, diabetes, history of angina, MI, and ventricular arrhythmias. CAD, coronary artery disease; CABG, coronary artery bypass graft; COPD, chronic obstructive pulmonary disease.

In another early series, Sundt and colleagues analyzed patients according to various risk factors classified as cardiovascular (angina, recent MI, congestive heart failure, severe hypertension, chronic obstructive pulmonary disease, age greater than 70), neurologic (progressive neurologic deficit, frequent TIAs, multiple strokes), or arteriographic (contralateral internal carotid artery occlusion, intracranial vascular disease, soft thrombus in the internal carotid artery). Patients with no risk factors had a stroke/MI risk of 1%. Patients with arteriographic risk factors had a risk of 2%, and those with cardiovascular risk factors, had a risk of 7% (primarily from perioperative MI). Patients with neurologic risk factors had the highest risk, at 10% (all from stroke).[49] These data confirmed that neurologic complications occur most frequently among patients presenting with unstable neurologic symptoms. A more recent multi-institutional review of more than 3000 CEAs confirmed a higher neurologic complication rate for patients with an unstable neurologic status, including progressing or recent stroke.[50]

Late Stroke Prevention

It is clear that technically proficient CEAs will lower the late stroke risk when performed in appropriate surgical candidates. The degree of stroke reduction, however, appears to vary with the clinical presentation of the patient. Asymptomatic patients, patients experiencing TIAs, and patients with stroke have successively higher rates of late stroke after CEA. When both retrospective and prospective data are examined in light of the preoperative status of the patients, the results are quite consistent (Table 46-2).

An early retrospective study by Thompson and colleagues documented a late stroke incidence of 2.3% after 167 CEAs performed for asymptomatic disease, with follow-up extending to 184 months. Asymptomatic patients managed medically had a stroke incidence of 17% at 124 months of follow-up.[51] The findings of this and other retrospective studies were in large measure confirmed by the ACAS data.

In a study of symptomatic patients (undergoing surgery for TIAs), Thompson et al reported that 81% had no further attacks during long-term follow-up, 16% had fewer attacks, and 3% were not improved.[52] In a more recent study of 211 symptomatic patients, 85 underwent CEA and 126 were managed nonoperatively. Among patients with stenoses of 70% or greater, the 5-year stroke rate was 31% in patients treated medically compared to 7& in patients treated surgically.[53] Although this was not a randomized study, the findings have been clearly confirmed by NASCET. Furthermore, the results of the early retrospective and later randomized trials compare favorably with the natural history of the disease, in which the *annual* incidence of stroke in the presence of hemodynamically significant carotid stenoses managed without surgery is 3 to 6%.[6,11,54]

Late Complications

The most common late complication of CEA is recurrent carotid stenosis. Recurrent stenosis appears to have two distinct etiologies: myointimal hyperplasia, which occurs relatively early (within 3 years) and is more likely to be asymptomatic, and secondary atherosclerosis, which occurs later, is more closely associated with smoking and hyperlipidemia, and is more likely to

Table 46-2.   Late Stroke Rates in Carotid Endarterectomy

Indication	Author	No. of Patients	Follow-up	Stroke (%)
Asymptomatic	Callow[67]	179	56 months	1.9% (annual)[*,†]
	Thompson[68]	132	55 months	4.7$[*]
	Hertzer[69]	126	14 years	9.0%
	Moneta[11]	56	2 years	4.0%[*,†]
	Hobson[27]	444	2 years	4.7%[*,†]
	ACAS[32]	1662	2.7 years	5.1% (5 year)[*,†]
TIA	Callow[67]	404	56 months	2.1% (annual)[8]
	Thompson[70]	293	156 months	4.7%[*,†]
	Hertzer[69]	123	10 years	6.0%[†]
	ECST[12]	778	3 years	12.3%[‡]
	NASCET[13]	659	2 years	9.0%[†]
Stroke	Thompson[70]	217	156 months	8.2%[*,†]
	Hertzer[69]	80	10 years	6.0%[†]

*Includes perioperative strokes.
‡Include perioperative strokes and perioperative deaths.
†Ipsilateral strokes only.

Table 46–3. Late Restenosis Rates in Carotid Endarterectomy

Author	No. of Operations	Follow-up	Restenosis (%)
Das[55]	1726	5 years	3.8%
Piepgras[62]	1992	12 years	1.7%
Stoney[56]	1654	13 years	1.2%
Baker[59]	133	4 years	9.7%
Zierler[58]	89	4 years	*14.6%*

*Diagnosed by noninvasive testing (others diagnosed by arteriography).

be symptomatic.[55] Although symptomatic restenosis appears to occur in only 1 to 2% of patients after CEA,[55,56] surveillance duplex data indicate that the true incidence of hemodynamically significant restenosis may be 10 to 15%, depending on the diagnostic modality used[57–59] (Table 46–3). Das and colleagues from the Cleveland Clinic found that 65 (3.8%) of 1726 CEAs required reoperation for recurrent stenosis, and approximately half of these patients were symptomatic.[55] Clagett et al compared patients with recurrent stenosis to matched controls and found no significant difference in the incidence of diabetes, hypertension, or hyperlipidemia but a striking difference in smoking rates. Specifically, 95% of patients with recurrent disease had continued to smoke compared to only 24% of control patients.[60] Other investigators have reported a higher incidence of recurrent stenosis in females, although it is unclear whether this complication is related to gender or to smaller vessel size.[61]

Patients with symptomatic recurrent carotid stenoses are best served by reoperation. Endarterectomy and patch angioplasty may be performed safely in many patients with recurrent stenosis, although if endarterectomy is technically difficult, particularly in cases of myointimal hyperplasia, patch angioplasty alone may be advisable. Piepgras and colleagues reported 57 operations for recurrent stenosis; myointimal hyperplasia accounted for 14 cases and recurrent atherosclerosis for 27. They recommended patch angioplasty without endarterectomy for hyperplastic lesions and either endarterectomy with patch angioplasty or interposition grafting for atherosclerotic lesions.[62]

While considerable data have been published regarding the role of patch angioplasty and its potential to reduce the incidence of recurrent stenosis, the issue remains unsettled. Clagett and coworkers, in two reports of a randomized prospective trial of patch angioplasty versus primary closure, found that the use of patch closure was actually associated with an increase in early restenosis, and they found no superiority in long-term results.[63,64] It should be noted, however, that randomization of this cohort of 136 patients took place only after exclusion of 30 patients who, because of small internal carotid arteries or anatomic consider-

ations, were converted to obligatory patch angioplasty and not included in the study.

However, another randomized prospective study by Ten Holter and colleagues found that recurrent stenosis was twice as common in women as in men and that patch angioplasty significantly reduced the indicence of recurrent stenosis.[65] In a study from the Cleveland Clinic, 917 patients with CEAs were randomized to patch versus primary closure. Recurrent stenosis of 30% or more (by diameter measurement) was found in 4.8% of arteries subjected to patch angioplasty versus 14% of arteries closed primarily.[66]

Though no consensus exists regarding routine versus selective patching, the results of these and other trials of patch angioplasty suggest that it is reasonable to consider patching all small carotid arteries (less than 5 mm in internal diameter) and those of patients with strong risk factors for recurrence, such as hyperlipidemia and continued tobacco use. In addition, the use of patch angioplasty in women undergoing CEA may be advisable.

REFERENCES

1. Fisher CM. Occlusion of the internal carotid artery. Arch Neurol Psychiatry 1951;65:346–377.
2. Fischer CM. Occlusion of the carotid arteries, further experiences. Arch Neurol Psychiatr 1951;72:187–204.
3. Eastcott HHG, Pickering GW, Rob CG. Reconstruction of internal carotid artery in a patient with intermittent attacks of hemiplegia. Lancet 1954;2:994–996.
4. DeBakey ME. Successful carotid endarterectomy for cerebrovascular insufficiency. Nineteen-year follow-up. JAMA 1975;233:1083–1085.
5. Wolf PA, Kannel WB, Sorlie P, McNamara P. Asymptomatic carotid bruit and risk of stroke. The Framingham study. JAMA 1981;245:1442–1445.
6. Norris JW, Zhu CZ, Bornstein NM, Chambers BR. Vascular risks of asymptomatic carotid stenosis. Stroke 1991;22:1485–1490.
7. Chambers BR, Norris JW. Outcome in patients with asymptomatic neck bruits. N Engl J Med 1986;315:860–865.
8. Easton JD, Sherman DG. Stroke and mortality in carotid endarterectomy: 228 consecutive operations. Stroke 1977;8:565–568.
9. Mattos MA, Mode JR, Mansour MA, et al. Evolution of carotid endarterectomy in two community hospitals: Springfield revisited—seventeen years and 2243 operations later. J Vasc Surg 1995;21:719–728.
10. Roderer GO, Langlois YE, Jager KA, et al. The natural history of carotid arterial disease in asymptomatic patients with cervical bruits. Stroke 1984;15:605–613.
11. Moneta GL, Taylor DC, Nicholls SC, et al. Operative versus nonoperative management of asymptomatic high-grade internal carotid artery stenosis: improved results with endarterectomy. Stroke 1987;18:1005–1010.
12. European Carotid Surgery Trialists' Collaborative Group. MRC European carotid surgery trial: interim results for symptomatic patients with severe (70–99%) or with mild (0–29%) carotid stenosis. Lancet 1991;337:1235–1243.
13. North American Symptomatic Carotid Endarterectomy Trial Collaborators. Beneficial effect of carotid endarter-

ectomy in symptomatic patients with high-grade carotid stenosis. *N Engl J Med* 1991;324:445–453.

14. Mayberg MR, Winn HR. Endarterectomy for asymptomatic carotid artery stenosis. Resolving the controversy (ed). *JAMA* 1995;273:1459–1461.

15. Gertler JP, Blankenstein JD, Brewster DC, et al. Carotid endarterectomy for unstable and compelling neurologic conditions: do results justify an aggressive approach? *J Vasc Surg* 1994;19:32–42.

16. Giordano JM, Trout HH, Kozloff L, DePalma RG. Timing of carotid artery endarterectomy after stroke. *J Vasc Surg* 1985;2:250–254.

17. Piotrowski JJ, Bernhard VM, Rubin JR, et al. Timing of carotid endarterectomy after acute stroke. *J Vasc Surg* 1990;11:45–51.

18. Pritz MB. Carotid endarterectomy after recent stroke: preliminary observations in patients undergoing early operation. *Neurosurgery* 1986;19:604–609.

19. Wardlaw JM, Warlow CP. Thrombolysis in acute ischemic stroke. Does it work? *Stroke* 1992;23:632–640.

20. Moore WS, Boren C, Malone JM, et al. Natural history of nonstenotic, asymptomatic ulcerative lesions of the carotid artery. *Arch Surg* 1987;113:1352–1359.

21. Dixon S, Pais SO, Raviola C, et al. Natural history of nonstenotic, asymptomatic ulcerative lesions of the carotid artery. A further analysis. *Arch Surg* 1982;117:1493–1498.

22. Eliasziw M, Streifler JY, Fox AJ, et al. Significance of plaque ulceration in symptomatic patients with high-grade carotid stenosis. *Stroke* 1994;25:304–308.

23. Bunt TJ. The clinical significance of the asymptomatic Hollenhorst plaque. *J Vasc Surg* 1986;4:559–562.

24. Bull DA, Fante RG, Hunter GC, et al. Correlation of ophthalmic findings with carotid artery stenosis. *J Cardiovasc Surg* 1992;33:401–406.

25. Chawluk JB, Kushner MJ, Bank WJ, et al. Atherosclerotic carotid artery disease in patients with retinal ischemic syndromes. *Neurology* 1988;38:858–863.

26. Schwarz TH, Eton D, Ellenby MI, et al. Hollenhorst plaques: retinal manifestations and the role of carotid endarterectomy. *J Vasc Surg* 1990;11:635–641.

27. Hobson RW II, Weiss DG, Fields WS, et al. Efficacy of carotid endarterectomy for asymptomatic carotid stenosis. *N Engl J Med* 1993;328:221–227.

28. Veterans Affairs Cooperative Study Group. Role of carotid endarterectomy in asymptomatic carotid stenosis. *Stroke* 1986;17:534–539.

29. Personal communication, Gilbert J. L'Italien, Ph.D.

30. Thompson JE, Austin DJ, Patman RD. Long-term results in 592 patients followed up to thirteen years. *Ann Surg* 1970;172:664–679.

31. Asymptomatic Carotid Atherosclerosis Study Group. Study design for randomized prospective trial of carotid endarterectomy for asymptomatic atheroscleerosis. *Stroke* 1989;20:844–849.

32. Executive Committee for the Asymptomatic Carotid Atherosclerosis Study. Endarterectomy for asymptomatic carotid artery stenosis. *JAMA* 1995;273:1421–1428.

33. Moneta GL, Edwards JM, Chitwood RW, et al. Correlation of North American Symptomatic Carotid Endarterectomy Trial (NASCET) angiographic definition of 70% to 99% internal carotid artery stenosis with duplex scanning. *J Vasc Surg* 1993;17:152–159.

34. Hertzer NR. A personal view: the Asymptomatic Carotid Atherosclerosis Study results—read the label carefully. *J Vasc Surg* 1996;23:167–171.

35. Call GK, Abbott WM, MacDonald NR, et al. Correlation of continuous-wave doppler spectral flow analysis with gross pathology in carotid stenosis *Stroke* 1988;19:548–588.

36. Mackey WC, O'Donnell TF, Callow AD. Cardiac risk in patients undergoing carotid endarterectomy: impact on perioperative and long-term mortality. *J Vasc Surg* 1990;11:226–234.

37. L'Italien GJ, Paul SD, Cambria RP, et al. Assessment of long-term cardiac risk after major vascular surgery: development and validation of a prognostic scoring system in a cohort of 914 patients. Submitted to *Circulation*.

38. Hertzer NR, Beven EG, Young JR, et al. Coronary artery disease in peripheral vascular patients. A classification of 1,000 coronary angiograms and results of surgical management. *Ann Surg* 1984;199:223–233.

39. Cohen SN, Hobson RW, Weiss DG, et al. Death associated with asymptomatic carotid artery stenosis: long-term clinical evaluation. *J Vasc Surg* 1993;18:1002–1011.

40. Gillespie DL, LaMorte WW, Josephs LG, et al. Characteristics of patients at risk for perioperative myocardial infarction after infrainguinal bypass surgery: an exploratory study. *Ann Vasc Surg* 1995;9:155–162.

41. Baron JF, Mundler O, Bertrand M, et al. Dipyridamole-thallium scintigraphy and gated radionuclide arteriography to assess cardiac risk before abdominal aortic surgery. *N Engl J Med* 1994;330:663–669.

42. Eagle KA, Singer DE, Brewster DC, et al. Dipyridamole-thallium scanning in patients undergoing vascular surgery. *JAMA* 1987;257:2185–2189.

43. Eagle KA, Coley CM, Newell JB, et al. Combining clinical and thallium data optimizes preoperative assessment of cardiac risk before major surgery. *Ann Intern Med* 1989;110:859–866.

44. Hertzer NR, Beven EG, Young JR, et al. Coronary artery disease in peripheral vascular patients. A classification of 1,000 coronary angiograms and results of surgical management. *Ann Surg* 1984;199:223–233.

45. Paul SD, Eagle KA, Kuntz KM, et al. Concordance of a validated clinical risk index with coronary arteriography prior to vascular surgery (VAS): The Cleveland Clinic (CCF) experience. Presented at the American Heart Association 67th Scientific Sessions Meeting, November 14–17, 1994.

46. Cambria RP, Ivarsson BL, Akins CW, et al. Simultaneous carotid and coronary disease: safety of the combined approach. *J Vasc Surg* 1989;9:56–64.

47. Akins CW, Moncure AC, Daggett WM, et al. Safety and efficacy of concomitant carotid and coronary artery operations. *Ann Thorac Surg* 1995;60:311–318.

48. Riles TS, Imparato AM, Jacobowitz GW, et al. The cause of perioperative stroke after carotid endarterectomy. *J Vasc Surg* 1994;19:206–216.

49. Sundt TM Jr, Sandok BA, Whisnant JP. Carotid endarterectomy. Complications and preoperative assessment of risk. *Mayo Clin Proc* 1975;50:301–306.

50. Fode NC, Sundt TM, Robertson JT, et al. Multicenter retrospective review of results and complications of carotid endarterectomy in 1981. *Stroke* 1986;17:370–376.

51. Thompson JE, Patman RD, Talkington CM. Long-term outcome of patients having endarterectomy compared with unoperated controls. *Ann Surg* 1978;188:308–316.

52. Thompson JE, Austen DJ, Patman RD. Carotid endarterectomy for cerebrovascular insufficiency: long-term results in 592 patients followed up to 13 years. *Ann Surg* 1970;172:663–679.

53. Hertzer NR, Flanagan RA, Beven EG, O'Hara PJ. Surgical versus nonoperative treatment of symptomatic carotid stenosis: 211 patients documented by intravenous arteriography. *Ann Surg* 1986;204:154–159.

54. Canadian Cooperative Study Group. A randomized trial of aspirin and sulfinpyrazone in threatened stroke. *N Engl J Med* 1978;299:53–59.

55. Das MB, Hertzer NR, Ratliff NB, et al. Recurrent carotid stenosis. A five-year series of 65 reoperations. *Ann Surg* 1985;202:28–35.

56. Stoney RJ, String ST. Recurrent carotid stenosis. *Surgery* 1976;80:705–710.

57. Hertzer NR, Martinez BD, Beven EG. Recurrent stenosis after carotid endarterectomy. *Surg Gynecol Obstet* 1979;149:360–364.

58. Zierler RE, Bandyk DF, Thiele BL, Strandness E Jr. Carotid artery stenosis following endarterectomy. *Arch Surg* 1982;117:1408–1415.

59. Baker WH, Hayes AC, Mahler D, Littooy FN, Durability of carotid endarterectomy. *Surgery* 1983;94:112–115.

60. Clagett GP, Rich NM, McDonald PT, et al. Etiologic factors for recurrent carotid artery stenosis. *Surgery* 1983;93:313–318.

61. Gelabert HA, el-Massry S, Moore WS. Carotid endarterectomy with primary closure does not adversely affect the rate of recurrent stenosis. *Arch Surg* 1994;120:648–654.

62. Piepgras DG, Sundt TM Jr, Marsh WR, et al. Recurrent carotid stenosis. Results and complications of 57 operations. *Ann Surg* 1986;203:205–213.

63. Clagett GP, Patterson CB, Fisher DF Jr, et al. Vein patch versus primary closure for carotid endarterectomy. a randomized prospective study in a selected group of patients. *J Vasc Surg* 1989;9:213–223.

64. Meyers SI, Valentine RJ, Chervu A, et al. Saphenous vein patch versus primary closure for carotid endarterectomy: long-term assessment of a randomized prospective study. *J Vasc Surg* 1994;19:15–22.

65. Ten Holter JBM, Ackerstaff RGA, Schwartzenberg GWST, et al. The impact of vein patch angioplasty on long-term surgical outcome after carotid endarterectomy. *J Cardiovasc Surg* 1990;31:58–68.

66. Hertzer NR, Beven EG, O'Hara PJ, Krajewski LP. A prospective study of vein patch angioplasty during carotid endarterectomy. Three-year results for 801 patients and 917 operations. *Ann Surg* 1987;206:628–635.

67. Callow AD, Mackey WC. Long-term follow-up of surgically managed carotid bifurcation atherosclerosis. *Ann Surg* 1989;210:308–316.

68. Thompson JE, Patman RD, Talkington CM. Asymptomatic carotid bruit: long-term outcome of patients having endarterectomy compared with unoperated controls. *Ann Surg* 1978;188:308–316.

69. Hertzer NR, Arison R. Cumulative stroke and survival ten years after carotid endarterectomy. *J Vasc Surg* 1985;2:661–670.

70. Thompson JE, Auston DJ, Patman RD. Carotid endarterectomy for cerebrovascular insufficiency: long-term results in 592 patients followed up to thirteen years. *Ann Surg* 1970;172:663–679.

47

The Surgical Treatment of Brachiocephalic Arterial Occlusive Disease

Kenneth J. Cherry, M.D.

Symptomatic atherosclerotic lesions of the innominate, carotid, and subclavian arteries require operation much less frequently than do similar lesions at the carotid bifurcation. In a large study of patients undergoing arch arteriography, only 17% of demonstrated lesions involved the innominate artery and proximal subclavian arteries.[1] In an early series detailing almost 2000 operations on the great vessels or carotid bifurcations, only 7.5% were performed for great vessel lesions.[2] These lesions occur in patients who are relatively younger than other patients with atherosclerosis, their mean or median ages ranging from 50 to 57 years.[3–10] Men predominate slightly, with women comprising 45 to 49% of patients.[3–5,7,10] In three series, women comprised a slight majority of patients.[6–9] Atherosclerosis is far and away the predominant etiology in North America, followed by Takayasu's arteritis and radiation-induced atherosclerosis. Smoking is the most important risk factor encountered, being present in over three-quarters of these patients.[4,7–10] Concomitant coronary artery disease is associated less frequently, being present in 27 to 65% of these patients.[4,7–10] Three of the largest series of aortic arch reconstructions reported a concomitant coronary disease rate of 45%.[4,7,8] Kieffer et al, in the largest study from a single institution on innominate artery atherosclerotic occlusive disease, including 148 patients, reported a concomitant coronary artery disease rate of 26%.[11]

INNOMINATE ARTERY

Symptomatic innominate artery lesions are distinctly uncommon. Wylie and Effeney reported that only 1.7% of 1961 operations performed for great vessel and carotid artery disease were directed at the innominate artery.[2]

Presentation

Innominate artery lesions may be asymptomatic. In the past, this was an uncommon indication for operative intervention.[3–6,8–10] However Kieffer et al reported that 22% of their 148 patients were operated on for asymptomatic disease.[11] Their results were excellent and justified that aggressive approach, at least in their hands. Many of those patients were undergoing sternotomy for coronary artery bypass grafting and were known to have innominate artery lesions. In the United States, the great majority of patients are operated on for symptomatic lesions. These symptoms include embolic and flow-reducing ischemia of the right upper extremity, cerebral anterior circulation symptoms, posterior circulation symptoms, combined anterior and posterior distribution symptoms (global ischemia), and combined upper extremity and neurologic symptoms. In the Mayo Clinic Series, 76.9% of patients had neurologic symptoms.[9] In the Texas Heart Institute series, 77.8% of patients had neurologic symptoms.[10] In contrast, Kieffer et al reported that only 39% of their patients had neurologic symptoms.[11] In the Mayo Clinic series, 50% of the symptoms were referrable to the anterior circulation, 40% to the posterior circulation, and 10% to both.[9]

Both the French and Texas Heart Institute studies reported very similar incidences of patients with right upper extremity symptoms: 14% and 14.8%, respectively.[10,11] In contrast, 54% of the patients in the Mayo Clinic series had right upper extremity symptoms, approximately one-third of them having microembolization and two-thirds experiencing pain with use of the extremity, that is upper extremity "claudication."[9] Combined upper extremity and neurologic symptoms occurred in 38.5% of the Mayo Clinic patients and 32% of the Texas Heart Institute patients.[9,10] Kieffer and co-workers did not tabulate their results in such a manner.

Diagnosis

The diagnosis of innominate artery occlusive disease rests on the history, physical examination, and results of arteriography. Unilaterality of symptoms in the upper extremity should alert the clinician to the probability of arterial disease in the subclavian or axillary arteries. Bilateral upper extremity symptoms are usually manifestations of collagen vascular disorders or other systemic illness. Unlike physical examination in patients with carotid bifurcation lesions, the physical examination in patients with great vessel lesions may be especially revealing. Physical examination should include palpation and auscultation of the *proximal* carotid as well as the midcervical carotid artery pulses, in addition to the superficial temporal, subclavian, brachial, radial, and ulnar artery pulses. Proximal bruits or thrills should raise the suspicion of such lesions, as should absent pulses or discrepancies in the blood pressure in the upper extremities. Careful examination may allow carotid or subclavian artery bruits to be distinguished from carotid bifurcation bruits and from referred cardiac murmurs. If pulses in the upper extremities are not present, the blood pressure in the arms should be compared to that of the lower extremities. Microembolization, or atheroembolization, presents as bluish, painful discolorations in the fingertips or subungual hemorrhages, or, less commonly, as levido reticularis. Both innominate and subclavian artery lesions may present in this manner. In young patients, and especially in young patients not likely to have premature atherosclerosis or having no manifestations of inflammatory arteritis, thoracic outlet syndrome with arterial involvement must be ruled out. Arch arteriography with four-vessel views of the carotid and vertebral arteries and runoff views of the upper extremity vessels is mandatory. This confirms the diagnosis and is very helpful in determining the etiology and in differentiating between the giant cell arteritides and atherosclerosis. It localizes and enumerates the lesions and, up to the present, has been necessary in planning surgery. Multiple lesions of the great vessels in atherosclerotic patients presenting with innominate artery disease seem to be the rule rather than the exception. Multiplicty of lesions including those of the carotid bifurcations and vertebral arteries, as well as those of the other great vessels, was found in 84.5% of the Mayo Clinic patients, in 84% of patients in the study by Kieffer et al, and in 61% of the Texas Heart Institute patients.[9–11]

Currently, magnetic resonance angiography (MRA) is a promising diagnostic modality, especially with gadolinium enhancement,[12] and may reduce the imperative for conventional arteriography in the future. Duplex scanning of the carotid and subclavian arteries may also be helpful. In follow-up, this technique is valuable in determining the patency of grafts or endarterectomized vessels and in detecting the presence of stenoses or impending occlusion. Waveform analysis may indicate proximal stenoses not directly accessible to the Doppler probe.

Assessment of cardiac function is important, especially as these patients may be undergoing median sternotomy. Kieffer et al routinely perform coronary angiography in all patients preoperatively.[11] At our institution, we have relied on a history of symptoms and on functional assessment of the heart, with coronary catherization reserved for patients with abnormal functional tests or for those whose symptoms warrant further evaluation.

Operative Approaches

Symptomatic innominate artery lesions may be approached indirectly via extra-anatomic methods, directly via arch reconstructions, or remotely via endovascular techniques. Endovascular techniques are discussed at the end of the chapter.

Extra-anatomic Methods

Extra-anatomic methods such as subclavian-subclavian or axillary-axillary artery bypass grafts became popular as a means of reducing the high morbidity and mortality encountered in the early experience with direct reconstructions.[13] It should be noted, however, that the extra-anatomic methods proposed by Crawford and colleagues in their report were carotid-subclavian and subclavian-carotid artery bypass grafts, and that those extra-anatomic methods have endured. They were proposed for subsets of patients with *localized* disease of the common carotid or subclavian arteries, and not for patients with innominate artery or multiple arch vessel lesions. Axillary-axillary artery bypass grafts are classically reported to have a 50% failure rate.[7] Criado reported that these grafts had the worst patency of any extra-anatomic bypass grafts.[14] Recent reports from selected series, on the other hand, have described excellent results, but most of these procedures were performed for the treatment of subclavian, not innominate, artery disease.[15–18] A recent report by Owens et al from the University of North Carolina included 3 patients with innominate artery disease in their series of 44 patients and noted good results in this small number of cases.[19]

The routes of extra-anatomic bypasses performed for innominate artery disease are in some ways unattractive, as they cross the trachea or sternum and are prone to skin erosion and infection. They complicate tracheostomy, subsequent coronary artery bypass grafting, or repeat arch reconstructions. Because 26 to 45% of patients may be expected to have associated coronary disease[4,7,8,11] and because these patients are relatively young, this is not simply a matter of academic concern. Furthermore, restenosis rates may range from 5.2 to 12%,[9,11] and a small group of patients do require reoperation.[9,20] Lesions giving rise to microemboli require direct repair to remove the atheroembolic source from circulation. And finally, *multiple* great vessel occlusive lesions are much more effectively treated by direct arch reconstruction, as the ascending aorta provides an excellent source of inflow, in contrast to diseased donor great vessels.

Direct Reconstruction

Direct reconstruction of the innominate artery is currently the treatment of choice for these lesions. Advocates of endovascular repair would certainly disagree with that opinion, but the long-term results of such interventions are still lacking, whereas both the short- and long-term results of innominate artery reconstructions have been well documented and are quite salutary.[3–11] The report from the Mayo Clinic found no early reconstructive failures for either bypass or endarterectomy, and late symptomatic failures occurred at similar rates with both techniques.[9] Whereas the bypass technique may be used in all patients with innominate artery disease, innominate artery endarterectomy is more limited in its applicability. The anatomic contraindications to endarterectomy include atherosclerotic disease of the aorta at the base of the innominate artery, precluding safe clamping of the arch without fear of embolization, dissection, or disruption; inadequate distance between the origins of the innominate artery and the left common carotid artery, precluding clamping of the innominate without also compromising flow into the left common carotid artery; and proximal innominate artery disease as opposed to mid- or distal innominate artery disease. The last is considered a contraindication by the Baylor group.[5] Interestingly, Kieffer and colleagues have all but abandoned endarterectomy for bypass surgery.[11] Physiologic or etiologic contraindications to endarterectomy include the presence of inflammatory arteritis, radiation-induced arteritis, and recurrent disease.

Aortic arch origin grafting to the innominate artery is accomplished using polyester grafts, usually 8–10 mm in size. These may be either woven or collagen coated. If grafting to the left common carotid artery is also indicated, a side arm may be added to this single limb graft, as first proposed by Crawford, et al.[5] Alternatively, a bifurcated graft may be used. If a bifurcated graft is used, the main trunk of the graft should be cut much longer than it would be for an infrarenal aortic reconstruction.[9,21] This prevents kinking and turbulence at the site of bifurcation and places the bifurcation in approximately the same location one would obtain with an added side arm. Mediastinal bulk has been recognized as one of the mechanisms of failure of these grafts in the past. The use of the single limb graft with a side arm may help reduce the amount of material in the mediastinum. Other maneuvers that reduce mediastinal bulk are resection of the diseased innominate artery and division and ligation of the left brachiocephalic vein. In our experience, division and ligation of the left brachiocephalic vein is a safe maneuver, with only transient problems of the upper extremity; this has also been the experience of Kieffer et al in their large series. However, they did note one death from hemorrhage from a venous stump.[11] Berguer, on the other hand (personal communication), reports problems with upper extremity venous obstruction in his patients and recommends against routine division and ligation of the left brachiocephalic vein. Obviously, monitoring lines should not be placed from the left upper extremity or left neck, whichever method of handling the left brachiocephalic vein is chosen, as extensive mobilization of the vein is necessary if division is not performed.

Innominate artery reconstruction is done through a full median sternotomy. Over time, this has proven to be a safe, well-tolerated incision. However, just as there is interest in minimally invasive cardiac surgery, minimally invasive great vessel reconstruction may also have appeal. In the case of innominate artery reconstruction, such minimally invasive surgery represents a case of rediscovering our past. The first endarterectomy of an innominate artery was reported by Davis et al in 1956 and was performed through a right anterior thoracotomy.[22] Takach, Reul, and Cooley have recently reported minimally invasive innominate artery graft reconstructions performed in two patients using these same techniques, with a right anterior thoracotomy and appropriately placed supraclavicular incisions.[21]

The Texas Heart Institute has been the leading proponent of the philosophy of repairing all diseased vessels, whether symptomatic or not. This approach results in placement of multiple grafts and has given excellent results at that institution. The philosophy of our group is to repair symptomatic lesions and those lesions needing repair on the basis of their anatomy, such as an asymptomatic left common carotid artery lesion or a left common carotid artery lesion arising from a common brachiocephalic trunk. Highly stenotic carotid bifurcation lesions are also usually repaired by the proponents of both philosophies. The real difference lies in the attention to asymptomatic left subclavian artery lesions. In the largest series to date, Kieffer et al employed selective repairs of these lesions.[11]

Results

The reported operative mortality in the two most recent series in this country were 0 and 3.8%.[9,10] The mortality rate in the study of Kieffer et al was 5.4%.[11] Early and long-term resuls of innominate artery reconstruction are excellent, with early relief of symptoms achieved in 95% of patients[3-10] and excellent long-term results in approximately 90% of patients. In the series from France, the probability of freedom from any neurologic event was 88.8% at 5 years and 80.4% at 10 years. The probability of freedom from an ipsilateral neurologic event was 92% and 84%, respectively, at those same time intervals. The probability of freedom from an ipsilateral stroke was 98.6% at both 5 and 10 years. The primary patency rate was 96% at 10 years.[11] These figures from France are obviously the gold standard that surgeons must try to attain.

COMMON CAROTID ARTERY

Common carotid lesions are relatively rare, accounting for 1.5% of carotid lesions undergoing reconstructions.[2,23,24] Lesions of the right common carotid artery are seen much less frequently than those of the left.

Diagnosis

The history, physical examination, and results of arteriography are the key elements in the diagnosis of common carotid artery lesions. Physical examination can also be quite instructive, as there may be proximal bruits or lack of pulses, depending on the degree of stenosis or occlusion. Not all of these lesions can be directly interrogated by duplex scanning, but one may expect a dampened waveform indicating a proximal flow disturbance with significant lesions. In addition to these modalities, especially conventional arteriography, other methods of investigation *must* be employed in assessing patients with occluded common carotid arteries who have persistent or recurrent symptoms. Conventional arteriography may fail to reveal patent external and/or internal carotid arteries distal to common carotid artery occlusions. Rapid-sequence computed tomography (CT) scanning, directional Doppler, and MRA have all been used successfully to delineate this more distal anatomy.[24-26] At our institution, we are currently using an approach combining duplex scanning and MRA.

Operative Approach

The operative approach to common carotid artery disease is quite simple if the ipsilateral subclavian artery is patent. In the absence of a healthy ipsilateral subclavian artery, bypass grafts may be originated from the contralateral carotid or subclavian arteries, from the ascending aorta, or from the descending aorta through a thoracotomy incision. Anecdotally and rarely, stenotic proximal common carotid artery stenoses with a widely patent distal artery may be treated by transposition of the carotid artery onto the subclavian artery with good results.[27] However, by and large, the standard reconstruction for localized common carotid artery stenoses or occlusions is a subclavian-carotid artery bypass graft using either a saphenous vein or prosthetic graft. Concomitant carotid bifurcation endarterectomy, if necessary, is performed at the same time.

Results

Fry and colleagues, reporting on 20 patients undergoing subclavian carotid artery grafting, had no strokes and one death.[28] Four of these patients had concomitant carotid bifurcation endarterectomies. In follow-up after 55 months, there were no reconstructive failures. In contrast to carotid-subclavian artery bypass grafts performed for subclavian artery disease, saphenous vein worked as well in these patients as did polyester or prosthetic grafts. All of the grafts in this series were placed to the carotid at or distal to the carotid bifurcation. The relative vertical orientation of the graft and the low cerebral vascular resistance were proposed as reasons for the better results achieved with saphenous vein grafting in this situation than are seen when it is used for carotid-subclavian artery bypass grafts.[28] The Emory group reported a 90% 3-year patency by life-table analysis in 29 patients in whom they performed reconstruction.[29]

SUBCLAVIAN ARTERY

Subclavian artery lesions are the most commonly encountered brachiocephalic lesions requiring operation. Wylie and Effeney found these lesions to account for 4.3% of the carotid, vertebral, and great vessel reconstructions they performed.[2] Crawford and colleagues reported that subclavian artery reconstructions constituted 56% of their 142 great vessel reconstructions.[5] The left subclavian artery is much more frequently involved than the right, being the site of involvement in about 70% of patients. Subclavian artery lesions are usually asymptomatic because of the abundant collateral blood supply about the head, neck, and shoulder. As a consequence, radiographic subclavian steal must be differentiated from clinical steal, as the vertebral artery may well act as a collateral blood source to the upper extremity, with no neurologic compromise. Subclavian artery lesions take on added significance in the presence of ipsilateral carotid bifurcation lesions, contralateral vertebral artery lesions, and other great vessel occlusive lesions. Patients with these multiple lesions are much more likely to have symptoms, and concomitant lesions are seen in 35 to 85% of symptomatic patients.[1,5,30,31] Walker and coworkers, in their study of 157 such patients, found 72% to have concomitant lesions.[31] There was no correlation between symptoms and the presence or absence of a radiographic steal. Symptomatic patients may present with vertebrobasilar insufficiency, in all its protean manifestations, or with the upper extremity symptoms such as "claudication" or ischemic rest pain, ulceration, digital necrosis, and atheroembolization. Microembolization is encountered with notable frequency in upper extremity ischemia.[32]

In constrast to the lower extremity, there are many etiologies of upper extremity ischemia, including vasospastic disorders, arteritides, autoimmune diseases, thoracic outlet syndrome, and cardiac source embolization. The presence of bilateral upper extremity ischemia should alert the physician to the higher probability of a systemic disorder, whereas unilateral symptoms usually indicate an arterial etiology.

Classically, the operation of choice in reconstructing the subclavian artery has been the carotid-subclavian bypass graft using prosthetic material. Prosthetics perform better than vein in his location. This difference is thought to be related to the axial forces at play in this region with movement of the head and shoulders and because of the size descrepancy between the saphenous vein and these arteries. Carotid-subclavian artery bypass grafting is performed through a supraclavicular incision. Operative results have been excellent, with many authors reporting no operative deaths[5,30,33,34] and stroke rates in the range of 1 to 2%.[30,33,34] The long-term patency rate have been in the range of 90% at 5 years and 85% at longer time intervals.[33] A peculiar mechanism of stroke in these patients is thrombosis of the synthetic graft, with protrusion of the thrombus into the common carotid artery and distal embolization.[5,30] As a consequence, patients who are known to have early occlusion of these grafts should undergo anticoagulation with heparin and warfarin to allow stabilization of that thrombus.

An alternative operation with even more appeal is transposition of the subclavian artery onto the common carotid artery. First introduced in 1964,[35] it is an excellent operation, with mortality rates in the range of 0 to 1.4%[36–38] and late patency rates of approximately 95% or better.[36] It would appear that the stroke rate of transposition is even lower than that associated with carotid-subclavian artery bypass grafting, with stroke rates in several series reported to be 0%.[34,36]

ENDOVASCULAR REPAIR OF BRACHIOCEPHALIC ARTERIES: A SURGEON'S PERSPECTIVE

The endovascular repair of brachiocephalic atherosclerotic lesions is being performed with increasing frequency by surgeons, cardiologists, and interventional radiologists.[39–41] Balloon angioplasty, angioplasty plus stenting, and stenting alone have all been used, with acceptable to excellent early success rates, ranging from 92 to 100%.[39–41] As in surgical series, the subclavian artery is the most commonly repaired brachiocephalic vessel when these techniques are employed, followed by the common carotid and innominate arteries. Despite the paucity of long-term follow-up data, some of these authors claim that endovascular repair is

the treatment of choice for symptomatic brachiocephalic lesions.[41] It would seem, from a review of the literature, that localized short-segment stenoses, or even short-segment occlusions, are the lesions best suited for such techniques, and indeed these are the lesions yielding the best results. Although most of the endovascular reports neglect to describe the status of the other brachiocephalic arteries, one infers that these patients do not have the multiplicity of lesions seen in surgical series of patients presenting with innominate artery disease. Isolated short-segment stenoses of the subclavian artery are no doubt well served in the early period by endovascular repair. One cannot help but be impressed by the large number of "symptomatic" patients identified in relatively short periods of time and reported on, such as 31 patients undergoing angioplasty of the left subclavian artery to prevent or treat coronary-subclavian steal syndrome,[42] 31 patients with "obstructed" subclavian arteries,[40] and 33 patients with symptomatic subclavian stenoses,[41] and wonder if the presence of the lesion and its accessibility, rather than its physiologic significance, played some part in the indication for intervention. In contrast, the largest series of endovascular repairs reported by surgeons involved in a very active and aggressive practice described 8 innominate artery, 6 common carotid artery, and 12 subclavian artery interventions.[39] These latter figures are more in keeping with the number of symptomatic brachiocephalic lesions reported in the surgical literature. Nevertheless, the very good to excellent early success rate for treatment of localized lesions is encouraging. The reported lack of neurologic and embolic complications is also heartening. The subclavian artery, as stated earlier, has been the brachiocephalic vessel most commonly treated by endovascular techniques, but there are reports of common carotid and innominate artery lesions also addressed, with excellent early success rates[39,43,44] (see Chapters 48 and 50).

The ultimate role of these endovascular techniques in treating patients with brachiocephalic artery occlusive lesions awaits long-term studies. I suspect that for isolated short-segment brachiocephalic artery stenoses these will be first-line options, whereas for multiple great vessel lesions with occlusions and long stenoses, operative intervention will remain the treatment of choice.

REFERENCES

1. Fields WS, Lemak NA. Joint study of extracranial arterial occlusion. VII. Subclavian steal—a review of 168 cases. *JAMA* 1972;222:1139–1143.
2. Wylie EJ, Effeney DJ. Surgery of the aortic arch branches and vertebral arteries. *Surg Clin North Am* 1979;59:669–680.

3. Carlson RE, Ehrenfeld WK, Stoney RJ, et al. Innominate artery endarterectomy: a 16-year history. *Arch Surg* 1977;112:1389–1393.

4. Vogt DP, Hertzer NR, O'Hara PJ, et al. Brachiocephalic arterial reconstruction. *Ann Surg* 1982;196:541–552.

5. Crawford ES, Stowe CL, Powers RW Jr. Occlusion of the innominate, common carotid, and subclavian arteries: long-term results of surgical treatment. *Surgery* 1983; 94:781–791.

6. Zelenock GB, Cronenwett JL, Graham LM, et al. Brachiocephalic arterial occlusions and stenoses: manifestations and management of complex lesions. *Arch Surg* 1985; 120:370–376.

7. Brewster DC, Moncure AC, Darling RC, et al. Innominate artery lesions: problems encountered and lessons learned. *J Vasc Surg* 1985;2:99–112.

8. Evans WE, Williams TE, Hayes JP. Aortobrachiocephalic reconstruction. *Am J Surg* 1988;156:100–102.

9. Cherry KJ Jr, McCullough JL, Hallett JW Jr, et al. Technical principles of direct innominate artery revascularization: a comparison of endarterectomy and bypass grafts. *J Vasc Surg* 1989;9:718–723.

10. Reul GJ, Jacobs MJHM, Gregoric ID, et al. Innominate artery occlusive disease: surgical approach and long-term results. *J Vasc Surg* 1991;14:405–412.

11. Kieffer E, Sabatier J, Koskas F, et al. Atherosclerotic innominate artery occlusive disease: early and long-term results of surgical reconstruction. *J Vasc Surg* 1995;21:326–337.

12. Cloft HJ, Murphy KJ, Prince MR, et al. 3D gadolinium-enhanced MR angiography of the carotid arteries. *Magnetic Resonance Imaging* 1996;14(6):593–600.

13. Crawford ES, De Bakey ME, Morris GC, et al. Surgical treatment of occlusion of the innominate, common carotid, and subclavian arteries: a 10-year experience. *Surgery* 1969;65:17–31.

14. Criado FJ. Extrathoracic management of aortic arch syndrome. *Br J Surg* 1982;69(suppl):45–51.

15. Posner MP, Riles TS, Ramirez AA, et al. Axilloaxillary bypass for symptomatic stenosis of the subclavian artery. *Am J Surg* 1983;145:644–646.

16. Schanzer H, Chung-Loy H, Kotok M, et al. Evaluation of axilloaxillary artery bypass for the treatment of subclavian or innominate artery occlusive disease. *J Cardiol Surg* 1987;28:258–261.

17. Rosenthal D, Ellison RG Jr, Clark MD, et al. Axilloaxillary bypass: is it worthwhile? *J Cardiol Surg* 1988;29:191–195.

18. Weiner RI, Deterling RA Jr, Sentissi J, et al. Subclavian artery insufficiency: treatment with axilloaxillary bypass. *Arch Surg* 1987;122:876–880.

19. Owens LV, Tinsley EA Jr, Criado E, et al. Extrathoracic reconstruction of arterial occlusive disease involving the supraaortic trunks. *J Vasc Surg* 1995;22:217–222.

20. Kieffer E, Petitjean C, Bahnini A. Surgery of failed brachiocephalic reconstructions. In: Bergan JJ, Yao JST, eds. *Reoperative Arterial Surgery.* Orlando, FL: Grune & Stratton; 1986:581–607.

21. Takach TJ, Reul GJ, Cooley DA. Transthoracic reconstruction of the great vessels using minimally invasive technique. *Tex Heart Inst J* 1996;23:284–288.

22. Davis JB, Grove WJ, Julian OC. Thrombic occlusion of the branches of the aortic arch. Martorell's syndrome: report of a case treated surgically. *Ann Surg* 1956;144:124–126.

23. Toole JF. Syndromes of the carotid artery and its branches. In: Toole JF, ed. *Cerebrovascular Disorders,* 3rd ed. New York: Raven Press; 1984:60–61.

24. Riles TS, Imparato AM, Postner MP, et al. Common carotid occlusion: assessment of the distal vessels. *Ann Surg* 1984;199:363–366.

25. Podore PC, Rob CG, DeWeese JA, et al. Chronic common carotid occlusion. *Stroke* 1981;12:98–100.

26. Keller HM, Valavanis A, Imhof HG, et al. Patency of external and internal carotid artery in the presence of an occluded common carotid artery: noninvasive evaluation with combined cerebrovascular Doppler examination and sequential computertomography. *Stroke* 1984;15:149–157.

27. Ehrenfeld WK, Chapman RD, Wylie EJ. Management of occlusive lesions of the branches of the aortic arch. *Am J Surg* 1969;118:236–243.

28. Fry WR, Martin JD, Clagett P, et al. Extrathoracic carotid reconstruction: the subvlavian-carotid artery bypass. *J Vasc Surg* 1992;15:83–88; discussion 88–89.

29. Salam TA, Smith RB III, Lumsden AB. Extrathoracic bypass procedures for proximal common carotid artery lesions. *Am J Surg* 1993;166:163–167.

30. Hallett JW, Knight CD Jr, Hollier LH, et al. Early and late results of carotid-subclavian grafts: A 26-year review. Unpublished report.

31. Walker PM, Paley D, Harris KA, et al. What determines the symptoms associated with subclavian artery occlusive disease? *J Vasc Surg* 1985;2:154–157.

32. Rapp JH, Reilly LM, Goldstone J, et al. Ischemia of the upper extremity: significance of proximal arterial disease. *Am J Surg* 1985;152:122–126.

33. Perler VA, Williams GM. Carotid-subclavian bypass–a decade of experience. *J Vasc Surg* 1990;12:716–722.

34. Kretschmer G, Teleky B, Marosi L, et al. Obliterans of the proximal subclavian artery: To bypss or to anastomose? *J Cardiol Surg* 1991;32:334–339.

35. Parrott JC. The subclavian steal syndrome. *Arch Surg* 1964;88:661–665.

36. Sandmann W, Kniemeyer HW, Jaeschock R, et al. The role of subclavian-carotid transposition in surgery for supra-aortic occlusive disease. *J Vasc Surg* 1987;5:53–58.

37. Sterpetti AV, Schultz RD, Farina C, et al. Subclavian artery revascularization: a comparison between carotid-subclavian artery bypass and carotid-subclavian transposition. *Surgery* 1989;106:624–631.

38. Weimann S, Willeit H, Flora G. Direct subclavian-carotid anastomosis for the subclavian steal syndrome. *Eur J Vasc Surg* 1987;1:305–310.

39. Queral LA, Criado FJ. The treatment of focal aortic arch branch lesions with Palmaz stents. *J Vasc Surg* 1996; 23:368–375.

40. Kumar K, Dorros G, Bates MC, et al. Primary stent deployment in occlusive subclavian artery disease. *Cathet Cardiovasc Diagn* 1995;34:281–285.

41. Bogey WM, Demasi RJ, Tripp MD. Percutaneous transluminal angioplasty for subclavian artery stenosis. *Am Surg* 1994;60(2):103–106.

42. Marques KMJ, Ernst SMKPG, Mast EG, et al. Percutaneous transluminal angioplasty of the left subclavian artery to prevent or treat the coronary-subclavian steal syndrome. *Am J Cardiol* 1996;78(6):687–690.

43. Urwin RW, Higashida RT, Halbach VV, et al. Endovascular therapy for the carotid artery. *Neuroimaging Clin North Am* 1996;6(4):957–973.

44. Watura R, Halpin SFS, Ruttley MST. Percutaneous transluminal angioplasty of an innominate artery occlusion. *Cardiovasc Intervent Radiol* 1995;18:396–398.

48

Subclavian and Vertebral PTA: Indications, Techniques, and Results

Donald E. Schwarten, M.D.
Katharine L. Krol, M.D.

SUBCLAVIAN ANGIOPLASTY

Etiologies of Subclavian Occlusive Disease Suitable for Angioplasty

Atherosclerosis is the most common cause of subclavian artery occlusive disease.[1] It tends to occur in the proximal subclavian arteries, most commonly proximal to the origin of the vertebral and internal mammary artery, and it tends to be relatively focal. The left subclavian artery is involved three to four times more commonly than the right. Approximately 12 to 15% of patients undergoing angiography for cerebral vascular symptoms are found to have subclavian lesions, and only 2 to 3% of patients demonstrate a subclavian steal phenomenon.[2]

Aortoarteritis (Takayasu's arteritis) is a relatively infrequent cause of subclavian occlusive disease in the United States. It can usually be distinguished from atherosclerosis by its tendency to occur in young female patients, approximately half of whom give a history of an acute inflammatory stage, which probably occurred years prior to the onset of symptoms related to the occlusive disease.[3] As with atherosclerosis, the left subclavian artery is more commonly affected than the right, but the differential is approximately 1.5 to 1.0. The angiographic appearance with a smoothly tapered, segmental stenosis should suggest the possibility of Takayasu's arteritis, particularly if other branches of the aortic arch have similar lesions.

Fibromuscular dysplasia is an uncommon cause of subclavian occlusive disease, but after the renal and internal carotid arteries, the 9% incidence of medial fibroplasia involving the subclavian artery makes it the next most common site.[4,5] The angiographic appear-ance of medial fibroplasia is identical to the "string of beads" appearance observed in other territories.

Radiation-induced occlusive disease of the subclavian artery is rare. However, it may produce symptoms at least 10 years following radiation therapy that may have included the subclavian artery within the field.[6]

Conditions Not Suitable for Angioplasty

The thoracic outlet syndrome is not suitable for percutaneous management. The underlying cause is extravascular, and therefore it should be treated surgically.[7]

Giant cell arteritis may involve the subclavian artery. It usually occurs in older women. These patients usually experience visual loss due to an ischemic optic neuritis. The complex of segmental smooth subclavian stenoses in a middle-aged or older female patient with a history of visual loss should prompt a trial of corticosteroid therapy, which leads to marked improvement.[8] The diagnosis can be confirmed by temporal artery biopsy.

Clinical Indications for Subclavian Angioplasty

The subclavian steal syndrome was first described[9] and named in 1961.[10] The symptom complex of this syndrome includes vertigo, syncope, ataxia, diplopia, transient perioral hypesthesia, motor deficits, and, in some patients, intermittent arm claudication. In addition to the subclavian steal syndrome, patients with symptoms of upper extremity ischemia, including lifestyle-limiting arm and hand claudication, evidence that digital events have occurred, and other evidence of hand and digital ischemia, are treatable by angioplasty.

Caution should be used when anticipating the treatment of a right subclavian lesion for digital ischemia secondary to embolic events. If the right subclavian has an anomalous origin, there is a relatively high incidence of aneurysm formation in the proximal portion of the anomalous subclavian artery. With current technology, this becomes a surgical lesion.[11]

Technical Aspects

Pharmacologic Adjuncts

Patients undergoing angioplasty start receiving antiplatelet therapy at least 24 hours prior to the anticipated procedure. A single 325-mg dose of aspirin daily is an effective platelet antagonist that we employ as our antiplatelet agent of choice and maintain indefinitely.

Patients should receive heparin and be anticoagulated to achieve therapeutic activated partial thromboplastin times for the angioplasty procedure. The authors choose to anticoagulate patients immediately prior to selective catheterization of the subclavian artery for angioplasty.

Catheter- and guidewire-induced vasospasm is rarely a problem when performing subclavian angioplasty. Manipulation-induced vasospasm responds promptly to 100- to 200-µg boluses of transcatheter nitroglycerin. It is neither necessary nor desirable to attempt to avoid manipulation-induced vasospasm by pretreating with calcium channel antagonists or transdermal nitroglycerin.

It has been shown that when the subclavian steal phenomenon is present, the reversal of flow in the ipsilateral vertebral artery may persist for as long as 20 minutes following successful subclavian angioplasty.[12,13] The retrograde flow protects the posterior fossa from angioplasty-induced embolic debris; therefore, when subclavian steal has been documented prior to angioplasty with arch aortography, it is not necessary to augment the flow. However, when retrograde vertebral flow is not present, the interventionalist must make every attempt to induce it for the angioplasty procedure by either pharmacologic or mechanical induction of reactive hyperemia in the ipsilateral upper extremity. We have seldom been successful in inducing retrograde vertebral flow with intra-arterial nitroglycerin and prefer to use 30 to 60 mg of papaverine to cause more profound peripheral vasodilatation. Papaverine is administered via the angioplasty catheter prior to balloon deflation. A mechanical alternative to papaverine is to simply place a blood pressure cuff on the ipsilateral upper extremity, maintaining suprasystolic pressure and then deflating the cuff immediately prior to deflation of the angioplasty balloon.

The widespread use of a left internal mammary artery as a conduit for bypass to the left anterior descending (LAD) or other left coronary artery has led to a number of reports of angioplasty for the management of coronary-subclavian steal.[14,15] Should the vertebral-subclavian steal phenomenon not accompany the coronary-subclavian steal phenomenon, every effort must be made to induce distal reactive hyperemia and retrograde vertebral flow.

The most desirable approach for subclavian angioplasty is the retrograde femoral approach. Whenever possible, the transaxillary access is to be avoided because of the inherently increased risk of transaxillary catheterization and the concern that this approach may adversely affect retrograde vertebral flow by reducing outflow from the subclavian artery.

The technical aspects of catheter and guidewire manipulation for angioplasty of subclavian stenoses are simpler than, and different from, the technical aspects of treating subclavian occlusions. The stenotic subclavian artery is treated rather simply with angioplasty by engaging the orifice of the vessel with an appropriately configured diagnostic catheter. A Headhunter I configuration catheter is usually placed easily into the left subclavian artery and frequently can be negotiated into the right subclavian artery, although a Simmons or other configuration may be necessary to traverse a proximal right subclavian artery stenosis. Placement of a (TAD) (Torsional Attenuating Diameter, Advanced Cardiovascular Systems, Inc., Santa Clara, CA) guidewire across the stenosis and into the axillary artery allows the interventionalist to advance the diagnostic catheter into the axillary artery. The TAD guidewire has a docking mechanism that can be extended from its nominal 145-cm length to an exchange length in seconds. The diagnostic catheter can be removed from the target vessel and the access vessel and replaced with an angioplasty catheter with an appropriately sized (diameter and length) balloon, which can be placed within the stenosis with the assistance of bony landmarks or road mapping. The balloon is inflated to its rated pressure until the deformity caused by the stenosis is obliterated. The balloon is then deflated, the catheter is advanced to well beyond the vertebral artery origin, and the TAD guidewire is removed and replaced by an 0.018-inch guidewire and a side arm adapter. This permits retraction of the angioplasty catheter to the orifice of the subclavian artery to obtain a documentary postangioplasty arteriogram. Tortuous anatomy may make it difficult to advance the angioplasty catheter over the TAD guidwire unless the weld in the TAD wire that demarcates the beginning of the 0.035-inch segment is in the distal subclavian or axillary artery. Then this guidewire is usually stiff enough to allow proper placement of the angioplasty balloon. When a stiffer wire is required, an exchange-length Rosen guidewire usually facilitates completion of the procedure from the transfemoral approach.

When the subclavian stenosis does not encroach on the vertebral artery, it has been clearly shown that it is safe to inflate a balloon across the origin of the vertebral artery.[16] However, when the vertebral artery origin is pathologic or is encroached on by the subclavian artery plaque, it is vulnerable to a noncolinear tear and the resultant dissection that might extend from the subclavian artery into the vertebral artery and place the vertebral artery at risk for occlusion. We believe it is not safe to perform the subclavian angioplasty without first protecting the vertebral artery with a safety guidewire to allow for immediate vertebral artery origin angioplasty if necessary (Fig. 48–1). This scenario may require dual access. If these guidelines are followed, the authors believe that subclavian angioplasty at any level of the subclavian artery can be safely performed. While transaxillary access for subclavian stenosis angioplasty is to be avoided if possible, subclavian occlusions frequently cannot be recanalized from the transfemoral approach. The occluded subclavian artery is successfully treated percutaneously less often than the stenotic subclavian artery; the complication rate is higher with occlusions, and the long-term patency rate is lower.[17] Therefore, when planning percutaneous management of occluded subclavian arteries, the authors believe the interventionalist should be prepared to access both the common femoral artery and the high brachial/axillary artery. The initial approach would be from the transfemoral access. If the occlusion can be traversed successfully with a guidewire, it would then be reasonable to perform the balloon angioplasty procedure much

the same way one would for a subclavian stenosis. However, in a situation somewhat analogous to coronary and common iliac occlusions,[18–21] the authors and others[22–24] believe that angioplasty alone will not give the desired long-term result; a stent should be deployed in the recanalized subclavian artery. This is an uncomplicated process from the transfemoral approach. An exchange is made for an appropriate guiding catheter and the stent is deployed in the usual fashion, taking care to avoid the orifice of the vertebral artery (Fig. 48–2). If the occluded subclavian artery cannot be recanalized from the transfemoral approach, then a transaxillary attempt is worthwhile. If the guidewire can be successfully placed across the occlusion and into the descending thoracic aorta, anticipating stent deployment, the guidewire placed from the axillary approach can be snared from the transfemoral approach and retracted into the femoral sheath. Then the angioplasty and stent placement can be completed entirely from the transfemoral approach, leaving only a relatively small 4 or 5 French puncture in the axillary artery to be managed.

Right Subclavian Angioplasty

There is the additional theoretical hazard of innominate artery bifurcation compromise if an extensive dissection occurs at the origin of the right subclavian

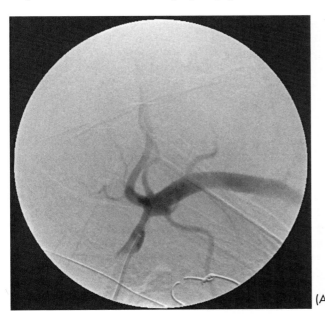

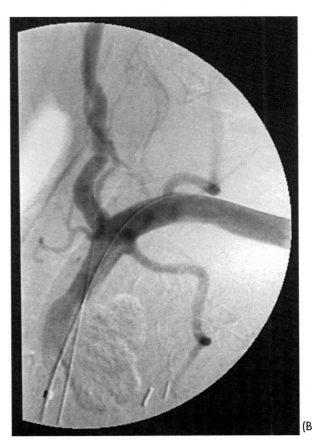

Figure 48–1. (A) Left subclavian stenosis adjacent to the vertebral origin. (B) Postangioplasty guidewires in subclavian and vertebral arteries.

(A)

(B)

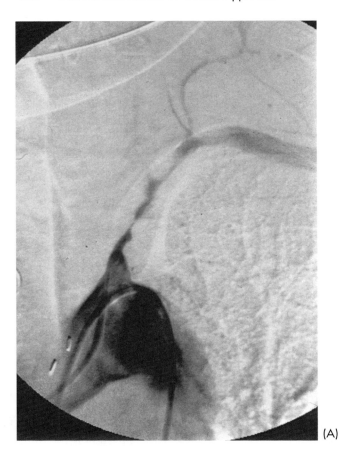

(A)

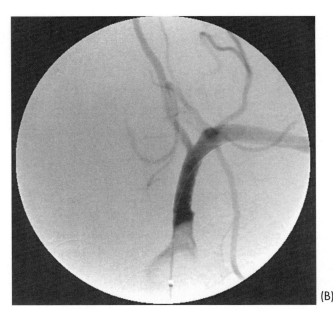

(B)

Figure 48–2.   (A) Recanalization of an occluded subclavian artery. (B) Poststent deployment.

artery during the angioplasty. A true orificial stenosis of the right subclavian artery should receive angioplasty with a safety wire in the right common carotid artery analogous to the previously described situation for subclavian plaque involving the vertebral artery origin. The safety wire can be placed from the ipsilateral common femoral approach as a second wire through the sheath, from the contralateral femoral approach, or the procedure can be performed as a combination of axillary approach (angioplasty) and transfemoral approach (safety wire).

Results of Subclavian Angioplasty

The subclavian artery is the most frequently angioplastied vessel of the brachiocephalic branches of the aortic arch. The majority of series report results in patients being treated for atherosclerotic disease. With 16 years of literature available for review, it is apparent that the technical success rates are high, ranging from 73 to 100%, with an average rate of 94%.[25–33] Previous reviews of subclavian angioplasty have noted the relative lack of long-term follow-up to document long-term patency rates, but it appears that the restenosis rate in patients treated with balloon angioplasty alone may be less than 10%.[34] One estimate of a 19% rate of clinical recurrence of symptoms included only series that were reported prior to 1987, and none of the treated vessels

had the benefit of stent deployment to optimize the anatomic result.[35] As noted earlier, the patency of subclavian occlusions to angioplasty is significantly worse than that of stenotic arteries treated with stenotic disease unless stents are deployed.[17] For the reasons reviewed earlier, successfully recanalized occluded or stenotic subclavian arteries treated to a less than optimal anatomic result with balloon angioplasty would be anticipated to have superior long-term patency rates following stent deployment.

The results of angioplasty and the management of the symptomatic patient with medial fibroplasia of the subclavian artery should be comparable to those seen in patients treated for renovascular hypertension with this etiology.

Data pertinent to the results of angioplasty of the subclavian artery in patients with Takayasu's arteritis are relatively limited, however, Joseph et al[36] reported the results in 26 arteries in which a technical success rate of 81% was achieved. During the mean 26-month follow-up time, six recurrences developed. The authors reported cumulative primary, secondary, and overall patency rates of 64%, 82%, and 65%, respectively. There was a significant difference in the results achieved with short- and long-segment lesions. There were no restenoses in short lesions, but half of the stenoses in long lesions recurred.

Complications related to subclavian angioplasty are uncommon, occurring in fewer than 5% of reported cases. Most complications are puncture site related. Embolic complications occur and, as observed previously, are more common when treating occluded subclavian arteries. All of the reported embolic complications have been in extracranial vessels. To our knowledge, there are no published reports of posterior fossa embolization occurring in association with subclavian angioplasty.

Conclusion

Carotid-subclavian bypass is the most commonly performed surgical procedure for patients with symptomatic subclavian occlusive disease. This procedure is associated with a 90 to 95% long-term patency rate. However, it is also associated with a stroke-mortality rate of 1 to 3% and an overall complication rate of up to 23%.[37–39]

In addition to the relatively low risk of stroke and/or death from surgical intervention for proximal subclavian disease, other complications include injury to the sympathetic chain resulting in Horner's syndrome, disruption of the thoracic duct, and injury to the phrenic nerve.

The high technical success rate associated with subclavian angioplasty, the low morbidity, and the lower cost, even if a stent is deployed, would seem to make percutaneous intervention the treatment of choice for symptoms associated with subclavian occlusive disease in the appropriate etiologic setting.

VERTEBRAL ANGIOPLASTY

The symptoms of vertebrobasilar insufficiency may be vague and poorly defined. Patients undergoing workup of these symptoms may be found to have hemodynamically significant disease at the carotid bifurcation, which, in turn, may lead (appropriately) to carotid endarterectomy and alleviation of the presenting symptoms.[40] The patient who has true vertebrobasilar insufficiency, exhibiting such symptoms as vertigo, syncope, ataxia, drop attacks, diplopia, or other visual disturbances, is at significant risk of posterior fossa stroke within 5 years of the onset of symptoms. This risk has been estimated to be 18% to 62%.[41,42]

The diagnostic imaging workup of patients suspected of harboring vertebrobasilar disease may begin with a duplex examination and should include magnetic resonance imaging, with or without magnetic resonance angiography. These studies may uncover pathology that would not ordinarily be treated by interventional or vascular surgical techniques, such as extrinsic compression by osteophytes or a mid basilar artery high-grade stenosis. In anticipation of percutaneous intervention, however, a complete four-vessel arteriogram is essential,

including examination of the entire course of both vertebral arteries. It has been shown that a unilateral vertebral stenosis may be the source of embolic debris resulting in posterior fossa symptoms.[43,44] In cases with embolic posterior fossa disease, magnetic resonance imaging examinations reveal multiple infarcts in the brain stem and cerebellum and occasionally in the distribution of the posterior cerebral arteries. Classic teaching would suggest that the vast majority of vertebral artery lesions are smooth and nonulcerated and cause transient ischemic attacks on a hemodynamic basis. These usually smooth, focal stenoses are optimal for angioplasty (Fig. 48–3). Therefore, in the presence of either bilateral vertebral disease or a unilateral lesion with a contralateralhypoplastic vertebral artery, angioplasty is a reasonable treatment. With regard to the use of angioplasty in the management of the potentially embolic vertebral artery lesion, embolic syndromes and other conditions have been successfully treated with angioplasty.[45] The smooth neointima that develops following a successful angioplasty may protect against future embolic events. Furthermore, it has been shown that the risk of embolization associated with carotid bifurcation angioplasty is low.[46]

More than 90% of vertebral artery pathology occurs at the origin of the vertebral artery, and this anatomy is involved in approximately 40% of all patients with symptoms of vertebrobasilar insufficiency.[47] Rarely, intrinsic atherosclerotic vertebral occlusive disease occurs in the middle and distal cervical segments or in the intracranial segment of the vertebral artery (Fig. 48–4). The segment of the vertebral artery above C1 is the second most common site for atherosclerotic disease in this vessel. All of these sites are amenable to balloon angioplasty if the pathology is proven to be intrinsic. Percutaneous transluminal angioplasty (PTA) of the vertebral artery has been regularly reported.[48,49] The majority of these reports have been confined to the treatment of the relatively smooth, concentric lesions originating in the vertebral artery.[50–52]

Indications for Vertebral Angioplasty

Vertebrobasilar insufficiency in the presence of appropriate anatomy is the principal indication for vertebral angioplasty. Patients with inoperable carotid occlusive disease who present with ipsilateral hemispheric symptoms, a widely patent posterior communicating artery, and a vertebral artery stenosis are also candidates for vertebral angioplasty, as are patients with global ischemic symptoms who have inoperable carotid disease.

ACAS[53] data suggest that a stenosis greater than 60% in the carotid bifurcation in a patient presenting with symptoms of vertebrobasilar insufficiency should undergo carotid endarterectomy to reduce the risk of

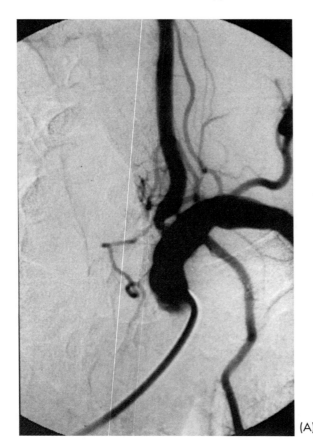
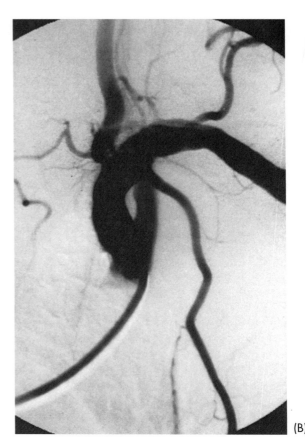

(A)   (B)

Figure 48–3.   (A) Stenosis near the origin of a dominant left vertebral artery. (B) After PTA.

a future hemispheric event. This, in turn, may result in resolution of the posterior fossa symptoms, eliminating the need for vertebral revascularization. Obviously, if the presenting symptoms persist, the patient deserves vertebral revascularization.

Technique of Vertebral Angioplasty

Pharmacologic adjuncts

As with subclavian angioplasty, antiplatelet therapy should be started 24 hours before the angioplasty procedure. The patient should be therapeutically heparinized during the procedure, and anticoagulation should not be reversed afterward.

Mild sedation is indicated for patients undergoing extracranial vertebral angioplasty, and more aggressive sedation is indicated for patients undergoing angioplasty of the intracranial segment of the vertebral artery. It is important to be prepared to manage procedure-related complications with aggressive sedation (the assistance of an anesthesiologist is most helpful) and to use all measures necessary for neurovascular rescue.

Vasospasm is easily induced in the vertebral artery and responds well to 100- to 200-µg boluses of transcatheter nitroglycerin (Fig. 48–5). Prophylaxis for vasospasm is achieved more safely with transdermal nitroglycerin than with oral or sublingual calcium antagonists.

Technique   While the transfemoral approach is most commonly employed, transbrachial and transaxillary approaches are available and, indeed, are occasionally preferable, particularly if the brachiocephalic anatomy is severely tortuous and a right vertebral artery must be treated with angioplasty.

With the transfemoral approach for lesions at the origin of the vertebral artery or even in the midcervical segment of the vertebral artery, the interventionalist has the option of using a guiding catheter or the guidewire exchange technique. The authors favor the use of a guiding catheter despite the increased diameter at the access site because it provides more sensitive catheter and guidewire control, easy manipulation, and easy intraprocedural pharmacologic manipulation and contrast material injections without guidewire removal. However, vertebral arteries more than 5 mm in diameter are more practically treated using the guidewire exchange technique (Fig. 48–5).

Before an angioplasty catheter is selected, the true size of the vertebral artery to be treated must be known. The vertebral artery is an extremely delicate, thin-walled

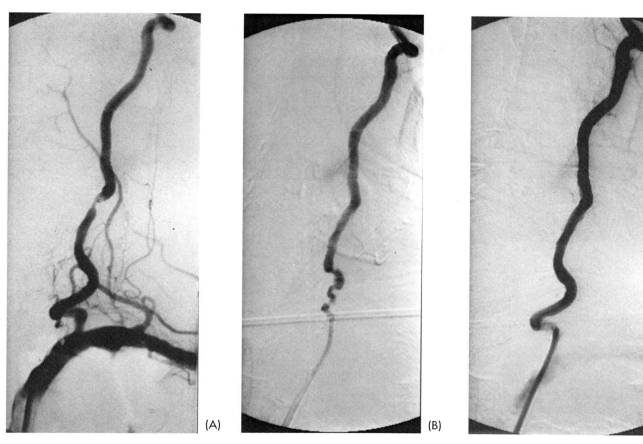

Figure 48–4. (A) Atherosclerotic stenosis in the midvertebral artery. (B) After PTA.

vessel that should not be subjected to overdilatation because of the risk of rupture. Once the guiding catheter has been placed adjacent to the orifice of the vertebral artery, images are obtained for precise measurement of the vertebral artery. Then the appropriately sized (length and diameter) balloon is chosen based on the known diameter of the vertebral artery. A 7 French guiding catheter that has an inner diameter of 0.074 inch or larger permits easy passage of the angioplasty catheter with a balloon diameter of up to 4.5 mm over a 0.014-inch guidewire. The left vertebral artery is more commonly dominant and, whenever possible, the left vertebral artery is chosen for angioplasty because it is usually much more easily accessed than the right vertebral artery from the transfemoral approach. The guiding catheter is placed at the orifice of the vertebral artery. A road map image may be obtained, although abundant bony landmarks and the use of a guiding catheter with small boluses of contrast material make this an unnecessary luxury. The lesion is traversed with the guidewire followed by the angioplasty catheter. Once the balloon has been placed within the stenosis, it is inflated to its maximum diameter and rated pressure until the balloon deformity is obliterated. This can usually be accomplished with a relatively short inflation time, so it is uncommon

to observe evidence of transient neurologic episode. Even inflation times of several minutes rarely provoke symptoms.

It is more difficult to achieve optimal anatomic results by balloon angioplasty of vertebral origin lesions than it is in midcervical vertebral artery lesions. This may be due, in part, to adjacent subclavian plaque encroaching on the orifice of the vertebral artery. This situation is somewhat analogous to that of renal artery ostial lesions. We resist the urge to employ noncompliant, rigid balloons in this location because of the course of the vertebral artery relative to the cervical vertebra, and because there is a high incidence of tortuosity in the first centimeter of the vertebral artery. The use of stents for resistant lesions of vertebral artery origin has been described.[54] This portion of the vertebral artery is vulnerable to trauma by external forces such as those of three-point seat belts and is frequently tortuous, and deployment of a rigid stent at this site may have undesirable consequences in the future. Stenting achieves a superior anatomic result and may well produce long-term results superior to those of balloon angioplasty, but the ideal stent for any segment of the vertebral artery is not yet available.

At the conclusion of an angioplasty procedure on the extracranial vertebral artery, the final documentary

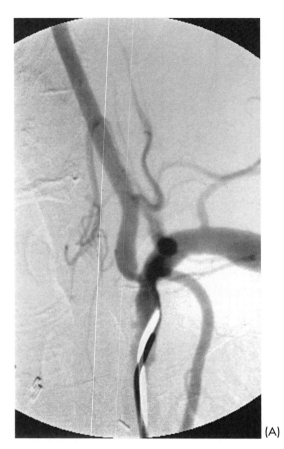
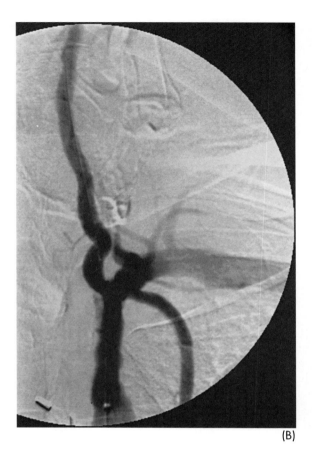

Figure 48–5. (A) Stenosis of large, dominant left vertebral origin. (B) Following PTA with a 5 French system.

arteriogram of the angioplasty site is performed, as is a complete study of the posterior fossa. Prior to sheath or catheter removal from the access site, it is best to observe the patient for approximately 30 minutes. If a complication occurs and rapid access to the angioplasty site or the intracranial vasculature is necessary, it can be accomplished without repuncture.

Angioplasty of the intracranial segment of the vertebral artery above the atlanto-occipital membrane is reserved for patients who have failed with maximum medical therapy and have ongoing symptoms of incapacitating vertebrobasilar insufficiency (Fig. 48–6). Angioplasty of the intracranial vertebral artery proximal to the posterior inferior cerebellar artery carries an approximately 15% risk of major morbidity or mortality; angioplasty distal to the posterior inferior cerebellar artery carries an approximately 30% risk.

Angioplasty of the intracranial segment of the vertebral artery requires advanced technical skills and a knowledge of neuroanatomy, neurophysiology, and neurology. It should be attempted only by interventionalists skilled in the use of devices for the management of intracranial pathology.

Results   The most common surgical procedure for the management of symptomatic vertebral disease is

transsection of the vertebral artery distal to the stenosis and reimplantation of the poststenotic vertebral artery into the ipsilateral common carotid artery,[55] the thyrocervical trunk, or the subclavian artery. Alternatives include endarterectomy and vein patch angioplasty. Surgical management of more distal vertebral artery disease is technically demanding and is employed regularly by a limited number of surgeons. Berguer most commonly employs a common carotid to vertebral artery bypass for any lesion above the C6 level. This is carried out at the C2 to C1 level. An alternative procedure is external carotid to distal vertebral bypass.[56]

A recent review of nearly 2000 angioplasty procedures performed for extracranial occlusive disease revealed reports of 268 vertebral angioplasty attempts that met with technical success in 95.1% of the cases, with no mortality, 0.7% morbidity, and "minor complications" of 3.3%. This review did not include any long-term follow-up data relevant to vertebral angioplasty.[57] In 1989 Becker et al,[35] in their comprehensive review of noncoronary angioplasty, concluded that there were insufficient data to state the proper role of vertebral artery PTA in the management of vertebrobasilar insufficiency. At the opposite end of the spectrum, Courtheoux et al[47] have proposed that vertebral angioplasty

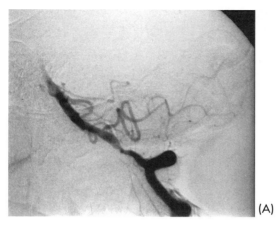 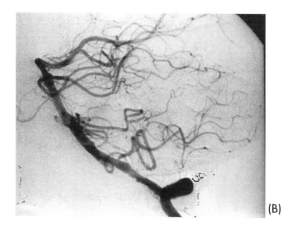

Figure 48-6. (A) Intracranial vertebral stenosis. (B) After PTA.

could be attempted therapeutically in the presence of uncertain vertebrobasilar insufficiency symptoms because of its low morbidity and mortality. Perhaps a more realistic and rational approach to extracranial vertebral angioplasty would be to accept the conclusion reported in the literature that balloon angioplasty of the vertebral artery can be technically successful in approximately 90% of attempts and that the risk of the procedure-associated adverse neurologic event will be less than 1%. From the limited long-term follow-up data, it appears that at least 75% of the patients treated experience clinical benefit at 1 to 2 years. This compares with Berguer's report of symptomatic cure or improvement in 83% of his patients undergoing proximal vertebral artery reconstruction.[58]

Long-term noninvasive or angiographic follow-up data are, for the most part, lacking. Surgical series have not withstood the test of prospective randomization that has proven the value of operative intervention for carotid bifurcation disease. Given its low risk and apparent clinical benefit for extracranial vertebral artery disease, balloon angioplasty is now our treatment of choice for patients with vertebrobasilar insufficiency.

REFERENCES

1. Perace WM, Yao JST. Upper extremity ischemia: overview. *Semin Vasc Surg* 1990;3:207.
2. Zelenock GH, Cronenvett JL, Graham LM, et al. Brachycephalic arterial occlusive and stenosis. *Arch Surg* 1985;120:370.
3. Pokrovsky AV. Nonspecific aortoarteritis. In: Rutherford RB, ed. *Vascular Surgery* 3rd ed. Philadelphia: WB Saunders; 1989.
4. Iwai T, Konno S, Hiejima K, et al. Fibromuscular dysplasia in the extremities. *J Cardiovasc Surg* 1985;26:496.
5. Drury JK, Pollock JG. Subclavian arteriopathy in the young patient. *Br J Surg* 1981;68:617.
6. Kretschmer G, Niederle B, Polterauer P, et al. Irradiation-induced changes in the subclavian and axillary arteries after radiotherapy for carcinoma of the breast. *Surgery* 1986;99:658.
7. Scher LA, Veith FJ, Samson RM, et al. Vascular complications of the thoracic outlet syndrome. *J Vasc Surg* 1986;3:565.
8. Joyce JW. The giant cell arteritides: diagnosis and the role of surgery. *J Vasc Surg* 1986;3:827.
9. Reivich M, Molling ME, Roberts B, et al. Reversal of blood flow through vertebral artery and its effect on cerebral circulation. *N Engl J Med* 1961;265:878–885.
10. Editorial: New vascular syndrome: "the subclavian steal." *N Engl J Med* 1961;265:912–913.
11. Akers DL, Fowl RJ, Plettner J, et al. Complications of anomalous origin of the right subclavian artery: case report and review of the literature. *Ann Vasc Surg* 1991;5:385.
12. Ringelstein EB, Zeumer H. Delayed reversal of vertebral artery blood flow following percutaneous transluminal angioplasty for subclavian steal syndrome. *Neuroradiology* 1984;25:189–198.
13. Tournade A, Zenglein JP, Braun JP, et al. Percutaneous transluminal angioplasty of the vertebral and subclavian arteries; an angiographic velocimetry comparison. *J Neuroradiol* 1986;13:95–110.
14. Ishi K, Horota Y, Kita Y, et al. Coronary subclavian steal corrected with percutaneous transluminal angioplasty. *J Cardiovasc Surg* 1991;32:275.
15. Souder MC, Sullivan KL. Subclavian artery angioplasty proximal to a left internal mammary–coronary artery bypass. *Cardiovasc Intervent Radiol* 1991;14:355.
16. Vitek JJ. Subclavian artery angioplasty and the origin of the vertebral artery. *Radiology* 1989;170:407.
17. Duber C, Klose KJ, Kopp M, et al. Percutaneous transluminal angioplasty for occlusion of the subclavian artery: short and long-term results. *Cardiovasc Intervent Radiol* 1992;15:205–210.
18. Goldberg SL, Columbo A, Maiello L, et al. Intracoronary stent insertion after balloon angioplasty for chronic total occlusions. *JACC* 1995;26(3):713–719.
19. Gunther RW, Vorweck D, Antonucci F, et al. Iliac artery stenosis or obstruction after unsuccessful balloon angioplasty: treatment with a self-expandable stent. *AJR* 1991;156:389.
20. Rees CR, Palmaz JC, Garcia O, et al. Angioplasty and stenting of completely occluded iliac arteries. *Radiology* 1989;172:953.
21. Gunther RW, Vorwerk D, Bohndorf K, et al. Iliac and femoral artery stenoses and occlusions: treatment with intravascular stents. *Radiology* 1989;172:725.

22. Sueoka BL. Percutaneous transluminal stent placement to treat subclavian steal syndrome. *JVIR* 1996;7:351–356.

23. Kuzelmass AD, Kim D, Kuntz RE, et al. Endoluminal stenting of subclavian artery stenosis for ischemia in the distribution of a patent left internal mammary graft. *Cathet Cardiovasc Diagn* 1994;33:175–177.

24. Mufti SIS, Young KR, Schulthesis T. Restenosis following subclavian artery angioplasty for treatment of coronary steal syndrome: definitive treatment with Palmaz stent placement. *Cathet Cardiovasc Diagn* 1994;33:172–174.

25. Bachman DM, Kim RM. Transluminal dilation for subclavian steal syndrome. *AJR* 1980;135:995–996.

26. Galichia JP, Bajaj AK, Vine DL, et al. Subclavian artery stenosis treated by transluminal angioplasty: six cases. *Cardiovasc Intervent Radiol* 1983;6:788–781.

27. Motarjeme A, Keifer JW, Zuska AJ, et al. Percutaneous transluminal angioplasty for treatment of subclavian steal. *Radiology* 1985;155:611–613.

28. Burke DR, Gordon RL, Miskin JD, et al. Percutaneous transluminal angioplasty of subclavian arteries. *Radiology* 1987;1164:699–704.

29. Theron J. Angioplasty of supra-aortic arteries. *Semin Intervent Radiol* 1987;4:331–342.

30. Erbtein RA, Wholey MH, Smoot S. Subclavian artery steal syndrome: treatment by percutaneous transluminal angioplasty. *AJR* 1988;151:919–924.

31. Mathias K. Catheter treatment of cerebrovascular disease. Program of the Cardiovascular and Interventional Rediology Society of Europe, Porto Cervo, Sardinia, Italy, May 27, 1987, pp 84–85. Abstract.

32. Gershong G, Basta L, Hagan AD. Correction of subclavian artery stenosis by percutaneous angioplasty. *Cathet Cardiovasc Diagn* 1990;21:165.

33. Nicholson AA, Kennan NM, Sheridan WG, et al. Percutaneous transluminal angioplasty of the subclavian artery. *Ann R Coll Surg* 1991;773:46.

34. Herbang A, Maskovic J, Tomac B. Percutaneous transluminal angioplasty of the subclavian arteries: long-term results in 52 patients. *AJR* 1991;156:1091–1094.

35. Becker GJ, Katzen BT, Dake MD. Noncoronary angioplasty. *Radiology* 1989;170:921–940.

36. Joseph S, Mandalam KR, Rao VRK, et al. Percutaneous transluminal angioplasty of the subclavian artery in nonspecific aortoarteritis: Results of long-term follow up. *JVIR* 1994;5:573–580.

37. Provan JL. Arteriosclerotic occlusive disease of brachycephalic and arch vessels. In: Rutherford RB, ed. *Vascular Surgery*. 3rd ed. Philadelphia: WB Saunders; 1989.

38. Herring M. The subclavian steal syndrome: a review. *Ann Surg* 1977;43:220–228.

39. Beebe HE, Stark R, Johnson ML, et al. Choices of operation for subclavian-vertebral arterial disease. *Am J Surg* 1980;139:616–623.

40. Humphries AW, Young YR, Bevan GG, et al. Relief of vertebrobasilar symptoms by carotid endarterectomy. *Surgery* 1965;57:48–52.

41. Baker RN, Carroll RJ, Schwartz WS. Prognosis in patients with transient cerebral ischemic attacks. *Neurology* 1968;18:1157–1165.

42. Cartlidge NEF, Whisnant JF, Elveback LR. Carotid and vertebral transient cerebral ischemic attacks. *Mayo Clin Proc* 1977;52:117–120.

43. Caplan LR, Tettenborn B. Embolism in the posterior circulation. In Berguer R, Caplan LR, eds. *Vertebrobasilar Arterial Disease*. St Louis: Quality Medical; 1992:52–65.

44. Pessin MS. Posterior cerebral artery disease and occipital ischemia. In: Berguer R, Caplan LR, eds. *Vertebrobasilar Arterial Disease*. St Louis: Quality Medical; 1992:66–75.

45. Kumpe DA, Zwerdlinger S, Griffin DJ. Blue digit syndrome: treatment with percutaneous transluminal angioplasty. *Radiology* 1988;166:37.

46. Highshida RT, Tsai FY, Halbach N, et al. Cerebral percutaneous transluminal angioplasty. *J Heart Dis Stroke* 1993;2:497–502.

47. Courtheaux P, Tournade A, Theron J, et al. Transcutaneous angioplasty of vertebral artery atheromatous ostial stricture. *Neuroradiology* 1984;27:259–264.

48. Higashida RT, Hieshima GB, Tsai FY, et al. Transluminal angioplasty of the vertebral and basilar artery. *Am J Neurol Radiol* 1987;8:745–750.

49. Ferguson RDG, Lee LI, Connoes JJ, et al. Angioplasty of the extracranial and intracranial vasculature. *Semin Intervent Radiol* 1994;11:64.

50. Motarjeme A, Keifer JW, Zuska AJ. Percutaneous transluminal angioplasty of the vertebral arteries. *Radiology* 1981;139:715–717.

51. Kachel R, Enbert G, Basche S, et al. Percutaneous transluminal angioplasty (dilatation) of carotid, vertebral and innominate artery stenosis. *Cardiovasc Intervent Radiol* 1987;110:142–146.

52. Kachel K. Percutaneous transluminal angioplasty (PTA) of supraaortic arteries especially of the carotid and vertebral artery. An alternative to vascular surgery. *J Mal Vasc* 1993;18:254–257.

53. ACAS—Executive Committee for the Asymptomatic Carotid Atherosclerosis Study. Endarterectomy for asymptomatic carotid artery stenosis. *JAMA* 1995;273:1421–1428.

54. Feldman RL, Rubin JJ, Kuykendall RC. Use of coronary Palmaz-Schatz stent in the percutaneous treatment of vertebral artery stenosis. *Cathet Cardiovasc Diagn* 1996;38:312–315.

55. Berguer R. Vertebrobasilar Ischemia: Indications, techniques and results of surgical repair. In: Rutherford RB, ed. *Vascular Surgery*. 4th ed. Philadelphia: WB Saunders; 1995:1574.

56. Berguer R. Vertebrobasilar ischemia: indications, techniques, and results of surgical repair. In: Rutheford RB, ed. *Vascular Surgery*. 4th ed. Philadelphia: WB Saunders; 1995:1581–1585.

57. Kachel R. Results of balloon angioplasty in carotid stenosis *J Endovasc Surg* 1996;3:22–30.

58. Berguer R. Vertebrobasilar ischemia: indications, techniques and results of surgical repair. In: Rutherford RB, ed. *Vascular Surgery*. 4th ed. Phildelphia: WB Saunders; 1995:1586.

49

A Surgeon's Perspective on Carotid Angioplasty/Stenting

Bruce A. Perler, M.D.

THE PAST

In 1987, based on a minimum of clinical experience, the Food and Drug Administration (FDA) approved the hot tip laser as a means of enhancing the role of percutaneous transluminal angioplasty (PTA) in the treatment of arterial occlusive disease. Almost immediately, many institutions in the United States acquired this technology and thousands of patients with lower extremity arterial occlusive disease were treated with laser angioplasty. Indeed, many health care facilities initiated very aggressive advertising campaigns to market this high-tech, minimally invasive method of treating peripheral occlusive disease. Some of these advertisements declared that laser angioplasty was a proven technology, and in some cases it was stated that this modality would replace conventional bypass surgery in the management of lower extremity arterial occlusive disease.

In the midst of this near-"laser hysteria," interventional radiologists and vascular surgeons at the Johns Hopkins Hospital collaborated in an investigation of femoropopliteal laser angioplasty. This study documented a poor initial recanalization rate and only a 14% 1-year primary patency rate in successfully treated patients.[1,2] Approximately 20% of the unsuccessfully treated patients were clinically worse after the procedure and required femoropopliteal bypass surgery. Based on this dismal experience, we concluded that laser angioplasty should be characterized purely as an investigational technique that was not appropriate for broad clinical use, and we stopped performing the procedure. In view of the investment that many institutions had made in this technology and the aggressive marketing associated with it, it is not surprising that our work generated a backlash of criticism. Subsequently, however, other workers began reporting suboptimal results.

Over the next 2 years, laser angioplasty largely disappeared from the therapeutic armamentarium of almost all peripheral vascular specialists in this country.

I think most would acknowledge that the laser angioplasty story represents an unfortunate "bump in the road" of what has generally been a rather impressive record of expansion and improvement in the endovascular treatment of circulatory disease over the last 20 years. Today, PTA and intravascular stent placement have become an accepted part of our therapeutic armamentarium in the management of atherosclerotic occlusive disease in diverse anatomic locations. At this 10th anniversary of its FDA approval, however, I remind the reader of the hot tip laser saga because I think it is important that we do not repeat the mistakes of the past. The most recent application of endovascular therapy has been in the treatment of carotid bifurcation occlusive disease, and I am concerned that the current enthusiastic advocacy of carotid angioplasty by some is strongly reminiscent of the laser era.

THE PROMISE

The endovascular treatment of carotid artery disease is clearly the most topical and controversial issue in vascular intervention today. While it is purely an investigational therapy at the present time, some of its proponents are already claiming that carotid angioplasty will supplant carotid endarterectomy (CEA) in many, if not most, patients with carotid artery disease. Just as with laser angioplasty, solid scientific support for carotid angioplasty is scant at best. To date, most information with respect to its safety and efficacy has been derived from limited clinical series typically presented in case report fashion at postgraduate courses and specialty seminars or in publications, most often in abstract form, of uncontrolled and imprecisely defined clinical experiences. This largely anecdotal information has raised many questions with respect to the selection of candidates for intervention and methods of outcome analysis; objective follow-up data have been almost non-existent.

THE FACTS

The interest in carotid PTA/stenting among endovascular and surgical specialists is not surprising. This is big business! CEA has become the most frequently performed peripheral vascular surgical operation in the United States, with more than 100,000 procedures carried out annually at an estimated cost of $2 billion. The frequency of this operation is not surprising because its purpose is the prevention of stroke, which is one of our most important health care problems. More than 500,000 strokes occur annually in the United States. Stroke is our third leading cause of death, as well as a cause of substantial morbidity and long-term disability. Stroke is responsible for 15% of all chronic care facility admissions and is the single leading cause of nursing home placement in this country. It is now estimated that the direct and indirect health care costs of stroke approach $30 billion annually in the United States. Furthermore, it is recognized that the most frequent etiology of stroke, especially among older individuals, is carotid artery disease. In view of this, it is reasonable to assume that CEA should be a very cost-effective means of preventing stroke, assuming that the operation can be performed with reasonable safety. The recently completed North American Symptomatic Carotid Endarterectomy Trial (NASCET) and the Asymptomatic Carotid Atherosclerosis Study (ACAS) have clearly affirmed the superiority of CEA to medical therapy in the management of symptomatic and asymptomatic patients with carotid artery disease, respectively.[3,4]

Despite the enthusiastic claims of some, however, it is premature to equate carotid angioplasty with CEA at the present time. On the one hand, the application of endovascular therapy to the treatment of cervical carotid atherosclerosis is quite logical. PTA has been associated with superior results in the treatment of short stenotic lesions. Therefore, carotid artery disease should be ideally amenable to angioplasty because carotid atherosclerotic plaques are typically focal in distribution, unlike the more diffuse atherosclerotic involvement of most other peripheral arteries. This is why endarterectomy is feasible in the management of carotid atherosclerotic disease. On the other hand, with the exception of the acutely thrombosed internal carotid artery (ICA), complete ICA occlusions are inoperable. Because there are no branches of the ICA in the neck, chronic occlusions involve the entire cervical ICA and extend into the cerebrum. Therefore, unlike the placement of stents in other anatomic sites such as in iliac, femoropopliteal, or coronary arteries, where one

can almost always construct a bypass graft to salvage the failed stented vessel, we do not know whether a surgical rescue will be possible in the patient who experiences a subacute or chronic ICA occlusion after stent placement. Furthermore, while the ICA can be surgically exposed over a length of several centimeters in the neck, the skull does impose a limit to that exposure, so that if a stenosis developed at the distal extent of a carotid stent, in some cases surgical repair might not be possible. In fact, I am not aware of a single published report documenting late operative repair of a carotid artery after placement of a stent.

Before carotid PTA/stenting can become an accepted part of our therapeutic armamentarium, therefore, I believe we need clear scientific evidence not only of its safety and efficacy acutely, but also of its long-term performance. Ultimately, a niche for carotid angioplasty will develop if it can be shown that it results in a comparable or superior outcome when compared to the conventional surgical management of carotid artery disease in terms of safety, durability, and cost. Within this context, the documented performance of CEA in contemporary practice suggests that it will be a difficult gold standard to displace. As noted above, the safety of CEA has been well demonstrated in several multicenter randomized clinical trials.[3,4] While some have argued that the performance of this operation reported in multicenter prospective trials or in publications from individual institutions of excellence may not reflect its track record in the community at large, recent work refutes this criticism.[5] CEA is an exceptionally safe procedure in contemporary practice today. Conversely, the safety of carotid angioplasty remains to be determined. Drs. Dietrich and Martinez are to be congratulated for their ongoing investigation of carotid angioplasty, as reported in this text (Chapter 50). However, a 30-day clinical failure rate of 11% and a periprocedural stroke and mortality rate of 8.1% are sobering.

As noted above, durability is another key parameter by which the performance of carotid angioplasty must be compared to conventional surgical management. Although early isolated reports demonstrated a rate of recurrent stenosis following CEA exceeding 10%, this experience is largely of historic interest today. Currently, most vascular surgeons close the carotid arteriotomy with a patch either routinely or selectively, and a growing body of clinical data suggests that this has dramatically reduced the rate of restenosis after endarterectomy. In a report from the Johns Hopkins Hospital, for example, the rate of restenosis after CEA among patients who underwent routine patching was 4.8%, with a mean follow-up of 18 months.[6] Furthermore, the vast majority of recurrent stenotic lesions consist of myointimal hyperplasia, are smooth, and in almost all cases are asympotomatic. Therefore, it is only a small minority of patients who require reoperation for these lesions. In fact, more than 95% of patients who undergo CEA never require another intervention on that vessel for the duration of their lives. While some have argued that carotid angioplasty should be more durable than CEA, no long-term resullts are currently available. Based on the long-term performance of stents in other small arteries, however, I am not optimistic. Coronary angioplasty is associated with as much as a 30% rate of restenosis within the first year. Renal and femoropopliteal stents have been associated with restenosis rates exceeding 30% and 40%, respectively, within 1 year. It will be crucial to determine whether the natural history of stents in the ICA is superior to this experience.

The appropriate role of carotid angioplasty, like that of so many procedures in medicine today, will ultimately be significantly influenced by economic considerations. Many have assumed that because it obviates a formal surgical procedure, carotid angioplasty should be a more cost-effective treatment for carotid artery disease. It must be emphasized, however, that significant progress is currently being made in reducing the cost of CEA. To reduce costs and avoid potential morbidity, for example, CEA is being increasingly performed in selected candidates without preoperative arteriography. Growing experience over the past decade has confirmed that operating based on a duplex scan, in some cases supplemented with magnetic resonance angiography, does not compromise the surgical outcome. Obviously, one cannot perform carotid angioplasty without a contrast study. Furthermore, through the performance of angiography and other diagnostic studies exclusively on an outpatient basis, same-day admission for surgery, and implementation of critical pathways, the hospital length of stay associated with CEA has been dramatically reduced in recent years. Today it is routine for many patients to be discharged within 24 hours postoperatively, and almost all patients are home by the second day following surgery.[7] When one considers the cost of balloon angioplasty catheters, stents, time in the catheterization suite and recovery room, and other associated expenses, it is uncertain whether the endovascular treatment of carotid disease will actu-

ally be less expensive than CEA. This is especially true if one considers the financial burden associated with repeat dilatations of stented arteries, as has been the coronary artery angioplasty experience.

THE FUTURE

In summary, I remain open-minded but skeptical about the endovascular treatment of carotid bifurcation disease. Some of the most prominent leaders in vascular surgery and endovascular therapy have presented scholarly statements regarding the need for careful documentation of the safety of carotid angioplasty so that scientifically valid and credible prospective studies may be undertaken to objectively assess the potential role of carotid angioplasty.[8,9] Until such investigations have been completed, however, carotid PTA/stenting must be viewed only as an investigational procedure. We must not repeat the mistakes of the laser era.

REFERENCES

1. Perler BA, Osterman FA, White RI Jr, et al. Percutaneous laser probe femoropopliteal angioplasty: a preliminary experience. *J Vasc Surg* 1989;10:351–357.
2. Perler BA. A plea for truth in advertising. *J Vasc Surg* 1990;12:373–374.
3. North American Symptomatic Carotid Endarterectomy Trial Collaborators. Beneficial effect of carotid endarterectomy in symptomatic patients with high-grade carotid stenosis. *N Engl J Med* 1991;325:445–453.
4. Executive Committee for the Asymptomatic Carotid Atherosclerosis Study. Endarterectomy for asymptomatic carotid artery stenosis. *JAMA* 1995;273:1421–1428.
5. Perler BA, Dardik A, Burleyson GP, et al. The influence of age and hospital volume on the results of carotid endarterectomy. A state-wide analysis of 9,918 cases. *J Vasc Surg* submitted.
6. Perler BA, Ursin F, Shanks U, et al. Carotid Dacron patch angioplasty; immediate and long-term results of a prospective series. *Cardiovasc Surg* 1995;3:631–636.
7. Perler BA. Does advanced age influence the results of carotid endarterectomy? An outcome analysis. *J Am Coll Surg* 1996;183:559–564.
8. Stanley JC, Abbott WM, Towne JB, et al. Statement regarding carotid angioplasty and stenting. *J Vasc Surg* 1996;24:900.
9. Beebe HG, Archie JP, Baker WH, et al. Concern about safety of carotid angioplasty. *Stroke* 1996;27:197–198.

50

The Role of Stents in the Management of Brachiocephalic and Carotid Occlusive Disease

Edward B. Diethrich, M.D.
Robert Martinez, M.D.

The treatment of coronary, peripheral, and renal vascular disease has been revolutionized by percutaneous transluminal angioplasty (PTA) and intraluminal stenting. In 1977, Mathias first proposed PTA for the treatment of proximal aortic arch vessel lesions,[1] and treatment of postsurgical stenosis in the common carotid artery with PTA was reported as early as 1983.[2] The advantages of brachiocephalic angioplasty compared to surgical intervention are evident: there is no cervical incision, the duration of induced occlusion is very short, surgically inaccessible lesions are amenable to treatment, general anesthesia is not required, and the hospitalization period and need for postoperative surveillance may be reduced.[3] Although application of the technique in the brachiocephalic vessels has been more cautious and controversial due to the potential for thromboembolic complications, investigations spanning nearly 20 years support the safety and efficacy of this application.[4] Currently, angioplasty is being increasingly performed to treat lesions of the aortic arch, and early reports from stenting in the carotid bifurcation region have begun to surface in the literature.[5]

Preliminary reports of small series of PTA of proximal brachiocephalic arteries suggest a high degree of technical success and acceptable complication rates.[6–9] A review of the published results on PTA of 774 supraaortic artery lesions (particularly those in the internal carotid artery) by Kachel and colleagues[10] found an overall technical success rate of 95.3%. The major and minor complication rates were 0.5% and 3.5%, respectively. In another review by Kachel[4] of more than 500 patients undergoing carotid angioplasty, there were no deaths and a 2.1% morbidity rate.

Intravascular specialists await the complete results of the Carotid and Vertebral Artery Transluminal Angioplasty Study (CAVATAS), an international multicenter, randomized trial aimed at determining the risks and benefits of carotid and vertebral artery transluminal angioplasty compared to surgery or medical treatment. A preliminary report including the first 100 patients indicates results comparable to those of carotid surgery, although longer, more detailed follow-up is necessary.[11]

Advances in stent technology and dilation techniques have led to the introduction of intravascular stenting in vessels above the arch. Stents have been used successfully in the subclavian and innominate arteries to maintain postdilation patency in these vessels.[12] Several investigators have reported early results of balloon angioplasty with stenting in the carotid artery and have speculated on the possibility that it may be safer and more effective than balloon angioplasty alone.[5,13] Although carotid stenting is relatively new, it clearly represents a natural progression of techniques that are less invasive than surgery.

STENT TECHNOLOGY

Stents have significantly influenced the outcome of endoluminal treatment and greatly expanded our therapeutic options over a broad range of pathologies and angioplasty-induced defects. For example, stents have reduced the rate of restenosis, compared to balloon angioplasty, in the treatment of iliac artery occlusive disease.

Stents were introduced to treat abnormal dilation characteristics (eg, resistance, recoil) and dilation failure (eg, persistent filling defect, dissection, intimal flaps).[14,15] In view of the performance of these devices in this setting, we now use stents routinely for infrarenal aortic stenoses and when treating complete iliac artery occlusions. The results of stent application in the arch vessel, cervical carotid, and renal arteries are more limited and, in general, less well documented. Palmaz stents (Johnson & Johnson Interventional Systems, Warren, NJ) and Wallstents (Schneider, Minneapolis, MN) have performed well in the brachiocephalic arteries arising from the aortic arch,[12,16] and one may surmise from early studies that similar results can be achieved in the extracranial carotid arteries.[5,17]

The Palmaz stent is a stainless steel tube with multiple rows of staggered rectangular slots that assumes a diamond shape when expanded, reducing to 10% the amount of metal in contact with the luminal surface. The Palmaz stent is available in lengths varying from 10 to 39 mm, with expansion ranges of 4 to 18 mm. Its longitudinal rigidity and large diameter make it ideal for straight vessels like the distal aorta, the renal and iliac arteries, and end-to-end graft anastomoses.

The Wallstent is a cylindrical device constructed by braiding multiple stainless steel monofilaments. Because of its spring-like structure, the Wallstent is flexible, compliant, and self-expanding, which makes it useful for delivery through curved arteries, implantation overlying the graft–artery junction in end-to-side anastomoses, and in vessels subject to flexion from adjacent joints or structures. The Wallstent comes in a variety of lengths ranging from 50 to 150 mm and in diameters ranging from 5 to 10 mm. Furthermore, it is anticipated that a variety of new stent designs will become available in the next few years, and several are currently undergoing clinical evaluation in a number of institutions throughout the world.

BRACHIOCEPHALIC STENTING

Techniques

Proximal Lesions

Balloon angioplasty of proximal arch vessel lesions is often accompanied by significant recoil and an inability to eradicate a pressure gradient periprocedurally. Recently, stenting in proximal lesions has been tried to address these deficiencies.[12,18,19] In a study at the Arizona Heart Institute, access was obtained through the brachial artery (Fig. 50–1), and balloon dilation and stent implantation were used to treat recurrent lesions in the arch vessels (Fig. 50–2). Ulcerated lesions were stented primarily to avoid embolic consequences.[12] Other investigators have described primary stenting in the subclavian and innominate arteries.[18,19] In patients with longer lesions where the stent might be affected by arm movement, we have preferred to use the more flexible Wallstent (Fig. 50–3). Femoral approaches have also been used in a number of cases.

Cervical Lesions

Experience gained with the techniques for direct carotid artery access may find use in the delivery of stents in the common and internal carotid arteries, in the cervical carotid bifurcation, and at the aortic arch. The majority of interventionists, however, will be more familiar and comfortable with the retrograde femoral access method, which has almost completely replaced the direct carotid stick for angiographic visualization of the arch and the cervical and intracranial arterial systems.

The preferred anesthesia for the percutaneous retrograde femoral approach is local with mild sedation. This allows the patient to communicate throughout the procedure so that immediate assessment of any neurologic change may be made.

The selection of the common femoral artery is based on the condition of the iliac artery. Because a sheath or guiding catheter is passed into the aortic arch, the side with the less tortuous and stenotic iliac artery is chosen. An 18-gauge, 2¹⁄₁₆-inch needle is inserted followed by a 0.035-inch guidewire (Glidewire, Meditech/Boston Scientific, Watertown, MA) and a No. 9 F sheath (Cordis, Miami, FL). Following intravenous heparin administration, a 260-cm, 0.035-inch angled hydrophilic guidewire (Medi-tech) is passed into the aortic arch, and a JB2 catheter (Cook, Inc., Bloomington, IN) is passed into the high ascending aorta. The wire is withdrawn a sufficient length to expose the angle of the JB2 catheter, which is then slowly pulled back to selectively engage either the brachiocephalic trunk or the origin of the left common carotid artery.

The angled guidewire is passed into the appropriate carotid artery, and the JB2 catheter is advanced over it to about the midlevel of the carotid artery. The wire is withdrawn, and a small bolus of contrast material is injected to secure a road-mapping image. The angled guidewire is then passed into the external carotid artery, followed by the JB2 catheter. This maneuver prevents a wire from crossing the lesion during insertion of the delivery sheath. The guidewire is removed and replaced with a 260-cm Super Stiff Amplatz wire (Cook), which is passed into the external carotid artery. The JB2 catheter is withdrawn, and the fluoroscope is panned from the cervical carotid artery across the arch to assess the angle and origin of the great vessel to be traversed by the delivery catheter. Too acute an angle at the carotid artery junction can produce kinking in the delivery sheath and require conversion to the direct stick approach.

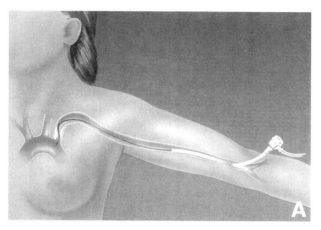

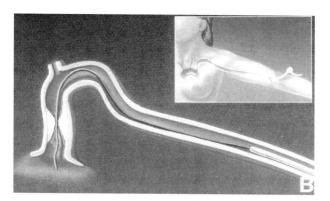

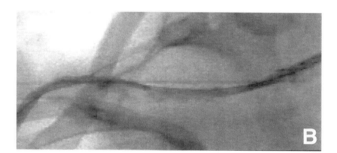

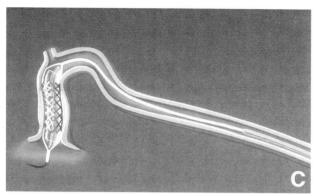

Figure 50–1.   (A) Brachial artery percutaneous approach using a No. 7 F sheath provides excellent access for proximal subclavian lesions. (B) Balloon angioplasty is performed prior to making the decision regarding the need for stent deployment. (C) Illustration of stent deployment in the proximal left subclavian artery.

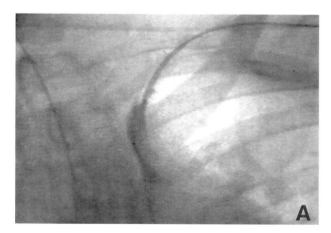

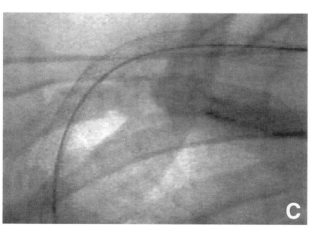

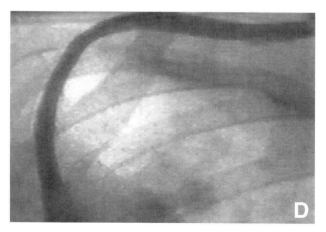

Figure 50–2.   (A) Angiogram showing occlusion of the left subclavian artery. (B) Following balloon angioplasty, a long, diffuse lesion was identified. (C, D) Two Wallstents were deployed, yielding a very satisfactory result.

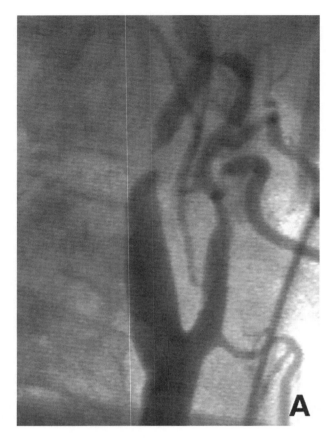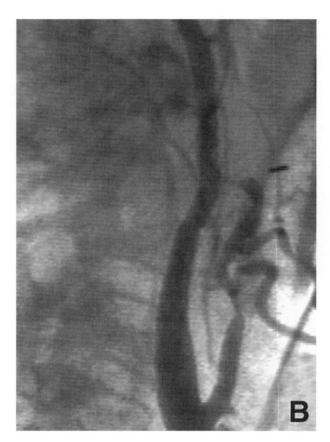

Figure 50–3. (A) Angiogram showing high-grade stenosis of the internal carotid artery. Due to its location, this type of lesion causes higher morbidity with the classical operation. (B) A stent was deployed to resolve the stenosis.

If the arch anatomy is favorable, the delivery catheter is passed into the midcarotid position, and either an Amplatz Super Stiff wire or an angled guidewire is positioned across the lesion in the internal carotid artery. If the Amplatz is selected, its positioning usually requires a wire exchange using an angled guidewire and a guiding catheter. Contrast material is injected to obtain a road-map image to determine the dimensions of the artery and the nature and length of the lesion. An appropriately sized balloon is selected for predilation, usually a 4- or 5-mm × 2-cm balloon with a 120-cm shaft length. At the same time, a stent is chosen and mounted on another balloon in preparation for delivery.

The predilation balloon is passed to the lesion, and after atropine has been administered, the balloon is inflated for 10 to 15 seconds at 12 atmospheres. A small bolus of contrast material is injected to assess the angioplasty result. The balloon with stent is then passed to the lesion, and a second contrast injection is used to confirm the proper location because patient movement is always a possibility. The stent is deployed with a 5-second balloon inflation.

The balloon catheter is used for a wire exchange to accommodate the 0.018-inch wire for the intravascular ultrasound (IVUS) catheter. If the IVUS analysis con-

firms perfect deployment, a final control angiogram is performed. If the IVUS image indicates incomplete stent deployment, additional dilation with larger balloon(s) should be undertaken until stent-wall apposition is adequate throughout.

The guiding catheter is then withdrawn into the descending thoracic aorta, where it is substituted for a short No. 9 F sheath in the groin. The patient is transferred to the intensive care unit for observation and duplex scanning. When the Activated Coagulation Time has returned to normal, the groin sheath is removed.

All carotid stent patients are placed on antiplatelet therapy (aspirin only) prior to treatment, and this is resumed the day following the procedure. No postprocedural anticoagulation is used. Neurologic changes are reported immediately, initiating neurology consultation and appropriate studies. Computed tomography (CT) is performed to assess any suspected embolic event. The majority of the patients are discharged the day following the procedure.

CLINICAL RESULTS

Proximal Lesions

Successful stenting of lesions in the subclavian and innominate arteries[12,18,19] has been reported in three small series reports. Results of primary stent deployment in the subclavian artery have been described by Kumar and colleagues.[18] Palmaz stent implantation was successfully performed in 27 consecutive patients with 31 obstructed subclavian arteries. A total of 50 stents were successfully deployed using the brachial ($n = 7$), femoral ($n = 16$), or combined ($n = 8$) approach. The percent diameter stenosis improved from $85 \pm 12\%$ to $6 \pm 7\%$ ($p < 0.001$). Peak and mean translesion pressure gradients decreased, respectively, from 56 ± 35 mm Hg to 3 ± 4 mm Hg ($p < 0.01$) and from 29 ± 18 mm Hg to 2 ± 2 mm Hg ($p < 0.01$). Complications were minor and procedural: one stent migration was treated uneventfully with deployment in the right external iliac artery, and two brachial arteries required repair. The investigators concluded that primary subclavian artery stent deployment was 100% successful in the immediate restoration of pulsatile flow.[18]

Experience with primary Palmaz stenting in 33 patients with lesions of the subclavian[31] and innominate arteries[2] resulted in technical success in 31 (94%) of patients.[19] Thirty (97%) of the 32 stented arteries were patent over a follow-up period of up to 2 years. Complications in this series included asymptomatic vertebral artery occlusion (one), entry site hematoma or pseudoaneurysm (four), and distal embolization (one). The investigators concluded that endovascular repair of symptomatic lesions in the subclavian and innominate arteries was a viable alternative to standard surgical repair.

Our experience in the treatment of brachiocephalic stenoses and recurrent lesions indicates that implantation success reaches 100% for stent placement in the subclavian and innominate arteries. Palmaz stents have been implanted in the majority of cases, although occasionally the Wallstent and Strecker stent (Boston Scientific, Watertown, MA) have been used as needed. Percutaneous access was normally gained through the brachial artery. Stents were ballooned except in the case of ulcerated lesions, where primary deployment was used to prevent embolic consequences. Follow-up ranging up to 4 years with duplex Doppler scans and/or arteriography has confirmed patency in the majority of cases.[12]

Cervical Lesions

Endovascular intervention in the cervical and carotid arteries is in its earliest stages, and clinicians are acutely aware of the opportunity for serious, debilitating, and lethal complications. A number of investigators have reported the preliminary results of their initial experiences with carotid stents.[12,13,17,20–24] Bergeron and colleagues were among the first to report the use of an intravascular stent in the carotid artery[24]; other case reports and small series have also been published.[12,13,17,20,22–24] The published results of the

larger series (>100 stent placements)[5,21] are discussed here in greater detail. Iyer and colleagues[21] reported their experience in 100 patients who underwent balloon angioplasty and a total of 157 stent placements (121 Palmaz biliary, 26 Gianturco-Roubin, 10 Wallstent) in 110 extracranial internal/common carotid arteries. Lesions in 64 of the vessels were symptomatic (18 strokes, 46 transient ischemic events [TIAs]), and 46 lesions were asymptomatic. Coronary artery disease was present in 80% of the patients. The study included independent neurologic assessments, with CT, magnetic resonance imaging (MRI), and carotid ultrasound studies at baseline and follow-up. In 10 patients, the contralateral carotid was occluded. Twenty-five lesions were severely ulcerated. Bilateral carotid procedures were performed during the same session in six patients. Following stent deployment, the mean baseline percent stenosis was reduced from $70\% \pm 12\%$ to $3\% \pm 16\%$. Five external carotid arteries required stenting. Procedures were successful in 97 of 100 patients. Inability to access the carotid artery transfemorally ($n = 2$) and suboptimal coverage of the dissection flap were the causes of the three failures.

Complications were not infrequent and included TIAs (three), minor strokes (six), major stroke (one), and death (one). The major stroke in this series occurred in a patient with severe mitral regurgitation and atrial fibrillation. The death resulted from a direct retrograde puncture of a carotid artery while the patient was under general anesthesia. Clinical follow-up in the 97 patients who received stents revealed two other deaths; one patient with severe aortic stenosis died from congestive heart failure, and one patient who had suffered a major stroke died from complications related to pneumonia 3 weeks after the procedure. There were no late neurologic events.

Angiographic follow-up in 38 vessels demonstrated one restenosis (2.6%), and deformation of a Palmaz stent was seen in eight vessels (21%). Three repeat angioplasties were successfully performed to correct one restenosis and two stent deformations. The investigators concluded that, based on their initial experience, carotid angioplasty with stenting appeared feasible and safe.

At the Arizona Heart Institute,[5] stent therapy was offered to symptomatic patients with ≥70% arteriographically defined carotid stenoses or ulcerative lesions. The procedure was performed on 110 nonconsecutive patients, and 72% were asymptomatic.[12] Lesions meeting the treatment criteria were in the proximal common ($n = 3$); midcommon ($n = 12$), distal common ($n = 8$), internal (carotid) ($n = 92$), and external ($n = 2$) carotid arteries. Seven patients had bilateral internal carotid artery stenoses, and 17 patients were treated for postsurgical recurrent disease. The mean lesion length and diameter stenosis for all lesions were 12.4 ± 9.2 mm and $86.5\% \pm 10.6\%$, respectively. The procedures were performed either via direct percutaneous access to the cervical common carotid artery or through a retrograde femoral artery approach.

A total of 109 patients were treated successfully with 129 stents (128 Palmaz, 1 Wallstent). One percutaneous procedure failed (0.9%) because the stent could not be deployed, and the patient underwent carotid endarterectomy. Minor complications included four cases of spasm (successfully treated with papaverine), one flow-limiting dissection (stented), and six access-site problems. There were seven strokes (two major, five reversible) (6.4%) and five minor transient events (4.5%) that resolved within 24 hours. Three patients (2.7%) were converted to endarterectomy prior to discharge. One stroke patient died (0.9%), and another patient died of an unrelated cardiac event in hospital. In the 30-day postprocedural period, two internal carotid artery stents were occluded (patients asymptomatic). Clinical success at 30 days (no technical failure, death, endarterectomy, stroke, or occlusion) was 89.1% (98/110). Life-table analysis showed an 89% cumulative primary patency rate.

Based on this early experience, we, like Iyer and colleagues,[21] concluded that carotid stenting appears feasible from a technical standpoint, with good early patency. However, the incidence of neurologic sequelae is clearly a serious problem. Technical enhancements and a more aggressive antiplatelet regimen warrant further study.

LESSONS LEARNED

Although stenting in the proximal brachiocephalic region has proved relatively straightforward and very successful, our experience with over 200 carotid stent procedures has illustrated several critical issues related to techniques for carotid stent deployment. The first is the selection of the access approach. In our early experience, we preferred the direct stick approach. Once long-shafted balloons and sheaths were available, we began using the retrograde femoral route preferentially. The use of systemic heparinization and scrupulous attention to factors influencing puncture site hemostasis has improved our success with the direct approach, however.

Another technical enhancement that has proven invaluable is the introduction of IVUS imaging. We have deployed more than 125 stents using IVUS monitoring and believe that inadequate stent expansion contributes to many complications, most notably stent occlusion and thrombus formation.

It is well known that as a stent is further dilated after its initial deployment, it not only expands in diameter but also shortens. Additionally, the interstices of the stent change their configuration and, in particular,

widen. In the carotid location, there may well be serious unacknowledged sequelae associated with further stent expansion.

As previously described, primary stent implantation has gained favor in other peripheral arteries, and some investigators have used it in the carotid arteries.[13] We believe this method is valuable in treating ulcerated lesions where dilation increases the likelihood of releasing embolic material. However, in the case of significant stenoses, if the stenosis is so tight that the stent might be dislodged from the balloon as it traverses the lesion, we consider it mandatory to predilate.

We have also elected not to use pacing wires during carotid stent implantation, as some investigators have done. We rely on atropine to control the baroreceptor response to balloon dilation within the carotid sinus. Clearly, blood pressure surveillance must be vigilant and the response to any deviation rapid.

We are encouraged by the durability of the successfully implanted devices but equally cognizant of potential complications. The techniques we described earlier in this chapter are being refined to reduce this potential, but we are in the earliest phases of our experience with carotid stenting and will certainly learn more about complications with further clinical experience. As we note in documenting the results in our first 110 patients,[5] this arterial territory in unique among the peripheral vessels. Although 200 iliac angioplasties would have elevated any operator to expert status, the same cannot be said for the cervical carotid arteries. Furthermore, the seriousness of ischemic injury cannot be overemphasized. Therefore, our challenge is to refine our techniques to bring the safety of the procedure into line with that of carotid endarterectomy so that we may pursue comparison against this gold standard.

CONCLUSION

Treatment of endovascular occlusive disease has been favorably affected by the introduction and application of transluminal angioplasty and intravascular stenting. Amid fears about the potential for significant thromboembolic complications associated with the use of these techniques above the arch, interventionists have treaded cautiously but steadily into these new territories, with promising results. Brachiocephalic angioplasty requires no general anesthesia or cervical incision and has been proven to be particularly safe in proximal lesions. The technique is now being applied to the treatment of cervical vessels. Advances in stent technology and technique have resulted in devices that maintain postdilation patency in a variety of brachiocephalic vessels. Experience with balloon angioplasty and stenting, as well as primary stenting in the subclavian and innominate arteries, has been very encouraging. The early results of balloon angioplasty with stenting in the carotid artery have led several interventionists to believe that stenting may be safer and more efficacious than balloon angioplasty alone. As technologies and techniques inevitably change and progress, it is paramount that we continually evaluate our successes and failures so that we may keep a clear perspective about their impact on our ability to provide optimal care to our patients.

REFERENCES

1. Mathias K. Ein neues Kathetersystem zur perkutanen transluminalen Angioplastie von Karotisstenosen. *Fortschr Med* 1977;95:1007–1011.

2. Tievsky AL, Druy EM, Mardiat JG. Transluminal angioplasty in postsurgical stenosis of the extracranial carotid artery. *AJNR* 1983;4:800–802.

3. Becquemin JP, Qvarfordt P, Castier Y, Melliere D. Carotid angioplasty: is it safe? *J Endovasc Surg* 1996;3:35–41.

4. Kachel R. Results of balloon angioplasty in the carotid arteries. *J Endovasc Surg* 1996;3:22–30.

5. Diethrich EB, Ndiaye M, Reid DB. Stenting in the carotid artery: initial experience in 110 patients. *J Endovasc Surg* 1996;3:42–62.

6. Mathias K, Schlosser V. Reinke MM. Katheterrekanalisation eines subklaviaverschlusses. *Fortschr Roentgenstr* 1980;132:346–347.

7. Motarjeme A, Keifer JW, Zuska AJ. Percutaneous transluminal angioplasty of the brachiocephalic arteries. *AJR* 1982;138:457–462.

8. Vitek JJ, Raymon BC, Oh SJ. Innominate artery angioplasty. *AJNR* 1984;5:113–114.

9. Hebrang A, Maskovic J, Tomac B. Percutaneous transluminal angioplasty of the subclavian arteries: long-term results in 52 patients. *AJR* 1991;156:1091–1094.

10. Kachel R, Basche S, Heerklotz I, Grossmann K, Endler S. Percutaneous transluminal angioplasty of supra-aortic arteries, especially the internal carotid artery. *Neuroradiology* 1991;33:191–194.

11. Gaines P. The European carotid angioplasty trial. *J Endovasc Surg* 1996;3:107. Abstract.

12. Diethrich EB. Initial experience with stenting in the innominate, subclavian, and carotid arteries. *J Endovasc Surg* 1995;2:196–221.

13. Bergeron P, Chambran P, Benichou H, Alessandri C. Recurrent carotid disease: will stents be an alternative to surgery? *J Endovasc Surg* 1996;3:76–79.

14. Palmaz JC, Garcia OJ, Schatz RA, et al. Placement of balloon-expandable intraluminal stents in iliac arteries: first 171 procedures. *Radiology* 1990;174:969–975.

15. Becker GJ. Intravascular stents. General principles and status of lower extremity arterial applications. *Circulation* 1991;83(suppl 11):1122–1136.

16. Diethrich EB, Cozacov JC. Subclavian stent implantation to alleviate coronary steal through a patent internal mammary artery graft. *J Endovasc Surg* 1995;2:77–80.

17. Diethrich EB, Rodriguez-Lopez JA, Lopez-Galarza LA. Stents for vascular reconstruction in the carotid arteries. *Circulation* 1995;92:1-383. Abstract.

18. Kumar K, Dorros G, Bates MC, Palmer L, Mathiak L, Dufek C. Primary stent deployment in occlusive subclavian artery disease. *Cathet Cardiovasc Diagn* 1995;34:281–285.

19. Sullivan TM, Bacharach M, Childs MB. PTA and primary stenting of the subclavian and innominate arteries. *Circulation* 1995;92:I-383. Abstract.

20. Mathias K. Stent placement in supra-aortic disease. In: Liermann DD, ed. *Stents. State of the Art and Future Developments.* Morin Heights, Canada: Polyscience Publication, Inc; 1995:87–92.

21. Iyer SS, Roubin G, Yadav S, et al. Elective carotid stenting. *J Endovasc Surg* 1996;3:105–106. Abstract.

22. Diethrich EB, Rodriguez-Lopez JA, Lopez-Galarza LA. Stents for vascular reconstruction in the carotid arteries. *Circulation* 1994;90:I-9. Abstract.

23. Diethrich EB, Gordon MH, Lopez-Galarza LA, Rodriguez-Lopez JA, Casses F. Intraluminal Palmaz stent implantation for treatment of recurrent carotid artery occlusive disease: a plan for the future. *J Intervent Cardiol* 1995;8(3):213–218.

24. Bergeron P, Rudondy P, Poyen V, et al. Experience with carotid angioplasty and the use of intravascular stents. *Angiology* 1993;44:28. Abstract.

51

Thrombolytic Therapy for Acute Stroke: Indications, Technique, and Results

Stanley L. Barnwell, M.D., Ph.D.
Wayne M. Clark, M.D.
Gary M. Nesbit, M.D.
Michael Horgan, M.D.

Stroke is a serious medical emergency with an incidence in the United States of 500,000 cases per year, resulting in 150,000 deaths yearly. This disease is the leading cause of long-term disability in adults, the second leading cause of dementia, and the primary reason patients are admitted to nursing homes. Stroke is the third leading cause of death following heart disease and cancer.[1] Thromboembolic occlusion is the most common cause of ischemic stroke.[2]

Even when a stroke is nonlethal, the temporary lack of blood flow in the brain often causes serious neurologic damage. To minimize mortality and morbidity, the American Heart Association recommends early intervention, preferably within 6 hours of the onset of symptoms.[3] However, stroke patients often seek medical care late: in the absence of a community awareness campaign, about 63% of stroke patients arrive at a hospital more that 24 hours after their symptoms begin.[4]

The degree of injury to the brain is reduced if recanalization is achieved early enough after stroke onset. Early recanalization is the goal of thrombolytic agents now being investigated for use in the treatment of stroke. Thrombolysis and recanalization can be achieved with urokinase, streptokinase, or recombinant tissue plasminogen activator (rt-PA).[5–10] The major concern in using thrombolytic therapy is the risk of hemorrhagic complications. These cerebral hemorrhagic transformations may or may not produce clinical effects and may occur spontaneously in the absence of therapy.

The use of streptokinase for acute stroke treatment has largely been abandoned due to hemorrhagic complications. In a randomized, multicenter, double-blind, controlled trial, treated patients with moderate to severe ischemia in the territory of the middle cerebral were infused with either placebo or streptokinase (1.5 million units over 1 hour). Treatment was given within 6 hours of stroke onset. The study was discontinued prematurely due to the higher rate of mortality 10 days after treatment, mainly caused by the greater rate of symptomatic cerebral hemorrhage (22%) seen in the group treated with streptokinase.[10]

Recent favorable experiences with other thrombolytic agents have suggested that they may play a role in acute stroke treatment.[11–13] A European Cooperative Acute Stroke Study (ECASS) tested thrombolytic therapy in a prospective, randomized, double-blind fashion.[6] Patients with moderate to severe neurologic deficits and without signs of major early infarct on initial computed tomography (CT) received either rt-PA or placebo within 6 hours of stroke symptoms. Therapy produced a better outcome than placebo in terms of three stroke outcome scales (Rankin Scale, Scandinavian Stroke Scale, and combine Barthel Index/Rankin Scale). For instance, 41% of patients treated with intravenous thrombolytics compared to 29% of those treated with placebo had an improved Rankin Scale score after 90 days. In the thrombolysis group there was a slight but not significant increase in the 30-day mortality rates and no significant difference in overall hemorrhagic events. The authors concluded that systemic thrombolysis in acute ischemic stroke is effective in improving some functional measures and neurologic outcomes in their defined patient group, but that such therapy could not be recommended in unselected patient groups.

A second large, randomized, placebo-controlled study in acute ischemic stroke was performed by the National Institute of Neurological Disorders and Stroke rt-PA Stroke Study Group.[14] Patients were selected for study according to the following criteria: acute ischemic stroke with defined time of onset within 180 minutes, significant neurologic deficit: NIH Stroke Scale ≥4, CT scan with no evidence of intracranial hemorrhage, and blood pressure readings below 185 mm Hg systolic and 110 mm Hg diastolic without aggressive blood pressure therapy. All patients were treated within 3 hours of stroke onset, and 302 of 624 were treated within 90 minutes of onset. Treatment consisted of either placebo or rt-PA (0.9 mg/kg body weight to a maximum dose of 90 mg).

In this study, patients receiving thrombolytic therapy within 3 hours of stroke onset were at least 30% more likely than patients on placebo to have minimal or no disability at 3 months.[14] Patient performance on all of the standard stroke scales, including Barthels's Index, the modified Rankin Scale, the Glasgow Outcome Score, and the NIH Stroke Scale, was significantly better in patients treated with thrombolytics than in those given placebo. Symptomatic intracerebral hemorrhage was more common in rt-PA patients (6.4%) than in placebo patients (0.6%), although 3-month mortality rates were comparable between these two groups (17% rt-PA, 21% placebo). Despite an increased incidence of symptomatic intracerebral hemorrhage, treatment of ischemic stroke within 3 hours of onset with rt-PA improved the clinical outcome and decreased the disability observed 3 months after treatment. Based on these results, the U.S. Food and Drug Administration recently approved rt-PA for treatment of acute stroke with symptoms of less than 3 hours' duration and a normal brain CT scan.

CATHETER-DIRECTED, LOCAL, INTRA-ARTERIAL THROMBOLYTIC THERAPY

Recent advances in the techniques of intracranial catheterization have made it possible to deliver thrombolytic agents intra-arterially directly into the thrombus. Experimental studies have demonstrated that intra-arterial administration produces more rapid thrombolysis at a lower dose than intravenous administration.[15] Clinical cardiac thrombolysis studies suggest that intra-arterial delivery may have less risk of systemic hemorrhagic complications.[16] Advantages of this approach include reliable delivery of highly concentrated drug and mechanical disruption of the thromboembolus by the catheter and guidewire.

Catheter-directed, local, intra-arterial thrombolysis for the treatment of acute stroke has been evaluated in several uncontrolled clinical studies.[9,11,17–22] In these studies, a total of 180 patients underwent thrombolytic treatment with rt-PA or urokinase, delivered either regionally into the carotid or vertebral artery, or locally directly into the thrombus at the site of the occlusion. Lysis of the clot, as demonstrated by angiography, occurred in 40 to 100% of cases, and clinical improvement correlated with vessel opening was noted in about 75% of patients. The rate of cerebral hemorrhage ranged from 0 to 17% in these studies. In one small, retrospective, controlled series, the efficacy of intra-arterial urokinase in vertebrobasilar occlusion was evaluated.[7] Seventy percent of the 19 patients successfully recanalized survived compared with 13% of 22 patients receiving conventional treatment.

Several additional uncontrolled studies using catheter-directed, local, intra-arterial thrombolysis have recently been reported. Higashida et al reported their experience with local thrombolytic therapy in 24 patients treated within 12 hours of stroke.[23] Successful clot lysis occurred in 80% of the patients. The authors reported that 15 patients (62%) showed neurologic improvement, although detailed quantification was not given. Clinically significant cerebral hemorrhage occurred in three cases (12%).

Given the apparent safety and efficacy of this approach to treating acute thromboembolic stroke, attention among neurointerventionalists has been turned catheter-directed, local, intra-arterial thrombolytic therapy.

TECHNIQUE OF CATHETER-DIRECTED THROMBOLYTIC THERAPY

Patients are first clinically evaluated by a stroke neurologist to determine the time period of stroke onset, involved cerebral vessel(s), and degree of deficit. A noncontrast CT scan is then obtained to rule out hemorrhage or new infarct. The criteria for evaluating the CT scan are strict and require an experienced person to rule out the subtle signs of mass effect suggestive of a completed infarct. Catheter-directed thrombolysis requires a limited diagnostic angiogram of the vessel with the suspected occlusion. Once location of the occlusion is confirmed by angiography, a microcatheter is navigated to the site of the occlusion, where the catheter tip is placed into the clot and repositioned as necessary to maintain its placement within the clot throughout thrombolytic infusion. A thrombolytic agent may be given by either a pulse-spray or a continuous-infusion technique. The course of thrombolysis is monitored using contrast injections through the guide catheter. A guiding catheter with a large inner diameter allows contrast material to be injected around the microcatheter so that the vessel can be studied during the thrombolytic therapy. When antegrade perfusion is restored in the vessel, the infusion is stopped (Fig. 51–1).

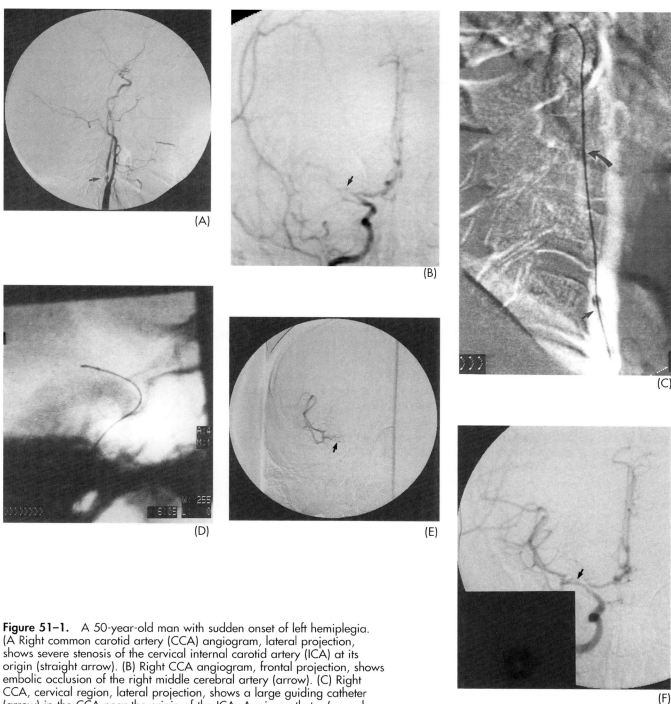

Figure 51–1. A 50-year-old man with sudden onset of left hemiplegia. (A Right common carotid artery (CCA) angiogram, lateral projection, shows severe stenosis of the cervical internal carotid artery (ICA) at its origin (straight arrow). (B) Right CCA angiogram, frontal projection, shows embolic occlusion of the right middle cerebral artery (arrow). (C) Right CCA, cervical region, lateral projection, shows a large guiding catheter (arrow) in the CCA near the origin of the ICA. A microcatheter (curved arrow) is easily navigated through the stenosis. (D) Skull X-ray, lateral projection, shows the microcather and guidewire in the right middle cerebral artery (MCA). (E) Right MCA angiogram, frontal projection, shows the tip of the microcatheter in the clot (arrow). Pressure injection of the contrast material fills the distal MCA branches. (F) Right ICA angiogram, frontal projection, after thrombolysis shows recanalization of the MCA (arrow). The patient's hemiparesis has almost completely resolved. The cervical ICA stenosis was successfully treated by endarterectomy 2 weeks later.

RESULTS OF CATHETER-DIRECTED, LOCAL, INTRA-ARTERIAL THROMBOLYTIC THERAPY

In a nonradomized trial, Sasaki et al compared the results of treatment of acute stroke within 8 hours with (1) catheter-directed urokinase or rt-PA (44 patients), (2) urokinase given via a local carotid infusion (18 patients), or (3) urokinase given by intravenous (33 patients) routes.[8] The rate of recanalization in the catheter-directed group was 84% compared with 11% in the local infusion group. In the patients with middle cerebral artery stroke, patients with catheter-directed therapy had a 44% rate of good recovery (correlated with early recanalization) compared with 19% in the locally treated patients and 31% in the intravenous group. The rate of hemorrhagic transformation was 22% (3% symptomatic) in the catheter-directed group, 28% in the cervical carotid or vertebral artery group, and not given for the intravenous group. Although the authors reported on a large number of patients, the various techniques were not performed consecutively (the intravenous group was treated up to 10 years previously), which makes direct comparisons difficult. The intravenous treatment group also did not have angiographic proof of large vessel occlusion.

Ueda et al reported their experience using either catheter-directed rt-PA or urokinase treatment in 34 patients with negative head CT scans treated within 6 hours of the stroke.[24] Twenty patients also had single photon emission computed tomography (SPECT) scans to measure blood flow prior to treatment. The authors reported a 94% rate of vessel recanalization. At 1 month, 65% of the patients showed improvement on a 5-point functional outcome scale. Seven of the patients (21%) showed hemorrhagic transformation (four symptomatic). Interestingly, the SPECT scans prior to treatment showed significantly lower cerebral blood flow in the patients who developed hemorrhages. In another series, Barr et al reported on 12 patients treated with catheter-directed intra-arterial urokinase within 8 hours of stroke.[25] Thrombolysis was angiographically successful in nine of the patients (75%), all of whom had neurologic improvement.

One study suggests that some of the "hemorrhages" reported with intra-arterial treatment may actually be contrast material.[26] Wildenhain et al examined 10 patients treated with intra-arterial urokinase within 8 hours of stroke. They found near-total clot lysis in eight patients (80%). Four of the patients showed immediate clinical improvement (all had clot lysis), and an additional four (total 80%) showed at least moderate improvement by 1 month. The authors did not quantify this improvement with standardized stroke scales. Six of the patients (60%) had high-intensity areas on their CT scans after treatment. However, in four of these cases, the areas had Hounsfield units (a measure of density on a CT scan to distinguish calcium, blood, and contrast material) higher than expected with hemorrhage, and the lesions resolved within 4 days. The authors conclude that in these cases the high-intensity areas represented contrast material from the angiogram.

Additional recent case reports suggest that catheter-directed urokinase can be given if needed after carotid endarterectomy complicated by stroke.[27] Stroke associated with internal carotid artery occlusion may also be reversed with catheter-directed, local, intra-arterial thrombolysis. Experience has shown that a catheter may be passed safely through an occluded cervical internal carotid artery and intracranial thrombolysis performed.[28-30]

We recently described our experience with intra-arterial urokinase treatment in 13 patients with acute ischemic stroke.[5] All patients had major neurologic symptoms before treatment, and the initial head CT scan was negative for acute ischemic changes. Initial angiographic studies revealed two basilar occlusions; one posterior cerebral artery, seven isolated middle cerebral artery (MCA) or combined internal carotid artery/MCA occlusions; and three distal branch MCA occlusions. The interval from the onset of symptoms to the start of intra-arterial urokinase therapy was 12 hours (range, 3 to 48 hours). Urokinase was directly infused into the occluded vessel. Repeat angiography performed 12 to 24 hours after treatment revealed recanalization of the symptomatic vessel in 77% of the patients. There were no cerebral hematomas, although, as previously reported, contrast material mimicked a hemorrhage.[26] Nine of 13 patients showed major neurologic improvement at 48 hours, as assessed by at least a 4-point improvement in the National Institutes of Health Stroke Scale.

Although intra-arterial thrombolysis should theoretically produce fewer systemic effects than intravenous thrombolysis, it does appear to induce changes in the coagulation factors. In a study using local intra-arterial urokinase in 34 patients, Ueda et al found that the levels of fibrinogen degradation products and n-dimer were higher in the seven patients who had cerebral hemorrhagic transformations.[31]

Catheter-directed thrombolysis appears to be a potentially efficacious method of restoring blood flow during stroke. Clinically beneficial results may be possible even after the standard 6-hour time window for thrombolytic treatment. Intracranial bleeding remains the most dreaded complication of thrombolytic stroke treatment. New imaging techniques including diffusion-weighted magnetic resonance imaging and SPECT scans may allow the identification of patients who can be safely treated.

REFERENCES

1. American Heart Association. Stroke: brain attack. *Heart and Stroke Facts: 1996 Statistical Supplement* 1996;1996:11.
2. Brott TG, Haley EC Jr, Levy DE, et al. Urgent therapy for stroke, I: pilot study of tissue plasminogen activator administered within 90 minutes. *Stroke* 1992;23:632–640.
3. Adams HP, Brott TG, Crowell RM, et al. Guidelines for the management of patients with acute ischemic stroke: A statement for healthcare professionals from a special writing group of the Stroke Council, American Heart Association. *Circulation* 1994;90:1588–1601.
4. Alberts MJ, Perry A, Dawson DV, Bertels C. Effects of public and professional education on reducing the delay in presentation and referral of stroke patients. *Stroke* 1992;23:352–356.
5. Barnwell SL, Clark WM, Nguyen TT, O'Neill OR, Wynn M, Coull B. Safety and efficacy of delayed intra-arterial urokinase therapy with mechanical clot disruption for thromboembolic stroke. *Am J Neuroradio* 1994;15:1817–1822.
6. Hacke W, Kaste M, Fieschi C, et al. Intravenous thrombolysis with recombinant tissue plasminogen activator for acute hemispheric stroke. The European Cooperative Acute Stroke Study (ECASS). *JAMA* 1995;274:1017–1025.
7. Hacke W, Zeumer H, Gerbert A, Brückmann H, del Zoppo G. Intra-arterial thrombolytic therapy improves outcome in patients with acute vertebrobasilar occlusive disease. *Stroke* 1988;19:1216–1222.
8. Sasaki O, Shigekazu T, Koike T, Koizumi T, Tanaka R. Fibrinolytic therapy for acute embolic stroke: intravenous, intracarotid, and intra-arterial local approaches. *Neurosurgery* 1995;36:246–253.
9. Del Zoppo GJ, Ferbert A, Otis S, et al. Local intra-arterial fibrinolytic therapy in acute carotid territory stroke. A pilot study. *Stroke* 1988;19:307–313.
10. Multicentre Acute Stroke Trial—Europe Study Group. Thrombolytic therapy with streptokinase in acute ischemic stroke. *N Engl J Med* 1996;335:145–150.
11. Mori E. Fibrinolytic recanalization therapy in acute cerebrovascular thromboembolism. In: Hacke W, del Zoppo GJ, Hirshberg M, eds. *Thrombolytic Therapy in Acute Ischemic Stroke.* Heidelberg: Springer-Verlag; 1991:137–146.
12. Von Kummer R, Hacke W. Safety and efficacy of intravenous tissue plasminogen activator and heparin in acute middle cerebral artery stroke. *Stroke* 1992;23:646–652.
13. Wardlaw JM, Warlow CP. Thrombolysis in acute ischemic stroke: does it work? *Stroke* 1992;23:1826–1839.
14. The National Institute of Neurological Disorders and Stroke rt-PA Stroke Study Group. Tissue plasminogen activator for acute ischemic stroke. *N Engl J Med* 1995;333:1581–1587.
15. Russell D, Madden KP, Clark WM, Zivin J. Tissue plasminogen activator induced cerebral thrombolysis: assessment of different dose rates using Doppler ultrasound. *Stroke* 1992;23:388–393.
16. de Bono D. Which thrombolytic agent? In: de Bono D, ed. *Practical Coronary Thrombolysis.* Oxford: Blackwell Scientific; 1990:42–52.
17. Zeumer H, Freitag HJ, Grzyska U, Neurnzig HP. Local intra-arterial fibrinolysis in acute vertebrobasilar occlusion. Technical developments and recent results. *Neuroradiology* 1989;31:336–340.
18. Möbius E, Berg-Dammer E, Kühne D, Ahser HC. Local thrombolytic therapy in acute basilar artery occlusion: experience with 18 patients. In: Hacke W, del Zoppo GJ, Hirschberg M, eds. *Thrombolytic Therapy in Acute Ischemic Stroke.* Heidelberg: Springer-Verlag; 1991:213–215.
19. Pfeiffer G, Thayssen G, Arlt A, Siepmann G, Zeumer H, Kunze K. Vertebrobasilar occlusion: outcome with and without local intra-arterial fibrinolysis. In: Hacke W, del Zoppo GJ, Hirschberg M, eds. *Thrombolytic Therapy in Acute Ischemic Stroke.* Heidelberg: Springer-Verlag; 1991:216–220.
20. Matsumoto K, Satoh K. Topical intra-arterial urokinase infusion for acute stroke. In: Hacke W, del Zoppo GJ, Hirshberg M, eds. *Thrombolytic Therapy in Acute Ischemic Stroke.* Heidelberg: Springer-Verlag; 1991:207–212.
21. Theron J, Courtheoux P, Casasco A, et al. Local intra-arterial fibrinolysis in the carotid territory. *Am J Neuroradiol* 1989;10:753–765.
22. Casto L, Moschini L, Camerlingo M, et al. Local intra-arterial thrombolysis for acute stroke in the carotid artery territories. *Acta Neurol Scand* 1992;86:308–311.
23. Higashida RT, Tsai FY, Halbach VV, Barnwell SL, Dowd CF, Hieshima GB. Interventional neurovascular techniques in the treatment of stroke—state-of-the-art therapy. *J Intern Med* 1995;237:105–115.
24. Ueda T, Hatakeyama T, Kumon Y, Sakaki S, Uraoka T. Evaluation of risk of hemorrhagic transformation in local intra-arterial thrombolysis in acute ischemic stroke by initial SPECT. *Stroke* 1994;25:298–303.
25. Barr JD, Horowitz MB, Mathis JM, Sclabassi RJ, Yonas H. Intraoperative urokinase infusion for embolic stroke during carotid endarterectomy. *Neurosurgery* 1995;36:606–611.
26. Wildenhain SL, Jungreis CA, Barr J, Mathis J, Wechsler L, Horton JA. CT after intracranial thrombolysis for acute stroke. *Am J Neuroradiol* 1994;15:487–492.
27. Barr JD, Mathis JM, Wildenhain SL, Wechsler L, Jungreis CA, Horton JA. Acute stroke intervention with intra-arterial urokinase infusion. *J Vasc Intervent Radiol* 1994;5:705–713.
28. Touho H, Karasawa J, Hideyuki O, et al. Successful intra-arterial fibrinolysis of the anterior choroidal artery in the acute stage of internal carotid artery occlusion: case report. *Surg Neurol* 1994;41:450–454.
29. Clark W, Barnwell SL, O'Neill OR, Ahuja A, Wynn M, Coull B. Successful middle cerebral artery thrombolysis by microcatheter navigation through an occluded internal carotid artery. *Stroke* 1995;26:167.
30. Nesbit GM, Clark WM, O'Neill OR, Barnwell SL. Intracranial intra-arterial thrombolysis facilitated by microcatheter navigation through an occluded cervical internal carotid artery. *J Neurosurg* 1996;84:387–392.
31. Ueda T, Hatakeyama T, Sakaki S, Ohta S, Kumon Y, Uraoka T. Changes in coagulation and fibrinolytic system after local intra-arterial thrombolysis in acute ischemic stroke. *Neurol Med Chir* 1995;35:136–143.

52

Intracerebral PTA: Indications, Technique, and Results

Robert A. Koenigsberg, D.O.
Fong Y. Tsai, M.D.

Stroke prevention and percutaneous transluminal angioplasty (PTA) specifically for the treatment of cerebrovascular diseases are rapidly gaining interest in the United States and abroad due to the high prevalence of stroke and stroke-related illnesses.[1-26] Currently, stroke is the third leading cause of death in the United States, with upwards of 500,000 strokes occurring yearly. The annual death toll is 150,000.[2,27]

PTA of the intracranial vessels has lagged behind angioplasty of other systems due to the fear of devastating neurologic complications. However, microcatheter and balloon technologies have advanced, so that the interventionalist now has a variety of balloons for intracranial use, several of which are shown in Figure 52–1. Therefore, intracranial vascular disorders previously considered incurable can now be evaluated for treatment.

The current goals of intracranial PTA are two: to prevent stroke and to reduce the ischemic penumbra surrounding an existing area of brain infarction so that potentially symptomatic regions of ischemic brain can be revascularized. This chapter focuses primarily on two intracranial problems amenable to PTA: vasospasm and atherosclerosis. Because the pathophysiology of these disorders is different, this chapter is divided into two sections, addressing these topics separately.

Intracranial angioplasty requires a cooperative effort between appropriate supportive services.[20] These may include the following fields: neurosurgery and vascular surgery, neurology, and/or cardiology and internal medicine. These services may interact with patients acutely or provide management for long-term patient care. Therefore, it is essential that these services be

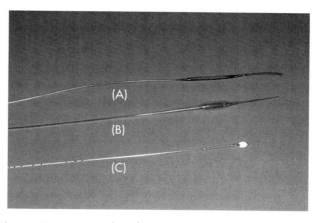

Figure 52–1. Examples of intracranial angioplasty balloons. (A) Stealth balloon, 2 mm (Target); (B) Stratus balloon, 3 mm (MIS); (C) Silicone balloon, 2 mm (ITC).

involved from the planning stages of intracranial PTA. In addition, anesthesia staffing is pivotal in maintaining patients motionless throughout the described neurointerventional procedures. Frequently, patients need to be paralyzed and intubated for microcatheter manipulations, as well as for optimal intracranial pressure control.[27]

EQUIPMENT

State-of-the-art angiography equipment is required for the diagnostic and neurointerventional procedures. The goal is to perform the diagnostic procedures quickly and accurate while keeping catheter time to a minimum. For interventions, the equipment should help facilitate safe microcatheter work, increasing the probability of utilizing the correct intracranial angioplasty balloon while keeping potential complications to a minimum. To this end, high-quality biplane or single-plane 1024 × 1024 matrix digital subtraction angiography (DSA) units. The equipment should allow rapid acquisition with high-resolution displays. The ability to measure stenoses rapidly and accurately is very helpful in quickly ascertaining the results of angioplasty. Units should also be equipped with rapid pixel shifting and additive road mapping capability. Another useful feature is rapid image recall on separate monitors, enabling the interventionalist to compare reference images to live fluoroscopic images for immediate decision making.

Magnetic resonance imaging (MRI) with state-of-the-art magnetic resonance angiography (MRA), computed tomographic angiography (CTA), single photon emission computed tomography (SPECT), and transcranial Doppler (TCD) are additional modalities useful in the evaluation of the intracranial vasculature and blood flow dynamics. Noninvasively, MRA and CTA can accurately detect and quantitate intracranial stenoses. SPECT may confirm focal areas of hypoperfusion, and TCD is particularly useful in quantitating flow velocity changes. TCD is especially useful in following flow changes associated with vasospasm secondary to subarachnoid hemorrhage. A discussion of specific imaging techniques is beyond the scope of this chapter.

INTRACRANIAL VASOSPASM

Arterial vasospasm is a relatively common complication of subarachnoid hemorrhage (SAH) following rupture of an intracranial aneurysm, occurring in at least 30% of cases. The precise mechanism of vasospasm is poorly understood. It has been postulated that the arterial narrowing occurs as a result of direct endothelial damage due to surrounding blood products.[27-29] Early, this results in thickening of both the arterial intima and media, as well as direct smooth muscle constriction. Delayed fibrosis may occur. These changes frequently result in arterial narrowing, which if left untreated may result in major zones of cerebral ischemia and stroke.

Vasospasm most commonly affects intracranial vessels where the concentration of subarachnoid blood is greatest. Typically vasospasm is seen in close proximity to the aneurysm that has bled. It may be recognized clinically by the delayed onset of neurologic symptoms and, with rare exceptions, is maximal 3 to 10 days after SAH. Invariably, patients present with delayed onset of a hemiparesis or, alternatively, a generalized decline in mentation.

TCD is currently the screening modality of choice in the early recognition of intracranial vasospasm.[30] In a noninvasive fashion, serial flow velocities of the circle of Willis vessels may be followed daily, allowing early recognition of velocity changes. Rising flow velocities, particularly above 180 to 220 cm/sec, or increasing velocities greater than 50 cm/sec above baseline suggest vasospasm. MRA and CTA may also provide useful information; however, diagnostic angiography remains the gold standard. A noncontrast CT examination is done prior to angiography to screen for significant areas of infarction or hemorrhage in the symptomatic regions of the brain.

The treatment of vasospasm at our institution is chemical with papaverine, mechanical with balloon angioplasty, or a combination of both. Table 52–1 lists common scenarios in which intracranial vasospasm is considered for intervention. Ultimately, the decision to treat any of our patients is made jointly by the appropriate clinical services.

Papaverine Therapy

Papaverine is an alkaloid of the opium group well known to cause vasodilatation of cerebral arteries through direct action on smooth muscle.[31] It is currently the drug of choice in the treatment of vasospasm, although its precise mechanism of action remains unknown. Current theories support inhibition of cyclic adenosine monophosphate (cAMP) and cyclic guanosine 3,5' monophosphate (cGMP) phosphodiesterase activity in smooth muscle cells. This increases intracellular cAMP and cGMP turnover, resulting in smooth muscle relaxation.

Chemical treatment utilizing papaverine may be initiated if, on the screening CT scan, there are no large infarcts or hemorrhages in the spastic vessel territory. We do not consider early areas of hypodensity a contraindication to therapy, as these zones may represent areas of reversible ischemia. We preferably infuse the spastic arteries superselectively. Following diagnostic angiography, a No. 6 or 7 Fr. guide catheter is placed within the cervical internal carotid artery. With continuous flushing, an infusion microcatheter is advanced into the intracranial vasculature.

Because vasospasm most commonly affects the anterior circulation, the internal carotid artery is catheterized at a level distal to the ophthalmic artery to maximize papaverine delivery to the vessels in greatest need. An example of typical microcatheter positioning is shown in Figure 52–2. Alternatively, the microcath-

Table 52–1. Indications for the Treatment of Intracranial Vasospasm

Delayed onset of new neurologic deficit or global decline in mental status.

Increasing TCD flow velocities greater than 200 cm/sec or serial increases in flow velocity greater than 50 cm/sec above baseline

Postoperative scenario in which angiographically documented critical vasospasm warrants treatment immediately following aneurysm clipping or coiling.

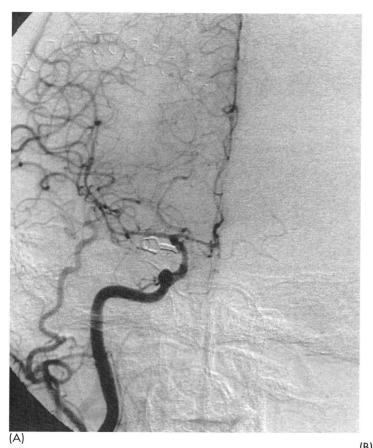

(A)

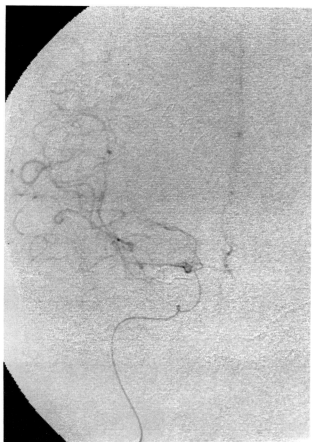

(B)

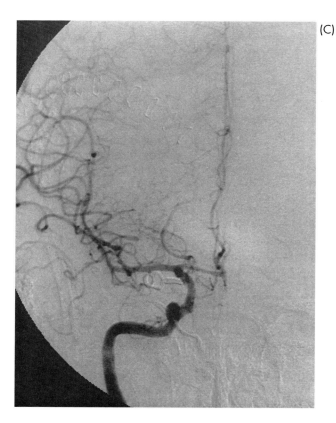

(C)

Figure 52–2. (A) Right internal carotid angiogram demonstrating intracranial vasospasm. Note significant narrowing of the distal internal carotid artery, M1, and multiple distal middle cerebral artery branches. (B) Microcatheter placement at the terminus of the internal carotid artery for papaverine infusion. (C) Right internal carotid artery injection after papaverine infusion. Note the improved caliber of all spastic vessels.

eter may be advanced into either the M1 or A1 segment for supraselective infusions.

We currently employ an infusion of 300 mg papaverine in 100 cc of normal slaine administered over 30 to 60 minutes. If no response is seen, the infusion is stopped. If a partial response is recognized, it may be appropriate to continue the infusion to a maximum of 600 mg per vessel. If necessary, additional doses of papaverine may be given superselectively to treat the internal carotid arteries bilaterally or to the posterior circulation. The vertebrobasilar system typically is infused with the catheter tip at the level of the vertebrobasilar junction. We consider 900 mg papaverine the maximum dose.

The chemical effect of papaverine lasts for approximately 24 hours. If symptoms recur, treatment may be repeated. We generally do not perform papaverine treatments for more than three sessions. We find, as reported in the literature, decreasing responsiveness of vasospasm to papaverine in subsequent treatment sessions.[2] If patients are not candidates for microcatheter placement, an infusion of papaverine directly through the diagnostic catheter at the level of the cervical internal carotid artery catheter may be useful.

Angioplasty

In cases where chemical angioplasty fails or severe vasospasm exists in accessible arteries of the circle of Willis, mechanical angioplasty is performed.[32,33] Here balloon inflation results in direct dilatation of the spastic artery, ideally returning the stenotic artery to its prestenotic diameter. Histologically, balloon inflation results in minimal disruption of the arterial intima and media. Furthermore, there is histologic evidence that stretching of the internal elastic membrane occurs.

The goal of treatment in the anterior circulation is to reestablish a reasonable caliber of either the internal carotid or the M1 segment of the middle cerebral arteries such that flow is improved. We currently do not consider spastic middle cerebral vessels distal to the trifurcation amenable to mechanical angioplasty. Similarly, vasospasm of the anterior cerebral artery may be difficult to treat due to its inherent unfavorable angle of origin.

Potential complications of intracranial vasospasm angioplasty include stroke secondary to distal embolization, vessel occlusion, and/or vessel rupture. The last may lead to massive intracranial hemorrhage and brain death. In addition, the posterior circulation may be particularly susceptible to brain stem ischemia or respiratory arrest during posterior circulation angioplasty.

Angioplasty is undertaken through a No. 6 or 7 Fr. guiding catheter placed within the appropriate carotid or vertebral artery. Full heparinization is accomplished utilizing a 3000- to 5000-unit bolus, followed by intermittent hourly doses of 1000 units.

Currently, there are two principal angioplasty methods. The first method employs soft, flow-directed balloons. The calibrated leak angioplasty balloon was first described by Berenstein and Lasjaunias.[34] It consists of a latex balloon mounted onto the end of a microcatheter. A tiny hole is made at the balloon tip prior to attachment, allowing the balloon to distend rapidly with the injection of contrast medium and then collapse when the injection stops. This provides an automatic protective mechanism, preventing balloon overdistention, and an automatic deflation mechanism. Figure 52–3 illustrates a case of internal carotid/middle cerebral artery vasospasm after middle cerebral artery aneurysm clipping successfully treated with this technique. The semipermeable silicone angioplasty balloon developed by Hieshima is currently manufactures by the Interventional Therapeutics Corporation (ITC). This balloon comes premounted on a Tracker microcatheter (Target Therapeutics), is soft, and inflates with low pressure. Both balloon types are effective, dilating intracranial vessels in the direction of greatest blood flow. They are typically utilized in the internal carotid, middle cerebral, vertebral, and basilar artery territories.

The second method of treatment utilizes a guidewire-directed angioplasty balloon catheter. The Stealth (Target) and Cirrus (Microinterventional Therapeutics—MIS) balloons typify this type of balloon. The design of these systems allows a steering capability that helps control the balloon's position. These balloon types are manufactured in varying sizes, with a minimum diameter of 2 mm. In the Stealth balloon, inflation is possible with a tip-occluding guidewire controlled by a manual balloon insufflation device. Deflation occurs by withdrawing the guidewire, which releases the balloon's contents through the end hole. The Cirrus balloon inflates with the manufacturer's guidewire in place without specific tip occlusion. Balloon choice is based on physician preference within this limited range of products.

The size of the balloon is determined by the size of the diseased vessel. Ideally, the diameter of the involved vessel is measured on an imaging study prior to the onset of vasospasm. Generally, a balloon 3 to 4 mm in diameter may be safely used in the internal carotid artery whereas a balloon 2 to 3 mm in diameter is used in the middle cerebral artery. Whenever possible, special care is taken to avoid performing angioplasty adjacent to an aneurysm clip due to the potential for clip dislodgment and vessel rupture.[35]

The vertebral and basilar arteries may be considered for angioplasty. This procedure is considered riskier due to the presence of critical perforating brain stem arteries arising directly from the basilar artery. Therefore, the potential for brain stem stroke or respiratory depression and/or arrest exists. However, the intracranial portions of the vertebral arteries may be angioplas-

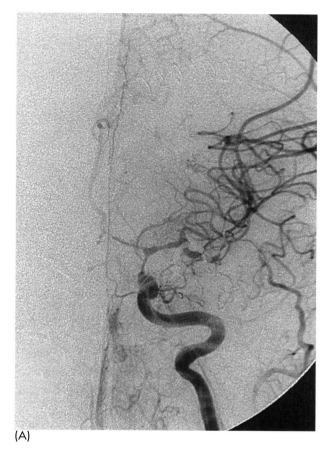

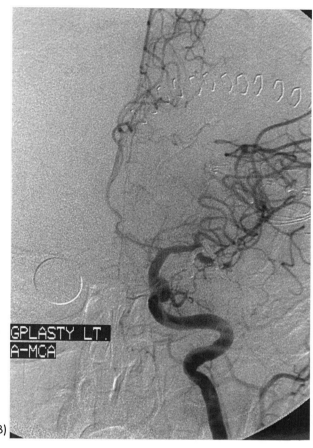

(A)   (B)

Figure 52–3. (A) Right internal carotid angiogram following left middle cerebral artery aneurysm clipping. Note the severe internal carotid artery/M1 segment vasospasm. (B) Right internal carotid artery angiogram after calibrated leak balloon angioplasy. (Courtesy Gerard Debrun, M.D., and Victor Aletich, M.D., University of Illinois at Chicago)

tied without such special concern. Generally, one vertebral artery, may be treated with or without treatment of the basilar artery.

Postangioplasty, we prefer to maintain the patient on heparin for at least 24 hours due to the potential for intimal damage. Patients are then generally maintained on 325 mg aspirin daily.

Results

Due to the availability of neurointerventional support at our institution, our neurosurgeons and neurointerventionalists tend to operate early rather than late in the treatment of ruptured intracranial aneurysms. This includes treatment either by surgical clipping or by endovascular coil embolization. The patient further benefits by avoiding the potentially dangerous waiting period for delayed surgery and the risk of rebleeding.

The superselective infusion of papaverine is highly effective alone in alleviating cerebral vasospasm in approximately 70 to 90% of cases. Kaku et al[31] described 10 patients treated with papaverine for spasm. Thirty-four of 37 territories were successfully dilated, and 8 of 10 patients showed neurologic improvement. Kassell et al reported on 12 patients, 4 of whom showed dramatic improvement following infusion.[36] They suggested that the middle cerebral and posterior circulations may be more responsive than the anterior circulation to papaverine. More recently, Clouston et al described 14 patients in whom 60 vascular territories were treated.[37] Angiographic improvement was shown in 18 of 19 treatment sessions, with 50% of patients showing clinical improvement. Potential limitations include transient new neurologic events and/or hemorrhages, severe thrombocytopenia, and cardiac arrhythmias. Despite these limitations, papaverine infusion has been well documented to be effective in the treatment of intracranial vasospasm.

Balloon angioplasty has been utilized in cases of severe symptomatic vasospasm or when supraselective papaverine infusion fails. Since the time of the first reports of vasospasm angioplasty by Zubkov et al,[38] angioplasty has been shown to be key in the management of severe vasospasm. During the past 5 years, additional authors have reported varying success with balloon angioplasty in the treatment of severe vasospasm.[2,8,19,28,39–40] The techniques are very effec-

Table 52–2. Criteria Used in Considering Angioplasty for Intracranial Atherosclerosis

Symptomatic atherosclerosis narrowing the parent vessel by more than 70% refractory to maximal conservative therapy

No intracranial bleed within 6 hours of treatment

Long-term candidate for anticoagulation

Intracranial plaque associated with recurrent thrombosis after thrombolysis.

tive; however, the risk of potential vessel rupture must be weighed in each case. Eskridge[27] described these techniques as complementary, a standard currently employed by practicing neurointerventionalists.

ATHEROSCLEROSIS

Intracranial Angioplasty

The North American Symptomatic Carotid Endarterectomy Trial (NASCET) trial, published in 1991, showed superior outcomes in the surgical versus medical management of carotid artery disease in cases of cervical carotid stenosis of 70% or greater.[41] The results have been extrapolated to the surgically inaccessible intracranial arteries. In particular, symptomatic patients, having failed conservative therapy, may have no other reasonable alternatives.

Table 52–2 lists several criteria most commonly used when considering a potential patient for angioplasty.

Most of the lesions considered for treatment are atherosclerotic in origin. However, stenosis may be secondary to other entities such as fibromuscular dysplasia, arteritis, vasculitis, dissection, intimal hyperplasia, or radiation-induced vasculopathy. When conservative measures fail, typical symptoms warranting intervention include repeated bouts of amaurosis fugax, transient ischemic attack, stroke, unremitting bruit or vascular headaches, and vascular steal. Patients with tandems lesion have a higher risk of ischemic events than those with intracranial stenoses alone.[13] These tandem intracranial lesions may be also considered for treatment. Additionally, there is a role for intracranial angioplasty in cases of intracranial atherosclerosis with recurrent cerebral thrombosis. In these cases, angioplasty may be necessary when thrombolytic agents alone fail[10,42] (Fig. 52–4).

Histologically, current research on angioplasty for intracranial atherosclerosis indicates that balloon inflation results in plaque disruption, including disruption of both the intima and media of the vessel. This leads to subintimal fissuring, delamination, disruption of the plaque, and dissection. Optimally, there is delayed healing with intimal retraction and neointima formation. This, theoretically, leads to a smooth intimal surface.[4,19]

Lesions considered for intracranial angioplasty most commonly involve either the internal carotid or proximal vertebral arteries. Rarely, stenoses involving the middle cerebral, anterior cerebral, distal vertebral, or

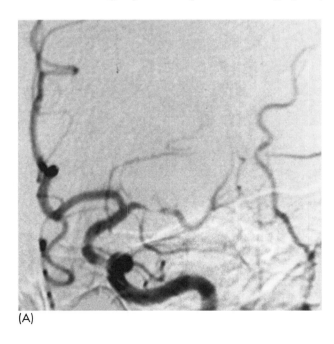

(A)

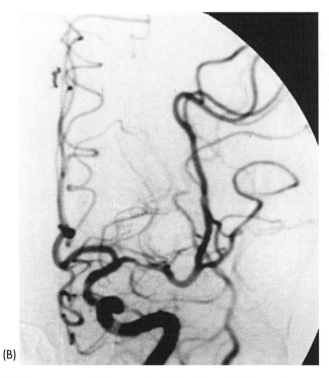

(B)

Figure 52–4. (A) Thrombosis of the left middle cerebral artery with short-segment M1 stenosis. (B) Postthrombolysis and angioplasty of the middle cerebral artery.

basilar arteries may be considered for treatment. More distal vessels are not considered within the realm of current intervention.

The goal of intracranial angioplasty, again, is to improve distal blood flow, thereby preventing stroke or reducing the ischemic penumbra surrounding a region of infarction. All intracranial angioplasty patients are considered high risk and must be handled with the greatest degree of caution. Intracranial hemorrhage within 6 hours of presentation is considered a contraindication for angioplasty, as systemic antiocoagulation is necessary to avoid thromboembolic complications.

Several balloons are currently manufactured for the treatment of intracranial atherosclerosis. These balloons are almost exclusively wire guided. The soft latex or silicone balloons have fallen out of vogue for the treatment of atherosclerosis because they lack the stability needed for precise positioning. Representative balloons include the Stealth (Target) and Stratus (MIS) balloons.

Intracranial angioplasty for an atherosclerotic lesion is typically an elective procedure. Antiplatelet therapy is begun 2 weeks prior to hospital admission. Again, the potential complications of any intracranial angioplasty must be considered.[43] These include vessel occlusion, vessel rupture, and distal embolization.

Angiography to depict the lesion is usually performed prior to the procedure date, and the scan is analyzed for plaque length and degree of stenosis. The normal caliber of the involved artery is measured, and an appropriate angioplasty balloon is chosen not to exceed the normal luminal width of the involved artery. Balloons measuring 2 to 4 mm are generally used for ICA stenoses, 2.5- to 3.0-mm balloons for basilar artery stenoses, and 3- to 6-mm balloons for vertebral artery stenoses. The balloon length is typically 1.0 to 1.5 cm longer than the area of stenosis.

Following appropriate common femoral arterial sheath placement, the patient is fully heparinized with a 5000-unit bolus, with additional hourly 1000-unit boluses. Utilizing coaxial technique, a guiding catheter is placed, typically within the ipsilateral carotid artery or VA. Again, care is taken to advance the guide catheter as high as possible within the neck while avoiding vasospasm and is placed to continuous flush. Nitroglycerine or papaverine may also be administered to avoid vasospasm; urokinase may be administered before angioplasty to lyse any associated clot. The doage range of the latter is from 250,000 to 1,000,000 units. The lesion is initially crossed by an appropriate 0.014- to 0.010-inch guidewire, followed by the angioplasty balloon. In the case of the Stealth balloon, the guidewire is then removed and replaced with the tip-occluding wire, allowing balloon inflation. Deflation occurs by withdrawing the tip-occluding wire. In the case of the Stratus balloon, the manufacturer's guidewire is left in

place during balloon inflation. Balloon inflation may be repeated as many as three or four times; however, we caution against repetitive angioplasties. A satisfactory result is obtained if the degree of stenosis improves to 50% of less. An example of a successful angioplasty of the vertebral artery utilizing the Stealth balloon is shown in Figure 52–5. After angioplasty, patients are maintained on heparin for 24 hours and then placed on 325 mg aspirin daily. Repeat angiography is performed at intervals ranging from 1 to 12 months to reevaluate the lesions.

Results

The literature supporting the treatment of symptomatic intracranial atherosclerotic lesions continues to grow. These reports describe preliminary results of both carotid and vertebrobasilar circulation angioplasties for atherosclerotic lesions. As microcatheter technology evolves, smaller vessels are becoming increasingly amenable to interventions.

Since the 1980s, isolated reports of successful intracranial angioplasties began to emerge in the literature. Sundt et al described angioplasty of a stenotic basilar artery via a surgical approach to the vertebral artery.[44] Purdy et al reported improved cerebral perfusion following successful middle cerebral artery angioplasty, and Rostomily et al described successful angioplasty of a focal petrous carotid lesion with a good outcome.[9,13] These and other early successes led to larger series.

Clark et al recently described a series of 17 patients with intracranial atherosclerotic stenoses.[18] In these patients, 22 vessels were treated. Successful angioplasty was defined as at least a 20% improvement in luminal diameter, with less than 50% residual stenosis. Utilizing these criteria, the authors reported an 82% rate of successful PTA, with a 9.1% major complication rate. Higashida et al described a series of 41 patients treated for posterior circulation atherosclerosis.[21] They reported 34 proximal vertebral, 5 distal vertebral, and 3 basilar artery stenoses. The authors noted three major complications, primarily related to distal vertebral and basilar artery treatments. They also classified those patients with distal vertebral and basilar artery stenoses as higher risk than patients with proximal vertebral lesions. McKenzie et al reported 17 intracranial angioplasties in 11 patients.[26] Although 16 of these patients improved angiographically, 6 continued to demonstrate moderate or severe residual stenoses after the procedure, and 1 patient with herpes vasculitis ultimately suffered occlusion despite repeated procedures. The authors suggested that nonatherosclerotic lesions related to inflammation may be at increased risk of dissection due to inflammatory weakening of the vessel wall. They further suggest that angioplasty may be contraindicated when vasculitis is in the acute phase.

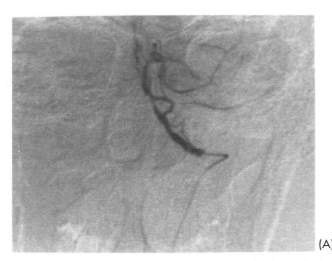
(A)

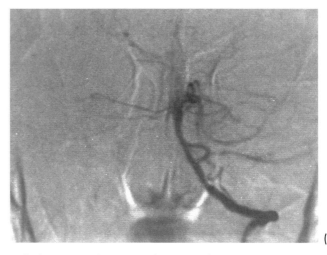
(B)

Figure 52–5. (A) Proximal left vertebral stenosis before angioplasty. (B) After angioplasty.

Intracranial angioplasty for atherosclerosis remains experimental but clearly is useful in selected cases, particularly in patients refractory to maximal medical therapy. It may be used as an adjunct to thrombolysis to prevent rethrombosis in patients suffering acute occlusion. As technological advances are made, smaller vessels will be amenable to treatment. Current research involves the development of new balloon catheters and small stents for intracranial use.[45,46]

REFERENCES

1. Dotter CT, Judkins MP. Transluminal treatment of arteriosclerotic obstruction: description of a new technique and preliminary report of its application. *Circulation* 1964;30:654–670.
2. Higashida RT, Halbach VV, Tsai FY, Dowd CF, Hieshima GB. Interventional neurovascular techniques for cerebral revascularization in the treatment of stroke. *AJR* 1994;163:793–800.
3. Theron J. Angioplasty of brachiocephalic vessels. In: Vinuela V, Halbach VV, Dion JE, eds. *Interventional Neuroradiology: Endovascular Therapy of the Central Nervous System.* New York: Raven Press; 1992:167–180.
4. Higashida RT, Tsai FY, Halbach VV, Dowd CF, Hieshima GB. Cerebral percutaneous transluminal angioplasty. *J Heart Dis Stroke* 1993;2:497–502.
5. Tsai FY, Matovich V, Hieshima G, et al. Percutaneous transluminal angioplasty of the carotid artery. *AJNR* 1986;7:349–358.
6. Kachel R, Basche ST, Heerklotz I, Grossmann K, Endler S. PTA of the supra-aortic arteries, especially the internal carotid artery. *Neuroradiology* 1991;33:191–194.
7. Millaire A, Trinca M, Marache P, de Groote P, Jabinet JL, Ducloux G. Subclavian angioplasty: immediate and late results in 50 patients. *Cathet Cardiovasc Diagn* 1993;29:8–17.
8. Higashida RT, Hieshima BG, Halbach VV. Advances in the treatment of complex cerebrovascular disorders by interventional neurovascular techniques. *Circulation* 1991;83(suppl I):I-196–I-206.
9. Purdy PD, Devous MD Sr, Unwin DH, Giller CA, Batjer HH. Angioplasty of an atherosclerotic middle cerebral artery associated with improvement in regional cerebral blood flow. *AJNR* 1990;11:878–880.
10. Tsai FY, Berberian B, Matovich V, Lavin M, Alfieri K. Percutaneous transluminal angioplasty adjunct to thrombolysis for acute middle cerebral artery rethrombosis. *AJNR* 1994;15:1823–1829.
11. Purdy PD, Devous MD Sr, Unwin DH, Giller CA, Batjer HH. Angioplasty of an atherosclerotic middle cerebral artery associated with improvement in regional cerebral blood flow. *AJNR* 1990;11:878–880.
12. Higashida RT, Hieshima GB, Tsai FY, Halbach VV, Norman D, Newton TH. Transluminal angioplasty of the vertebral and basilar artery. *AJNR* 1987;8:745–749.
13. Rostomily RC, Mayverg MR, Eskridge JM, Goodkin R, Winn HR. Resolution of petrous internal carotid artery stenosis after transluminal angioplasty. *J Neurosurg* 1992;76:520–523.
14. Theron J, Courtheoux P, Henriet JP, et al. Angioplasty of supraaortic arteries. *J Neuroradiol* 1984;11:187–200.
15. Hasso AN, Bird CR, Zinke DE, et al. Fibromuscular dysplasia of the internal carotid artery. Percutaneous transluminal angioplasty. *AJR* 1981;136:955–960.
16. Wiggli U, Gratzl O. Transluminal angioplasty of stenotic carotid arteries: case reports and protocol. *AJNR* 1983;4:793–795.
17. O'Leary DH, Clouse ME. Percutaneous transluminal angioplasty for the cavernous carotid artery for recurrent ischemia. *AJNR* 1984;5:644–645.
18. Clark WM, Barnwell SL, Nesbit G, O'Neill OR, Wynn ML, Coull BM. Safety and efficacy of percutaneous transluminal angioplasty for intracranial atherosclerotic stenosis. *Stroke* 1994;26:1200–1204.
19. Higashida RT, Tsai FY, Halbach VV, Barnwell SL, Dowd CF, Hieshima CB. Interventional neurovascular techniques in the treatment of stroke—state of the art therapy. *J Int Med* 1995;237:105–115.
20. Higashida RT, Tsai FY, Halbach V, Dowd CF, Hieshima GB. Cerebral percutaneous transluminal angioplasty. *Heart Dis Stroke* 1993;2:497–502.
21. Higashida RT, Tsai F, Halbach VV, et al. Transluminal angioplasty for atherosclerotic disease of the vertebral and basilar arteries. *J Neurosurg* 1993;78:192–198.
22. Tsai FY, Matovich VB, Hieshima GB, et al. Practical aspects of percutaneous transluminal angioplasty of the carotid artery. *Acta Radiol—Suppl* 1986;369:127–130.

23. Higashida RT, Hieshima GB, Tsai FY, Bentson JR, Halbach VV. Percutaneous transluminal angioplasty of the subclavian and vertebral arteries. *ACTA Radiol—Suppl* 1986;369:124–126.

24. Kachel R, Basche ST, Heerdlotz I, Grossmann K, Endler S. Percutaneous transluminal angioplasty of supra-aortic arteries, especially the internal carotid artery. *Neuroradiology* 1991;33:191–194.

25. Brown MM. Balloon angioplasty for cerebrovascular disease. *Neurol Res* 1992;14:159–163.

26. McKenzie JD, Wallace RC, Dean BL, Flom RA, Khayata MH. Preliminary results of intracranial angioplasty for vascular stenosis caused by atherosclerosis and vasculitis. *AJNR* 1996;17:263–268.

27. Eskridge JM, McAuliffe W. Intracranial angioplasty and thrombolysis. In: Maciunas RJ, ed. *Endovascular Neurological Intervention.* American Association of Neurological Surgeons; 1994:105–110.

28. Eckard DA, Siegel EL, Batnitzky S. Angioplasty of the supra-aortic vessels. In: Rumbaugh CL, Wang A, Tsai FY, eds. *Cerebrovascular Disease: Imaging and Treatment Options.* New York: Igaku-Shoin; 1995:487–501.

29. Macdonald RL, Wallace MC, Montanera WJ, Glen JA. Pathological effects of angioplasty on vasospastic carotid arteries in a rabbit model. *J Neurosurg* 1995;83:111–117.

30. Hurst RW, Schnee C, Raps EC, Farber R, Flam ES. Role of transcranial Doppler in neuroradiological treatment of intracranial vasospasm. *Stroke* 1993;24:299–303.

31. Kaku Y, Yonekawa Y, Tsukahara T, Kazekawa K. Superselective intra-arterial infusion of papaverine for the treatment of cerebral vasospasm after subarachnoid hemorrhage. *J Neurosurg* 1992;77:842–847.

32. Kobayashi H, Ide H, Aradachi H, Arai Y, Handa Y, Kubota T. Histological studies of intracranial vessels in primates following transluminal angioplasty for vasospasm. *J Neurosurg* 1993;78:481–486.

33. Pile-Spellman J, Berenstein A, Bun T, et al. Angioplasty of canine cerebral vessels. *AJNR* 1987;8:938. Abstract.

34. Berenstein A, Lasjaunias P. Newer developments in endovascular surgery in the CNS. In: Berenstein A, Lasjaunias P, eds. *Surgical Neuroangiography*, Vol 5. *Endovascular Treatment of Spine and Spinal Cord Lesions.* New York: Springer-Verlag; 1992:149–205.

35. Linskey ME, Horton JA, Rao GR, Yonas H. Fatal rupture of the intracranial carotid artery during transluminal angioplasty for vasospasm induced by subarachnoid hemorrhage. *J Neurosurg* 1991;74:985–990.

36. Kassell NF, Helm G, Simmons N, Phillips CD, Cail WS. Treatment of cerebral vasospasm with intra-arterial papaverine. *J Neurosurg* 1992;77:848–852.

37. Clauston JE, Numaguchi Y, Zoarski GH, Aldrich EF, Simard JM, Zitnay KM. Intraarterial papaverine infusion for cerebral vasospasm after subarachnoid hemorrhage. *AJNR* 1995;16:27–38.

38. Zubkov YN, Nikiforv BM, Shustin VA. Balloon catheter technique for dilatation of constricted cerebral arteries after aneurysmal SAH. *Acta Neurochir* 1984;70:65–79.

39. Higashida RT, Halbach VV, Cahan LD, et al. Transluminal angioplasty for treatment of intracranial arterial vasospasm. *Neurosurg* 1989;71:648–653.

40. Newell DW, Eskridge JM, Mayberg MR, et al. Angioplasty for the treatment of symptomatic vasospasm following subarachnoid hemorrhage. *J Neurosurg* 1989;71:654–660.

41. North American Symptomatic Carotid Endarterectomy Trial Collaborators. Beneficial effect of carotid endarterectomy in symptomatic patients with high-grade carotid stenosis. *N Engl J Med* 1991;325:445–453.

42. Touho H, Ohnishi H, Karasawa J, Furuoka N, Komatsu T. Percutaneous transluminal angioplasty for acute stroke due to stenosis of major cerebral vessels: report of two cases. *Surg Neurol* 1994;41:362–367.

43. Ferguson R, Ferguson J, Schwarten D, et al. Immediate angiographic results and in hospital central nervous system complications of cerebral percutaneous trans luminal angioplasty (CPTA). *Circulation* 1993;1:1–393. Abstract.

44. Sundt T, Smith HC, Campbell JK, Vlietstra RE, Cucchiara RF, Stanson AW. Transluminal angioplasty for basilar artery stenosis. *Mayo Clin Proc* 1980;55:673–680.

45. Marks, M, Duke M, Steinberg G, Norbash AM, Lane B. Stent placement for arterial and venous cerebrovascular disease: preliminary experience. *Radiology* 1994;191:441–446.

46. Becker GJ. Should metallic vascular stents be used to treat cerebrovascular occlusive diseases? *Radiology* 1994;191:309–312.

Section 5

Visceral Vascular Disease

53

Chronic Mesenteric Arterial Occlusive Disease: Clinical Presentation and Diagnostic Evaluation

Lewis B. Schwartz, M.D.
Bruce L. Gewertz, M.D.

The fact that chronic occlusion or critical stenosis of the mesenteric arteries can cause abdominal pain was not recognized until the end of the nineteenth century.[1-3] At that time, the suggestion that patients could experience postprandial *abdominal angina* analogous to the newly described *angina pectoris* was controversial. Indisputable evidence was finally provided by J.E. Dunphy, a surgical resident at the Peter Bent Brigham Hospital in Boston, who described the clinical course of a 47-year-old male laborer with postprandial periumbilical pain and weight loss who was thought to be exaggerating his symptoms.[4] He was admitted to the hospital during an exacerbation but died suddenly after 3 days. Postmortem examination revealed chronic occlusion of the superior and inferior mesenteric arteries and fresh thrombus completely occluding the celiac trunk. Because of the absence of coronary artery disease, this was the first demonstration of abdominal pain originating solely from mesenteric artery pathology. More than 20 years later, the first successful cases of surgical treatment for chronic mesenteric ischemia were reported.[5,6]

Since that time, chronic mesenteric ischemia has been recognized as an uncommon but unequivocal cause of chronic abdominal pain. Although its incidence is estimated at only 1 case per 100,000 population,[7] its lethal nature requires vigilance and high clinical suspicion. This chapter will consider the anatomy, pathophysiology, clinical presentation, natural history, and diagnostic evaluation of chronic mesenteric ischemia.

ANATOMY

The mesenteric circulation (Fig. 53–1) consists of three named arteries: the celiac trunk, superior mesenteric artery (SMA), and inferior mesenteric artery (IMA). The stomach and upper half of the duodenum comprise the foregut and are supplied by the celiac trunk. The lower half of the duodenum, the jejunum, ileum, cecum, appendix, ascending colon, and proximal two-thirds of the transverse colon are midgut structures and are supplied by the SMA. Finally, the left third of the transverse colon, descending colon, sigmoid colon, rectum, and upper part of the anal canal comprise the hindgut and are supplied by the IMA. The mesenteric

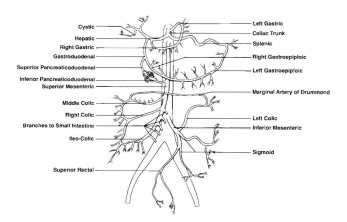

Figure 53–1. The mesenteric circulation. (Reprinted from Schwartz LB, Davis RD Jr, Heinle JS, Purut CM, Taylor DC, Brown WC. The vascular system. In: Lyerly HK, Gaynor JW Jr, eds. *The Handbook of Surgical Intensive Care,* 3rd ed. St Louis: Mosby Year Book; 1992:287 with permission.)

517

circulation has the potential to form extensive collateral pathways that may preserve blood flow even when the main trunks are compromised. The celiac trunk and SMA communicate primarily via the superior and inferior pancreaticoduodenal arteries (via the gastroduodenal artery; Fig. 53–1). The SMA and IMA communicate via the *Arc of Riolan* (also called the *meandering mesenteric artery*), as well as by a large peripheral branch following the course of the entire colon called the *marginal artery of Drummond*. In addition to these collateral pathways between the three mesenteric arteries, multiple other branches of the aorta may contribute to intestinal perfusion, including the lumbar intercostal arteries, internal mammary arteries (via the deep epigastric), middle sacral artery, and internal iliac arteries (via collaterals between the inferior and superior rectal arteries). Because of the redundancy of these extensive collaterals, at least two of the three major mesenteric orifices must be occluded or critically stenotic for ischemia to occur.

PHYSIOLOGY

The gut mucosa is among the most metabolically active tissues in the body. Measurements of mean blood flow in revascularized celiac arteries and SMA vary from 300 to 1200 ml/min (about 10 to 30% of cardiac output).[8–10] These mean values are among the highest for any type of bypass graft, which may account for their high patency.[11] Furthermore, the ratio of characteristic impedance (high-frequency component) to resistance (low-frequency component) in the mesenteric circulation is much higher than in any other peripheral bypass graft.[10] Thus, the resistance to the mean and oscillatory components of flow is nearly equivalent, giving rise to the notion of a low-resistance, *privileged* outflow bed.

As in skeletal muscle beds, mesenteric blood flow may increase 25 to 30% during periods of increased metabolic demand.[12] Control of mesenteric blood flow is complex, with contributions from neural, humoral, and local axes. The dependance of flow on sympathetic discharge and levels of circulating catecholamines and vasoactive peptides has been well described.[13,14] More recently recognized are the intrinsic mechanisms regulating flow, including local release of mediators such as adenosine and nitric oxide.[15] These serve to maintain blood flow despite drops in systemic blood pressure up to the "autoregulatory limit" of about 50 mm Hg.[16] This phenomenon, combined with the increased capacity for oxygen extraction with decreased flow, maintains mucosal viability despite wide perturbations in input pressure.

PATHOLOGY

The clinical syndrome of chronic mesenteric ischemia is generally the result of critical stenosis or occlusion of two or all of the celiac artery, SMA, and IMA. The lesions are usually extensions of aortic atheroma as opposed to intrinsic disease of the mesenteric branches. Over 90% of the cases of chronic mesenteric ischemia are due to atherosclerosis. Risk factors for its development parallel those of atherosclerosis in general and include family history, smoking, hypertension, and hypercholesterolemia. There is experimental evidence that chronic digitalis administration leads to altered mesenteric hemodynamics.[17] Nonatherosclerotic causes of chronic mesenteric ischemia include thrombosis associated with thoracoabdominal aneurysm,[18–22] aortic coarctation,[23–25] mesenteric arteritis,[22,24–26] fibromuscular dysplasia,[22,25,26] neurofibromatosis,[27] middle aortic syndrome,[28] Buerger's disease,[29,30] celiac artery compression (by the median arcuate ligament),[24–26,31–34] vasospasm,[35] and radiation arteritis.[36] Embolic disease, aortic dissection, mesenteric venous thrombosis, trauma, and aortic reconstruction with IMA exclusion are more common causes of acute mesenteric ischemia and occasionally may lead to chronic symptoms if the patient survives the initial catastrophic event.

CLINICAL PRESENTATION

Chronic mesenteric ischemia most often occurs in the sixth decade, with a slight female preponderance. Over 70% of patients are smokers. Abdominal pain is rarely the only manifestation of atherosclerosis, as a significant percentage of patients have hypertension, coronary artery disease, and/or peripheral vascular disease, with nearly 50% having undergone previous vascular surgery. About 12% of affected patients have diabetes mellitus.

The sine qua non of chronic mesenteric ischemia is abdominal pain (Table 53–1). The abdominal pain is variable in character but most often is dull and crampy, occurring primarily in the epigastrium or midabdominal area and frequently radiating to the back. The discomfort results from activation of visceral afferent nerves that are responsive to distention and ischemia but that poorly localize pain. Peritoneal inflammation is rare. Over 80% of patients note the relationship of pain and caloric intake. Abdominal pain classically occurs 15 to 45 minutes after eating and abates within 1 to 2 hours. This mimics the increased metabolic demand of the enterocyte following a meal; the larger the meal, the worse the pain.[24] Interestingly, some authors have reported that squatting or explosive diarrheal movements afford temporary relief.[9,30]

Table 53–1. Clinical Presentation of Chronic Mesenteric Ischemia

Author	Year	n	Abd Pain (%)	Postprand (%)	Weight Loss (%)	Diarrhea (%)	N/V %	Constipation (%)
University of Chicago*	1995	21	71%	71%	67%	33%	43%	19%
McMillan[11]	1995	25	100	NR	84	40	25	12
Harward[44]	1993	18	100	100	94	61	18	11
Calderon[45]	1992	20	100	80	65	40	20	NR
Cormier[22]	1991	20	100	100	90	60	0	NR
Geelkerken[46]	1991	14	100	79	75	NR	0	NR
MacFarlane[26]	1989	23	74	74	NR	38	0	NR
Rheudasil[47]	1988	41	100	100	90	32	41	26
Rapp[8]	1986	67	93	84	79	19	67	6
Rogers[33]	1982	13	85	85	62	23	0	NR
Connelly[48]	1981	28	100	100	80	25	0	43
Crawford[20]	1977	40	98	NR	68	33	40	NR
Buchardt Hansen[9]	1976	12	100	100	100	50	0	50
McCollum[21]	1976	33	100	88	55	9	33	12
Jaumin[49]	1975	7	86	71	71	29	0	43
Reul[25]	1974	25	92	56	36	16	25	NR
Total (weighted percent)		407	94%	86%	74%	33%	31%	19%

*1985–1995 (unreported).
Abbreviation: NR, not reported.

Weight loss is the second classic symptom of chronic mesenteric ischemia. Although malabsorption can contribute to weight loss in severe cases, loss of weight is primarily due to the patient's anticipation of postprandial pain or *food fear* (sitophobia), which leads to decreased caloric intake. Loss of weight is variable, however, and some patients are able to maintain their weight despite significant disease. Many patients lose so much weight that they undergo extensive evaluations for occult neoplasms. The emaciated habitus of patients with chronic mesenteric ischemia has been described as *starvation, torture,* and *premature aging.*[9]

Ischemia and malabsorption can lead to other significant symptoms, including diarrhea, nausea and vomiting, and constipation. About half of the patients have normal stool patterns, however. The variability of presenting signs and symptoms probably depends on the region of the gut affected. Foregut (celiac) ischemia is usually heralded by nausea, vomiting, and bloating, while midgut (SMA) ischemia causes classic postprandial abdominal pain and weight loss. The infrequent findings of constipation, occult blood in the stool, and histologic evidence of ischemic colitis reflect hindgut (IMA) involvement.[21,37]

Physical examination of the abdomen in patients with chronic mesenteric ischemia is usually not revealing. An abdominal bruit (70% of patients) and a scaphoid appearance suggest the diagnosis but are nonspecific. Even during an attack, the physical examination is usually unimpressive, consistent with the characteristic presentation of *pain out of proportion to the physical exam.* As stated previously, physical examination is more likely to reveal other manifestations of atherosclerosis, such as carotid bruits and/or decreased peripheral pulses.

Routine laboratory evaluation is rarely helpful, although the patient may exhibit a low hematocrit or immunoincompetence due to malnutrition.[38] Malnutrition may also be manifested by hypoalbuminemia, hypoproteinemia, and hypocholesterolemia.[9] More specific tests for panmalabsorption may be revealing, including measurement of stool fat, D-xylose tolerance, or vitamin B_{12} absorption.[9,39] Electrocardiograms often show signs of past episodes of myocardial infarction or ischemic dysrhythmia. Plain abdominal films are usually nonspecific but may show calcification in the course of arterial vessels.

NATURAL HISTORY

Atherosclerosis of the mesenteric circulation is, surprisingly, a common finding. In autopsy series of unselected patients, the incidence of significant narrowing of the celiac artery, SMA, and IMA is approximately 50%, 30%, and 30%, respectively.[6,40] In patients undergoing aortography for aneurysmal or occlusive disease, significant stenosis of the celiac artery or SMA may be found in up to one-third of cases.[20] Most lesions are of no clinical consequence, as most patients are asymptomatic. The natural history of patients with *symptomatic* mesenteric atherosclerosis is largely unknown but is sus-

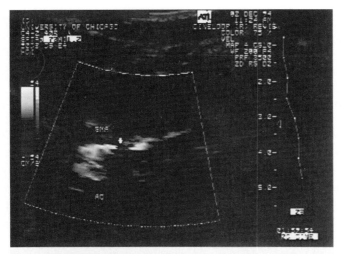

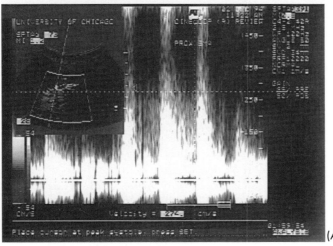

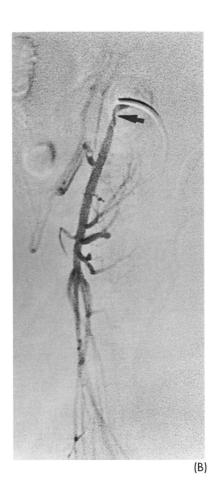

(A)

(B)

Figure 53–2. Mesenteric duplex ultrasonography. (A) Mesenteric duplex scan in a 63-year-old female with severe weight loss. Note the Peak Systolic Velocity of >500 cm/sec and the color flow image of the proximal SMA stenosis (SMA, superior mesenteric artery; AO, aorta). (B) Lateral SMA injection with digital subtraction confirming high-grade SMA stenosis (arrow).

pected by most clinicians to be grave. Although the incidence of symptomatic disease that progresses to frank intestinal infarction is debatable, approximately 50 to 80% of patients who die from acute mesenteric ischemia have previously suffered some form of premonitory abdominal symptomatology.[9,30,41]

DIAGNOSTIC EVALUATION

Neither intestinal contrast studies nor endoscopic evaluation are helpful in making the diagnosis of chronic mesenteric ischemia, although they are important in eliminating other causes of abdominal pain. Occasionally, biopsy of the jejunum or colon will reveal some sequelae of ischemia, including villous atrophy, epithelial cell flattening, and/or chronic inflammation.

As with most diseases of the vascular system, considerable effort has been devoted to the development of noninvasive methods of diagnosis. The ability to screen patients with chronic abdominal pain without incurring

the risk of contrast arteriography would be a significant advance in the early diagnosis of chronic mesenteric insufficiency. As early as 1986, attempts were made to visualize the mesenteric circulation via abdominal ultrasonography.[42] Ultrasound detection of mesenteric lesions is technically difficult, however, due to the requirement for deep abdominal sound penetration. Nevertheless, using peak systolic velocity criteria of ≥275 cm/sec for the SMA and ≥200 cm/sec for the celiac artery, Moneta et al. achieved positive predictive values of 80% and 63% for ≥70% angiographic stenosis or occlusion of the SMA and celiac artery, respectively, in 100 patients.[43] More important, perhaps, is that the sensitivity for significant SMA and celiac lesions was 92% and 87%, respectively. Thus, it would appear that duplex ultrasound may be a reliable screening test for the presence of mesenteric atherosclerosis (Fig. 53–2). The test is highly operator dependent, however, and independent confirmation of accuracy is necessary

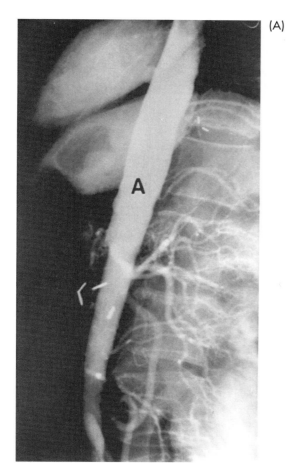

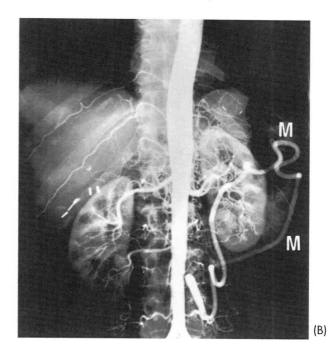

Figure 53–3 Chronic mesenteric ischemia. Aortogram in a 66-year-old female with postprandial pain and weight loss. (A) Lateral projection with absence of filling of the celiac or SMA (A, aorta). (B) The viscera are supplied by a meandering mesenteric artery (M) originating from an IMA with proximal high-grade stenosis and poststenotic dilatation.

Table 53–2. Vessel Involvement in Chronic Mesenteric Ischemia

Author	Year	n	Celiac SMA IMA (%)	Celiac SMA (%)	SMA IMA (%)	Celiac IMA (%)	Celiac Alone (%)	SMA Alone (%)
University of Chicago*	1995	21	24%	52%	14%	0%	0%	10%
Harward[44]	1993	18	61	22	17	0	0	0
Calderon[45]	1992	20	25	25	10	15	10	15
Cormier[22]	1991	20	85	10	0	0	0	5
Geelkerken[46]	1991	14	50	21	7	21	0	0
MacFarlane[26]	1989	23	20	NR	NR	NR	0	0
Rheudasil[47]	1988	41	74	23	0	0	0	3
Rapp[8]	1986	67	46	49	0	3	0	4
Rogers[33]	1982	13	46	NR	NR	NR	NR	NR
Connelly[48]	1981	28	75	NR	NR	NR	NR	NR
Buchardt Hansen[9]	1976	12	75	25	0	0	0	0
Jaumin[49]	1975	7	57	0	0	0	0	14
Reul[25]	1974	25	NR	NR	NR	NR	NR	NR
Total (weighted percent)		342	55%	32%	4%	4%	1%	5%

*1985–1995 (unreported).
Abbreviation: NR, not reported.

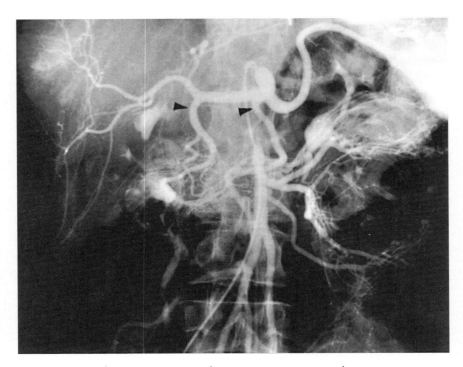

Figure 53–4. Chronic mesenteric ischemia. Anteroposterior celiac injection in a 67-year-old female with nausea, vomiting, and weight loss. Note the high-grade stenosis of the celiac axis, with extensive collateralization to the distribution of an occluded SMA (arrows).

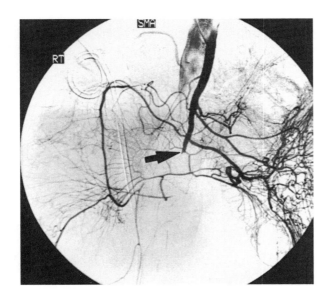

Figure 53–5. Acute mesenteric ischemia. Anteroposterior digital subtraction SMA injection in a 65-year-old female with stage IV cervical cancer, intracardiac mural thrombus, and sudden onset of abdominal pain. Note the abrupt occlusion of the mid-SMA (arrow), with relative lack of collateralization. RT, right; SMA, superior mesenteric artery injection.

for each noninvasive vascular laboratory employing this technique.

The gold standard for the diagnosis of chronic mesenteric ischemia is selective mesenteric arteriography. Full anteroposterior views of the aorta are required to evaluate the aorta and the renal and iliac arteries. In addition, lateral aortic views are essential to delineate the origins of the three mesenteric vessels en face. Recently, digital subtraction arteriography has

been employed in an attempt to limit the volume of contrast dye.

Occlusion of two or three of the celiac artery, SMA, and IMA is strongly suggestive of chronic mesenteric ischemia (Table 53–2). Additionally, large collateral vessels and/or poststenotic dilatation often accompany chronic stenoses. A large, winding collateral vessel combined with occlusion or stenosis of the celiac artery and SMA is pathognomonic (Figs. 53–3 and 53–4). Con-

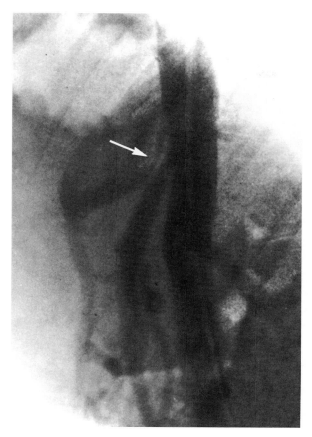

Figure 53–6. Median arcuate compression syndrome. Lateral aortogram in a 27-year-old female with postprandial abdominal cramping, bloating, and occasional nausea and vomiting. Note the compression of the celiac artery and SMA (arrow). Her twin sister had similar complaints and similar arteriographic findings. (Reprinted from Bech F, Loesberg A, Rosenblum J, Glagov S, Gewertz BL. Median arcuate ligament compression syndrome in monozygotic twins. *J Vasc Surg* 1994;19:935 (with permission.)

versely, occlusion of SMA in the *absence* of collateralization suggests an acute process, and immediate intervention will likely be required (Fig. 53–5). Lastly, celiac trunk compression by the median arcuate ligament may occasionally be the cause of chronic mesenteric ischemia, especially in younger patients[32] (Fig. 53–6).

REFERENCES

1. Schnitzler J. Zur symptomatologie des darmarterienverschlesses. *Wien Med Wochenschr* 1901;51:505–511.
2. Goodman EH. Angina abdominis. *Am J Med Sci* 1918;155:524–528.
3. Councilman WT. Three cases of occlusion of the superior mesenteric artery. *Boston Med Surg J* 1894;130:410–411.
4. Dunphy JE. Abdominal pain of vascular origin. *Am J Med Sci* 1936;192:109–113.
5. Shaw RS, Maynard EP III. Acute and chronic thrombosis of the mesenteric arteries associated with malabsorption. *N Engl J Med* 1958;258:874–878.
6. Derrick JR, Pollard HS, Moore RM. The pattern of atherosclerotic narrowing of the celiac and superior mesenteric arteries. *Ann Surg* 1959;149:684–689.
7. Marston A. Diagnosis and management of intestinal ischemia. *Ann R Coll Surg Engl* 1972;50:29–41.
8. Rapp JH, Reilly LM, Qvarfordt PG, Goldstone J, Ehrenfeld WK, Stoney RJ. Durability of endarterectomy and antegrade grafts in the treatment of chronic visceral ischemia. *J Vasc Surg* 1986;3:799–806.
9. Buchardt Hansen HJ. Abdominal angina. Results of arterial reconstruction in 12 patients. *Acta Chir Scand* 1976;142:319–325.
10. Schwartz LB, Purut CM, Craig DM, Smith PK, McCann RL. Input impedance of revascularized skeletal muscle, renal, and mesenteric vascular beds. *Vasc Surg* 1996;30:459–470.
11. McMillan WD, McCarthy WJ, Bresticker MR, et al. Mesenteric artery bypass: objective patency determination. *J Vasc Surg* 1995;21:729–741.
12. Granger DN, Richardson PDI, Kvietys PR, Mortillaro NA. Intestinal blood flow. *Gastroenterology* 1980;78:837–863.
13. Clark ET, Gewertz BL. Mesenteric ischemia. In: Hall J, Schmidt G, Wood LDH, eds. *Principles of Critical Care.* New York: McGraw-Hill; 1992:2043–2049.
14. Clark ET, Gewertz BL. Glucagon potentiates intestinal reperfusion injury. *J Vasc Surg* 1990;11:270–277.
15. Umans JG, Levi R. Nitric oxide in the regulation of blood flow and arterial pressure. *Annu Rev Physiol* 1995;57:771–790.
16. Desai TR, Sisley AC, Brown S, Gewertz BL. Defining the critical limit of oxygen extraction in human small intestine. *J Vasc Surg* 1996;23:832–838.
17. Kim EH, Gewertz BL. Chronic digitalis administration alters mesenteric vascular reactivity. *J Vasc Surg* 1987;5:382–389.
18. Svensson LG, Crawford ES, Hess KR, Coselli JS, Safi HJ. Thoracoabdominal aortic aneurysms associated with celiac, superior mesenteric, and renal artery occlusive disease: methods and analysis of results in 271 patients. *J Vasc Surg* 1992;16:378–390.
19. Schwartz LB, Belkin M, Donaldson MC, Mannick JA, Whittemore AD. Improvement in results of repair of type IV thoracoabdominal aneurysms. *J Vasc Surg* 1996;24:74–81.
20. Crawford ES, Morris GC Jr, Myhre HO, Roehm JO Jr. Celiac axis, superior mesenteric artery, and inferior mesenteric artery occlusion: surgical considerations. *Surgery* 1977;82:856–866.
21. McCollum CH, Graham JM, DeBakey ME. Chronic mesenteric arterial insufficiency: results of revascularization in 33 cases. *South Med J* 1976;69:1266–1268.
22. Cormier JM, Fichelle JM, Vennin J, Laurian C, Gigou F. Atherosclerotic occlusive disease of the superior mesenteric artery: later results of reconstructive surgery. *Ann Vasc Surg* 1991;5:510–518.
23. Meacham PW, Dean RH. Chronic mesenteric ischemia in childhood and adolescence. *J Vasc Surg* 1985;2:878–885.
24. Rob C. Surgical diseases of the celiac and mesenteric arteries. *Arch Surg* 1966;93:21–32.
25. Reul GJ Jr, Wukasch DC, Sandiford FM, Chiarillo L, Hallman GL, Cooley DA. Surgical treatment of abdominal angina: review of 25 patients. *Surgery* 1974;75:682–689.
26. MacFarlane SD, Beebe HG. Progress in chronic mesenteric arterial ischemia. *J Cardiovasc Surg* 1989;30:178–184.
27. Zochodne D. Von Recklinghausen's vasculopathy. *Am J Med Sci* 1984;287:64–65.

28. Messina LM, Goldstone J, Ferrell LD, Reilly LM, Ehrenfeld WK, Stoney RJ. Middle aortic syndrome: effectiveness and durability of complex arterial revascularization techniques. *Ann Surg* 1986;204:331–339.

29. Lye CR. Chronic mesenteric ischemia. *Can J Surg* 1988;31:159–161.

30. Fry WJ, Kraft RO. Visceral angina. *Surg Gynecol Obstet* 1963;117:417–424.

31. Mulder DS, Rubush J, Lawrence MS, Ehrenhaft JL. Celiac axis compression syndrome. *Can J Surg* 1971;14:122–126.

32. Bech F, Loesberg A, Rosenblum J, Glagov S, Gewertz BL. Median arcuate ligament compression syndrome in monozygotic twins. *J Vasc Surg* 1994;19:934–938.

33. Rogers DM, Thompson JE, Garrett WV, Talkington CM, Patman RD. Mesenteric vascular problems: a 26-year experience. *Ann Surg* 1982;195:554–565.

34. Dunbar JD, Molnar W, Beman FF, Marable SA. Compression of the celiac trunk and abdominal angina. *Am J Roentgenol* 1965;95:731–744.

35. Gewertz BL, Zarins CK. Postoperative vasospasm after antegrade mesenteric revascularization: a report of three cases. *J Vasc Surg* 1991;14:382–385.

36. Moneta GL. Diagnosis of chronic intestinal ischemia. *Semin Vasc Surg* 1990;3:176–185.

37. Friedman G, Sloan WC. Ischemic enteropathy. *Surg Clin North Am* 1972;52:1001–1012.

38. Tilson MD, Stansel HC. Abdominal angina. Intestinal absorption eight years after successful mesenteric revascularization. *Am J Surg* 1976;131:366–368.

39. Bergan JJ. Recognition and treatment of intestinal ischemia. *Surg Clin North Am* 1967;47:109–126.

40. Reiner L, Jimenez FA, Rodriquez FL. Atherosclerosis in the mesenteric circulation. Observations and correlations with aortic and coronary atherosclerosis. *Am Heart J* 1963;66:200–209.

41. Watt JK. Arterial disease of the gut. *Br Med J* 1968;3:231–233.

42. Nicholls SC, Kohler TR, Martin RL, Strandness DE Jr. Use of hemodynamic parameters in the diagnosis of mesenteric ischemia. *J Vasc Surg* 1986;3:507–510.

43. Moneta GL, Lee RW, Yeager RA, Taylor LM Jr, Porter JM. Mesenteric duplex scanning: a blinded prospective study. *J Vasc Surg* 1993;17:79–86.

44. Harward TR, Brooks DL, Flynn TC, Seeger JM. Multiple organ dysfunction after mesenteric artery revascularization. *J Vasc Surg* 1993;18:459–469.

45. Calderon M, Reul GJ, Gregoric ID, et al. Long-term results of the surgical management of symptomatic chronic intestinal ischemia. *J Cardiovasc Surg* 1992;33:723–728.

46. Geelkerken RH, van Bockel JH, de Roos WK, Hermans J, Terpstra JL. Chronic mesenteric vascular syndrome. Results of reconstructive surgery. *Arch Surg* 1991;126:1101–1106.

47. Rheudasil JM, Steward MT, Schellack JV, Smith RB 3rd, Salam AA, Perdue GD. Surgical treatment of chronic mesenteric arterial insufficiency. *J Vasc Surg* 1988;8:495–500.

48. Connelly TI, Perdue GD, Smith RB, Ansley JD, McKinnon WM. Elective mesenteric revascularization. *Am Surg* 1981;47:19–25.

49. Jaumin P, Fastrez J, Goenen M, Kestens-Servaye Y, Schoevaerdts J, Dautrebande J. Revascularization of the superior mesenteric artery. *J Cardiovasc Surg* 1975;16:548–551.

54

The Presentation, Diagnosis, and Management of Acute Mesenteric Ischemia

Robert P. Smilanich, M.D.
Robert G. Atnip, M.D.

Abrupt interruption of splanchnic blood flow causes an often fatal sequence of events progressing from visceral ischemia to bowel infarction. The numerous disease pathways that lead to acute mesenteric ischemia are so variable as to preclude the use of a universal diagnostic and therapeutic formula. In all instances, however, successful treatment begins with prompt recognition of the onset of the ischemic state. Early confirmation of the diagnosis and immediate therapy by qualified surgeons and interventional radiologists offer the patient the best chance of survival. As with many other vascular catastrophes, delay in any phase of management will yield a poor outcome.

ANATOMY

Intestinal blood flow is derived from three arteries that correspond to the principal embryologic segments of the gut: the celiac trunk supplies the foregut, the superior mesenteric artery (SMA) supplies the midgut, and the inferior mesenteric artery (IMA) supplies the hindgut. Receiving 25% of total cardiac output, the celiac and mesenteric arterial beds are highly metabolically active and have a low capacity for anaerobic metabolism. The gut is therefore supplied by specific collateral pathways that connect the major axial vessels to one another and to the internal iliac arteries. The celiac branches and SMA are linked by the pancreaticoduodenal arcades; the SMA and IMA in turn share collaterals such as the Arc of Riolan and the marginal artery of Drummond. In the setting of sudden occlusion of either the celiac or SMA, however, splanchnic collaterals are seldom capable of meeting the total visceral oxygen demand. In this situation, the midgut is the most vulnerable to ischemia and necrosis (Fig. 54–1).

PATHOPHYSIOLOGY

The majority of cases of acute mesenteric ischemia result from either embolic arterial occlusion, arterial thrombosis, venous thrombosis, or nonocclusive hypoperfusion (Fig. 54–2).

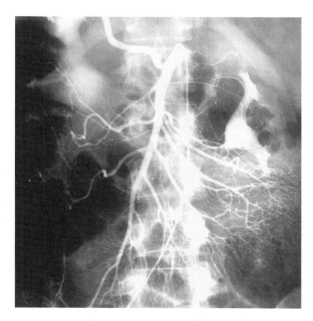

Figure 54–1. Selective arteriogram of a normal SMA, which supplies the entire midgut, including the jejunum, ileum, right colon, and much of the transverse colon.

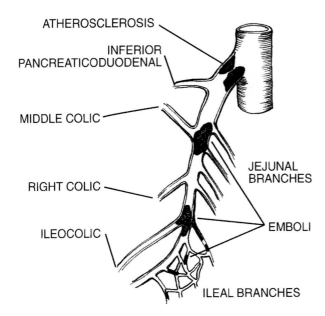

Figure 54–2. The SMA and its major branches, with depiction of the most common sites for thrombosis and embolism. Note that thrombosis is likely to occur at the origin of the SMA, where atherosclerotic plaque causes luminal stenosis. Emboli tend to lodge more distally at branch points.

Embolism

Arterial embolism is the most common cause of acute mesenteric ischemia, accounting for about 45% of cases.[1] Embolic sources include thromboemboli from the heart or aorta, cholesterol emboli from the aorta, septic emboli from heart valves, tumor emboli such as atrial myxoma, mural thrombus from arterial aneurysms, and paradoxical emboli from the venous system. The heart is the source of about 80% of peripheral emboli, largely because of the high prevalence of atherosclerotic heart disease. Atrial fibrillation is a risk factor found in three-fourths of patients with arterial emboli, and recent myocardial infarction is diagnosed in 24%. Approximately 5% of cardiogenic emboli involve the visceral vessels.[2]

The incidence of thromboembolism related to rheumatic valvular heart disease has decreased dramatically over the past few decades. Improved treatment of ischemic heart disease and arrhythmias, along with the more prevalent use of chronic anticoagulant therapy, has also lowered the incidence of thromboembolism in some patient populations. These gains may be offset somewhat by the rapid expansion of our aging population and by an increase in iatrogenic emboli due to surgical and catheter-induced arterial trauma.

Thrombosis

Arterial thrombosis accounts for 12% of cases of acute mesenteric ischemia, and venous thrombosis causes approximately 8%.[1] The conditions that lead to the development of mesenteric arterial or venous thrombosis are those described originally by Virchow: stasis, endothelial injury, and hypercoagulability.

Stasis (reduction of flow) may be caused by intrinsic or extrinsic vascular disease. Atherosclerotic occlusive disease is by far the most common intrinsic occlusive disease, but nonatherosclerotic vascular diseases such as fibromuscular dysplasia and the various forms of arteritis have also been implicated. *Iatrogenic* arterial stasis is common in the hospitalized patient due to vasopressor drugs or intravascular catheters. Extrinsic vascular compression may occur with either neoplastic or nonneoplastic masses. Portal or mesenteric venous stasis results from various mechanical, neoplastic, inflammatory, congenital, traumatic, or fibrotic processes. Pyelophlebitis resulting from intraperitoneal sepsis is the most common cause of mesenteric venous thrombosis. Nonocclusive stasis phenomena include severe congestive heart failure, valvular disease, aortic coarctation, and splanchnic arteriovenous fistula.

Endothelial injury contributes to acute mesenteric thrombosis. Endothelial erosion or ulceration in atherosclerotic vessels and cytokine-mediated endothelial damage in response to injury and inflammation may precipitate thrombosis. Guidewire and catheter manipulation of the aorta and its branches is an increasingly common cause of endothelial injury and subsequent thrombosis.

Hypercoagulable states (thrombophilia) are being recognized with growing frequency in a variety of thrombotic conditions. The majority of patients presenting with intestinal ischemia due to mesenteric vein thrombosis have a history of lower extremity venous thrombosis that is consistent with the presence of hypercoagulability.[3] Known hypercoagulable conditions include protein S and C deficiencies, antithrombin III deficiency, antiphospholipid antibodies, heparin-induced thrombocytopenia, thrombocytosis, malignancy, pregnancy, use of oral contraceptives, and polycythemia. New defects have recently been discovered, such as activated protein C resistance (Leiden Factor V), which is present in about 5% of the general population.[4,5] Its clinical significance is still being assessed.

Nonocclusive Ischemia

The term *nonocclusive mesenteric ischemia* refers to a state of hypoperfusion that exists in the absence of thrombotic or embolic vascular occlusion. In practical terms, it is synonymous with splanchnic vasoconstriction. The most common causes are cardiac failure, sepsis, and other severe systemic illnesses that result in shock. The combination of poor pump function, hypovolemia, maximal endogenous sympathetic tone, and exogenous vasopressor support is often present in these patients. Endogenous vasopressin exerts its most potent vasoconstrictive effects in the mesenteric circulation, providing improved cerebral and cardiac blood flow at the expense of poor intestinal perfusion. Angiotensin II also causes a potent mesenteric vasoconstrictor response that is largely resistant to local metabolic autocrine control.

In addition to endogenous mediators and exogenous catecholamines, other drugs have been implicated in severe visceral vasoconstriction, including the ergot alkaloids[6] and cocaine.[7] An association between acute mesenteric ischemia and digitalis use has often been described in textbooks, but it is unclear whether this is a specific drug-related phenomenon or a result of confounding variables in the high-risk patient population being treated with digitalis. In an animal model, digitalis alters mesenteric vascular reactivity in response to increased intestinal venous pressures, suggesting at least a contributory risk for mesenteric ischemia.[8] A rare cause of nonocclusive mesenteric ischemia that is probably mediated by endogenous pressor agents is that seen after repair of aortic coarctation in children.[9]

Nonocclusive mesenteric ischemia is most likely to occur in patients with critical multisystemic illness, in whom numerous comorbidities make the diagnosis more difficult to establish. In some cases, multiple etiologic factors may be involved, although none of them would necessarily result by itself in intestinal ischemia. Nonocclusive etiologies of acute mesenteric ischemia account for approximately 20% of cases.[1] This may in fact represent a slight decrease in incidence over the past decade due to recent improvements in intensive care monitoring and intervention for cardiogenic shock.

Iatrogenic causes of acute mesenteric ischemia warrant special mention because of the potential for prevention. Acute mesenteric ischemia following cardiopulmonary bypass has been reported in up to 0.36% of pump cases and has been associated with mortality in 60 to 100% of cases.[10,11] Either diffuse microembolism or hypoperfusion due to inadequate pump function (heart or bypass machine) may be responsible. Vasopressor agents and intraaortic balloon counterpulsation are contributing risk factors. Common iatrogenic causes of *large bowel* ischemia include inadequate mesenteric revascularization following aortic aneurysm repair and compromise of mesocolic collaterals due to colonic resection.

The remaining 15% of cases not attributable to embolism, nonocclusive ischemia, arterial thrombosis, or venous thrombosis are designated *idiopathic*. Some of these cases likely represent a failure to diagnose the previously discussed mechanisms. A complex mix of factors may be present in others.

EPIDEMIOLOGY

In a recent review, Taylor and Moneta[12] noted that acute mesenteric embolism was associated with a mean age of 67 years and a male:female ratio of 1.7:1. This is quite different from acute mesenteric arterial thrombosis, with a male:female ratio of 1:1.7 and a mean age of 74. Mesenteric venous thrombosis has a slightly younger age distribution (64 years) and a slight male predilection. Patients with nonocclusive ischemia had a mean age of 72 and no significant gender bias.

Risk factors for acute mesenteric ischemia are essentially the general risk factors for atherosclerosis, thromboembolism, and shock, and include tobacco use, diabetes mellitus, hypercholesterolemia, family history, cardiac disease (congenital, acquired, or ischemic, including valve disease, endocarditis, and arrhythmias), and hypercoagulable conditions. Other risk factors include steroids, digitalis, ergots (typically used for migraine headaches), radiation injury, various collagen vascular diseases, cocaine abuse, and iatrogenic causes such as aortic surgery and bowel resection with injury to the mesenteric blood supply. Chronic mesenteric ischemia (*intestinal angina*) was recognized as a risk factor for subsequent acute intestinal infarction by Dunphy in 1936.[13] In two small series reviewed by Taylor and Moneta,[12] 58% of patients dying of acute mesenteric ischemia (and all eight patients undergoing operation for acute mesenteric arterial thrombosis) had a history consistent with chronic mesenteric ischemia. The subset of patients with postoperative acute mesenteric ischemia has its own set of risk factors, including emergent operations,[14,15] use of intraaortic balloon pump counterpulsation,[15–17] use of vasopressors,[1,16] cardiopulmonary bypass, and advanced age.[10]

DIAGNOSIS

The differential diagnosis is that of the acute abdomen. Intestinal ischemia may be misdiagnosed as anything from gastroenteritis to perforated duodenal ulcer. Perhaps the most common cause for delay in diagnosis is the failure to seriously consider the possibility of acute mesenteric ischemia in the patient with abdominal pain.

Clinical Presentation

Abdominal pain is the presenting complaint of virtually all patients with acute mesenteric ischemia. Intestinal angina was first recognized as a symptom of mesenteric ischemia by Bacelli, as credited by Goodman in 1918.[17] Due to the sudden onset and severity of the pain, patients tend to present early for evaluation. *Pain out of proportion to abdominal tenderness* is the classic description of the clinical presentation of acute mesenteric ischemia. The pain is often described as the worst pain ever experienced, and the patient is typically restless and distressed. Actual signs and symptoms vary markedly, depending on the etiology, acuity, adequacy of collaterals, and anatomic distribution of ischemia.

The pain is usually poorly localized and is described as a severe, dull ache or cramps. Diarrhea with or without blood may be reported. Vomiting is reported by the majority of patients following the onset of pain.

One-third of patients with embolic occlusion have a history of prior peripheral emboli. The patient may experience simultaneous embolic symptoms in other vascular locations, most commonly the lower extremities. Of the various causes of mesenteric ischemia, embolic occlusion is characterized by an extremely acute onset and a rapidly progressive course because of the usual lack of collateral flow.

Approximately 50% of patients with SMA thrombosis report prior symptoms of chronic mesenteric ischemia such as postprandial pain, weight loss, and vague gastrointestinal complaints. These patients typically report a sudden exacerbation of their prior symptoms when thrombotic occlusion supervenes. The acuity of onset is typically intermediate between the catastrophic onset of embolic occlusion and the more indolent course of nonocclusive ischemia or mesenteric venous thrombosis. Most patients with thrombotic occlusion have other end-organ manifestations of atherosclerotic occlusive disease involving the heart, brain, or peripheral vessels.

Patients with mesenteric venous thrombosis and nonocclusive intestinal ischemia tend to have a slower onset and a more protracted course, but the signs and symptoms are otherwise similar. The typically subacute nature of these cases often results in delays in presentation and diagnosis. Patients with a cardiogenic etiology (low flow state) may exhibit masking of the abdominal symptoms owing to chest pain, altered mental status, or multisystem end-organ ischemia.

Physical findings vary with the duration of the ischemic process but are often few in the early hours. Acute loss of bowel perfusion tends to cause initial peristaltic spasms (accounting for the typical diarrhea), followed by adynamic ileus. Bowel sounds are thus hypoactive even early in the course, and after 2 hours the abdomen is usually distended and silent. Ascites is a common late finding, and the abdomen is generally dull to percussion rather than tympanitic owing to fluid sequestration in the flaccid bowel loops. Occult blood in gastric or rectal specimens is found in 25% of patients.[18] The physical exam will initially reveal surprisingly little indication of peritonitis, hence the disproportion between pain and tenderness. An initial lack of impressive abdominal tenderness should heighten rather than reduce the suspicion of gut ischemia. Inflammation of the visceral peritoneum does not seem to develop until later in the evolution of ischemia, and its presence may actually signify the onset of bowel necrosis. Failure of the clinician to understand this phenomenon leads to missed diagnoses and a poor patient outcome.

Laboratory Evaluation

Although no single laboratory test or combination of tests is diagnostic of acute mesenteric ischemia, certain assays can provide valuable supportive evidence. Perhaps more important, they can serve as parameters to guide the resuscitative component of treatment and to gauge the prognosis. Acidemia is one of the few relatively consistent laboratory findings, but it may be absent early in the ischemic process. Severe acidemia is a poor prognostic factor and generally reflects the duration, severity, and extent of ischemia. Serum lactate levels correspond roughly with the course of the acidemia. Leukocytosis and hyperamylasemia are common findings, but are not sufficiently sensitive or specific to be useful in making a firm diagnosis. By the same token, *normal* laboratory assays do not exclude the diagnosis and should not deter the clinician from persuing the other studies to be described.

Duplex Scanning

Duplex scanning has found an increasingly important niche in the diagnosis of *chronic* mesenteric ischemia, with good positive predictive values compared to arteriography using criteria established by the Oregon Health Sciences University[19] and others.[20] Conversely, duplex ultrasound has not proven useful in diagnosing *acute* mesenteric ischemia, due in part to the technical difficulty of imaging the visceral arteries in a distended abdomen. Moreover, the accuracy of duplex is greater with vascular *stenosis* than with *occlusion*.

Radiography

Plain abdominal films are rarely diagnostic of mesenteric ischemia, and their primary value is in excluding other diagnoses. Pneumatosis intestinalis, air in the biliary tree, and free peritoneal air, although nonspecific, indicate necrosis or perforation. Bland, nonspecific findings such as small bowel distention, bowel wall thickening, and "thumbprinting" may be seen in acute splanchnic ischemia but are of little help in guiding therapeutic decisions. Barium contrast gastrointestinal studies are contraindicated when intestinal ischemia is suspected, both because of the risk of perforation and because retained barium will interfere with attempts at angiography.

Computed tomographic (CT) scans may be helpful in making the difficult diagnosis of mesenteric venous thrombosis by revealing thrombus within the mesenteric and portal veins (Fig. 54–3). The age of the thrombus cannot be determined, and its presence, though highly suggestive, is not pathognomonic. The triad of hypodensity in the superior mesenteric vein (representing clot), thickening of the small bowel wall, and the presence of significant peritoneal fluid has been proposed as diagnostic of intestinal infarction.[21]

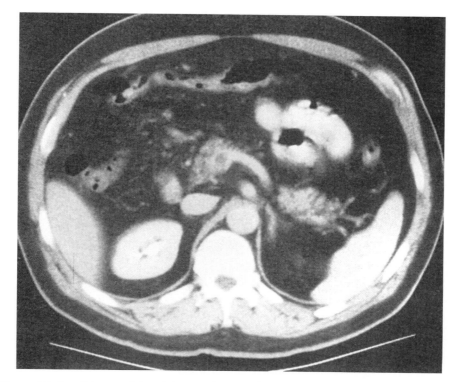

Figure 54–3.   CT scan of the abdomen showing thrombus in the superior mesenteric vein.

Magnetic resonance imaging (MRI) seems to offer no significant advantage over CT.

Angiography

Angiography (including lateral and anteroposterior aortograms and selective mesenteric and celiac catherization) can confirm the diagnosis, demonstrate the extent and severity of disease, and at times enable nonoperative treatment. For patients without signs of peritonitis and with an atypical or mild clinical presentation, arteriography may actually speed diagnosis and treatment. An arteriogram can be extremely helpful in operative planning by localizing occlusions and identifying other areas of embolic or atherosclerotic disease. Several reports have shown improved outcomes with a policy of aggressive, early (emergent) angiography. Nevertheless, the surgeon must weigh the benefits of visceral angiography against the potential delays that can occur in obtaining it. If signs and symptoms strongly support a clinical diagnosis of thromboembolic mesenteric ischemia, *particularly if peritonitis is present,* long delays in the angiography suite should be avoided in favor of immediate laparotomy.

The most common angiographic finding in cases of embolic occlusion is an abrupt cutoff in an otherwise nondiseased SMA just distal to the takeoff of the middle colic or first jejunal branch vessel (Fig. 54–4). The embolic occlusion often has a characteristic meniscus. Thrombotic arterial occlusion is usually seen at the origin of the SMA in the presence of a diffusely dis-

eased aorta (Fig. 54–5). Extensive collateral development suggests chronic occlusive disease. In the patient with acute abdominal pain, the arteriographic demonstration of an occluded vessel is powerful evidence for the diagnosis of acute visceral ischemia, especially if collaterals are scant.

Nonocclusive mesenteric ischemia exhibits a characteristic angiographic pattern of narrowing of the origins of major branches of the SMA (Fig. 54–6). Additionally, there may be tapering, beading, or narrowing of intestinal branches and spasm of intestinal arcades, with reduced or absent filling of intramural vessels.[15] Direct SMA infusion of papaverine (typically a bolus of 60 mg followed by continuous infusion of 30 to 60 mg/hr if indicated) has been shown to relieve vasoconstriction even in low-flow states, and may be both diagnostic and therapeutic.[15] Tolazoline (as a 25-mg/10-cc intra-arterial bolus followed by a continuous infusion of 12.5 to 25 mg/hr) appears to be as effective as papaverine, but its use has not been as thoroughly studied.

Venous phase films during selective arteriography may visualize mesenteric venous thrombosis. A characteristically prolonged arterial phase and spasm in the SMA branches are also consistent with mesenteric venous thrombosis. Reflux of contrast material into the aorta and dense opacification of thickened bowel wall are other diagnostic radiographic signs of mesenteric venous thrombosis. Small bowel luminal contrast stud-

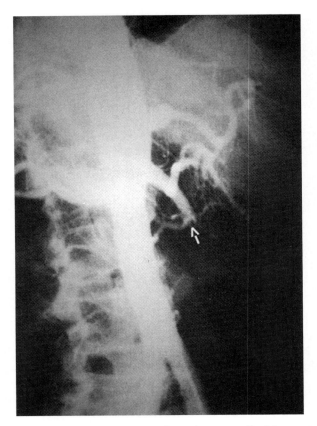

Figure 54–4.   Aortogram revealing abrupt cutoff of the SMA with meniscus, characteristic of SMA embolus (arrow).

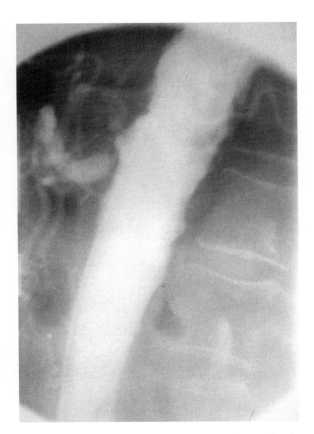

Figure 54–5.   Lateral aortogram showing a diseased celiac trunk and total occlusion (nonvisualization) of the SMA.

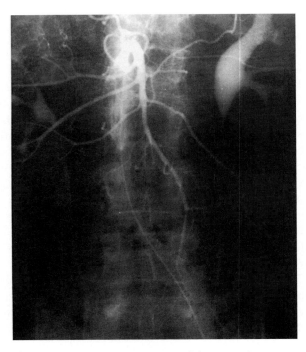

Figure 54–6.   Selective angiogram of the SMA showing pruning and tapering of the SMA branches typical of nonocclusive ischemia.

ies often show edema and "thumbprinting" of the bowel wall (Fig. 54–7).

Endoscopy

Endoscopy of the upper gastrointestinal tract is not generally helpful, except in ruling out other diagnoses, because ischemia rarely extends proximal to the ligament of Treitz. Colonoscopy is an accurate method for revealing colonic ischemia and infarction, but the insufflation required for adequate visualization can also cause perforation. Moreover, the presence of an entirely normal colon does not exclude the possibility of lethal small bowel ischemia.

Peritoneal lavage

Peritoneal lavage may sometimes be useful, such as in the patient with a decreased level of consciousness and equivocal peritoneal signs.[22] Diagnostic sensitivity will vary with the degree and duration of ischemia. A positive lavage by standard criteria (based on assays of white blood cells, red blood cells, amylase, bacteria, or vegetative matter) is nonspecific but indicates the need for laparotomy. Unfortunately, a positive peritoneal lavage is usually a late finding and indicates progression to gangrene.

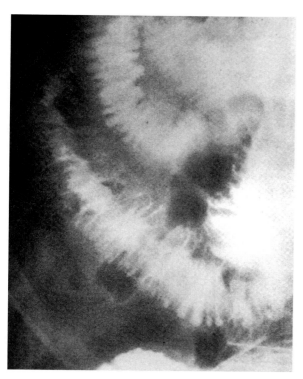

Figure 54–7. Small bowel contrast series showing marked wall thickening and mucosal edema suggestive of intestinal ischemia.

TREATMENT

Treatment begins with resuscitation, which includes the identification and management of concurrent diseases (pulmonary, cardiac, renal, hepatic, etc.), as well as initiation of therapy for the primary disease process. Diagnosis and resuscitation often proceed in parallel, followed by implementation of the most appropriate definitive treatment.

Medical Treatment

For a small percentage of patients, treatment can be limited to supportive measures. This is particularly true of patients with arteriographically demonstrated nonocclusive mesenteric ischemia in whom it is believed that bowel ischemia is not yet irreversible. In other infrequent cases, primary supportive therapy should be considered when the best available evidence indicates a mild, transient ischemic event with no suggestion of necrosis. Among the etiologies discussed, venous thrombosis and nonocclusive ischemia tend to have a less aggressive course that may be amenable to medical treatment under selected circumstances. This may avoid laparotomy in some patients and allow elective rather than emergent revascularization in others. The success of such an approach is, of course, closely linked to careful monitoring of the patient's clinical course.

Systemic anticoagulation with heparin is efficacious in the treatment of mesenteric ischemia caused by SMV or portal vein thrombosis. It appears to minimize the progression of stasis-related thrombosis until adequate collateral venous flow develops. Long-term anticoagulation is indicated in patients with identifiable hypercoagulable states. Anticoagulation may also be a useful adjunct to radiologic or operative treatment to limit extension of thrombus and prevent recurrence after successful revascularization. The benefits of anticoagulation do not overshadow a substantial risk of hemorrhage from ischemic intestinal mucosa or remote sites, especially if hepatic and bowel ischemia has already produced a coagulopathy. Similar considerations apply to the use of thrombolytic agents, which have enjoyed some anecdotal success in selected cases of SMA thrombosis. The risk of hemorrhage is significant, and long-term success is unlikely without correction of the underlying stenosis by catheter-based (angioplasty or stent) or operative revascularization. At best, this regimen may convert an emergent procedure into an elective procedure, but not without considerable risk of undetected bowel infarction.

Broad-spectrum antibiotics with anaerobic coverage should be employed in cases of suspected mesenteric ischemia. Nasogastric decompression and, in some cases, sigmoidoscopic decompression may be useful to improve perfusion and decrease the risk of perforation in distended viscera. Liberal volume resuscitation is usually necessary because of the extensive sequestration that occurs with ischemic bowel. Especially in cases of nonocclusive ischemia, the correction of intravascular volume deficits may be therapeutic in restoring normal perfusion. Captopril, nitroglycerin, and other vasodilators and afterload reducers may improve mesenteric blood flow by improving cardiac function and relieving intestinal vasospasm in cases of cardiogenic ischemia. Vasopressor agents should be discontinued if possible.

Invasive hemodynamic monitoring should be instituted and used to guide resuscitation. Pulmonary artery catheters provide reliable volume and cardiac performance parameters to moniter resuscitation further, although controversy about their ultimate benefit is increasing. Supplemental oxygen should be administered. If needed, transfusion to correct severe anemia may be warranted. Parenteral nutrition should be considered early in the course.

Interventional Radiology

Directed SMA infusion of papaverine as a 60-mg bolus followed by continuous selective infusion at a rate of 30 to 60 mg/hr has been found to be efficacious, especially in cases of nonocclusive mesenteric ischemia. (Tolazoline appears to be a reasonable substitute for papaverine, as previously noted.) Infusion may be required for 24 hours or more, concurrent with best medical management and monitoring for evidence of bowel necrosis. Papaverine infusion may also be used as an adjunct to surgical treatment, as will be described.

Boley and colleagues[23] demonstrated that selective SMA catheterization with intra-arterial injection of papaverine resulted in improved survival in patients with documented mesenteric ischemia. An overall survival of 54% in a series of 35 patients was achieved. A subset of patients with nonocclusive acute mesenteric ischemia had a 60% survival rate, but another subset with peritoneal signs had a lower survival rate (40%), as might be expected. A subsequent study by Boley et al[24] compared operative treatment with a regimen of intra-arterial papaverine followed by selective operation in patients with SMA embolism. Mortality was decreased from 80% to 55% with the selective combined approach.

The obvious limitation of percutaneous interventional techniques is that they provide no means of differentiating ischemic from infarcted bowel, a distinction that is critical to patient survival and can be made with absolute reliability only by laparotomy. There may be a role for diagnostic laparoscopy combined with catheter-based techniques, but this remains to be shown in clinical trials.

Operative Treatment

Operative treatment guided by angiography and complemented by aggressive medical support is the gold standard to which other forms of therapy must be compared. The surgeon should determine the etiology of ischemia, revascularize viable bowel, and resect nonviable bowel. Grossly necrotic bowel should be resected early in the procedure to avert sepsis and cardiovascular collapse. To preserve overall bowel length, intestinal segments of borderline viability should not be resected until after revascularization and careful reassessment, as such bowel can improve dramatically in appearance with reperfusion. A common mistake for the surgeon is to focus only on resection, with inadequate consideration of the value of revascularization. Bowel resection with optimal preservation of length may require a staged or planned second-look operation.

Assess the Etiology

The clinical presentation frequently suggests the etiology of ischemia. When arteriography is not available, the anatomic pattern of ischemia can help differentiate thrombotic from embolic occlusion of the SMA. In the setting of arterial thrombotic occlusion, the entire small bowel as well as the right colon may be involved, without sparing or skip areas. Ischemia due to venous thrombosis is often patchy and is usually limited to mid-small intestine, with sparing of the entire colon. Embolic occlusion typically occurs distal to the first branches of the SMA and thus often spares the proximal

jejunum. A pattern of segmental ischemia is seen with multiple small emboli, as may occur from an ulcerated aortic plaque or aneurysm.

Venous thrombosis is distinguished at laparotomy by a palpable SMA pulsation and pronounced mesenteric and bowel wall edema. The bowel is cyanotic, and on resection clot may be seen in the divided mesenteric veins. Concurrent findings may include varices and splenomegaly, in addition to those related to the primary underlying pathologic state.

Direct assessment of the mesenteric vessels is performed by standard surgical exposure. The SMA can be located at the junction of the transverse mesocolon and the small bowel mesentery. The celiac trunk can be found by dividing the gastrohepatic ligament or, alternatively, by medial visceral rotation.

Revascularize

Revascularization may involve thrombectomy, embolectomy, bypass, endarterectomy or rarely thrombolysis.

For embolic occlusions, the proximal SMA is dissected out at the root of the mesentery as it emerges from the inferior border of the pancreas. The transverse colon is moved cephalad and the mesocolic peritoneum incised at the base, exposing the SMA proximal to the first jejunal branch and just distal to the middle colic branch. The point of embolic occlusion can be palpated by the loss of pulse. Proximal and distal control of the SMA is obtained through gentle dissection. A transverse arteriotomy is made, through which No. 2 Fr to No. 4 Fr embolectomy catheters are passed antegrade and retrograde, using gentle technique so as not to injure the fragile mesenteric vessels. With small vessels, a longitudinal arteriotomy may be necessary, with subsequent patch angioplasty for closure. In the case of multiple small peripheral emboli, complete embolectomy is not likely to be successful and the affected segments of bowel may require resection. Successful embolectomy may be followed by irrigation with heparin, papaverine, low molecular weight dextran, urokinase, or a combination of these agents prior to closure. If it appears that primary closure of the arteriotomy will compromise the lumen, vein patch closure can be performed. After a brief period of reperfusion, the bowel is reassessed for viability.

In the patient who has experienced a thrombotic arterial occlusion, the SMA is carefully exposed distal to the point of obstruction, and a relatively nondiseased segment is selected for a bypass graft anastomosis. The most favorable site for distal anastomosis is usually inferior to the pancreas at the level of the middle colic and jejunal branches, but in severely diseased arteries it may be further distally. Complete revascularization may require multiple bypasses if both the celiac trunk and SMA are occluded.

Choice of inflow is controversial, but the authors prefer antegrade bypass from the supraceliac aorta. The supraceliac abdominal aorta is approached by dividing the gastrohepatic ligament and the right crus of the diaphragm. Alternatively, medial visceral rotation provides excellent high aortic exposure and control. The choice of approach may depend on patient-specific factors such as prior abdominal operations, obesity, and the condition of the supraceliac aorta. The aorta is controlled with adequate exposure for either partial or full cross-clamping, depending on the quality of the aorta at this level and the surgeon's preference. Clamp time should be as short as possible to minimize complications.[25] After the aortic anastomosis has been performed, the graft is either sewn to the mobilized portion of the SMA posterior to the pancreas (medial visceral rotation) or passed through a retropancreatic tunnel to the root of the mesocolon (anterior approach).

Other surgeons prefer the technique of retrograde aortomesenteric bypass from the infrarenal aorta, citing the relative ease of exposure and the reduced morbidity with infrarenal aortic clamping. Potential disadvantages of this method include the need to contend with severe atherosclerosis or aneurysmal disease of the infrarenal aorta (which may require separate graft replacement) and the tendency of retrograde grafts to kink or twist if the length and position of the graft are not optimal.

The choice of conduit depends on the degree of contamination of the surgical field. In the absence of frank gangrene, perforation, or purulent ascites, prosthetic material may be used, with an acceptably small risk of graft infection. A 12 × 6 mm or even a 14 × 7 mm bifurcated Dacron graft works well when both the SMA and the celiac artery require bypass. In the presence of gross contamination or a small-diameter outflow vessel, the proximal greater saphenous vein is preferable.

For purely nonocclusive mesenteric ischemia surgical revascularization is not feasible, and if laparotomy becomes necessary the focus is on resection of nonviable bowel. The surgeon should ascertain by angiography that correctable vascular pathology does not coexist. Similarly, surgery for mesenteric venous thrombosis is aimed primarily at resection of affected bowel. Since venous thrombectomy fails to address or correct the inciting disease process, it has been associated with predictably poor results and has largely been abandoned.

Resect

A colostomy is usually necessary following resection of unprepared or grossly contaminated colon, but the small bowel can often be managed with primary anastomosis. Surgical experience and judgment must be exercised to determine which segments of bowel may be preserved and whether reanastomosis or diversion should be performed.

Signs of bowel infarction include lack of peristalsis, dilatation, wall edema, discoloration, and hemorrhage into the mesentery. Intraoperative determination of bowel viability can be extremely challenging and usually requires more than simple visual inspection. Most surgeons resect short segments of marginal viability; when bowel involvement is extensive, adjunctive methods of predicting viability may help avoid unnecessary massive bowel resection. Doppler ultrasound,[26,27] photoplethysmography,[28] fluorescein,[27] pulse oximetry,[29] and surface oximetry[30] have been used to help predict viability. In a prospective controlled study of 28 patients, Bulkley and associates[27] found clinical judgment to be 89% accurate in predicting intestinal viability compared to 84% for Doppler ultrasound and 100% for fluorescein injection. Other clinical evaluations of fluorescein have failed to reproduce this high accuracy rate because interpretation of the intensity and pattern of fluorescence under Wood's lamp illumination is rather subjective. Methods for quantitative interpretation of fluorescence have not found clinical utility.

Second-look laparotomy should be employed whenever the viability of any segment of intestine cannot be accurately judged at the original operation. The decision to perform a second-look operation should not be reversed on the basis of a seemingly benign postoperative course. Postoperative bowel necrosis and anastomotic leakage cannot be detected by clinical parameters until they are irreversible. Therefore, morbidity and mortality will be minimized with the early detection that a second laparotomy provides. If doubt still remains at the time of the second look, additional exploratory laparotomies can be planned.

Perioperative Management

Perhaps the most challenging aspect of caring for the patient with acute mesenteric ischemia is the nonoperative component. Massive fluid, electrolyte, and acid-base shifts are the rule rather than the exception. Hemodynamic lability should be expected. Significant comorbid diseases are common in this patient population.

Preoperative care should focus on expeditious volume resuscitation, correction of significant electrolyte abnormalities, and general hemodynamic support. Volume requirements are frequently underestimated: the capacity of ischemic bowel for massive fluid sequestration leads to major but covert losses of extracellular fluid. Large-bore peripheral IV access is essential, and urine output should be monitored hourly as a guide to volume replacement. The choice of a balanced crystalloid solution should be based on specific electrolyte abnormalities. Lactated Ringer's solution is a reasonable initial fluid for resuscitation pending laboratory electrolyte analysis.

In the operating room, therapy proceeds along two parallel courses: the surgeon identifies and corrects the pathologic state of the bowel, and the anesthesiologist provides ongoing and aggressive supportive care, assisted by liberal use of hemodynamic monitoring. Support of blood pressure and cardiac performance may require inotropic and pressor agents, but volume replacement should be the first line of treatment. Blood and blood products are administered as needed to ensure optimal oxygen delivery and to correct consumptive coagulopathies. All available measure should be employed to prevent and/or treat hypothermia.

Postoperative care includes ongoing volume replacement and correction of any metabolic derangements. Anticoagulation therapy may be indicated, depending on the etiology of the ischemic event. Nutritional support is critical, and typically must be administered parenterally over the first few days and longer if bowel resection has been performed. In spite of the recognized advantages of early enteral nutrition, it has been the authors' experience that enteral feeding is seldom tolerated by patients with acute and often chronic mucosal injury.

COMPLICATIONS

Multisystemic organ failure is the most feared complication following successful revascularization of ischemic bowel. Reperfusion injury, mediated by reactive oxygen intermediates and multiple cytokines, is a contributing factor. Reperfusion effects are not limited to the previously ischemic organ but are wide-ranging. Turnage and coworkers demonstrated that reperfusion of acutely ischemic bowel causes hepatic injury characterized by decreased bile flow rates, increased release of hepatocellular enzymes, and increased hepatic white blood cell infiltration.[31] Although this hepatic injury is generally reversible, it may result in a significant vitamin K–resistant coagulopathy or contribute to severe metabolic derangement. Schmeling and coworkers[32] demonstrated acute lung injury following reperfusion of acutely ischemic bowel in an animal model. Reperfusion after 2 hours of bowel ischemia resulted in lung adenosine triphosphate levels decreasing by 60% and lung neutrophil accumulation increasing by sevenfold above baseline. Pulmonary microvascular permeability increased threefold. Pulmonary physiologic shunting and increased peak inspiratory pressures are also characteristic lung effects of reperfusion injury. In a study of reperfusion effects with chronically ischemic bowel, Harward et al noted a high incidence of early postoperative hepatic, renal, and pulmonary insufficiency despite their technique of partial occlusion clamping of the aorta.[33] In that study, 16 of 18 patients had acute pulmonary insufficiency on postoperative day 2. This

high-risk time period is notable clinically as a frequent point of reintubation after successful early extubation. Renal effects of reperfusion may be a direct result of toxic mediators or secondary to hepatic dysfunction, as in the hepatorenal syndrome.

Aside from reperfusion, a number of complications are associated with the medical, radiologic, or operative treatment of acute mesenteric ischemia. Acute renal failure, myocardial infarction, hepatic failure with coagulopathy, acute respiratory distress syndrome, sepsis (possibly from bacterial translocation), synthetic graft infection, graft thrombosis, and intraperitoneal hemorrhage occur not uncommonly.

Postoperative hemorrhage is often precipitated or aggravated by coagulopathy, which itself often results from ischemic hepatic dysfunction, as characterized by Cohen.[25,34] Surgically correctable bleeding may also contribute to the development and persistence of coagulopathy and must not be overlooked either during or after surgery. Intraoperative use of the "cell saver," in the absence of contamination from gangrenous or perforated bowel, may help reduce the transfusion requirement.

OUTCOME

In a review of the recent literature on acute mesenteric ischemia, Taylor and Monetta[12] found a cumulative mortality of 70% in 120 patients with embolism and 92% in 86 patients with arterial thrombosis. Nonocclusive intestinal ischemia was associated with a 92% mortality rate. Death from mesenteric venous thrombosis occurred less commonly, and was 35% in these authors' report.[35] In fact, autopsy series have shown that portomesenteric venous thrombosis results in bowel infarction in less than half of cases.[36]

SUMMARY

The key to reducing the high mortality of acute mesenteric ischemia is preventive efforts targeted at the specific etiologic risk factors. Specifically, this includes therapeutic anticoagulation for the patient with uncorrectible embolic risk factors, early diagnosis and elective revascularization for the patient with chronic mesenteric ischemia, anticoagulation and decompression to relieve stasis when warranted for the patient at risk for venous thrombosis, and aggressive treatment of low flow states such as congestive heart failure.

Furthermore, early diagnosis, prompt referral, angiographic confirmation in selected cases, and aggressive medical, radiologic, and operative treatment will afford the best chance of survival. Revascularization strategies must not be overlooked in favor of simple resection. Advances in perioperative intensive care over the past decade have resulted in improved outcomes following intervention, but the emphasis must be on prevention and earlier diagnosis to further lower mortality rates.

REFERENCES

1. Rivers S. Acute nonocclusive mesenteric ischemia. *Semin Vasc Surg* 1990;3:172.

2. Elliott JP Jr, Hageman JH, Szilagyi E, et al. Arterial embolization: problems of source, multiplicity, recurrence and delayed treatment. *Surgery* 1980;88:833–845.

3. Clavien PA, Durig M, Harder F. Venous mesenteric infarction, a particular entity. *Br J Surg* 1988;75:252–255.

4. Svensson PJ, Dahlback B. Resistance to activated protein C as a basis for venous thrombosis. *N Engl J Med* 1994;330:517–522.

5. Greengard JS, Eichinger S, Griffin JH, Bauer KA. Brief report: variability of thrombosis among siblings with resistance to activated protein C due to an Arg to Gln mutation in the gene for factor 5. *N Engl J Med* 1994;331:1559–1562.

6. Greene FL, Ariyan S, Stausel HC Jr. Mesenteric and peripheral vascular ischemia secondary to ergotism. *Surgery* 1977;81:176–179.

7. Nalbandian H, Sheth N, Dietrich R, et al. Intestinal ischemia caused by cocaine ingestion: report of two cases. *Surgery* 1985;97:374–376.

8. Kim EH, Gewertz BL. Chronic digitalis administration alters mesenteric vascular reactivity. *J Vasc Surg* 1987;5:382–389.

9. Kawauchi M, Tada Y, Asano K, et al. Angiographic demonstration of mesenteric arterial changes in postcoarctectomy syndrome. *Surgery* 1985;98:602–604.

10. Gennaro M, Ascer E, Matano R, Jacobowitz IJ, Cunningham JN Jr, Uceda P. Acute mesenteric ischemia after cardiopulmonary bypass. *Am J Surg* 1993;166:231–236.

11. Allen KB, Salam AA, Lumsden AB. Acute mesenteric ischemia after cardiopulmonary bypass. *J Vasc Surg* 1992;16:391–396.

12. Taylor LM, Moneta GL. Basic data underlying decision-making in vascular surgery. Intestinal ischemia. *Ann Vasc Surg* 1991;5:403–406.

13. Dunphy JE. Abdominal pain of vascular origin. *Am J Med Sci* 1936;192:109–113.

14. Leitman IM, Paull DE, Barie PS, Isom OW, Shires GT. Intra-abdominal complications of cardiopulmonary bypass operations. *Surg Gynecol Obstet* 1987;165:251–254.

15. Siegelman SS, Sprayregan S, Boley SJ. Angiographic diagnosis of mesenteric arterial vasoconstriction. *Sprayregen Radiology* 1974;112:533.

16. Ohri SK, Desai JB, Gaer JAR, et al. Intra-abdominal complications after cardiopulmonary bypass. *Ann Thorac Surg* 1991;52:226–231.

17. Goodman EH. Angina abdominis. *Am J Med Sci* 1918;155:524–528.

18. Ottinger LW. The surgical management of acute occlusion of the superior mesenteric artery. *Ann Surg* 1978;188:72L–736.

19. Moneta GL, Yeager RA, Dalman R, Antonovic R, Hall LD, Porter LM. Duplex ultrasound criteria for diagnosis of splanchnic artery stenosis or occlusion. *J Vasc Surg* 1991;14:511–520.

20. Bowersox JC, Zwolak RM, Walsh DB, et al. Duplex ultrasonography in the diagnosis of celiac and mesenteric artery occlusive disease. *J Vasc Surg* 1991;14:780–788.

21. Clavien PA, Huber O, Mirescu D, Rohner A. Contrast enhanced CT scan as a diagnostic procedure in mesenteric ischaemia due to mesenteric venous thrombosis. *Br J Surg* 1989;76:93–94.

22. Richardson J, Flint LM, Polk LM. Peritoneal lavage: a useful diagnostic adjunct for peritonitis. *Surgery* 1983;93:826–829.

23. Boley SJ, Sprayregen S, Siegelman SS, Veith FJ. Initial results from an aggressive roentgenological and surgical approach to acute mesenteric ischemia. *Surgery* 1977;82:848–855.

24. Boley SJ, Feinstein FR, Sammartano R, Brandt LJ, Sprayregen S. New concepts in the management of emboli of the superior mesenteric artery. *Surg Gynecol Obstet* 1981;153:561–569.

25. Cohen JR, Augus L, Asher A, Chang JB, Wise L. Disseminated intravascular coagulation as a result of supraceliac clamping: implications for thoracoabdominal aneurysm repair. *Ann Vasc Surg* 1987;1:522–557.

26. Wright CB, Hobson RW. Prediction of intestinal viability using Doppler ultrasound technique. *Am J Surg* 1975;129:642–645.

27. Bulkley GB, Zuidema GD, Hamilton SR, et al. Intraoperative determination of small bowel viability following ischemic injury. A prospective, controlled trial of two adjuvant methods (Doppler and fluoroscein) compared with standard clinical judgment. *Ann Surg* 1981;193:628–637.

28. Pearce WH, Joness DN, Warren GH, et al. The use of infrared photoplethysmography in identifying early intestinal ischemia. *Arch Surg* 1987;193:628–637.

29. Denobile J, Guzzetta P, Patterson K. Pulse oximetry as a mean of assessing bowel viability. *J Surg Res* 1990;48:21–23.

30. Ferrara J, Dyess D, Lasecki M, et al. Surface oximetry: a new method to evaluate intestinal perfusion. *Am Surg* 1988;54:10–14.

31. Turnage RH, Bagnasco J, Berger J, Guice KS, Oldham KT, Hinshaw DB. Hepatocellular oxidant stress following intestinal ischemia-reperfusion injury. *J Surg Res* 1991;51:467–471.

32. Schmeling DJ, Caty MG, Oldham KT, Guice KS, Hinshaw DB. Evidence for neutrophil-related acute lung injury after intestinal ischemia-reperfusion. *Surgery* 1989;106:195–202.

33. Harward TRS, Brooks DL, Flynn TC, Seeger JM. Multiple organ dysfunction after mesenteric artery revascularization. *J Vasc Surg* 1993;18:459–469.

34. Cohen JR, Schroder W, Leal J, Wise L. Mesenteric shunting during thoracoabdominal aortic clamping to prevent disseminated intravascular coagulation in dogs. *Ann Vasc Surg* 1988;2:261–267.

35. Abdu RA, Zakhour BJ, Dallis DJ. Mesenteric venous thrombosis 1911 to 1984. *Surgery* 1987;101:383–388.

36. Johnson CC, Baggenstoss AH. Mesenteric venous occlusion. Study of 99 cases of occlusion of veins. *Mayo Clin Proc* 1949;24:628.

55

Surgical Treatment of Chronic Mesenteric Arterial Occlusive Disease: Options and Results

Paul DiMuzio, M.D.
Ronald J. Stoney, M.D.

Chronic mesenteric ischemia is caused by atherosclerosis of the paravisceral aorta and the proximal portions of the unpaired major aortic branches, the celiac axis (CA) and superior mesenteric artery (SMA). Frequently the minor visceral aortic branch, the inferior mesenteric artery (IMA), is also occluded or narrowed, and the hypogastric arteries provide critical flow to the upper abdominal viscera via the mesenteric and gastroduodenal collateral pathways. These collateral branches originate beyond the obstructing disease in the proximal aortic visceral branches (Fig. 55–1).

Impairment of the visceral circulation develops gradually, and eventually symptoms of mesenteric ischemia appear secondary to inadequate blood flow. Postprandial abdominal pain, weight loss, food aversion, and intestinal dysmotility are seen. The patient is frequently suspected of having peptic ulcer disease, malignancy, or another nonspecific disorder. The diagnosis is often delayed for months or even years, and intensive gastrointestinal evaluations exclude even remote diagnostic possibilities. Finally, a biplane aortogram is performed, revealing the distribution of disease and the collateral pathways classic for this disease. If untreated, the patient may develop visceral gangrene, which is often fatal.[1–3]

This chapter focuses on our preferred treatment strategies at the University of California, San Francisco (UCSF), for patients with chronic mesenteric ischemia caused by atherosclerosis. The exposure, approach, and surgical technique, refined over nearly 40 years, and the long-term results of transaortic visceral endarterec-

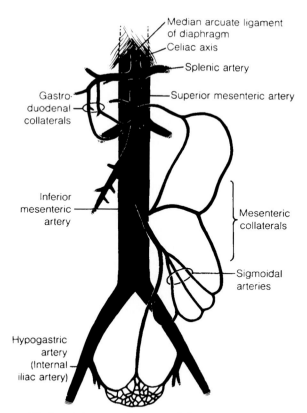

Figure 55–1. Schematic drawing of the visceral circulation demonstrating the collateral pathways between the CA, SMA, IMA, and pelvic circulation.

tomy and antegrade aortovisceral prosthetic bypass will be described.

CLINICAL PRESENTATION

The typical patient is female, in her sixth or seventh decade, who complains of significant postprandial abdominal pain. The pain usually occurs 15 to 30 minutes following food ingestion and is located in the epigastrium. The consistent and chronic nature of this pain leads to food aversion, or *food fear*. Loss of up to 20% of body weight ensues, depending on the duration of symptoms. Symptoms of intestinal dysmotility, usually diarrhea, are also common. Mikkelson in 1957 named this clinical syndrome *intestinal angina*,[4] and that term or *abdominal angina* persists today. Physical examination reveals a scaphoid abdomen, and an epigastric bruit is heard frequently (50 to 80% of patients).[5-11] Associated findings of peripheral vascular and coronary artery disease are common.[12]

It is important to remember that atherosclerosis of the aortic visceral branches is frequently found incidentally at autopsy in patients dying of other causes; symptomatic chronic mesenteric ischemia is rare.[13-15] Often these lesions are not hemodynamically significant, but even when they are, the collateral circulation between the mesenteric vessels provides abundant visceral blood flow. Most authors state that two of the three major visceral arteries must be significantly obstructed or stenosed to produce symptoms of chronic visceral ischemia.[5-11,16-24] A rarer pattern of upper aortic atherosclerosis, termed *coral reef* atheroma, may cause chronic mesenteric ischemia.[25] These large, calcified, polypoid lesions originate in the posterior surface of the upper abdominal aorta and impair blood flow through the lumen of the aorta. This can impair circulation to the gastrointestinal viscera, kidneys, or lower extremities, together or singly. The anatomic distribution of disease will obviously dictate the most appropriate surgical treatment.

The pathophysiologic mechanism of the postprandial pain in chronic mesenteric ischemia is presumed to be an inability to increase intestinal blood flow, as required for intestinal metabolism following ingestion of food. The occurrence of pain 15 to 30 minutes postprandially, before the food has reached the small bowel, is the result of a "gastric steal." The hyperemic response of the stomach mandates an increase in blood flow that cannot be achieved by the diseased visceral arteries. The increased flow comes completely or partly from the SMA via the gastroduodenal collaterals, resulting in decreased small intestine perfusion and subsequent acidosis and pain.[26]

DIAGNOSTIC EVALUATION

Although chronic visceral ischemia is rare, the clinical presentation, as just outlined, is well defined. Patients frequently, however, undergo an extensive workup for abdominal pain consisting of barium studies, endos-copy, axial scanning, and other imaging studies. A high index of suspicion of vascular disease explaining the patient's complaints will help establish the diagnosis early, before the patient becomes nutritionally depleted. Even when the diagnosis of chronic visceral ischemia is suspected, selected studies should be performed to exclude other diseases, such as pancreatic neoplasm. The most useful screening test for suspected chronic mesenteric ischemia is duplex ultrasound, as described in Chapter 53.[27]

Biplane aortography is the gold standard test for establishing the diagnosis of chronic mesenteric ischemia and for planning revascularization. The lateral view of the aorta is necessary to visualize the visceral branch lesions in profile, and therefore is the most important view. The posteroanterior view allows visualization of the collateral pathways, which provide evidence of the hemodynamic significance of the visceral branch orifice disease.

The goal for the patient undergoing elective visceral revascularization is to restore a normal, durable circulation to the viscera without harm to the related vascular beds involved. The goal of an anesthesiologist faced with managing the patient intraoperatively is to maintain the required pain-free setting of general anesthesia that permits the surgical strategies needed to achieve the surgical goals.[28] The anesthesiologist should preserve myocardial, pulmonary, central nervous system, renal, and visceral function by ensuring adequate oxygenation of the heart and perfusion of all organs at risk. Careful systemic arterial, venous, and pulmonary pressure monitoring and selective use of two-dimensional transesophageal echocardiography are valuable adjuncts in this patient population with systemic atherosclerotic disease. These can increase the safety of supraceliac cross-clamping—a formidable myocardial strain that occurs during visceral revascularization.

INDICATIONS FOR TREATMENT

The treatment objectives in chronic mesenteric ischemia are two: (1) relief of the symptoms of chronic visceral ischemia and (2) prevention of visceral gangrene. As the natural history of symptomatic chronic visceral ischemia places patients in danger of fatal visceral infarction, all symptomatic patients should undergo visceral revascularization.

Prophylactic revascularization of the viscera is a more controversial subject. Most authorities agree that the presence of mesenteric atherosclerosis alone, in the absence of symptoms of intestinal angina, is not an indication for revascularization.[5-11,16-24] Collateral pathways play an important part in maintaining bowel viability, and even patients with occlusion of all three mesenteric vessels may be asymptomatic.[13]

Prophylactic revascularization is recommended in several selected circumstances, however. Patients undergoing an aortic operation who have coexisting severe occlusive disease involving the CA and SMA branches and collateral flow from the IMA require some form of revascularization. Examples include patients undergoing thoracoabdominal aneurysm repair, combined renal artery and aortic reconstruction, and infrarenal aortoiliac reconstruction. The prophylactic operations useful in these patterns of disease include transaortic thromboendarterectomy, antegrade aortovisceral bypass, and vessel reimplantation. Connolly and Kwaan[29] and Rheudasil et al[20] have reported their experiences with patients undergoing prophylactic revascularization during aortic surgery. At long-term follow-up, none of these patients developed intestinal infarction and there was no increase in operative mortality.

Prophylactic revascularization should be more liberally used in young patients with severe atherosclerosis of the visceral branches and in patients in whom crucial visceral collateral circulation may be disrupted by a planned gastroduodenal or left colonic resection.

TREATMENT STRATEGIES AND OUTCOME

Mesenteric revascularization began with transarterial endarterectomy of the SMA performed by Shaw and Maynard.[30] Other techniques, including reimplantation, retrograde bypass, and transarterial endarterectomy, have been abandoned by us due to an unacceptably high rate of failure, either early or late.[17]

Transaortic Visceral Endarterectomy

Atherosclerosis of the upper abdominal aorta may involve the major visceral branches (CA and SMA) or may include the paired renal arteries. Typically, the atherosclerotic plaque involves the aortic wall and extends a short distance into the aortic branch origins, producing stenosis or occlusion. Extraction endarterectomy of the aortic branches through an aortotomy in the renal arteries was perfected at UCSF in the early 1950s. It was logical to extend these techniques to the major visceral branches, which are similar in size and arise from the adjacent upper abdominal aorta.

Because the overlying pancreas obscures access to the aorta anteriorly, we began our search for an ideal exposure. Originally this involved a transthoracic, retroperitoneal approach. This required left-to-right medial visceral rotation, which provided exposure of the entire upper abdominal aorta. This approach mandated a left thoracotomy that proved to be unnecessary to treat this pattern of atherosclerosis, and furthermore, added significant pulminary morbidity to the patient's post operative course. However, we now employ a transperitoreal left-to-right medial visceral rotation to perform visceral revascularization. Although there is an increased incidence of splenic injury and, rarely, transient pancreatitis, the pulmonary morbidity of left thoracotomy is eliminated.[31,32]

The abdomen is explored through a full-length midline incision. The left colon, spleen, and pancreas are rotated to the right side of the abdomen, leaving the left kidney in situ. After division of the left crus of the diaphragm, the autonomic ganglion tissue is mobilized and displaced beyond the midline. Circumferential mobilization of the upper aorta and all its branches is performed. Mannitol is given to promote diuresis, and the patient is anticoagulated with 3500 U of heparin. The distal thoracic aorta above and the juxtarenal aorta below are clamped, as are all intervening aortic branches, including the posterior paired intercostal and lumbar arteries.

Transaortic visceral thromboendarterectomy is peformed through an anterior "trapdoor" aortotomy surrounding the orifices of the CA and SMA (Fig. 55–2). An endarterectomy plane is established in the roof of the trapdoor. The ventral aortic atheroma is mobilized in continuity with the extensions of the plaque within the orifices of the visceral branches. Endpoints within the branches themselves are achieved via the extraction technique aided by simple eversion of each visceral branch. If the SMA is occluded, the distal endpoint and trailing thrombus may be extracted through the aorta or through a separate SMA arteriotomy for direct visualization, with subsequent patch closure (Fig. 55–3). Aortic ischemia time averages 25 minutes for the visceral branch endarterectomy alone and 30 minutes when renal endarterectomy is included.

Aortovisceral Bypass (Antegrade)

The method of revascularization used in approximately one-third of our patients at UCSF is aorta-visceral prosthetic bypass.[6,7] Although others use the retrograde orientation of the graft,[8,10,16,18,21] we prefer the antegrade prosthetic bypass using short segments of woven Dacron, 6 or 7 mm in diameter, in a bifurcated or occasionally a single-limb configuration. These originate from an undiseased part of the ventral, supraceliac aorta and are attached end-to-end to the visceral branch beyond the extend of the disease. This avoids the turbulence associated with retrograde graft orientation and end-to-side anastomosis. Antegrade alignment and configuration are also less prone to kinking or to contact with overlying viscera.

Exposure of the supraceliac aorta for antegrade grafting can be performed via a transperitoneal, transcrural approach (Fig. 55–4). The CA and proximal SMA exposure requires division of the median arcuate ligament and mobilization and caudad displacement of the superior border of the pancreas. A flanged or bifurcated graft originates from an appropriately sized aortotomy on the anterior supraceliac aorta and is anastomosed end-to-end to the CA and SMA beyond the disease.

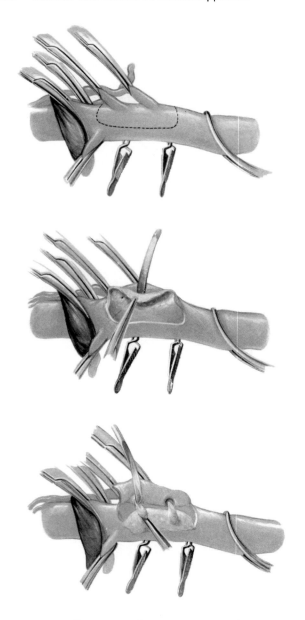

Figure 55–2. Illustrations of transaortic visceral endarterectomy. Top: the trapdoor aortotomy surrounding the visceral orifices is outlined. Middle: an endarterectomy plane is established in the roof of the trapdoor. Bottom: the Halle elevator gently displaces the arterial wall from the atheroma until the endpoint is visualized and separates in the SMA. The CA endarterectomy is complete.

While the transcrural approach allows access to the supraceliac aorta, the exposure is vertically oriented, and aortic mobilization can be awkward and incomplete. As described for transaortic endarterectomy, we now prefer to expose the upper abdominal aorta for aortovisceral bypass using left medial visceral rotation. This exposure simplifies both the proximal aortic and distal SMA anastomoses, and it allows uncompromised antegrade graft placement.

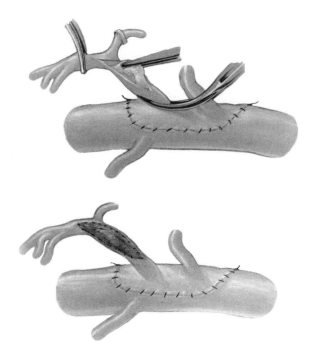

Figure 55–3. Top: following a transaortic visceral thromboendarterectomy, flow is restored in the aorta. A persistent distal thrombus occluding the SMA remains. A distal SM arteriotomy allows precise removal of this lesion, ensuring a satisfactory endpoint. Bottom: The completed repair is shown, with a saphenous vein patch applied to the SM arteriotomy to prevent narrowing.

If contamination or bowel necrosis is found at exploration, we avoid the use of prosthetic material for antegrade bypass. In this situation, transaortic endarterectomy or an autogenous graft conduit for bypass are appropriate choices for visceral revascularization.

Although several authors agree that single-vessel revascularization may be sufficient to relieve symptoms and prevent bowel ischemia,[6,7,16,17] many believe that multivessel revascularization is preferred in the event of late occlusion of a graft.[5,8–11,21,23,24] This implies that visceral revascularization is prone to failure, an event that is rare in our experience. When single-vessel revascularization is chosen, we prefer CA rather than SMA revascularization. We have observed that among patients who had simultaneous revascularization of the CA and SMA, symptoms recurred when the CA repair failed, despite patency of the SMA repair.[6,7] Conversely, patients whose SMA repair occluded remained asymptomatic as long as CA revascularization functioned. If neither the CA nor the SMA can be directly reconstructed, a situation we have observed only in reoperative visceral procedures, revascularization of the IMA alone will provide effective symptom relief through the important mesenteric collateral pathways (W.K. Ehrenfeld, unpublished series).

Reoperation for recurrent chronic visceral ischemia is effective, safe, and employs the strategies discussed in

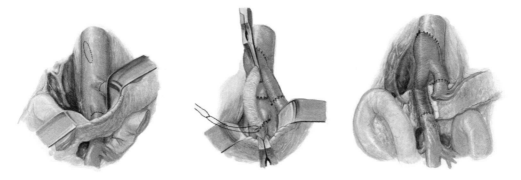

Figure 55–4. Illustrations of antegrade aortovisceral bypass. Left: exposure of the supraceliac and paravisceral aorta, with proposed aortotomy and transection sites of the CA and SMA. Middle: anastomoses to the aorta and CA are complete, while the remaining graft limb is anastomosed to the SMA beyond the extent of the disease. Right: the aortovisceral bypass is completed.

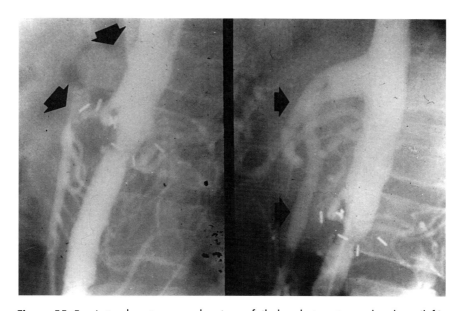

Figure 55–5. Lateral aortograms showing a failed endarterectomy elsewhere (left) and following subsequent aortovisceral bypass to the CA and SMA (right).

this chapter. In general, the diagnosis is established early, usually within a month, rather than over a year, as in primary cases, solely because the patient is known to have had a visceral revascularization. Aortography defines the failed original repair, and the operative strategy involves left medial visceral rotation and the reconstructive technique not used at the original visceral revascularization. For example, Figure 55–5 presents the aortogram at a patient who developed recurrent visceral ischemia after a previous endarterectomy occluded at 3 months. Aortovisceral bypass rescued the patient by restoring normal visceral circulation. The pre- and postoperative angiograms reveal the visceral artery problem and solution. Twenty patients have undergone repairs for recurrent chronic

visceral ischemia at UCSF, with 19 survivors being free of symptoms.

Assurance of Technical Success

Following visceral revascularization by either method, intraoperative duplex scanning is performed to examine the endarterectomy endpoints or graft anastomoses.[33] Any major defects are then repaired. Prior to discharge from the hospital, a postoperative aortogram is obtained to confirm the status of the repaired visceral arteries (Figs. 55–5 and 55–6).

Results of Treatment

The long-term survival for patients undergoing elective visceral revascularization largely depends on their inter-

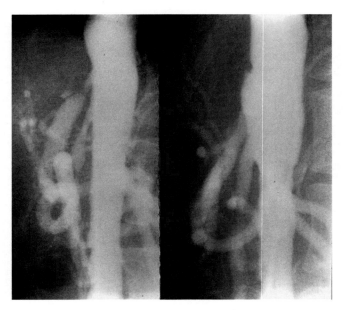

Figure 55–6. Lateral aortograms before (left) and after (right) transaortic visceral thromboendarterectomy.

current health problems. In this population, which generally averages the seventh decade of life, 5- and 10-year survival has been reported to be 68% and 50%, respectively, and deaths are predominantly cardiac in origin.[5,24]

Surgical Results

Visceral revascularization for chronic mesenteric ischemia has generally been highly successful. Despite advanced age, nutritional debility, and concomitant other vascular diseases, operative mortality in recent and larger experiences averages 8% (range, 0 to 15%).[5–11,16–24] Early reconstruction failure is always due to technical causes, occurs in less than 10% of patients, and is usually correctable. Patients who undergo successful revascularization are relieved of their symptoms and subsequently gain weight. Long-term symptom relief has been excellent with 5-year follow-up revealing that 86 to 90% of patients remain symptom free.[5,6]

Our preferred methods of revascularization have evolved over the past three decades and consist of transaortic visceral endarterectomy or antegrade prosthetic bypass.[6] A total of 74 patients (two-thirds endarterectomy, one-third bypass) were followed for an average of 71 months. Early failure was seen in 3% of reconstructions, and 86% of the patients were asymptomatic at long-term follow-up. These results support our continuing use of these methods of visceral revascularization in patients with chronic visceral ischemia, and there are no differences in the durability of these two procedures.

SUMMARY

Chronic visceral ischemia is an uncommon disorder resulting from the atherosclerotic narrowing or occlusion of the major visceral branches of the upper abdominal aorta. Abdominal angina is characterized by postpradial pain, weight loss, and intestinal dysmotility. This diagnosis is rarely considered in the initial workup for abdominal pain. A high index of suspicion of visceral ischemia as the etiology of this pain and the use of visceral duplex sonography are necessary to make the diagnosis early. The diagnosis of chronic mesenteric ischemia is confirmed when biplane aortography demonstrates the typical collateral patterns of visceral circulation and occlusion or stenosis of the CA and SMA. Visceral revascularization is indicated in symptomatic patients to relieve their symptoms, reverse their nutritional wasting, and prevent fatal visceral gangrene.

Surgical revascularization is accomplished in our institution using antegrade aortovisceral bypass or transaortic visceral endarterectomy, although others prefer retrograde aortovisceral bypass. Operative mortality is low in primary and reoperative patients, and long-term symptom-free survival is achievable in over 80% of cases. The revascularization procedure should include both the CA and SMA, whenever possible, to maximize the chance for long-term symptom relief.

ACKNOWLEDGMENT

Supported in part by Pacific Vascular Research Foundation, San Francisco.

REFERENCES

1. Dunphy JE. Abdominal pain of vascular origin. *Am J Med Sci* 1936;192:109–112.
2. Perdue GD Jr, Smith RB III. Intestinal ischemia due to mesenteric arterial disease. *Am Surg* 1970;36:152–6.
3. Williams LF Jr. Vascular insufficiency of the intestines. *Gastroenterology* 1971;61:757–77.
4. Mikkelson WP. Intestinal angina: its surgical significance. *Am J Surg* 1957;99:262.
5. McAfee MK, Cherry KJ, Naessens JM, et al. Influence of complete revascularization on chronic mesenteric ischemia. *Am J Surg* 1992;164(3):220–224.
6. Cunningham CG, Reilly LM, Rapp JH, Schneider PA, Stoney RJ. Chronic visceral ischemia. Three decades of progress. *Ann Surg* 1991;214(3):276–287.
7. Rapp JH, Reilly LM, Qvarfordt PG, Goldstone J, Ehrenfeld WK, Stoney RJ. Durability of endarterectomy and antegrade grafts in the treatment of chronic visceral ischemia. *J Vasc Surg* 1986;3(5):799–806.
8. Baur GM, Millay DJ, Taylor LM, Porter JM. Treatment of chronic visceral ischemia. *Am J Surg* 1984;148(1):138–144.
9. Hollier LH, Bernatz PE, Pairolero PC, Payne WS, Osmundson PJ. Surgical management of chronic intestinal ischemia: a reappraisal. *Surgery* 1981;90(6):940–946.

10. Eidemiller LR, Nelson JC, Porter JM. Surgical treatment of chronic visceral ischemia. *Am J Surg* 1979;138(2):264–268.
11. Crawford ES, Morris GC, Myhre HO, Roehm JOF. Celiac axis, superior mesenteric artery, and inferior mesenteric artery occlusion: surgical considerations. *Surgery* 1977;82(6):865–866.
12. Hansen KJ, Connelly DP, Stoney RJ. Visceral ischemic syndromes. In: Loscalzo J, Creager MA, Dzau VJ, eds. *Vascular Medicine.* Boston: Little, Brown; 1992:887–902.
13. Cheine, J. Complete obliteration of the celiac and mesenteric arteries: viscera receiving their blood supply through extraperitoneal system of vessel. *J Anat Physiol* 1868;3:65–66.
14. Reiner L, Jimenez FA, Rodriguez FL. Atherosclerosis in the mesenteric circulation. Observations and correlations with aortic and coronary atherosclerosis. *Am Heart J* 1963;66:200–209.
15. Derrick JR, Pollard HS, Moore RM. The pattern of arteriosclerotic narrowing of the celiac and superior mesenteric arteries. *Ann Surg* 1959;149:684–689.
16. Hertzer NR, Beven EG, Humphries AW. Chronic intestinal ischemia. *Surg Gynecol Obstet* 1977;145(3):321–328.
17. Stoney RJ, Ehrenfeld WK, Wylie EJ. Revascularization methods in chronic visceral ischemia caused by atherosclerosis. *Ann Surg* 1977;189(4):468–476.
18. Rogers DM, Thompson JE, Garrett WV, Talkington CM, Patman RD. Mesenteric vascular problems. A 26-year experience. *Ann Surg* 1982;195(5):554–565.
19. Beebe HG, MacFarlane S, Raker EJ. Supraceliac aortomesenteric bypass for intestinal ischemia. *J Vasc Surg* 1987;5(5):749–754.
20. Rheudasil JM, Stewart MT, Schellack JV, Smith RB, Salam AA, Perdue GD. Surgical treatment of chronic mesenteric arterial insufficiency. *J Vasc Surg* 1988;8(4):495–500.
21. Calderon M, Reul GJ, Gregoric ID, et al. Long-term results of the surgical management of symptomatic chronic intestinal ischemia. *J Cardiovasc Surg (Torino)* 1992;33(6):723–728.
22. Gentile AT, Moneta GL, Taylor LM, Park TC, McConnell DB, Porter JM. Isolated bypass to the superior mesenteric artery for intestinal ischemia. *Arch Surg* 1994;129(9):926–931.
23. McMillan WD, McCarthy WJ, Bresticker MR, et al. Mesenteric artery bypass: objective patency determination. *J Vasc Surg* 1995;21(5):729–740.
24. Johnston KW, Lindsay TF, Walker PM, Kalman PG. Mesenteric arterial bypass grafts: early and late results and suggested surgical approach for chronic and acute mesenteric ischemia. *Surgery* 1995;118(1):1–7.
25. Qvarfordt PG, Reilly LM, Sedwitz MM, Ehrenfeld WK, Stoney RJ. "Coral reef" atherosclerosis of the suprarenal aorta. *J Vasc Surg* 1984;1:903–909.
26. Poole JW, Sammartano RJ, Boley SJ. Hemodynamic basis of the pain of chronic mesenteric ischemia. *Am J Surg* 1987;153:171–176.
27. Moneta GL, Yeager RA, Dalman R, et al. Duplex ultrasound criteria for diagnosis of splanchnic artery stenosis or occlusion. *J Vasc Surg* 1991;14:511–520.
28. Roizen MF. Anesthesia goals for surgery to relieve or prevent visceral ischemia. In: Roizen MF, ed. *Anesthesia for Vascular Surgery.* New York: Churchill Livingstone; 1990:171–196.
29. Connolly JE, Kwaan JHM. Prophylactic revascularization of the gut. *Ann Surg* 1979;190:514–522.
30. Shaw RS, Maynard EP. Acute and chronic thrombosis of mesenteric arteries associated with malabsorption. *N Engl J Med* 1958;258:874–875.
31. Murray SP, Kuestner LM, Stoney RJ. Transperitoneal medial visceral rotation. *Ann Vasc Surg* 1995;9(2):209–216.
32. Reilly LM, Ramos TK, Murray SP, Cheng WK, Stoney RJ. Optimal exposure of the proximal abdominal aorta: a critical appraisal of transabdominal medial visceral rotation. *J Vasc Surg* 1994;19(3):375–390.
33. Okuhn SP, Reilly LM, Bennett JB, et al. Intraoperative assessment of renal and visceral artery reconstruction. *J Vasc Surg* 1987;5:137–147.

56

Mesenteric Angioplasty and Stenting for Chronic Mesenteric Ischemia

Alan H. Matsumoto, M.D.
John F. Angle, M.D.
Charles J. Tegtmeyer, M.D.

INTRODUCTION

The rarity of clinically apparent chronic mesenteric ischemia is a reflection of the abundant collateral circulation that exists among the visceral vessels. Gradual progressive stenosis of one or more of the major visceral arteries is generally well tolerated as long as adequate collateralization exists. Indeed, all three main vessels supplying the mesenteric circulation may become totally occluded without creating symptoms.[1] Although many authors feel that severe disease in at least two of the three main vessels is necessary to produce symptoms, it is now fairly well accepted that obstruction of one, two, or a combination of the three main visceral vessels can result in intestinal hypoperfusion and mesenteric ischemia. Therefore, correlating the symptoms of mesenteric ischemia with the degree of narrowing and the number of obstructed visceral vessels is not always straightforward.

Symptoms of chronic mesenteric ischemia include postprandial abdominal pain and eventually weight loss. A history of fear of food can sometimes be elicited. Nausea, vomiting, and diarrhea can also occur but are neither common to nor specific for this entity.[2,3] All symptomatic patients in whom the diagnosis is entertained should have a biplane abdominal aortogram to thoroughly evaluate the origins of the celiac artery, superior mesenteric artery (SMA), and inferior mesenteric artery (IMA). If proximal disease is not seen, selective catheterization and filming of each of these arteries is necessary to define the anatomy of the branch vessels (Fig. 56–1). Lesions with at least 70% narrowing of the cross-sectional area are hemodynamically significant. Stenoses of 50 to 70%, when associated with a peak-to-peak systolic blood pressure gradient greater than 10 mm Hg, should be considered significant. Stenoses of less than 50% are usually not flow limiting.

Patients with signs and symptoms consistent with intestinal angina and a hemodynamically significant stenosis in one or more of the mesenteric arteries should undergo a revascularization procedure. Unless mesenteric perfusion is restored, patients develop progressive symptoms and ultimately intestinal infarction.[4] Vascular lesions that can lead to chronic mesenteric ischemia are potentially amenable to treatment using endovascular techniques. However, percutaneous treatment has not been widely utilized.[5–20] This is probably because intestinal angina is relatively rare, and when it is present, it frequently remains undiagnosed until acute deterioration occurs.

Atherosclerosis is the most common cause of occlusive mesenteric vascular disease, but fibromuscular dysplasia (FMD) and vasculitides have also been known to cause chronic mesenteric ischemia.[21,22] Intimal hyperplasia can also lead to narrowing of bypass grafts to the mesenteric vessels, resulting in recurrent intestinal ischemia (Fig. 56–2).

ENDOVASCULAR TECHNIQUES

The technique for percutaneous transluminal angioplasty (PTA) of the mesenteric arteries is similar to that used in the renal arteries.[23] The femoral artery approach is usually employed. However, in patients with severe weight loss, the mesenteric arteries often originate at a steep caudad angle from the aorta, so that a high left brachial artery approach affords a

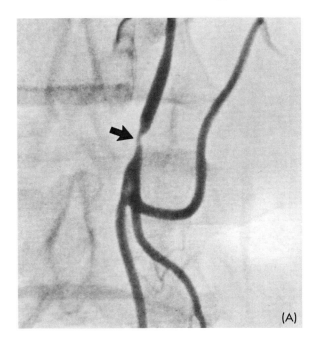

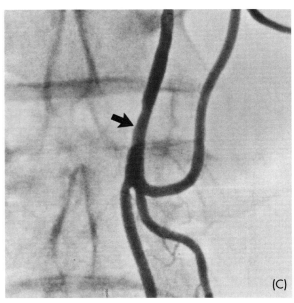

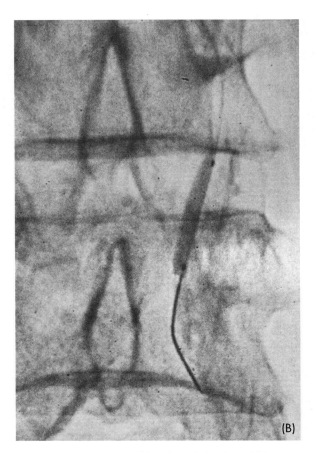

Figure 56–1. A 61-year-old male with bright red blood per rectum and endoscopically proven ischemic colitis underwent diagnostic angiography. The proximal celiac artery, SMA, and IMA were widely patent. (A) Selective catheterization and injection of the IMA revealed a tight stenosis of the IMA beyond its origin (arrow). (B) With the use of a 3-mm TEGwire balloon (Boston Scientific, Natick, MA), the lesion was dilated. (C) Control arteriogram after the PTA shows a good result (arrow). The patient's ischemic colitis resolved following the procedure. An angiogram 68 months after the PTA showed the treated site to be widely patent, and he remains asymptomatic. (Reprinted with permission from Tegtmeyer CJ, Matsumoto AH, Angle JF. Percutaneous transcatheter therapy of visceral ischemia. In: Ernst CB, Stanley JC, eds. Current Therapy in Vascular Surgery, 3rd ed. St. Louis: Mosby Year Book; 1995:689–693.)

mechanical advantage for endovascular interventions over the femoral approach.

With the standard over-the-wire balloon system, the high left brachial artery approach provides better control for crossing the stenosis and subsequent positioning of the balloon and/or stent. A better result in resistant lesions may also be achieved because the balloon is more parallel to the axis of the mesenteric vessel. The drawback to a high brachial approach is the increased risk of damage to the nerves to the upper extremity from a hematoma. The proximal brachial artery also tends to be smaller in diameter than the common femoral artery and may not tolerate the use of a 7 F or 8 F introducer sheath.

We usually begin the interventional portion of the procedure after placement of a 6 F introducer sheath. When approaching the lesion from the brachial artery, a preshaped 5 F catheter (multipurpose or H1H shape) facilitates catheterization. A reverse-curve catheter, such as a shepherd's crook, RC 1, or Simmonds 1, is preferred from the femoral approach. A floppy-tipped guidewire (Bentson wire, Cook, Inc., Bloomington, IN) or a steerable guidewire (Glidewire, Terumo Corp., Tokyo, Japan) is used to traverse the lesion. Once the guidewire is across the lesion, the catheter is advanced beyond the stenosis and contrast material is injected to confirm the intraluminal location. We routinely administer 2000 to 3000 units of heparin during the proce-

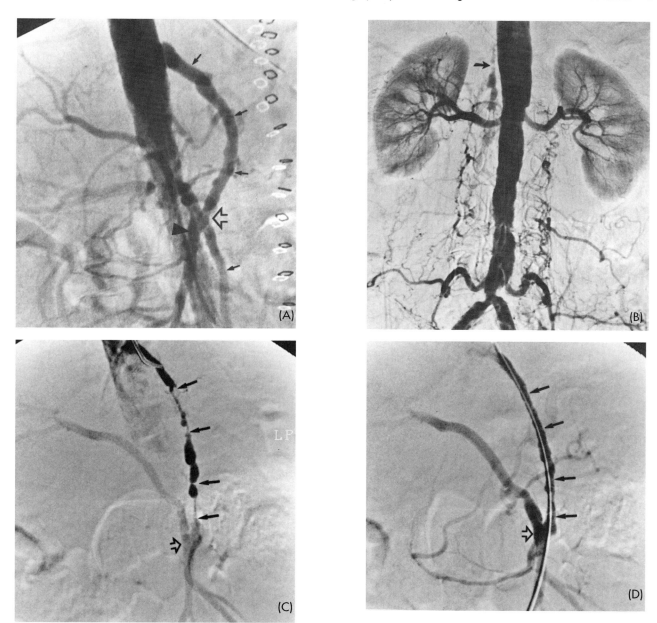

Figure 56–2. A 61-year-old female with postprandial abdominal pain and weight loss had a diagnostic arteriogram, which revealed complete occlusion of the celiac artery, SMA, and IMA, with reconstitution of these vessels via internal iliac artery collaterals. (A) The patient underwent a side-to-side anastomosis (open arrow) between the venous bypass graft (small arrows) and the SMA (arrowhead), with extension of the graft to the IMA in an end-to-side fashion. The patient was asymptomatic for 12 months. (B) She presented 15 months later with a 3-month history of recurrent symptoms, a 10-lb weight loss, and an abdominal bruit. An aortogram revealed diffuse disease of the bypass graft (arrow), with no antegrade flow into the SMA or IMA. The internal iliac arteries reconstituted the mesenteric circulation via collaterals. (C) Selective catheterization of the venous bypass graft demonstrates diffuse disease of the venous conduit (closed arrows) to the level of the side-to-side anastomosis with the SMA (open arrow). (D) Following PTA with a 5-mm-diameter balloon, the venous bypass graft is widely patent (closed arrows). The patient's symptoms resolved, and she has remained asymptomatic for 8 months of follow-up. (Reprinted with permission from Matsumoto AH, Tegtmeyer CJ, Angle JF. Endovascular interventions for chronic mesenteric ischemia. In: Baum S, Pentecost MJ, Eds. Abrams Angiography: Interventional Radiology, Vol. III. Boston: Little, Brown; 1997; 326–328.

dure. Vasodilating agents are not given unless spasm is identified. A 200-cm Rosen wire (Cook, Inc.) is used to exchange the diagnostic catheter for an appropriately-sized balloon catheter. The balloon diameter is chosen according to the size of the artery on the lateral cut-film arteriogram; no allowance is made for magnification. This results in a slight but fairly consistent (about 30% at our institution) overdilatation of the artery. If there is a question about balloon size, it is prudent to choose the smaller balloon.

The balloon is inflated for approximately 30 to 60 seconds to a pressure sufficient to eliminate any "waist" on the balloon. The patient may experience some abdominal, chest, or back pain during balloon inflation, but the pain should rapidly abate on balloon deflation. If the pain does not decrease following balloon deflation, a repeat arteriogram should be performed to exclude vessel rupture. If the patient experiences severe pain during balloon inflation, a smaller balloon should be used.

Following balloon dilatation, the balloon catheter is removed and a 6 F nontapered catheter with a radiopaque marker at its tip and an 0.061-inch ID (Microvena Corp., Vadnais, MN) can be fitted with a side arm adapter and advanced over the 0.035-inch exchange wire. A control arteriogram is then performed.

Whenever possible, the endpoint of the procedure should be complete ablation of the lesion. Residual stenoses greater than 30% or residual pressure gradients greater than 10 mm Hg are associated with higher recurrence rates. If a balloon with an appropriate diameter has been used but elastic recoil or a dissection leads to a suboptimal PTA result, placement of a vascular stent is helpful. Vascular stents are not currently Food and Drug Administration (FDA) approved for use in the mesenteric circulation, but both the Palmaz balloon-expandable stent (Johnson & Johnson Interventional Systems, Warren, NJ) and the self-expanding Wallstent (SchneiderUSA, Inc., Minneapolis, MN) have been used in this vascular bed.

The Palmaz stent requires the use of a long, reinforced 7 F sheath (Super Arrow-Flex, Arrow International, Inc., Reading, PA) or a short 8 F sheath with an 8 F guiding catheter. The guiding catheter that we have found to be most useful is a hockey stick–shaped guiding catheter (Cordis Corp., Miami, FL) with an 0.086-inch ID. The guiding catheter should be at least 80 cm in length. The shaft of the balloon catheter on which the Palmaz stent is loaded should be at least 20 cm longer than the guiding catheter. Insertion of a Palmaz stent is facilitated by a high left brachial artery approach, but the accessed artery must be large enough to tolerate insertion of a 7 F or 8 F introducer sheath. Indeed, we have had two patients in whom the brachial artery was used to place a mesenteric artery stent develop thrombosis after the procedure.

Insertion of a Wallstent requires a 7 F introducer sheath but no guiding catheter. The Wallstent is more flexible than the Palmaz stent. Therefore, it can be inserted from either a femoral or a high left brachial artery approach. The delivery catheter for the standard Wallstent is only 75 cm in length and may be too short to allow its insertion into a mesenteric artery from a high left brachial artery approach. The Wallstent is also available on longer delivery catheters (135 cm) for use in the tracheobronchial system. The deployment mechanism of the Wallstent requires unrestricted retraction of the constraining sleeve to allow exposure and expansion of the Wallstent. If the mesenteric vessel is angled acutely caudad from the abdominal aorta, withdrawal of the constraining sleeve of the delivery device from a femoral artery approach can be problematic secondary to friction and prevent the Wallstent from being properly deployed.

RESULTS

Following the initial description of SMA angioplasty in 1980 by Furrer et al,[5] there have been scattered case reports on the use of PTA for the treatment of mesenteric ischemia.[6–10] More recently, several series have been published on this topic[2,11–20] (Table 56–1). A meta-analysis of these 11 reports reveals a mean initial technical success rate of 86% (108 of 126 patients). Excluding the initial technical failures, the mean initial clinical success rate (as measured by resolution of symptoms) is 90%. Long-term primary and secondary clinical success rates are 76% and 92%, respectively. The mean follow-up period varied between 9 to 39 months, with follow-up as long occurring as 101 months after the procedure. Major complications occurred in 6.0% of the patients, and the 30-day mortality rate was 3.0%.

Since the time of our initial report,[17] we have treated a total of 32 patients with endovascular therapy: 22 for classic symptoms of chronic mesenteric ischemia, 6 for symptoms atypical for mesenteric ischemia, and 4 to prevent the development of mesenteric ischemia. Of the 22 patients with classic symptoms of chronic mesenteric ischemia, 10 were male and 12 were female. Their mean age was 65 years. Risk factors included smoking, hypertension, diabetes, and coronary artery disease. Postprandial abdominal pain and either weight loss (n = 15; range of weight loss, 6 to 80 pounds; mean, 23 pounds), surgical or endoscopic findings of ischemic bowel, or angiographic demonstration of more than 70% stenosis in at least two of the three visceral arteries were present in 21 of the 22 patients. The 26 lesions treated in the 22 patients were all stenoses (1 fibromuscular dysplasia, 22 atherosclerotic, and 3 related to intimal hyperplasia in bypass grafts).

Our initial technical success rate was 91% (20 of 22 patients). Initial technical failures were related to the median arcuate ligament in one patient and to a combination of the median arcuate ligament and an occult malignancy in the second patient. Excluding the initial technical failures, our initial clinical success rate was 90% (18 of 20 patients). In the two clinical failures, one patient was subsequently diagnosed with an occult carcinoma metastatic to the porta hepatis. The other patient underwent successful PTA of the celiac artery but had total occlusion of both the SMA and IMA. An

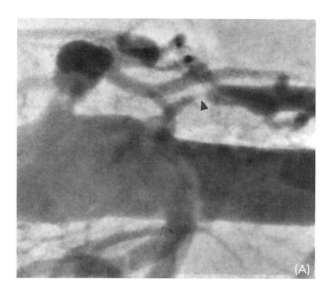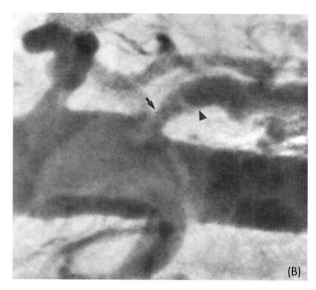

Figure 56–3. A 60-year-old female presented with postprandial abdominal pain and a 40-lb weight loss. (A) A diagnostic arteriogram revealed an occluded IMA, 50% stenosis of the celiac artery, and 95% stenosis of the SMA (arrowhead). (B) An arteriogram following the PTA showed no residual stenosis at the site of 95% narrowing (arrowhead). A residual 30% ostial narrowing (arrow) was seen. The patient had immediate relief of her pain and has gained 50 lb at 33 months of follow-up. (Reprinted with permission from Matsumoto AH, Tegtmeyer CJ, Fitzcharles EJ, et al. Percutaneous transluminal angioplasty of visceral arterial stenoses: results and long-term clinical follow-up. (see Ref #17) *J Vasc Intervent Radiol* 1995;6:165–174.)

IMA endarterectomy at the time of an aortobifemoral bypass graft 4 days after PTA resulted in complete relief of symptoms. Of the 18 patients who had both a technically and a clinically successful PTA, recurrent stenosis occurred in 2. Repeat PTA was successful in one of these patients. Therefore, our long-term primary clinical success rate was 89% (16 of 18 patients) (Fig. 56–3), with a secondary clinical success rate of 94% (17 of 18 patients). Clinical follow-up was obtained in all patients, with a mean follow-up of 30 months (range, 1 to 101 months).

In general, we refer most patients with complete mesenteric artery occlusions for surgical revascularization. However, there have been reports documenting the successful use of endovascular therapy for patients with mesenteric artery occlusions.[7–10,16] Simonetti et al published a series on seven patients with either acute, chronic, or acute on chronic mesenteric ischemia and complete arterial occlusions.[16] Five of these seven patients (71%) were successfully revascularized with a combination of thrombolysis and balloon angioplasty.

There have also been isolated reports on the use of vascular stents in the treatment of mesenteric arterial disease. In the largest series to date, 12 patients with classic symptoms of chronic mesenteric ischemia underwent placement of a Strecker balloon-expanded tantalum stent following a suboptimal balloon PTA.[24] A stent was placed in the celiac artery in three patients and in the SMA in nine patients. All patients had immediate improvement in symptoms. Four patients developed restenoses within the stent (one patient at 6 months and three patients at more than 24 months)

but were successfully retreated with PTA. Therefore, the long-term primary clinical benefit was 67%, with a secondary clinical benefit of 100%. The mean follow-up period was 28 months (range, 6 to 48 months).

We have successfully placed mesenteric arterial stents to supplement endovascular therapy in four patients with chronic mesenteric ischemia. In all cases, a suboptimal PTA result was the indication for stent placement (Fig. 56–4). Two patients also had a second mesenteric vessel balloon dilated. All patients are asymptomatic at a mean follow-up period of 15 months (range, 3 to 32 months).

There are relatively few indications for revascularization in patients with asymptomatic mesenteric arterial disease. However, in certain patients with tenuous mesenteric circulation who are undergoing procedures involving the abdominal aorta, prophylactic mesenteric artery revascularization may be indicated to reduce the incidence of postoperative mesenteric ischemia.[25,26] Division of the IMA during reconstruction of the abdominal aorta, in conjunction with disease of the SMA and iliac arteries, predisposes the patient to the development of postoperative mesenteric ischemia.[25] In one study, bowel infarction that occurred after reconstructive abdominal aortic surgery was associated with a 100% mortality rate.[26]

Although little has been written about prophylactic mesenteric revascularization, we have treated four patients with mesenteric artery PTA for this indication. Two of these patients had significant disease of the SMA, IMA, abdominal aorta, and both common and internal iliac arteries. Because of concern about the

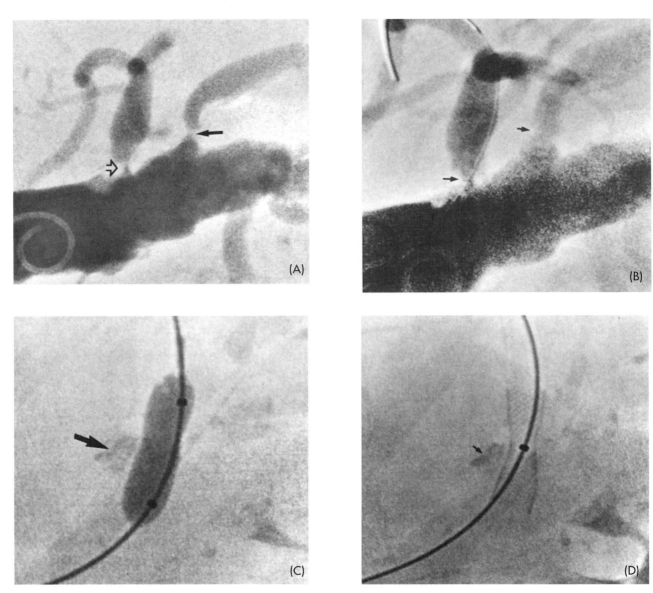

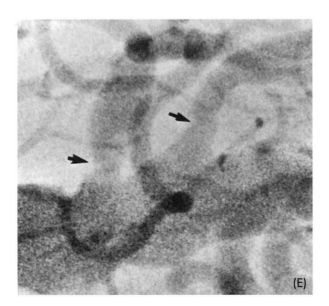

Figure 56–4.   A 60-year-old female presented with an 11-lb weight loss and a 4-month history of vague abdominal pain associated with eating solid food. She had had a prior aortobifemoral bypass graft. (A) A diagnostic arteriogram demonstrated an 80% stenosis of the SMA (straight arrow) and a 95% stenosis of the celiac artery (open arrow). The IMA was occluded. (B) Following balloon dilatation of the SMA and celiac artery, the SMA had a satisfactory appearance (short arrow), but the celiac artery remained narrowed (long arrow). (C) The resistant lesion involving the celiac artery was related to a calcified plaque (arrow), which was easily visualized at the time of balloon dilatation. (D) An 8-mm-diameter, 20-mm-long Wallstent was deployed in the celiac artery, and balloon dilated to 9 mm in diameter. A residual "waist" on the stent secondary to the calcified plaque (arrow) could not be completely obliterated. (E) Despite this, the control arteriogram demonstrated a satisfactory appearance of the celiac artery (short arrow) and SMA (long arrow). The patient had resolution of her symptoms and is asymptomatic at 22 months of follow-up. (Reprinted with permission from Matsumoto AH, Tegtmeyer CJ, Angle JF. Endovascular interventions for chronic mesenteric ischemia. In: Baum S, Pentecost MJ, eds. *Abrams Angiography: Interventional Radiology*, Vol III. Boston: Little, Brown; 1997:326–338.

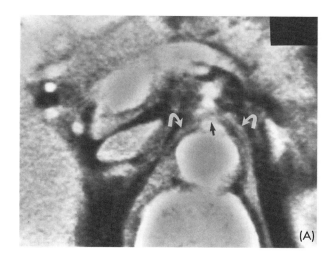

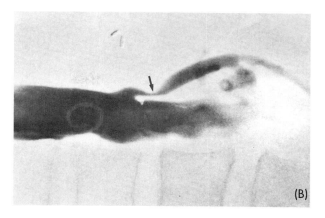

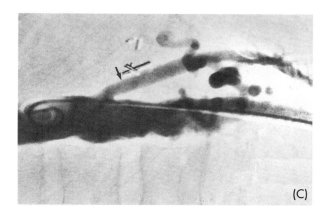

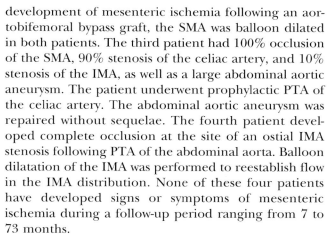

Figure 56–5. (A) A computed tomography scan demonstrates the crura of the diphragm (curved arrows) joining centrally to form the median arcuate ligament and compressing the SMA (straight arrow). This 56-year-old female presented with weight loss and postprandial abdominal pain and represents one of the failures of PTA in the subset of patients with "classic" symptoms of chronic mesenteric ischemia. (B) A diagnostic angiogram on the patient in (A) shows extrinsic compression of the SMA and total occlusion of the celiac artery. PTA of the SMA resulted in no change in appearance. (C) An angiogram done several days after surgical release of the median arcuate ligament shows a widely patent SMA. The patient became asymptomatic and has continued to do well at follow-up. (Reprinted with permission from Matsumoto AH, Meuhle C, Cassada D, et al. Compression of the superior mesenteric artery by the median arcuate ligament: a cause for mesenteric ischemia. (see Ref #28) Vasc Surg 1994;28:489–493.)

development of mesenteric ischemia following an aortobifemoral bypass graft, the SMA was balloon dilated in both patients. The third patient had 100% occlusion of the SMA, 90% stenosis of the celiac artery, and 10% stenosis of the IMA, as well as a large abdominal aortic aneurysm. The patient underwent prophylactic PTA of the celiac artery. The abdominal aortic aneurysm was repaired without sequelae. The fourth patient developed complete occlusion at the site of an ostial IMA stenosis following PTA of the abdominal aorta. Balloon dilatation of the IMA was performed to reestablish flow in the IMA distribution. None of these four patients have developed signs or symptoms of mesenteric ischemia during a follow-up period ranging from 7 to 73 months.

We have also treated six patients with a clinical or angiographic presentation suggestive of, but not classic for, mesenteric ischemia. Symptoms usually included atypical abdominal pain unrelated to eating and greater than 70% stenosis of at least two visceral arteries. None of these patients experienced weight loss, and no other etiology for their abdominal pain had been diagnosed at the time of the procedure. There were two (33%) immediate technical failures in this group. Both of these patients had angiographic findings consistent with extrinsic compression of the celiac artery by the median arcuate ligament. Following median arcuate ligament release at surgery, both patients had resolution of their symptoms (Fig. 56–5). Of the four patients with immediate technical successes, only two (50%) had resolution of symptoms. One patient had abdominal bloating unrelated to meals. This patient did not improve or deteriorate following SMA angioplasty. Another patient had mild improvement in symptoms after a successful SMA angioplasty but became completely asymptomatic following a surgical bypass of a totally occluded celiac artery. Therefore, of the six patients with symptoms atypical of mesenteric ischemia, only two (33%) benefited from the endovascular procedure.

In our series, 28 patients initially underwent dilatation of a single mesenteric vessel. We evaluated the success rates of PTA in terms of which visceral vessel was treated. We found that PTA of 15 of 18 (83%) SMAs, 3 of 6 (50%) celiac arteries, and 4 of 4 (100%) IMAs was both technically and clinically successful. Two of the three failures of celiac artery PTA were secondary to compression by the median arcuate ligament. Although compression of a mesenteric artery by the median arcuate ligament can lead to mesenteric ischemia or cause

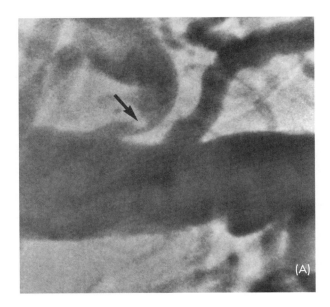
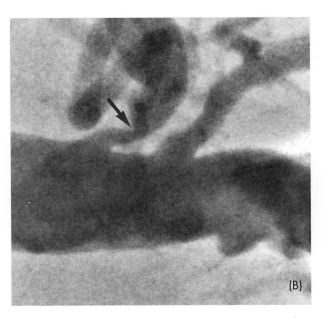

Figure 56–6.   Narrowing of a mesenteric artery by the median arcuate ligament is characterized by an asymmetric, nonostial stenosis that varies with respiration. (A) On expiration, the celiac artery stenosis is 80% (arrow). (B) On inspiration, the celiac artery is only 50% narrowed (arrow). (Reprinted with permission from Matsumoto AH, Tegtmeyer CJ, Fitzcharles EJ, et al. Percutaneous transluminal angioplasty for visceral artery stenoses: results and long-term follow-up. *J Vasc Intervent Radiol* 1995;6:165–174.) (Reprinted with permission: Matsumoto AH et al. *Vasc Surg* 1994;28:489–493.)

symptoms that mimic it,[27,28] PTA is ineffective in dilating vessels narrowed by extrinsic compression.

Narrowing of a mesenteric vessel by the median arcuate ligament should be suspected when an asymmetric, nonstial stenosis involving the superior and anterior aspects of either the celiac artery or SMA is present, especially if the stenosis increases with expiration and decreases with inspiration[28,29] (Fig. 56–6). If balloon inflation is easy and if rapid arterial recoil occurs during balloon deflation, extrinsic compression of the mesenteric artery is even more likely. Although stenting such a lesion seems attractive, a Palmaz stent may be permanently deformed by the extrinsic pressure and occlude the vessel. In addition, there is some evidence to suggest that some of the symptoms caused by the median arcuate ligament are related to compression of the adjacent celiac nerve plexus.[26] Therefore, vascular stents for the treatment of symptoms related to the median arcuate ligament compression of a mesenteric vessel cannot currently be advocated.

When we compared our PTA results in the treatment of nonstial (20 lesions) versus ostial (14 lesions) versus combined ostial and nonstial (2 lesions) visceral artery stenoses, we found no statistical significant difference in the clinical success rates (65% versus 86% versus 100%, respectively). Intuitively, one might expect nonstial lesions to respond better to PTA, but the median arcuate ligament causes a nonstial narrowing. Since we treated several lesions related to the median arcuate ligament, our data may be biased toward an unfavorable PTA result for nonstial lesions.

Lesions caused by FMD should respond favorably to balloon dilatation.[21] We have treated one patient with FMD of the SMA. Balloon dilatation was successful, and the patient remains asymptomatic at 15 months of follow-up.

The response of vasculitic lesions to PTA is variable. In general, the longer the lesion and the higher the sedimentation rate, the less favorable the PTA response will be in a patient with an arteritis.[22]

Complications associated with mesenteric arterial PTA are similar to those encountered in patients with diffuse vascular disease who are undergoing peripheral PTA.[30] We have treated a total of 32 patients and have had 5 (15.6%) major complications. All of the complications were related to the arterial access site when large balloon catheters were used (early in our experience) or larger sheaths were used to allow introduction of a vascular stent (more recent experience). There is no question that the use of larger devices (such as stents) is associated with a higher risk in this patient population with severe peripheral vascular disease. Our most serious complication required a patient to undergo an amputation when one limb of an aorto-bifemoral bypass graft occluded at the access site in the femoral artery. Although our 30-day mortality rate is zero, four deaths have been reported in the literature in the 126 patients treated (Table 56–1).

About 5% of patients with an acute aortic dissection develop mesenteric ischemia. These patients experience an operative mortality of about 90%. When an aortic dissection occurs, the true lumen usually com-

Table 56–1.　Summary of the 11 Largest Visceral PTA Series

Study Authors	No. of Patients Treated	Initial Technical Success	Initial Clinical Success	No. of Patients with Recurrence	Primary Long-Term Clinical Success	Successful Repeat PTA	Secondary Long-Term Clinical Success	Follow-up (Mo)*	Major Complications†
Matsumoto et al[17]	19	15/19 79%	12/15 80%	2/12 17%	10/12 83%	1/2 50%	11/12 92%	4–73 (25)	3/19 (0) 16%
Sniderman et al[2]	13	11/13 85%	11/11 100%	5/11 45%	6/11 54%	3/3 100%	9/11 82%	1–96 (N/A)	0/12 (1) 0%
Simonetti et al[16]	22‡	21/22 95%	18/21 86%	2/18 11%	16/18 89%	2/2 100%	18/18 100%	24–36 (N/A)	0/22 (0) 0%
Mcshane et al[15]	6	5/6 83%	5/5 100%	3/5 60%	2/5 40%	2/2 100%	4/5 80%	7–24 (16)	0/5 (1) 0%
Levy et al[14]	4	4/4 100%	4/4 100%	2/4 50%	2/4 50%	2/2 100%	4/4 100%	8–42 (25)	0/4 (0) 0%
Wilms et al[13]	8	7/8 88%	7/7 100%	0/7 0%	7/7 100%	—	—	1–15 (N/A)	1/8 (0) 12%
Roberts et al[12]	4	4/4 100%	4/4 100%	2/4 50%	2/4 50%	2/2 100%	4/4 100%	16–28 (22)	1/4 (0) 25%
Rose et al[19]	8	3/8 38%	6/8 75%	2/6 33%	4/6 67%	0/1 0%	4/6 67%	4–19 (9)	1/8 (1) 13%
Hallisey et al[18]	16	14/16 88%	14/14 100%	3/12 25%	9/12 75%	3/3 100%	12/12 100%	4–60 (28)	1/16 (0) 6%
Golden et al[11]	7	6/7 85%	6/6 100%	0/6 0%	6/6 100%	—	—	N/A–28 (28)	0/7 (0) 0%
Allen et al[20]	19	18/19 95%	15/18 83%	3/15 20%	12/15 80%	2/3 67%	14/15 93%	4–101 (39)	1/19 (1) 5%
Totals	126	108/126 86%	102/113 90%	24/100 24%	76/100 76%	17/20 85%	80/87 92%	1–101 (N/A)	8/124 (4) 6%

N/A = Not available
*Ranges are given, with mean values in parentheses.
†Numbers given do not include 30-day mortality, which is given in parentheses.
‡Includes only patients with chronic mesenteric ischemia.

municates with the false lumen via multiple fenestrations in the dissection septum (flap). Mesenteric ischemia may develop when the pressure and flow in the aortic lumen (either true or false) supplying the SMA or IMA are not enough to meet the physiologic demands of the bowel or when the dissection flap directly extends into the SMA or IMA and compromises intestinal perfusion. Because balloon PTA alone is usually ineffective in "tacking down" dissection flaps, stents have been used to reestablish vascular patency. Creating de novo fenestrations and enlarging naturally occurring fenestrations between the true and false lumens have also been performed by inflating PTA balloons (8 to 20 mm in diameter) directly across the dissection flap.[31]

We have treated one patient with a type I aortic dissection using endovascular stents. In this patient, the SMA and celiac artery were originating from the true lumen. There was compression of the true aortic lumen by the false channel, beginning just cephalad to the celiac artery. This narrowing was associated with a 40 mm Hg gradient. The dissection also extended directly into the left renal artery, and the right renal artery was

supplied by the false lumen. The patient developed abdominal pain and deteriorating renal function. The risk associated with surgical repair was considered to be prohibitive. A Gianturco Z-stent (modified tracheobronchial Z-stent, Cook, Inc.) 30 mm in diameter by 50 mm in length was placed just cephalad to the origin of the celiac artery. This resulted in a decrease in the gradient to 15 mm Hg. Access to the false lumen was obtained from the true lumen. The right renal artery was then catheterized, and a Palmaz stent was deployed in the right renal artery, bridging the true and false lumens. Subsequently, a Wallstent was placed to reapproximate the dissection flap in the left renal artery (Fig. 56–7). The patient's abdominal pain resolved, and his renal function returned to normal. He is doing well at 4 months of follow-up.

DISCUSSION

A variety of surgical techniques have been used in the treatment of mesenteric arterial occlusive disease. The nature of the surgical procedure is determined by the surgeon's experience, the anatomic distribution of the disease, and the institutional bias. The overall techni-

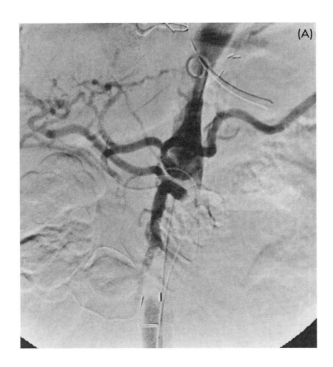

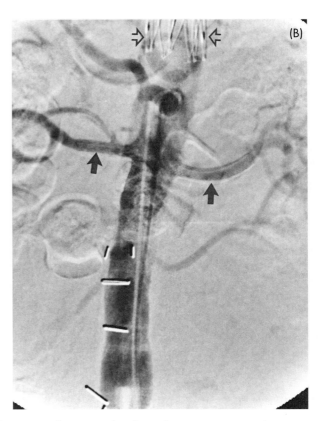

Figure 56–7. (A) A 60-year-old male with a prior coronary artery bypass graft presented 4 days after a type I aortic dissection with abdominal pain and deteriorating renal function. A diagnostic arteriogram showed a compromised true aortic lumen and diminished flow to the mesenteric and renal arteries. (B) Following placement of stents in the abdominal aorta (open arrows) above the celiac artery and both renal arteries (straight arrows), perfusion was restored to the mesenteric and renal vascular beds.

cal success rates reported with surgical revascularization have varied between 90% and 98%, with long-term clinical success rates of 61 to 100%. Morbidity rates range from 20 to 54%, with a 30-day mortality rate of 0 to 8%.[3,32–36]

Although clinical studies comparing surgical and endovascular techniques in the treatment of mesenteric ischemia are lacking, based on our experience and a review of the literature, endovascular therapy represents an effective alternative to surgery in patients with chronic mesenteric ischemia. In addition, the endovascular procedures did not compromise subsequent surgical intervention in any of our technical or clinical failures. For complete arterial occlusions, surgical revascularization remains the mainstay of therapy at our institution. However, patients at high risk for surgery may benefit from an initial attempt at percutaneous therapy as long as immediate surgical backup is available.

The adequacy of collateral mesenteric blood flow is difficult to determine. Therefore, the issue of when to perform prophylactic PTA on the mesenteric vessels is hard to determine. What is known is that the development of mesenteric ischemia following reconstructive surgery on the abdominal aorta is associated with a high mortality rate.[25,26] Therefore, PTA may be justi-

fied in some asymptomatic patients with tenuous visceral arterial circulation, especially if the patients will be undergoing a revascularization procedure involving the abdominal aorta.

Mesenteric PTA in patients with symptoms atypical for intestinal ischemia or with an isolated, nonstial stenosis of the celiac artery appears to be less effective. This is partly due to the prevalence of extrinsic arterial compression by the median arcuate ligament or, less frequently, by an occult malignancy. Since the symptoms of an occult abdominal or retroperitoneal malignancy can mimic those of chronic mesenteric ischemia, it is important to be alert to this diagnostic possibility. Therefore, a clinical failure despite a technically successful PTA should raise the possibility of an occult malignancy.[17] An immediate technical failure of mesenteric artery PTA unrelated to a technical complication should raise the suspicion of vascular compression by the median arcuate ligament, especially if there are characteristic angiographic findings.

With continued improvements in fluoroscopic equipment, balloon catheters, guidewire technology, and intravascular ultrasound, endovascular techniques will undergo further refinement and become even more effective for treating mesenteric arterial insufficiency.

Although the long-term efficacy of stents in the mesenteric vessels is still unknown, vascular stenting clearly complements balloon PTA in achieving excellent technical results. As in other vascular beds, the Palmaz stent should be used cautiously where extrinsic vascular compression (ie, the median arcuate ligament) can cause collapse or distort the stent and lead to abrupt vascular occlusion.

REFERENCES

1. Fisher D, Fry W. Collateral mesenteric circulation. *Surg Gynecol Obstet* 1987;164:487–492.
2. Sniderman KW. Transluminal angioplasty in the management of chronic intestinal ischemia. In: Strandness DE, van Breda A, eds. *Vascular Diseases: Surgical and Interventional Therapy*. New York: Churchill Livingstone; 1994:803–809.
3. Baxter BT, Pearce WH. Diagnosis and surgical management of chronic mesenteric ischemia. In: Strandness DE, van Breda A, eds. *Vascular Diseases: Surgical and Interventional Therapy*. New York: Churchill Livingstone; 1994:795–802.
4. Kalaya RN, Sammartano RJ, Boley SJ. Aggressive approach to acute mesenteric ischemia. *Surg Clin North Am* 1992;72:157–182.
5. Furrer J, Gruntzig A, Kugelmeier J, Goebel N. Treatment of abdominal angina with percutaneous dilatation of an arteria mesenterica superior stenosis. *Cardiovasc Intervent Radiol* 1980;3:43–44.
6. Uflacker R, Goldany MA, Constant S. Resolution of mesenteric angina with percutaneous transluminal angioplasty of a superior mesenteric artery stenosis using a balloon catheter. *Gastrointest Radiol* 1980;5:367–369.
7. Novelline RA. Percutaneous transluminal angioplasty: newer applications. *AJR* 1980;135:983–988.
8. Birch SJ, Colapinto RF. Transluminal dilatation in the management of mesenteric angina: a report of two cases. *J Can Assoc Radiol* 1982;33:46–47.
9. Crotch-Harvey MA, Gould DA, Green AT. Case report: percutaneous transluminal angioplasty of the inferior mesenteric artery in the treatment of chronic mesenteric ischaemia. *Clin Radiol* 1992;46:408–409.
10. Warnock NG, Gaines PA, Beard JD, Cumberland DC. Treatment of intestinal angina by percutaneous transluminal angioplasty of a superior mesenteric artery occlusion. *Clin Radiol* 1992;45:18–19.
11. Golden DA, Ring EJ, McLean GK, Freiman DB. Percutaneous angioplasty in the treatment of abdominal angina. *AJR* 1982;139:247–249.
12. Roberts L, Wertman DA, Mills SR, Moore AV, Heaston DK. Transluminal angioplasty of the superior mesenteric artery: an alternative to surgical revascularization. *AJR* 1983;141:1039–1042.
13. Wilms G, Baert AL. Transluminal angioplasty of superior mesenteric artery and celiac trunk. *Ann Radiol* 1986; 29:535–538.
14. Levy PJ, Haskell L, Gordon RL. Percutaneous transluminal angioplasty of splanchnic arteries: an alternative method to elective revascularization in chronic visceral ischemia. *Eur J Radiol* 1987;7:239–242.
15. McShane MD, Proctor A, Spencer P, Cumberland DC, Welsh CL. Mesenteric angioplasty for chronic intestinal ischemia. *Eur J Vasc Surg* 1992;6:333–336.
16. Simonetti G, Lupattelli L, Urigo F, et al. Interventional radiology in the treatment of acute and chronic mesenteric ischemia. *Radiol Med* 1992;84:98–105.
17. Matsumoto AH, Tegtmeyer CJ, Fitzcharles EJ, et al. Percutaneous transluminal angioplasty of visceral arterial stenoses: results and long-term clinical follow-up. *JVIR* 1995;6:165–174.
18. Hallisey MJ, Deschaine J, Illescas FF, et al. Angioplasty for the treatment of visceral ischemia. *JVIR* 1995;6:165–174.
19. Rose SC, Qurgley TM, Rakev EJ. Revascularization for chronic mesenteric ischemia: comparison of operative arterial bypass grafting and percutaneous transluminal angioplasty. *JVIR* 1995;6:339–349.
20. Allen RC, Martin GH, Rees CR, et al. Mesenteric angioplasty in the treatment of chronic intestinal ischemia. *J Vasc Surg* 1996;24:415–423.
21. Tegtmeyer CJ, Selby JB Jr, Hartwell GD, Ayers C, Tegtmeyer V. Results and complications of angioplasty in fibromuscular disease. *Circulation* 1991;83(Suppl I):I-155–I-161.
22. Tanimoto A, Hiramatsu K. Percutaneous transluminal angioplasty for Takayasu's arteritis. *Semin Intervent Radiol* 1993;10:1–7.
23. Tegtmeyer CJ, Sos TA. Techniques of renal angioplasty. *Radiology* 1986;161:577–586.
24. Liermann DD, Strecker EP. Tantalum stents in the treatment of stenotic and occlusive diseases of abdominal vessels. In: Liermann DD, ed. *Stents: State of the Art and Future Developments*. Watertown, MA: Boston Scientific Corp; 1995:127–134.
25. Gonzalez LL, Jaffe MS. Mesenteric arterial insufficiency following abdominal aortic resection. *Arch Surg* 1996; 93:10–20.
26. Rogers DM, Thompson JE, Garrett WV, Talkington CM, Patman RD. Mesenteric vascular problems: a 26-year experience. *Ann Surg* 1982;195:554–565.
27. Tribble CG, Harman PK, Mentzer RM Jr. Celiac artery compression syndrome: report of a case and review of current opinion. *Vasc Surg* 1986;20:120–129.
28. Matsumoto AH, Meuhle C, Cassada D, Navid F, Tegtmeyer CJ, Tribble CG. Compression of the superior mesenteric artery by the median arcuate ligament: a cause for mesenteric ischemia. *Vasc Surg* 1994;28:489–493.
29. Reuter SR, Bernstein EF. The anatomic basis for respiratory variation in median arcuate ligament compression of the celiac artery. *Surgery* 1973;73:381–385.
30. Becker GJ, Katzen BT, Dake MD. Noncoronary angioplasty. *Radiology* 1989;170:921–940.
31. Slonim SM, Nyman VR, Semba CP, Miller DC, Mitchell RS, Dake MD. True lumen obliteration in complicated aortic dissection: endovascular treatment. *Radiology* 1996;210:161–166.
32. McMillan WD, McCarthy WJ, Bresticker MR, et al. Mesenteric artery bypass: objective patency determination. *J Vasc Surg* 1995;21:729–741.
33. Calderon M, Reul GH, Gregoric ID, et al. Long-term results of the surgical management of symptomatic chronic intestinal ischemia. *J Cardiovasc Surg* 1992;33:723–728.
34. Rheudasil JM, Stewart MT, Schellack JV, Smith RB III, Salam AA, Perdue GD. Surgical treatment of chronic mesenteric arterial insufficiency. *J Vasc Surg* 1988;8:495–500.

35. Rapp JH, Reilly LM, Qvarfordt PG, Goldstone J, Ehrenfeld WK, Stoney RJ. Durability of endarterectomy and antegrade grafts in the treatment of chronic visceral ischemia. *J Vasc Surg* 1986;3:799–806.

36. Reul GJ Jr, Wukasch DC, Sandiford FM, Chiarillo L, Hallman GL, Cooley DA. Surgical treatment of abdominal angina: review of 25 patients. *Surgery* 1974;75:682–689.

57

Diagnostic Evaluation of Renovascular Hypertension and Dysfunction: Patient Selection for Evaluation

Marshall E. Benjamin, M.D.
Richard H. Dean, M.D.

The evaluation of the patient with renovascular occlusive disease has evolved through several screening methods. During this evolution, rapid-sequence intravenous pyelography, peripheral plasma renin activity, infusion of angiotensin II antagonists, and radionuclide renography have been suggested as valuable screening methods to detect functionally significant renal artery disease. However, none of these methods has emerged as the dominant screening modality due to a lack of sensitivity, specificity, or both.

Without doubt, the most important screening tests for patients presenting with hypertension are the medical history, physical examination, and routine blood studies. With this simple approach, selected patients can be referred for more complex screening tests to identify possible renal artery occlusive disease. Currently, the most popular screening tests are renal duplex sonography and isotope renography before and after captopril ingestion or exercise. Prior to review of their use, however, a brief discussion of which hypertensive patients require such diagnostic screening studies is relevant.

Renovascular hypertension is a severe form of hypertension and probably represents only 1 to 5% of the entire hypertensive population.[1] Because the renovascular form tends to be relatively severe, its prevalence among the population of severely hypertensive individuals is much greater. For example, among 85

patients evaluated at Vanderbilt University for malignant hypertension, Davis and colleagues reported a 31% incidence of renovascular hypertension.[2]

In our experience, severe hypertension at the two extremes of life has the highest probability of being of renovascular origin. Review of the causes of hypertension in 74 children admitted to Vanderbilt University for diagnostic evaluation over a 5-year period showed that 78% of those patients less than 5 years old had a correctable renovascular etiology.[3] Interestingly, after childhood, the age group most likely to have renovascular hypertension is the elderly. Thirty-three percent of patients over the age of 60 admitted for evaluation during the same time period had disease of the renal artery as the responsible etiology.

It is clear that the probability of finding a renovascular origin correlates with the severity of the hypertension. Accordingly, the search for the disease should be directed to the subset of patients with the higher degree of hypertension. It must be remembered, however, that severity of hypertension is based on its level without medication and does not take into account the difficulty of its control by drug therapy.

Because of the relative infrequency of renovascular hypertension in the entire hypertensive population, many reports have focused on the value of demographic factors, physical findings, and screening tests to discriminate between it and essential hypertension as a

Table 57–1. Clinical Considerations in Hypertension and Renovascular Hypertension

	Essential Hypertension (339 Cases)		Renovascular Hypertension			
			Arteriosclerotic (91 Cases)		Fibromuscular (84 Cases)	
	Percent	Years	Percent	Years	Percent	Years
History						
Average age		41		48		35
Less than 20 years	2		1		14	
Average duration		3.1		1.9		2.0
Less than 1 year	10		23		19	
More than 10 years	23		12		10	
Average age at onset		35		36		33*
More than 50 years	7		39		3*	
Less than 20 years	12		2		16*	
Sex (female)	40		34		81	
Race (black)	29		7		10	
Acceleration of hypertension	13		23		14	
Family history						
Hypertension	67		68*		41	
Stroke	37		44*		22	
Neither of foregoing	19		30*		46	
Symptoms						
Nocturia	38		55		35	
Weakness, fatigue	32		49		42*	
Angina						
Headache						
All of foregoing	0		14		10	
Previous vascular occlusive disease	10		20		6	
Physical examination						
Body habitus						
Obese	38		17		11	
Thin	6		13*		30	
Fundi (grades 3 and 4)	12		26		10*	
Bruit						
Abdomen	6		38		55	
Flank	1		8		20	
Abdomen or flank	7		41		57	

Source: Cooperative Study of Renovascular Hypertension (see Ref. 4).
*Differences are statistically different at the 5% level except where so designated.

basis for deciding to pursue further diagnostic study. The most frequently quoted factors are recent onset of hypertension, young age, lack of family history of hypertension, and the presence of an abdominal bruit. The most complete study comparing the clinical characteristics of patients with renovascular hypertension and those with essential hypertension was the Cooperative Study of Renovascular Hypertension.[4] In that study, the prevalence of certain clinical characteristics in 339 patients with *essential hypertension* was compared with their prevalence in 175 patients with *renovascular hypertension* secondary to atherosclerotic lesions (91 patients) and fibromuscular dysplasia (84 patients). A summary of the differential points identified in that study is presented in Table 57–1. Although several characteristics show significant differences in prevalence between the two disorders, *none* of them has sufficient discriminative value to be useful in excluding patients from further diagnostic investigation for renovascular hypertension. Unquestionably, the finding of an epigastric bruit in a young white woman with malignant hypertension is strongly suggestive of a renovascular origin of the hypertension. However, the absence of such criteria does not exclude the presence of the disease, and such criteria should not be used to eliminate patients from further diagnostic study. The key clinical

Table 57–2.   Typical Assessment of Patients with Hypertension

1. History and physical examination
2. Blood count, SMA-12, urinalysis, urine culture, serum potassium (three times)
3. Electrocardiogram and chest x-ray
4. Analysis of 24-hour urine collection for creatinine clearance, electrolytes, catecholamines, vanillylmandelic acid, and 17-hydroxysteroids and ketosteroids
5. Creatinine clearance
6. Renal duplex sonography (RDS)

feature on which to base the decision on further diagnostic study is the severity of hypertension. The more severe the hypertension, the greater the probability that it is secondary to a correctable cause. We therefore submit all patients who have diastolic blood pressure above 115 mm Hg, and who would be acceptable candidates for operation, to evaluation for a correctable origin of hypertension.

DIAGNOSTIC EVALUATION

The general evaluation of all hypertensive patients is outlined in Table 57–2. Electrocardiography is important to gauge the extent of secondary myocardial hypertrophy or associated ischemic heart disease. Serum electrolytes and serial serum potassium determinations can effectively exclude patients with primary aldosteronism if potassium levels are above 3.0 mg/dL. One must remember, however, that hypokalemia is most often due to salt-depleting diets and previous diuretic therapy. Estimation of renal function is requisite. An approximate gauge of excretory impairment can be obtained simply by measuring the serum creatinine level. When it is abnormal, a 24-hour creatinine clearance measurement is appropriate. Finally, assessment of the urinary 17-hydroxysteroid, ketosteroid, and vanillylmandelic acid levels, will effectively identify the rare patient with a pheochromocytoma or a functioning adrenal cortical tumor. These latter studies are performed only when some component of the initial assessment hints at the presence of these conditions.

Renal Duplex Sonography

Renal duplex sonography (RDS) has been used at our center as a screening test to identify those patients who would benefit from further invasive study, that is, arteriography. Through continued improvements in probe design and duplex sonographic technology, imaging and Doppler-shift interrogation of deep abdominal vasculature have been introduced as a potentially accurate screening method to identify and quantify visceral and renal artery occlusive disease. Our clinical experience with its use has centered on evaluation of renovascular disease. We have evaluated the role of duplex sonogra-

phy as an initial surface screening test, as an intraoperative study to confirm the technical success of reconstructive procedures, and as a postoperative surveillance method to follow progression of disease and endurance of reconstructions.

With regard to initial screening, we have evaluated the sensitivity and specificity of this method for the identification of renal artery disease. The study population consisted of 74 consecutive patients who had 77 comparative renal duplex examinations and standard angiographic studies in the arterial anatomy of 148 kidneys. In 122 kidneys with single renal arteries, RDS correctly identified 67 of 68 kidneys without significant stenosis and 35 of 39 kidneys with 60 to 99% renal artery stenosis (Table 57–3). All 15 renal artery occlusions were correctly identified by the failure to obtain a Doppler-shifted signal from an imaged renal artery. Using this methodology and criteria for interpretation, RDS was 93% sensitive and 98% specific, with a positive predictive value of 98% and a negative predictive value of 94%. Overall accuracy was 96% when compared prospectively with cut-film angiography. Technically successful studies were defined as a complete main renal artery interrogation from aortic origin to renal hilum, and were obtained in 95% of cases.[5,6]

RDS criteria for critical renal artery stenosis are depicted in Table 57–4. Assuming that Renal Artery Peak Systolic Velocity (RA-PSV) varied with the degree of renal artery stenosis and aortic PSV (i.e., inflow), most authors have advocated the use of the ratio of RA-PSV to aortic PSV (the renal-aortic ratio) to define critical renal artery stenosis.[7,8] In contrast, we have found no relationship between RA-PSV and aortic PSV in the presence or absence of disease (Fig. 57.1). In our patient population, a focal increase in the RA-PSV to 2 m/sec or more in combination with distal poststenotic turbulence has proved to correlate highly with the angiographic presence of a 60% or greater diameter-reducing stenosis of the renal artery.[5,6]

Multiple or polar renal arteries pose a potentially serious limitation for surface RDS. Nineteen percent of the patients presenting to our institution for evaluation of renovascular hypertension have had polar renal arteries on angiography. Among these patients, 43% have had multiple vessels to both kidneys, and 40% of all these vessels have demonstrated 60% or greater diameter-reducing stenosis or occlusion. Because of the variable polar vessel origin, small vessel size, and compromised image quality associated with low-frequency probes, identification of polar vessels and their associated disease is difficult. In our analysis of surface RDS, we identified only 1 of 43 polar arteries. Although Doppler color flow has enhanced recognition of multiple renal arteries, failure to identify these polar vessels and their associated disease constituted the largest single source of false-negative studies.

Table 57–3. Comparative Analysis Parameter Estimates and Their 95% Confidence Intervals

Group	N	Measure	Estimate	95% Confidence Interval
All kidneys	142 (kidneys)	Sensitivity	0.88	(0.84, 0.92)
		Specificity	0.99	(0.97, 1.00)
		PPV	0.98†	(0.96, 0.99)
		NPV	0.92‡	(0.89, 0.95)
		Accuracy	0.91	(0.87, 0.95)
Kidneys with single renal artery	148 (kidneys) 122 (kidneys)	Sensitivity	0.93	(0.90, 0.96)
		Specificity	0.98†	(0.96, 1.00)
		PPV	0.98‡	(0.96, 1.00)
		NPV	0.94	(0.91, 0.97)
		Accuracy	0.91	(0.87, 0.95)
Kidneys with multiple renal arteries	148 (kidneys) 21 (arteries)	Sensitivity	0.67	(0.53, 0.81)
		Specificity	1.00*	——
		PPV	1.00*†	——
		NPV	0.79‡	(0.68, 0.90)
		Accuracy	0.86	(0.76, 0.96)
All patients	74 (subjects)	Sensitivity	0.93	(0.87, 0.99)
		Specificity	1.00*	——
		PPV	1.00*†	——
		NPV	0.91‡	(0.84, 0.98)
		Accuracy	0.96	(0.91, 1.00)

*Estimated standard error is zero; confidence level is inestimable.
†PPV, positive predictive value.
‡NPV, negative predictive value.

Table 57–4. Duplex Ultrasound Criteria for the Diagnosis of Renal Artery Stenosis

Defect	Criteria
< 60% diameter-reducing RA lesion	RA-PSV from entire RA <2.0 m/sec
≥ 60% diameter-reducing RA lesion	Focal RA-PSV ≥2.0 m/sec and distal turbulent velocity waveform
Occlusion	Absent Doppler-shifted signal from renal artery B-scan image
Inadequate study for interpretation	Failure to obtain Doppler samples from entire main renal artery

The pertinence of RDS insensitivity to polar vessel disease is related to the prevalence of such disease within the patient population examined and the clinical indication for surface RDS. Fourteen percent of our patients who underwent repair for unilateral renovascular disease and presumed renovascular hypertension had only polar branch disease. We believe this group constitutes a significant minority of patients. Therefore, we proceed with conventional angiography in patients less than 60 years of age with poorly controlled hypertension despite multidrug therapy, even in the presence of a negative surface RDS. When RDS is used to screen for ischemic nephropathy and renal insufficiency, however, a negative RDS study effectively excludes significant renovascular disease because polar vessel disease alone does not account for renal insufficiency.[9]

Captopril Renal Scintigraphy

To comprehend the basis of captopril renal scintigraphy (CRS), one must understand some of the components of renal excretory physiology and the importance of the renin-angiotensin system in the maintenance of homeostasis (Fig. 57.2). Glomerular filtration is governed partially by the relative tone of the afferent and efferent arterioles. During periods recognized by the juxtaglomerular apparatus as reduced blood pressure (eg, proximal renal artery stenosis), increased renin is released, which ultimately leads to an increase in the level of angiotensin II. Angiotensin II acts predominantly to vasoconstrict the efferent arteriole to maintain renal glomerular perfusion pressure and filtration. When an angiotensin II converting enzyme (ACE) inhibitor such as captopril is given in this circumstance, an acute reduction in the amount of angiotensin II

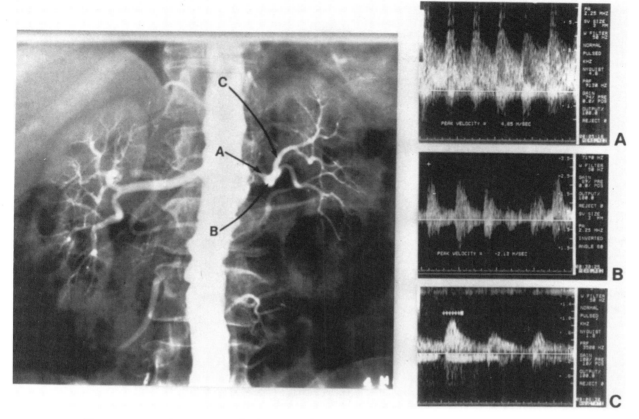

Figure 57–1.   Cut-film angiogram demonstrating high-grade left renal artery stenosis. (A) At the site of stenosis, the Doppler spectral analysis demonstrates a focal increase in RA-PSV (4.6 m/sec). (B) Beyond the stenosis, a turbulent spectral waveform is displayed: decreased RA-PSV with a ragged spectral envelope and spontaneous bidirectional signals. (C) Spectral analysis of the distal renal artery demonstrating return of a near-normal waveform.

occurs. This results in diminished vasoconstriction of the efferent arteriole and a decrease in the glomerular filtration pressure. Hence, CRS is a study composed of a baseline renogram and a repeat renogram performed after a dose of captopril is administered. The test is considered positive when a normal baseline scan becomes abnormal after captopril administration either by an increase in the time to peak activity to more than 11 minutes or by a normal glomerular filtration rate ratio between the two sides increasing to more than 1.5:1 (Fig. 57.3). In experienced hands, this study is reported to be highly reliable.[10] Unfortunately, it is less reliable when significant parenchymal disease is present. For that reason, we have found reliance on activation of the renin-angiotensin system leads to an unacceptably high incidence of false-negative results, especially in azotemic patients.

Renal Arteriography

There continues to be controversy over the use of aortography and renal arteriography in the routine screening of hypertensive individuals. Although some believe that it should be reserved for selected groups of patients, we do not concur and proceed with arteriography in any patient who would be a candidate for renal revascularization if a treatable lesion were found. Both aortography and selective renal arteriography using multiple projections are typically necessary to adequately examine the entire renal artery. The proximal third of the left renal artery usually courses anteriorly, the middle third transversely, and the distal third posteriorly, whereas the right renal artery pursues a more consistently posterior course. Lesions in the renal artery that are coursing anteriorly or posteriorly are frequently not seen or may appear insignificant in an anteroposterior (AP) aortogram. Oblique aortography or oblique selective renal arteriography will project these portions of the vessels in a profile more likely to demonstrate the stenosis. Similarly, delicate septal lesions of fibromuscular dysplasia may be unrecognizable or appear insignificant in the AP projection, whereas in the oblique projection their true severity is more likely to be demonstrated.

The introduction of digital subtraction angiography (DSA) has increased enthusiasm for the use of angiography as an outpatient screening procedure for renovascular disease. Although the intravenous route of

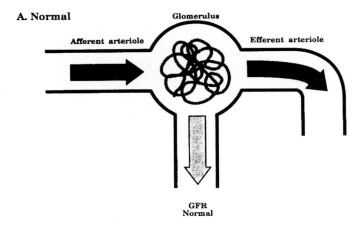

A. Normal

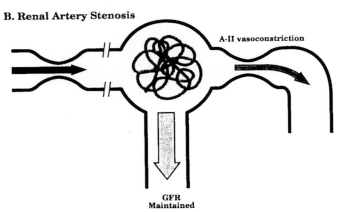

B. Renal Artery Stenosis

Figure 57–2. Drawing of the afferent arteriole. glomerulus, and efferent arteriole showing the juxtaglomerular region, the site of effect of angiotensin II.

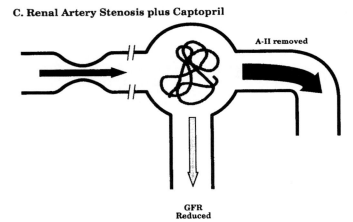

C. Renal Artery Stenosis plus Captopril

contrast injection for DSA was initially thought to be useful for this evaluation, this method provides such poor delineation that many fibromuscular dysplastic lesions are missed and one cannot evaluate branch vessels with sufficient accuracy. In addition, the amount of contrast material used for intravenous DSA is contraindicated in patients with reduced renal function. In contrast, intra-arterial DSA can be performed as an outpatient procedure and is useful in some patients. However, in our experience, adequate assessment of the renal vasculature and juxtarenal aorta requires mul-

tiple injections, and branch disease can be missed or inadequately defined. A single midstream flush aortagram requires no more contrast material than is required for multiple intra-arterial DSA studies. Moreover, we are not aware of any patient who required permanent dialysis as a result of contrast nephropathy. For these reasons, we continue to rely primarily on standard cut-film arteriography for most evaluations, and believe the potential benefit derived from the identification and correction of a functionally significant lesion exceeds the risk of arteriography.

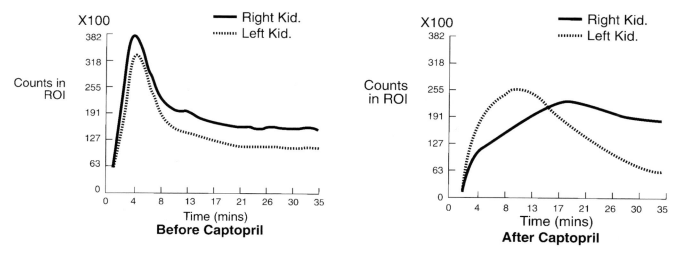

Figure 57–3. Captopril renal scintigraphy before (left) and after (right) captopril ingestion demonstrating the positive finding of a slowing of the rate of isotope clearance and the time to peak radioactivity after captopril ingestion.

DEFINITIVE FUNCTION STUDIES

Functional assessment of lesions found on arteriography remains an important component of the diagnostic evaluation. Two tests, renal vein renin assays and split renal function studies, have proven valuable in confirming the functional significance of renal artery stenosis. Neither has great value, however, when severe bilateral disease or disease in the renal artery supplying a solitary kidney is present. In these circumstances, the decision on whether to operate is based clinically, on the severity of hypertension and the magnitude of associated renal insufficiency.

Renal Vein Renin Assays

When a unilateral obstructive lesion is found by renal arteriography, its functional significance should be evaluated. Most centers now rely on renal vein renin assays (RVRAs) to establish the diagnosis of renovascular hypertension. Understanding the specifics of RVRAs is imperative to achieve valid results. Many factors affect the results of RVRAs that, if not properly managed, lead to erroneous results.

The effect of antihypertensive medications and unrestricted sodium intake on renin release, and thereby RVRAs, is widely recognized. Many antihypertensive medications, especially those that function through beta-adrenergic blockade or suppress renin output, can lead to false nonlateralization of RVRAs. Before one can conclude that there is no drug interference in the release of renin, all such medications must have been withheld for at least 5 days prior to performing RVRAs. Similar effects on renin levels are seen when sodium intake is not restricted. For this reason, the patient must be on a diet containing no more than 2 g sodium for at least 2 weeks prior to the study.

Probably the most common situation currently producing erroneous results of RVRAs is the chronic use of ACE inhibitors. Because these drugs block angiotensin II production, they also block the negative feedback mechanism controlling renin production. As a result, renin activity will be too high to interpret in the effluent from both kidneys, regardless of the presence or absence of renal artery lesions. For this reason, the use of ACE inhibitors should be stopped at least 5 days prior to RVRAs. The preparation of patients for RVRAs in our center is summarized in Table 57–5.

The technical aspects of performing RVRAs cannot be overemphasized as a potential source of error. Because the left renal vein contains not only renal venous effluent but also adrenal, gonadal, and lumbar venous effluent, misplacement of the venous catheter in the origin of any of these nonrenal branches of sampling in the proximal renal vein where a mixture from these other sources is present may dilute the renin activity from the kidney. This will lead to erroneously low measurements of renin activity and produce a false interpretation of the RVRAs.

The time of sampling the two renal veins for renin activity is also a potential source of error in RVRAs. In studies performed with a single catheter, several min-

Table 57–5. Patient Preparation for RVRAs at the Wake Forest Medical Center

1. Chronic salt restriction (20-g sodium diet)
2. Discontinue all interfering antihypertensive drugs for at least 5 days prior to study
3. Oral furosemide (40 mg) duresis night before the study
4. Nothing by mouth for 8 hours prior to study
5. Strictly flat bed rest for 4 hours before and during study
6. Prestudy sedation with intramuscular Valium (5 mg)

utes may elapse between sampling of the two renal veins as the catheter is switched from one side to the other. Furthermore, catheter manipulation and patient discomfort may affect renin release. It is not surprising, therefore, that when the single catheter is employed, both false-positive and false-negative renal vein renin ratios are frequent.

Vaughn et al have stressed the importance of expressing RVRAs in relation to systemic renin activity rather than simply evaluating the ratio of renin activity between the two renal veins.[11] In patients with renovascular hypertension secondary to unilateral renal artery stenosis, one should find hypersecretion of renin from the ischemic kidney and suppression of renin secretion from the normal kidney. Applying this theory, Stanley and Fry have shown a statistically significant difference in the renal-systemic renin indices in patients who were cured of renovascular hypertension by operation compared to those who were only improved.[12] Although this method has appeal as a predictor of the extent of benefit, its value in patients with bilateral renal artery lesions is limited. Because both lesions may be producing renovascular hypertension, this method in particular, as well as the use of RVRAs in general, have reduced validity as predictors of response to operation. What's more, the long-term systemic sequelae of hypertension are more directly related to its severity rather than its presence or absence. If one bases the decision for operative management solely on whether or not an absolute cure is to be expected, many patients who would receive the benefit of reduction in the severity of hypertension to a mild, easily controlled level would be ruled out as operative candidates. Therefore, this method of RVRA interpretation should be considered only as an additional predictive tool, and not as an alternative to the evaluation of renal vein renin ratios.

SUMMARY

In summary, each patient should be handled on an individual bases with respect to the screening and diagnostic evaluation for renovascular hypertension. In general, we limit our screening to patients with recent onset or accelerated hypertension, those with poorly controlled hypertension, and those with diastolic blood pressures above 115 mm Hg with no antihypertensive medication. Although we may perform RDS in any of these circumstances, in almost all such instances we proceed to arteriography. When hypertension is less severe but azotemia is present, we are guided by the results of RDS. In this situation, we contend that renal insufficiency requires global ischemia from a main renal artery stenosis to be present to explain the azotemia. RDS is highly accurate for identification or exclusion of such lesions of the main renal artery and can be used to dictate further evaluation.

When renovascular disease is identified by arteriography, RVRAs are used to investigate the importance of unilateral lesions. As a general rule, we would not recommend revascularization of unilateral disease unless RVRAs lateralize to the involved side. In contrast, the decision to intervene for bilateral lesions is dictated clinically, by the severity of the hypertension or by the presence of azotemia.

REFERENCES

1. Tucker RM, Labarthe DR. Frequency of surgical treatment for hypertension in adults at the Mayo Clinic from 1973 through 1975. *Mayo Clin Proc* 1977;52:549.
2. Davis BA, Crook JE, Vestal RE, et al. Prevalence of renovascular hypertension in patients with grade III or IV hypertensive retinopathy. *N Engl J Med* 1979;301:1273–1276.
3. Lawson JD, Boerth RK, Foster JH, et al. Diagnosis and management of renovascular hypertension in children. *Arch Surg* 1977;112:1307–1316.
4. Simon N, Franklin SS, Bleifer KH, et al. Clinical characteristics of renovascular hypertension. *JAMA* 1972;220:1209.
5. Hansen KJ, Tribble RW, Reavis S, et al. Renal duplex sonography: Evaluation of clinical utility. *J Vasc Surg* 1990;12:227–236.
6. Hansen KJ, Reavis SW, Dean RH. Use of duplex scanning in renovascular hypertension. *Technol Vasc Surg* 1992;15:174–184.
7. Kohler TR, Zierler RE, Martin RL, et al. Noninvasive diagnosis of renal artery stenosis by ultrasonic duplex scanning. *J Vasc Surg* 1986;4:450–456.
8. Taylor DC, Kettler MD, Moneta GL, et al. Duplex ultrasound scanning in the diagnosis of renal artery stenosis: a prospective evaluation. *J Vasc Surg* 1988;7:363–369.
9. Dean RH. Renovascular hypertension: an overview. In: Rutherford R.B. ed. *Vascular Surgery,* 4th ed. Philadelphia: WB Saunders; 1995:1371–1376.
10. Meier GH, Sumpio B, Black HR, Gusberg RJ. Captopril renal scintigraphy: an advance in the detection and treatment of renovascular hypertension. *J Vasc Surg* 1990;11:770–777.
11. Vaughn ED, Buhler FR, Larach JH, et al. Renovascular hypertension: renin measurements to indicate hypersecretion and contralateral suppression, estimate renal plasma flow, and score for surgical curability. *Am J Med* 1973;55:402–404.
12. Stanley JC, Fry WJ. Surgical treatment of renovascular hypertension. *Arch Surg* 1977;112:1291–1297.

58

Surgical Treatment of Renovascular Occlusive Disease: Options and Results

James C. Stanley, M.D.

Renovascular hypertension is the most common cause of surgically correctable high blood pressure. The treatment of patients with renovascular occlusive disease and secondary hypertension has markedly improved during the past three decades. Salutory outcomes are influenced most by the proficient performance of properly chosen operations. Operative details vary among the renal artery disease subgroups treated, and discussion of specific interventions must be individualized.[1,2]

OPERATIVE EXPOSURE

Adequate exposure is essential to the successful performance of arterial reconstructions for all forms of renal artery disease. The author prefers the use of a transverse supraumbilical abdominal incision in which both rectus muscles are transected, extending from the opposite midclavicular line to the posterior axillary line on the side of the renal artery reconstruction. This incision includes transection, not muscle splitting, of the ipsilateral internal and external abdominal oblique musculature. Such a transverse abdominal incision provides a distinct technical advantage in the greater ease of handling instruments parallel to the longitudinal axis of the renal artery during complex operations. Exposure is facilitated by placing a rolled pack under the flank and lumbar spine. Alternatively, midline vertical incisions may be used for renal artery reconstructions, and many surgeons routinely use this type of transabdominal approach. After the peritoneal cavity has been entered and its contents explored, the intestines are retracted to the opposite side of the abdomen. In certain instances, exposure of the renal vasculature is more easily obtained if the intestines are displaced outside the confines of the abdominal cavity. The exact dissection of the renal artery depends on the specific revascularization to be performed.

ENDARTERECTOMY

Two principal means of endarterectomy for arteriosclerotic renal artery disease exist: (1) transaortic renal endarterectomy through either an axial aortotomy or the transected infrarenal aorta and (2) direct renal artery endarterectomy. The use of one or the other of these procedures depends on the extent of the aortic and renal artery arteriosclerosis.[2-5]

Dissection of the renal arteries for most endarterectomy procedures is the same. Exposure of the renal artery affected with arteriosclerotic disease is usually direct, through the retroperitoneum at the base of the mesocolon in the midline over the aorta. Dissection of the renal artery should begin proximally, with complete skeletonization of the vessel at its aortic origin, and proceed toward the midportion of the vessel. The dissection should continue distally well beyond the obvious extent of arteriosclerotic plaque. This is necessary to allow extensive renal artery eversion during the course of the endarterectomy. The renal vein should be mobilized from its exit at the renal hilum to the vena cava. This necessitates ligation and transection of the adrenal and gonadal branches, as well as of the posterior coursing lumbar vein on the left.

The perirenal aorta should be dissected about its circumference to a level usually above the superior mesenteric artery. This requires incision of surrounding neural and fibrous tissue enveloping the aorta, the latter being especially prominent along the left posterior aspect of the aorta. Transection of the periaortic diaphragmatic crus facilitates this dissection and provides for greater ease in placement of the proximal aortic clamp. Ligation and transection of lumbar arteries may be necessary to completely free the aorta from surrounding tissue, although these vessels are usually occluded with microvascular clamps. Following this exposure, systemic anticoagulation is achieved by intravenous administration of heparin, 150 units/kg, and diuresis is established by intravenous administration of mannitol, 12.5 g.

Transaortic renal artery endarterectomy is a common direct method of restoring renal blood flow in cases of renal arteriosclerotic occlusive disease[2] (Fig. 58–1). The aorta is occluded above the superior mesenteric artery and below the renal artery origins. Backflow from the renal arteries should be controlled with microvascular clamps. The superior mesenteric artery, which is usually dissected for approximately 1 cm beyond its origin, is similarly occluded with a microvascular clamp. An axial aortotomy is then made, extending from the left anterolateral side of the aorta adjacent to the superior mesenteric artery, being curved to the anterior midline as the renal arteries are approached. The aortotomy is extended inferiorly approximately 2 cm below the renal vessels. A plane is developed between the diseased and normal aortic media and extended circumferentially. The plaque is transected just below the origin of the superior mesenteric artery. The renal artery endarterectomy is accomplished by maintaining gentle traction on the extension of aortic plaque into the renal artery while pushing the everted renal artery wall away from the plaque. Usually a well-defined endpoint is easily established, with feathering of the distal plaque occurring in the more normal distal renal

artery. The aortotomy is closed with a continuous 4-0 Teflon or polypropylene suture after vigorous irrigation of the endarterectomized aortic segment and renal arteries. Once the aortotomy has been closed, the aortic clamp and then the renal artery clamps are removed and antegrade flow to the kidneys is reestablished.

If the former type of renal endarterectomy is to be accompanied by an aortic procedure, an infrarenal clamp may be reapplied across the aortotomy closure, using a soft-jaw clamp to prevent fracture or crushing of the suture. Transaortic renal artery endarterectomy in other patients undergoing concomitant aortic reconstruction may be performed in a slightly different manner.[2,5] In these instances, dissection of the aorta and renal arteries is undertaken as previously noted. The aorta is transected just below the renal arteries, and endarterectomy of the diseased aorta and prolapsed renal arteries is undertaken through the divided aorta. Subsequently, the aortic reconstruction is completed in a conventional manner.

Transaortic endarterectomy is appropriate therapy for several forms of atherosclerosis. This is particularly true when disease is limited to the proximal renal artery. Poststenotic dilation in these circumstances is usually indicative of relative ease in obtaining a well-defined endarterectomy endpoint. Transaortic renal artery endarterectomy is often favored in the management of patients having multiple renal arteries where a

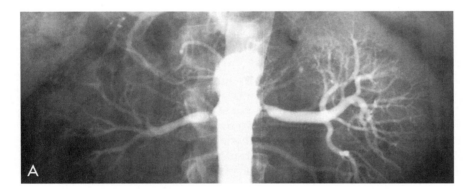

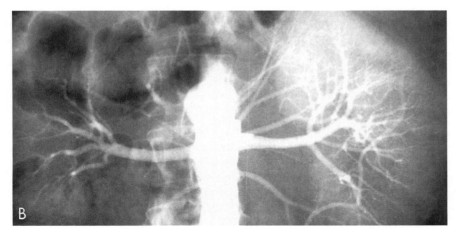

Figure 58–1. Transaortic bilateral renal endarterectomy. Preoperative (A) and postoperative (B) aortography. (Reprinted from Ref. 2 with permission.)

complex reconstruction would otherwise be required if a conventional bypass were undertaken. The adequacy of renal artery blood flow following endarterectomy may be documented with the use of directional Doppler or intraoperative duplex scanning. If the presence of an intimal flap within the renal artery is suspected, a separate axial incision in this vessel should be made beyond the plaque's endpoint, followed by tacking of the distal plaque and closure of the rental artery with or without a vein patch.

Direct renal artery endarterectomy is often undertaken in patients without extensive perirenal aortic atherosclerosis, especially in those with unilateral proximal lesions. In these cases, an anterior renal arteriotomy is performed, being extended for a short distance onto the aorta. A direct endarterectomy of the focal renal artery lesion may then be undertaken, with either simple primary closure or patch graft closure of the renal arteriotomy. This approach is also applicable for bilateral renal artery disease, although in many of the latter instances a transaortic endarterectomy is preferred because closure of lengthy renal artery incisions often requires time-consuming placement of a renal artery patch graft. In such cases, if the stenotic disease affecting one kidney is not preocclusive, with adequate collateral vessels to the kidney, ischemic renal injury may follow prolonged interruption of renal blood flow.

ANATOMIC BYPASS AND AORTIC REIMPLANTATION

Aortorenal Bypass

The right renal artery and aorta are usually exposed for most bypass procedures by incising the lateral parieties from the hepatic flexure to the cecum and reflecting the overlying right colon, duodenum, and pancreas medially with an extended Kocher-like maneuver. The left renal vascular pedicle is exposed using a similar retroperitoneal dissection, with medial reflection of the viscera, including the left colon. Such an approach provides better visualization of the middle and distal renal vessels than exposure gained through the retroperitoneum at the root of the mesocolon and mesentery.

Dissection of the right renal artery should be initiated in its midportion lateral to the vena cava. Initial dissection of the distal renal artery is more likely to result in troublesome injury to small arterial and venous branches. Renal artery dissection is facilitated by retraction of the renal vein, which should be dissected carefully from surrounding tissues, with small branches such as those to the adrenal gland being ligated and transected. In a similar manner, adequate exposure of the left renal artery usually requires mobilization of the overlying renal vein. Certain proximal atherosclerotic or developmental ostial lesions of the right renal artery may be exposed at the origin of the

vessel by dissection between the aorta and vena cava through the retroperitoneal tissue at the base of the mesocolon. Under these circumstances, the distal renal vessels remain undisturbed during the reconstructive procedure.

The aortic bypass graft anastomosis is undertaken before the renal artery anastomosis. As with endarterectomy procedures, patients are anticoagulated with intravenous administration of heparin, 150 units/kg. A side-biting vascular clamp is used to occlude the aorta. A lateral or anterolateral aortotomy is made, with its length approximately two times the bypass graft diameter. The saphenous vein is the preferred graft for most reconstructions. It is harvested with a branch included at its caudal end whenever possible. This branch is incised along its lumen adjacent to the parent vein so that a common orifice is created, connecting the branch lumen to the lumen of the main trunk. The generous circumference created by this "branch patch" maneuver lessens the likelihood of anastomatic narrowing and allows for a relatively perpendicular origin of the vein graft from the aorta. The graft-to-aorta anastomosis is usually performed using 4-0 or 5-0 polypropylene suture.

The most direct route for right-sided aortorenal grafts is in a retrocaval position. However, some renal grafts are less likely to kink when originating from the anterolateral surface of the aorta and carried in front of the inferior vena cava, then posteriorly to the renal vessels. The choice of antecaval or retrocaval graft positioning must be individualized in each patient. Grafts to the left kidney are almost always positioned beneath the left renal vein.

The renal artery anastomosis is fashioned after the aortic anastomosis is completed. The proximal renal artery is clamped, transected, and ligated in preparation for performance of the renal anastomosis. As in other renal revascularization procedures, a sustained diuresis should be established by intravenous administration of 12.5 g mannitol prior to interrupting antegrade renal artery blood flow. Preformed collateral vessels usually provide enough blood flow to maintain kidney viability during the period of operative renal artery occlusion. Microvascular clamps, developing tensions ranging from 30 to 70 g, are favored for occluding distal renal vessels over conventional macrovascular clamps or elastic slings. They have less potential to cause vessel injury, and because of their very small size, they do not obscure the operative field.

The graft-to-renal artery anastomosis, performed in an end-to-end fashion, is facilitated by spatulation of the graft posteriorly and the renal artery anteriorly. This allows visualization of the artery's interior, such that inclusion of its intima with each stitch is easily accomplished. Stay sutures are placed at the apex of each spatulation, being continued to the tongue of the

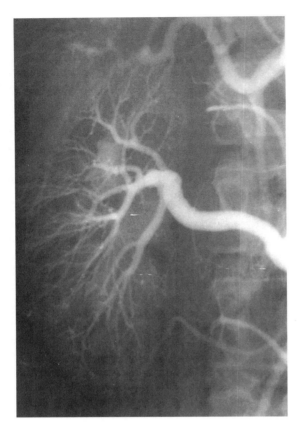

Figure 58-2. Autogenous saphenous vein aortorenal graft. (Reprinted from Stanley JC, Graham LM. Renovascular hypertension. In: Miller DC, Roon AJ, eds. *Diagnosis and Management of Peripheral Vascular Disease.* Menlo Park, CA: Addison-Wesley; 198:231–253 with permission.)

opposite conduit. In adults, the anastomosis is completed using a continuous suture of 5-0 or 6-0 polypropylene. In pediatric patients, multiple 6-0 or 7-0 polypropylene sutures are interrupted to provide for anastomotic growth. These spatulated anastomoses are ovoid, and with healing are less likely to develop later strictures.

After the anastomoses are completed, the vascular clamps are removed and antegrade renal blood flow is reestablished. Anticoagulation is reversed with slow intravenous administration of 1.5 mg protamine sulfate for each 100 units of previously given heparin. The reconstruction is assessed by duplex scanning or flow evaluation with directional Doppler scanning.

Autologous saphenous vein grafts are usually preferred for reconstructions in adults with fibrodysplastic renal artery disease[6–9] (Fig. 58–2). Dacron or expanded polytetra fluroethylene conduits may be used for main renal artery reconstructive procedures, especially when originating from an aortoiliac or aortofemoral graft in the treatment of arteriosclerotic renal artery disease[2,10,11] (Fig. 58–3). However, synthetic grafts are less compliant and technically more difficult to use when revascularizations involve small, dysplastic segmental vessels. Hypogastric artery grafts are preferred when undertaking an aortorenal bypass in a child (Fig. 58–4A).[12,13] Vein grafts should not be used in children because of their propensity to undergo aneurysmal dilation.[14]

Management of stenotic disease affecting multiple renal arteries or segmental branches often requires separate implantations of the renal arteries into a single

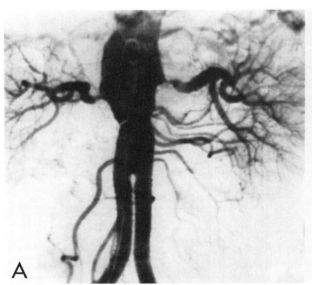

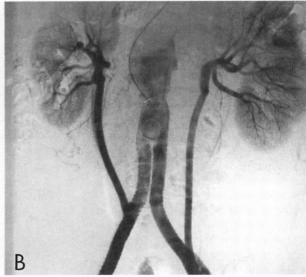

Figure 58-3. (A) Preoperative arteriographic demonstration of bilateral severe orificial artery stenoses. (B) Postoperative arteriogram of bilateral renal revascularization with PTFE grafts originating from limbs of a previously placed aortobifemoral graft. (Reprinted from Messina LM, Zelenock GB, Yao KA, Stanley JC. Renal revascularization for recurrent pulmonary edema in patient with poorly controlled hypertension and renal insufficiency: a distinct subgroup of patients with arteriosclerotic renal artery occlusive disease. *J Vasc Surg* 1992;15:73–82 with permission.)

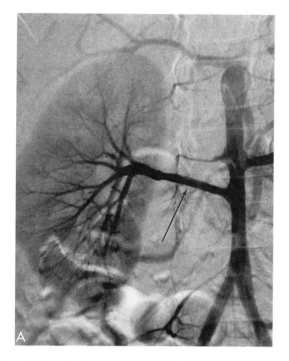

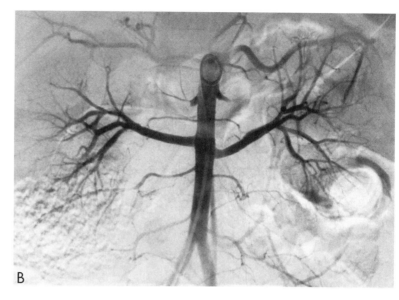

Figure 58–4. (A) Autogenous iliac artery aortorenal graft in a pediatric patient. (B) Aortic reimplanation of main renal arteries beyond orificial stenoses in a pediatric patient. (Reprinted from Ref. 13 with permission.)

graft.[15] This may be accomplished with an end-to-side anastomosis of one artery into the side of the proximal graft and an end-to-end anastomosis of the second artery to the distal graft. If a nonreversed branching segment of saphenous vein in which the valves have been cut or a hypogastric artery with its branches intact is used as the bypass conduit, then multiple end-to-end, graft-to-artery anastomoses may be undertaken. In some patients, it may be easier to perform an in situ anastomosis of the involved arteries in a side-to-side manner so as to form a single channel, with the graft then anastomosed to this common orifice. In complex reconstructions the surgeon should be capable of performing an ex vivo renal revascularization.[16–19]

Aortic Reimplantation

Renal artery reimplantation of the normal renal artery into the aorta, or into an adjacent undiseased renal artery, after transection beyond its stenotic segment, is an important alternative to conventional aortorenal bypass, especially in children with proximal orificial disease[13] (Fig. 58–4B). In these circumstances, the transected renal artery should be spatulated anteriorly and posteriorly to create a generous anastomotic patch. A lateral aortotomy or arteriotomy in an adjacent renal artery, with its length twice the diameter of the artery to be implanted, will provide for a sufficiently large anastomosis. These anastomoses are performed using monofilament suture in an interrupted fashion in the case of small vessels in children and with continuous

sutures in larger arteries in adults. Reimplantations in adults are not commonly performed because of the presence of aortic arteriosclerosis that may lead to anastomotic complications. This is not an issue in pediatric patients, in whom reimplantation is the currently preferred manner of renal revascularization when treating ostial disease.

NONANATOMIC BYPASS

In extensive aortic atherosclerosis where an endarterectomy or a direct aortic origin of the renal graft might prove hazardous, an indirect reconstruction should be considered.[20–24] In some situations, the splenic or hepatic arteries may serve as adequate inflow sites, provided that preoperative lateral aortography has documented the absence of significant celiac artery stenotic disease. In other instances, an iliorenal bypass may be fashioned with minimal technical difficulties. Specific comments on these individual nonanotomic bypasses deserve note.

Splenorenal Bypass

In the case of left-sided renal artery lesions in adults, an in situ splenorenal bypass is an alternative to an endarterectomy or aortorenal bypass.[23,24] Parenthetically, splenorenal bypass in pediatric patients should be avoided because of poor outcomes, often due to occult or progressively overt celiac artery narrowing that evolves as the child grows older.[12]

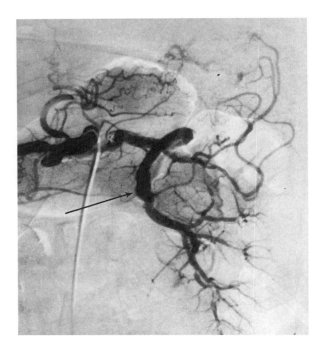

Figure 58–5. Splenorenal bypass. Direct end-to-end anastomosis (arrow) of the left renal artery-to-splenic artery. (Reprinted from Stanley JC, Messina LM. Renal revascularization for recurrent pulmonary edema in patients with poorly controlled renovascular hypertension and renal insufficiency. In: Veith FJ, ed. *Current Critical Problems in Vascular Surgery*, Vol 5. St Louis: Quality Medical; 1993:309–315 with permission.)

Splenorenal bypasses are usually performed following either a retroperitoneal exposure of the renal artery through a thoracoabdominal incision from the 10th intercostal space into the flank or an abdominal incision with an extraperitoneal reflection of the left colon, spleen, and distal pancreas to the right. The splenic artery is easily identified in its midportion along the superior margin of the pancreas and is dissected far enough medially to allow a sufficient length of this vessel to be transposed to the region of the renal artery. Careful identification, transection, and ligation of small splenic artery branches should be undertaken as the dissection proceeds. Following exposure of the left renal artery in a conventional manner, the splenic artery is divided, leaving the distal vessel undissected so as to not disturb existing collateral vessels to the spleen. The mobilized splenic artery is brought down and anastomosed in an end-to-side fashion to the renal artery beyond the stenosis (Fig. 58–5). These vessels are spatulated to form an ovoid anastomosis. It is important to avoid redundancy in these vessels because when the viscera are allowed to resume their normal position, kinking is more likely to occur in the presence of excessive lengths of the splenic and renal arteries.

Hepatorenal Bypass

In certain circumstances in which the aorta is not amenable to an aortorenal endarterectomy or is an unacceptable site for origination of an aortorenal graft due to extensive atherosclerotic disease, the hepatic artery may be used as an inflow source.[22–24] This presumes that there is no proximal celiac artery stenotic disease. In these circumstances, the common hepatic artery is identified and dissected distally a few centimeters beyond its gastroduodenal artery branching. This necessitates freeing the artery from the common duct, which lies lateral to the vessel in this region, and the underlying portal vein. In most instances, the hepatic artery is occluded following systemic anticoagulation, and a segment of autogenous saphenous vein is anastomosed to the hepatic artery in an end-to-side manner in the region of the gastroduodenal artery. The latter vessel is often ligated and transected at its origin. The hepatic artery is incised at this point to create a generous end-to-side, graft-to-hepatic artery anastomosis. Following the completion of the hepatic-graft anastomosis, the right renal artery, having been exposed in a conventional manner, is then divided and the graft is anastomosed to its distal portion beyond the stenotic disease. This is performed in an end-to-end fashion. In most instances, the hepatorenal graft assumes a gentle course over the common duct, passing in an inferoposterior direction to the renal hilum. In certain circumstances, such as with a long renal artery or replaced hepatic artery originating from the superior mesenteric artery, a direct end-to-side implantation of the renal artery may be performed without the use of a graft (Fig. 58–6). Occasionally, the gastroduodenal artery may be used as an in situ graft to the renal artery.

Iliorenal Bypass

When a diseased aorta precludes its clamping or when minimal aneurysmal disease exists, not warranting aortic replacement but sufficient to be hazardous if aortic clamps are applied, renal artery bypass grafts may be originated from the lateral or anterolateral aspects of the common iliac artery.[2] Autogenous saphenous vein as well as synthetic prostheses may be used for these reconstructions. The iliac anastomosis is fashioned first, with subsequent completion of an end-to-end graft to renal artery anastomosis. Although such grafts are associated with acute changes in blood flow direction at their origin and are downstream from proximal aortic disease that may progress, they have actually proven to be quite durable. In instances where more conventional reconstructions, including nonanatomic bypasses involving the splenic or hepatic circulations, are not possible, iliorenal grafts are an acceptable means of treating renovascular hypertension.

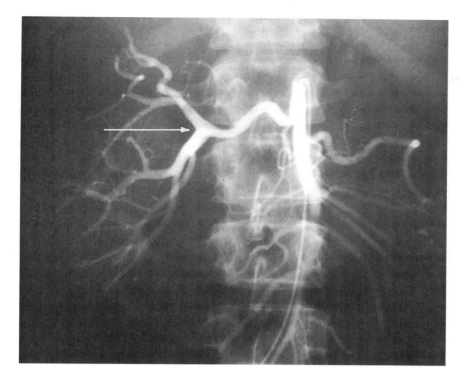

Figure 58–6. Hepatorenal bypass, constructed by direct implantation in an end-to-side fashion, of the right renal artery into a replaced common hepatic artery (arrow) originating from the superior mesenteric artery. A contralateral nephrectomy was also undertaken. (Reprinted from Stanley JC, Messina LM. Renal revascularization for recurrent pulmonary edema in patients with poorly controlled renovascular hypertension and renal insufficiency. In: Veith FJ, ed. *Current Critical Problems in Vascular Surgery*, Vol 5. St Louis: Quality Medical; 1993:309–315 with permission.)

Table 58–1.   Results of Surgical Treatment of Renovascular Hypertension in Specific Patient Subgroups: University of Michigan Experience

Subgroup	Number of Patients	Postoperative Status*†			Operative Mortality Rate
		Cure	Improvement	Failure	
Pediatric disease	34	85%	12%	3%	0
Arterial fibrodysplasia	144	55%	39%	6%	0
Arteriosclerosis					
Focal renal artery disease	64	33%	58%	9%	0
Overt extrarenal disease	71	25%	47%	28%	8.5%

*Represents outcomes of 415 operations (346 primary, 59 secondary), including initial nephrectomy in 17 patients.
† Cure: blood pressures were 150/90 mm Hg or less for a minimum of 6 months postoperatively, during which time no antihypertensive medications were administered. *Improvement*: normotensive while on drug therapy, or if diastolic blood pressure ranged between 90 and 100 mm Hg but were at least 15% lower than preoperative levels: *Failures*: diastolic blood pressure above 90 mm Hg but less than 15% lower than preoperative levels or above 110 mm Hg. Lower pressure standards were used in evaluating pediatric patients.
Source: Ref. 7.

RESULTS OF OPERATIVE THERAPY

Renal preservation and maintenance of renal function are important in assessing clinical outcomes following operative therapy. Nephrectomy may provide good early results but obviously leaves the patient at considerable risk if contralateral disease occurs later. An appropriately performed primary revascularization is exceedingly relevant in that reoperations are often associated with loss of the kidney.[25] Cumulative primary and secondary nephrectomy rates in any given practice should not exceed 10%. Improved renal function after revascularization is well recognized and is most likely to occur among patients exhibiting arteriosclerotic dis-

ease with marked impairment in preoperative renal function.[26–28]

Surgical treatment of renovascular hypertension affords excellent outcomes.[60,61] Differences among many reported experiences reflect variations in the prevalence of different renovascular disease categories. These differencs are most evident when analyzing outcomes in an individual practice (Table 58–1). Arteriosclerotic renovascular hypertension appears to occur in two subgroups: (1) those with focal renal artery disease whose only clinical manifestation of arteriosclerosis is secondary hypertension and (2) those with clinically overt extrarenal arteriosclerosis affecting the coronary,

Table 58–2. Pediatric Renovascular Hypertension

Institution	No. of Patients	Operative Outcome (%)			Surgical Mortality %
		Cured	Improved	Failed	
University of Michigan	57	79	19	2	0
Cleveland Clinic	27	59	18.5	18.5	4
University of California, Los Angeles	26	84.5	7.5	4	4
Vanderbilt University	21	68	24	8	0
University of Pennsylvania	17	76.5	23.5	0	0
Argentinian Institute, Buenos Aires, Argentina	15	53	13	27	7
University of California, San Francisco	14	86	7	0	7

Source: Modified from Ref. 1.

Table 58–3. Fibrodysplastic Renovascular Hypertension in Adults

Institution	No. of Patients	Operative Outcome (%)			Surgical Mortality %
		Cured	Improved	Failed	
University of Michigan	144	55	39	6	0
Baylor College of Medicine	113	43	24	33	0
Cleveland Clinic	92	58	31	11	Unstated
University of California, San Francisco	77	66	32	1.3	0
Mayo Clinic	63	66	24	10	Unstated
University Hospital Leiden, Leiden, the Netherlands	53	53	34	13	2
Vanderbilt University	44	72	24	4	2.3
Columbia University	42	76	14	10	Unstated
Bouman Gray	40	33	57	10	0
University of Lund, Malmo, Sweden	40	66	24	10	0

Source: Modified from Ref. 1.

Table 58–4. Arteriosclerotic Renovascular Hypertension in Adults

Institution	No. of Patients	Operative Outcome (%)			Surgical Mortality %
		Cured	Improved	Failed	
Baylor College of Medicine	360	34	31	35	2.5
Bowman Gray	152	15	75	10	1.3
University of Michigan	135	29	52	19	4.4
University of California, San Francisco	84	39	23	38	2.4
Cleveland Clinic	78	40	51	9	2
Columbia University	67	58	21	21	Unstated
University of Lund, Malmo, Sweden	66	49	24	27	0.9
Hospital Aiguelongue, Montpellier, France	65	45	40	15	1.1
Vanderbilt University	63	50	45	5	9

Source: Modified from Ref. 1.

carotid, aorta, or extremity vessels. The severity and duration of hypertension, age, and sex distribution in these two subgroups exhibiting arterioslcerosis are similar, yet the surgical outcome regarding amelioration of hypertension is worse in those with overt extrarenal arteriosclerotic disease.

Pediatric renovascular hypertension is most likely to exhibit a salutory outcome after restoration of normal renal blood flow (Table 58–2). Arterial fibrodysplastic renovascular hypertension (Table 58–3) is more likely to benefit from operation than is arteriosclerotic renovascular hypertension (Table 58–4). This is likely a reflection of coexistent essential hypertension in older patients with arteriosclerotic disease. Salutary outcomes in contemporary surgical experiences justify operative intervention in properly selected patients with renovascular hypertension.

REFERENCES

1. Stanley JC. The evolution of surgery for renovascular occlusive disease. *Cardiovasc Surg* 1994;2:195–202.
2. Stanley JC, Messina LM, Wakefield TW, et al. Renal artery reconstruction. In: Bergan JJ, Yao JST, ed. *Techniques in Arterial Surgery* Philadelphia: WB Saunders; 1990:247–263.
3. Dougherty MJ, Hallett JW Jr, Naessens J, et al. Renal endarterectomy vs. bypass for combined aortic and renal reconstruction: is there a difference in clinical outcome? *Ann Vasc Surg* 1995;9:87–94.
4. McNeil JW, String ST, Pfeiffer RB Jr, et al. Concomitant renal endarterectomy and aortic reconstruction. *J Vasc Surg* 1994;20:331–337.
5. Stoney RJ, Messina LM, Goldstone J, et al. Renal endarterectomy through the transected aorta: a new technique for combined aortorenal arteriosclerosis. A preliminary report. *J Vasc Surg* 1989;9:224–233.
6. Novick AC, Stewart BH, Straffon RA. Autogenous arterial grafts in the treatment of renal artery stenosis. *J Urol* 1977;118:919–922.
7. Stanley JC, Whitehouse WM Jr, Graham LM, et al. Operative therapy of renovascular hypertension. *Br J Surg* 1982;69(suppl):S63–S66.
8. Anderson CA, Hansen KJ, Benjamin ME, et al. Renal artery fibromuscular dysplasia: results of current surgical therapy. *J Vasc Surg* 1995;22:207–216.
9. Hansen KJ, Starr SM, Sands RE, et al. Contemporary surgical management of renovascular disease. *J Vasc Surg* 1992;16:319–330.
10. Kaufmann JJ. Long-term results of aortorenal Dacron grafts in the treatment of renal artery stenosis. *J Urol* 1974;111:298–304.
11. Lagneau P, Michel JB, Charrat JM. Use of polytetrafluoroethylene grafts for renal bypass. *J Vasc Surg* 1987;5:738–742.
12. Novick AC, Straffon RA, Stewart BH, et al. Surgical treatment of renovascular hypertension in the pediatric patient. *J Urol* 1978;119:794–805.
13. Stanley JC, Zelenock GB, Messina LM, et al. Pediatric renovascular hypertension: a thirty-year experience of operative treatment. *J Vasc Surg* 1995;21:212–227.
14. Stanley JC, Ernst CB, Fry WJ. Fate of 100 aortorenal vein grafts: characteristics of late graft expansion, aneurysmal dilatation, and stenosis. *Surgery* 1973;74:931–944.
15. Ernst CB, Stanley JC, Fry WJ. Multiple primary and segmental renal artery revascularization utilizing autogenous saphenous vein. *Surg Gynecol Obstet* 1973;137:1023–1026.
16. Brekke IB, Sodal G, Jakobsen A, et al. Fibro-muscular renal artery disease treated by extracorporeal vascular reconstruction and renal autotransplantation: short- and long-term results. *Eur J Vasc Surg* 1992;6:471–476.
17. Kent KC, Salvatierra O, Reilly LM, et al. Evolving strategies for the repair of complex renovascular lesions. *Ann Surg* 1987;206:272–278.
18. Murray SP, Kent KC, Salvatierra O, et al. Complex branch renovascular disease: management options and late results. *J Vasc Surg* 1994;20:338–346.
19. van Bockel JH, van den Akker PJ, Chang PC, et al. Extracorporeal renal artery reconstruction for renovascular hypertension. *J Vasc Surg* 1991;13:101–111.
20. Cambria RP, Brewster DC, L'Italien G, et al. Simultaneous aortic and renal artery reconstruction: evolution of an eighteen-year experience. *J Vasc Surg* 1994;21:916–925.
21. Cambria RP, Brewster DC, L'Italien GJ, et al. The durability of different reconstructive techniques for atherosclerotic renal artery disease. *J Vasc Surg* 1994;20:76–87.
22. Chibaro EA, Libertino JA, Novick AC. Use of the hepatic circulation for renal revascularization. *Ann Surg* 1984;199:406–411.
23. Khauli RB, Novick AC, Ziegelbaum M. Splenorenal bypass in the treatment of renal artery stenosis: experience with 69 cases. *J Vasc Surg* 1985;2:547–551.
24. Moncure AC, Brewster DC, Darling RC, et al. Use of the splenic and hepatic arteries for renal revascularization. *J Vasc Surg* 1986;3:196–203.
25. Stanley JC, Whitehouse WM Jr, Zelenock GB, et al. Reoperation for complications of renal artery reconstructive surgery undertaken for treatment of renovascular hypertension. *J Vasc Surg* 1985;2:133–144.
26. Hallett JW Jr, Textor SC, Kos PB, et al. Advanced renovascular hypertension and renal insufficiency: trends in medical comorbidity and surgical approach from 1970 to 1993. *J Vasc Surg* 1995;21:750–760.
27. Hansen KJ, Thomason RB, Craven TE, et al. Surgical management of dialysis-dependent ischemic nephropathy. *J Vasc Surg* 1995;21:197–211.
28. Whitehouse WM Jr, Kazmers A, Zelenock GB, et al. Chronic total renal artery occlusions: effects of treatment on secondary hypertension and renal function. *Surgery* 1989;89:753–763.

59

Renal Artery Angioplasty and Stent Placement: Indications and Results

David W. Trost, M.D.
Thomas A. Sos, M.D.

It has been estimated that 1 to 5% of hypertension is due to occlusive renal artery disease.[1] Recently, it has been recognized that ischemic nephropathy can produce renal failure even without accompanying hypertension.[2,3]

SCREENING AND DIAGNOSIS OF PATIENTS WITH SUSPECTED RENOVASCULAR HYPERTENSION (Algorithm 1)

Clinical Characteristics (Tables 59–1 and 59–2)

The clinical characteristics and diagnosis of renovascular hypertension have been described in detail elsewhere.[4]

Most diagnostic and screening tests are somewhat unreliable, especially in the presence of bilateral renal artery disease or renal dysfunction. For these reasons, a diagnostic arteriogram should be obtained sooner rather than later. Conventional cut-film arteriography requires relatively large amounts of contrast material for adequate visualization of the renal arteries; this frequently results in transient or even permanent renal failure, especially in patients with compromised renal function.[5] We now use intra-arterial digital subtraction angiography (IADSA) and only 15 to 20 mL of 30% ionic contrast medium for aortography, and renal failure has been almost completely eliminated. A single frontal aortogram allows the diagnosis of significant renal artery disease in virtually all patients.

Experimental studies have demonstrated that flow is decreased when the cross-sectional area stenosis reaches 80 to 90%.[6] Most clinically significant renal artery stenoses compromise 80% of the vessel diameter

Table 59–1. Clinical Characteristics of Renovascular Hypertension

1. Recent onset of hypertension
2. Relatively difficult to control hypertension
3. Retinopathy
4. Onset of hypertension after age 55 (etiology most likely atherosclerosis)
5. History of smoking
6. Presence of vascular disease in other organ systems
7. Renal dysfunction
8. Continuous systolic/diastolic abdominal bruit
9. Onset of hypertension at a relatively young age, particularly in women (etiology most likely fibromuscular dysplasia)
10. Recurrent pulmonary edema even in the absence of severe coronary disease

Table 59–2. Diagnostic Tests for Renovascular Hypertension

1. Radionuclide renal scanning with and without angiotensin-converting enzyme (ACE) inhibition (insensitive and inaccurate in the presence of renal dysfunction and/or bilateral disease)
2. Selective renal vein renin sampling and assay with and without ACE inhibition (insensitive and inaccurate in the presence of renal dysfunction and/or bilateral disease)
3. Magnetic resonance angiography
4. Renal artery duplex sonography
5. Helical (spiral) computed tomography (contraindicated in patients with renal dysfunction)

and are not difficult to recognize as being very severe. When in doubt, the stenosis is usually *not* considered clinically important, and in some of these cases, meas-

ALGORITHM 1
Algorithm for the Evaluation and Treatment of patients with suspected Renovascular Hypertension

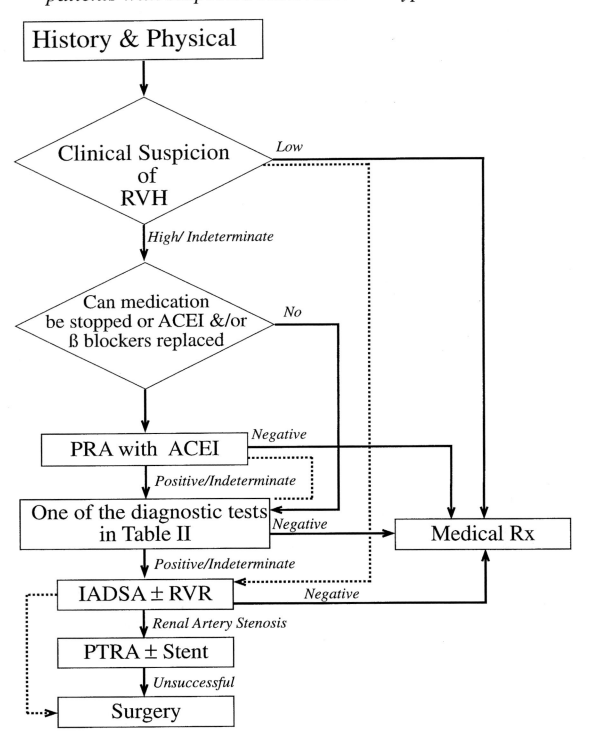

Algorithm 1 Evaluation and treatment of patients with suspected renovascular hypertension. ACEI, angiotensin-converting enzyme inhibitor; IADSA, intra-arterial digital subtraction angiography; PRA, peripheral plasma renin activity; PTRA, percutaneous transluminal renal angioplasty; RVH, renovascular hypertension; RVR, renal vein sampling for renin assay; Rx, therapy; solid lines, preferred and accepted; dashed lines, optional based on individual patient and on physician's judgment.

ALGORITHM 2
Algorithm for the Evaluation and Treatment of
patients with suspected Ischemic Nephropathy

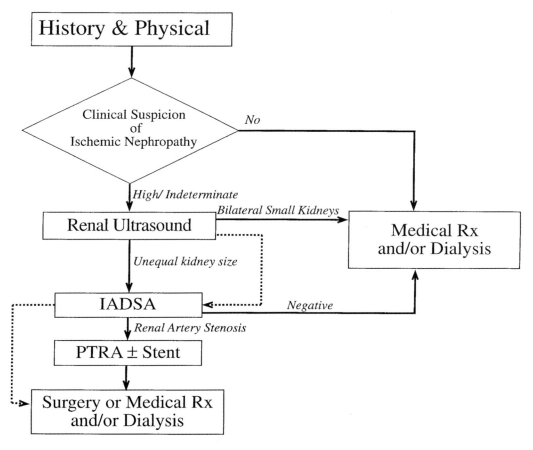

Algorithm 2 Evaluation and treatment of patients with suspected ischemic nephropathy. For abbreviations, see legend of Algorithm 1.

uring the arterial pressure beyond the stenosis (recognizing that even a No. 4 Fr catheter will contribute to the transstenotic gradient) is recommended.

SCREENING AND DIAGNOSIS OF PATIENTS WITH SUSPECTED ISCHEMIC NEPHROPATHY (Algorithm 2)

Clinical Characteristics (Table 59–3)

Renal artery stenosis is the cause of renal failure in only a significant minority of patients. However, it is one of the few *reversible* causes of azotemia. Patients without clearly documented medical renal parenchymal disease, particularly those who have other vascular disease, those who smoke, and those with relatively recent onset

and rapid progression of renal dysfunction and who have kidneys of unequal size should be suspected of having renal artery stenosis as the cause of their azotemia.

Table 59–3. Clinical Characteristics Suggestive of Ischemic Nephropathy

1. Presence of vascular disease in other organ systems
2. Absence of documented renal parenchymal disease
3. Recent onset of renal dysfunction
4. History of smoking
5. Unequal kidney size
6. Rapid progression of renal dysfunction
7. Presence of hypertension

Physiologically significant renal arterial occlusive disease can produce renovascular hypertension with or without ischemic nephropathy. Although the pathophysiologic basis of renovascular hypertension (renin-angiotensin-aldosterone axis) is now well understood, applications of tests based on these physiologic principles have been disappointing. We strongly urge the early use of intra-arterial digital subtraction angiography for confirmation of the diagnosis. We believe that no patient should be treated by dialysis unless a reversible cause has been looked for and eliminated. It is far less expensive and less dangerous to perform intra-arterial digital subtraction arteriography than to dialyze a patient with reversible renal artery disease. If angioplasty or stenting is the initial procedure of choice, then a significant lesion should be treated immediately rather than subjecting the patient to the risk of a repeat catheterization. Prior to performing an angioplasty, the surgical options should also be discussed in case the angioplasty or stent fails or produces a complication. If the surgical procedure of choice is a bypass graft from the branches of the celiac axis, then prior to the angioplasty the celiac axis should be selectively catheterized to determine whether there is a pressure gradient rather than using additional contrast material for a lateral aortogram. If the surgeon's preferred operation is an aortorenal endarterectomy, then a stent should be placed in the ostium only if it is accepted that this surgical option probably would not be available. A stent should not be deployed near the renal hilum because it may interfere with a subsequent aortorenal bypass graft.

Treatment Options

Although there has never been a randomized, prospective study to compare medical therapy, surgery, and angioplasty with stents, many physicians intuitively believe that revascularization and salvage of the ischemic kidney is preferable to long-term systemic antihypertensive therapy. If this assumption is accepted, then it is reasonable to perform angioplasty or stent deployment initially because these rarely interfere with a subsequent surgical revascularization.

RENAL ANGIOPLASTY

The concept of percutaneous transluminal angioplasty (PTA) for the treatment of vascular obstructive disease was first described by Dotter and Judkins in 1964.[7] The initial technique consisted of advancing rigid coaxial Teflon dilators over a guidewire sequentially, one over the other, and was applicable only to relatively straight arteries. Developments in technology culminated in Gruntzig's design of a double-lumen balloon dilation catheter in 1974. This catheter had a flexible, thin shaft and a cylindrical balloon at its tip that could be inflated in the stenotic area. Gruntzig reported the first renal balloon angioplasty (percutaneous transluminal renal angioplasty [PTRA]) in 1979.[8,9] An example of a PTRA is illustrated in Figure 59–1.

COMPLICATIONS AND THEIR PREVENTION

Complications are reported to occur in 5 to 10% of patients.[5] The most frequent major complications in

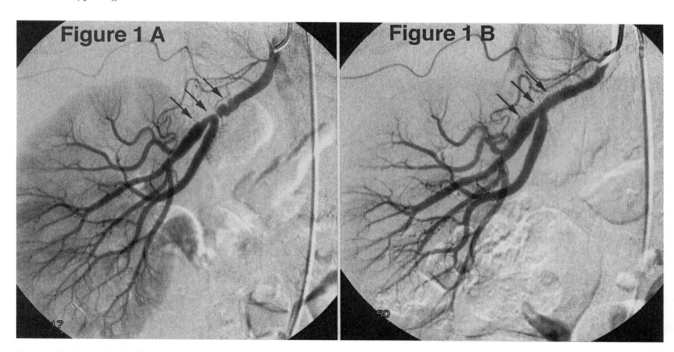

Figure 59–1.   (A) The classic beaded appearance of the medial form of fibromuscular dysplasia is seen in the right renal artery (arrows). (B) The appearance of the artery immediately after balloon angioplasty (arrows).

PTRA are initiated by thrombosis and spasm of the renal artery. Macroembolization of atheroma and microcholesterol crystal embolization of the kidneys and other organs can occur. Mechanical perforation and frank rupture of the renal artery are infrequent complications in experienced hands.

Careful technique and the use of adjunctive antispasmotic medications can prevent or diminish the incidence and severity of complications.

RESULTS OF PTRA

The overall technical success rate is approximately 90 to 95%.[10–13] Technical success is highest in the Fibro Muscular Dysplasia (FMD) and unilateral nonostial atheroma. Technical success in occlusions is obtainable about 50% of the time.[14] The hypertensive benefit after PTRA is about 70 to 90% overall; for atheroma, 65 to 95%; and for FMD, 85 to 100%[10–13] (Table 59–4). Hypertensive benefit is about 70%[10–13,15,16] in unilateral, nonostial, atheromatous stenosis (Table 59–5), 46% in bilateral atheroma,[13] and only 25% in ostial

lesions. Patients in whom renal vein renins lateralize can expect a higher therapeutic benefit rate than those in whom they do not.[11] The hypertensive benefit rates for various subsets of patients are as follows: arteritis 86%,[17] azotemia 43%[18] renal allografts 76%[18] and pediatric age group almost 100%.[19]

PTRA has also been shown to be useful in the treatment of renal artery stenoses due to Takayasu's arteritis,[20] and case reports have shown benefit in lesions due to neurofibromatosis.[21]

RESTENOSIS

Recurrences within the first couple of weeks to the first few months are probably due to inadequate and incomplete dilations (especially in ostial lesions), which stretch the elastic vessel but fail to rupture the plaque and inadequately overdilate the adventitia. In recurrences at or after 6 months, the pathophysiology is more complicated. The initial controlled trauma of angioplasty results in platelet deposition and activation at the dilation site followed by fibrocellular prolifera-

Table 59–4.   Immediate and Long-Term Clinical Results of Renal Angioplasty in Fibromuscular Dysplasia

Author	No. of Patients	Successfully Dilated (%)	Cured (%)	Improved (%)	Follow-up (mos) Mean (Range)
Sos[10]	31	27 (87)	16 (59)	9 (33)	16 (4–40)
Tegtmeyer[12]	27	27 (100)	10 (37)	17 (63)	NA (2–51)
Geyskes[15]	21	21 (100)	10 (48)	10 (48)	NA (12–48)
Martin[18]	20	20 (100)	5 (25)	12 (60)	16 (3–36)
Jensen[31]	30	29 (97)	11 (39)	13 (47)	12 (12)
Martin[32]	11	8 (73)	5 (63)	1 (13)	13 (NA)
Grim[16]	10	9 (90)	5 (56)	4 (44)	10 (1–14)
Total	150	141 (94)	62 (41)	66 (44)	

Abbreviation: NA, not available.

Table 59–5.   Immediate and Long-Term Clinical Results of Renal Angioplasty in Unilateral, Nonostial Atheroma

Author	No. of Patients	Successfully Dilated (%)	Cured (%)	Improved (%)	Follow-up (mos) Mean (Range)
Tegtmeyer[12]*†	65	61 (94)	15 (25)	129 (55)	NA (1–60)
Grim[16]	16	16 (100)	1 (7)	8 (50)	10 (3–24)
Schwarten[33]	54	49 (91)	23 (47)	25 (51)	NA (1–18)
Martin[18]†	38	?38 (100)?	10 (25)	19 (47)	19 (3–36)
Martin[32]	15	13 (87)	2 (15)	4 (31)	13 (NA)
Sos[10]	20	15 (75)	4 (27)	9 (60)	16 (4–40)
Geyskes[15]*	44	44 (100)	4 (9)	19 (43)	NA (12–48)
Total	252	236 (94)	59 (25)	130 (55)	

*Includes some patients with bilateral disease.
†Includes some patients with ostial stenoses.
Abbreviation: NA, not available.

tion leading to neointimal hyperplasia. Smoking and hyperlipidemia also contribute to the frequency and severity of restenosis.[22,23]

In most PTRA series, the recurrence rate is reported to be 15 to 20%. Unfortunately, most authors combine atheromatous and fibromuscular recurrences, and because recurrences in fibromuscular disease are rare, the combined recurrence rate is significantly lower than it would be for atheromatous disease alone. Additionally, most authorities base recurrence data on clinical follow-up or angiographic examination of only those patients clinically suspected of having restenosis. There are very few studies and very few patients in whom routine follow-up angiography was performed. These studies indicate that some patients with clinical suspicion of recurrence do indeed have recurrent stenoses; however, not infrequently, the dilated renal artery is normal, while the contralateral, previously normal artery has developed a stenosis. In other instances, there is angiographic recurrence with no clinical manifestation of hypertension.[24] For these reasons, only recurrence data based on nonselected angiographic follow-up are statistically valid.

We attempted to restudy by angiography 36 patients with unilateral, nonostial atheromatous disease. At follow-up after approximately 30 months (mean), half of these patients have been restudied, and the restenosis rate was 17%.

RENAL ARTERY STENTING

Angioplasty of the renal ostium does not work well because in ostial stenoses the sheet of atheroma surrounding the renal artery ostium is acted on in a longitudinal rather than a radial fashion by the dilating balloon. Soon the deflation of the balloon, the atheroma recoils and the stenosis recurs.

To solve this problem, several large multicenter renal artery stent trials have been completed or are underway in Europe, Australia, and the United States (although none of the stent designs have been approved by the Food and Drug Administration for use in renal arteries). Renal artery stents are probably best used for ostial stenoses, restenoses following PTRA, complications of PTRA, and for other lesions that responded poorly to conventional angioplasty. From the published data, it appears clear that stenting of ostial stenoses has a higher initial success rate[25] and a greatly improved intermediate-term patency rate over balloon angioplasty alone. These data justify primary placement of stents for ostial disease.

TECHNICAL CONSIDERATIONS

Placing renal stents is similar but not identical to angioplasty. While angioplasty does not usually affect subsequent surgical renal artery revascularization, stenting

can. Stents prevent the performance of an aortic endarterectomy, a procedure that is again gaining popularity. A proximally placed stent will not usually affect most bypass procedures unless the stent extends too far toward the renal hilum. Correctly positioning the stent in an ostial stenosis is of the utmost importance. It is essential that the artery origin is imaged in the proper oblique so that it is exactly in profile, allowing accurate deployment of the stent so that it extends slightly (~1 to 2 mm) into the aorta and covers the entire lesion. An example of a stent procedure is illustrated in Figure 59–2.

COMPLICATIONS

Potential problems with stent placement include malpositioning, migration, embolization of the stent, and difficulty removing the balloon from the stent. Malpositioning can be minimized by performing the procedure in the proper oblique and taking the time to position the stent carefully. The other complications can be minimized only by using careful technique and sizing the stent and balloon properly.

RESULTS OF STENTING

Early reports of stenting of the renal arteries are now being published. Rees et al presented the results of a multicenter trial of the Palmaz-Schatz stent at the 1994 meeting of the Cardiovascular and Interventional Radiological Society of Europe.[26] A total of 304 stents were placed in 296 arteries in 263 patients. The technical success rate was 95%, 98% of lesions were atherosclerotic, and 80% were ostial. At the 6-month follow-up, 64% of patients had improvement or cure of hypertension. In 123 patients with renal insufficiency (creatinine level >1.5 mg/dL), there was improvement in 34%, stabilization in 39%, and deterioration in 27%. Angiographic follow-up at 6 months was performed in 150 patients. Angiographic restenosis (residual luminal diameter <50%) occurred in 32.7%. Restenosis was lower in males 23% (p <0.05), lower for stents dilated to >6 mm (26%, p <0.05), and lowest for males with stents dilated to >6 mm (10.5%).

Similar results have been reported by Dorros et al[27]; 92 arteries were stented in 76 patients. 62 (82%) patients were hypertensive and 39 (51%) patients had renal dysfunction. Repeat angiography at 6 months was performed in 45 of 62 eligible arteries (73%). Restenosis was seen in 14 (25%). In patients with chronic renal failure, benefit was observed in 55%. Blood pressure was improved in the entire cohort.

At The New York Hospital, we have stented 60 arteries in 53 patients using Palmaz stents; 55 of these stents were placed for atheromatous ostial stenoses. All patients were hypertensive; 32 had serum creatinine levels ≥1.5 mg/dL and 24 had levels ≥2.0 mg/dL.

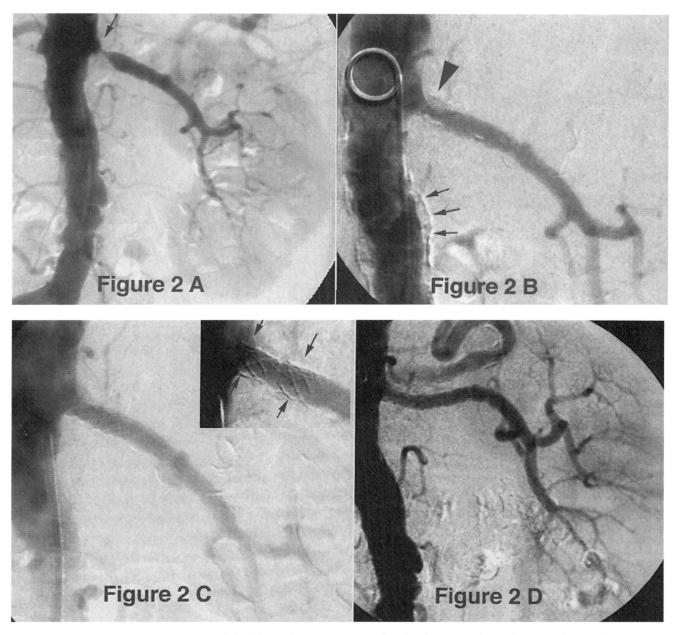

Figure 59—2.   (A) Severe ostial stenosis of the left renal artery. (B) Immediately after angioplasty, there is still a significant stenosis (large arrowhead). Note the calcium in the thickened aortic wall (arrows), which suggests that the stenosis is due to ostial atheromatous disease. (C) After stent placement, the arterial lumen is normal. (D) The metallic stent is more clearly seen on the inset (small arrows). The follow-up arteriogram at 17 months shows the stented artery to be widely patent.

Thirty percent of the patients were functionally or anatomically uninephric. Ninety-seven percent of the procedures were technically successful. Repeat angiography was performed in 22 (39%) of the eligible stented arteries after a mean interval of 11 months. Five (23%) of the stents had 60% or greater luminal diameter restenosis; however, in only two patients was this accompanied by deterioration of renal function and worsening of hypertension. The mean clinical follow-up interval was 15.8 months, with a range of 0 to 43 months; however, 22 patients were followed for at least

15 months. No patients were cured, but 51% of patients had reduction of hypertension. All patients with serum creatinine levels ≤1.5 mg/dL were stable at the last clinical follow-up. Of 24 patients with serum creatinine levels ≥2.0 mg/dL, 13 were improved, 7 were stable and 4 deteriorated (one of whom had microcholesterol embolization).

In 1994, Hennequin et al reported the long-term follow-up of 25 Wallstents placed in 21 patients.[28] Thirteen were placed for restenosis after previous balloon angioplasty and eight following an inadequate immediate postangioplasty response. Clinical indications were hypertension in all patients and renal preservation in seven. The stenoses were atheromatous in 15 patients and involved the ostium in only 7. Initial stent placement was successful in 91% (19/21) of patients. In two patients, the first stent did not cover the lesion and an additional stent was placed at two and three months. At follow-up angiography (range, 12 to 60 months; mean, 29th ± 14.22 months), four patients (20%) had restenosis. Of these four, three had undergone stenting for restenosis after angioplasty and three had ostial lesions. The cumulative primary patency rate was 95%, 85%, and 77% at 7, 9, and 15 months, respectively. The cumulative secondary patency rate was 92% at 15 months. Hypertension was improved in all cases and cured in three. Renal function was improved in one patient, worsened in one patient, and unchanged in the remainder. There were three complications: thrombosis of a small branch vessel ($n = 1$), renal hilar hemorrhage ($n = 1$), and progressive renal dysfunction thought to be secondary to cholesterol embolization ($n = 1$).

Also in 1994, Raynaud et al reported their experience with the Wallstent.[29] Twenty-five stents were deployed in 18 renal arteries in 18 patients. Fifteen were atheromatous lesions, only four of which were ostial. Thirteen were placed for PTRA failures, and the others were placed for post-PTRA dissections. Five patients required a second stent because the initial stent was malpositioned. There were two stent-related complications: one acute thrombosis 15 days after placement and an early restenosis. Hypertension at 6 months was cured in one patient, improved in eight, and unchanged in eight. Sixteen of 18 patients had follow-up angiograms at a mean interval of 11 months. One artery had a restenosis greater than 50%, and one was occluded.

In 1992 Kuhn et al reported their use of the Strecker flexible balloon-expandable tantalum stent for treatment of renal artery stenosis.[30] Indications were an inadequate immediate postangioplasty response ($n = 16$) and obstructing intimal flaps following transaortic endarterectomy ($n = 2$). Seventeen patients were hypertensive and one was normotensive. In two patients, renal artery stenosis had developed after kidney transplantation. Stent placement was technically successful, and patency was preserved in 14 patients. Midterm results (mean, 12 to 13 months) in 11 patients showed restenoses (greater than 50%) in two patients and improvement of hypertension in eight patients.

The immediate and intermediate results of stenting in the renal arteries are encouraging; however, longer follow-up is needed to compare the durability of stents to the results of surgical reconstruction. Currently available stent designs are clearly adequate, but there is room for improvement in the stents and the delivery systems.

REFERENCES

1. Gifford R. Evaluation of the hypertensive patient with emphasis on detecting curable causes. *Millbank Mem Fund Q* 1969;47:170–173.
2. Mailloux LU, Bellucci AG, Mossey RT, et al. Predictors of survival in patients undergoing dialysis. *Am J Med* 1988;84(5):855–862.
3. Dean RH, Tribble RW, Hansen KJ, O'Neil E, Craven TE, Redding JF 2nd. Evaluation of renal insufficiency in ischemic nephropathy. *Ann Surg* 1991;213:446–456.
4. Mann SJ, Pickering TG. Detection of renovascular hypertension: state of the art 1992. *Ann Intern Med* 1992;117:845–853.
5. Trost D, Sos TA, Complications of renal angioplasty and stenting. *Semin Intervent Radiol* 1994;11:150–160.
6. May AG, DeBerg LV, DeWeese JA, Rob CG. Critical arterial stenosis. *Surgery* 1963;54:250–259.
7. Dotter CT, Judkins MP. Transluminal treatment of arteriosclerotic obstruction: description of a new technique and a preliminary report of its applications. *Circulation* 1964;30:654.
9. Gruntzig A, Hopff H. Perkutane rekanalisation chronischer arterieller verschlusse mit einem neuen dilatationskatheter. Modifikation der Dotter-Technik. *Deutsch Med Wochenschr* 1974;99:2502–2511.
10. Sos TA, Pickering TG, Sniderman KW, et al. Percutaneous transluminal renal angioplasty in renovascular hypertension due to atheroma or fibromuscular dysplasia. *N Engl J Med* 1983;309:274–279.
11. Schwarten DE. Transluminal angioplasty of renal artery stenosis: 70 experiences. *AJR* 1980;135:969–974.
12. Tegtmeyer CJ, Kellum CD, Ayers C. Percutaneous transluminal angioplasty of the renal artery. *Radiology* 1984;153:77–84.
13. Martin LG, Price RB, Casarella WJ, et al. Percutaneous angioplasty in the clinical management of renovascular hypertension: initial and long term results. *Radiology* 1985;155:629–633.
14. Sniderman KW, Sos TA. Percutaneous transluminal recanalization and dilatation of totally occluded renal arteries. *Radiology* 1982;142(3):607–610.
15. Geyskes GG, Puylaert CBA, Dei HY, et al. Follow-up study of 70 patients with renal artery stenosis treated by percutaneous transluminal dilatation. *Br Med J* 1983;287–333.
16. Grim CE, Luft FC, Yune HY. Percutaneous transluminal dilatation in the treatment of renal vascular hypertension. *Ann Intern Med* 1981;95:439–442.
17. Dong ZJ, Li S, Lu X. Percutaneous transluminal angioplasty for renovascular hypertension in arteritis: experience in China. *Radiology* 1987;162:477–479.
18. Martin LG, Casarella WJ, Gaylor GM. Azotemia caused by renal artery stenosis: treatment by percutaneous angioplasty. *AJR* 1988;150:839–844.
19. Sos TA, Saddekni S. Pediatric renovascular hypertension: the role of renal angioplasty. Dialogues in *Pediatr Urol* 1985;8(12):7–57. Mahler F, Triller J, Weidmann P, et al. Complications in percutaneous transluminal dilatation of renal arteries. *Nephron* 1986;44(1):60–63.
20. Tyagi S, Singh B, Kaul UA, et al. Balloon angioplasty for renovascular hypertension in Takayasu's arteritis. *Am Heart J* 1993;125(5 pt 1):1386–1393.
21. Fossali E, Minoja M, Intermite R, et al. Percutaneous transluminal renal angioplasty in neurofibromatosis. *Pediatr Nephrol* 1995;9(5):623–625.
22. Kent KM. Restenosis after percutaneous transluminal coronary angioplasty. *Am J Cardiol* 1988;61(14):67G–70G.

23. Wolinsky H. Insights into coronary angioplasty-induced restenosis from examination of atherogenesis. *Am J Cardiol* 1987;60(3):65B–67B.

24. Schwarten DE. Percutaneous transluminal angioplasty of the renal arteries: intravenous digital subtraction angiography for follow-up. *Radiology* 1984;150:369–373.

25. Dorros G, Prince C, Mathiak L. Stenting of a renal artery stenosis achieves better relief of the obstructive lesion than balloon angioplasty. *Cathet Cardiovasc Diagn* 1993; 29:191–198.

26. Rees CR, Niblett R, Snead D. United States Multicenter study of Palmaz-Schatz stents in the renal arteries. Presented at the CIRSE annual meeting and postgraduate course of the Cardiovascular and Interventional Radiological Society of Europe, Crete, June 1994.

27. Dorros G, Jaff M, Jain A, Dufek C, Mathiak L. Follow-up of primary Palmaz-Schatz stent placement for atherosclerotic renal artery stenosis. *Am J Cardiol* 1995; 15;75(15):1051–1055.

28. Hennequin LM, Joffre FG, Rousseau HP, et al. Renal artery stent placement: long-term results with theWallstent endoprosthesis: *Radiology* 1994;191(3):713–719.

29. Raynaud AC, Beyssen BM, Turmel-Rodigues LE, et al. Renal artery stent placement: immediate and midterm technical and clinical results: *JVIR* 1994;5:849–858.

30. Kuhn FP, Malms J, Kutkuhn B, Furst G, Torsello G, Modder U. Renal stent implantation. The current indications, 2-year results and the possibilities for percutaneous stent recovery. *Rofo Fortschr Geb Rontgenstr Neuen Bildgeb Verfahr* 1992;157(1):65–71.

31. Jensen G, Zachrisson B, Delin K, et al. Treatment of renovascular hypertension: one year results of renal angioplasty. *Kidney Int* 1995;48:1936–1945.

32. Martin ED, Mattern RF, Baer L, Fankuchen EL, Casarella WJ. Renal angioplasty for hypertension: predictive factors for long-term success. *Am J Radiol* 1981;137(5):921–924.

33. Schwarten DE, Yune HY, Klatte EC, et al. Clinical experience with percutaneous transluminal angioplasty (PTA) of stenosed renal arteries. *Radiol* 1980;135:601.

60

The Role of PTA, Stents, and Thrombolytic Therapy in the Management of Dialysis Access Sites

Scott O. Trerotola, M.D.

Currently, over 150,000 patients undergo chronic hemodialysis in the United States. For these patients, their vascular access is their lifeline, and maintenance of this access is of paramount importance to the patients as well as their physicians. Interventional radiology (IR) plays an important role in the multidisciplinary effort (along with nephrologists and surgeons) to maintain such vascular access. IR's role in hemodialysis access management can include preoperative venography and/or ultrasound, as well as screening procedures to detect impending access failure. These screening procedures are described in detail elsewhere.[1,2] IR plays the most significant role in the treatment of vascular access complications for which fistulography, angioplasty, atherectomy, thrombolysis, and/or stent placement may become necessary. In addition, interventionalists may place percutaneous temporary and tunneled hemodialysis catheters and treat complications of such catheters.

The sometimes confusing anatomy of hemodialysis fistulae and grafts is beyond the scope of this chapter but is discussed in detail elsewhere.[1,3] Briefly, there are currently two forms of permanent hemodialysis access: the native arteriovenous fistula and the synthetic bridge graft. Arteriovenous fistulae are considered the optimal initial vascular access due to superior patency to synthetic grafts, yet due to an aging population and numerous other factors, only approximately 17% of vascular accesses created in this country are native fistulae.[4] The remainder are synthetic grafts, which have a higher complication rate and lower patency.

Venous outflow stenosis accounts for the majority of vascular access failures. It is the response of the venous stenosis to a given treatment modality that ultimately determines the long-term results of therapy, whether balloon angioplasty, atherectomy, surgical revision, thrombectomy, or thrombolytic therapy. Most graft failures begin with stenosis at the graft–vein anastomosis due to intimal hyperplasia, with progressive increases in graft pressure and reduction in flow. If screening modalities do not detect these abnormalities to allow treatment, the graft will ultimately thrombose. After thrombosis, if simple thrombectomy is performed without treatment of the outflow stenosis, rapid rethrombosis will usually occur.[5,6] The accumulation of venous anastomotic intimal hyperplasia is thought to be due to shear-induced intimal injury, compliance mismatch, and possibly upstream release of platelet-derived growth factor.[7] The material is a firm, rubbery, whitish material consisting primarily of smooth muscle and extracellular matrix. Although the nature of this material is relatively well characterized, efforts to prevent its development (and ensuing graft failures) have to date been fruitless. Until some means are developed to prevent intimal hyperplasia, therapies aimed at treating the resulting venous stenosis will remain the mainstay of percutaneous and surgical management.

Arterial stenoses account for only approximately 5% or less of lesions in grafts,[8,9] although the reported incidence of arterial stenosis is higher in series describing radiologic[10,11] rather than surgical[12,13] treatment of clotted grafts. This discrepancy is probably accounted for by interpretation of residual thrombus at the arterial anastomosis as a stenosis (see the following discussion of thrombolysis) in radiologic series. Approximately 10% of all stenoses are intragraft,[8,12] most commonly at frequent needle puncture sites; they are due to a buildup of intimal hyperplasia at these sites.[14] Such "intra-access" stenoses are also seen in native fistulae, also at the sites of frequent punctures. Graft–graft anastomosis or graftotomy sites are other causes of intragraft stenosis. Stenoses also occur central to the venous anastomosis, at sites of prior trauma such as catheter insertion sites as well as hypertrophied valves.[8,15–17] Occult central venous stenosis occurs in up to 40% of patients who have had prior central venous catheters placed.[18]

TREATMENT OF STENOSIS

Surgical revision,[5,6,10–21] which usually involves patch angioplasty and/or the placement of an interposition graft, continues to be the mainstay in many institutions. Acceptable patency rates are achieved with surgery, with resulting cumulative patency rates of 4 years or more. Surgical revision, however, has the distinct disadvantage of depleting a segment of vein with each subsequent procedure. Multiple revisions may rapidly result in no further usable vein in a given extremity, and access must be sought elsewhere.

The primary advantage of percutaneous management (Fig. 60–1) is that it does not deplete vein. In the early era of percutaneous management of venous outflow stenosis, it was discovered that while initial results were favorable, restenosis was common.[3,8,12,15,17,22–32] Glanz et al (Table 60–1) showed a range of patencies, depending on the location of the lesion, with 50% 1-year patency for graft anastomotic stenoses, 35% for downstream venous and central venous stenoses, and 38% for native fistula anastomotic stenoses.[12] Although many changes in catheter materials and improvements in technique have occurred, the results of venous angioplasty have changed little since that study over a decade ago. More recently, Beathard reported a series of 536 venous angioplasty procedures,[33] showing an overall 61% 6-month patency rate and a 38% 1-year patency rate. Beathard showed that repeated angioplasty of the same lesion for restenosis demonstrated identical patency on subsequent angioplasties (up to five procedures), although Kanterman et al,[34] in a smaller series, had conflicting results, showing results similar to those of Beathard for the first percutaneous transluminal angioplasty (PTA) but a reduction to 50% 6-month patency and 25% 1-year patency for the second PTA. Beathard's findings contrast with the surgical literature, where progressively decreasing patencies with revision of the same access are reported. Etheridge et al reported 30-day patency after the first revision of 65%, after the second revision of 53%, and after the third revision of 44%.[19]

The relative roles of surgical and percutaneous techniques have been debated. Brooks et al compared PTA to surgical repair and showed better patency and slightly lower cost for the latter.[20] This study has been widely quoted in the surgical literature supporting surgical revision over PTA. However, the series is fairly small (19 in the surgical group and 24 in the PTA group), and angioplasty was performed with outdated equipment. Dapunt et al reported exactly opposite results in a group of 37 angioplasties compared to 37 surgical procedures.[21] Five-month (41.2% for PTA and 28.9% for surgery) and 1-year (31.3% for PTA and 19.3% for surgery) patencies were significantly superior for PTA. Currently, percutaneous management is increasing because it is an outpatient procedure, the patient can undergo dialysis immediately after the procedure (unlike many surgical revisions) and the procedure may be used repeatedly on the same lesion without further loss of vein, and technical and long-term success rates are acceptable.

It should be noted that there is even debate as to whether venous stenoses should be treated at all prior to graft thrombosis. Schwab et al provided the most convincing evidence in favor of stenosis treatment,[35] with a study documenting the utility of venous pressure measurement as a screen for venous stenosis. A subset of their patients refusd fistulography despite evidence of outflow stenosis by pressure measurement. The rate of graft thrombosis was significantly higher in the 15 patients who refused fistulography when compared to the 50 patients treated with angioplasty. Besarab et al showed that over a 7-year period at their institution, vigorous screening and PTA of stenoses >50% yielded a dramatic reduction in the thrombosis rate (70% reduction) and in the access replacement rate (79% reduction). They found an increase in the average age of patent, usable accesses, from 1.97 to 2.98 years.[36] Burger et al reported a 50% reduction in operations for stenosis with an average prolongation of access life of 1 year using PTA in hemodialysis access.[26] Nonetheless, some surgeons remain skeptical about the role of prophylactic treatment of venous stenosis.[37] Despite the controversies surrounding venous angioplasty, it is one of the most rapidly growing areas in interventional radiology. Further prospective, randomized clinical trials are needed to assess the relative efficacy and cost effectiveness of PTA versus surgery for venous stenosis.

Few complications are associated with venous angioplasty. Both acute[15,33] and delayed venous rupture[38] have been reported. In our experience, access rupture during angioplasty is most often associated with performing the angioplasty procedure too soon (less than 1 month) after surgical revision or creation of the access. Generally, stenoses that occur at an anastomosis within a month of creation of the access are due to technical problems and should not be treated with balloon angioplasty.[12] When rupture does occur, it is usually self-limited; in rare cases, placement of a stent across the ruptured vessel may contain the rupture. Once stent-grafts become available, they may become the treatment of choice for this complication.

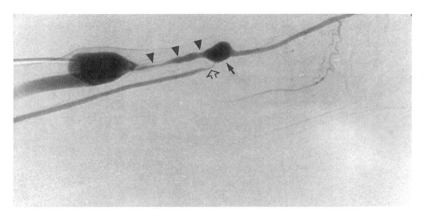

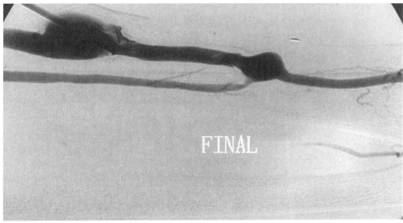

Figure 60–1. (A) Angioplasty of venous and arterial stenosis in a Brescia-Cimino fistula. This patient was experiencing low pressures on the arterial needle during hemodialysis. Dialysis fistulography with a blood pressure cuff inflated to allow reflux of contrast material across the anastomosis (arrow) shows high-grade stenoses of the cephalic vein (arrowheads) and radial artery just proximal to the anastomosis (open arrow). The cephalic vein just beyond the stenosis is dilated from repeated punctures with the arterial dialysis needle. (B) After angioplasty of the radial artery to 3 mm and the cephalic vein to 6 mm, there is marked improvement. The patient's pressures during dialysis returned to normal.

Table 60–1. Patency Rates of Percutaneous Angioplasty

Site	Initial		6 Months		1 Year		2 Years		3 Years		5 Years	
Arterial anastomotic stenosis	2/3	(67%)	2/2	(100%)	1/2	(50%)	0/2		0/2		0/2	
Direct arteriovenous fistula												
Anastomotic venostenosis	9/15	(60%)	4/9	(44%)	3/8	(38%)	1/7	(14%)	0/7		0/4	
Graft anastomotic venostenosis	80/93	(86%)	42/71	(59%)	32/64	(50%)	16/50	(32%)	6/38	(16%)	0/20	(0%)
Far proximal venous stenosis (graft and direct arterio-venous fistula)	25/30	(83%)	13/25	(52%)	8/23	(35%)	2/20	(10%)	1/18	(6%)	0/14	
Total	116/141	(82%)	61/107	(57%)	44/98	(45%)	19/79	(24%)	7/63	(11%)	0/40	(0%)

Source: Adapted from Ref. 12.

THE ROLE OF ATHERECTOMY

Because venous angioplasty is prone to early restenosis, use of atherectomy devices in the treatment of venous stenosis has been investigated.[39–42] The term *atherectomy* in this instance is a misnomer because neointima, not atheroma, is being removed. Most authors have concluded that atherectomy is probably comparable to angioplasty for venous outflow stenoses, although it may be superior to angioplasty for intragraft stenoses. Gaylord et al reported a slight benefit for atherectomy over angioplasty in the initial percutaneous treatment of venous stenosis, but this benefit was

no longer present for the second procedure.[41] To date, there have been no randomized studies comparing atherectomy to angioplasty, but it appears that use of the atherectomy device offers only marginal, if any, benefit. We use the Simpson atherectomy device in selected (rare) instances in which lesions fail to respond to venous angioplasty (ie, the waist on the balloon cannot be effaced). Using the atherectomy device to "nick" the lesion prior to angioplasty usually results in subsequent successful balloon angioplasty. We have also found the atherectomy device to be helpful in excising intimal hyperplasia from stents (Fig. 60–2).

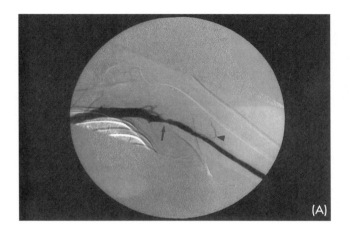

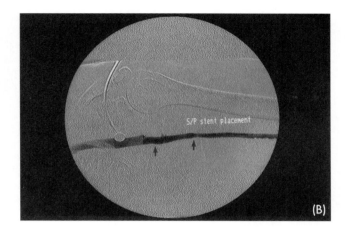

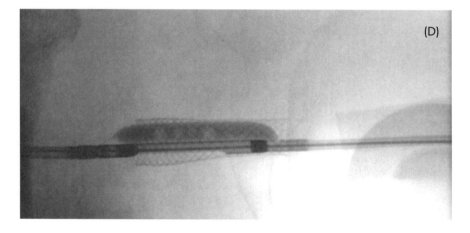

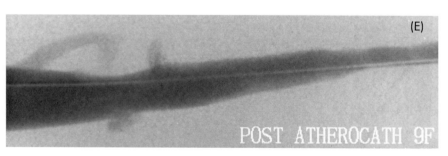

Figure 60–2. (A) This patient, with a left forearm loop dialysis graft that had been extended to the axillary vein, developed graft thrombosis. After mechanical thrombolysis, a venous outflow stenosis was identified just beyond the anastomosis (arrow). It was initially treated with balloon angioplasty, but the stenosis was elastic. This postangioplasty radiograph demonstrates persistent stenosis, as well as collateralization (arrowhead) around the stenosis. (B) Because this stenosis was in an area poorly accessible to surgical revision, a metallic stent was placed. A fistulogram after stent placement shows no residual stenosis (arrows indicate margins of stent). (C) One-year follow-up fistulogram shows moderate restenosis within the stent, which had resulted in graft thrombosis. (D) An atherectomy catheter is used to remove intimal hyperplasia from within the stent. (E) After use of the atherectomy catheter, there is no residual stenosis.

Because of the significant cost of these devices (about $1000), even if they do have a slight benefit over angioplasty alone, the cost-benefit ratio almost certainly falls in favor of balloon angioplasty. If a less expensive, more flexible atherectomy device were to become avail-able, based on the slightly improved results listed in the previous series, atherectomy could assume a more significant role in the treatment of hemodialysis-related venous stenosis. Presently, however, its role is limited to stent maintenance (see the following section) and treatment of PTA-resistant venous stenosis. Although it is probably more expensive than surgical revision, it will preserve vein.

THE ROLE OF STENTS

A variety of stent designs have been used in hemodialysis access. None are approved by the Food and Drug Administration (FDA) for use in the venous system at this time. It must be emphasized, therefore, that venous use of metallic stents in the United States is limited to compassionate "off-label" use or clinical trials.

Although the Palmaz stent (Johnson & Johnson Interventional Systems, Warren, NJ) is the most commonly used stent for arterial applications, it has a very limited role in hemodialysis access. This rigid stent is not self-expanding, so if it is exposed to an extrinsic crushing force, the expanded stent may collapse. This feature renders it unsuitable for use in the superficial veins associated with hemodialysis access. Although the Palmaz stent has been used in the treatment of central venous stenoses, such use has been associated with stent migration[43] and compression[44]; therefore, its role in the central veins should be considered limited or nonexistent.

The Gianturco Z stent (Cook, Inc., Bloomington, IN) consists of a zigzag configuration of stainless steel wire. It is self-expanding, and therefore, if exposed to extrinsic force, will resume its shape once the force is removed. The Z-stent design has a potential advantage over other stents in that it has the lowest metallic surface area, which has been shown to offer increased patency when used at the venous anastomosis in a hemodialysis access model.[45–47]

The Wallstent (Schneider, Inc., Minneapolis, MN) is a self-expanding, woven stainless steel alloy stent. This flexible stent is well suited to use in curved vessels. It has slightly higher metallic surface area than some other stent designs. Due to its commercial availability, self-expanding nature, flexibility, and acceptable delivery system size, this has been the preferred stent in the treatment of hemodialysis-related venous stenosis among most investigators.

It is useful to separate peripheral applications of stents in hemodialysis access from central venous applications because of differences in technique, possible differences in patency, and differences in philosophy with respect to alternatives for the patient. Since Zollikofer et al reported the first clinical application of percutaneously placed metallic stents in 1988,[48] multiple reports and small series describing the use of stents in hemodialysis access have been published.[45,46,49–61] In most series, stents were reserved as a means of access salvage after all other percutaneous means (PTA, atherectomy) were exhausted. Wallstents have been used most commonly, although use of the Gianturco[45,46] and Strecker[56] stents has been

reported. Although technical success rates for stent placement are in excess of 90%, the use of stents in peripheral venous lesions has been hampered by significant problems with restenosis. Vorwerk et al used Wallstents to treat venous outflow stenoses in 18 patients and reported primary patency at 18 months of only 27%.[58] Using aggressive reintervention, the group was able to achieve 77% cumulative patency, but this required multiple stent maintenance procedures (thrombolysis, PTA, additional stents). The same group, reporting their 7-year experience with stents in hemodialysis access, reported cumulative shunt function of 86% at 1 year, 77% at 2 years, and 70% at 3 years, with aggressive reintervention.[62] They concluded that stents should be reserved for failures of PTA in peripheral lesions. Many other investigators have reported similar results. Quinn et al, reporting a combination of central and peripheral stents, found a 2-year primary patency of 25%, secondary patency of 34%, and tertiary patency of 42%.[45] In general, the patency of stents used peripherally in hemodialysis access has been no better than that of angioplasty alone. Two randomized studies have compared angioplasty to Gianturco stents. Beathard showed no difference in patency between grafts treated with stents or PTA.[46] The 1-year primary patency was 17%. Cumulative patency was not reported. Quinn et al randomized 47 patients to PTA and 40 to PTA and stent placement.[63] For peripheral lesions the primary patency was 10% and 11% at 1 year, with secondary patencies of 71% and 64%, respectively. For central lesions the primary patency was 12% and 11%, and secondary patency was 100% and 78%, respectively. There was no significant difference between any of these values.

Although acceptable cumulative patency can be achieved by aggressive treatment of restenosis within stents, with significant prolongation of access life, the cost and effort involved must be weighed against the satisfactory results of surgical revision. Because of this, surgical revision of peripheral venous stenoses will remain the mainstay of therapy when PTA fails, for several reasons. First, stent cost ($1000 per device) may erase any potential cost savings of the percutaneous approach over the surgical approach. Second, stents can be damaged if punctured with dialysis needles; thus, they have limited use in Brescia-Cimino fistulae. Third, stents, like surgical revision, use up some normal vein and therefore may also deplete veins. For these reasons, the relative role of stents in peripheral lesions in hemodialysis access compared with surgical revision remains unclear. Control of restenosis will be necessary before widespread use of stents in peripheral venous lesions can occur.

We reserve stents for failures of angioplasty in patients in whom surgical revision is either not possible or undesirable. Such patients include those with high axillary vein anastomoses that are no longer accessible to surgical treatment and patients in whom cessation of hemodialysis (conversion to chronic ambulatory peritoneal dialysis or transplant) is anticipated in the near future and therefore relatively short-term prolongation of access life is needed. In patients with limited or no remaining access sites, stents can be used to prolong the existing access life almost indefinitely, using the aggressive stent maintenance approach described. One group has reported a 71% cumulative patency at 3 years using this approach.[64]

In contrast to peripheral lesions, stents have a very significant role in the treatment of hemodialysis related central venous stenosis (Fig. 60–3) because there may be limited surgical options for central venous stenosis and restenosis may be less significant in central stents. Although restenosis occurs in all stents as the stent is incorporated into the vessel wall and healing occurs,[65] the larger initial stent lumen will be less significantly compromised by the intimal hyperplasia. Unfortunately, while intimal hyperplasia in arterial and non-hemodialysis-related venous stenoses appears to peak after a few months and then regress, in the hemodialysis population it appears to be a relentlessly progressive process; thus, even central stents eventually require stent maintenance. Despite restenosis, central venous

stents offer substantial prolongation of patency after angioplasty failure. As with all hemodialysis-related venous stenoses, stents should be reserved for failure of angioplasty. Unfortunately, in central lesions, angioplasty results are inferior to those achieved in peripheral lesions, with 10 to 35% 1-year patency.[12,33] On the other hand, PTA is less costly, does not involve implantation of a permanent device, can be repeated on an outpatient basis, and offers long-term benefit in some patients. For these reasons, PTA should be the primary treatment modality for all venous lesions. When central venous PTA fails, however, surgical options are limited to bypasses or abandonment of access in that limb. Thus, in contrast to peripheral lesions, stents offer an intermediate option and can be used to preserve access in the affected limb for months to years. To date, no comparative studies of stents versus angioplasty in central venous stenosis have been performed. Few large series describing central stents in hemodialysis access have been published. In Quinn's series, central stents appeared to have less restenosis than peripheral stents.[45] Vorwerk et al, describing brachial and central stents in 33 patients, reported 40% 1-year patency and 77% 1-year assisted patency.[59] In their follow-up report, the same group suggested that central stents had better patency than PTA and proposed "liberal" use of

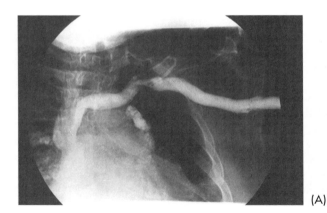

(A)

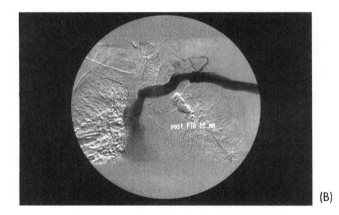

(B)

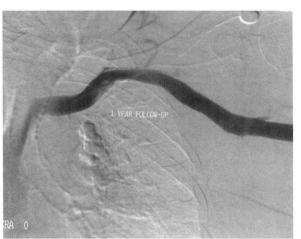

(C)

Figure 60–3.   Central venous angioplasty and stent. (A) This patient has a functioning dialysis graft in the left arm and presented with left arm swelling. Previously, she had had left subclavian vein catheters. Fistulography demonstrates a moderate left subclavian stenosis with collateral flow around it. (B) This lesion was expanded with angioplasty to 12 mm, with an excellent postangioplasty result. However, the lesion recurred after 1 month. Repeat angioplasty was unsuccessful due to elasticity; therefore, a Wallstent was placed, with an excellent angiographic result. (C) Fistulography at 1 year of follow-up shows an excellent angiographic appearance with very little intimal hyperplasia.

stents in central venous lesions.[61] Gray et al described a series of 32 central and 24 peripheral stents, with 20% 1-year primary patency and 33% 1-year cumulative patency.[60] The results for central and peripheral lesions were not separated. These authors suggested stent use only when PTA failed. Schoenfeld et al reported 68% primary and 93% secondary patency for central stents at 17 months, although, venographic follow-up was not performed in these patients.[57] Because stent thrombosis may occur and may be clinically asymptomatic, presumably due to the development of collaterals,[52] the lack of venographic follow-up in Schoenfeld's series casts doubt on the reported patency. Kovalik et al, reporting a small series of stents in central venous stenosis, suggested that only elastic lesions should be treated with stents due to early restenosis with "nonelastic lesions."[55] The results indicate that stents should be reserved for failures of angioplasty and that angioplasty should be used as long as possible before stent placement. The results of central venous stents described by these authors and others indicate initial success in treating lesions that no longer respond to angioplasty, but reintervention is needed frequently.

The role of stents in hemodialysis access remains unclear. Further carefully controlled, randomized studies are needed to compare the relative value of stents and angioplasty. The introduction of larger (up to 24-mm Wallstent, 40-mm Gianturco stent) stents may enhance their role in central venous stenosis. It is obvious that venous stents are not the panacea they were once thought to be. Initial enthusiasm for these devices has been tempered by the observation that they are much more prone to restenosis than was anticipated. If new stent designs and/or stent treatments can prevent restenosis, their role in hemodialysis access will increase. Until such newer devices become available, judicious use of stents in selective patients and lesions should be the rule.

THE ROLE OF PHARMACOLOGIC AND MECHANICAL THROMBOLYSIS

Despite our best efforts to detect and treat venous stenosis before access thrombosis occurs, patients continue to present with a clotted grafts. Although venous stenosis accounts for the majority of access thromboses, other causes include faulty compression technique, hypotension, compression of the graft during sleep, and other causes. In surgical series no cause for access thrombosis is found in at least 50% of cases, whereas in radiologic series a cause for thrombosis is identified approximately 90% of the time. This difference can be explained by radiologists' routine performance of post-thrombolysis fistulography, which reveals the underlying etiology. In contrast, intraoperative fistulography is not routinely performed by all access surgeons, and thus the underlying cause of thrombosis may go unde-

tected. For this reason, after surgical thrombectomy/revision, postoperative fistulography should be performed in all patients to exclude occult lesions.

Hemodialysis access thrombosis is a major contributor to cost, morbidity, and hospitalization for hemodialysis patients. Treatment options include surgical thrombectomy, surgical thrombectomy with revision, percutaneous infusion, pharmacologic thrombolysis, percutaneous pharmacomechanical thrombolysis and percutaneous mechanical thrombolysis.

Initially, percutaneous thrombolytic therapy in clotted dialysis access used streptokinase, but clinicians soon converted to infusion of urokinase due to high complication rates, especially bleeding.[11,66–70] In addition, the inability to repeat streptokinase therapy within 6 months due to antibody formation rendered it less useful for grafts that may clot frequently. Early investigators using urokinase either directly injected the graft with needles[71,72] or used angled catheters.[69] Urokinase was then infused for several hours. These approaches led to reasonable technical success, but significant bleeding complications commonly occurred due to opening up of multiple puncture sites along the graft or fistula.[69,70] In addition, the expense of an overnight hospital stay, usually in the intensive care unit, was prohibitive. Most interventional radiologists no longer use infusion thrombolysis; but rather use pulse-spray pharmacomechanical thrombolysis (PSPMT). PSPMT, first reported by Valji et al,[10] is probably the most widely practiced percutaneous thrombolytic technique. It involves using two multi-side-slit or sidehole catheters (crossed catheter technique) and forceful injection of small aliquots of highly concentrated urokinase mixed with heparin into the clotted access. Initially, this approach required an average of 299,000 ± 125,000 units of urokinase and took a mean of 46 ± 21 minutes to complete. The authors had 93% initial success, with 1-year primary patency of 26% and 1-year cumulative patency of 51%.[10] Further refinements of this technique have reduced the time of thrombolysis to 23 ± 13 minutes (overall procedure time, 67 ± 26 minutes),[73] and now often only a single vial of urokinase (250,000 units) is used. After the urokinase is pulsed, regardless of whether flow is restored, a balloon is passed beyond the arterial anastomosis, inflated, and pulled back into the graft to dislodge the arterial plug (see the following discussion) and usually restore flow in the graft. After this mechanical procedure, any residual clot in the graft or fistula is macerated using an angioplasty balloon, and underlying stenoses are treated. This approach has been technically successful in up to 92% of cases, with excellent long-term patency.[74] Results with the pulse-spray technique have been replicated by other authors using slight modifications in technique.[75] Brunner et al described the "ultrarapid urokinase" technique, using infusion via multi-side-hole catheters to achieve 1-hour lysis in 79% of grafts.[76] Berger et al showed that PSPMT could be used after recent surgery (previously thought to be a contraindication) without significant complications.[77] Twelve procedures performed within 30 days after surgical thrombectomy yielded a clinical success rate of 75%, with a mean primary patency of 94 days.

PSPMT has proliferated greatly since its initial description, but the concept has recently been challenged by Beathard.[78] In a randomized study, this author compared PSPMT using Valji's most recent technique[73] ($n = 48$) to pulse-spray *mechanical* lysis using heparinized saline alone ($n = 55$). Procedure success rates for the mechanical and PSPMT groups were 92.8% and 93.8%, respectively, with 30-day patencies of 65% and 72%, respectively, and 90-day patencies of 37% and 46%, respectively. No statistically significant difference was found between the groups in terms of technical results, clinical success, or complication rates. The only statistically significant difference was a shorter procedure time in the mechanical group (48 versus 58 minutes). This well-designed trial casts significant doubt on the concept of PSPMT. The results, however, are not particularly surprising. The volume of clot in an average dialysis graft is small (mean, 3.3 cc).[79] The primary impediments to restoration of flow in an access are the underlying stenosis, usually in the venous outflow, and the arterial plug. The arterial plug consists of lamellated white thrombus with alternating layers of erythrocytes, leukocytes, and fibrin[79] and has a characteristic appearance when removed surgically, consisting of a cylindrical piece of white clot with a concave surface facing the artery, leading some surgeons to describe it as a "bullet." Removal of the arterial plug is essential, and failure to do so results in decreased patency after thrombectomy.[19] The plug is well documented to be extremely resistant to thrombolysis,[10] which is what led to the use of balloon mobilization of the arterial plug in the current PSPMT procedure. The resistance to lysis was previously thought to be due to the high platelet content[10] but is more likely due to the densely lamellated nature of the plug.[79] It is acknowledged that the urokinase used in PSPMT does not affect the arterial plug,[10] and it obviously does not affect the venous outflow stenosis, yet these are the two most important determinants of the success of the procedure. Thus it is not surprising that pulse-spray heparinized saline was found by Beathard to be equivalent to PSPMT. This concept forms the basis for other forms of mechanical thrombolysis (vide infra).

In addition to pulse-spray saline, a variety of other mechanical thrombolytic techniques have been described. The balloon technique of mechanical declotting originally reported by Trerotola et al involves placement of crossed sheaths and the use of a balloon catheter to push the clot into the central circulation.[80] The arterial plug is dislodged with a Fogarty balloon catheter and then also pushed centrally. This technique is relatively quick, taking far less than 1 hour for the entire procedure. Technical success was 94%, with 52% 30-day patency. Symptomatic pulmonary emboli have not been reported; however, the procedure is contraindicated in patients with known significant pulmonary disease or right-to-left shunts. Middlebrook et al compared balloon mechanical declotting to PSPMT and found the balloon procedure to be faster and cheaper, with comparable results.[81] We have also used a modified technique in which thromboaspiration is performed using a 7 F venous sheath; this results in removal of approximately half of the expected clot volume. Thromboaspiration was previously reported, with relatively good results in conjunction with fibrinolysis.[82]

A number of devices have been used to perform mechanical thrombolysis in dialysis access grafts. The Arrow-Trerotola percutaneous thrombolytic device (Arrow International, Reading, PA) consists of a rotating metal fragmentation cage that pulverizes the clot and effectively strips it from the walls of the graft. The resulting slurry can be aspirated through a 5 F sheath. In a clinical pilot study, this 5 F device was highly effective, with complete lysis in 16 of 17 grafts and partial lysis in 1 of 17.[83] In an animal study, clotted grafts were randomized to PSPMT or the Arrow-Trerotola device ($n = 11$ each). Technical success was 100% in both groups, with 100% 30-day patency.[84] Interestingly, pulmonary arteriograms documented pulmonary emboli in 100% of the PSPMT group versus 27% of the device group ($p < 0.001$).

The Amplatz mechanical thrombectomy device (Microvena, White Bear Lake, MN) has been used successfully in dialysis grafts.[85] This 8 F device consists of a gas-driven, high-speed (150,000 rpm) cam that creates a vortex that pulverizes the clot. In a randomized series comparing surgical thrombectomy ($n = 10$) to the device ($n = 10$), 100% success was achieved in the device group and 70% in the surgery group. Forty-eight-hour and 30-day patencies were comparable (70%/60% with the device, 70%/70% with surgery). However, the device group contained secondary and partial successes; the primary 30-day patency was approximately 50%. Adjunctive urokinase was required in some cases.

Vorwerk et al described the use of the Hydrolyser catheter (Cordis, Miami, FL) in native ($n = 8$) and synthetic ($n = 7$) access.[86] This 7 F device is driven using a conventional angiographic injector to create a Venturi effect to achieve mechanical thrombolysis. Although thrombectomy was successful in 15 of 16 instances, rethrombosis occurred in 5 cases within the first 24 hours. Cumulative patency was 41% at 6 months. Given the inclusion of native fistulae (which have poorer results with thrombolysis), these results are encouraging.

The rheolytic catheter,[87] (AngioJet, Possis Medical, Minneapolis, MN) which uses high-velocity saline jets to pulverize clot as well as aspirate the particulate using the Venturi effect, is currently being used in clinical trials. This device consists of a 5 F catheter used over a 0.018-inch wire. It is connected to an external drive unit. In a study of clotted dialysis grafts, successful recanalization was achieved in nine of nine patients. One patient required adjunctive urokinase. As with the Amplatz device, some hemolysis occurs with the rheolytic catheter.

The Trac-Wright catheter has been used in clotted dialysis access, and has been shown to be faster and more effective than pulse-spray chemical thrombolysis.[88] Only two of the devices described (AngioJet and Amplate device) are currently available in the United States. Mechanical thrombolytic devices have some significant drawbacks. Some devices are large (8 F or more) and perform poorly in curved vessels, which limits their use in hemodialysis access. Other devices aspirate significant amounts of blood and/or result in hemolysis. Importantly, while the concept of mechanical thrombolysis with devices is attractive, financial considerations will prohibit the development of mechanical thrombolysis unless device costs are kept to an absolute minimum.

COMPLICATIONS OF THROMBOLYSIS

Complications associated with mechanical and pharmacomechanical thrombolysis have been limited. Bleeding complications may occur when thrombolytic agents are used, particularly with infusion technique. Urokinase may cause a pyrogen-type reaction consisting of shaking chills and fever; these usually respond well to meperidine and Tylenol.[77] Emboli to the arterial circulation have been reported[10,11,66,72,83,86] but can usually be treated percutaneously. Pulmonary emboli represent a serious potential complication of both mechanical and pharmacomechanical thrombolysis. Although many proponents of PSPMT believe that the procedure does not result in pulmonary emboli, the work of Trerotola et al, described earlier, proves otherwise. In addition, the only reported symptomatic pulmonary emboli in the dialysis access thrombolysis literature have occurred with pharmacologic and pharmacomechanical thrombolysis.[10,71,72] A recent study by Swan et al used pulmonary perfusion scanning after modified PSPMT to document pulmonary emboli in a significant number of patients.[89] Two of their patients died of pulmonary emboli, both with severe preexisting pulmonary disease. A further argument has been made that clot that is embolized to the lungs with PSPMT is somehow more likely to lyse than clot that has not been pre-

treated with urokinase, but there are no data to support this hypothesis. Although pulmonary emboli are known to occur secondary to the balloon mechanical technique, symptomatic emboli have not been reported, probably because the small clot burden is well tolerated by the patient.[80] Because pulmonary emboli are known to occur with *both* mechanical and pharmacomechanical thrombolysis, significant pulmonary disease and right-to-left shunts should be considered contraindications to *any* percutaneous thrombolytic technique. Whether refinements in mechanical devices will make the issue of pulmonary emboli moot remains unclear.

CONCLUSIONS

As discussed previously, the advantage of percutaneous treatment compared to surgical revision is preservation of vein. Beathard, in a time-based comparison of percutaneous and surgical techniques, showed no significant difference between rates of thrombosis during the time in which surgery and the time when percutaneous declotting was performed. Long-term patency with thrombolysis was superior to that achieved with thrombectomy alone and identical to revision.[90] Schwartz et al compared PTA to surgical revision in clotted grafts and also found no differences in acute or long-term patency.[91] Percutaneous thrombolytic techniques, whether mechanical or chemical, can effectively and rapidly restore flow in dialysis grafts. However, while percutaneous thrombolysis is possible in native fistulae, success rates are generally lower in this form of access than with synthetic grafts.

Clearly, interventional radiology plays an important role in the care of the hemodialysis patient, ranging from diagnostic (fistulography) to therapeutic (treatment of stenosis and thrombosis). Participating in the care of hemodialysis patients can be rewarding, but may also be time-consuming, demanding, and frustrating due to the recurrent nature of problems in these patients' access sites. However, as an integral part of the access management team along with access surgeons and nephrologists, the interventional radiologist can play a pivotal role in the overall management of these patients.

ACKNOWLEDGMENTS

I wish to thank Kathie Pedersen for her outstanding secretarial assistance. In addition, I wish to acknowledge the tireless dedication of our technologists, without whom we would not be able to provide the interventional support described herein.

REFERENCES

1. Trerotola, SO. Interventional radiologic approach to hemodialysis access management. In: Savader SJ, Trero-

tola SO, eds. *Venous Interventional Radiology: With Clinical Perspective.* New York: Thieme; 1995.

2. Depner TA. Techniques for prospective detection of venous stenosis. *Adv Renal Replacement Ther* 1994; 1(2):119–130.

3. Zijlstra J. *Percutaneous Transluminal Angioplasty in Vascular Access for Hemodialysis.* Dordrecht, the Netherlands; ICG Printing; 1989.

4. Windus DW. In-depth review: permanent vascular access: a nephrologist's view. *Am J Kidney Dis* 1993;21(5):457–471.

5. Brotman D, Fandos L, Faust G, Doscher W, Cohen J. Hemodialysis graft salvage. *J Am Coll Surg* 1994;178:431–434.

6. Palder S, Kirkman R, Whittemore A, Hakim R, Lazarus M, Tilney N. Vascular access for hemodialysis: patency rates and results of revision. *Ann Surg* 1985;202:235–239.

7. Swedberg S, Brown B, Sigley R, Wight T, Gordon D, Nicholls S. Intimal fibromuscular hyperplasia at the venous anastomosis of PTFE grafts in hemodialysis patients: clinical, immunocytochemical, light and electron microscopic assessment. *Circulation* 1989; 80(6):1726–1736.

8. Glanz S, Bashist B, Gordon DH, Butt K, Adamsons R. Angiography of upper extremity access fistulas for dialysis. *Radiology* 1982;143:45–52.

9. Cada E, Karnel F, Mayer G, Langle F, Schurawitzki H, Graf H. Percutaneous transluminal angioplasty of failing arteriovenous dialysis fistulae. *Nephrol Dial Transplant* 1989;4:57–61.

10. Valji K, Bookstein J, Roberts A, Davis G. Pharmacomechanical thrombolysis and angioplasty in the management of clotted hemodialysis grafts: early and late clinical results. *Radiology* 1991;178:243–247.

11. Zeit R. Arterial and venous embolization: declotting of dialysis shunts by direct injection of streptokinase. *Radiology* 1986;159:639–641.

12. Glanz S, Gordon D, Butt K, Hong J, Lipkowitz G. The role of percutaneous angioplasty in the management of chronic hemodialysis fistulas. *Ann Surg* 1987;206(6):777–786.

13. Munda R, First M, Alexander J, Linnemann C Jr, Fidler J, Kittur D. Polytetrafluoroethylene graft survival in hemodialysis. *JAMA* 1983;249(2): 219–222.

14. Puckett J, Lindsay S. Medgraft curettage as a routine adjunct to salvage operations for thrombosed polytetrafluoroethylene hemodialysis access grafts. *Am J Surg* 1988;156:139–143.

15. Glanz S, Gordon D, Lipkowitz G, Butt K, Hong J, Sclafani J. Axillary and subclavian vein stenosis: percutaneous angioplasty. *Radiology* 1988;168:371–373.

16. Koga N, Sato T, Baba T, et al. Angioscopy in transluminal balloon and laser angioplasty in the management of chronic hemodialysis fistulae. *ASAIO Trans* 1989;35:193–196.

17. Glanz S, Gordon D, Butt K, Hong J, Adamson R, Sclafani S. Dialysis access fistulas: treatment of stenoses by transluminal angioplasty. *Radiology* 1984;152:637–642.

18. Surratt R, Picus D, Hicks M, Darcy M, Kleinhoffer M, Jendrisak M. The importance of preoperative evaluation of the subclavian vein in dialysis access planning. *AJR* 1991;156:623–625.

19. Etheredge E, Haid S, Maeser M, Sicard G, Anderson C. Salvage operations for malfunctioning polytetrafluoroethylene hemodialysis access grafts. *Surgery* 1983;94(3):464–470.

20. Brooks J, Singley R, May K Jr, Mack R. Transluminal angioplasty versus surgical repair for stenosis of hemodialysis grafts: a randomized study. *Am J Surg* 1987;153:530–531.

21. Dapunt O, Feurstein M, Rendl K, Prenner K. Transluminal angioplasty versus conventional operation in the treatment of haemodialysis fistula stenosis: results from a 5-year study. *Br J Surg* 1987;74:1004–1005.

22. Hunter D, So S, Castaneda-Zuniga W, Coleman C, Sutherland D, Amplatz K. Failing or thrombosed Brescia-Cimino arteriovenous dialysis fistulas. *Radiology* 1983; 149:105–109.

23. Hunter D, Castaneda-Zuniga W, Coleman C, et al. Failing arteriovenous dialysis fistulas: evaluation and treatment. *Radiology* 1984;152:631–635.

24. Gordon D, Glanz S, Butt K, Adamsons R, Koenig M. Treatment of stenotic lesions in dialysis access fistulas and shunts by transluminal angioplasty. *Radiology* 1982; 143:53–58.

25. Bohndorf K, Gunther R, Vorwerk D, Gladziwa U, Kistler D, Sieberth H. Technical aspects and results of percutaneous transluminal angioplasty in Brescia-Cimino dialysis fistulas. *Cardiovasc Intervent Radiol* 1990;13:323–326.

26. Burger H, Zijlstra J, Kluchert S, Scholten A, Kootstra G. Percutaneous transluminal angioplasty improves longevity in fistulae and shunts for haemodialysis. *Nephrol Dial Transplant* 1990;5:608–611.

27. Glanz S, Gordon D, Butt K, Hong J et al. Stenotic lesions in dialysis-access fistulas: treatment by transluminal angioplasty using high-pressure balloons. *Radiology* 1985; 156:236.

28. Ingram T, Reid S, Tisnado J, Cho S, Posner M. Percutaneous transluminal angioplasty of brachiocephalic vein stenoses in patient with dialysis shunts. *Radiology* 1988;166:45–47.

29. Saeed M, Newman G, McCann R, Sussman S, Braun S, Dunnick N. Stenoses in dialysis fistulas: treatment with percutaneous angioplasty. *Radiology* 1987;164:693–697.

30. Spinowitz B, Carsen G, Meisell R, Charytan C. Percutaneous transluminal dilatation for vascular access. *Nephron* 1983;35:201–204.

31. Trerotola S, McLean G, Burke D, Meranze S. Treatment of subclavian venous stenoses by percutaneous transluminal angioplasty. *J Intervent Radiol* 1986;1:15–18.

32. Gmelin E, Winterhoff R, Rinast E. Insufficient hemodialysis access fistulas: late results of treatment with percutaneous balloon angioplasty. *Radiology* 1989;171:647–660.

33. Beathard G. Percutaneous transvenous angioplasty in the treatment of vascular access stenosis. *Kidney Int* 1992;42:1390–1397.

34. Kanterman RY, Vesely TM, Pilgram TK, Guy BW, Windus DW, Picus D. Dialysis access grafts: anatomic location of venous stenosis and results of angioplasty. *Radiology* 1995;195:135–139.

35. Schwab S, Quarles D, Middleston J, Cohan R, Saeed M, Dennis V. Hemodialysis-associated subclavian vein stenosis. *Kidney Int* 1988;33:1156–1159.

36. Besarab A, Sullivan KL, Ross RP, Moritz MJ. Utility of intra-access pressure monitoring in detecting and correcting venous outlet stenoses prior to thrombosis. *Kidney Int* 1995;47:1364–1373.

37. Kirkman R. Can diagnostic testing help prolong access function? A prophylactic approach to graft thrombosis is not yet justifiable. *Semin Dialysis* 1993;6(3):1993:203–205.

38. Bourne E. Late venous rupture after angioplasty of an arteriovenous dialysis fistula. *AJR* 1988;150:797–798.

39. Zemel G, Katzen B, Dake M, Benenati J, Lempert T, Moskowitz L. Directional atherectomy in the treatment of stenotic dialysis access fistulas. *JVIR* 1990;1:35–38.

40. Gray R, Dolmatch B, Buick M. Directional atherectomy treatment for hemodialysis access: early results. *JVIR* 1992;3:497–503.

41. Gaylord G, Taber T, Ehrman K, Brown P. Angioplasty versus directional atherectomy of dialysis graft venous anastomotic stenoses. *JVIR* 1994;5:49. Abstract.

42. Castaneda F, Herrera MA, Mendez A, Mancera JL. Comparison of percutaneous angioplasty, atherectomy and vascular stent placement in failing hemodialysis grafts. *JVIR* 1994;5(1):49. Abstract.

43. Gray R, Dolmatch B, Horton K, Romolo J, Zarate A. Migration of Palmaz stents following deployment for venous stenoses related to hemodialysis access. *JVIR* 1994;5:117–120.

44. Bjarnason H, Hunter D, Crain M, Ferral H, Miltz-Miller S, Wegryn S. Collapse of a Palmaz stent in the subclavian vein. *AJR* 1993;160:1123–1124.

45. Quinn S, Schuman E, Hall L, et al. Venous stenosis in patients who undergo hemodialysis: treatment with self-expandable endovascular stents. *Radiology* 1992;183:499–504.

46. Beathard G. Gianturco self-expanding stent in the treatment of stenosis in dialysis access grafts. *Kidney Int* 1993;43:872–877.

47. Trerotola S, Fair J, Davidson D, Samphilipo M, Magee C. Comparison of Gianturco Z stents and Wallstents in a hemodialysis access graft animal model. *JVIR* 1995;6:387–396.

48. Zollikofer C, Largiader I, Bruhlmann W, Uhlschmid G, Marty A. Endovascular stenting of veins and grafts: preliminary clinical experience. *Radiology* 1988;167:707–712.

49. Antonucci F, Salomonowitz E, Stuckmann G, Stiefel M, Largiader J, Zollikofer C. Placement of venous stents: clinical experience with self-expanding prosthesis. *Radiology* 1992;183:493–497.

50. Antonucci F, Salomonowitz E, Stuckmann G, Stiefel M, Hugentobler M, Zollikofer C. Hemodialysis related venous stenoses: treatment with self-expanding endovascular prostheses. *Eur J Radiol* 1992;14:195–200.

51. Dondelinger R, Goffette P, Kurdziel J, Roche A. Expandable metal stents for stenoses of the venae cavae and large veins. *Semin Intervent Radiol* 1991;8(4):252–262.

52. Ehrman K, Reed J, Gaylord G, Harris V. Use of the Palmaz balloon-expandable stent in subclavian/brachiocephalic vein stenosis. *JVIR* 1992;3(1):13. Abstract.

53. Gunther R, Vorwerk D, Klose K, et al. Self-expanding stents for the treatment of a long venous stenosis in a dialysis shunt: case report. *Cardiovasc Intervent Radiol* 1989;12:29–31.

54. Gunther R, Vorwerk D, Bohndorf K, et al. Venous stenoses in dialysis shunts: treatment with self-expanding metallic stents. *Radiology* 1989;170:401–405.

55. Kovalik E, Newman G, Suhocki P, Knelson M, Schwab S. Correction of central venous stenoses: use of angioplasty and vascular Wallstents. *Kidney Int* 1994;45:1177–1181.

56. Petar B, Tomislav I, Miodrag I, Snezana A. Strecker stent in stenotic hemodialysis: Brescia-Cimino arteriovenous fistulas. *Cardiovasc Intervent Radiol* 1992;15:217–220.

57. Shoenfeld R, Hermans H, Novick A, Brener B, et al. Stenting of proximal venous obstructions to maintain hemodialysis access. *J Vasc Surg* 1994;19:532–539.

58. Vorwerk D, Gunther R, Bohndorf K, Kistler D, Gladziwa U, Sieberth H. Follow-up results after stent placement in failing arteriovenous shunts: a three-year experience. *Cardiovasc Intervent Radiol* 1991;14:285–289.

59. Vorwerk D, Guenther R, Bohndorf K, et al. Self-expanding stents in peripheral and central veins used for arteriovenous shunts: five years of experience. *Radiology* 1993;189(P):174. Abstract.

60. Gray RJ, Horton KM, Dolmatch BL, et al. Use of Wallstents for hemodialysis access-related venous stenoses and occlusions untreatable with balloon angioplasty. *Radiology* 1995;195:479–484.

61. Zollikofer C, Antonucci F, Stuckmann G, Mattias P, Bruhlmann W, Salomonowitz E. Use of the Wallstent in the venous system including hemodialysis-related stenoses. *Cardiovasc Intervent Radiol* 1992;15:334–341.

62. Vorwerk D, Gunther RW, Mann H, et al. Venous stenosis and occlusion in hemodialysis shunts: follow-up results of stent placement in 65 patients. *Radiology* 1995;195:140–146.

63. Quinn SF, Schuman ES, Demlow TA, et al. Percutaneous transluminal angioplasty versus endovascular stent placement in the treatment of venous stenoses in patients undergoing hemodialysis: intermediate results. *JVIR* 1995;6:851–855.

64. Turmel-Rodrigues L, Pengloan J, Blanchier D, et al. Insufficient dialysis shunts: improved long-term patency rates with close hemodynamic monitoring, repeated percutaneous balloon angioplasty and stent placement. *Radiology* 1993;187:273–278.

65. Palmaz J. Intravascular stents: tissue–stent interactions and design considerations. *AJR* 1993;160:613–618.

66. Rodkin RS, Bookstein JJ, Heeney DJ, Davis GB. Streptokinase and transluminal angioplasty in the treatment of acutely thrombosed hemodialysis access fistulas. *Radiology* 1983;149:425–428.

67. Zeit RM, Cope C. Failed hemodialysis shunts: one year of experience with aggressive treatment. *Radiology* 1985;154:353–356.

68. Goldberg JP, Contiguglia RC, Mishell JL, Klein MH. Intravenous streptokinase for thrombolysis of occluded arteriovenous access. *Arch Intern Med* 1985;145:1405–1408.

69. Young A, Hunter D, Castadneda-Zuniga W, et al. Thrombosed synthetic hemodialysis access fistulas: failure of fibrinolytic therapy. *Radiology* 1985;154:639–642.

70. Kumpe D, Cohen M. Angioplasty/thrombolytic treatment of ailing and failed hemodialysis access sites: comparison with surgical treatment. *Prog Cardiovasc Dis* 1992;34(4):263–278.

71. Mangiarotti G, Canavese C, Thea A, et al. Urokinase treatment for arteriovenous fistulae declotting in dialyzed patients. *Nephron* 1984;36:60–64.

72. Schilling J, Eiser A, Slifkin R, Whitney J, Neff M. The role of thrombolysis in hemodialysis access occlusion. *Am J Kidney Dis* 1987;10(2):92–97.

73. Valji K, Bookstein JJ, Roberts AC, Oglevie SB, Pittman C, O'Neill MP. Pulse-spray pharmacomechanical thrombolysis of thrombosed hemodialysis access grafts: long-term experience and comparison of original and current techniques. *AJR* 1995;164:1495–1500.

74. Valji K. Transcatheter treatment of thrombosed hemodialysis access grafts. *AJR* 1995;164:823–829.

75. Ehrman K, Gaylord G. Thrombolytic therapy for occluded dialysis access grafts. *Semin Intervent Radiol* 1992;9(3):190–194.

76. Brunner M, Matalon T, Patel S, McDonald V, Jensik S. Ultrarapid urokinase in hemodialysis access occlusion. *JVIR* 1991;2:503–506.

77. Berger M, Aruny J, Skibo L. Recurrent thrombosis of polytetrafluoroethylene dialysis fistulas after recent surgical thrombectomy: salvage by means of thrombolysis and angioplasty. *JVIR* 1994;5:725–730.

78. Beathard G. Mechanical versus pharmacomechanical thrombolysis for the treatment of thrombosed dialysis access grafts. *Kidney Int* 1994;45:1401–1406.

79. Winkler TA, Trerotola SO, Davidson DD, Milgrom ML. Study of thrombus from thrombosed hemodialysis access grafts. *Radiology* 1995;197:461–465.

80. Trerotola S, Lund G, Scheel P, Savader S, Venbrux A, Osterman F. Thrombosed dialysis access grafts: percutaneous mechanical declotting without urokinase. *Radiology* 1994;191:721–726.

81. Middlebrook MR, Amygdalos MA, Soulen MC, et al. Thrombosed hemodialysis grafts: percutaneous mechanical balloon declotting versus thrombolysis. *Radiology* 1995;196:73–77.

82. Poulain F, Raynaud A, Bourquelot P, Knight C, Rovani X, Gaux J. Local thrombolysis and thromboaspiration in the treatment of acutely thrombosed arteriovenous hemodialysis fistulas. *Radiology* 1991;14:98–101.

83. Trerotola SO, Lund GB, Savader SJ, et al. New device for mechanical thrombectomy of dialysis access grafts. *JVIR* 1992;3:25. Abstract.

84. Trerotola SO, Johnson MS, Schauwecker D, et al. Pulmonary emboli from pulse-spray versus mechanical thrombolysis in an animal dialysis graft model. Submitted to *Radiology*, 1996;200:169–176.

85. Uflacker R, Rajagopalan PR, Vujic I, Chita MA, Stutley JE, Kilpatrick PS. Percutaneous mechanical thrombectomy of dialysis fistulas: a randomized study. *JVIR* 1995;6(1):9. Abstract.

86. Vorwerk D, Sohn M, Schurmann K, Hoogeveen Y, Gladziwa U, Guenther R. Hydrodynamic thrombectomy of hemodialysis fistulas: first clinical results. *JVIR* 1994;5:813–821.

87. Drasler WJ, Jenson ML, Wilson GJ, et al. Rheolytic catheter for percutaneous removal of thrombus. *Radiology* 1992;182:263–267.

88. Gaylord GM, Ehrman KO, Peltzer M, Taber TE. Mechanical thrombolysis versus urokinase for treatment of acutely occluded dialysis access grafts: randomized prospective comparison. *JVIR* 1993;4(1):56. Abstract.

89. Swan TL, Smyth SH, Ruffenach SJ, Berman SS, Pond GD. Pulmonary embolism following hemodialysis access thrombolysis/thrombectomy. *JVIR* 1995;6:683–686.

90. Beathard GA. Thrombolysis versus surgery for the treatment of thrombosed dialysis access grafts. *J Am Soc Nephrol* 1995;6:1619–1624.

91. Schwartz CI, McBayer CV, Sloan JH, Meneses P, Ennis WJ. Thrombosed dialysis grafts: comparison of treatment with transluminal angioplasty and surgical revision. *Radiology* 1995;194:337–341.

61

The Clinical Evaluation and Nonoperative Management of Portal Hypertension

James Farrell, M.D.
H. Franklin Herlong, M.D.

Portal hypertension develops when there is an increase in the gradient between the portal and systemic circulations. While pre and posthepatic disorders can produce portal hypertension, intrahepatic liver diseases, particularly cirrhosis, account for the majority of cases (Table 61–1). As the portal pressure rises, splanchnic venous blood is redirected through portal-systemic collaterals, the most important of which are the submucosal veins in the esophagus. In prehepatic causes of portal hypertension, the portal pressure is high, but sinusoidal pressure is normal or low. Variceal bleeding is common in these patients, but ascites and hepatic encephalopathy are rare. With posthepatic and hepatic causes of portal hypertension, the sinusoidal pressure is elevated. When the increase in sinusoidal pressure results in hepatic lymph formation at a rate exceeding the hepatic lymphatic capacity for removal, ascites accumualtes.[1] The most common clinical sequelae of por-

Table 61–1. Causes of Portal Hypertension

Prehepatic
  Splenic vein thrombosis, portal vein thrombosis
  Splenic artery arteriovenous malformation
Hepatic
  Presinusoidal
    Schistosomiasis, congenital hepatic fibrosis
  Sinusoidal
    Cirrhosis, myelofibrosis, granulomata tumor
  Postsinusoidal
    Alcohol-induced perivenular fibrosis, veno-occlusive
      disease
Posthepatic
  Right heart failure, constrictive pericarditis, Budd-Chiari
    syndrome

tal hypertension are bleeding from portosystemic collaterals, ascites, hepatic encephalopathy, and hypersplenism. The first three complications will be discussed in this chapter.

MANAGEMENT OF VARICEAL HEMORRHAGE

The management of gastroesophageal variceal hemorrhage requires a concerted effort involving critical care specialists, internists, therapeutic endoscopists, surgeons, interventional radiologists, and trained nursing personnel. There are four main goals in the management of variceal bleeding: maintenance of hemodynamic stability, treatment of complications relating to bleeding and therapy, achievement of hemostasis, and finally, prevention of recurrent bleeding. The general measures for treating patients with variceal hemorrhage are the same as those used in other patients with upper gastrointestinal bleeding. Reliable, adequate venous access is followed by initial resuscitation with normal saline in an effort to maintain a central venous pressure between 5 and 8 cm of water. Overexpansion of the intravascular volume should be avoided because a concomitant rise in portal pressure may induce further bleeding. Intravenous colloid is reserved for immediate infusion until blood becomes available. The gelatin-based colloid solutions are preferred because they have less effect on platelet and clotting factor function. Platelet infusions are indicated when the platelet count is less than 50,000, and fresh frozen plasma is used when the prothrombin time ratio is greater than 1.5. Clotting factor deficiency is common in patients with advanced liver disease and may be worsened by hemodilution or disseminated intravascular coagulation. Thus, supplemental frozen plasma should be given with every 5 units of transfused blood, and supplemental platelets should be given with every 8 units transfused. Parenteral vitamin K is given routinely.

A nasogastric tube is inserted both to detect active bleeding and to prepare the patient for endoscopy. Evacuation of the stomach also reduces the risk of aspiration. Once the nasogastric tube aspirate clears, emergency endoscopy is indicated, preferably with a dual-chamber endoscope. Endoscopy is necessary to confirm a variceal source of hemorrhage because as many as half of patients with chronic liver disease and upper gastrointestinal bleeding are bleeding from nonvariceal sites. It is rare to see direct bleeding from esophageal varices; instead, one often sees cherry red spots over the blue-colored varix. In patients with recent hematemesis in whom nonbleeding varices are seen at endoscopy and no other obvious source of bleeding is identified, a presumed variceal source of hemorrhage should be treated. Patients should undergo endotracheal intubation when there is a risk of aspiration during active hematemesis or when balloon tamponade is used. When possible, sedatives should be avoided because of the risk of precipitating encephalopathy.

As soon as active bleeding stops, lactulose should be administered via the nasogastric tube to prevent encephalopathy. The management of alcoholic patients requires thiamine, multivitamin therapy, and folate therapy, as well as close observation for the development of alcohol withdrawal symptoms and delirium tremens. Along with aspiration and hepatic encephalopathy, other major contributors to the high mortality associated with acute variceal hemorrhage include renal failure, sepsis, multiorgan failure, and exsanguination.

Pharmacologic and nonpharmacologic approaches are used to obtain hemostasis. Pharmacologic agents can be useful in the treatment of gastroesophageal variceal hemorrhage by reducing portal blood flow or by decreasing hepatic resistance. These agents are particularly important when emergent endoscopy or interventional radiology is not available. The vasoconstrictors vasopressin, glypressin, somatostatin, and octreotide decrease mesenteric arterial blood flow and hence portal pressure. Trials of vasopressin in portal hypertensive bleeding have yielded disappointing results, however. In addition, serious side effects including myocardial ischemia or infarction, peripheral ischemia, and cerebrovascular accidents limit the use of this agent. Glypressin, which is converted to lysine vasopressin in vivo, has effects similar to those of vasopressin. Somatostatin is equivalent to or better than vasopressin in controlling initial bleeding and is associated with fewer side effects. A similar amino acid peptide, octreotide (50 μg/hr), has a longer half-life and is widely used in the acute setting. The role of vasodilators like nitroglycerin in combination with vasoconstrictors in the management of acute variceal hemorrhage has not yet been established, although there is a potential role for nitroglycerin to counteract the adverse hemodynamic effects of vasoconstrictors.

Balloon tamponade has been highly effective in controlling bleeding from distal esophageal and gastric varices, achieving initial hemostasis in 90% and permanent hemostasis in 30 to 50% of cases. Controlled studies have shown that in experienced hands, balloon tamponade is superior to pharmacologic agents and equivalent to sclerotherapy for immediate control of bleeding. However, because morbidity and mortality may be unacceptably high in inexperienced hands, balloon tamponade is best reserved for the management of life-threatening bleeding where endoscopic intervention is not feasible. In view of the high rate of rebleeding after balloon deflation, an alternative method to prevent further bleeding should be available.

Immediate therapeutic endoscopy plays a central role in the management of emergent variceal bleeding. Sclerotherapy and endoscopic ligation are the two techniques most commonly utilized. The goal of endoscopic sclerotherapy is to inject a sclerosant material that will provoke an intense inflammatory reaction in the varix, resulting in fibrosis and ultimate obliteration. The agents most commonly used are sodium tetradecyl, sodium morrhuate, and ethnolamine oleate. No single agent has consistently proved superior. Reports of cerebral toxicity associated with the use of polymers like cyanoacrylate prevent their widespread use. Intravariceal injection has been compared with paravariceal injection in the control of acute variceal bleeding, and both procedures have their advocates. Whichever method is chosen, injection should be restricted to the distal 4 to 5 cm of the esophagus, where virtually all variceal hemorrhages occur. Injection should not be made above 30 cm from the teeth to avoid possible spinal injury. Gastric varices within 3 cm of the gastroesophageal junction may also be injected. A maximum dose of 20 mL is recommended to minimize complications. Ideally, one should inject an actively bleeding site; however, if no site is visible, the initial injection is begun at the gastroesophageal junction, moving proximally using 1 to 2 mL per varix. The actual dose used depends on the effects of injection, including ballooning of the varix, mucosal blanching, and resistance to injection.

Sclerotherapy should be instituted at the initial diagnostic endoscopy unless massive bleeding precludes it. The technique is successful in arresting bleeding in 90% of cases and decreases the risk of early rebleeding from 70% in untreated patients to 30 to 40%. If bleeding persists after an initial course of endoscopic sclero-

Table 61–2. Complications Associated with Endoscopic Sclerotherapy

Esophageal
    Ulceration, perforation, bleeding, wall necrosis, mediastinitis
    Stricture requiring dilatation
    Nonspecific motility disorders
    Pseudodiverticula
    Distal esophageal mucosal bridges
Regional
    Pleural effusions
    Pulmonary infiltrates and atelectasis
    Noncardiac chest pain, esophageal spasm
    Acute respiratory distress syndrome
    Bronchoesophageal fistulae
    Chylothorax
    Pneumothorax
    Subcutaneous emphysema
    Portal vein thrombosis
Remote
    Bacteremia
    Sepsis

therapy, a second procedure may be performed within 24 hours. Four to six endoscopic sessions are usually required before variceal obliteration is achieved. Significant complications develop in 10 to 30% of patients undergoing endoscopic sclerotherapy and are summarized in Table 61–2. The routine use of prophylactic antibiotics in endoscopic sclerotherapy is controversial, although antibiotics should be given to patients with prosthetic heart valves, with mitral valve prolapse, and possibly to immunosuppressed patients.

Endoscopic ligation of varices is an increasingly utilized alternative to sclerotherpay in controlling acute variceal hemorrhage. The procedure is initiated by passing a standard endoscope along with a 25-cm overtube. The endoscope is then removed, and the ligating device is attached to the tip of the endoscope. The endoscope is then reinserted through the outer tube and passed to the distal esophagus or stomach, where the variceal channel in the distal esophagus or gastric fundus is identified. The varix is pulled into the outer cylinder. The device is then used to deploy a band around a portion of the mucosa containing the varix. Ligations are repeated around the circumference of the esophagus in a spiral fashion. One can usually perform five ligations per sessions, ideally placing a band near a bleeding site. The banding of varices results in venous obstruction, mucosal inflammation, necrosis, and scar formation. After 1 or 2 days, the band and strangulated tissue slough off, and as the ulcer heals, fibrous tissue replaces the varix. Complications from variceal ligations are fewer than those reported with endoscopic sclerotherapy. Both procedures result in superficial ulcers; however, perforation is less common with variceal ligation. Endoscopic variceal ligation, like sclerotherapy, can be difficult when a patient is actively bleeding, especially when the chamber at the end of the endoscope fills with blood. Although the choice of endoscopic procedure is institution dependent, esophageal variceal ligation is rapidly becoming the treatment of choice in the management of acute variceal bleeding.

Interventional radiology also plays a significant role in the management of acute variceal hemorrhage using embolization techniques and, with increasing frequency, transjugular intrahepatic portosystemic shunts (TIPS). When hemostasis cannot be achieved by pharmacologic, endoscopic, or interventional radiologic techniques, surgical options include portosystemic shunting, devascularization, transection procedures, and liver transplantation (see Chapters 62 and 63).

PREVENTION OF VARICEAL BLEEDING AND REBLEEDING

Once an episode of acute variceal hemorrhage has been controlled, attention should be directed toward preventing recurrent hemorrhage. Approximately two-thirds of patients will bleed again, most frequently within the first 6 weeks after the initial bleed. Beta blockers are the most commonly used pharmacologic agents in preventing recurrent variceal hemorrhage. Beta blockers reduce cardiac output, mediated by beta$_1$ receptors, and allow unopposed catecholamine-mediated alpha-adrenergic splanchnic vasoconstriction. Thus, nonselective beta blockers such as nadolol or propranolol are more effective than selective beta blockers like atenolol. The dose should be titrated to maintain a heart rate between 50 and 60 beats per minute. Nonselective beta blockers are also first-line therapy for prophylaxis against initial variceal bleeding and for reducing acute and chronic bleeding from portal hypertensive gastropathy. Some studies have reported benefit from the addition of isosorbide-5-mononitrate in reducing the frequency of initial bleeding and preventing rebleeding.

In patients who rebleed despite maintenance pharmacologic therapy, endoscopic variceal ligation is the treatment of choice. Ligation is associated with lower rates of rebleeding, complications, and mortality than sclerotherapy. Recurrent variceal hemorrhage despite pharmacologic, endoscopic, or radiologic therapy is an indication for liver transplantation in otherwise suitable candidates.

ASCITES

Ascites is a poor prognostic sign in the cirrhotic patient; fewer than half the patients who develop ascites live for more than 2 years.[2] Diagnostic paracentesis should be performed when ascites is initially detected or if there is unexplained deterioration in an otherwise well-compensated cirrhotic patient with ascites. If the physical examination is inconclusive about the presence of ascites, blind paracentesis should not be attempted because of the risk of inadvertent bowel puncture. Computed tomography scanning, magnetic resonance imaging scanning, or, more practically, ultrasonographic examination can more reliably detect small amount of ascites and can locate a site for safe paracentesis.

A cell count with differential, Gram stain and culture for bacteria, and quantitation of total protein and albumin concentrations should be obtained in the analysis of ascitic fluid. The serum:ascitic fluid albumin gradient is helpful in determining the etiology of ascites; specifically, a gradient between the serum and ascitic fluid albumin concentrations of more than 1.1 g/dL suggests portal hypertension, whereas a smaller gradient indicates an alternative cause when portal pressure is normal, such as tuberculous peritonitis, peritoneal malignancy, pancreatic ascites, or the nephrotic syndrome. If the serum:ascitic fluid albumin concentration gradient is low, or if there is other clinical evidence of tuberculosis or tumor, then fluid culture for Acid Fast Bacilli or cytopathologic examination should be obtained. An ascitic fluid amylase, bilirubin, or triglyceride level greater than the corresponding serum level is suggestive of pancreatic ascites, bile ascites, or chylous ascites, respectively (Table 61–3).

Clinically significant ascites should be treated to increase the patient's comfort and to reduce the risk of ascitic fluid infection or cardiopulmonary compromise. Restriction of dietary salt intake and diuretic therapy are the cornerstones of ascites management, although fluid restriction is not necessary unless the serum sodium concentration falls below 130 mEq/L. Diuretic therapy mobilizes ascites primarily because of a decrease in the rate of formation rather than an increase in the rate of reabsorption. Weight loss of 0.5 to 1.0 kg/day should be the goal of diuretic therapy.

Measurement of urinary sodium excretion is helpful in assessing the efficacy of diuretic therapy. A diuretic regimen that results in urinary sodium excretion greater than dietary sodium intake (a negative sodium balance) will control ascites in most patients with cirrhosis. Assessing urinary sodium excretion can also help determine the diuretic regimen needed to mobilize ascites. If urinary sodium excretion is greater than 50 mEq/24 hr on a 1-g sodium diet, salt restriction alone may be sufficient. When sodium excretion is between 25 and 50 mEq/24 hr, spironolactone should be added. An initial 50-mg dose may be increased to a maximum dose of 300 mg/day to achieve the desired daily weight loss. If sodium excretion is less than 25 mEq/24 hr or if overall fluid loss is not sufficient, a loop diuretic (eg, furosemide) or a thiazide diuretic (eg, hydrochlorothiazide) should be added. These agents decrease sodium reabsorption in the proximal nephron, resulting in an increase in the sodium load to the distal nephron, where the aldosterone antagonists work. If there is inadequate fluid loss and urinary sodium excretion remains less than 10 mEq/24 hr after a trial of dietary sodium restriction and diuretic combinations, the patient is deemed to have refractory ascites. This usually reflects advanced liver disease and occurs in only a small percentage of patients with ascites. In these patients, repeated therapeutic paracentesis, a portosystemic shunt, a peritoneovenous shunt, or liver transplantation will likely be necessary.

Therapeutic paracentesis effectively controls tense ascites and is well tolerated. Up to 5 L of ascitic fluid can be safely removed, with no more frequent electrolyte abnormalities than with diuretic therapy. Repeated large-volume paracentesis is rarely associated with acute risks such as hemorrhage or infection, although the administration of 6 to 8 g of intravenous albumin per liter of ascites removed may be indicated in patients with renal insufficiency or edema.

Peritoneovenous shunts have been used to treat refractory ascites. However, a number of complications limit their usefulness. In approximately a third of patients, the shunt fails for mechanical reasons. Occasionally, repositioning the distal end of the shunt may restore function. In some patients, the valve becomes clogged and needs to be replaced. In patients with underlying heart disease, right ventricular overload

Table 61–3. Ascitic Fluid Analysis

Etiology	S-A Gradient	Cell Count (Predominant)	Other
Cirrhosis	>1.1	<250 (mononuclear)	—
Nephrotic syndrome	<1.1	<250 (mononuclear)	—
Pancreatic	<1.1	>500 (PMN)	↑ Fluid amylase
SBP*	<1.1	>250 (PMN)	+ Fluid culture
Tuberculosis*	<1.1	>500 (mononuclear)	
Tumor	<1.1	>250 (mononuclear)	+ Fluid cytology ↑ Fluid lactic dehydrogenase
Chylous	<1.1	>500 (mononuclear-PMN)	↑ Fluid triglyceride

*Gradient may be high in patients with portal hypertension.
Abbreviations: S-A, serum:ascites gradient; PMN, polymorphonuclear leukocyte.

may induce congestive heart failure. The most significant complication of a peritoneovenous shunt is a coagulopathy, with resulting hemorrhage often from esophageal varices. While surgical side-to-side portosystemic shunts will control ascites, the morbidity and mortality from shunt surgery restrict the usefulness of this form of therapy in most patients with cirrhosis and ascites (see Chapter 62). TIPS have been used in some patients as an alternative to surgical shunts, but the long-term efficacy of this therapy is yet to be determined (see Chapter 63). Refractory ascites is an indication for liver transplantation in patients who are otherwise good candidates for the procedure.

SPONTANEOUS BACTERIAL PERITONITIS

Bacterial infection complicates ascites in approximately 10% of patients with cirrhosis and is associated with an estimated inpatient mortality of 40%.[3] Perforation of the bowel or leakage of bacteria into the ascitic fluid from localized pockets of infection such as subhepatic abscesses can cause peritonitis and is designated *secondary bacterial peritonitis*. In most patients, however, bacterial infection of ascites occurs with no identifiable "inoculation" site and is called *spontaneous bacterial peritonitis (SBP)*.[3] Patients with a low level of total ascitic fluid protein (<1.5 g/dL) are at increased risk of developing SBP due to reduced ascitic complement levels and opsonic activity. Symptoms and signs of SBP are neither sensitive nor specific, and up to 50% of patients with SBP have no signs of peritonitis. Likewise, it is not possible to differentiate SBP from secondary peritonitis on the basis of symptoms and signs alone. Therefore, all cirrhotic patients with ascites should be considered for paracentesis to analyze ascitic fluid. Antibiotic therapy should be instituted if the ascitic fluid level of polymorphonuclear leukocytes (PMNs) is greater than 250 cells/mm. Directly inoculating ascitic fluid into blood culture bottles at the bedside increases the sensitivity of ascitic fluid culture. Peripheral blood cultures should be obtained, and are positive in 25% of cases. Empiric antibiotic therapy is based on the epidemiology of SBP. A single gram-negative enteric organism is most often responsible for the infection, with *Escherichia coli* being the most common. *Klebsiella pneumoniae* and enterococci are also common pathogens. Anaerobic infection is rare. We use cefotaxime, a third-generation cephalosporin, in the empiric treatment of suspected SBP. Intravenous administration of 2 g of cefotaxime every 8 hours for 7 days should be sufficient. Antibiotic coverage may be altered, depending on organism sensitivity. Because of the high rate of nephrotoxicity in cirrhotic patients, aminoglycosides should be avoided.

Occasionally, a positive ascitic fluid culture will be obtained with fewer than 250 PMNs in the ascitic fluid. If the patient is asymptomatic, a repeated paracentesis

with cell count and culture should be performed. If the repeat culture is negative and the cell count remains low, then no therapy is indicated. The prophylactic administration of a daily oral quinolone (eg, norfloxacin, 400 mg/day) may reduce the incidence of gram-negative SBP and is particularly indicated in cirrhotic patients with low ascitic protein content.

SBP must be distinguished from secondary peritonitis because the latter usually requires surgical intervention. An ascitic fluid protein level greater than 1 gm/dL, a glucose concentration less than 50 mg/dL, or polymicrobial infection suggests secondary peritonitis. If secondary peritonitis is suspected, metronidazole in addition to cefotaxime should be used as initial therapy. An aggressive search for evidence of colonic perforation, biliary tract infection, or another localized abdominal infection should be initiated and treated appropriately.

Ultimately, because of the high in-hospital mortality associated with SBP and because of its common recurrence within a year, liver transplantation should be considered in all patients who survive SBP and are otherwise suitable candidates.

HEPATIC ENCEPHALOPATHY

Hepatic encephalopathy is a complex and usually reversible neuropsychiatric syndrome that develops in about 10% of patients with cirrhosis and portal hypertension.[4] The spectrum of clinical manifestations of hepatic encephalopathy ranges from minor personality changes and abnormal psychometric tests results to coma. Asterixis and with other alterations in neuromuscular transmission are common. While the most common form of hepatic encephalopathy in cirrhosis is reversible, a small minority of patients develop a severe motor disorder known as *hepatocerebral degeneration*, which may progress to spastic paralysis. This variant of hepatic encephalopathy is refractory to therapy. The diagnosis of hepatic encephalopathy is made on clinical grounds because no single laboratory test is diagnostic. However, the diagnosis should be questioned in patients with a normal plasma ammonia concentration, and other diagnoses should be pursued (Table 61–4).

Hepatic encephalopathy results from exposure of the central nervous system to portal blood containing toxic compounds produced by the action of colonic flora on nitrogenous substrates and shunted around the diseased liver. Hepatic encephalopathy can be precipitated by factors that increase toxin production or increase cerebral sensitivity to toxic agents. Azotemia, gastrointestinal bleeding, hypoglycemia, systemic infection, alkalosis, and sedative drugs are common precipitants of encephalopathy. When the precipitating agent can be identified and corrected, the prognosis for recovery is usually better than when encephalopathy is caused by worsening liver function.

Table 61–4. Differential Diagnosis of Hepatic Encephalopathy

Intracranial lesions
  Hemorrhage
  Infarct
  Tumor
  Abscess

Infection
  Meningitis
  Encephalitis
  Sepsis

Metabolic encephalopathy
  Hyperglycemia or hypoglycemia
  Uremia
  Acidosis
  Electrolyte imbalances
  Hypoxia
  Hyperammonemia without liver failure
    Inborn errors of urea cycle
    Reye's syndrome
    Ureterosigmoidostomy

Alcohol-related disorders
  Intoxication
  Withdrawal
  Wernicke's encephalopathy

Drug toxicity
  Sedatives
  Psychoactive drugs
  Salicylates

Postictal encephalopathy

Primary neuropsychiatric disorders

Empiric therapy for hepatic encephalopathy is initiated after precipitating factors have been eliminated or treated.[4] Initially, dietary protein should be restricted to less than 20 g/day. Protein intake can be increased gradually as symptoms improve. Protein administered intravenously does not precipitate hepatic encephalopathy. Some patients with hepatic encephalopathy tolerate vegetable protein better than animal sources. The administration of branched chained amino acids, intended to restore the normal plasma ratio of branched chained to aromatic amino acids, has been advocated for the treatment of hepatic encephalopathy but is not widely used due to the high cost.

The drug of choice in the treatment of hepatic encephalopathy is lactulose, which functions by decreasing ammoniagenesis by enteric flora and by decreasing ammonia absorption from the gastrointestinal tract. A dose of 30 mL of lactulose is given orally every hour until diarrhea develops. Once symptoms improve, the dose is tapered. In comatose patients who cannot take oral medications, lactulose may be given via a nasogastric tube or as an enema. Toxin production by gut flora may also be suppressed by the administration of oral antibiotics. Neomycin (1 to 2 g orally four times a day) was used for many years but is being increasingly replaced by metronidazole (250 mg orally three times a day) because of the potential for neomycin-associated ototoxicity, nephrotoxicity, and diarrhea.

Benzodiazepine-like compounds, originating in the gut and acting at the benzodiazepine receptor complex in the brain, may play a role in the etiology of hepatic encephalopathy. Several reports using benzodiazepine antagonists (eg, flumazenil) have shown improvement in patients with hepatic encephalopathy. This form of therapy is still considered experimental. If medical management fails to improve hepatic encephalopathy, liver transplantation should be considered.

REFERENCES

1. Alam I, Bass N. Hemodyamis and pathophysiology of portal hypertension. In: Sleisenger M, ed. *Gastrointestinal and Disease Update.* Philadelphia: WB Saunders; 1996:1–20.
2. Rector W. Sodium retention and ascites formation. In: *Complications of Chronic Liver Disease.* St Louis: Mosby Year Book; 1992:68–82.
3. Hoefs J, Runyon B. Spontaneous bacterial peritonitis. *Dis Mon* 1985;31(9):1–48. Editor: Roger Bone Mosby Year Book.
4. Capocaccia L, Merli M, and Riggio O, eds. *Advances in Hepatic Encephalopathy and Metabolic Nitrogen.* Boca Raton, FL: CRC Press; 1995.

62

Surgical Treatment of Portal Hypertension: Patient and Procedure Selection

David R. Holt, M.D.
Andrew S. Klein, M.D.

Portal hypertension (PH) is defined as portal vein pressure that exceeds the normal value of 3 to 6 mm Hg. In the splanchnic circulation, as in any fluid system, the pressure gradient is a product of flow and resistance to flow. Two hypotheses have been proposed to explain the development of increased portal pressure—the *forward flow theory* (increased portal venous blood flow secondary principally to increased production of vasodilating agents) and the *backward flow theory* (increased resistance to flow due to fibrosis, granuloma, tumors, or thrombosis). Currently, it is generally accepted that increased resistance to flow is the *initial* event in most patients with PH, and increased splanchnic blood flow is an important factor in the maintenance and progression of elevated portal venous pressure. PH is often classified by referring to the primary location of abnormally increased resistance: prehepatic, intrahepatic, and posthepatic. Alternatively, PH may be defined by the site of resistance with respect to the hepatic sinusoid: presinusoidal, sinusoidal, and postsinusoidal PH. Table 62–1 lists the common causes of PH in each category. There is prognostic utility in this classification in that patients with presinusoidal hypertension tolerate the complications of PH, such as variceal bleeding, better than do patients with sinusoidal or postsinusoidal lesions. In the United States, the most common etiology of PH is hepatic cirrhosis secondary to alcohol abuse, which is thought to have

components of both sinusoidal and postsinusoidal resistance.

It is not PH per se that demands therapeutic intervention, but rather the complication of this pathophysiologic state—hemorrhage from gastroesophageal varices, ascites, spontaneous bacterial peritonitis, hepatic encephalopathy, and hypersplenism. Of these potential complications, bleeding from ruptured varices accounts for the greatest morbidity and mortality. This chapter will therefore focus on the surgeon's role in the prophylaxis and treatment of this complication.

CLINICAL PRESENTATION

The symptoms and signs that lead to the diagnosis of PH are generally those produced by its causes (ie, hepatic cirrhosis) or its complications, as discussed above. Most often, upper gastrointestinal hemorrhage or the new onset of ascites precipitates further evaluation. Because cirrhosis is the most common cause of PH in the United States, inquiry should be made to determine alcohol consumption patterns; a history of jaundice, hepatitis, or blood transfusion; or exposure to hepatotoxins. In cirrhotic individuals, the physical examination may reveal jaundice, hepatic enlargement or shrinkage, gynecomastia, ascites, peripheral edema, muscle wasting, testicular atrophy, splenomegaly, spi-

Table 62–1. Anatomic Classification of PH

Presinusoidal	Sinusoidal	Postsinusoidal
Portal or splenic vein occlusion	Cirrhosis	Veno-occlusive disease
Schistosomiasis	Alcoholic Hepatitis	Budd-Chiari syndrome
Congenital hepatic fibrosis		Constrictive pericarditis
Sarcoidosis		

der angiomata, Dupuytren's contractures, parotid enlargement, or palmar erythema. In response to PH, collateral blood vessels between the portal and systemic venous systems dilate and hypertrophy. These collateral varices, the formation of which may be potentiated by active angiogenesis, may develop throughout the body. Decompression of the hypertensive portal system occurs via the coronary vein to esophageal collaterals, the superior rectal vein to the middle and inferior rectal veins, the paraumbilical veins, and splenic or pancreatic tributaries. Due to a lack of valves in these veins, portal blood is free to flow into these collaterals, resulting in hemorrhoids, caput medusa, and most importantly, esophageal varices. Clinically significant bleeding from varices occurs most commonly in the distal esophagus due to the submucosal location of these poorly supported, thin-walled vessels, as well as the turbulent flow that is present at the gastroesophageal junction.

The laboratory workup of patients with PH should include a routine battery of liver function tests, specifically aminotransferases, lactate dehydrogenase, bilirubin, albumin, fibrinogen, cholesterol, and prothrombin time. In patients with a presinusoidal cause of PH, biochemical measures of hepatic synthetic function, biotransformation, detoxification, and excretory function are often normal or minimally abnormal. Patients with underlying cirrhosis, however, often have evidence of some degree of hepatocellular dysfunction.

NATURAL HISTORY

The prognosis of patients with PH depends on the underlying etiology. Patients with sinusoidal or postsinusoidal PH most often have concomitant parenchymal liver disease and thus less hepatic reserve. The physiologic implications of this observation are illustrated by comparing mortality rates among patients who bleed from esophageal varices. The initial variceal hemorrhage is fatal in 30 to 80% of all patients who sustain this complication of PH. If, however, patients are stratified according to the primary location of increased resistance to portal venous flow, those with portal vein occlusion (presinusoidal PH) are found to have a substantially lower risk of death (5 to 10% than those with sinusoidal obstruction due to cirrhosis (40 to 70%).[1]

A useful system for assessing hepatocellular dysfunction is the Childs-Pugh classification. This categorization is based on degree of encephalopathy, ascites, serum bilirubin, serum albumin, and prothrombin time. The prognosis following variceal hemorrhage has been shown to be directly related to the patient's Childs class (A, B, or C).[2]

Not all cirrhotic patients suffer variceal bleeding. Indeed, only about half of these patients develop gastroesophageal varices, and of this subgroup, approximately 20 to 33% bleed.[3] If untreated, 70% of these patients rebleed within 1 year.[3] This can be further stratified by Child's category. At 1 year, 68% of Childs class C, 48% of Childs class B, and 28% of Childs class A patients can be expected to rebleed.[2]

The decision to perform a procedure to control bleeding or to reduce PH must be based on the overall plan for management of the patient. In patients with preserved liver function, portal-systemic shunting and the resulting portal decompression may cure the PH. However, similar procedures in patients suffering from liver failure do not change the prognosis. Portal decompression may lessen or alleviate the risk of variceal bleeding, but it will not change the mortality rate, which is due to liver failure and/or sepsis. The 5-year survival rate for cirrhotic patients who have suffered a variceal bleed is 0 to 35%.[4] Thus, total liver replacement in those patients suitable for such an operation is the only therapy that will alter the otherwise grim prognosis.

DIAGNOSIS

The only physical finding pathognomonic for PH is the presence of a caput medusa. Indirect evidence of PH includes the presence of ascites, encephalopathy, splenomegaly, purpura, thrombocytopenia, and leukopenia. Nonbleeding varices require more invasive procedures for diagnosis. Barium swallow has been used as a noninvasive screening test, although the diagnostic accuracy of this study is only 60%.[5] Modifications of a simple barium swallow using cineradiography, Müller and Valsalva maneuvers, upper esophageal balloon occlusion, or administration of Pro-Banthine can increase the yield somewhat.[6,7]

Another noninvasive method for diagnosing portal hypertension is magnetic resonance imaging (MRI).[8] This technique is useful in identifying gastroesophageal as well as intra-abdominal and retroperitoneal varices. Because MRI does not distinguish between intraluminal (esophageal) and extraluminal (eg, retroperitoneal) varices, the procedure has a high false-positive rate. Another drawback is the expense of MRI. Rarely, actual measurement of portal venous pressure is required to establish the diagnosis of PH. This can be performed indirectly by measuring wedged hepatic venous pressure (WHVP) or by direct measurement of portal vein pressure (PVP). PVP can be quantified by (1) direct cannulation of the portal vein or superior mesenteric vein at laparotomy, (2) percutaneous or transjugular transhepatic portal vein cannulation,[9] (3) splenic pulp catheterization,[10] or (4) umbilical vein catheterization.[11] Abnormal elevations in PVP may be inferred from determinations of esophageal variceal pressures obtained by endoscopic needle puncture or placement of a pressure transducer on esophageal varices.[12,13] Portal flow velocity measured by duplex

Doppler ultrasonography has been shown to correlate with PVP and thus represents a noninvasive means of assessing PVP.[14] WHVP can be measured by placing a balloon-tipped catheter directly into a hepatic vein, inflating the balloon, and measuring the wedged pressure via a transducer at the tip of the catheter, thus measuring pressure at the level of the hepatic sinusoids.[15] These various techniques allow for discrimination between presinusoidal and sinusoidal/postsinusoidal PH. Presinusoidal PH results in an elevated PVP and a normal WHVP, whereas sinusoidal and postsinusoidal PH cause elevation of both PVP and WHVP. It should be emphasized, however, that few patients require invasive measurement of PVP to establish the presence of PH, which is often diagnosed on the basis of a careful history and physical examination.

TREATMENT: PROPHYLAXIS

Gastroesophageal varices are the source of upper gastrointestinal bleeding in 80 to 90% of cirrhotics.[16] Although 30 to 80% of patients who bleed from varices die from the initial hemorrhage, only 20% of patients with PH and gastroesophageal varices develop bleeding. Therefore, efforts have been made to identify the patients in this group who are at high risk for bleeding and which methods are effective in preventing the first bleed among this population. It appears that patients with varices due to alcoholic cirrhosis have the highest incidence of hemorrhage, especially if they continue to abuse alcohol.[17] This is probably explained by the observation that bleeding is directly related to the degree of hepatocellular dysfunction, which deteriorates with continued drinking but which may improve in patients who permanently abstain from alcohol consumption.[18]

Endoscopy has been shown to be the most useful method for directly identifying varices most likely to bleed. Large varices, tortuous varices, "cherry red spots" or "red wale" markings, varices on varices, and gastric varices are all signs indicating a greater likelihood of hemorrhage.[18,19] One group has used a combination of endoscopic findings and liver function to assess the risk of bleeding; patients at highest risk have Childs class C liver dysfunction, large varices, and "red wale" markings.[20]

A number of prophylactic options are available for patients at high risk for bleeding. Clearly, nonselective portal-systemic shunt procedures have been shown to be of no survival benefit.[21] Though bleeding may be reduced in shunted patients, this is negated by death due to operative mortality, as well as encephalopathy, liver failure, and sepsis. While shunting procedures play no role in prophylaxis, nondecompression procedures might confer a survival benefit.[22] Inokuchi showed an advantage for patients treated with either variceal interruption procedures or selective shunts compared to those treated medically. These data must be looked at cautiously, however, due to the highly selected group of patients and the multiple different procedures used in the surgical arm. Prophylactic sclerotherapy or variceal banding has been investigated by several groups. The results of these studies vary, and no conclusive benefit has been shown for patients treated endoscopically. For patients with high-risk stigmata, as defined above, the use of beta blockers (propranolol) has been shown to be effective in reducing the risk of hemorrhage.

TREATMENT: ACUTE BLEEDING

Medical treatment of acutely bleeding gastroesophageal varices has evolved rapidly over the last two decades, but an extensive discussion is beyond the scope of this chapter (see Chapter 61). Briefly, initial pharmacologic therapy involves intravenous infusion of various drugs intended to lower PVP. These include vasopressin with or without simultaneous nitroglycerin infusion, terlipressin, and somatostatin. For patients who continue to bleed despite aggressive pharmacologic measures, invasive radiologic and endoscopic techniques have become the treatment of choice. Although surgical options are often considered only for those patients who fail minimally invasive therapy, there are instances in which operative procedures are most appropriate for primary management.

Invasive Radiologic Techniques

Invasive radiologic therapy can be divided into embolic and shunting procedures. Transhepatic embolization of portosystemic collaterals was introduced in the early 1970s.[23] Access to a branch of the portal vein is gained by percutaneous puncture of the liver using a Teflon-sheathed needle. A guidewire is then threaded through a portal vein branch into the desired collaterals, such as the coronary vein. A sclerosing agent such as Gelfoam, thrombin, autologous thrombus, hypertonic glucose, bucrylate, or sodium tetradecyl sulfate can then be injected. This procedure is most useful in the setting of an acute bleed, with the expectation that it will be followed by definitive portal decompression either surgically or by percutaneous shunting using the transjugular intrahepatic portosystemic shunt (TIPS) procedure (see Chapter 63). Percutaneous variceal obliteration may also be useful as a minimally invasive therapy for bleeding mesenteric varices.[24]

Endoscopic Techniques

Endoscopy has come to play a very important role in the diagnosis and management of acute variceal bleeding. Sclerotherapy was first used in the late 1930s but subsequently was overshadowed by surgical shunting procedures. Enthusiasm for the use of this technique in acute episodes of bleeding returned in the 1970s.

Today it is used extensively for acute variceal bleeding, as well as for prevention of recurrent bleeding.

There are several techniques for endoscopic sclerotherapy using either a rigid or a flexible endoscope (see Chapter 61). The resurgent interest in endoscopic sclerotherapy began with the use of a rigid endoscope in children.[25] This instrument was used to inject varices directly with a variety of sclerosants, including sodium morrhuate, ethanolamine, and sodium tetradecyl sulfate. In 1973, Johnston et al published their 15-year experience with endoscopic sclerotherapy, reporting a 93% success rate for control of variceal bleeding.[26] In 1979, use of the flexible endoscope for sclerotherapy was described.[27] Flexible endoscopy has the advantage of being portable, and because it may be performed using topical anesthesia alone, it does not require an operating room setting.

Injection technique can be classified as intravariceal, paravariceal, or a combination of both. Direct intravariceal injection introduces the sclerosant into the varix, causing thrombosis. With the paravariceal approach, the sclerosing agent is injected into the submucosa between varices, inducing a fibrotic reaction that thickens the wall of the varix and lessens the propensity to rupture. The latter technique has the potential to produce deep or even transmural ulceration of the esophagus. Its theoretic advantage is maintenance of collateral blood flow, thus reducing the chance of new variceal formation. A randomized study comparing intravariceal versus paravariceal injection demonstrated a higher rate of control of bleeding with intravariceal injection but a lower rate of late rebleeding using the paravariceal technique.[28] A combination of intravariceal and paravariceal injection has also been reported, with a 4.9% rebleeding rate in 17 patients.[29]

An alternative to endoscopic variceal sclerosis is endoscopic variceal ligation. This was first reported in 1988[30] and is similar to rubber band ligation of internal hemorrhoids. Several reported studies suggest that endoscopic variceal ligation is at least as effective as sclerotherapy, with the advantages of fewer complications, better initial control of acute bleeding, and fewer sessions necessary for variceal obliteration.[31] However, there is a higher incidence of bleeding from gastric varices after ligation.

Surgical Techniques

Among the surgical procedures employed to control acute variceal hemorrhage, the most widely used are portal-systemic shunts. These operations have proven to be very effective in controlling acute variceal bleeding, albeit associated with high rates of morbidity and mortality. Portal-systemic shunts can be separated into two basic types: nonselective (total) shunts and selective shunts. Total shunts are designed to divert portal blood flow away from the liver. These shunts include end-to-

side portacaval shunts, side-to-side portacaval shunts, interposition portacaval shunts, splenorenal shunts, and mesocaval shunts. Of these, the end-to-side shunt is unique in that the portal vein is divided and the distal (hepatic) end is ligated, thus anatomically preventing any portal venous perfusion of the liver. While this procedure effectively reduces blood flow to varices, it also eliminates transport of hepatotrophic hormones and gut metabolites to the liver. In addition, end-to-side shunts do not decompress the hepatic sinusoids. Theoretically, these factors could result in more rapid liver failure, worsened encephalopathy, and poor control of ascites. There have been several studies comparing end-to-side and side-to-side portacaval shunts.[32–34] The results are difficult to interpret with respect to postoperative encephalopathy and survival due to the lack of stratification of patients based on degree of liver failure and variable follow-up periods. Side-to-side shunts do appear to be effective in reducing ascites and are preferable in patients with this complication who require a nonselective surgical shunt. It is generally agreed that patients with refractory ascites, reversal of portal vein flow, and Budd-Chiari Syndrome are best served by side-to-side shunts or the equivalent to decompress the portal system. From a practical standpoint, while end-to-side and side-to-side shunts are equally effective in controlling variceal bleeding, the end-to-side shunt is technically simpler and is recommended in the emergency situation.

Other studies have compared total shunts to selective shunts (distal splenorenal shunts).[35–38] Such comparisons have failed to show a persistent, statistically significant difference in postoperative encephalopathy, suggesting that maintenance of portal blood flow is not protective against subsequent encephalopathy or, alternatively, that portal venous flow is indeed shunted from the liver in patients undergoing a supposedly selective decompression of their gastroesophageal varices (eg, via the *pancreatic sump*). Studies comparing full-diameter (14- to 18-mm) total shunts with small-diameter interposition portacaval shunts or side-to-side shunts have in some instances shown a decreased incidence of encephalopathy in the latter group, implying that preservation of portal blood flow does indeed help reduce postoperative encephalopathy.[39,40] Such a distinction is not uniformly accepted and remains an area of considerable controversy.[34,41,42]

Several therapeutic shunt trials have been undertaken in an effort to delineate further the usefulness of shunting procedures compared to medical treatment.[43–46] No statistically significant difference in survival or encephalpathy was noted in any of these studies. However, spontaneous encephalopathy did occur in the shunted patients, whereas in the medically treated patients there was usually a precipitating event. In addition, while there was a markedly lower incidence of recurrent bleeding in the surgically treated groups, shunting was not completely effective in preventing hemorrhage. It is not well documented whether recurrent variceal bleeding is consistently associated with shunt occlusion.

Nonshunting operations have been used, with variable degrees of success, in the treatment of bleeding esophageal varices. These procedures interrupt collateral pathways between the splanchnic and systemic venous circulations, decreasing blood flow to gastroesophageal varices. Several approaches have been utilized, including splenectomy,[47] splenic artery and coronary vein occlusion,[48] esophagogastrectomy,[49] and esophageal transection with esophagogastric devascularization and splenectomy.[50] There are three basic indications for nonshunting procedures: (1) emergency control of bleeding varices; (2) treatment of extrahepatic portal occlusion with anatomy unfavorable for a shunting procedure; and (3) to avoid shunt-induced encephalopathy. Currently, the most popular nonshunting procedure is the Sugiura procedure.[50] This operation requires both thoracic and abdominal incisions, and involves extensive devascularization of the esophagus and proximal stomach. This is done in such a manner that the periesophageal-azygous vein collaterals remain intact to preserve portal-systemic flow. In addition, splenectomy, vagotomy, and pyloroplasty are performed. The results of this operation have been encouraging in Japan[51] but less successful in the United States.[52]

Finally, an important consideration in electing to perform a procedure for PH is an appreciation of the patient's potential candidacy for orthotopic liver transplantation (OLT). OLT should be reserved as a therapeutic option for patients suffering from PH associated with cirrhosis and liver failure. It has even been suggested that liver transplantation may be useful as a primary treatment for such patients who develop bleeding esophageal varices.[53] The Pittsburgh group demonstrated an equal or better survival for patients with a history of variceal bleeding undergoing liver transplantation compared to reported survival in several other studies in which shunt or nonshunt procedures were performed for variceal bleeding. Furthermore, when the subset of Childs class C patients was considered, a marked survival advantage was conferred on the transplanted patients. If an operation for control of bleeding gastroesophageal varices is required prior to OLT, one must consider that dissection of the porta hepatis prior to liver transplantation results in a more difficult operation, with greater blood loss and a longer operating time.[54] In view of this, many transplant surgeons recommend that patients who may at some point become candidates for OLT, but who require interim management of complications of PH, undergo either the TIPS procedure, distal splenorenal shunting, or mesocaval shunting with an interposition graft.

REFERENCES

1. Vorrhees AB Jr, Price JB Jr. Extrahepatic portal hypertension: a retrospective analysis of 127 cases and associated clinical implications. *Arch Surg* 1974;108:338–341.
2. Sherlock S. Esophageal varices. *Am J Surg* 1990;160:9–13.
3. Grace ND. A hepatologist's view of variceal bleeding. *Am J Surg* 1990;160:26–31.
4. Powell WJ Jr, Klatskin G. Duration of survival in patients with Laennec's cirrhosis. *Am J Med* 1968:44:406–420.
5. Peternel WW, Dagardi AE, Rogers AI, Nadal HM, Perrin EB, Jackson FC. Clinical investigation of the portacaval shunt III: the diagnosis of esophageal varices. *JAMA* 1967;202:1081–1084.
6. Conn HO, Greenspan RH, Clemett AR, Mitchell JR, Brodoff M. Balloon tamponade in the radiological diagnosis of esophageal varices. *Gastroenterology* 1966;50:29–40.
7. Dalinka MK, Smith EH, Wolfe RD, Goldenberg D, Langdon DE. Pharmacologically enhanced visualization of esophageal varices by pro-banthine. *Radiology* 1972;102:281–282.
8. Johnson CD, Ehman RL, Rakela J, Ilstrup DM, MR angiography in portal hypertension: detection of varices and imaging techniques. *Am J Roentgenol* 1991;15:578–584.
9. Smith-Liang G, Camilo ME, Dick R, Sherlock S. Percutaneous transhepatic portography in the assessment of portal hypertension: clinical correlations and comparison of radiographic techniques. *Gastroenterology* 1980;78:197–205.
10. Leger LH. *Splenoportography Diagnostic Phlebography of the Portal Venous System.* Springfield, IL: Charles C Thomas; 1966.
11. Reynolds TB, Ito S, Iwatsuki S. Measurement of portal pressure and its clinical application. *Am J Med* 1970;49:649–657.
12. Mosimann R. Nonaggressive assessment of portal hypertension using endoscopic measurement of variceal pressure: preliminary report. *Am J Surg* 1982;143:212–214.
13. Staritz M, Meyer BKH. The endoscopic measurement of intravascular pressure and flow in oesophageal varices. *J Hepatol* 1988;7:126–131.
14. Cioni G, D'Alimonte P, Zerbinati F, et al. Duplex-Doppler ultrasonography in the evaluation of cirrhotic patients with portal hypertension and in the analysis of their response to drugs. *J Gastroenterol Hepatol* 1992;7:388–392.
15. Groszmann RJ, Glickman M, Blei AT, Storer E, Conn HO. Wedged and free hepatic venous pressure measured with a balloon catheter. *Gastroenterology* 1979;76:253–258.
16. Tabibian N, Graham DY. Source of upper gastrointestinal bleeding in patients with esophageal varices seen at endoscopy. *J Clin Gastroenterol* 1987;9:279–282.
17. Grace ND. Prevention of initial variceal hemorrhage. *Gastroenterol Clin North Am* 1992;21:149–161.
18. de Franchis R, Primignani M. Why do varices bleed? *Gastroenterol Clin North Am* 1992;21:85–101.
19. Galambos JT. Evaluation of patients with portal hypertension. *Am J Surg* 1990;160:14–18.
20. MacMathunda P, Westaby D, Williams R. Taking the tension out of the portal system. An approach to the management of portal hypertension in the 1990's. *Scand J Gastroenterol* 1990;25:131–145.
21. Collini FJ, Brener B. Portal hypertension. *Surg Gynecol Obstet* 1990;170:177–192.

22. Inokuchi K. Improved survival after prophylactic portal nondecompression surgery for esophageal varices: a randomized clinical trial. Cooperative Study Group of Portal Hypertension of Japan. *Hepatology* 1990;12:1–6.

23. Lunderquist A, Vang J. Transhepatic catheterization and obliteration of the coronary vein in patients with portal hypertension and esophageal varices. *N Engl J Med* 1974;291:646–649.

24. Ozaki CK, Hansen M, Kadir S. Transhepatic embolization of superior mesenteric varices in portal hypertension. *Surgery* 1989;105:446–448.

25. Fearon B, Sass-Kortsak A. The management of esophageal varices in children by injection of sclerosing agents. *Ann Otol Rhino Laryngol* 1959;68:906–915.

26. Johnston GW, Rodgers HW. A review of 15 years' experience in the use of sclerotherapy in the control of acute haemorrhage from oesophageal varices. *Br J Surg* 1973; 60:797–800.

27. Williams KG, Dawson JL. Fibreoptic injection of oesophageal varices. *Br Med J* 1979;2:766–767.

28. Sarin SK, Nanda R, Sachdev G, Chari S, Anand BS, Broor SL. Intravariceal versus paravariceal sclerotherapy: a prospective, controlled, randomised trial. *Gut* 1987;28:657–662.

29. Kitano S, Koyanagi N, Iso Y, Higashi H, Sugimachi K. Prevention of recurrence of esophageal varices after endoscopic injection sclerotherapy with ethanolamine oleate. *Hepatology* 1987;7:810–815.

30. Van Stiegmann G, Goff JS. Endoscopic esophageal varix ligation: preliminary clinical experience. *Gastrointest Endosc* 1988;34:113–117.

31. Laine L, el-Newihi HM, Migikovsky B, Sloane R, Garcia F. Endoscopic ligation compared with sclerotherapy for the treatment of bleeding esophageal varices. *Ann Intern Med* 1993;119:87–88.

32. Reynolds TB, Hudson NM, Mikkelsen WP, Turrill FL, Redeker AG. Clinical comparison of end-to-side and side-to-side portacaval shunt. *N Engl J Med* 1966;274:706–710.

33. Turcotte JG, Wallin VW Jr, Child CG III. End to side versus side to side portacaval shunts in patients with hepatic cirrhosis. *Am J Surg* 1969;117:108–116.

34. Zuidema GD, Kirsh MM. Hepatic encephalopathy following portal decompression: evaluation of end-to-side and side-to-side anastomosis. *Am Surg* 1965;31:567–569.

35. Langer B, Taylor BR, Mackenzie DR, Gilas T, Stone RM, Blendis L. Further report of a prospective randomized trial comparing distal splenorenal shunt with end-to-side portacaval shunt. An analysis of encephalopathy, survival, and quality of life. *Gastroenterology* 1985;88:424–429.

36. Millikan WJ Jr, Warren WD, Henderson JM, et al. The Emory Prospective Randomized Trial: selective versus nonselective shunt to control variceal bleeding. Ten year follow-up. *Ann Surg* 1985;201:712–722.

37. Harley HA, Morgan T, Redecker AG, et al. Results of a randomized trial of end-to-side portacaval shunt and distal splenorenal shunt in alcoholic liver disease and variceal bleeding. *Gastroenterology* 1986;91:802–809.

38. Grace ND, Conn HO, Resnick RH, et al. Distal splenorenal vs. portal-systemic shunts after hemorrhage from varices: a randomized controlled trial. *Hepatology* 1988;8:1475–1481.

39. Sarfeh IJ, Rypins EB. Partial versus total portacaval shunt in alcoholic cirrhosis. Results of a prospective, randomized clinical trial. *Ann Surg* 1994;219:353–361.

40. Bismuth H, Franco D, Hepp J. Portal-systemic shunt in hepatic cirrhosis: does the type of shunt decisively influence the clinical result? *Ann Surg* 1974;179:209–218.

41. Iwatsuki S, Mikkelsen WP, Redeker AG, Reynolds TB, Turrill FL. Clinical comparison of the end-to-side and side-to-side portacaval shunt: ten year follow-up. *Ann Surg* 1973;178:65–69.

42. Keighley MR, Ionescu MI, Wooler GH. Late results of elective and emergency portacaval anastomosis. *Ann J Surg* 1973;126:601–605.

43. Jackson FC, Perrin EB, Felix WR, Smith AG. A clinical investigation of the portacaval shunt. V: survival analysis of the therapeutic operation. *Ann Surg* 1971;174:672–701.

44. Resnick RH, Iber FL, Ishibara AM, Chalmers TC, Zimmerman H. A controlled study of therapeutic portacaval shunt. *Gastroenterology* 1974;67:843–857.

45. Reynolds TB, Donovan AJ, Mikkelsen WP, Redeker AG, Turrill FL, Weiner JM. Results of a 12-year randomized trial of portacaval shunt in patients with alcoholic liver disease and bleeding varices. *Gastroenterology* 1981; 80:1005–1011.

46. Rueff B, Prandi D, Degos F, et al. A controlled study of therapeutic portacaval shunt in alcoholic cirrhosis. *Lancet* 1976;1:655–659.

47. Pemberton J, Kiernan P. Surgery of the spleen. *Surg Clin North Am* 1945;25:880–890.

48. Del Guercio LR, Hodgson WJ, Morgan JC, Berman HL, Kinkhabwalla MN. Splenic artery and coronary vein occlusion for bleeding esophageal varices. *World J Surg* 1984;8:680–687.

49. Phemister DB, Humphreys EM. Gastro-esophageal resection and total gastrectomy in the treatment of bleeding varicose veins in Banti's syndrome. *Ann Surg* 1947; 126:397–410.

50. Sugiura M, Futagawa S. A new technique for treating esophageal varices. *J Thorac Cardiovasc Surg* 1973;66:677–685.

51. Sugiura M, Futagawa S. Results of six hundred thirty-six esophageal transections with parasophagogastric devascularization in the treatment of esophageal varices. *J Vasc Surg* 1984;1:254–260.

52. Barbot DJ, Rosato EF. Experience with the esophagogastric devascularization procedure. *Surgery* 1987;101:685–690.

53. Iwatsuki S, Starzl TE, Todo S, et al. Liver transplantation in the treatment of bleeding esophageal varices. *Surgery* 1988;104:697–705.

54. Brems JJ, Hiatt JR, Klein AS, et al. Effect of a prior portasystemic shunt on subsequent liver transplantation. *Ann Surg* 1989;209:51–56.

63

TIPS: Indications, Technique, and Results

Richard R. Saxon, M.D.[1]
Paul C. Lakin, M.D.

HISTORY

A transjugular, minimally invasive approach to decompressing the portal venous system was initially conceptualized and described by Rösch et al in 1969.[1] Through a series of animal experiments, they demonstrated the feasibility of creating a connection from the portal to the hepatic vein using a transjugular approach. The procedure was limited by available technology to maintain patency of the resultant parenchymal tract. Initially, tract patency was maintained with Silastic tubing connecting hepatic and portal veins.[2] Rapid advances in medical technology during the late 1970s and early 1980s, however, brought the transjugular intrahepatic portosystemic shunt (TIPS) from concept to clinical reality. The most important of these advances was the introduction of angioplasty balloon catheters and expandable metallic stents. Angioplasty balloons allowed creation of a shunt 8 to 10 mm in diameter, adequate to decompress the portal system.[3] Metallic endoprostheses provided a buttress for the tract through the liver, helping to maintain patency of the shunt.[4–6] Preliminary attempts to create TIPS in patients were carried out by Colapinto et al.[7] Prolonged balloon inflation was used to create a connection from the portal to the hepatic vein and only moderate success was achieved.

In 1989, Richter described the initial experience with TIPS creation in patients using a metallic stent.[8] Early TIPS were performed from both a transhepatic and a transjugular approach and were long, difficult procedures. The technique has undergone extensive improvement, application, and clinical evaluation. We estimate that well over 15,000 TIPS have been performed worldwide. Currently, most operators experienced in TIPS can perform the procedure in well under 1.5 hours. The purpose of this chapter is to describe the current indications for TIPS, outline techniques for performing the procedure in an expeditious fashion, and review the expected results.

INDICATIONS AND CONTRAINDICATIONS

TIPS for Variceal Bleeding

Not surprisingly, the first TIPS procedures performed clinically were accomplished in desperate situations. The patients had severe liver disease and massive variceal bleeding and were very poor candidates for surgical portosystemic decompression.[9–11] These cases demonstrated the technical safety of the TIPS procedure and documented its ability to relieve severe portal hypertension and treat variceal hemorrhage. The relative success of these initial attempts led to large clinical series that have established TIPS as a viable procedure in the care of patients with complications of portal hypertension.[12–17] The Food and Drug Administration has since approved use of the Wallstent endoprosthesis (Schneider, Minneapolis, MN) for TIPS creation. In addition, a diagnostic and therapeutic technology assessment committee of the American Medical Association (DATTA) recently evaluated the procedure. The committee, composed of medical, surgical, and interventional specialists with stated expertise in liver disease and varices, concluded that "TIPS is a promising or established procedure for treating both acute and chronic variceal bleeding and for portal decompression prior to liver transplant. The positive health outcomes are reduction in variceal bleeding and ascites."[18] Recommendations concerning the appropriate role of TIPS were also developed at a consensus conference sponsored by the National Digestive

Table 63-1.   TIPS: Indications and Contraindications

Accepted Indications
   Uncontrolled acute variceal bleeding despite medical and
      endoscopic intervention
   Recurrent variceal bleeding after endoscopic therapy
Probable Indications Requiring More Evaluation
   Refractory ascites
   Budd-Chiari syndrome
   Cirrhotic hydrothorax
Contraindications
   Absolute
      Severe hepatic failure
      Severe right heart failure
   Relative
      Hepatic neoplasm
      Polycystic liver disease
      Hepatic encephalopathy
      Portal vein thrombosis

Disease Advisory Board of the National Institutes of Health (ML Shiffman et al, presented February 1994).[19] The recommendations are listed in Table 63-1.

TIPS is most useful in the treatment of patients with uncontrolled acute variceal bleeding and in those with recurrent variceal bleeding refractory to conventional medical or endoscopic management (Fig. 63-1). Medications such as propranolol, vasopressin, and somatostatin are first-line therapies for both emergent and recurrent variceal bleeding in unstable patients.[20-22] Most patients should be initially treated with these medications and stabilized in an intensive care unit set-

ting. The addition of balloon tamponade in hemodynamically unstable patients can be helpful as a temporizing measure.[23] Unfortunately, the rapid development of rebleeding is extremely common when medical management and balloon tamponade are stopped. Endoscopic therapy (sclerotherapy or banding) has been demonstrated to be an efficacious means of treating both acute and recurrent bleeding from esophageal varices.[24-26] However, these therapies can fail to control both acute and recurrent variceal bleeding, which has led to the widespread application of TIPS. TIPS is also indicated in circumstances in which endoscopic therapy is not effective, such as in patients who are bleeding from gastric varices and ectopic intestinal or peristomal varices, and possibly in severe portal hypertensive gastropathy.[27,28]

The role of TIPS in relation to emergent and elective surgical portosystemic shunts remains to be clarified. Although Orloff et al have reported reasonable survival rates for patients with emergent portacaval shunt creation, most series suggest that surgical shunts in actively bleeding patients are associated with very high morbidity and mortality (≥50% 30-day mortality), particularly in Child's class C patients.[29-31] As the survival appears to be substantially better, it is our practice to perform TIPS prior to surgical shunts in all Child's class B and C patients. This is especially true in transplant candidates, as the indwelling TIPS does nothing to alter the extrahepatic vascular anatomy or interfere with the transplant procedure. In well-

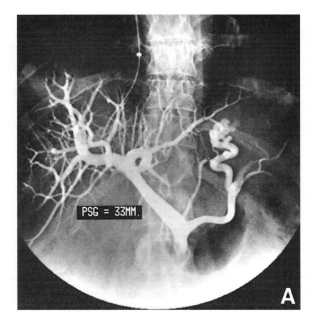
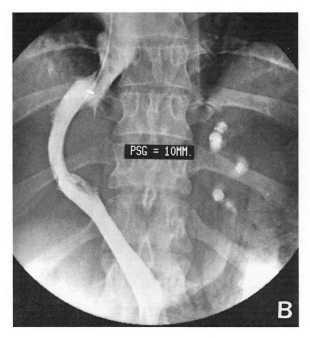

Figure 63-1.   Radiographs from a 45-year-old female with alcoholic cirrhosis who had uncontrollable bleeding from gastric varices. (A) The pre-TIPS portal venogram demonstrates gastric varices and a portosystemic gradient of 33 mm hg. (B) After TIPS placement, the portosystemic gradient has been reduced to 10 mm Hg and the varices have been eliminated by embolization.

compensated Child's A patients, a selective surgical shunt (such as a distal splenorenal shunt) should certainly be considered as a viable alternative to TIPS. At least for the time being, surgical shunts are associated with more durable primary patency.

TIPS for Ascites

TIPS has been used successfully to treat both intractable ascites and cirrhotic hydrothorax.[32,33] The use of TIPS in the treatment of refractory ascites remains controversial. Standard treatment includes multiple large-volume paracentesis or peritoneovenous shunting.[34,35] Initial series of patients with TIPS for variceal bleeding demonstrated a dramatic improvement in ascites after the procedure.[12,13] For example, 77% of our patients with clinically apparent ascites had a dramatic improvement by 3 months after TIPS.[36] This does not mean, however, that treating patients for intractable ascites who do not have variceal bleeding will lead to similarly positive results. Careful evaluation will have to be done to determine which patients are most likely to benefit from TIPS placement. We will discuss this further in the Results section.

Prophylactic TIPS Placement

Placing TIPS in patients awaiting liver transplantation as prophylaxis against bleeding or to improve the surgical outcome has been suggested. Although TIPS is extremely useful in controlling refractory esophageal variceal hemorrhage, initial reports suggesting that the decrease in portal hypertension after TIPS placement may facilitate surgery and minimize blood loss during transplantation have not been supported by subsequent investigations. The prophylactic preoperative performance of a TIPS procedure cannot be recommended.[37,38]

Contraindications

Although TIPS is relatively safe, with minimal procedure-related morbidity and mortality, several relative and absolute contraindications exist[19] (see Table 63–1). In patients with severe hepatic failure, hepatic function may be further compromised by any type of portosystemic shunt. The benefits of TIPS must be weighed against the potential for deterioration in hepatic synthetic function. Therefore, TIPS should not be considered in patients with severe, acute, or progressive hepatic failure except as a life-saving measure for severe, uncontrollable variceal hemorrhage. One is truly caught "between a rock and a hard place" when treating such patients.

In patients with elevated central venous pressure due to severe right-sided heart failure, TIPS may be of little benefit. TIPS successfully treats variceal hemorrhage by reducing portal pressure. Failure of TIPS to relieve variceal bleeding has been reported in patients with elevated central venous pressures.[39] More important, deaths have been reported after TIPS due to acute decompensation and right-sided heart failure. Therefore, known right-sided heart failure should be viewed as an absolute contraindication to TIPS placement.

Relative contraindications to TIPS include primary hepatic neoplasms, chronic hepatic encephalopathy, hepatic metastasis, and polycystic liver disease. One should carefully weigh the marginal benefit in some of these patients against the potential risk. For example, placing a TIPS through a liver with multiple large cysts might lead to severe hemorrhage into the cysts. On the other hand, Haskal et al have reported successfully treating variceal bleeding with a TIPS in a number of patients with known hepatomas.[40]

Patients with substantial chronic hepatic encephalopathy generally should not have a TIPS placed. Further diversion of blood flow from the portal system to the hepatic vein will likely cause worsening of the chronic encephalopathy. However, if the patient has relatively acute encephalopathy associated with variceal hemorrhage, then a TIPS may lead to improved mental status by decreasing hemorrhage into the gastrointestinal tract.[13,14,36]

Although portal vein thrombosis is considered a relative contraindication to TIPS, several authors have reported successful recanalization of portal vein thrombosis.[41,42] In patients with acute thrombosis, the thrombus can be lysed, stented, and/or displaced into the intrahepatic portal vein branches, allowing creation of an excellent shunt. On occasion, patients who would not have been transplant candidates prior to TIPS placement due to occlusion of the entire portal vein (Fig. 63–2) can have transplantation after such a shunt. TIPS can also be quite useful in the treatment of severe hepatic vein occlusion and Budd-Chiari syndrome.[43] The creation of a TIPS in a patient with extensive hepatic, portal, mesenteric, and splenic vein occlusion, although technically challenging, is also sometimes possible and can be a lifesaving procedure.

A distinction between relatively acute and chronic portal vein thrombosis has been made.[42] Chronic portal vein thrombosis significantly increases the difficulty of the procedure. Creating TIPS in patients with cavernous transformation of the portal vein is extremely difficult and can sometimes be impossible. Evaluation of patients with portal vein thrombosis prior to TIPS through a careful history, cross-sectional imaging,[44] arterial portography, and/or wedged hepatic venography is essential in an attempt to differentiate between acute and chronic portal vein occlusion.

PRE-PROCEDURE CONSIDERATIONS

It is imperative that the source of the bleeding be known with certainty before a TIPS procedure is undertaken. Therefore, endoscopy is performed prior to

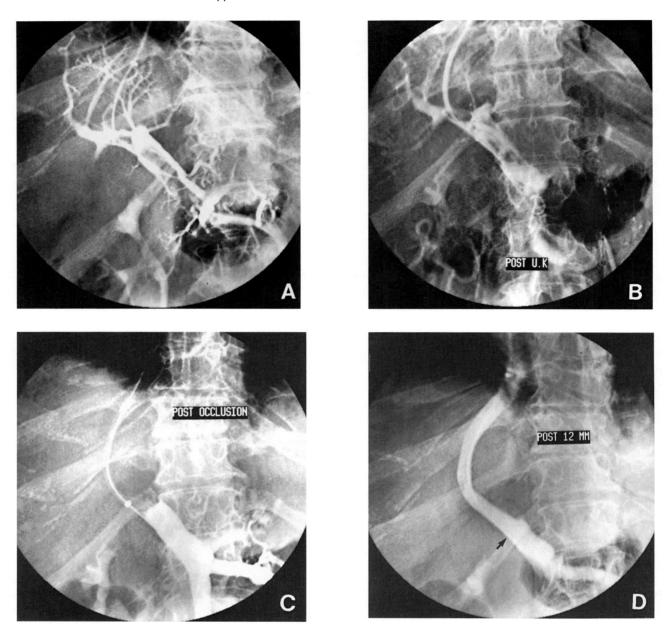

Figure 63–2.   Portal venograms form a 43-year-old male who underwent TIPS after failing sclerotheraphy for esophageal varices. (A) The initial portal venogram shows extensive portal vein thrombosis that was suspected on the basis of a preprocedure ultrasound scan. (B) After variceal embolization, 500,000 units of urokinase were administered using a pulse-spray technique. The venogram demonstrates moderate improvement in the appearance of the thrombus.
(C) Portal venogram obtained after a 11.5-mm occlusion balloon was used to ''sweep'' the residual thrombus out of the superior mesenteric vein and portal vein into the intrahepatic portal vein. This allowed TIPS creation in a standard fashion.
(D) The post-TIPS venogram demonstrates an excellent shunt using a 12-mm Wallstent. Note that the Wallstent ends high in the portal vein (arrow), allowing subsequent transplantation.

TIPS in all bleeding patients. Ultrasound evaluation is useful to document patency of the hepatic veins, portal vein, and hepatic artery. It can also help to exclude intrahepatic neoplasms and polycystic liver disease. In patients with isolated gastric varices, splenic vein patency should be established. If this cannot be done by ultrasound, portography utilizing a splenic artery injection can be performed. Isolated splenic vein

thrombosis can rarely lead to gastric variceal bleeding in the absence of portal hypertension. This is well treated by splenectomy.

Preprocedure clinical and laboratory evaluations include an assessment of the degree of encephalopathy, cardiovascular status, need for airway protection, or possible tube tamponade of actively bleeding varices. Bleeding patients should be stabilized in an intensive

Table 63–2. Modified Child's-Pugh Classification of Cirrhosis

Clinical Assessment	Score		
	1	2	3
Encephalopathy	None	Moderate	Severe
Ascites	None	Moderate	Severe
Bilirubin (mg/dL)	<2	2–3	>3
Albumin (g/dL)	≥3.5	2.8–3.4	<2.8
Prothrombin time	≤14	15–17	≥18

Note: Childs-Pugh scores are determined by adding the five scores and are related to Child's class in the following way: C ≥10, B = 7–9, A ≤6. This is in accordance with the recommendations of Dimagno EP, Zinmeister AR, Larson DE, et al. *Mayo Clin Proc* 1985;60(3):149–57.

care unit setting, with fluid resuscitation and blood products prior to TIPS. The Child's-Pugh score, a measure of the severity of liver disease, should be calculated (Table 63–2). Finally, laboratory values routinely obtained include the complete blood count, prothrombin time, partial thrombo-plastin time, creatinine, electrolytes, and liver functions studies. In patients with a platelet count below 50,000 or a prothrombin time over 18 seconds, we initiate appropriate platelet or fresh frozen plasma transfusion.

All patients at Oregon Health Sciences University (OHSU) are treated with a single prophylactic dose of intravenous broad-spectrum antibiotics such as Unasyn 1.5 g (Roerig, New York, NY). Both conscious sedation and general anesthesia have been advocated for TIPS creation. We believe that a TIPS can be performed with conscious sedation in most patients, although it requires careful patient monitoring and excellent assistance by a nurse with knowledge of the procedure. We continue to be concerned that general anesthesia in patients with severe liver disease may represent an unnecessary risk and expense. However, intubation and airway protection in unconscious patients with active

bleeding are certainly warranted, and uncooperative patients require general anesthesia.

TECHNIQUE

Many different approaches to TIPS creation have been described.[10–12] This section will concentrate on highlights of the techniques currently in use at the Dotter Interventional Institute at OHSU. The approach we use has been developed in treating more than 280 patients over the last 6 years, and a number of "tips on TIPS" have been developed that may prove useful to those new to the procedure. It is important to remember that performing a TIPS in a patient with difficult portal and hepatic venous anatomy can be quite a challenge to any interventional radiologist. Moreover, experience is quite important, as mortality has been shown to be lower at institutions where >150 TIPS have been performed when compared to institutions with less experience.[45] There is a long learning curve to this procedure.

A TIPS is best performed from a right internal jugular vein approach. Secondary access sites include the left internal jugular and large external jugular veins. TIPS creation from a femoral vein has been reported.[46] We have utilized the Rösch-Uchida portal access set (RUPS-100 Cook, Inc., Bloomington, IN) to create all but one of our TIPS.[47] A long No. 10 Fr. angiographic sheath with a side port and a radiopaque tip is first placed into the internal jugular vein. A No. 10 Fr. Teflon tapered catheter covering a blunt, long 14-gauge metal stiffening cannula (that comes with a preshaped 30° angulation) is introduced inside the No. 10 Fr. sheath (Fig. 63–3). Through this, a No. 5 Fr. catheter is placed, as well as a needle that locks to the back of the catheter. The No. 5 Fr. catheter and needle are used to puncture from the hepatic vein to the portal vein across the liver. This results in a relatively atrau-

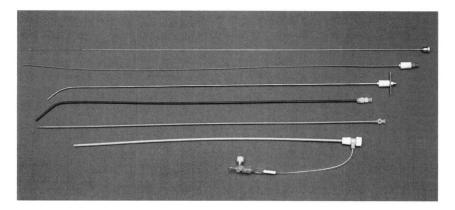

Figure 63–3. Components of the RUPS-100 portal venous access set. From the bottom of the photograph to the top, the set includes: a 41-cm-long No. 10 Fr. angiographic sheath with a side port and a radiopaque tip, a dilator that can be used to introduce the sheath, a No. 10 Fr. Teflon tapered catheter that fits through the No. 10 Fr. sheath and over a blunt, angled 51.5-cm-long, 14-gauge metal stiffening cannula, and a No. 5 Fr. catheter with a matched puncture needle. The needle is designed to protrude from the tip of the catheter when they are locked together.

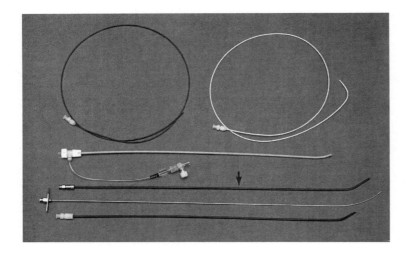

Figure 63–4. Components of the Ring Transjugular intrahepatic access set. The set includes two 80-cm-long angiographic catheters (one curved and one straight), a 38.5-cm No. 9 Fr. angiographic sheath with a side port and introducer, and a No. 9 Fr. Teflon 45.5-cm-long catheter (arrow) that covers the 16-gauge transjugular needle. Also included but not shown are two 0.035-inch, 190-cm-long guidewires: one 15-mm "J" and one Amplatz extra stiff.

matic puncture because of the pencil point tip of the sheathed needle when compared to the angular, cutting Colapinto needle.

The alternative access set most often used for TIPS in the United States is the Ring transjugular set, which uses a modified Colapinto transjugular biopsy needle (RTPS-100 Cook, Inc., Bloomington, IN).[13,48] This system (Fig. 63–4) is relatively simple to use. However, the puncture is made with the larger 16-gauge Colapinto needle. One advantage of this system is that the needle can be "steered" toward the expected position of the portal vein during its course through the liver. This may be helpful in very hard, cirrhotic livers.

The Richter-Angiomed catheter needle set (Angiomed, Karlsruhe, Germany) has achieved popularity in Europe and is similar to the RUPS transjugular set. The Cope-Ring portal vein access set (Cook, Inc., Bloomington, IN) utilizes an open 21-gauge needle for the portal vein puncture. Although we believe that both the Rösch-Uchida set and the Cope-Ring set are less traumatic systems than the Colapinto needle for puncturing the portal vein, no morbidity benefit has been demonstrated for the smaller portal vein access sets.[49]

The first step in TIPS creation is catheterizing an adequate hepatic vein. Care must be taken to determine which hepatic vein has been entered. Generally, the right hepatic vein is preferred unless the angle of origin off of the inferior vena cava (IVC) is too acute to accept the guiding cannula or Colapinto needle. The middle hepatic vein is usually the second choice. The right hepatic vein enters the IVC posteriorly, whereas the middle hepatic vein enters it anteriorly (Fig. 63–5A). On the frontal projection, both veins extend to the right of the spine (Fig. 63–5B). Therefore, it can be hard to determine which vein has been catheterized. If possible, it is important to determine which vein one is starting from, as the right portal vein lies anterior to the right hepatic vein and posterior to the middle hepatic vein (Fig. 63–5C). After the cannula has been advanced into the hepatic vein, the arrow on the back

of the Colapinto needle or RUPS-100 cannula is often a clue. For orientation, imagine that you are looking at this arrow from the head of the table. If the arrow points between 3:00 and 5:00 o'clock (posterior to the horizontal line), then the tip of the catheter is likely placed in the right hepatic vein. If it points between 1:00 and 3:00 o'clock (anterior to the horizontal line), it is likely in the middle hepatic vein. This simple-minded approach is a quick way to determine one's position relative to the goal: the central right portal vein.

Once the hepatic vein has been catheterized and evaluated, we turn our attention to localizing and puncturing the portal vein. As this remains the most difficult and potentially the most time-consuming part of the procedure, several different guidance methods have been advocated. These include real-time ultrasound guidance,[50] placement of a portal venous guidewire,[51] placement of a microcoil next to the portal vein percutaneously,[52] arterial portography, placement of a wire in the hepatic artery during the procedure,[53] and catheterizing the paraumbilical vein[54] (just to mention a few). We believe that these approaches tend to add needless time, complexity, and risk to the procedure without improving our ability to gain access to the portal vein. After some experience has been gained with the anatomy, knowing where the portal vein is located is usually much less of a problem then steering the needle along the appropriate path required to gain entry into the portal vein.

Wedged hepatic venography is the only technique we routinely use to evaluate and localize the portal vein during a TIPS. Wedged venography is an excellent technique due to its simplicity, speed, and accuracy. Although a No. 5 Fr. catheter or the No. 10 Fr. sheath of the RUPS-100 set can be advanced to a wedged position, better results are achieved if a 11.5-mm occlusion balloon (Boston Scientific, Watertown, MA) is used to temporarily obstruct flow in a moderately sized branch of the hepatic vein. Occlusion balloons may also help

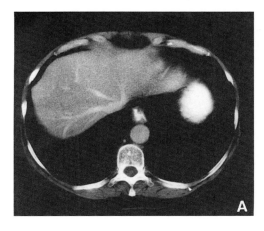

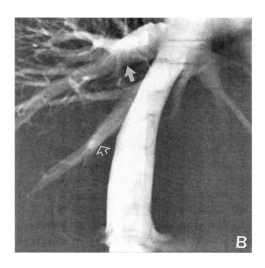

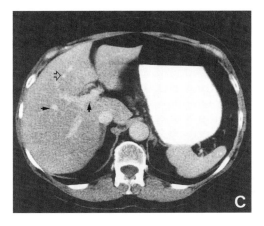

Figure 63–5. (A) Transverse image from a computed tomography (CT) scan at the confluence of the hepatic veins. Note that the right hepatic vein tends to arise posteriorly and the middle hepatic vein anteriorly, but both extend to the right of the spine.
(B) Radiograph from an inferior vena cavagram demonstrating reflux into the hepatic veins. Note that the course of both the right (arrow) and middle (open arrow) hepatic veins is almost identical on this frontal projection.
(C) Image from a CT scan demonstrating that the main right portal vein (arrow) lies anterior to the right hepatic vein (arrowhead) but posterior to the middle hepatic vein (open arrow).

to prevent capsular perforation and intraperitoneal bleeding, which have rarely been reported from wedging a small catheter into a peripheral vein branch.[55] Occlusion balloons are especially useful when CO_2 is used as the contrast for wedged venography. CO_2 tends to reflux around wedged catheters into the right atrium, and occlusion balloons seem to form a better seal with the wall of the hepatic vein.

Although we performed most of our TIPS using iodinated, liquid contrast material (5 cc/sec for a total of 25 cc) for wedged venography, we have recently found CO_2 (60 cc, rapidly hand injected) to be the contrast material of choice. First described for portal vein localization during TIPS by Rees et al,[56] CO_2 appears to traverse the hepatic sinusoids easily, often opacifying the entire portal venous system (Fig. 63–6). Rapid digital filming ($\geq$3f/sec) is essential. Using CO_2 and an occlusion balloon, we can opacify the intrahepatic portal vein in >85% of patients. Once the location of the portal vein is identified relative to bony landmarks, portal vein catheterization is often easily achieved, and other, more complex techniques for localizing the vein become unnecessary.

When puncturing the portal vein, we usually attempt to exit the hepatic vein in its proximal portion (within

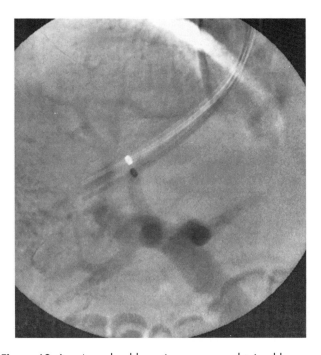

Figure 63–6. A wedged hepatic venogram obtained by injecting 50 cc of CO_2 through an 11.5-mm occlusion balloon that had been inflated in the right hepatic vein. Note that the entire portal vein has been opacified.

about 3 or 4 cm of the IVC). This helps to ensure that one is cephalad to the desired portal vein entry site. Using the RUPS-100 set, the guiding cannula covered by the Teflon catheter is rotated ventrally (counterclockwise) if one is in the right hepatic vein and advanced so that it is wedged against the wall of the hepatic vein (Fig. 63–7). The No. 5 Fr. catheter and puncture needle are then advanced with short, forceful thrusts in the direction of the right portal vein. Usually fewer than five passes with the needle through the liver are required to gain access to the portal vein. Entry into the vein is achieved by slowly withdrawing the No. 5 Fr. catheter while suction is applied with a contrast-filled syringe. When blood is aspirated, an injection is performed to confirm entry into a portal vein branch, and then a guidewire is advanced into either the superior mesenteric or splenic vein. The No. 5 Fr. catheter is subsequently advanced into the main portal vein. If there is any doubt about which vessel has been entered, a test injection can then be performed to confirm the position in the portal vein. Enlarged, replaced right hepatic arteries can masquerade as the portal vein when small injections of contrast material are made in intrahepatic branches prior to advancing a catheter into the main portal vein. Our only fatality that clearly resulted from a procedural complication at the time of TIPS placement was caused by inadvertent passage of the No. 10 Fr. catheter into the hepatic artery, which led to intraperitoneal bleeding, hepatic

artery embolization, and subsequent liver necrosis. Significant hepatic artery injury is an avoidable complication of TIPS.

Ideally, the portal vein is entered within 3 cm of the bifurcation. The more peripheral the puncture, the more curved the tract, which can make stent placement more difficult. Conversely, puncturing the main portal vein may result in an extrahepatic entry with minimal reinforcement from surrounding connective tissue.[57] A few severe bleeding complications have been reported secondary to portal vein rupture, which likely occurs when the extrahepatic portal vein has been punctured.[58] These access sites are better abandoned once recognized, if possible.

After portal vein catheterization, we predilate the parenchymal tract using a "Dottering" technique by advancing the No. 10 Fr. Teflon catheter over the wire through the portal vein wall (Fig. 63–8). Holding the metal cannula firmly in the same position that was used to puncture the portal vein facilitates this maneuver. Doing this can be extremely helpful in hard livers, in which it is sometimes difficult to advance the angioplasty balloon past the portal vein wall. Subsequently, all parts of the RUPS-100 set are removed except for a wire in the portal vein (we use a .035-inch, 180-cm Amplatz Super Stiff guidewire, Medi-Tech, Watertown, MA) and the No. 10 Fr. sheath. We then place a No. 5 Fr. pigtail catheter into the portal vein, obtaining a portal venogram and simultaneous pressure measurements

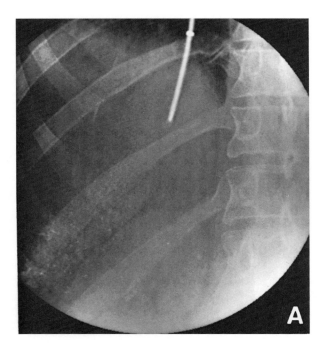
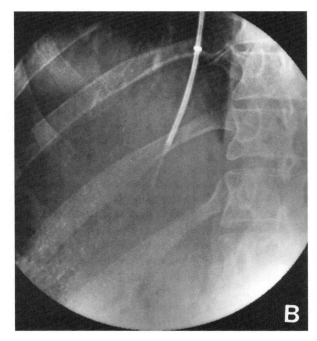

Figure 63–7.   (A) Radiograph demonstrating the position of the RUPS-100-covered No. 14 Fr. cannula prior to puncture of the portal vein. Note that the cannula has been rotated anteriorly and is forced against the hepatic vein wall, pointing at the location of desired portal vein entry.
(B) Radiograph after the puncture has been made through the expected position of the portal vein by the No. 5 Fr. catheter and needle. The needle has been removed, and the catheter is slowly withdrawn as suction is applied.

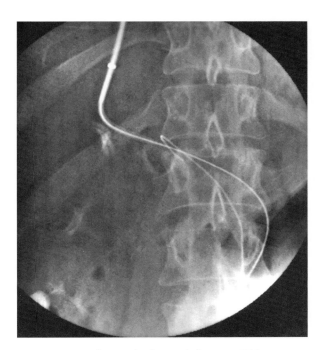

Figure 63–8. Radiograph obtained during a TIPS demonstrating the No. 10 Fr. Teflon catheter being advanced over a guidewire through the portal vein off of the metal cannula. This maneuver predilates the portal vein wall.

(from the pigtail in the portal vein and from the No. 10 Fr. sheath with its tip in the IVC).

The TIPS is created by first dilating the parenchymal tract with an angioplasty balloon. Although an argument can be made for starting with an 8-mm-diameter balloon, our patient population tends to have relatively severe portal hypertension, and we have elected to begin with a 10-mm-diameter balloon in all cases. It is helpful to obtain a digital spot film during inflation of the balloon. When the balloon is partially inflated, a waist is invariably present at the point where the balloon traverses the wall of the hepatic and portal veins (Fig. 63–9). Noting the location where this occurs relative to bony landmarks allows fairly accurate stent placement.

Many different stents have been utilized for TIPS. Most U.S. institutions, including our own, currently utilize the Wallstent (Schneider USA, Inc., Minneapolis, MN). Some institutions, especially in Europe, continue to utilize the Palmaz stent (Johnson & Johnson Co., Warren, NJ).[12] TIPS creation using the Strecker and Gianturco-Rösch Z-stent has also been described.[59,60] Wallstents are deployed such that at least 1.5 to 2 cm extend into both the hepatic and portal veins. This is due to some continued shortening and expansion of Wallstents after placement. We utilize medium-length (60- to 68-mm) stents only. The longer stents are difficult to place accurately and difficult to expand. Frequently, a second Wallstent needs to be deployed proximally or distally. It is important to remember that

stents extending too far into either the portal vein or the IVC can interfere with subsequent liver transplantation. If this occurs, stents can be shortened by overdilation and usually do not need to be removed. Migrated stents and stents extending into the right atrium can be removed using a Nitinol snare (Microvena, White Bear Lake, MN).[61,62]

A clear recommendation on whether to use 10- or 12-mm-diameter stents cannot be made based on available information. Although there was initial optimism that 12-mm stents would lead to improved primary patency by compensating for pseudointimal formation, this has not been proven. In fact, some investigators have reported a greater problem with stent shortening and acute thrombosis after TIPS creation using 12-mm stents.[63] We have not experienced substantial difficulty with compression or early occlusion of 12-mm stents. Consequently, we take what we believe to be a pragmatic approach when deciding which stent to use. If the patient has a markedly elevated portosystemic gradient (>30 mm Hg), hepatofugal flow, very large varices, and/or a large portal vein, we use a 12-mm stent. If not, we tend to use a 10-mm stent. One must weigh the advantages of adquate reduction of portal pressure against the possible risk of increased encephalopathy from excessive shunting.

Regardless of which size stent is used, we always dilate the stent with a 10-mm balloon first and then measure the portosystemic gradient. If utilized, a

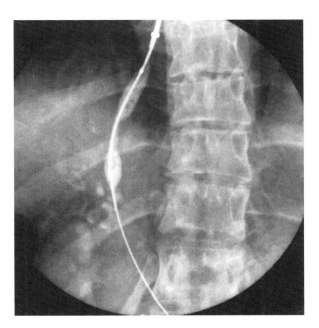

Figure 63–9. Radiograph obtained after partial inflation of a 10 mm × 6 cm long angioplasty balloon at the time of TIPS. The impression on the balloon made by the portal and hepatic veins serves as a very useful road map for subsequent stent placement. In this case, one could be relatively sure of creating an adequate shunt if the stent was centered on the 10th rib.

12-mm Wallstent can be further dilated as necessary to reduce portal pressure to ≤12 mm Hg. If 12-mm stents are not used in cases of severe portal hypertension with hepatofugal flow, then adequate portal decompression may not be obtained and a parallel TIPS may be required.[64] One can attempt to overdilate 10-mm stents with 12-mm balloons, but this can break parts of the stent, cause a great deal of shortening, and is not always successful. Through judicious use of 12-mm stents, we believe that this time-consuming and difficult task can be avoided. We have had to create a second, dual TIPS on only one occasion in order to obtain adequate portal decompression. On the other hand, 12-mm stents dilated to 10 mm have substantially less hoop strength compared to 10-mm stents, which may lead to collapse of the stent and early occlusion.[65]

No clear indication for variceal embolization at the time of TIPS placement has been determined. Some investigators have advocated variceal embolization based on variceal filling on the venogram after shunt creation.[13,66] We believe that variceal filling is heavily influenced by catheter position and injection rates. It is likely of little predictive value in deciding who will benefit from embolization. Consequently, in those patients who have bled in the 3 to 5 days preceding TIPS, we normally embolize visualized gastroesophageal varices at the time of the procedure, regardless of the post-TIPS venographic appearance.

In our first 55 patients, we did not embolize varices. It was our belief that patients with adequate portal decompression (<12 to 15 mm Hg) would stop bleeding. However, a number of patients who were actively bleeding continued to do so after TIPS. At follow-up venography their shunts were patent, with adequate portal decompression (≤12 mm Hg). All of these patients stopped bleeding after we embolized their varices. The reason for continued bleeding after "adequate" portal decompression remains unclear. It may be secondary to continued severe coagulopathy despite administration of blood products. In any event, we believe the pragmatic approach is to embolize varices at the time of TIPS in patients with acute or subacute bleeding. We tend to use a combination of embolic materials, including Gelfoam (Upjohn Co., Kalamazoo, MI), Sotradecol (Elkins-Sinn, Inc., Cherry Hill, NJ), and/or Gianturco coils (Cook, Inc., Bloomington, IN.).

Immediately after TIPS placement, repeat manometrics and a final portal venogram are obtained. One needs to be sure that the stents are appropriately positioned and that there is good flow through the shunt. Ideally, the portosystemic gradient should be ≤12 mm Hg. There is invariably a rise in central venous pressure following TIPS placement that is usually transient and is thought to be secondary to a rapid increase in venous return to the right side of the heart. Careful monitoring is necessary in patients with compromised cardiac status, possibly including Swan-Ganz catheter placement.

The procedure's duration is related to the learning curve. Once experience is gained, the procedure usually takes 30 to 90 minutes. Difficult portal vein anatomy including thrombosis, significant hepatic vein distortion from cirrhosis, and variceal embolization can lengthen the procedure substantially.

RESULTS

The short-term results of the TIPS procedure have been well documented in a number of large series, including one multicenter trial.[12,13,36,67] Technical success ranges from 93 to 100%, with procedure-related mortality of 1 to 3%. Immediate clinical success is achieved in 85 to 95% of patients. At OHSU, we had a 100% technical success in our first 100 patients, with one procedural death. The mean portal pressure was decreased from 34 to 21 mm Hg after TIPS, with a decrease in the portosystemic gradient from 24 mm Hg (range, 7 to 43 mm Hg) to 11 mm Hg (range, 0 to 22 mm Hg). The mean duration of the hospital stay was 3 days.

Complications

Morbidity and mortality associated with the TIPS procedure can be significant, although most poor clinical outcomes are dictated by the patient's underlying status and are not caused by complications occurring at the time of shunt placement. Thorough reviews of the complications of TIPS have been reported.[58,68] Procedural complications are usually self-limited and include intraperitoneal hemorrhage (1 to 6%), hemobilia (1 to 4%), sepsis, and transient renal failure. Stent migration during the procedure has been encountered occasionally, usually after placing a second stent to extend the shunt into the hepatic vein. By keeping the guidewire through the stent and running a loop snare over the wire, it can generally be removed.[62,69] In our first 100 patients, major complications within 30 days of the procedure occurred in 11 and included pulmonary edema in 4, hepatic artery injury in 2, sepsis in 2, portal vein thrombosis in 1, acute renal failure in 1, and hepatorenal syndrome in 1. These results are very similar to those of other large series.[12,13,36,67]

Survival

Cumulative survival at 30 days ranges from 97% to 85%. Survival after TIPS is directly related to the patient's status prior to TIPS. The majority of patients who die within 30 days of the procedure are critically ill and have a mean Acute Physiologic or Chronic Health Evaluation II (APACHE II) score of more than 18.[70] The majority are also Child's C cirrhotics with a Child's-

Pugh score of ≥12. Liver failure and multiorgan system failure are the most common causes of death within 30 days of TIPS.

Cumulative long-term survival after TIPS at OHSU is 85% at 30 days, 71% at 1 year, and 56% at 2 years. This is similar to the results of LaBerge et al, who reported a cumulative survival at 2 years of 75%, 55%, and 43% for Child's class A, B, and C patients, respectively.[14] Cumulative survival is directly related to Child's class.[67] At both OHSU and the University of California at San Francisco, cumulative survival is significantly worse for patients with Child's-Pugh scores ≥12. Eleven of 15 patients who died within 30 days of TIPS at OHSU were Child's C patients. The most common cause of death more than 30 days after TIPS remains hepatic failure.

Recurrent Bleeding

Recurrent upper gastrointestinal bleeding occurs in approximately 15 to 30% of patients. About one of out of every five bleeding episodes after TIPS, however, is secondary to something other than varices. Common causes include post-sclerotherapy ulcers, gastric ulcers, duodenal ulcers, and Mallory Weiss tears. Among our first 100 patients at OHSU, 20% rebled at a mean of 7.3 months after TIPS. Thirteen of these patients had an endoscopic evaluation. Nine of them bled from varices, while four bled from other causes. Despite poor primary TIPS patency (discussed below), only about 10% of the fatalities after TIPS are due to recurrent variceal bleeding.[12,13,36,67]

Encephalopathy

Hepatic encephalopathy is a frequent complication of severe cirrhosis that is exacerbated by the placement of any type of portosystemic shunt. Assessment of encephalopathy rates before and after TIPS is somewhat complicated by the fact that acute bleeding episodes can cause acute mental status alterations that resolve after the bleeding stops. In general, approximately 20 to 30% of patients develop new or worsening encephalopathy after TIPS, but about the same percentage experience an improvement in their encephalopathy. Usually, encephalopathy is well controlled by medical therapies, but in about 5% of patients it can be intractable and incapacitating.[71,72] Severe encephalopathy very rarely requires intentional shunt narrowing[73,74] or occlusion, which is most easily performed by inflating an occlusion balloon within the shunt and allowing it to thrombose over 12 to 24 hours.[75] The incidence and severity of encephalopathy after TIPS approximate those of selective surgical shunts (such as the distal splenorenal shunt) and appear to be far less than in nonselective portacaval shunts. This may be due to the relatively small caliber of a TIPS.

Ascites

All series on TIPS for variceal bleeding have demonstrated a dramatic improvement in ascites after the procedure.[12,13,36,67] Sahagun et al demonstrated marked clearing of ascites 3 months following TIPS placement in 36 patients.[76] Ochs et al reported similar results in 50 patients with refractory cirrhotic ascites, with total remission at 3 months in 74% of the patients.[33] However, patients with ascites are prone to liver failure after TIPS placement. In addition, when patients are specifically treated for refractory ascites, the mortality rate appears to be higher than when they are treated for variceal bleeding.[77] Among our patients treated for refractory ascites, alcoholics who continued to drink after TIPS had an extremely high mortality rate (80% at 1 month). Independent risk factors for death after TIPS placement included alcohol use, creatinine and total bilirubin. Other investigators have raised the concern that TIPS may not be an appropriate therapy for a subset of ascites patients with severe Child's C liver disease.[78] Currently, we believe that TIPS should be considered only for patients who are truly refractory to conventional therapy, are capable of abstaining from further alcohol consumption, and probably have adequate hepatic reserve to tolerate a portosystemic shunt.

TIPS Patency

Impaired long-term patency of TIPS has been reported in every series, with shunt stenosis or occlusion occurring in 17 to 50% of patients within 6 months of insertion and in 23 to 87% by 12 months.[12,13,14,67,79,80] We recently completed a thorough review of TIPS patency at OHSU.[81] The high incidence of stenosis has raised concerns about the long-term efficacy of TIPS.

Making clinical judgments based on TIPS patency data is a complex issue. The exact prevalence of TIPS malfunction reported varies widely, and is heavily dependent on the degree of surveillance and the definition of malfunction. Moreover, the situation is not analogous to older surgical series in which patients were not screened for patency. Often shunts were assumed to be patent unless the patient rebled. In many current series on TIPS, asymptomatic patients are screened with either ultrasound or venography, increasing the detection of early shunt stenosis. These high stenosis rates may be leading to a negative view of the long-term efficacy of the procedure that is unwarranted. For example, in our patients who have undergone angiographic evaluation, shunt stenosis or occlusion was present in 52% at 6 months, in 70% at 1 year, and in 83% at 2 years. However, 80% of our first 100 patients treated for variceal bleeding remained free of rebleeding at 1 year by Kaplan-Meier analysis. Therefore, a "shunt malfunction" does not necessarily portend a clinical failure. In our patient population, two out of three angiographically or ultrasound-detected stenoses have occurred in asymptomatic patients who may or may not have bled if their shunt malfunction was not detected and revised.

That being said, poor TIPS patency is still a significant problem that is responsible for over 80% of variceal rebleeding after TIPS. Three basic types of shunt malfunction are seen: (1) acute thrombosis within 30 days after TIPS placement, (2) exuberant pseudointimal hyperplasia within the parenchymal tract of the shunt through the liver, and (3) intimal hyperplasia within the outflow hepatic vein (Fig. 63–10). We have recently completed an evaluation of shunt patency in 113 patients who had follow-up venography after TIPS, as well as a histologic evaluation of both human and swine shunts, from which we were able to draw a number of interesting conclusions.[82,83] Both shunt thromboses and parenchymal tract stenoses are associated with underlying biliary fistulae in a majority of cases. Moreover, these two types of shunt malfunction account for over 75% of symptomatic shunt failures in our patient population, a third of which had documented fistulae between the shunt and the biliary tree. Whether there is an etiologic link—and the specific link, if there is one—between transection of a substantial bile duct and shunt stenosis or occlusion remain unclear. The proliferation of a metaplastic biliary epithelium along the lumen of these abnormal shunts has been observed histologically and may play a role through the secretion of mucin (a very thrombogenic substance).[83] Although hepatic vein stenoses were responsible for well over half of the shunt abnormalities seen (similarly to other reports on TIPS patency[63,79]), this type of stenosis was seldom responsible for recurrent variceal bleeding. The late onset of hepatic vein stenosis (generally somewhere between 3 months and 1 year after TIPS placement) may mean that these stenoses are detected and revised by shunt surveillance prior to the development of recurrent variceal bleeding.

The vast majority of shunt stenoses can be revised from a transjugular approach on an outpatient basis, leading to a relatively high secondary patency rate of (over 80%) in almost all series.[14,79,80,81] For this reason, we currently view TIPS as a multistage procedure requiring routine shunt surveillance with duplex ultrasonography and revision of stenotic or occluded shunts. A number of recent studies have confirmed the utility of duplex ultrasonography. In experienced hands, ultrasound is approximately 85% accurate for the detection of shunt stenosis and close to 100% accurate for the detection of occlusion.[84–87]

The fact that symptomatic shunt failures often occur in patients with early shunt thrombosis or stenosis associated with underlying biliary fistulae suggests the possibility that symptomatic TIPS failures may be well suited to treatment and/or prevention through the use of stent-grafts to create or revise TIPS. We have demonstrated improved TIPS patency using polytetrafluoroethylene (PTFE)-convered stent-grafts in a swine model.[88] Stent-grafts made of PTFE prevent transected

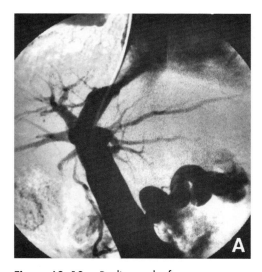 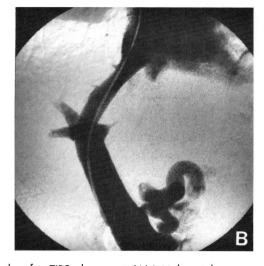

Figure 63–10. Radiographs from an asymptomatic patient 6 months after TIPS placement. (A) Initial portal venography demonstrates a >60% stenosis of the hepatic vein outflow. The portosystemic gradient was 18 mm Hg. (B) The stenosis did not respond well to angioplasty, and therefore an additional Wallstent was placed. The portosystemic gradient dropped to 9 mm Hg. Note that the top of the Wallstent extended to the junction of the IVC with the right atrium. Extending stents into the IVC and right atrium can be a major problem at transplantation. This patient was not a transplant candidate.

bile ducts from leaking into the lumen of the shunt, at least over the short term.

CONCLUSION

The difficulty of managing patients with severe variceal bleeding has fueled the rapid introduction and acceptance of the TIPS procedure as routine in the armamentarium of clinical medicine. Surgeons and gastroenterologists have accepted TIPS as having a vital role in the management of patients with the complications of severe cirrhosis and portal hypertension. However, as with any new medical procedure, it will take much more study to refine the procedure, improve the patency, improve the outcome, and determine appropriate indications.

The relative roles of TIPS and surgical portosystemic decompression will be determined only by further study. The mortality of surgical decompression appears to be more dependent than is TIPS on the patient's clinical status. For example, mortality rates for emergent portosystemic shunt surgery in actively bleeding Child's B and C cirrhotics range up to 90%. TIPS will likely have a survival benefit over surgery in the sickest patients with Child's B and C cirrhosis. On the other hand, the rebleeding rate in Child's A patients may be less over the long term for selective surgical shunts. A recent retrospective comparison demonstrated that TIPS placed in liver transplant candidates with variceal bleeding was associated with a somewhat more favorable outcome when compared with a previous distal splenorenal shunt.[89] Therefore, TIPS appears to be a preferable means of decompressing the portal system in symptomatic patients who are likely to progress to liver transplantation (perhaps even in Child's A patients). Multicenter, randomized trials are needed to decide the relative merits of surgical and percutaneous portal decompression.

Endoscopic therapy and TIPS for the prevention of recurrent variceal bleeding also require further comparison. Although not yet published, initial reports from ongoing randomized trials have all shown similar results.[90,91] TIPS has led to a significantly lower rebleeding rate than sclerotherapy, with both procedures having similar complication rates. No clear differences in mortality have been demonstrated. If these results prove true in large series comparing TIPS with sclerotherapy, then other factors (overall cost, quality of life) will have to be assessed to determine which procedure is most appropriate as the initial mode of therapy in patients with variceal bleeding. If patency is improved, TIPS may well become the most cost-effective and least invasive means of initially treating a large proportion of the patient population presenting with clinical manifestations of portal hypertension.

REFERENCES

1. Rösch J, Hanafee WN, Snow H. Transjugular portal venography and radiologic portacaval shunt. *Radiology* 1969;92:1112.
2. Rösch J, Hanafee W, Snow H, Barenfus M, Gray R. Transjugular intrahepatic portacaval shunt: an experimental study. *Am J Surg* 1971;121:588–592.
3. Burgener FA, Gutierrez OH. Nonsurgical production of intrahepatic portosystemic venous shunts in portal hypertension with the double lumen balloon catheter. *ROFO* 1979;130:686.
4. Palmaz JC, Sibbitt R, Reuter SR, et al. Expandable intrahepatic portacaval shunt stents: early experiences in the dog. *AJR* 1985;145:821.
5. Palmaz JC, Garcia F, Sibbitt RR, et al. Expandable intrahepatic portacaval shunt stents in dogs with chronic portal hypertension. *AJR* 1986;147:1251.
6. Rösch J, Uchida BT, Putnam JS, Buschman RW, Law RD, Hershey AL. Experimental intrahepatic portacaval anastomosis: use of expandable Gianturco stens. *Radiology* 1987; 162:481–485.
7. Colapinto RF, Stronell RD, Gildiner M, et al. Formation of intrahepatic portosystemic shunts with a balloon dilatation catheter. Preliminary clinical experience. *AJR* 1983;140:708.
8. Richter GM, Palmaz JC, Nöldge G, et al. Der transjugulare portosystemiche stent-shunt (TIPSS). *Radiologe* 1987;29:406.
9. Richter GM, Noeldge G, Palmaz JC, et al. Transjugular intrahepatic portacaval stent shunt: preliminary clinical results. *Radiology* 1990;174:1027–1030.
10. LaBerge JM, Ring EJ, Lake JR. Transjugular intrahepatic portosystemic shunts (TIPS): preliminary results in 25 patients. *J Vasc Surg* 1992;16:258–267.
11. Rösch J, Barton RE, Keller FS, Uchida B. Transjugular intrahepatic portosystemic shunt, *Prob Gen Surg* 1992; 9:502–512.
12. Rössie M, Haag K, Ochs A, et al. The transjugular intrahepatic portosystemic stent-shunt procedure for varicela bleeding. *N Engl J Med* 1994;330:165–171.
13. LaBerge JM, Ring EJ, Gordon RL, et al. Creation of transjugular intrahepatic portosystemic shunts with the Wallstent endoprosthesis: reuslts in 100 patients. *Radiology* 1993; 187:413–420.
14. LaBerge JM, Somberg KA, Lake JR, et al. Two year outcome following transjugular intrahepatic portosystemic shunt for varicela bleeding: results in 90 patients. *Gastroenterology* 1995;108:1143–1151.
15. Martin M, Zajko AB, Orons PD, et al. Transjugular intrahepatic portosystemic shunt in the management of variceal bleeding: indications and clinical results. *Surgery* 1993; 114:719–727.
16. Helton WS, Belshaw A, Althaus S, Park S, Coldwell D, Johansen K. Critical appraisal of the angiographic portacaval shunt (TIPS). *Am J Surg* 1993:165:566–571.
17. Zemel G. Katzen BT, Becker GJ, Benenanti JF, Sallee DS. Percutaneous transjugular portosystemic shunt. *JAMA* 1991; 226:390–393.
18. Miller-Catchpole R. Diagnostic and therapeutic technology assessment. Transjugular intrahepatic portosystemic shunt (TIPS) *JAMA* 1995;273(23):1824–1830.
19. Shiffman ML, Jeffers L, Hoofnagle JH, Traika TS. The role of transjugular intrahepatic portosystemic shutns (TIPS) for treatment of portal hypertension and its complications. Presented at the National Digestive Diseases Conference 1994.

20. Gimson AE, Westaby D, Hegarty J, et al. A randomized trial of vasopressin and vasopressin plus nitroglycerin in the control of acute variceal hemorrhage. *Hepatology* 1986;6:410–413.

21. Burroughs AK, McCormick PA, Hughes MD, et al. Randomized, double-blind, placebo controlled trial of somatostatin for variceal bleeding: emergency control and prevention of early variceal bleeding. *Gastroenterology* 1990;99:1388–1395.

22. Sanyal AJ, Purdum PP III, Luketic VA, Shiffman ML. Bleeding gastroesophageal varices. *Semin Liver Dis* 1993;13:328–342.

23. Panes J, Teres J, Bosch J, et al. Efficacy of balloon tamponade in treatment of bleeding gastric and esophageal varices: results in 151 consecutive episodes. *Dig Dis Sci* 1988;34:454–459.

24. Sorensen T, Andersen B, Backer O, et al. Sclerotherapy after first variceal hemorrhage in cirrhosis. *N Engl J Med* 1984;311:1594–1600.

25. Westaby D, Polson RJ, Gimson AES, Hayes PC, Haylian K, Williams RA. Controlled trial of oral propranolool as compared with injection scierotherapy for long-term management of variceal bleeding. *Hepatology* 1990; 11:353–339.

26. Fleig WE, Stange EF, Hunecke R, et al. Prevention of recurrent bleeding in cirrhosis with recent variceal hemorrhage: prospective randomized comparison of propranolol and sclerotherapy. *Hepatology* 1987;7:355–361.

27. Haskal ZJ, Scott M, Rubin RA, Cope C. Intestinal varices: treatment with the tranjugular intrahepatic portosystemic shunt. *Radiology* 1994;191:183–187.

28. Conn HO. Transjugular intrahepatic portal-systemic shunts: the state of the art. *Hepatology* 1993;17:148–157.

29. Orloff MJ, et al. Emergency portacaval shunts for bleeding varices. *J Am Coll Surg* 1995;180:257–272.

30. Villeneuve JP, Pomier-Layrargues G, Dugay L, et al. Emergency portacaval shunt for variceal hemorrhage: a prospective study. *Ann Surg* 1987;206:48–52.

31. Bomman PC, Terblanche J, Kahn D, et al. Limitation of multiple injection sclerotherapy sessions for acute variceal bleeding. *S Afr Med J* 1986;70:34–36.

32. Strauss RM, Martin LG, Kaufman SL, Boyer TD. Transjugular intrahepatic portal systemic shunt for the management of symptomatic cirrhotic hydrothorax. *Am J Gastroenterol* 1994;89:1520–1522.

33. Ochs A, Rössle M, Haag K, et al. The transjugular intrahepatic portosystemic stent-shunt procedure for refractory ascites. *N Engl J Med* 1995;332:1192–1197.

34. Gines P, Arroyo V, Vargas V, et al. Paracentesis with intravenous infusion of albumin as compared with peritoneovenous shunting in cirrhosis with refractory ascites. *N Engl J Med* 1991;325:829–835.

35. Smith HL, Triger DR. A randomized prospective trial comparing daily paracentesis and intravenous albumin with recirculation in diuretic refractory ascites. *Hepatology* 1990;10:191–197.

36. Sahagun G, Benner KG, Saxon RR, et al. Clinical outcome of 100 patients after transjugular intrahepatic portosystemic shunt (TIPS) for variceal hemorrhage. Submitted to *Am J Gastroenterol*.

37. Ring EJ, Lake JR, Roberts JP, et al. Using transjugular intrahepatic portosystemic shunts to control variceal bleeding before liver transplantation. *Ann Intern Med* 1992;116:304–309.

38. Somberg KA, NIDDK Liver Transplantation Database (LTD). Transjugular intrahepatic portosystemic shunts (TIPS) have a limited impact on the liver transplant operation *Gastroenterology* 1994;106:989A. Abstract.

39. Hudes BK, Sanyal AJ, Shiffman ML. Recurrent variceal hemorrhage despite a patient transjugular intrahepatic portosystemic shunt (TIPS). *Am J Gastroenterol* 1993;88:1615.

40. Haskal ZJ, Cope C, Shlansky-Goldberg RD, Baum RA, Pentecost MJ, Soulen MC. Three-year outcome in patients undergoing TIPS placement. *JVIR* 1996;7(S):152. Abstract.

41. Radosevich PM, Ring EJ, LaBerge JM, et al. Transjugular intrahepatic portosystemic shunts in patients with portal vein occlusion. *Radiology* 1993;186:523–527.

42. Blum U, Haag K, Rossie M, et al. Noncavernomatous portal vein thrombsis in hepatic cirrhosis: treatment with transjugular intrahepatic portosystemic shunt and local thrombolysis. *Radiology* 1995;195:153–157.

43. Peltzer MY, Ring EJ, LaBerge JM, Haskal ZJ. Radosevich PM, Gordon RL. Treatment of Budd-Chian syndrome with a transjugular intrahepatic portosystemic shunt. *J Vasc Intervent Radiol* 1993;4:263–267.

44. Parvey HR, Raval B, Sandler CM. Portal vein thrombosis: imaging findings. *AJR* 1994;162:77–81.

45. Barton RE, Rosch J, Saxon RR, Lakin PC, Petersen BD, Keller FS. TIPS: short- and long-term results: a survey of 1750 patients. *Semin Intervent Radiol* 1995;12:364–367.

46. LaBerge JM, Ring EJ, Gordon RL. Percutaneous intrahepatic portosystemic shunt from a femoral approach. *Radiology* 1991;181:679–681.

47. Rösch J, Uchida BT, Barton RE, Keller FS. Coaxial catheter-needle system for transjugular portal vein entrance. *JVIR* 1993;4:145–147.

48. Zemel G, Becker GJ, Bancroft JW, Benenati JF, Katzen BT. Technical advances in transjugular intrahepatic portosystemic shunts. *Radiogrpahics* 1992;12:615–622.

49. Haskal ZJ, Cope C, Shlansky-Goldberg RD, et al. Transjugular intrahepatic portosystemic shunt-related arterial injuries: prospective comparison of large- and small-gauge needle systems. *JVIR* 1995;6:911–915.

50. Longo JM, Bilbao JI, Rousseau HP, et al. Color Doppler US guidance in transjugular placement of intrahepatic portosystemic shunts. *Radiology* 1992;184:281–284.

51. Teitelbaum GP, Van Allan RJ, Reed RA, Hanks S, Katz MD. Portal venous branch targeting with a platinum-tipped wire to facilitate transjugular intrahepatic portosystemic shunt (TIPS) procedures. *Cardiovasc Intervent Radiol* 1993;16:198–200.

52. Harman JT, Reed JD, Kopecky KK, Harris VJ, Haggerty MF, Strzembosz AS. Localization of the portal vein for transjugular catheterization: percutaneous placement of a metallic marker with real-time US guidance. *JVIR* 1992;3:545–547.

53. Warner DL, Owens CA, Hibbeln JF, Ray CE Jr. Indirect localization of the portal vein during a transjugular intrahepatic portosystemic shunt procedure: placement of a radiopaque marker in the hepatic artery. *JVIR* 1995;6:87–90.

54. Wenz F, Nemcek AA, Tischier HA, Minor PL, Vogelzang RL. US-guided paraumbilical vein puncture: an adjunct to transjugular intrahepatic portosystemic shunt (TIPS) placement. *JVIR* 1992;3:549–551.

55. Semba CP, Saperstien L, Nyman U, Dake MD. Hepatic laceration from wedged venography performed before transjugular intrahepatic portosystemic shunt palcement.

56. Rees CR, Niblett RL, Lee SP, Diamond NG, Crippin JS. Use of carbon dioxide as a contrast medium for trans-

jugular intrahepatic portosystemic shunt procedures. *JVIR* 1994;5:383–386.

57. Schultz SR, LaBerge JM, Gordon RL, Warren RS. Anatomy of the portal vein bifurcation: intravenous extrahepatic location—implications for transjugular intrahepatic portosystemic shunts. *MVIR* 1994;5:457–459.

58. Freedman A, Sanyal A, et al. Complications of transjugular intrahepatic portosystemic shunts: a comprehensive review. *Semin Intevent Radiol* 1994;11:161–177.

59. Matsuzaka S, Kanazawa H, Kobayashi M, Kumazaki T. An experience of transjugular intrahepatic portosystemic shunt in the treatment of gastro-esophageal varices. *Jpn J Gastroenterol* 1994;91:257–266.

60. Echenagusia AJ, Camunez F, Simo G, et al. Variceal hemorrhage: efficacy of transjugular intrahepatic portosystemic shunts created with Strecker stents. *Radiology* 1994;192:235–240.

61. Sanchez R, Roberts A, Valji K, et al. Wallstent misplaced during transjugular intrahepatic portosystemic shunt: retrieval with a loop snare. *AJR* 1992;159:129–130.

62. Cekirge S, Foster R, Wiess J, et al. Percutaneous removal of an embolized Wallstent during a transjugular intrahepatic portosystemic shunt procedure. *JVIR* 1993;4:559–560.

63. Hausegger KA, Sternthal HM, Klein GE, Karaic R, Stauber R, Zenker G. Transjugular intrahepatic portosystemic shunt: angiographic follow-up and secondary interventions. *Radiology* 1994;191:177–181.

64. Haskal ZJ, Ring EJ, LaBerge JM, et al. Role of parallel transjugular intrahepatic portosystemic shunts in patients with persistent portal hypertension. *Radiology* 1992;185:813–817.

65. Kuhn-Fulton J, Terotola SO, Harris VJ, et al. Transjugular intrahepatic portosystemic shunt procedure: efficacy of 10 mm versus 12 mm Wallstents. *Radiology* 1996;199:658–644.

66. Kerlan RK, LaBerge JM, Gordon RL, Ring EJ. Transjugular intrahepatic portosystemic shunts: Current status. *AJR* 1995; 164:1059–1066.

67. Coldwell DM, Ring EJ, Rees CR, et al. Multicenter investigation of the role of transjugular intrahepatic portosystemic shunt in the management of portal hypertension. *Radiology* 1995;196:335–340.

68. Petersen BD, Saxon RR, Barton RE, Lakin PC. TIPS: management of major procedural complications. *Semin Intervent Radiol* 1995;12:335–363.

69. Cohen GS, Ball DS. Delayed Wallstent migration after a transjugular intrahepatic portosystemic shunt prcoedure: relocation with a loop snare. *MVIR* 1993;4:561–563.

70. Rubin RA, Haskal ZJ, OBrien CB, Cope C, Brass CA. Transjugular intrahepatic portosystemic shunting: decreased survival for patients with high APACHE II scores. *Am J Gastroenterol* 1995;90:556–563.

71. Sanyal AJ, Freedman AM, Shiffman ML, Purdum PP III, Luketic VA, Cheatham AK. Portosystemic encephalopathy after transjugular intrahepatic portosystemic shunt: results of a prospective controlled study. *Hepatology* 1994;20:46–55.

72. Somberg KA, Riegler JL, Doherly M, et al. Hepatic encephalopathy following transjugular intrahepatic portosystemic shunts (TIPS): incidence and risk factors. *Hepatology* 1992;16:122A. Abstract.

73. Hauenstein KH, Haag K, Ochs A, Langer M, Rossie M. The reducing stent: treatment for transjuglar intrahepatic portossytemic shunt-induced refractory heaptic encephalopathy and liver failure. *Radiology* 1995;194:175–179.

74. Haskal ZJ, Middlebrook MR. Creation of a stenotic stent to reduce flow through a transjugular intrahepatic portosystemic shunt. *JVIR* 1994;5:827–830.

75. Kerlan RK, Laberge JM, Baker EL, et al. Successful reversal of hepatic encephalopathy with intentional occlusion of transjugular intrahepatic portosystemic shunts. *JVIR* 1995;6:917–921.

76. Sahagun G, Benner KG, Barton RE, Keller FS, Rösch J. Encephalopathy, ascites, and hepatic synthetic function after TIPS for variceal hemorrhage. *Hepatology* 1992; 16:80A. Abstract.

77. Fillmore DJ, Miller FJ, Fox LF, Disario JA, Tietze CC. Transjugular intrahepatic portosystemic shunt: midterm clinical nad angiographic follow-up. *JVIR* 1996;7:255–261.

78. Ferral H, Bjarnason H, Wegryn SA, et al. Refractory ascites: early experience in treatment with transjugular intrahepatic portosystemic shunt. *Radiology* 1993;189:795–801.

79. Haskal ZJ, Pentecost MJ, Soulen MC, et al. Transjugular intrahepatic portosystemic shunt stenosis and revision: early and midterm results. *AJR* 1994;163:439–444.

80. Lind CD, Malisch TW, Chong WK, et al. Incidence of shunt occlusion or stenosis following transjugular intrahepatic portosystemic shunt placement. *Gastroenterology* 1994: 106;1277–1283.

81. Saxon RR, Barotn RE, Keller FS, Rosch J. Prevention, detection and treatment of TIPS stenosis and occlusion. *Semin Intervent Radiol* 1995;12:357–383.

82. Saxon RR, Benner KG, Barton RE, Rabkin J, Keller FS. TIPS: results of long-term venographic follow-up in symptomatic and asymptomatic patients. *JVIR* 1996;7(S):153. Abstract.

83. Saxon RR, Mendel-Hartvig J, Nishimine K, et al. Comparative histopathologic analysis of human and swine TIPS: evidence for bile duct injury as a major cause of TIPS stenosis and occlusion. *JVIR* in press.

84. Chong WK, Malisch TA, Mazer MJ, Lind CD, Worrell JA, Richards WO. Transjugular intrahepatic portosystemic shunt: US assessment with maximum flow velocity. *Radiology* 1993;189:789–793.

85. Dodd GD, Zajko AB, Orons PD, Martin MS, Eichner LS, Santaguida LA. Detection of transjugular intrahepatic portosystemic shunt dysfunction value of duplex Doppler sonography. *AJR* 1995;164:1119–1124.

86. Foshager MC, Ferral H, Finlay DE, Castaneda-Zuniga WR, Letourneau JG. Color Doppler sonography of transjugular intrahepatic portosystemic shunts (TIPS). *AJR* 1994;163:105–111.

87. Koslin DB, Mizutani PA. Noninvasive evaluation of TIPS. *Semin Intrvent Radiol* 1995;12:368–375.

88. Nishimine K, Saxon R, Kichikawa K, et al. Improved TIPS patency using PTFE covered stent-grafts: experiemtnal results in swine. *Radiology*, 1995;196:341–347.

89. Abouljoud MS, Levy MF, Rees CR, et al. A comparison of treatment with transjugular intrahepatic portosystemic shunt or distal splenorenal shunt in the management of variceal bleeding prior to liver transplantation. *Transplantation* 1995;59:226–229.

90. Maynar MA, Cabera J, Gorriz E, et al. TIPS versus sclerotherapy in elective treatment of variceal hemorrhage: a randomized controlled trial. *JVIR* 1996;7(S):152. Abstract.

91. Rossi P, Bezzi M, Capocaccia L, Riggio O, Ziparo V, Bolognese A. Transjugular portosystemic shunt versus endoscopic sclerotheraphy for the prevention of variceal bleeding: preliminary result of a randomized controlled trial. *RSNA* 1994;193(P):130.

64

The Non-Surgical Management of Patients with Budd-Chiari Syndrome

Anthony C. Venbrux, M.D.

Budd-Chiari syndrome is an infrequent but often fatal condition with a wide range of clinical presentations from acute hepatic failure to portal hypertension and chronic hepatic dysfunction. Previously, it was thought that the majority of patients who developed the Budd-Chiari syndrome had no predisposing illness; however, a greater understanding of predisposing factors, improved diagnostic imaging, and improved laboratory analysis have shown a lower incidence of idiopathic Budd-Chiari syndrome, ranging from 0 to 30%.[1–4]

ETIOLOGY AND CLINICAL PRESENTATION

The Budd-Chiari syndrome is a major cause of postsinusoidal portal hypertension. This condition, first described by Budd in 1845 and further characterized by Chiari in 1899, is a result of hepatic venous and/or inferior vena cava (IVC) outflow obstruction. The etiologies are multiple. Predisposing factors include the following:

1. hypercoagulable states and systemic illnesses (eg, polycythemia vera, paroxysmal nocturnal hemoglobinuria, idiopathic thrombocytopenia, systemic lupus erythematosus, juvenile rheumatoid arthritis, Behcet's disease, essential thrombocytosis, circulating lupus anticoagulant, myeloproliferative diseases).
2. Malignant obstruction due to neoplasms in the liver, adrenal glands, kidneys, and IVC.[5]
3. Trauma.
4. Infection. Recently, an unusually high incidence of positive hepatitis B surface antigen has been documented in patients who develop hepatic vein or retrohepatic IVC obstruction, suggesting that preexisting cirrhosis and hepatitis may be risk factors.[1,6–7]

5. Drug ingestion and/or conditions involving changes in hormonal levels (eg, oral contraceptive and estrogen use, pregnancy, and the postpartum state).
6. Progressive occlusion of veins of the liver. Veno-occlusive disease, the most infrequently reported etiology of Budd-Chiari syndrome, may be seen following ingestion of herbal teas containing pyrrolizidine alkaloids found in the species of *Heliotropium, Senecio, Crotolaria* and *Comfrey* leaves and roots.[8] Prior to allogenic bone marrow transplantation, veno-occlusive disease of the liver may occur in 20 to 50% of patients receiving both chemotherapy and radiation therapy.[9–12] In this subgroup of patients, the mortality rate can be as high as 53%.[13] Lastly, veno-occlusive disease of the liver with involvement of both large and small vessels may be seen in 3% of patients receiving the chemotherapeutic agent dacarbazine (DTIC).[14]
7. Anatomic causes including membranes or webs of the IVC or hepatic veins.

As listed above, associated conditions may predispose a patient to Budd-Chiari syndrome, a devastating condition in which, overall, approximately 50% of patients die within 2 years of the onset of symptoms.[15] Given that medical therapy alone has achieved poor success,[16,17] a multidisciplinary approach is required for managing patients with Budd-Chiari syndrome. To manage such patients, effectively, the radiologist is involved at multiple levels, from diagnostic imaging to interventions. Interventional procedures may be used to treat patients acutely at initial clinical presentation (eg, thrombolytic therapy) or at a later date, such as in the patient requiring angioplasty for a failing surgically created decompressive portosystemic shunt. Recently, interventional radiologists have become involved in the direct application of definitive endovascular therapy ranging from venous stent placement to the transjugular intrahepatic portosystemic shunt procedure.

CLINICAL PRESENTATION

Because the onset of Budd-Chiari syndrome may be gradual and the symptoms nonspecific, an accurate diagnosis is frequently not made. Abdominal pain, hepatomegaly, and ascites are characteristic. Rarely do patients present with hepatic failure and encephalopathy.[18]

More commonly, the initial presentation is characterized by normal or mildly elevated values of serum transaminases, alkaline phosphatase, bilirubin, and prothrombin time. Serum albumin may be decreased, due to both impaired hepatic synthesis and loss of protein into the ascites.[1,3,19] If unrecognized, progressive portal hypertension with clinical sequelae of esophageal variceal hemorrhage, coagulopathy, end-stage hepatic failure, encephalopathy, and death may result.[1,3,20] The syndrome may be misdiagnosed as cirrhosis with portal hypertension, hepatitis, or possibly congestive heart failure. Results of medical therapy alone are poor. In an article by McCarthy et al[21] describing the results of medical therapy alone, 14 patients were treated with diuretics, anticoagulants, and intensive supportive measures. Of these, 12 patients died. The mean survival was only 6 months. Similarly, Ahn et al[20] retrospectively reported results of 12 patients managed with medical therapy alone. Two years after diagnosis, there was only one survivor (9%). Thus surgical and interventional therapeutic options must also be considered to treat the sequelae of portal hypertension in patients with Budd-Chiari syndrome. Given the difficulty of making the diagnosis clinically, diagnostic imaging studies are essential.

DIAGNOSTIC IMAGING AND INTERVENTIONAL PROCEDURES

Noninvasive Imaging

It is essential that the diagnosis of Budd-Chiari syndrome be made promptly so that therapy may be instituted. Noninvasive imaging may assist in clarifying a confusing clinical picture. Diagnostic imaging studies include nuclear scintigraphy, ultrasonography, computed tomography, and magnetic resonance imaging.

The more invasive procedures performed by the radiologist will be discussed in greater detail later in this chapter.

Scintigraphy

The classic nuclear medicine finding of a caudate lobe "hot spot" occurs in only 17 to 63% of patients with Budd-Chiari syndrome.[22,23] This appearance on a nuclear medicine scan is believed to be due to independent venous drainage into the IVC from the caudate, which is typically spared from thrombotic occlusion even when the three main hepatic veins are involved.[3] Early in Budd-Chiari syndrome, the radionuclide liver scan may be normal or demonstrate only minimal hepatocyte dysfunction.[3] An enlarged liver with inhomogeneous uptake may be seen, with progressive right and left lobe congestion and an eventual decrease in hepatic function as the size and activity of the caudate lobe increase. A pattern of diffuse, symmetrically decreased uptake with increased splenic medullary uptake may be seen if the IVC is occluded. Such a pattern may be indistinguishable from that of cirrhosis.[3] The scan may also appear normal if multiple sets of accessory hepatic veins are present despite occlusion of all three main hepatic veins.[23]

Ultrasonography

Color flow and Doppler ultrasound (US) may assist in the diagnosis of Budd-Chiari syndrome. However, limitations include the inability to image through bowel gas, operator dependency, and difficulty in imaging structures if there is massive hepatomegaly due to the compression of vascular structures. The addition of color flow Doppler ultrasound may allow confirmation of hepatic vein flow based on the auditory signal even if direct hepatic vein visualization is not possible.[24] The advantage of US includes its noninvasive nature, multiplanar imaging capability, ready availability, and relatively low cost.[3] US also uses no ionizing radiation.

Computed Tomography

Computed tomography (CT) frequently demonstrates enlargement of the caudate lobe and lack of visualization of the hepatic veins. The IVC may be markedly narrowed in its intrahepatic portion (Fig. 64–1). Ascites is easily visualized, and on contrast-enhanced imaging, the liver generally has a patchy, inhomogeneous enhancement pattern, with the greatest intensity identified centrally and decreasing enhancement noted in the periphery. The inhomogeneous enhancement is thought to be due to slow flow from venous outflow obstruction and collateral circulation in the liver.[3]

Magnetic Resonance Imaging

Magnetic resonance imaging (MRI) may be extremely useful in making the diagnosis of Budd-Chiari syndrome. Simultaneous multiplanar imaging is advantageous. Not only is multiplanar anatomic information obtained, MRI has the ability to detect blood flow. MRI can depict inhomogeneous liver enhancement (particularly on T2-weighted images),[3] varices, ascites, hepatomegaly, and collateral blood flow. Park et al correlated MRI with vena cavography in nine patients with obstruction of the IVC.[25] They found that MRI accurately demonstrated membranous obstruction of the

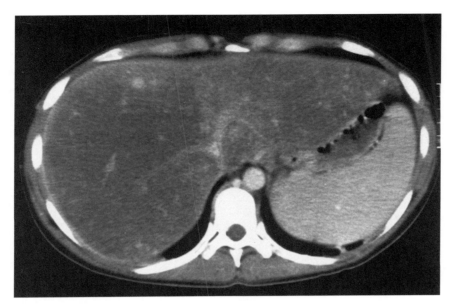

Figure 64–1. Intravenous contrast-enhanced axial CT scan in a patient with chronic Budd-Chiari syndrome. Note the inhomogeneous enhancement of the liver and the obliteration of the lumen of the IVC by the enlarged caudate lobe and swollen liver.

IVC. Stark et al[26] found that high-quality imaging is produced with a T1-weighted spin-echo sequence (TR/TE 260 milliseconds/18 milliseconds) which results in a reduction of respiratory, cardiac, and peristaltic motion artifacts. With obstruction of the IVC or hepatic vein, a small, thin, curvilinear soft tissue membrane may be visualized using T2-weighted spin-echo imaging (TR/TE 2000 milliseconds/60 to 150 milliseconds).[25] On T2-weighted images or even echo rephasing, thrombus typically stands out as high signal intensity against the low signal intensity background of flowing blood.[3,25] The hepatic veins may simply not be visualized, indicating thrombosis.[25,27] Such imaging is accomplished without ionizing radiation. Despite its advantages, MRI is not universally available and is costly.

The history, physical examination, laboratory analysis, and frequently noninvasive imaging studies suggest the diagnosis of Budd-Chiari syndrome. Confirmation of the diagnosis and hemodynamic evaluation are then obtained by the radiologist through invasive procedures.

ANGIOGRAPHY AND INTERVENTIONAL RADIOLOGY IN BUDD-CHIARI SYNDROME

Diagnostic Angiography and Hemodynamic Pressure Measurements

Celiac and superior mesenteric arteriography are generally nonspecific. Depending on the stage of the disease, the hepatic arterial branches on a selective celiac injection may be stretched due to the swollen liver, and the hepatic parenchymal staining may be inhomogeneous. The spleen is frequently enlarged, with progressive disease and advanced portal hypertension. Angiographically, hepatofugal flow and esophageal varices may also be identified.

Accurate evaluation of the patient with Budd-Chiari syndrome is derived from transvenous studies. Because percutaneous punctures are frequently accomplished from either a femoral or a jugular approach, inferior vena cavography and selective hepatic venography not only provide accurate anatomic definition but allow hemodynamic pressure measurements to be made to assist in planning subsequent interventional and/or surgical therapy.

Biplane vena cavography is generally performed. One classically sees a "steeple" or "pencil point" configuration of the intrahepatic IVC; the latter is considered to be due to compression by the swollen liver and the enlarged caudate lobe (Fig. 64–2A). Occasionally, one may identify thrombus in the IVC. Webs of the hepatic vein orifice or IVC may be missed unless the diagnostic catheter is placed directly adjacent to the web. Even then it may be difficult to image a web accurately on contrast venography. This is particularly true if blood flow in an obstructed IVC is reversed. Webs may be missed during routine cavography unless the catheter is advanced (eg, cephalad from a femoral approach) to a point directly inferior to the point of obstruction (Fig. 64–2B).

If a web is present, either at the hepatic vein orifice or at the IVC, and has not caused complete obstruction, a marked change in hemodynamic pressures is noted as the catheter is withdrawn across the lesion.

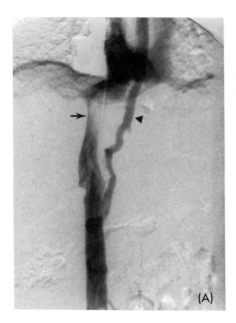

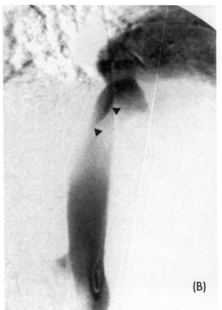

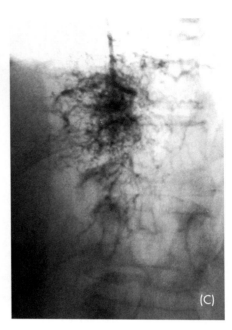

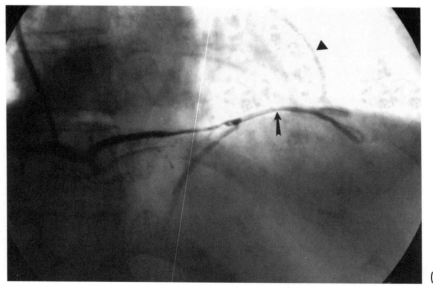

Figure 64-2. A 66-year-old female with progressive liver deterioration, ascites, abnormal liver function tests, and polycythemia. (A) Digital subtraction venogram in the frontal projection performed with a pigtail catheter placed through the right internal jugular vein. Note the narrowing of the IVC in its intrahepatic portion (arrow) with a large collateral vein (arrowhead). The narrowing of the IVC is believed to be due to the enlarged caudate lobe. (B) Digital subtraction inferior vena cavogram in the lateral projection, with the pigtail catheter withdrawn more cephalad. Contrast material is seen opacifying the IVC. A focal reduction in vena cava pressure was noted as the catheter was withdrawn across an oblique lucency (arrowhead). This lucency is believed to represent an IVC web. Mean IVC pressure at the level of L1 was 16 mm Hg; right atrial pressure was 2 mm Hg. (C) Selective catheterization of the "stump" of the junction of the middle and left hepatic veins. Note the "spider web" appearance, a classic finding in chronic Budd-Chiari syndrome. (D) Selective catheterization of the hepatic vein orifice, believed to represent the left hepatic vein. Irregular collateral veins are identified in this patient with chronic Budd-Chiari syndrome. As seen in this patient, unusual venous collaterals may be identified. Blood flows along the diaphragmatic surface (arrow) and courses along the epicardium (arrowhead). Angioplasty of the narrowed intrahepatic segment of the IVC web was performed with an 18-mm-diameter balloon. The mean pressure gradient between the IVC below the level of the liver and the right atrium changed by only 2 mm Hg after angioplasty of the narrowed intrahepatic IVC and web (not shown).

This technique is possible only with invasive procedures (eg, percutaneous puncture of the femoral or jugular vein, use of a diagnostic catheter connected to a pressure transducer).

The hepatic veins are selectively catheterized from either a superior (ie, jugular) or inferior (ie, femoral) approach. A diligent search for the hepatic veins must be made in patients with suspected Budd-Chiari syndrome. This is not always easy given the marked narrowing of the intrahepatic segment of the IVC and the occluded or narrowed hepatic veins. A number of techniques have been described for selective catheterization of the hepatic veins.

During selective catheterization of the hepatic veins in patients with suspected Budd-Chiari syndrome, one may occasionally identify thrombus on the hepatic venogram. However, one frequently sees a chronic picture of a "spider web" pattern of collateral veins and/or lymphatics, with absence of normal hepatic sinusoidal filling (Fig. 64–2C). Unusual collateral venous pathways may be identified (Fig. 64–2D). If a hepatic vein is found (not always possible), wedged and free hepatic vein pressure measurements are obtained and recorded. These provide baseline pressure measurements and allow calculation of the corrected sinusoidal pressure. A pullback pressure across the hepatic vein orifice is essential to determine whether or not a hemodynamically significant web exists. A sharp drop in pressure indicates an ostial web. Such patients may benefit from venous percutaneous transluminal angioplasty. If this fails, stenting may be used. It is important that IVC pressure measurements be obtained to determine whether a significant gradient exists between the IVC below the level of the liver and the right atrium. If excessive pressures are found in the infrahepatic portion of the IVC, a surgically created mesocaval shunt, although technically feasible, would generally not remain patent. A patient is not believed to be a candidate for a mesocaval shunt if the caval diameter is decreased more than 75% or there is a pressure gradient between the right atrium and intrahepatic IVC exceeding 20 mm Hg.[28] Other alternatives, such as a surgically created mesoatrial shunt or possibly a transjugular intrahepatic portosystemic shunt (TIPS), may be considered.

The corrected sinusoidal pressure is equal to the wedged hepatic vein pressure minus the IVC pressure. Normal corrected sinusoidal pressures are 0 to 5 mm Hg (0 to 7 cm of saline); mild portal hypertension, 6 to 10 mm Hg (8 to 13.6 cm of saline); moderate portal hypertension, 11 to 15 mm Hg (15.0 to 20.4 cm of saline); and severe portal hypertension, over 15 mm Hg (over 20.4 cm of saline). (1.36 cm of saline = 1 mm Hg).[29] In patients with Budd-Chiari syndrome, one should see abnormal corrected sinusoidal pressures because the obstruction is postsinusoidal.

A percutaneous transhepatic injection of contrast material into the liver through a skinny needle will demonstrate the classic "spider web" collateral venous pattern if hepatic veins cannot be selectively catheterized from the jugular or femoral approach.[30] This percutaneous procedure, however, carries an added risk in patients with coagulopathies and ascites due to advanced liver disease.

Occasionally, a transvenous biopsy of the liver may be performed by the radiologist, either from a transjugular approach using a Colapinto needle or from a femoral approach using flexible "clam-shell" biopsy forceps. Both techniques require protective sheaths to avoid damage to other mediastinal (jugular approach) or pelvic/abdominal (femoral approach) structures. However, transvenous hepatic biopsy assumes that selective catheterization of the hepatic veins will be successful. If these veins cannot be selectively catheterized, a transvenous biopsy via a central venous approach from either the jugular or femoral approach is not possible.

A percutaneous transhepatic biopsy may be the only alternative and is associated with a risk of bleeding complications. In such instances, needle tract embolization after biopsy has been advocated by some investigators.

THROMBOLYTIC THERAPY

If thrombus is identified during inferior vena cavography or selective hepatic venography, attempts to lyse it are warranted, using catheter-directed infusions of Urokinase similar to those used in arterial thrombolysis procedures. Occasionally, streptokinase may be used; however, most interventional radiologists prefer use of urokinase because the enzyme is of human renal cell origin and is less antigenic than Streptokinase. Streptokinase is derived from streptococcal bacteria. When diffuse, generalized hepatic venous thrombosis occurs (as opposed to IVC thrombosis), case reports suggest that systemic levels of thrombolytic therapy, rather than catheter directed, may be used given the extensive clot burden. In general, focal IVC thrombosis is treated with catheter-directed thrombolytic therapy.[3,31–33] Catheter-directed thrombolytic therapy may also be used occasionally to treat individual thrombosed hepatic veins.

PERCUTANEOUS TRANSLUMINAL ANGIOPLASTY

Segmental IVC stenosis or occlusion or hepatic vein orifice stenosis is currently treated with percutaneous transluminal angioplasty (PTA) rather than the invasive abdominal surgical procedures previously used to break up caval webs or segmental caval obstruction. PTA offers an initial high success rate with improved hemodynamics. One-year patency rates have been reported to be as high as 80 to 100%, but frequent repeat angioplasty is required due to restenosis.[34–36]

When angioplasty from the jugular or femoral approach is not technically feasible, a transhepatic approach may be used. This involves a percutaneous transhepatic puncture and may be risky in patients with coagulopathies. On completion of the percutaneous transhepatic interventional procedure, embolization of the tract with spring coils (Cook, Inc., Bloomington, IN) or Gelfoam (Upjohn, Kalamazoo, MN) is appropriate to reduce the risk of intraperitoneal bleeding. The author believes that angioplasty should be tried first. Should this fail, intravascular stents may then be considered. A more durable result may be a surgical mesocaval shunt, but this is not always possible due to the increased IVC pressures.

INTRAHEPATIC STENTS

A number of case reports have described the percutaneous application of stents to treat patients with Budd-Chiari syndrome. This procedure is particularly useful in patients who have failed angioplasty (Fig. 64–3). Restenosis, however, remains a problem in certain patients.

At the author's institution, self-expanding Z-stents have been used to maintain the patency of the IVC in two female patients with Budd-Chiari syndrome. Both patients underwent mesocaval shunt surgery, and IVC stents were placed percutaneously to maintain the patency of the surgically created portosystemic shunts. One patient developed IVC restenosis in the stented segment 10 months after placement and required multiple IVC balloon dilations until eventual hepatic dysfunction necessitated hepatic transplantation. The second patient eventually required orthotopic liver transplantation; however, no significant restenosis occurred in the IVC. In the second patient, IVC stents were placed as an alternative to mesoatrial stenting. At the time of transplantation, her intrahepatic IVC was widely patent.[37] In contrast, other authors have had excellent long-term patency results with the Gianturco Z-stents. Lopez et al[38] reported the successful treatment of a 26-year-old male with marked ascites, lower extremity edema, and preserved hepatic function in whom a self-expanding stainless steel Rosch-modified Gianturco Z-stent in the IVC and a hepatic vein served as a primary means of therapy. This patient remains com-

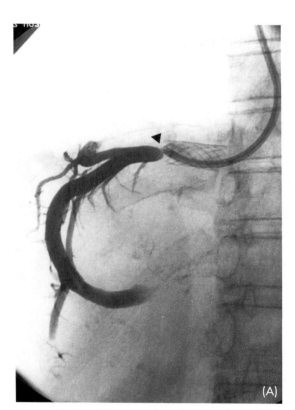

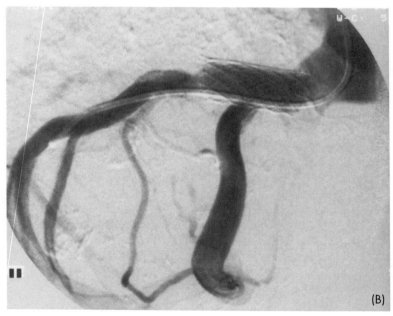

Figure 64–3. Selective catheterization of a right hepatic vein in a patient with polycythemia vera, Budd-Chiari syndrome, and a known hepatic vein ostial web. (A) Multiple PTA procedures were performed to maintain patency in this single remaining hepatic vein. PTA eventually failed, and a Palmaz stent (Johnson & Johnson Interventional Systems, Warren NJ) was deployed, with initial excellent results. However, stenosis at the end of the stent occurred (arrowhead), requiring repeat PTA. (B) Selective right hepatic venogram after PTA of the stenotic region. Although there is still moderate stenosis, hemodynamic improvement was noted during catheterization. Clinically, this resulted in elimination of ascites and improved liver function. (Case courtesy of Sally E. Mitchell, M.D., Gunnar B. Lund, M.D., and Floyd A., Osterman, Jr., M.D., The Johns Hopkins Hospital)

pletely asymptomatic at 40 months of follow-up after Z-stent placement in the IVC and hepatic vein. The author believes that maintaining patency of a hepatic vein is necessary if interventional techniques (eg, stenting) are to serve as the primary means of therapy. In the two female patients described above, no hepatic veins could be selectively catheterized due to advanced disease. However, other investigators have deployed stents to maintain hepatic vein patency.[38,39]

TRANSJUGULAR INTRAHEPATIC PORTOSYSTEMIC SHUNTS

In the patient treated with a transjugular intrahepatic portosystemic shunt (TIPS), as reported by Peltzer et al,[40] the procedure served as a "bridge" to transplantation. Similarly, in the author's institutional experience, TIPS has been used to treat three patients with Budd-Chiari syndrome (Fig. 64–4). Excellent clinical results have been achieved in two patients (one patient required multiple additional PTA and restenting procedures for TIPS shunt restenosis) and minimal if any benefit in the third patient. Thus, despite initial encouraging results, long-term shunt patency and survival rates using TIPS in patients with Budd-Chiari syndrome are unknown.

INTERVENTIONAL MANAGEMENT OF PATIENTS WITH BUDD-CHIARI SYNDROME WHO HAVE HAD PRIOR SURGERY

Secondary interventions in patients who have undergone prior surgical portosystemic shunt procedures (eg, mesocaval, mesoatrial) may be necessary to improve long-term patency. These interventions include PTA, stenting, and thrombolytic therapy and serve to re-establish normal shunt function.

Also to be included in the discussion of nonsurgical therapeutic options are those interventional procedures performed in patients who have had liver transplantation due to Budd-Chiari syndrome. Orthotopic liver transplantation is described as both a primary and a secondary treatment option for patients with Budd-Chiari syndrome, with 3-year survival rates ranging from 45 to 88%.[1,3,41–43] Portal vein stenosis at a surgical anastomosis in a liver transplant can occur in 0.6 to 6.5% of patients, and two-thirds of these patients may present with gastrointestinal hemorrhage from esophageal varices.[44,45] Thus portal vein angioplasty may be considered a nonsurgical therapeutic option in patients who are at risk for reoperation.

During percutaneous interventional procedures in patients who are hypercoagulable, it is advisable to achieve systemic anticoagulation with heparin during

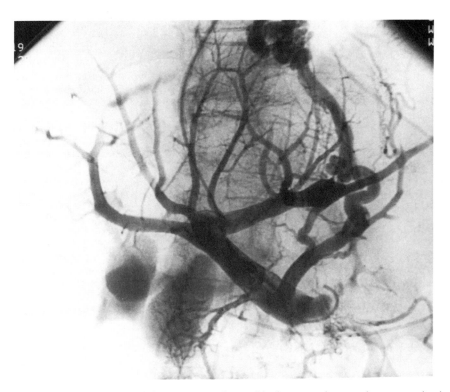

Figure 64–4. Direct portal venogram performed during a TIPS for Budd-Chiari syndrome. This patient had marked ascites. After the TIPS procedure, ascites disappeared. A small hepatic vein "stump" was found as the point of origin for the hepatic vein end of the TIPS shunt (not shown). Though TIPS is technically difficult, a limited number of patients have successfully undergone this procedure for Budd-Chiari syndrome.

interventions. In general, concomitant intravenous heparin therapy and follow-up warfarin therapy are used in patients who have Budd-Chiari syndrome due to a hypercoagulable state.

CONCLUSION

The multidisciplinary approach to the patient with Budd-Chiari syndrome requires a well-thought-out plan. The interventional radiologist provides the surgeon, gastroenterologist, and internal medicine specialist with therapeutic options including (1) diagnostic confirmation through imaging; (2) selective catheterization of the hepatic veins and IVC, with hemodynamic pressure measurements for baseline evaluation and for planning surgical/interventional treatment; (3) specific interventions including PTA, thrombolytic therapy, stenting, and TIPS; and (4) assistance in maintaining the patency of previously created surgical portosystemic shunts or in patients with problems associated with liver transplantation.[3,46] Prospective, randomized, multicenter trials are needed to establish the long-term efficacy of interventional procedures. Initial results suggest that percutaneous interventions provide an adjuvant therapeutic option and, in some cases, may serve as the primary means for treatment in patients with this complex and potentially lethal condition.

REFERENCES

1. Klein AS, Sitzmann JV, Coleman J, Herlong FH, Cameron JL. Current management of the Budd-Chiari syndrome. *Ann Surg* 1990;212(2):144–149.
2. Mitchell MC, Boitnett JK, Kaufman S, Cameron JL, Madrey WC. Budd-Chiari syndrome: etiology, diagnosis and management. *Medicine* 1982;61(4):199–218.
3. Klein AS, Cameron JL. Diagnosis and management of the Budd-Chiari syndrome. *Am J Surg* 1990;160:128–133.
4. Savader SJ, Venbrux AC, Kelin AS, Osterman FA. Percutaneous intervention in portosystemic shunts in Budd-Chiari syndrome. *JVIR* 1991;2:489–495.
5. Simson IW. Membranous obstruction of the inferior vena cava and hepatocellular carcinoma in South Africa. *Gastroenterology* 1982;82:171.
6. Lehmann H, Kaiserling E, Schlaak M. Left hepatic lobe artrophy and partial Budd-Chiari syndrome in a patient with alcoholic liver cirrhosis. *Hepatogastroenterology* 1982;29:3–5.
7. Cameron JL, Herlong F, Sanfey H. The Budd-Chiari syndrome: treatment by mesenteric systemic venous shunts. *Ann Surg* 1983;198:82:335–346.
8. Bach N, Thung SN, Schaffner F. Comfrey herb tea-induced hepatic veno-occlusive disease. *Am J Med* 1989;87:97–99.
9. McDonald GB, Hinds M, Fisher L, Schoch HG, Ballard B. Liver disease following cytoreductive therapy for marrow transplantation: risk factors, incidence, and outcome. Presented at the annual meeting of the American Association for the Study of Liver Diseases, Chicago, November 1991.
10. Hommeyer SC, Teefey SA, Jacobson AF, Higano CS, Bianco JA, Colacucio CJ. Veno-occlusive disease of the liver: prospective study of US evaluation. *Radiology* 1992;184:683–686.
11. Jones RJ, Lee KS, Beschorner WE. Veno-occlusive disease of the liver after allogeneic bone marrow transplantation. *Transplantation* 1987;44:778–783.
12. McDonald GB, Sharma P, Matthews DE, Shulman HM, Thomas ED. Veno-occlusive disease of the liver after bone marrow transplantation: diagnosis, incidence, and predisposing factors. *Hepatology* 1984;4:116–122.
13. Ganem G, Saint-Marc-Girardin MD, Kuentz M. Veno-occlusive disease of the liver after allogeneic bone marrow transplantation in man. *Int J Radiat Oncol Biol Phys* 1988;14:879–884.
14. Marsh JC. Hepatic vascular toxicity of dacarbazine (DTIC): not a rare complication. *Hepatology* 1989;9:790–792.
15. Ahn SS, Yellin A, Sheg FC, Colonna JO, Goldstein LI, Busuthl RW. Selective surgical therapy of the Budd-Chiari syndrome provides superior survivor rates than conservative medical management. *J Vasc Surg* 1987;5:20–36.
16. Lois JF, Hartzman S, Mcglade CT, et al. Budd-Chiari syndrome: treatment with percutaneous transhepatic recanalization and dilatation. *Radiology* 1989;170:791–793.
17. Sato M, Yamada R, Tsuji K, et al. Percutaneous transluminal angioplasty in segmental obstruction of the hepatic inferior vena cava: long-term results. *Cardiovascular Intervent Radiol* 1990;13:189–192.
18. Powell-Jackson PR, Ede RJ, Williams R. Budd-Chiari syndrome presenting as fulminant hepatic failure. *Gut* 1986;27:1101–1105.
19. Henderson JM, Warren WD, Millikan WJ Jr, et al. Surgical options, hematological evaluation, and pathologic changes in Budd-Chiari syndrome. *Am J Surg* 1990; 159:41–50.
20. Ahn SS, Yellin A, Sheng FC, Colonna JO, Goldstein LI, Busuttil RW. Selective surgical therapy of the Budd-Chiari syndrome provides superior rates than conservative medical management. *J Vasc Surg* 1987;5(1):28–37.
21. McCarthy PM, vonHeerden JA, Adson MA, Schaffer LW, Wisner RH. Budd-Chiari syndrome: medical and surgical management of thirty patients. *Arch Surg* 1985;120:657–662.
22. Powwell-Jackson PR, Karari J, Ede RJ, Hylton M. Ultrasound scanning and ^{99m}Tc sulphur colloid scintigraphy in diagnosis of Budd-Chiari syndrome. *Gut* 1986;27:803–809.
23. Picard M, Carrier L, Chartrand R, Franchebois, Picard D, Guimond J. Budd-Chiari syndrome: typical and atypical scintigraphic aspects. *J Nucl Med* 1987;28:803–809.
24. Grant EG, Percella R, Tessler FN, Lois J, Busuttil R. Budd-Chiari syndrome: the results of duplex and color Doppler imaging. *AJR* 1989;152:377–381.
25. Park JH, Han KJ, Choi BI, Han MC. Membranous obstruction of the inferior vena cava with Budd-Chiari syndrome: MR imaging findings. *JVIR* 1991;2:463–469.
26. Stark DD, Hahn PF, Trey C, Clouse MB, Ferrucci JT Jr. MRI of the Budd-Chiari syndrome. *AJR* 1986;146:1141–1148.
27. Friedman AC, Ramchandani P, Black M, Caroline DF, Radecki PD, Heeger P. Magnetic resonance imaging diagnosis of Budd-Chiari syndrome. *Gastroenterology* 1986;91:1289–1295.
28. Klein A. Budd-Chiari syndrome. In: Cameron JL, ed. *Current Surgical Therapy*, 5th ed. Baltimore: CV Mosby; 1995:323–331.
29. Kadir S. Pressure measurements and hemodynamics. In: *Diagnostic Angiography*. W.B. 377–444.

30. Reuter SR, Redman HC, Cho KJ. Cirrhosis and portal hypertension. In: *Gastrointestinal Angiography*. Philadelphia: WB Saunders; 1986:382–445.

31. Greenwood LH, Yrizarry JM, Hallett JW Jr, Scoville GS Jr. Urokinase treatment of Budd-Chiari syndrome. *AJR* 1983;141:1057–1059.

32. Cassel GA, Morley JE. Hepatic vein thrombosis treated with streptokinase. *S Afr Med J* 1974;48:2319–2320.

33. Sholar PW, Bell WR. Thrombolytic therapy for inferior vena cava thrombosis in paroxysmal nocturnal hemoglobinuria. *Ann Intern Med* 1985;103:539–541.

34. Martin LG, Henderson JM, Millikan WJ, Casarella WJ, Kaufman SL. Angioplasty for long-term treatment of patients with Budd-Chiari syndrome. *AJR* 1990;154:1007–1010.

35. Uflacker R, Francisconi CF, Rodriguez MP, Amaral NM. Percutaneous transluminal angioplasty of hepatic veins for treatment of Budd-Chiari syndrome. *Radiology* 1984;153:641–642.

36. Ida M, Arai K, Yoshikawa J, et al. Therapeutic hepatic vein angioplasty for Budd-Chiari syndrome. *Cardiovasc Intervent Radiol* 1986;9:187–190.

37. Venbrux AC, Mitchell SE, et al. Long-term results with the use of metallic stents in the inferior vena cava for treatment of Budd-Chiari syndrome. *JVIR* 1994;5:411–416.

38. Lopez RR Jr, Benner KG, Hall L, Rosch J, Pinson CW. Expandable venous stents for treatment of the Budd-Chiari syndrome. *Gastroenterology* 1991;100:1435–1441.

39. Walker HS, Rholl KS, Register TE, van Breda A. Percutaneous placement of a hepatic vein stent in the treatment of Budd-Chiari syndrome. *JVIR* 1990;1:23–27.

40. Peltzer MY, Ring EJ, LaBerge JM, Haskal ZJ, Radosevich PM, Gordon RL. Treatment of Budd-Chiari syndrome with a transjugular intrahepatic portosystemic shunt. *JVIR* 1993;4:263–267.

41. Campbell DA Jr, Rolles K, Jamieson N, et al. Hepatic transplantation with perioperative and long term anticoagulation as treatment for Budd-Chiari syndrome. *Surg Gynecol Obstet* 1988;166:511–518.

42. Halff G, Todo S, Tzakis AG, Gordon RD, Starzl TE. Liver Transplantation for the Budd-Chiari syndrome. *Ann Surg* 1990;211(1):43–49.

43. Scharschmidt BF. Human liver transplantation: analysis of data on 540 patients from four centers. *Hepatology* 1984;4:955–1015.

44. Wozney P, Zajko AB, Bron KM, Point S, Starzl TE. Vascular complications after liver transplantation: a 5-year experience. *AJR* 1986;147:657–663.

45. Scantlebury VP, Zajko AB, Esquivel CO, Marino IR, Starzl TE. Successful reconstruction of late portal vein stenosis after hepatic transplantation. *Arch Surg* 1989;124:503–505.

46. Savader SJ, Venbrux AC, Klein AS, Osterman FA Jr. Percutaneous intervention in portosystemic shunts in Budd-Chiari syndrome. *JVIR* 1991;2:489–495.

Section 6

Venous Disease

65

Venous Thromboembolic Disease: Clinical Presentation, Epidemiology, and Medical Management

John J. Bergan, M.D., FACS, FRCS (Hon.), Eng.
Niren Angle, M.D.

It is now widely accepted that the clinical diagnosis of venous thrombosis is nonspecific. Therefore, clinical decisions made on the basis of physical findings, without corroboration by objective testing, are potentially dangerous. A false-negative clinical evaluation of a patient with suspected thromboembolic disease may be rewarded with death of the patient. A false-positive diagnosis made on clinical grounds may unnecessarily submit the patient to long-term anticoagulant therapy and the consequences of being labeled as a thrombotic cripple. This impacts directly on his or her subsequent life in undergoing medical interventions such as surgery, pregnancy, and even contraception. Because of the importance of accurate diagnosis in venous thromboembolic disease and because treatment of this condition is constantly changing, these elements of clinical practice will be the subject of this chapter.

CLINICAL MANIFESTATIONS

In the introductory teaching of clinical diagnosis, venous thrombosis is described as a syndrome consisting of pain, warmth, and swelling of the lower extremity. Vast experience has emphasized these findings. Pain may be due to venous wall inflammation, perivascular inflammation, or distention of the vein itself, with stretching of pain receptors as well as pressure on pain receptors in adjacent tissues. Limb swelling may be due to inflammation of the vein or the perivenous tissues. In addition, venous outflow obstruction may contribute to an increase in limb girth. Swelling accompanied by warmth may be caused by release of vasoactive substances and shunting of blood from the muscular compartment of superficial veins through perforating veins rendered incompetent by the venous dilatation. Erythematous discoloration, when present in a limb with venous thromboembolic disease, may also be caused by vasoactive substances and diversion of venous blood from deep to superficial veins.

FORMS OF THROMBOSIS

Venous thrombosis may appear clinically in a variety of ways (Table 65–1). The presence of a palpable cord suggests superficial venous thrombosis, with a thrombosed vein or thickened vein wall being responsible for the physical finding. Perivenous inflammation may stimulate periarterial sympathetic nerve fibers, causing subsequent arterial spasm. This leads to pallor of the affected limb and the term *phlegmasia alba dolens* (white leg, milk leg).

In more advanced forms of venous thrombosis with occlusion approaching totality, cyanosis may be present in the most distal parts of the extremity. This is a stagnant anoxia caused by slowing of venous flow and desaturation of venous blood. As the venous thrombosis becomes more extensive and total venous obstruction is approached, massive swelling will develop due to proximal iliofemoral venous occlusion, fluid extravasation because of increased hydrostatic pressure, and the inflammatory response mentioned above. A mottled cyanosis will indicate sludging and cessation of flow, and bursting pain will be caused by increased compartmental pressure. As pressure is exerted on motor and sensory nerves, numbness, paresthesias, anesthesia, and motor weakness will supervene.

Table 65–1. Forms of Venous Thrombosis

Superficial thrombophlebitis	Palpable cord, erythema
Bland, deep venous thrombosis	Unilateral edema, local tenderness
Phlegmasia alba dolens	Weak pulses, pallor
Phlegmasia cerulea dolens	Cyanosis, marked edema
Venous gangrene	Marked edema, pain, gangrene

CLINICAL TESTING

When pressure is exerted on a thrombosed venous segment, pain may be increased. This leads to *Louvel's sign*, which is pain in the region of a venous thrombosis worsened by coughing or sneezing.[1] When pain is produced by upward compression of the gastrocnemius muscles again the posterior surface of the tibia, the pain is termed *Mose's sign*.[2] A particularly useful clinical sign is elicited by placing a sphygmomanometer cuff around the thigh and inflating the cuff above diastolic pressure. The pain produced is due to congestion at the site of venous thrombosis and is termed *Lowenberg sign*.[3] Pain in the region of venous thrombosis when the patient stands is a similar phenomenon.

Perhaps the most popular and best-known sign is *Homans' sign*. This is demonstrated by flexing the knee to 30 degrees and then suddenly dorsiflexing the foot at the ankle. A positive sign is discomfort elicited in the upper calf. It is well known that this is a very nonspecific sign and may be caused by a number of conditions, including superficial thrombophlebitis, a gastrocnemius muscle tear, a plantaris muscle tear, a ruptured Baker's cyst, and even a herniated lumbosacral disk.[4] Finally, the Peabody sign, which is indicative of calf muscle spasm, is elcited by placing the thumbs on the soles of the feet over the ends of the second metatarsal bones. Enough pressure is applied to elevate both feet to 20 inches. In affected individuals, spasm in calf muscles caused by the deep venous thrombosis supposedly prevents elevation of the affected leg.[2]

Important findings in a limb with deep venous thrombosis may be elicited by close inspection in addition to the palpation tests discussed above. Unilateral leg swelling at the ankle is a common manifestation of deep venous thrombosis. It may be pitting or not, and involves the calf and dorsum of the foot. The earliest finding is loss of the normal concavity in the retromalleolar area at the ankle. Such edema may be painless, and the location of the edema has no relationship to the segment of vein or veins involved. If documentation of the degree of limb enlargement is thought necessary, the circumference of the calf and ankle should be measured at the same distance from a reference point each day. The tibial tuberosity and the medial malleolus are useful reference points, and the circumference can be measured 10 cm below the tibial tuberosity and 10 cm above the medial malleolus. A difference of 1 cm between the two legs is considered significant.

The subjective and objective sensation of warmth in the involved extremity may be a prominent manifestation of deep venous thrombosis.[5] Clearly, the release of vasoactive amines and the increase in superficial venous flow may be responsible for the increase in skin temperature, but these are not specific. Such increased warmth may occur in association with conditions as widely divergent as cellulitis, arthritis, vasculitis, or any other inflammatory process. When rubor is present, such redness may be due to a variety of conditions, including a ruptured Baker's cyst. Nevertheless, this is a useful clinical sign because, in practice, it narrows the differential diagnosis to deep venous thrombosis, cellulitis, or a ruptured Baker's cyst.

Further inspection may reveal superficial venous dilation. This is probably caused by diversion of venous flow from the deep to the superficial venous system. Pretibial venous distention is characteristic of proximal venous thrombosis, and an increased pattern of superficial veins in the upper thigh and groin suggests iliofemoral venous thrombosis. The pretibial venous distention may be termed *Pratt's sign* to honor the New York surgeon who discovered its significance.

SPECIAL TERMS IN VENOUS THROMBOSIS

The term *phlegmasia alba dolens* has been referred to above. This condition is infrequently seen, possibly because it is caused by arterial spasm, a manifestation of iliofemoral venous thrombosis that occurs only in the first few hours after the development of venous thrombosis. This is manifested by reduction or absence of the arterial pulsations in femoral, popliteal, and ankle areas, as well as a decreased skin temperature of the foot and lower leg.

Phlegmasia cerulea dolens has been known by a number of terms, including *blue phlebitis, gangrene of venous origin,* and *acute massive venous occlusion*. Haimovici has named this condition *ischemic venous thrombosis,* but few have used that term.[6] His classification of this condition is useful. He has stressed that phlegmasia cerulea dolens is a reversible form of ischemic venous thrombosis and venous gangrene is that form in which the changes are, by definition, irreversible. The overall incidence of phlegmasia cerulea dolens in deep venous thrombosis ranges from 1 to 6%. However, the relation-

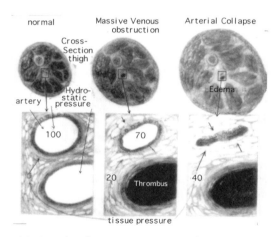

Figure 65–1. This diagram summarizes the progression of deep venous thrombosis from normal to venous gangrene. Arterial occlusion and collapse are caused by increased tissue pressure due to massive venous outflow occlusion. (Source: Ref. 7.)

ship of phlegmasia cerulea dolens to venous gangrene is dramatically different. Venous gangrene may occur in 65 to 90% of cases of phlegmasia cerulea dolens.

Initial explanations of phlegmasia cerulea dolens stated that the ischemia was due to arterial spasm. However, experimental work by Vasko showed that the acknowledged arterial insufficiency in phlegmasia cerulea dolens was due to mechanical venous blockage and not vasospasm (Fig. 65–1). Using a canine hind limb model, Vasko and his collaborators obliterated venous outflow by a combination of ligation and infusion of barium sulfate. While this was being accomplished, arterial pressure and blood flow were measured; the reduction of arterial flow was clearly seen to be a secondary phenomenon. An early change was collapse of small ramifications of the arterial tree caused by critical closing pressure being exceeded by the pressure of surrounding tissue.[7] Others have measured muscular compartment pressure in humans and have confirmed the theory advanced by Vasko. Eklöf's group confirmed that wick catheter measurements of compartment pressure exceeded 50 mm Hg.[8]

Phlegmasia cerulea dolens frequently involves more than one extremity, and occurs in association with malignancy in 50 to 100% of cases and in Trosseau's syndrome. The associated tumors include carcinoma of the lung, stomach, gallbladder, biliary tree, pancreas, and urinary bladder.

SUMMARY: CLINICAL MANIFESTATIONS OF DEEP VENOUS THROMBOSIS

This review of the clinical signs and symptoms of deep venous thrombosis suggests accuracy of diagnosis that is actually erroneous. Unfortunately, as shown in Table 65.2, the clinical diagnosis of deep venous thrombosis

has both low specificity and low sensitivity. Clearly, the only two venous thromboembolic conditions that can be diagnosed reliably on clinical grounds are superficial thrombophlebitis and phlegmasia cerulea dolens.

EPIDEMIOLOGY OF VENOUS THROMBOEMBOLIC DISEASE

It is recognized that venous thromboembolic disease is an important cause of morbidity as well as mortality in hospitalized patients. Epidemiology of the condition must refer to two elements. The first is how frequently venous thrombosis and pulmonary embolization are recognized in hospitalized versus outpatient populations. The second factor is the clinical situations that predispose to such venous thromboembolic disease.

The Malmö group has published an extensive autopsy-verified study of venous thromboembolic disease over a 30-year period. This excellent study serves as a summary of other, less complete observations. In Malmö, a continuing high frequency of pulmonary embolism observed at autopsy was documented during the entire 30-year period of study. Pulmonary embolism was associated with 20.3% of deaths and 31.7% of autopsies. Of the 391 pulmonary embolism cases verified at autopsy between 1981 and 1988, the pulmonary embolism was considered to be the actual cause of death in 28.9% of patients. In an additional 26.6%, the pulmonary thromboembolism contributed to death, and in 44.5% the emboli found at autopsy were thought to be incidental. The overall frequency of major pulmonary embolism in surgical patients was stable at 0.3%. When a longitudinal comparison was made, the frequency of major postoperative pulmonary embolism increased throughout the 1950s and 1960s but decreased in the second half of the 1970s. This decrease continued throughout the 1980s. The maximum observed incidence was 0.4% and the minimum, reached in the late 1980s, was 0.2% ($p < 0.05$).[10]

An American study involving 16 short-stay hospitals in metropolitan Worcester, MA was performed by Wheeler's group,[11] encompassing the period between

Table 65–2. Clinical Diagnosis of Deep Venous Thrombosis

Conditions	Sensitivity	Specificity
Calf pain	66–91%	3–19%
Calf tenderness	56–82%	26–74%
Ankle edema	40–76%	23–52%
Leg swelling	35–97%	8–88%
Redness	15–26%	90–91%
Superficial venous distention	27–33%	30–91%
Homans' sign	13–43%	39–84%

Source: Modified from Ref. 2, Table 13-2.

July 1, 1985, to December 31, 1986. The average annual incidence of deep vein thrombosis was 48 per 100,000, and the incidence of pulmonary embolism, with or without diagnosed deep venous thrombosis, was 23 per 100,000. The in-hospital case fatality rate due to venous thromboembolism was 12%.

More recently, the incidence of postoperative pulmonary embolism in the general surgical department of the Bispebjerg Hospital in Copenhagen has been reported.[12] The incidence of postoperative pulmonary embolism was found to be 0.6% ± 0.2%. The incidence of fatal pulmonary embolism was 0.4% ± 0.1%, and fatal pulmonary embolism was found in 8.6% of patients in whom an autopsy was performed.

CLINICAL RISK FACTORS

The factors that influence the clinical decision to employ deep venous thrombosis prophylaxis range from crucial, as in patients with a previously diagnosed hypercoagulability state, to controversial, such as ethnicity or varicose veins.

While the blood group type may or may not be important in the development of deep venous thrombosis, there is no question that hypercoagulability provides a very strong risk. Studies have shown a predominance of blood group A and a deficit of blood group O in patients with thromboembolic disease.[13] While a majority of reports suggests this conclusion, Nicolaides' prospective study has challenged it.[14]

The various coagulopathies considered important are discussed elsewhere in this volume. These include resistance to activated protein C, anticardiolipin antibody, protein C deficiency, protein S deficiency, antithrombin III deficiency, congenital plasminogen deficiency, and dysplasminogenemia. Reduced fibrinolytic activity has been implicated, as has a deficiency in heparin cofactor II. Patients with known coagulopathy are at high risk for recurrent thromboembolic disease, and serious consideration must be given to prolonged or lifetime treatment with anticoagulants.

Among the strongest risk factors for the development of venous thromboembolic disease is a history of previous venous thrombosis or pulmonary embolization.[15] In taking this aspect of a patient's history, the method of documentation of the deep venous thrombosis must be recorded. A clinical diagnosis alone is unacceptable, whether or not the patient has been treated with anticoagulant therapy.

Other clinical risk factors are also relevant. Several studies support the association of increasing age with an increased incidence of venous thromboembolic disease. Evidence regarding obesity is conflicting. Immobilization is important historically, as it is part of Virchow's triad. Surgical intervention, especially for malignancy, is another important risk factor.

MEDICAL TREATMENT OF VENOUS THROMBOEMBOLIC DISEASE

If the diagnosis of venous thromboembolic disease is definite, treatment includes immediate anticoagulation with heparin and longer-term anticoagulation with an oral anticoagulant such as coumadin.

Only about one-third of heparin binds to antithrombin III, and this is responsible for most of its anticoagulant effect. The remaining two-thirds has minimal anticoagulant activity at therapeutic concentrations. The two preferred routes of heparin administration are continuous intravenous infusion and subcutaneous injection. If the subcutaneous route is selected, the initial dose must be high enough to compensate for the reduced bioavailability.[16] In administering the continuous intravenous dose, a bolus of 5000 units is given for immediate effect, and the average maintenance dose of 32,000 units per 24 hours is generally accepted.[17,18] Habitually, many physicians order 1000 units per hour until the monitoring values of activated partial thromboplastin time are received, and then the dose is adjusted. If the subcutaneous route is utilized, a bolus dose of 5000 units is given, and an average maintenance dose of 35,000 units per 24 hours has been found to be effective.[19]

Audits have shown that heparin is frequently given inadequately. A standard protocol, empirically based, should be utilized in writing orders. For example, if the activated partial thromboplastin time is less than 60 seconds, the dose should be increased, and if the monitoring time is more that 85 seconds, the dose should be decreased. The amount of change ordered will depend on the concentration of heparin in the intravenous solution.

The time-honored approach used frequently in the past was a 7- to 10-day course of heparin, with a 4- to 5-day overlap period with oral anticoagulants. This, fortunately, has been vigorously challenged. Two randomized studies in patients with proximal vein thrombosis showed that a short course of 4- to 5-day intravenous heparin was effective.[20,21] This is appealing both from a time and an economic viewpoint.

EARLY TREATMENT WITH FRACTIONATED HEPARIN

Since 1986, a number of reports have documented the efficacy of low molecular weight heparin in the treatment of established venous thromboembolic disease. These supplement studies comparing the prophylaxis of thromboembolism with unfractionated and fractionated heparin. Studies that document the efficacy of low molecular weight heparin suggest that many patients with venous thrombosis may be treated in the future on an outpatient basis.[22–25] A single daily injection, with no need for anticoagulant monitoring, has great appeal.[26] Outpatient therapy of deep venous thrombosis allows early mobilization of the patient, a quick return to physical activity and occupation, and an increased feeling of well-being.[27]

Because long-term anticoagulation is necessary to effectively treat venous thromboembolic disease, oral anticoagulants must be used. Warfarin is the most widely used oral anticoagulant in North America because its onset and duration of action are predictable and because it has excellent bioavailability.[28] Now the prothrombin time has been standardized.[29–31] The calibration system, known as the *International Normalized Ratio (INR)*, has been in increasing use since it was adopted by the World Health Organization in 1982. In general, the optimal therapeutic range for laboratory evaluation of oral anticoagulant therapy has been modified downward based on the results of randomized studies. Current guidelines were proposed by an advisory group to the American College of Chest Physicians in late 1989.[32]

Two levels of intensity of anticoagulant therapy have been recommended. A less intense range corresponds to an INR of 2.0 to 3.0, and a more intense range corresponds to an INR of 2.5 to 3.5. The lower range is used for prophylaxis of venous thrombosis and in the treatment of established venous thrombosis and/or pulmonary embolism. The higher INR has been advocated in high-risk patients such as those with mechanical prosthetic valves. Studies have shown that the less intense regimen of INR (2.0 to 3.0) is safer and as effective as a higher-intensity regimen.

A study of physician practices in the management of venous thromboembolism has been conducted by the Worcester group.[33] In their survey of 16 short-stay hospitals, they found that 97% of 1231 clinically recognized cases of venous thromboembolism were treated with intravenous heparin. This was given as a mean bolus of 6674 IU for a mean duration of 6.6 days. The modern therapy of overlapping oral anticoagulant doses earlier was followed, and a mean delay of 2.3 days in starting warfarin was revealed by this survey. This resulted in a decreased hospital stay and appreciable cost savings. However, a recognized in-house recurrence of venous thromboembolism during treatment was found in 2% of patients.

THROMBOLYTIC THERAPY FOR VENOUS THROMBOEMBOLIC DISEASE

Thrombolytic agents dissolve thrombi by activating plasminogen to plasmin. Steptokinase, urokinase, and tissue plasminogen activator (tPA) are the three thrombolytic agents currently available for clinical use. Neither streptokinase nor urokinase is specific for thrombi, and each may lyse fresh platelet fibrin hemostatic plugs. tPA is more fibrin specific and activates plasminogen associated with thrombi or, unavoidably, hemostatic plugs. It does this in preference to acting on circulating plasminogen and may not cause the marked in vitro hemostatic abnormalities associated with the use of streptokinase or urokinase. However, tPA appears to cause at least as much bleeding as the other two agents.[34,35]

The optimum application of thrombolytic therapy in the treatment of deep venous thrombosis and pulmonary embolism remains undefined. Currently, appropriate indications include patients with upper extremity axillary-subclavian venous thrombosis and young patients with iliofemoral venous thrombosis when the diagnosis has been made within 5 days. Thrombolytic therapy followed by heparin has achieved early resolution of pulmonary thromboembolism and has done so more rapidly than heparin alone.[36] However, there is no proven decrease in short-term mortality with any thrombolytic agent used in the treatment of pulmonary embolism.[37]

Although the optimum dose and duration of thrombolytic therapy have not been established, there is agreement that the agents given by intravenous infusion activate fibrinolysis in more than 90% of patients. A loading dose is followed by maintenance therapy, and the duration of therapy is ideally limited to 24 to 48 hours. Heparin is infused concurrently only to prevent catheter thrombosis, not to achieve a systemic anticoagulant effect. There is no good correlation between in vitro tests of fibrinolysis and thrombolysis. However, activated partial thromboplastin times should be monitored during therapy.

Lytic therapy, with or without venoplasty and stenting, is not within the guidelines of this chapter, but it should be recognized that even very old thrombi may be manipulated by direct catheter infusion of lytic therapy followed by percutaneous transluminal angioplasty and stenting.

CONCLUSIONS

Clinical findings of venous thromboembolic disease are important to every physician. However, clinical findings that suggest venous thromboembolic disease must be corroborated by objective testing, as described elsewhere in this volume. When such corroboration has been achieved, immediate therapy must be begun. Today, this therapy consists of intravenous heparinization followed by oral anticoagulation. In the future, outpatient treatment with low molecular weight heparins will be feasible. The duration of oral anticoagulation will depend on the primary and secondary factors that induced the venous thrombosis initially.

REFERENCES

1. Lawrence ED. The cough-pain sign in acute superficial thrombophlebitis. *J Med Soc NJ* 1950;47:164–165.

2. LeClerc JR, Illescas F, Jarzem P. Diagnosis of deep vein thrombosis. In: LeClerc JR (ed). *Venous Thromboembolic Disorders*. Philadelphia and London: Lea & Febiger; 1991.

3. Lowenberg RL. Early diagnosis of phlebothrombosis with aid of a new clinical test. *JAMA* 1954;155:1566–1567.

4. Homans J. Venous thrombosis and pulmonary embolism. *N Engl J Med* 1947;236:196–201.

5. Provnan JR. Raised skin temperature in the early diagnosis of deep vein thrombosis of the legs. *Br Med J* 1965;2:334–337.

6. Haimovici H. In: Bergan JJ, Yao JST, eds. *Surgery of the Veins*. Orlando, FL: Grune & Stratton; 1985:

7. Brockman SK, Vasko JS. The pathologic physiology of phlegmasia cerulea dolens. *Surgery* 1966;59:997–1007.

8. Qvarfordt P, Eklöf B, Ohlin P. Intramuscular pressure in the lower leg in deep vein thrombosis and phlegmasia cerulea dolens. *Ann Surg* 1983;197:450–453.

9. Lindblad B, Sternby NH, Bergqvist D. Incidence of venous thromboembolism verified by necropsy over 30 years. *Br Med J* 1991;302:709–711.

10. Lindblad B, Eriksson A, Bergqvist D. Autopsy-verified pulmonary embolism in a surgical department: analysis of the period from 1951 to 1988. *Br J Surg* 1991;78:849–852.

11. Anderson FA Jr, Wheeler HB, Goldberg RJ, et al. A population-based perspective of the hospital incidence and case-fatality rates of deep vein thrombosis and pulmonary embolism: The Worcester DVT study. *Arch Intern Med* 1991;151:933–938.

12. Rasmussen MS, Wille-Jorgensen P, Jorgensen LN. Postoperative fatal pulmonary embolism in a general surgical department. *Am J Surg* 1995;169:214–216.

13. Jick H, Westerholm B, Vessey MP, et al. Venous thromboembolic disease and ABO blood type. *Lancet* 1969;1:539–540.

14. Nicolaides AN, Irving D. Clinical factors and the risk of deep venous thrombosis. In: Nicolaides AN, ed. *Thromboembolism: Aetiology, Advances in Prevention, and Management*. Lancaster, England: MPT Press; 1975:??.

15. Kakkar VV. Deep vein thrombosis of the leg: Is there is a "high risk" group? *Am J Surg* 1970;120:527–530.

16. Hirsh J, Fuster V. Guide to anticoagulant therapy. Part I: heparin. *Circulation* 1994;89:1449–1468.

17. Hull R, Delmore T, Genton E, et al. Warfarin sodium versus low-dose heparin in the long-term treatment of venous thrombosis. *N Engl J Med* 1979;301:855–858.

18. Lagerstedt CT, Olsson CG, Fagher BO, et al. Need for long-term coagulant treatment in symptomatic calf vein thrombosis. *N Engl J Med* 1979;2:515–518.

19. Pini M, Pattachini C, Quintavalla R, et al. Subcutaneous vs. intravenous heparin in the treatment of deep venous thrombosis: a randomized clinical trial. *Thromb Haemost* 1990;64:222–226.

20. Hull RD, Raskob GE, Rosenbloom D, et al. Heparin for five days as compared with ten days in the initial treatment of proximal venous thrombosis. *N Engl J Med* 1990;322:1260–1264.

21. Gallus A, Jackaman J, Tillett J, et al. Safety and efficacy of warfarin started early after submassive venous thrombosis or pulmonary embolism. *Lancet* 1986;2:1293–1296.

22. Holm HA, Ly B, Handeland GF, et al. Subcutaneous heparin treatment of deep venous thrombosis: a comparison of unfractionated and low-molecular-weight heparin. *Haemostasis* 1986;16(suppl 2):30–37.

23. Albada J, Nieuwenhuis HK, Sixma JJ. Treatment of acute venous thromboembolism with low-molecular-weight heparin (Fragmin). Results of a double-blind, randomized study. *Circulation* 1989;80:935–940.

24. Bratt G, Aberg W, Johannson M, et al. Two daily subcutaneous injections of Fragmin and compared with standard heparin in the treatment of deep venous thrombosis (DVT). *Thromb Haemost* 1990;64:506–510.

25. Holmström M, Berglund MC, Granqvist S, et al. Fragmin once or twice daily subcutaneously in the treatment of deep venous thrombosis of the leg. *Thromb Res* 1992;67:49–55.

26. Lindmarker P, Holmström M, Granqvist S, et al. Comparison of once-daily subcutaneous Fragmin with continuous intravenous unfractionated heparin in the treatment of deep vein thrombosis. *Thromb Haemost* 1994;72:186–190.

27. Blättler W, Linder C, Bergan JJ. Outpatient versus conventional treatment of acute deep vein thrombosis: a randomized, prospective trial. Presented at the 8th meeting of the American Venous Forum, February 1996, San Diego, CA.

28. Hirsh J, Fuster V. Guide to anticoagulant therapy. Part II: oral anticoagulants. *Circulation* 1994;89:1469–1480.

29. Kirkwood TBL. Calibration of reference thromboplastins and standardization of the prothrombin time ratio. *Thromb Haemost* 1983;49:238–244.

30. Hirsh J. Oral anticoagulant drugs. *N Engl J Med* 1991;324:1865–1875.

31. Poller L. Progress in standardization in anticoagulant control. *Hematol Rev* 1987;1:225–241.

32. Second ACCP Conference on Antithrombotic Therapy, June 21, 1988. *Chest* 1989;95(suppl):1S-169S.

33. Anderson FA Jr, Wheeler HB. Physician practices in the management of venous thromboembolism: a communitywide survey. *J Vasc Surg* 1992;16:707–714.

34. Goldhaber SZ, Vaughn DE, Markis JE, et al. Acute pulmonary embolism treated with tissue plasminogen activator. *Lancet* 1986;2:886–889.

35. Come PC, Ducksoo K, Parker JA, et al. Early reversal of right ventricular dysfunction in patients with acute pulmonary embolism after treatment with intravenous tissue plasminogen activator. *J Am Coll Cardiol* 1987;10:971–978.

36. Sharma GVRK, Burleson VA, Sasahara AA, et al. Effect of thrombolytic therapy on pulmonary capillary blood volume in patients with pulmonary embolism. *N Engl J Med* 1980;303:842–845.

37. Hyers TM, Hull RD, Weg JG. Antithrombotic therapy for venous thromboembolic disease. Fourth ACCP Consensus Conference on Antithrombotic Therapy. *Chest* 1995(suppl);108:335–351.

66

The Role of the Vascular Laboratory in the Diagnosis of Deep Venous Thrombosis

Robert W. Barnes, M.D.
M. Lee Nix, B.S.N, R.V.T.
Eric S. Williams, M.D.

Despite the introduction of venography by Bauer[1] in 1940, most physicians relied on a clinical diagnosis of deep vein thrombosis (DVT) until the development of noninvasive diagnostic techniques in the 1970s. These techniques included Doppler ultrasound, various forms of venous outflow or volume plethysmography, and I-125 fibrinogen leg scanning. Of these so-called physiologic techniques, the last was instrumental in heightening clinicians' awareness of the incidence of DVT in certain high-risk groups of patients and the efficacy of prophylactic measures. However, over the past decade, real-time B-mode ultrasonic imaging, especially when coupled with Doppler ultrasound (duplex scanning) or colorflow imaging, has become the diagnostic procedure of choice for the diagnosis or surveillance of DVT. This chapter will review the principles, diagnostic techniques, interpretation, reported accuracy, limitations, clinical applications, and cost effectiveness of ultrasonic diagnosis of DVT.

PRINCIPLES

Real-time B-mode imaging involves the generation of a pulsed beam of ultrasound from a linear array of piezoelectric crystals that is transmitted into the tissues through a coupling of acoustic gel on the skin. Sound reflected from tissue interfaces is received by the transducer and, after appropriate signal processing, is displayed on a gray-scale oscilloscope with a brightness proportional to the amplitude of the reflected signal. Transducers in clinical practice emit ultrasound with frequencies varying between 2 and 10 megahertz (MHz). Transducers with higher frequencies have greater image resolution but less depth of tissue pen-

etration, while the opposite is true of lower-frequency transducers.

Duplex scanners combine real-time B-mode imaging with Doppler detectors to record blood movement. The Doppler transducer detects the frequency shift in the reflected ultrasound from moving targets such as red blood cells moving toward or away from the transducer. The frequency shift, which is in the audible range, is proportional to the velocity of the blood flow. Doppler frequency shifts may be detected as an audible signal or may be recorded by analog tracings or sound spectral analysis. The latter technique involves oscilloscopic or recorded displays of frequency (representing blood flow velocities) on the vertical axis, time on the horizontal axis, and amplitude (representing the number of blood cells moving at a given velocity) displayed as the degree of brightness or density on the recording.

Colorflow ultrasonic scanning combines real-time B-mode imaging with superimposed Doppler frequency information on blood flow direction and velocity information depicted as color within the vascular lumen. Flow direction relative to the transducer is depicted conventionally by either a red or blue color, and Doppler frequencies, reflecting blood velocities, are represented by varying shades of color, with lighter shades indicating higher frequencies.

TECHNIQUES

Lower Extremity

Our preference is to use duplex ultrasound for venous exams, incorporating a hybrid of methods used in real-time B-mode imaging, duplex scanning, and colorflow imaging.[2,3] The patient initially is positioned supine, with the head of the examination table elevated about 15°. The lower extremity should be relaxed, with external rotation of the hip and slight flexion of the hip and knee. A 5-MHz transducer is positioned transversely over the common femoral vessels at the inguinal crease. The femoral vein is identified next to the pulsatile artery. Confirmation is made with either Doppler interrogation or colorflow imaging of the lumen. The transducer is then rotated to provide a longitudinal image of the common femoral vein. When the transducer is moved cephalad, the proximal common femoral vein is imaged, and occasionally even the iliac vessels or the inferior vena cava may be examined although intestinal gas often obscures visualization.

The imaged venous segments are interrogated for thrombus by several maneuvers. In our experience, the most reliable method is to exert mild probe pressure to attempt to coapt the venous walls on a transverse image.[4] Failure to obliterate the lumen suggests intraluminal thrombus, the extent of which is inversely proportional to the degree of lumen obliteration. Thrombus can also be recognized by alteration of the normally spontaneous and phasic venous Doppler signal, which waxes and wanes with respiration.[5] Such interrogation is our preferred method of indirectly assessing the patency of the iliocaval system, which infrequently can be imaged. Finally, the presence (and extent) or absence of intraluminal thrombus may be assessed by longitudinal colorflow imaging, although the reliability of this technique requires careful setting of the color and velocity gains on the scanner.

After the interrogation of the common femoral vein is completed, the probe is moved sequentially down the anteromedial thigh in a transverse plane, carrying out similar imaging compression and flow detection maneuvers. Attention should be paid to the presence of duplicate superficial femoral veins, which occur in up to one-third of individuals and may be at greater risk of harboring DVT.[6] The distal superficial femoral vein may be difficult to compress where it passes through the adductor hiatus. Adequate interrogation of this segment may require probe repositioning, scanning from the posterior aspect of the distal thigh, and correlating Doppler flow signals or color imaging with the B-mode information.

The popliteal and posterior crural (tibioperoneal, posterior tibial, and peroneal) veins are examined from the posterior aspect of the extremity, with the patient in the lateral or prone position and the knee slightly flexed. The distal popliteal and crural veins may be difficult to visualize in patients with extensive edema, obesity, or large gastrocnemius muscles. The distal posterior tibial veins may be examined with the patient supine and the transducer positioned over the medial leg posterior to the tibia. The anterior tibial veins, while seldom a site of DVT, may be examined over their course along the lower leg anterior to the interosseous membrane. Colorflow imaging may be helpful in identifying crural veins, but color and frequency settings must be carefully adjusted to avoid false-positive or false-negative diagnoses of tibial DVT. The greater and lesser saphenous veins may be examined for superficial thrombophlebitis.

Upper Extremity

The examination of the internal jugular, subclavian, axillary, brachial, cephalic, and basilic veins may be carried out using maneuvers similar to those in the lower extremity.[3,7] However, the subclavian vein lies posterior and caudad to the clavicle, which limits the extent of venous imaging, so that much of the diagnostic information relies on interpretation of Doppler flow velocity signals. Similarly, indirect evaluation of innominate veins and the superior vena cava depends on Doppler signal assessment. The remaining veins of the upper extremity may be more directly visualized with compression B-mode studies and colorflow imaging.

INTERPRETATION

The interpretation of venous ultrasonography involves collation of information provided by the B-mode image, the Doppler signal, and the colorflow scan. The B-mode image of a normal vein in cross section reveals a relatively echo-free, circular lumen adjacent to the corresponding pulsatile artery (Fig. 66–1A). Light probe pressure should obliterate the venous lumen while not affecting the arterial lumen (Fig. 66–1B). Spectral recording of the Doppler frequency shifts from a sample volume within the lumen should reveal spontaneous signals that are phasic with respiration (Fig. 66–1C) and augmented by manual compression of the limb distal to the site of examination (Fig. 66–1D). Flow velocity in calf veins may not be sufficient to result in spontaneous audible Doppler frequency shifts, but it should be elicited by augmentation maneuvers such as foot compression. Pulsatile venous signals that are cyclic with each heartbeat are normal in the upper extremity but, when present in the lower extremity, often signify venous hypertension, as in congestive heart failure or fluid overload. Competence of venous valves should result in cessation of the venous Doppler signal in response to proximal limb compression or a Valsalva maneuver. The latter maneuver should also result in a significant increase in the diameter of the common femoral vein (50 to 200%).[8] This test, and the character of the Doppler signal in the common femoral vein, are indirect indicators of patency of the iliocaval venous system, which often cannot be directly visualized. Finally, in the presence of a normal vein, the colorflow scan should fill in the entire venous lumen on longtudinal section (Fig. 66–1C).

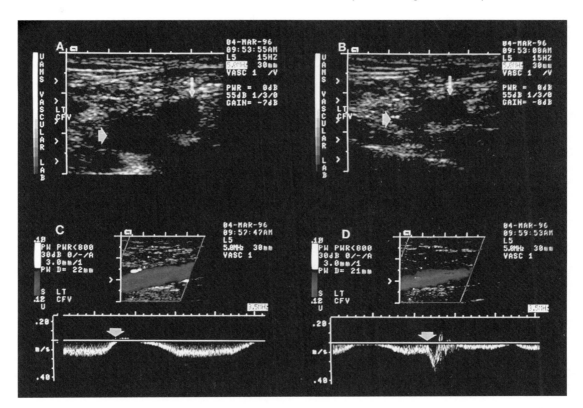

Figure 66–1. (A) B-mode ultrasonic cross-sectional view of a patent left common femoral vein (broad arrow) and artery (narrow arrow). (B) Same view as (A) during compression with the transducer, showing normal collapse of the common femoral vein (broad arrow) and patent artery (narrow arrow). (C) Longitudinal colorflow scan of the common femoral vein shown in (A) and (B), with normal phasic Doppler signal attenuated by inspiration (arrow). (D) Same view as (C), with normal augmentation of the femoral venous Doppler signal during calf compression (arrow).

Venous thrombosis may be detected by the presence of intraluminal echogenic or echolucent filling defects (Figs. 66–2 and 66–3). In vitro studies[9] suggest that clots initially (within 24 hours) are echogenic, but as the red blood cells lyse during the next few days and the thrombus becomes an aggregate of platelets and fibrin, the clot appears more echolucent. As the thrombus organizes with time, echogenicity may increase. Echolucent thrombi may be detected by probe compression, which partially or completely fails to obliterate the venous lumen, depending on the extent of thrombosis (Figs. 66–2B and 66–3B). With nonocclusive thrombi, the venous Doppler signal may be of higher frequency and more continuous (Fig. 66–2D), and augmentation of the signal may be attenuated or absent, particularly if there is obstruction between the site of examination and the site of distal limb compression. In the presence of occlusive venous thrombosis, no Doppler signal will be present. Colorflow scanning will reveal filling defects in the presence of nonocclusive venous thrombosis (Figs. 66–2C, D and 66–3C, D), and color will be absent if the thrombus is occlusive. Occasionally, free-floating thrombi can be identified either as intraluminal echos that move with respiration (Fig. 66–4A) or by colorflow scanning. Although such

thrombi may pose an increased risk of thromboembolism, there have been few reports of documented emboli at the time of compression ultrasonography.[10,11]

Chronic venous thrombi are occasionally identified by increased echogenicity of the organized clot[9,12–18] (Fig. 66–4B). Other indications of chronicity include incompetence of venous valves, narrower veins or irregular and thickened vein walls, recanalized veins with one or more flow channels on the colorflow scan, or prominent collateral veins around occluded venous segments. Recurrent venous thrombosis may be diagnosed if new venous segments demonstrate clots that were not present on previous ultrasonic exams.[19] However, if symptoms recur at the site of previous involvement, ultrasonography may not be diagnostic unless a nonocclusive or free-floating thrombus can be demonstrated (Fig. 66–4A).

VALIDATION

The published results of venographic validation of ultrasonic diagnosis of DVT in symptomatic and asymptomatic patients using real-time B-mode imaging, duplex scanning, and colorflow imaging are shown in

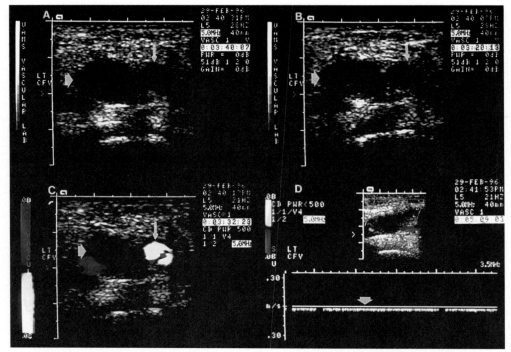

Figure 66–2. (A) Cross-sectional B-mode image of the left common femoral vein (broad arrow), harboring acute echolucent thrombus, and the corresponding artery (narrow arrow). (B) Same view as (A) during probe compression, with failure to collapse the common femoral vein (broad arrow). Artery indicated by narrow arrow. (C) Cross-sectional colorflow scan of the vessels in (A) and (B), showing a large, nonocclusive thrombus in the common femoral vein (broad arrow) and a patent artery (narrow arrow). (D) Longitudinal colorflow scan of the vein in (A–C) showing nonocclusive thrombus and an abnormal continuous Doppler signal unaffected by inspiration (arrow).

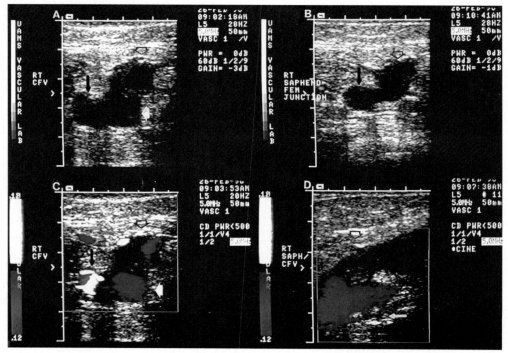

Figure 66–3. (A) Cross-sectional B-mode image of echogenic thrombus in the right greater saphenous vein (hollow arrow) at its junction with the common femoral vein (white arrow) adjacent to the femoral artery (black arrow). (B) Same view as (A) during probe compression showing failure to collapse the greater saphenous vein (hollow arrow), incomplete collapse of the common femoral vein (white arrow), and a patent artery (black arrow). (C) Same view as (A), with colorflow scan showing a large thrombus in the greater saphenous vein (hollow arrow) encroaching on the anterior lumen of the common femoral vein (white arrow) adjacent to the artery (black arrow). (D) Longitudinal view with colorflow scan of the same patient showing a thrombus in the greater saphenous vein (hollow arrow) encroaching on the lumen of the common femoral vein (white arrow).

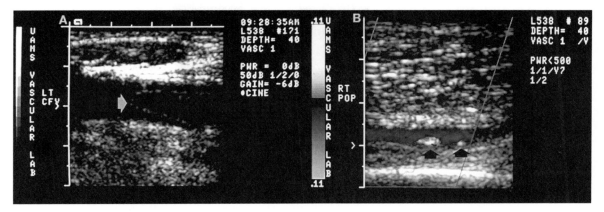

Figure 66–4. Longitudinal B-mode image of the echogenic surface of a free-floating thrombus (arrow) in the left common femoral vein. (B) Longitudinal colorflow scan showing a nonocclusive, densely echogenic, chronic thrombus in the right popliteal vein.

Tables 66–1, 66–2, and 66–3, respectively. During the past 11 years, there have been at least 50 such reports,[8,12,14–16,20–64] in which both venous ultrasonography and venography have been carried out and independently analyzed on over 5600 limbs. The overall reported sensitivity of ultrasonography in detecting DVT is 88%, and the specificity is 95%. With a mean reported prevalence of venous thrombosis of 27%, the positive and negative predictive values of venous ultrasonography are 95% and 93%, respectively, with an overall diagnostic accuracy of 93%. The sensitivity in detecting proximal DVT of the femoropopliteal system, 93%, is significantly higher than the 70% reported sensitivity of detecting calf vein thrombosis. The overall sensitivity of ultrasonography for diagnostic studies of symptomatic patients is 94%, compared to 50% for surveillance studies of asymptomatic patients. Presumably, this difference is due to the smaller size and extent of thrombi in the latter group of patients. Also, the lower prevalence of DVT in asymptomatic individuals (13%) compared to symptomatic patients (33%) explains the lower positive predictive value of surveillance ultrasonography (68%) compared to that of diagnostic studies (95%).

The reported overall diagnostic accuracy rates of B-mode, duplex, and colorflow imaging are not significantly different (90%, 95%, and 92%, respectively). However, the reported overall sensitivity of B-mode imaging, 76%, is significantly lower than that of duplex and colorflow imaging, 94% and 88%, respectively. This appears to reflect the poor sensitivity of B-mode imaging of calf veins (31%), when compared to that of duplex (85%) and colorflow imaging (83%). The sensitivity of B-mode, duplex, and colorflow imaging in detecting proximal DVT is similar and relatively good (91%, 97%, and 93%, respectively).

CLINICAL APPLICATIONS

Acute DVT

The most common use of venous ultrasonography is for diagnostic evaluation of symptomatic patients with suspected DVT.[8,12,14,15,20–32,35–51,55–63] For the past 25 years, the clinical diagnosis has been considered both insensitive and nonspecific,[65–67] and most clinicians realize the importance of objective diagnosis of DVT. The established accuracy of ultrasound has resulted in its replacement of venography as the diagnostic standard for detection of DVT in most centers today. In the past few years, the value of defining the probability of DVT based on clinical criteria (pretest probability) has increased the likelihood of correctly predicting the presence or absence of DVT after venous ultrasonography (posttest probability).[68–71] The authors' algorithm for evaluating patients with suspected DVT is shown in Figure 66–5.

A patient with suspected DVT is given an intravenous bolus of heparin (unless contraindicated) and then is evaluated by venous duplex or colorflow ultrasonic imaging. If the study is abnormal, the patient is treated with anticoagulants for DVT. In this regard, involvement of the superficial femoral vein (which is a deep vein) is best reported as femoral DVT to avoid the common misunderstanding that it is a superficial vein not requiring anticoagulation.[72] If the ultrasonic study is equivocal, a venogram is performed and the patient is managed based on the results of that study. If the ultrasonogram is normal, management of the patient is based on the clinical presentation.[68,71] However, if the clinical probability of DVT is high, a venogram should be considered to clarify the diagnosis or the ultrasound study can be repeated; management of the patient is based on serial diagnostic studies. If the clinical probability of DVT is intermediate, serial venous ultrasonog-

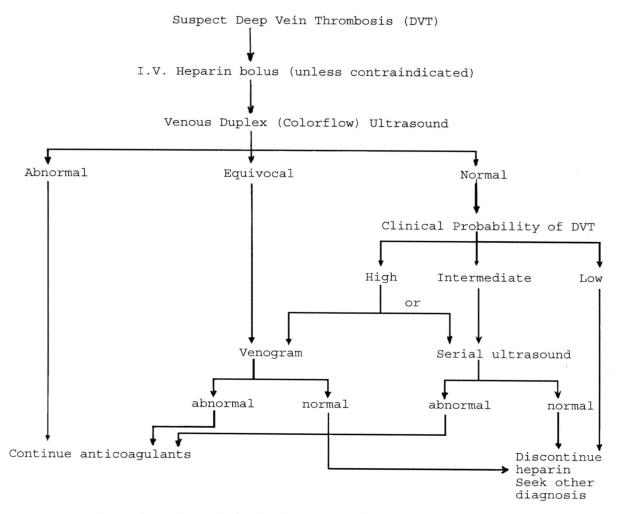

Figure 66–5. Diagnostic algorithm for evaluation of a patient with suspected DVT.

raphy is recommended and the patient is treated based on the outcome of those studies. If the clinical likelihood of DVT is low, anticoagulation is discontinued and the workup focuses on other conditions, such as a Baker's cyst or muscle hematoma.[20,21,23,35,38,48,63,73–75]

During the past decade, venous ultrasonography has been used for prospective surveillance of certain asymptomatic, high-risk patients, such as those undergoing hip or knee replacement, operation for malignancy, or neurosurgical procedures.[16,27,31,33,34,44,52,54,59,64,76–86] However, as mentioned previously, the accuracy of such surveillance studies is significantly lower than that of diagnostic ultrasonography of symptomatic patients, particularly in the detection of calf vein thrombosis. The clinical significance of calf DVT remains unclear, with reports both supporting and questioning the value of anticoagulation of these patients.[87–93] If calf DVT is not treated, most physicians recommend serial diagnostic studies to identify that minority of patients (about 20%) who develop extension of thrombosis into the popliteal or more proximal veins and who require anticoagulation or other treatment.

Venous ultrasonography has permitted longitudinal studies of the outcome of DVT.[93–103] Most patients develop partial or complete thrombolysis of the obstructed venous segments, presumably from endogenous fibrin degradation. In many individuals, recanalization is associated with damage to the venous valves, with resulting venous incompetence. Such retrograde venous flow can be quantified by duplex scanning and is associated with the clinical development of postthrombotic sequelae such as hyperpigmentation, stasis dermatitis, or cutaneous ulceration, particularly with venous incompetence below the knee. Early postthrombotic edema is often due to venous outflow obstruction, while late swelling is often the result of venous valvular incompetence.

Because of the increasing use of ultrasonography for the diagnosis of DVT, several laboratories have recommended techniques to limit the extent of the study to

Table 66–1. Results of Real-Time B-Mode Ultrasonic Imaging of DVT

Author	Year	No. of Limbs	% Sensitivity			% Specificity	% PPV	% NPV	% Accuracy
			Proximal	Calf	Total				
Diagnostic (Symptomatic) Studies:									
Effency et al[18]	1984	37	83 (19/23)			86 (12/14)	90 (19/21)	75 (12/16)	84 (31/37)
Sullivan et al[12]	1984	30			100 (14/14)	94 (15/16)	93 (14/15)	100 (15/15)	97 (29/30)
Raghavendra et al[20]	1986	20	100 (14/14)			100 (6/6)	100 (14/14)	100 (6/6)	100 (20/20)
Dauzat et al[21]	1986	145	94 (94/100)			100 (45/45)	100 (45/45)	88 (45/51)	96 (139/145)
Cronan et al[22]	1987	51	89 (25/28)			100 (23/23)	100 (25/25)	88 (23/26)	94 (48/51)
Aitken & Godden[23]	1987	42	94 (15/16)			100 (26/26)	100 (15/15)	96 (26/27)	98 (41/42)
Appelman et al[24]	1987	112	94 (48/52)			97 (58/60)	96 (48/50)	94 (58/62)	95 (106/112)
Rollins et al[25]	1988	46			100 (40/40)	100 (6/6)	100 (40/40)	100 (6/6)	100 (46/46)
Lensing et al[26]	1989	220	100 (66/66)	36 (4/11)	89 (70/77)	99 (142/143)	99 (70/71)	94 (142/149)	96 (212/220)
Monreal et al[27]	1989	69	93 (40/43)	0 (0/5)	83 (40/48)	86 (18/21)	98 (40/41)	71 (20/28)	84 (58/69)
Habscheid et al[28]	1990	174	98 (59/60)	87 (20/23)	95 (79/83)	100 (91/91)	100 (91/91)	98 (171/174)	98 (170/174)
Mussurakis et al[29]	1990	94	100 (24/24)	50 (6/12)	83 (30/36)	100 (58/58)	100 (30/30)	91 (58/64)	94 (88/94)
Pederson et al[30]	1991	218	89 (101/113)			97 (74/76)	98 (101/103)	86 (74/86)	93 (175/189)
Ginsberg et al[31]	1991	98	92 (35/38)			95 (57/60)	92 (35/38)	95 (57/60)	94 (92/98)
Heijboer et al[32]	1993	89	100 (84/84)				94 (84/89)		
Surveillance (Asymptomatic) Studies:									
Borris et al[33]	1989	60	63 (15/24)	29 (4/14)	54 (15/28)	91 (29/32)	83 (15/18)	69 (29/42)	73 (44/60)
Monreal et al[27]	1989	39	50 (3/6)	0 (0/3)	33 (3/9)	97 (29/30)	75 (3/4)	83 (29/35)	82 (32/39)
Ginsberg et al[31]	1991	247	52 (11/21)	13 (5/40)	26 (16/61)	99 (184/186)	89 (16/18)	80 (184/229)	81 (200/247)
Jongbloets et al[34]	1994	100	38 (5/13)	50 (8/16)	50 (13/26)	74 (55/74)	41 (13/32)	81 (55/68)	68 (68/100)

Abbreviations: PPV, positive predictive value; NPV, negative predictive value.

Table 66–2. Results of Duplex Ultrasonic Scanning of DVT

Author	Year	No. of Limbs	% Sensitivity			% Specificity	% PPV	% NPV	% Accuracy
			Proximal	Calf	Total				
Diagnostic (Symptomatic) Studies:									
Oliver[35]	1985	30			90 (9/10)	95 (19/20)	90 (9/10)	95 (19/20)	93 (28/30)
Langsfeld et al[36]	1987	19			100 (10/10)	78 (7/9)	83 (10/12)	100 (7/7)	89 (17/19)
George et al[37]	1987	50			92 (22/24)	100 (26/26)	100 (22/22)	93 (26/28)	96 (48/50)
Vogel et al[38]	1987	54		0 (0/4)	96 (24/25)	100 (29/29)	100 (24/24)	97 (29/30)	98 (53/54)
Elias et al[39]	1987	854	100 (241/241)	92 (85/92)	98 (326/333)	96 (500/521)	94 (326/347)	99 (500/507)	97 (826/854)
Comerota et al[40]	1988	37			96 (21/22)	93 (14/15)	96 (21/22)	93 (14/15)	95 (35/37)
O'Leary et al[41]	1988	50			88 (22/25)	96 (24/25)	96 (22/23)	89 (24/27)	92 (46/50)
Rosner & Doris[42]	1988	32	90 (9/10)			100 (22/22)	100 (9/9)	96 (22/23)	97 (31/32)
Killewich et al[43]	1989	50			92 (35/38)	92 (11/12)	97 (35/36)	79 (11/14)	92 (46/50)
Comerota et al[44]	1990	72	100 (37/37)	86 (6/7)	98 (43/44)	86 (24/28)	98 (43/47)	96 (24/25)	93 (67/72)
Wright et al[15]	1990	71		57 (4/7)	91 (31/34)	95 (35/37)	94 (31/33)	92 (35/38)	93 (66/71)
Lee et al[45]	1990	90	100 (30/30)	84 (36/43)	87 (41/47)	93 (40/43)	93 (41/44)	87 (40/46)	90 (81/90)
Cavaye et al[46]	1990	56	95 (20/21)	89 (24/27)	91 (30/33)	91 (21/23)	94 (30/32)	88 (21/24)	91 (51/56)
Ezekowitz et al[47]	1990	34	73 (8/11)			83 (19/23)	67 (8/12)	86 (19/22)	79 (27/34)
Mitchell et al[48]	1991	64	96 (23/24)	81 (17/21)	85 (25/29)	80 (28/35)	78 (25/32)	88 (28/32)	83 (53/64)
Ramshorst et al[49]	1991	120	91 (58/64)			95 (53/56)	95 (58/61)	90 (53/59)	93 (111/120)
Abu Rahma et al[50]	1992	53			91 (20/22)	87 (27/31)	83 (20/24)	93 (27/29)	89 (47/53)
Size et al[51]	1993	56	95 (18/19)	85 (11/13)	100 (25/25)	90 (28/31)	89 (25/28)	100 (28/28)	95 (53/56)
Surveillance (Asymptomatic) Studies:									
Froehlich et al[52]	1989	40	100 (5/5)			97 (34/35)	83 (5/6)	97 (34/35)	98 (39/40)
Comerota et al[44]	1990	38	100 (7/7)	50 (1/2)	89 (8/9)	100 (29/29)	100 (8/8)	97 (29/30)	87 (37/38)
Barnes et al[53]	1991	428			80 (16/20)	98 (400/408)	67 (16/24)	99 (400/404)	97 (416/428)
Grady-Benson et al[54]	1994	102	100 (7/7)	60 (3/5)	83 (10/12)	99 (89/90)	91 (10/11)	98 (89/91)	97 (99/102)

Abbreviations: PPV, positive predictive value; NPV, negative predictive value.

Table 66–3. Results of Colorflow Ultrasonic Imaging for DVT

Author	Year	No. of Limbs	% Sensitivity			% Specificity	% PPV	% NPV	% Accuracy
			Proximal	Calf	Total				
Diagnostic (Symptomatic) Studies:									
Foley et al[55]	1989	47	100 (12/12)	71 (5/7)		100 (35/35)	100 (12/12)	100 (35/35)	100 (47/47)
Persson et al[14]	1989	30	100 (21/21)	100 (21/21)	100 (21/21)	100 (9/9)	100 (21/21)	100 (9/9)	100 (30/30)
Rose et al[56]	1990	75	96 (25/26)	73 (22/30)	79 (27/34)	88 (36/41)	84 (27/32)	84 (36/43)	84 (63/75)
Ezekowitz et al[47]	1990	27	88 (7/8)			84 (16/19)	70 (7/10)	94 (16/17)	85 (23/27)
Schindler et al[57]	1990	94	98 (54/55)			100 (39/39)	100 (54/54)	98 (39/40)	99 (93/94)
Yucel et al[58]	1991	44		88 (15/17)		96 (26/27)	94 (15/16)	93 (26/28)	93 (41/44)
Mattos et al[59]	1992	77	100 (32/32)	94 (33/35)	100 (40/40)	73 (27/37)	80 (40/50)	100 (27/27)	87 (67/77)
Kalodiki et al[60]	1992	100			93 (43/46)	91 (45/54)	89 (43/48)	94 (49/52)	92 (92/100)
Baxter et al[61]	1992	40	100 (15/15)	95 (19/20)	95 (19/20)	100 (20/20)	100 (19/19)	95 (20/21)	98 (39/40)
Bradley et al[62]	1993	100	97 (33/34)	100 (16/16)	98 (49/50)	100 (50/50)	100 (49/49)	98 (50/51)	99 (99/100)
Labropoulos et al[63]	1995	112	100 (30/30)	88 (28/32)	93 (51/55)	96 (55/57)	96 (51/53)	93 (55/59)	95 (106/112)
Surveillance (Asymptomatic) Studies:									
Cronan et al[16]	1991	76	100 (12/12)			100 (64/64)	100 (12/12)	100 (64/64)	100 (76/76)
Mattos et al[59]	1992	190	67 (2/3)	56 (24/43)	55 (24/44)	98 (143/146)	89 (24/27)	88 (143/163)	88 (167/190)
Davidson et al[64]	1992	319	38 (8/21)			92 (275/298)	26 (8/31)	95 (275/288)	89 (283/319)

Abbreviations: PPV, positive predictive value; NPV, negative predictive value.

reduce both the duraton of the examination and its cost.[15,26,48,91,104-109] A complete examination of all venous segments of both lower extremities, including calf veins, requires 30 minutes to 1 hour. We[105] have recommended limiting the examination to the symptomatic extremity in patients with suspected unilateral DVT. In a retrospective review of 215 patients (430 limbs), duplex scanning of both lower extremities detected DVT in 67 patients (31%), and in 10 it was bilateral. However, among the patients with unilateral thrombus, it was limited to the symptomatic extremity in 97%, suggesting that the examination need not be bilateral in patients with unilateral symptoms. Bilateral ultrasonography is recommended for patients with suspected uplmonary embolism, with bilateral extremity symptoms, or at high risk for venous thromboembolism. A recent study [104] of the distribution of DVT in the lower extremity suggested that venous ultrasonography may be limited to examination of the common femoral and popliteal veins. While such limited studies will reduce the time and cost of the examination, further investigation is necessary to validate the accuracy of attenuated exams.[91,109]

Recurrent DVT

The development of recurrent symptoms of leg pain, tenderness, edema, or inflammation in a patient with a prior history of DVT may pose a diagnostic dilemma: The patient may have true recurrent active DVT, although these symptoms and signs are typical of patients with venous valvular incompetence, with or without persistent, chronic venous obstruction secondary to inactive thrombosis. In the past, the I-125 fibrinogen leg scan was sensitive and specific for active DVT. In the absence of this test, patients with recurrent symptoms should initially be evaluated with duplex or colorflow ultrasonography.[99] If the deep veins are patent and competent, prior diagnosis of DVT may have been incorrect. A venogram may be recommended to establish the fact that the patient does not have venous disease (pseudophlebitis), and other disorders should be sought. If the deep veins are patent but the venous valves are incompetent, the patient should be treated for the postthrombotic (postphlebitic) syndrome, which does not require anticoagulation unless indicated for secondary prophylaxis in patients with factors predisposing to DVT. If the duplex or colorflow scan reveals venous obstruction, attempts should be made to identify the age of the thrombus, if possible. If a venous segment is involved that was not affected on a prior study, the patient may be treated for recurrent DVT. Likewise, if a nonocclusive or free-floating thrombus is identified, treatment for acute recurrent DVT is warranted. If the age of the venous obstruction cannot be so identified, venography is recommended to clarify the problem.

Superficial Thrombophlebitis

The diagnosis of superficial thrombophlebitis usually can be made on clinical grounds by the presence of a tender, inflamed induration along the course of the greater or lesser saphenous vein, especially in the presence of a predisposing varicosity or above the site of an indwelling venous catheter. On the other hand, this diagnosis may be confused with other inflammatory conditions, such as cellulitis or lymphangitis.[110] Venous ultrasonography is indicated in such instances, particularly because venography may be painful and even nondiagnostic in superficial thrombophlebitis. Duplex or colorflow imaging will rapidly define (or exclude) the presence and extent of superficial thrombophlebitis (Fig. 66–3), as well as the presence of associated DVT. Such information will assist the physician in choosing therapy, which may include anti-inflammatory agents (isolated superficial thrombophlebitis), ligation (if the thrombosis approaches the saphenofemoral junction; Fig. 66–3C, D), anticoagulation (for associated DVT), or antibiotics (for cellulitis or lymphangitis).

Pulmonary Embolism

Noninvasive venous evaluation of the lower extremities, particularly venous ultrasonography, is often used in conjunction with ventilation-perfusion lung scanning to evaluate patients with suspected pulmonary embolism.[16,111-117] While a normal lung scan essentially excludes the diagnosis (because of the high sensitivity of the test), an abnormal lung scan is less specific and frequently is falsely positive. Venous ultrasonography may be used to increase the specificity of lung scanning. Many physicians treat patients with a high-probability lung scan for pulmonary embolism, but the diagnosis is more firm in the presence of an abnormal venous ultrasonogram. By contrast, in the presence of a low-probability lung scan and a negative venous ultrasonogram, pulmonary embolism is unlikely. For other cases in which venous ultrasonography is negative and the lung scan is of intermediate or high probability, pulmonary angiography is recommended to clarify the diagnosis.

COST EFFECTIVENESS

Several reports have documented the cost benefit or cost effectiveness of objective, noninvasive venous examinations in the diagnosis and therapy of DVT, both in terms of disease detection and deaths averted.[111,113,116,118-120] Originally, such studies supported the value of less expensive tests such as impedance plethysmography and I-125 fibrinogen scanning.[118] Recent studies have suggested that venous ultrasonography has similar cost effectiveness, despite its increased cost, when compared to venography. All objective diagnostic studies, including venography, are cost effective when compared to clinical diagnosis alone because the latter may be incorrect at least 50% of the time. Conversely, the value of such studies for surveillance of high-risk but asymptomatic patients remains unproven.

At present, the Health Care Financing Administration (HCFA) will not reimburse laboratories for screening high-risk Medicare patients for DVT. Indeed, the reimbursement of vascular laboratories for noninvasive vascular studies in general has become of increasing concern,[121–125] and in some cases the reimbursement fails to support the acquisition and maintenance costs of the diagnostic equipment and the expenses for experienced technologists and other personnel necessary to operate a quality diagnostic facility. Certainly, the past has seen many abuses of the noninvasive vascular laboratory. Questionable practices have included routine screening studies of asymptomatic patients, repeated follow-up studies, mobile laboratories, and lack of quality control of both tests and examiners. During the past decade, several steps have been taken to eliminate these problems. Examination of technologists and physicians working in noninvasive vascular laboratories has been developed by the Registry of Diagnostic Medical Sonography (RDMS), leading to the certificate of Registered Vascular Technologist (RVT). Accreditation of vascular laboratories has been established by the Intersocietal Commission on the Accreditation of Vascular Laboratories (ICAVL). This process has led to the development of standards of practice, quality controls, and periodic recertification to ensure optimal application of noninvasive vascular diagnostic studies to clinical practice.

SUMMARY

Venous ultrasonography has become the method of choice in most vascular laboratories for the noninvasive diagnosis of DVT. The test may involve real-time B-mode ultrasonic imaging, combined B-mode and Doppler ultrasonic scanning (duplex), or B-mode and Doppler displayed as a colorflow image. The quality of the study is highly dependent on the technical skills of the examiner. With attention to procedural details, the accuracy of venous ultrasonography compared to venography has exceeded that of any other noninvasive method, and the exam is cost effective. The sensitivity and specificity of the examination usually exceed 90 to 95% for detection or exclusion of DVT in the proximal (femoropopliteal) veins of the lower extremity in patients with suspected disease (diagnostic study). However, lower accuracy has been reported in detecting calf vein thrombosis and in surveillance studies of asymptomatic, high-risk patients. Venous ultrasonography is useful to detect proximal DVT in symptomatic patients, evaluate patients with suspected recurrent DVT or the postthrombotic syndrome, differentiate superficial thrombophlebitis from inflammatory conditions, and assess patients with suspected pulmonary embolism for a possible thrombotic source.

ACKNOWLEDGMENTS

The authors express their appreciation to Rhonda Troilett, R.T., R.D.M.S., R.V.T., Vicki Morris, L.P.N., R.V.T., and Michael Morris for their technical assistance.

REFERENCES

1. Bauer G. A venographic study of thrombo-embolic problems. *Acta Chir Scand* 1940;84 (Suppl):61:1–73.
2. Stewart JH, Grubb M. Understanding vascular ultrasonography. *Mayo Clin Proc* 1992;67:1186–1196.
3. Nix ML, Troillet RD. The use of color in venous duplex examination. *J Vasc Technol* 1991;15:123–128.
4. Talbot SR. Use of real-time imaging in identifying deep venous obstruction: a preliminary report. *Bruit* 1982;6:41–42.
5. Barnes RW, Russell HR, Wilson MR. *Doppler Ultrasonic Evaluation of Venous Disease.* Iowa City: University of Iowa Press; 1975:1–251.
6. Liu G, Ferris EJ, Reifsteck JR, Baker ML. Effect of anatomic variations on deep venous thrombosis of the lower extremity. *AJR* 1986;146:845–848.
7. Froehlich JB, Zide RS, Persson AV. Diagnosis of upper extremity deep venous thrombosis using color Doppler imaging system. *J Vasc Technol* 1991;15:251–253.
8. Effeney DJ, Friedman MB, Gooding GAW. Iliofemoral venous thrombosis: real-time ultrasound diagnosis, normal criteria, and clinical application. *Radiology* 1984;150:787–792.
9. Coelho JCU, Sigel B, Ryva JC, Machi J, Renigers SA. B-mode sonography of blood clots. *J Clin Ultrasound* 1982;10:323–327.
10. Schroder WB, Bealer JF. Venous duplex ultrasonography causing acute pulmonary embolism: a brief report. *J Vasc Surg* 1992;15:1082–1083.
11. Feld R. Pulmonary embolism caused by venous compression ultrasound examination. *J Vasc Surg* 1993;17:450.
12. Sullivan ED, Peter DJ, Cranley JJ. Real-time B-mode venous ultrasound. *J Vasc Surg* 1984;1:465–471.
13. Semrow CM, Friedell M, Buchbinder D, Rollins DL. Characterization of lower extremity venous disease using real-time B-mode ultrasonic imaging. *J Vasc Technol* 1987;9:187–191.
14. Persson AV, Jones C, Zide R, Jewell ER. Use of the triplex scanner in diagnosis of deep venous thrombosis. *Arch Surg* 1989;124:593–596.
15. Wright DJ, Shepard AD, McPharlin M, Ernst CB. Pitfalls in lower extremity venous duplex scanning. *J Vasc Surg* 1990;11:675–679.
16. Cronan JJ, Dorfman GS. Advances in ultrasound imaging of venous thrombosis. *Semin Nucl Med* 1991;21:297–312.
17. Parsons RE, Sigel B, Feleppa EJ, et al. Age determination of experimental venous thrombi by ultrasonic tissue characterization. *J Vasc Surg* 1993;17:470–478.
18. Kolecki RV, Sigel B, Justin J, et al. Determining the acuteness and stability of deep venous thrombosis by ultrasonic tissue characterization. *J Vasc Surg* 1995;21:976–984.
19. Meissner MH, Caps MT, Bergelin RO, Manzo RA, Strandness DE. Propagation, rethrombosis and new thrombus formation after acute deep venous thrombosis. *J Vasc Surg* 1995;22:558–567.

20. Raghavendra BN, Horii SC, Hilton S, Subramanyam BR, Rosen RJ, Lam S. Deep venous thrombosis: detection by probe compression of veins. *J Ultrasound Med* 1986;5:89–95.

21. Dauzat MM, Larouche JP, Charras C, et al. Real-time B-mode ultrasonography for better specificity in the non-invasive diagnosis of deep venous thrombosis. *J Ultrasound Med* 1986;5:625–631.

22. Cronan JJ, Dorfman GS, Scola FH, Schepps B, Alexander J. Deep venous throbosis: US assessment using vein compression. *Radiology* 1987;162:191–194.

23. Aitken AGF, Godden DJ. Real-time ultrasound diagnosis of deep vein thrombosis: a comparison with venography. *Clin Radiol* 1987;38:309–313.

24. Appelman PT, DeJong TE, Lampmann LE. Deep venous thrombosis of the leg: US findings. *Radiology* 1987; 163:743–746.

25. Rollins DL, Semrow CM, Friedell ML, Calligaro KD, Buchbinder D. Progress in the diagnosis of deep venous thrombosis: the efficacy of real-time B-mode ultrasonic imaging. *J Vasc Surg* 1988;7:638–641.

26. Lensing AWA, Prandoni P, Brandjes D, et al. Detection of deep-vein thrombosis by real-time B-mode ultrasonography. *N Engl J Med* 1989;320:342–345.

27. Monreal M, Montserrat E, Salvador R, et al. Real-time ultrasound for diagnosis of symptomatic venous thrombosis and for screening of patients at risk: correlation with ascending conventional venography. *Angiology* 1989;6:527–533.

28. Habscheid W, Hohmann M, Wilhelm T, Epping J. Real-time ultrasound in the diagnosis of acute deep venous thrombosis of the lower extremity. *Angiology* 1990;7:599–608.

29. Mussurakis S, Papaioannou S, Voros D, Vrakatselis T. Compression ultrasonography as a reliable imaging monitor in deep venous thrombosis. *Surg Gynecol Obstet* 1990;171:233–239.

30. Pedersen OM, Aslaksen A, Vik-Mo H, Bassoe AM. Compression ultrasonography in hospitalized patients with suspected deep venous thrombosis. *Arch Intern Med* 1991;151:2217–2220.

31. Ginsberg JS, Caco CC, Brill-Edwards PA, et al. Venous thrombosis in patients who have undergone major hip or knee surgery: detection with compression US and impedance plethysmography. *Radiology* 1991;181:651–654.

32. Heijboer H, Buller HR, Lensing AWA, Turpie AGG, Colly LP, Wouter Ten Cate J. A comparison of real-time compression ultrasonography wit impedance plethysmography for the diagnosis of deep-vein thrombosis in symptomatic outpatients. *N Engl J Med* 1993;329:1365–1369.

33. Borris LC, Christiansen HM, Lassen MR, Olsen AD, Schott P. Comparison of real-time B-mode ultrasonography and bilateral ascending phlebography for detection of postoperative deep vein thrombosis following elective hip surgery. *Thromb Haemost* 1989;61:363–365.

34. Jongbloets LMM, Lensing AWA, Koopman MMW, Buller HR, W ten Cate J. Limitations of compression ultrasound for the detection of symptomless postoperative deep vein thrombosis. *Lancet* 1994;343:1142–1144.

35. Oliver MA. Duplex scanning in venous disease. *Bruit* 1985;9:206–209.

36. Langsfeld M, Hershey FB, Thorpe L, et al. Duplex B-mode imaging for the diagnosis of deep venous thrombosis. *Arch Surg* 1987;122:587–591.

37. George JE, Smith MO, Berry RE. Duplex scanning for the detection of deep venous thrombosis of lower extremities in a community hospital. *Curr Surg* 1987;44:202–204.

38. Vogel P, Laing FC, Jeffrey RB Jr, Wing VW. Deep venous thrombosis of the lower extremity: US evaluation. *Radiology* 1987;163:747–751.

39. Elias A, LeCorff G, Bouvier JL, Benichou M, Serradimigni A. Value of real time B mode ultrasound imaging in the diagnosis of deep vein thrombosis of the lower limbs. *Int Angiol* 1987;6:175–182.

40. Comerota AJ, Katz ML, Grossi RJ, et al. The comparative value of noninvasive testing for diagnosis and surveillance of deep vein thrombosis. *J Vasc Surg* 1988;7:40–49.

41. O'Leary DH, Kane RA, Chase BM. A prospective study of the efficacy of B-scan sonography in the detection of deep venous thrombosis in the lower extremities. *J Clin Ultrasound* 1988;16:1–8.

42. Rosner NH, Doris PE. Diagnosis of femoropopliteal venous thrombosis: comparison of duplex sonography and plethysmography. *AJR* 1988;150:623–627.

43. Killewich LA, Bedford GR, Beach KW, Strandness DE. Diagnosis of deep venous thrombosis: a prospective study comparing duplex scanning to contrast venography. *Circulation* 1989;79:810–814.

44. Comerota AJ, Katz ML, Greenwald LL, Leefmans E, Czeredarczuk M, White JV. Venous duplex imaging: should it replace hemodynamic tests for deep venous thrombosis? *J Vasc Surg* 1990;11:53–61.

45. Lee B, Lea Thomas M, Burnand KG, Browse NL. Comparative trial of ascending phlebography versus duplex ultrasonography in the diagnosis of deep venous thrombosis. *Br J Surg* 1990;77:A701.

46. Cavaye D, Kelly AT, Graham JC, Appleberg M, Briggs GM. Duplex ultrasound diagnosis of lower limb deep venous thrombosis. *Aust NZ J Surg* 1990;60:283–288.

47. Ezekowitz MD, Migliaccio F, Farlow D, et al. Comparison of platelet scintigraphy, impedance plethysmography gray scale and color flow duplex ultrasound and venography for the diagnosis of venous thrombosis. *Prog Clin Biol Res* 1990;355:23–27.

48. Mitchell DC, Grasty MS, Stebbings WSL, et al. Comparison of duplex ultrasonography and venography in the diagnosis of deep venous thrombosis. *Br J Surg* 1991;78:611–613.

49. van Ramshorst B, Legemate DA, Verzijibergen JF, et al. Duplex scanning in the diagnosis of acute deep vein thrombosis of the lower extremity. *Eur J Vasc Surg* 1991;5:255–260.

50. AbuRahma AF, Kennard W, Robinson PA, Boland JP, Young LL, Alberts S. The judicial use of venous duplex imaging and strain gauge plethysmography (single or combined) in the diagnosis of acute and chronic deep vein thrombosis. *Surg Gynecol Obstet* 1992;174:52–58.

51. Size GP, Peterson DL, Laubach M, et al. Our experience with venous duplex imaging for the diagnosis of symptomatic deep vein thrombosis. *J Vasc Technol* 1993;17:87–89.

52. Froehlich JA, Dorfman GS, Cronan JJ, Urbanek PJ, Herndon JH, Aaron RK. Compression ultrasonography for the detection of deep venous thrombosis in patients who have a fracture of the hip. *J Bone Joint Surg* 1989;71-A:249–256.

53. Barnes CL, Nelson CL, Nix ML, McCowan TC, Lavender RC, Barnes RW: Duplex scanning versus venography as a screening examination in total hip arthroplasty patients. *Clin Orthop* 1991;271:180–189.

54. Grady-Benson JC, Oishi CS, Hanson PB, Colwell CW Jr, Otis SM, Walker RH. Routine postoperative duplex ultrasonography screening and monitoring for the detection of deep vein thrombosis. *Clin Orthop* 1994;307:130–141.

55. Foley WD, Middleton WD, Lawson TL, Erickson S, Quiroz FA, Macrander S. Color Doppler ultrasound imaging of lower-extremity venous disease. *AJR* 1989;152:371–376.

56. Rose SC, Zwiebel WJ, Nelson BD, et al. Symptomatic lower extremity deep venous thrombosis: accuracy, limitations and role of color duplex flow imaging in diagnosis. *Radiology* 1990;175:639–644.

57. Schindler JM, Kaiser M, Gerber A, Vuilliomenet A, Popovic A, Bertel O. Colour coded duplex sonography in suspected deep vein thrombosis of the leg. *Br Med J* 1990;301:1369–1370.

58. Yucel EK, Fisher JS, Egglin TK, Geller SC, Waltman AC. Isolated calf venous thrombosis: diagnosis with compression US. *Radiology* 1991;179:443–446.

59. Mattos MA, Londrey GL, Leutz DW, et al. Color-flow duplex scanning for the surveillance and diagnosis of acute deep venous thrombosis. *J Vasc Surg* 1992;15:366–376.

60. Kalodiki E, Marston R, Volteas N, et al. The combination of liquid crystal thermography and duplex scanning in the diagnosis of deep vein thrombosis. *Eur J Vasc Surg* 1992;6:311–316.

61. Baxter GM, Duffy P, Partridge E. Colour flow imaging of calf vein thrombosis. *Clin Radiol* 1992;46:198–201.

62. Bradley MJ, Spencer PA, Alexander L, Milner GR. Colour flow mapping in the diagnosis of the calf deep vein thrombosis. *Clin Radiol* 1993;47:399–402.

63. Labropoulos N, Leon M, Kalodiki E, Al Kutoubi A, Chan P, Nicolaides AN: Colour flow duplex scanning in suspected acute deep vein thrombosis; experience with routine use. *Eur J Vasc Endovasc Surg* 1995;9:49–52.

64. Davidson BL, Elliott CG, Lensing AWA. Low accuracy of color Doppler ultrasound in the detection of proximal leg vein thrombosis in asymptomatic high-risk patients. *Ann Intern Med* 1992;117:735–738.

65. Haeger K. Problems of acute deep venous thrombosis. *Angiology* 1969;20:219–223.

66. Barnes RW, Wu KK, Hoak JC. Fallibility of the clinical diagnosis of venous thrombosis. *JAMA* 1975;234:605–607.

67. Cranley JJ, Canos AJ, Sull WJ. The diagnosis of deep venous thrombosis. *Arch Surg* 1976;111:34–36.

68. Landefeld CS, McGuire E, Cohen AM. Clinical findings associated with acute proximal deep vein thrombosis: a basis for quantifying clinical judgement. *Amer J Med* 1990;88:382–388.

69. Nypaver TJ, Shepard AD, Kiell CS, McPharlin M, Fenn N, Ernst CB. Outpatient duplex scanning for deep vein thrombosis: parameters predictive of a negative study result. *J Vasc Surg* 1993;18:821–826.

70. Rosenow EC III. Venous and pulmonary thromboembolism: an algorithmic approach to diagnosis and management. *May Clin Proc* 1995;70:45–49.

71. Wells PS, Hirsh J, Anderson DR, et al. Accuracy of clinical assessment of deep-vein thrombosis. *Lancet* 1995;345:1326–1330.

72. Bundens WP, Bergan JJ, Halasz NA, Murray J, Drehobl M. The superficial femoral vein: a potentially lethal misnomer. *JAMA* 1995;274:1296–1298.

73. Aronen HJ, Pamilo M, Suoranta HT, Suramo I. Sonography in differential diagnosis of deep venous thrombosis of the leg. *Acta Radiol* 1987;28:457–459.

74. Cronan JJ, Dorfman GS, Grusmark J. Lower-extremity deep venous thrombosis: further experience with and refinements of US assessment. *Radiology* 1988;168:101–107.

75. Sluzewski M, Koopman MMW, Schuur KH, van Vroonhoven Th. JMV, Ruijs JHJ. Influence of negative ultrasound findings on the management of in- and outpatients with suspected deep-vein thrombosis. *Eur J Radiol* 1991;13:174–177.

76. Barnes RW, Nix ML, Barnes CL, et al. Perioperative asymptomatic venous thrombosis: role of duplex scanning versus venography. *J Vasc Surg* 1989;9:251–260.

77. Flinn WR, Sandager GP, Cerullo LJ, Havey RJ, Yao JST. Duplex venous scanning for the prospective surveillance of perioperative venous thrombosis. *Arch Surg* 1989;124:901–905.

78. White RH, Goulet JA, Bray TJ, Daschbach MM, McGahan JP, Hartling RP. Deep-vein thrombosis after fracture of the pelvis: assessment with serial duplex-ultrasound screening. *J Bone Joint Surg* 1990;72A:495–500.

79. Babcock SL, Villemure PA, Erlandson EE, et al. Duplex venous imaging for surveillance of patients undergoing total joint arthroplasty. *J Vasc Technol* 1991;15(1):11–14.

80. Woolson ST, Watt M. Intermittent pneumatic compression to prevent proximal deep venous thrombosis during and after total hip replacement. *J Bone Joint Surg* 1991;73-A:507–512.

81. Winkler JL, Lohr JM, Lutter KS, Spirtoff K, Cranley JJ. Lower extremity venous duplex imaging of asymptomatic patients: our one-year experience. *J Vasc Technol* 1992;16:167–171.

82. Kraay MJ, Goldberg VM, Herbener TE. Vascular ultrasonography for deep venous thrombosis after total knee arthroplasty. *Clin Orthop* 1993;286:18–26.

83. Babcock SL, Higginbotham CC, Lampman RM, et al. Venous duplex imaging for surveillance of patients undergoing total joint arthroplasty: a three-year study. *J Vasc Technol* 1994;18:75–79.

84. Wells PS, Lensing AWA, Davidson BL, Prins MH, Hirsh J. Accuracy of ultrasound for the diagnosis of deep venous thrombosis in asymptomatic patients after orthopedic surgery. *Ann Intern Med* 1995;122:47–53.

85. Tremaine MD, Choroszy CJ, Menking SA, et al. Duplex ultrasound evaluation for acute deep venous thrombosis in 962 total joint arthroplasty patients. *J Vasc Technol* 1995;19:25–29.

86. Meyer CS, Blebea J, Davis K Jr, Fowl RJ, Kempczinski RF. Surveillance venous scans for deep venous thrombosis in multiple trauma patients. *Ann Vasc Surg* 1995;9:109–114.

87. Meibers DJ, Baldridge ED, Ruoff BA, Karkow WS, Cranley JJ. The significance of calf muscle venous thrombosis. *J Vasc Technol* 1988;12:143–149.

88. Semrow CM, Friedell ML, Buchbinder D, Rollins DL. The efficacy of ultrasonic venography in the detection of calf vein thrombosis. *J Vasc Technol* 1988;12:240–244.

89. van Bemmelen PS, Bedford G, Strandness DE. Visualization of calf veins by color flow imaging. *Ultrasound Med Biol* 1990;16:15–17.

90. Solis MM, Ranval TJ, Nix ML, et al. Is anticoagulation indicated for asymptomatic postoperative calf vein thrombosis? *J Vasc Surg* 1992;16:414–419.

91. Messina LM, Sarpa MS, Smith MA, Greenfield LJ. Clinical significance of routine imaging of iliac and calf veins by color flow duplex scanning in patients suspected of having acute lower extremity deep venous thrombosis. *Surgery* 1993;114:921–927.

92. Lohr JM, James KV, Deshmukh RM, Hasselfeld KA. Calf vein thrombi are not a benign finding. *Am J Surg* 1995;170:86–90.

93. Giannoukas AD, Labropoulos N, Burke P, Katsamouris A, Nicolaides AN. Calf deep venous thrombosis: a review of the literature. *Eur J Vasc Endovasc Surg* 1995;10:398–404.

94. Strandness DE Jr, Langlois Y, Cramer M, Randlett A, Thiele BL. Long-term sequelae of acute venous thrombosis. *JAMA* 1983;250(10):1289–1292.

95. Killewich LA, Bedford GR, Beach KW, Strandness DE Jr. Spontaneous lysis of deep venous thrombi: rate and outcome. *J Vasc Surg* 1989;9:89–97.

96. Krupski WC, Bass A, Dilley RB, Bernstein EF, Otis SM. Propagation of deep venous thrombosis identified by duplex ultrasonography. *J Vasc Surg* 1990;12:467–475.

97. Murphy TP, Cronan JJ. Evolution of deep venous thrombosis: a prospective evaluation with US. *Radiology* 1990;177:543–548.

98. Mantoni M. Deep venous thrombosis: longitudinal study with duplex US. *Radiology* 1991;179:271–273.

99. Meissner MH, Manzo RA, Bergelin RO, Markel A, Strandness DE Jr. Deep venous insufficiency: the relationship between lysis and subsequent reflux. *J Vasc Surg* 1993;18:596–608.

100. van Ramshorst B, van Bemmelen PS, Hoeneveld H, Eikelboom BC. The development of valvular incompetence after deep vein thrombosis: a follow-up study with duplex scanning. *J Vasc Surg* 1994;19:1059–1066.

101. Johnson BF, Manzo RA, Bergelin RO, Strandness DE Jr. Relationship between changes in the deep venous system and the development of the postthrombotic syndrome after an acute episode of lower limb deep vein thrombosis: a one- to six-year follow-up. *J Vasc Surg* 1995;21:307–313.

102. Caprini JA, Arcelus JI, Hoffman KN, et al. Venous duplex imaging follow-up of acute symptomatic deep vein thrombosis of the leg. *J Vasc Surg* 1995;21:472–476.

103. Caps MT, Manzo RA, Bergelin RO, Meissner MH, Strandness DE Jr. Venous valvular reflux in veins not involved at the time of acute deep vein thrombosis. *J Vasc Surg* 1995;22:524–531.

104. Cogo A, Lensing AWA, Prandoni P, Hirsh J. Distribution of thrombosis in patients with symptomatic deep vein thrombosis. *Arch Intern Med* 1993;153:2777–2780.

105. Nix ML, Blackburn D. Should bilateral venous duplex imaging be performed in a patient with unilateral leg symptoms? *J Vasc Technol* 1994;18:211–212.

106. Blackburn D. Bilateral examination. *J Vasc Technol* 1994;18:213–214.

107. Lohr JM, Hasselfeld KA, Byne MP, Deshmukh RM, Cranley JJ. Does the asymptomatic limb harbor deep venous thrombosis? *Am J Surg* 1994;168:184–187.

108. Strothman G, Blebea J, Fowl RJ, Rosenthal G. Contralateral duplex scanning for deep venous thrombosis is unnecessary in patients with symptoms. *J Vasc Surg* 1995;22:543–547.

109. Poppiti R, Papanicolaou G, Perese S, Weaver FA. Limited B-mode venous imaging versus complete color-flow duplex venous scanning for detection of proximal deep venous thrombosis. *J Vasc Surg* 1995;22:553–557.

110. Barnes RW, Wu KK, Hoak JC. Differentiation of superficial thrombophlebitis from lymphangitis by Doppler ultrasound. *Surg Gynecol Obstet* 1976;143:23–25.

111. Sainte-Luce P, Dauzat M, Laroche JP, et al. Social and economical effectiveness of non-invasive vascular examinations in the clinical management of thrombo-embolic disease. *Int Angiol* 1987;6:203–208.

112. Kelley MH, Carson JL, Palevsky HI, Schwartz JS. Diagnosing pulmonary embolism: new facts and strategies. *Ann Intern Med* 1991;114:300–306.

113. Oudkerk M, van Beek EJR, van Putten WLJ, Buller HR. Cost-effectiveness analysis of various strategies in the diagnostic management of pulmonary embolism. *Arch Intern Med* 1993;153:947–954.

114. Killewich LA, Nunnelee JD, Auer AI. Value of lower extremity venous duplex examination in the diagnosis of pulmonary embolism. *J Vasc Surg* 1993;17:934–939.

115. Dalen JE. When can treatment be withheld in patients with suspected pulmonary embolism? *Arch Intern Med* 1993;153:1415–1418.

116. Beecham RP, Dorfman GS, Cronan JJ, Spearman MP, Murphy TP, Scola FH. Is bilateral lower extremity compression sonography useful and cost-effective in the evaluation of suspected pulmonary embolism? *AJR* 1993;161:1289–1292.

117. Smith LL, Knoedler J, Hollerman JJ. Calf vein duplex imaging in the work-up of patients with clinically suspected pulmonary embolism. *J Vasc Technol* 1994;18:9–13.

118. Hull R, Hirsh J, Sackett DL, Stoddart G. Cost effectiveness of clinical diagnosis, venography, and noninvasive testing in patients with symptomatic deep-vein thrombosis. *N Engl J Med* 1981;304:1561–1567.

119. Paiement GD, Wessinger SJ, Harris WH. Cost-effectiveness of prophylaxis in total hip replacement. *Am J Surg* 1991;161:519–524.

120. Hillner BE, Philbrick JT, Becker DM. Optimal management of suspected lower-extremity deep vein thrombosis: an evaluation with cost assessment of 24 management strategies. *Arch Intern Med* 1992;152:165–175.

121. Strandness DE Jr, Andros G, Baker JD, Bernstein EF. Vascular laboratory utilization and payment: report of the Ad Hoc Committee of the Western Vascular Society. *J Vasc Surg* 1992;16:163–170.

122. Fillinger MF, Zwolak RM, Musson AM, Cronenwett JL. Vascular laboratory cost analysis and the impact of the Resource-Based Relative Value Scale payment system. *J Vasc Surg* 1993;17:267–279.

123. Baker JD. Costs of duplex scanning and the impact of the changes in Medicare reimbursement. *J Vasc Surg* 1993;18:702–707.

124. Baker JD. The vascular laboratory: regulations and other challenges. *J Vasc Surg* 1994;19:901–904.

125. Lohr JM, James KV, Hasselfeld KA, Deshmukh RM, Winkler JL. Vascular laboratory personnel on-call: effect on patient management. *J Vasc Surg* 1995;22:548–552.

67

Upper Extremity Venous Thrombosis

Herbert I. Machleder, M.D.

Upper extremity venous thrombosis usually becomes evident in one of two clinically distinct situations. These two categories have generally been referred to as *primary* and *secondary axillosubclavian vein thrombosis*. Primary venous thrombosis has also been described as spontaneous, or effort-related, thrombosis or by the eponym *Paget-Schroetter syndrome*. Secondary venous thrombosis is a more heterogeneous entity, and in modern clinical practice is a not uncommon consequence of upper extremity venous catheterization for either temporary or permanent central venous or cardiac access. Venous access for dialysis or central lines, for chronic alimentation, antibiotic, or chemotherapy delivery, as well as chronic pacemaker wires have a high incidence of asymptomatic or symptomatic axillosubclavian vein thrombosis.

The development of catheter-directed thrombolytic therapy and transvascular angioplastic techniques, coupled with surgical techniques based on a better understanding of underlying anatomic abnormalities, has led to a dramatic evolution in the treatment of upper extremity venous thrombosis. This evolution combines the newer vascular interventional methods with more traditional surgical techniques and has resulted in significantly better success in dealing with upper extremity venous thrombosis.

HISTORICAL BACKGROUND

After 100 years of sporadic reports on spontaneous thrombosis of the axillary-subclavian vein, Hughes undertook the first significant analysis of the problem in 1949. He wrote in the *International Abstracts of Surgery*, "The association of a more or less acute venous obstruction in the upper extremity of an otherwise perfectly healthy person constitutes a syndrome which, in the absence of accurate knowledge of the etiology and pathology, can be called the 'Paget-Schroetter syndrome,' after the first two to describe it as a clinical entity." He also credited Professor Ranzi of Pisa (1849) as the first to suggest "effort" as the cause of the thrombosis. Over the course of subsequent investigations, it became evident that in contrast to the apparently spontaneous nature of the event, there is an underlying chronic venous compressive anomaly at the thoracic outlet.[1]

In 1985 a clinical management strategy based on contemporary concepts of pathophysiology and a multidisciplinary approach to therapy was initiated at the UCLA Medical Center and subsequently applied to 50 consecutive patients. The results of this therapeutic approach were reported in 1989, then updated and extensively analyzed in 1992.[2,3]

As in other thrombotic venous disorders, the ultimate outcome is to a considerable extent determined by the effectiveness of the initial therapy. Consequently, the following discussion will outline a successful interventional algorithm for the initial thrombotic event and definitive management of the underlying anatomic abnormality.

PATHOLOGIC ANATOMY AND PHYSIOLOGY

The acute thrombosis most often occurs in an area of chronic compression and stricture of the axillosubclavian vein at the costoclavicular space (Figs. 67–1 and 67–2). The vein is compressed between a hypertrophied scalene or subclavius tendon and the first rib, with a large exostosis often found at the costoclavicular junction. (Fig. 67–3).

The natural history of the disease reflects the development of venous hypertension due to chronic venous compression, with acute symptoms resulting from sudden thrombosis and obstruction of collateral veins.

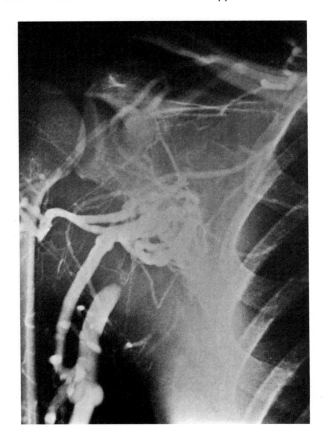

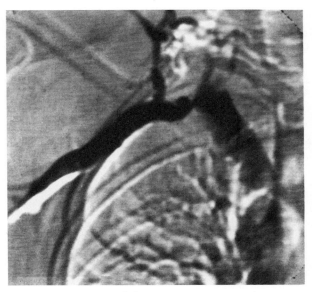

Figure 67–2. Area of chronic compression at the costoclavicular (thoracic outlet) portion of the subclavian vein. This compressive abnormality is revealed after successful lytic therapy for the acute thrombosis.

Figure 67–1. Acute, spontaneous thrombosis of the axillosubclavian vein.

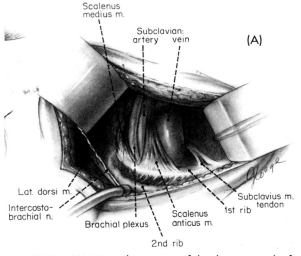

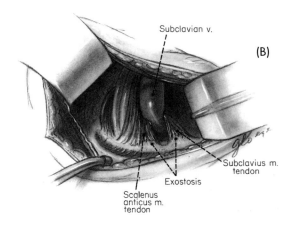

Figure 67–3. (A) Normal anatomy of the thoracic outlet from the transaxillary surgical approach. (B) Typical deformity seen in patients with the Paget-Schroetter syndrome. (Compare it with the radiologic picture in Fig. 67–2).

MANAGEMENT

Clinical Presentation

The typical presentation includes the sudden onset of a feeling of heaviness, with noticeable swelling and mild cyanosis of the affected extremity. Some patients report premonitory symptoms of transitory swelling with resolution, occurring within several months of the presenting symptoms. Increased venous prominence, collateral vein appearance, and axillary tenderness are characteristic.

Laboratory Evaluation

To confirm the diagnosis, all patients should have venography, with the arms in the neutral and abducted positions. Ninety-three percent of patients in our series had complete thrombotic obstruction, and 7% had evidence of external compression or stricture without evidence of residual thrombus. High-grade stenosis, with probable intermittent occlusion, was suspected in 14 of Hughes' collected cases and was analyzed later in more detail by McLeery et al.[4] A surprising finding in the UCLA series, not previously reported, was the high incidence (68%) of thrombosis or compressive stricture of the contralateral vein. Routine hematologic, serum chemistry, and coagulation studies are generally unremarkable in this group of patients.

Treatment

The algorithm for management that we follow includes verification of the diagnosis by venography followed by local thrombolytic therapy and anticoagulation for up to 4 weeks. After that time, patients with stable occlusion of the axillosubclavian vein are evaluated for residual symptoms. For those patients with significant disability, decompression of the costoclavicular space by transaxillary first rib resection is recommended. Patients with patent but compressed axillosubclavian veins are likewise treated with first rib resection. Following that procedure, percutaneous transluminal balloon angioplasty is utilized to correct residual venous stenosis or stricture when this is demonstrated on follow-up venography.

Local Thrombolytic Therapy

In recent years, the superiority of local thrombolytic therapy over systemic infusion of fibrinolytic agents has been demonstrated, particularly for the treatment of axillosubclavian vein thrombosis.[5–7] Venography should be performed via the basilic vein of the affected extremity. A separate retrograde innominate or superior vena caval injection from a transfemoral approach can be utilized in selected cases to obtain better visualization of the central veins.

When thrombus is visualized in the brachial, axillary, or subclavian veins, a small catheter is positioned in the clot via the percutaneous basilic vein approach. An attempt is made to traverse the clot with either a guidewire or a catheter to establish a channel prior to infusion. A loading dose of 250,000 IU urokinase is infused into the clot over 1 hour (4000 IU/minute). Infusion at this rate can be continued for an additional hour and then reduced to 1000 IU/minute for up to 24 hours.[8,9]

A recent review of our experience with 76 patients has clarified certain elements of diagnosis and treatment that we consider axiomatic.[10] The UCLA approach can be outlined as follows:

1. Any individual with swelling of the arm without an obvious cause (eg, cellulitis, insect bite, hematoma) should have a venogram. If the subclavian vein is patent, the venogram should be done in the neutral as well as the stress position (hand behind the head). In this way, a positionally compressive abnormality will not be overlooked.

2. If a thrombus is encountered, catheter-directed lytic therapy is the most effective way to restore patency. Heparin is used concomitantly. Then anticoagulation with Coumadin is established prior to discharge from the hospital.

3. We recommend avoiding the temptation to dilate the narrow segment. The external compression cannot be corrected by balloon dilatation. For a convincing demonstration, place the arm in the stress position and repeat the venogram. Dilation in the acute situation further damages the intima of the vein and invites rethrombosis in a high percentage of patients. (Fig. 67–4).

4. Avoid the temptation to place a stent in the costoclavicular portion of the subclavian vein. The repetitive compressing forces of the clavicle and first rib lead to deformity or fragmentation of the stent, rethrombosis, and a very unsatisfactory situation.

5. Correction of the thoracic outlet compression immediately after the transluminal procedure will often lead to rethrombosis. We initially delayed repair for 3 months based on very basic studies of vein healing. In cases of expeditious treatment and rapid clot lysis, we now often proceed, after a 4-week period, to surgical correction of the thoracic outlet compression.

6. Unless the thrombosis occurred in a very unusual setting, in a generally sedentary patient, it is recommended that the patient undergo definitive correction of the thoracic outlet compression. Thirty-six percent of our surgically uncorrected patients had recurrent episodes of venographically demonstrated thrombosis. No patient has had recurrence of

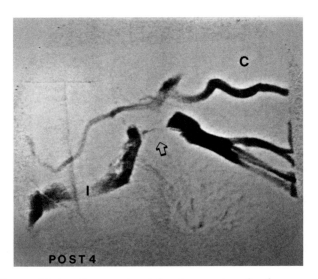

Figure 67–4. Compressive deformity remains after four attempts at balloon dilatation following successful lytic therapy but prior to surgical decompression.

thrombosis after surgical correction during 10 years of follow-up.

7. Transaxillary resection of the first rib provides the best access to decompress this portion of the thoracic outlet and permits full visualization of the axillosubclavian venous segment, with a minimum of disruption of other tissue planes. There are excellent reviews of the surgical approach.[11,12]

UCLA EXPERIENCE

Demographics

From 1985 until the present, 76 patients have been treated in accordance with the original algorithm. This group of patients includes 45 men with a mean age of 27 years and 31 women with a mean age of 31 years. Seventy-one of the patients were right hand dominant and the remaining five were left hand dominant. In 48 patients the side of the thrombosis was the right arm and in 28 patients it was the left arm.

In classifying their major daily activities; 21 of the patients were professional or student athletes, 21 were laborers, and 3 were white-collar workers. Seven of these patients were engaged in sedentary activity at the onset of thrombosis, and 69 were directly engaged in some vigorous upper extremity activity just prior to the onset of edema and cyanosis. In further characterizing their usual daily activities, 19 would be considered relatively sedentary individuals and the remaining 57 very active. Thirty-two were avid recreational athletes. Five were weight lifters, and three were rowers. There were two basketball players, baseball players, skiers, swimmers, and aerobic exercisers. There was one representative of the following sports: gymnastics, jogging, cycling, golfing, handball, boxing, soccer, tennis, volleyball, and wrestling.

Clinical Presentation

The most common presentation is the young student athlete with sudden swelling of the upper extremity. The treatment of this group illustrates the most direct therapeutic approach. We have treated 17 student athletes, the average age of the 14 boys being 18 years and that of the 3 girls 21 years. Amont the young men there were four baseball players, two basketball players, two rowers, one swimmer, and five weight lifters. Of the young women, two were competitive swimmers and one was on a rowing crew. The presentation of sudden edema and cyanosis is characteristic, with patients appearing expeditiously for treatment. Clot lysis is usually prompt, within 24 hours, and the vein appears quite satisfactory in the neutral position. Venography in the stress position demonstrates the site of the compressive abnormality. Surgical repair is usually delayed for 4 weeks while the patient remains on Coumadin.

Another group of individuals, usually somewhat older, typically presents with a chronic thrombus that resists lysis. Initially, an explanation for the sudden onset of edema was perplexing. After repetitive study of several patients during acute exacerbations of edema, it became evident that older individuals develop chronic fibrosis in the area of compression, often with a small attached chronic thrombus. Collateral venous circulation develops over a period of time and results in minimal transient symptoms during vigorous activity. These episodes are often overlooked by the patient. On unexpected occasions the area destabilizes and the thrombus propagates, blocking the collateral veins, which are often in close proximity to the compressed area. With thrombus propagation and obstruction of collaterals, the arm becomes edematous and swollen. With rapid sequential studies we have seen spontaneous clot lysis and return to the baseline situation in two patients.

In patients who do not experience spontaneous remission, the initial lytic therapy dissolves the new thrombus, revealing the well-developed collateral veins and the usually very discrete area of chronic thrombus. Unfortunately, these patients remain at risk for recurrent events. Following surgical correction, with the use of serial venography we have observed the vein recanalize and respond to transluminal dilatation. We have managed 30 patients with residual chronic occlusions of the subclavian vein. Four of these patients remained relatively asymptomatic and nondisabled for their usual occupation. We have recommended no further therapy. Nine of these patients continue to be symptomatic and may yet benefit from a surgical approach. We have proceeded with thoracic outlet decompression in 17 patients with residual occlusion. Ten are asymptomatic and unrestricted, and seven have residual symptoms.

There is another group of patients with stable occlusion of the axillosubclavian vein whose progress we have followed. Some of them complain of very transient episodes of cyanosis, lasting for minutes, occasionally followed by swelling lasting for minutes or up to an hour. Initially, these patients were referred for venous bypass or had a venous reconstructive procedure. Based on careful observations, we have come to recognize that these patients have more extensive thoracic outlet compression. Their symptoms reflect autonomic instability rather than transient venous hypertension. These symptoms derive from sympathetic stimulation from compression of the inferior trunk of the brachial plexus, the source of sympathetic innervation of the arm. Decompression of the thoracic outlet with specific attention to the brachial plexus area, particularly the C8–T1 nerve roots, will relieve these symptoms. Venous reconstruction will usually provide no benefit.

In this regard, it is essential to recognize that a significant number of patients with effort thrombosis will have some symptoms based on coincidental arterial or brachial plexus compression. We have found the most useful way of evaluating the neurogenic component to be assessment of somatosensory evoked responses or the electromyography-guided scalene muscle block. When the anterior scalene muscle is identified by its characteristic electromyographic response, with the use of a shielded needle, the muscle can be infiltrated with a small amount of local anesthetic. This avoids a brachial plexus or sympathetic block. In affected patients, there is prompt and profound relief of symptoms and reversal of the provocative tests findings. Relaxation of the anterior scalene muscle permits the first rib to descend, relieving costoclavicular compression. In addition, there is relief of compression in the interscalene triangle, where the subclavian artery and brachial plexus pass between the anterior and middle scalene muscles.

Percutaneous Transluminal Angioplasty

We have avoided dilating the vein following successful lytic therapy based on considerable experience with the complications of this strategy. One exception to that rule has been in cases of very-high-grade stricture associated with external compression. In these instances, where the postlytic venogram suggests very poor flow across the damaged area, we have dilated the stricture with a 4-mm balloon. This tends to rupture some of the synichia without unduly damaging the remaining intima. Better flow is then evident across the stenosed area during the healing process. We have resorted to this tactic on two occasions.

Following surgical decompression we restudy the vein usually at about 1 month. If a hemodynamically significant stricture remains on cross-sectional area assessment, corroborated by residual large collaterals, we dilate the vein to 1 cm and maintain the patient on 4 additional weeks of anticoagulant protection with Coumadin (Fig. 67–5). We have never stented the area and discourage this practice. Long-term venographic follow-up of our patients has demonstrated the transluminal angioplasty to be durable in this situation. Fourteen (22%) of our patients, who satisfied the above criteria, underwent postoperative transluminal angioplasty.

We have encountered two young patients with recurrent edema and cyanosis with a normal-appearing venogram. After somewhat exasperating follow-up, very careful restudy by venography demonstrated a fine web or diaphragm at the costoclavicular portion of the subclavian vein. This likely represented some residual valve leaflet fusion, barely discernible on conventional venography. There was no evidence of residual compression in the stress position. Inflation of a transluminal balloon revealed the thin diaphragm. This was followed by complete relief of symptoms.

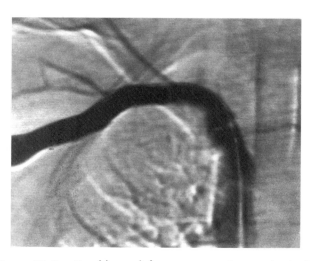

Figure 67–5. Durable result from postoperative transluminal angioplasty. Stents were not necessary in this group of patients.

The Contralateral Vein

Sixty-one percent of our patients studied with bilateral venography had thrombosis or compression of the contralateral vein. Consequently, we recommend study of the contralateral vein whenever this is possible. When a patient presents with thrombosis in the nondominant arm, we recommend subsequent elective repair of the contralateral side when the vein in the dominant arm demonstrates the potential for thrombosis and the patient is in an occupation that predisposes to further risk. In 41 patients we obtained full bilateral venographic studies. Eleven of these patients had a normal contralateral vein. Twenty patients demonstrated evidence of compression and stricture in the neutral position, and five had evidence of hemodynamically significant compression in the stress position. Five patients underwent occlusion of the contralateral vein during the course of our initial review. Seventy-three percent of the patients studied had a bilateral abnormality, and 12% went on to bilateral thrombosis.

Results

In reviewing the results of treatment in this group of patients, there were 63 surgical procedures at the thoracic outlet, including five patients who were treated bilaterally. We have classified the results into seven general categories. Four patients with occluded veins were not treated surgically and remained essentially asymptomatic (5%). Nine patients had chronic occlusion of the subclavian vein, declined surgical correction, and remained symptomatic or disabled (12%). Seven patients had chronic venous occlusion and underwent surgical correction but remained symptomatic (9%). A similar group of 10 patients, with chronic subclavian vein occlusion, underwent surgical decompression and remained essentially asymptomatic when returned to their usual activity (13%). In 46 patients we were able to restore normal patency. Five of these patients did not have surgical correction, and remained patent and asymptomatic (7%). One patient had a patent vein but remained symptomatic postoperatively. Forty patients with restoration of normal patency were asymptomatic and returned to normal activity after surgical correction (53%). No patient treated surgically experienced an episode of rethrombosis during the 10 years of medical follow-up.

Sixty-four of the patients returned to their usual activity without restriction (84%). Seven workers required retraining for a less physically stressful occupation. Five individuals remained disabled for their usual work or accustomed recreational activity.

Based on the outcome of 76 patients, treated over a 10-year period, it remains evident that an algorithm directed toward treating the acute event and then correcting the underlying anatomic abnormality yields excellent results with very low risk. This approach appropriately utilizes well-established contemporary techniques from the disciplines of medicine, surgery, and interventional radiology.

REFERENCES

1. Daskalakis E, Bouhoutsos J. Subclavian and axillary vein compression of musculoskeletal origin. *Br J Surg* 1980;67:573–576.
2. Kunkel JM, Machleder HI. Treatment of Paget-Schroetter syndrome; a staged, multidisciplinary approach. *Arch Surg* 1989;124:1153–1158.
3. Machleder HI. Evaluation of a new treatment strategy for Paget-Schroetter's syndrome: spontaneous thrombosis of the axillary-subclavian vein. *J Vasc Surg* 1993;17:305–317.
4. McCleery RS, Kesterson JE, Kirtley JA. Subclavius and anterior scalene muscle compression as a cause of intermittent obstruction of the subclavian vein. *Arch Surg* 1981;133:588–602.
5. Zimmerman R, Morl H, Harenberg J, et al. Urokinase therapy of subclavian-axillary vein thrombosis. *Klin Wochenschr* 1981;59:851–856.
6. Becker GJ, Holden RW, Rabe FE, et al. Local thrombolytic therapy for subclavian and axillary vein thrombosis. *Radiology* 1983;149:419–423.
7. Machleder HI. The role of thrombolytic agents for acute subclavian vein thrombosis. *Semin Vasc Surg* 1992;2:82–88.
8. McNamara TO, Fischer JR. Thrombolysis of peripheral arterial and graft occlusions: improved results using high-dose urokinase. *AJR* 1985;144:769–755.
9. Machleder HI. Upper extremith venous thrombosis. *Semin Vasc Surg* 1990;3:219–226.
10. Machleder HI. Thrombolytic therapy and surgery for primary axillosubclavian vein thrombosis: current approach. *Semin Vasc Surg* 1996;9:46–49.
11. Roos DB. Essentials and safeguards of surgery for thoracic outlet syndrome. *Angiology* 1981;32:187–193.
12. Machleder HI. Transaxillary operative management of thoracic outlet syndrome. In: C. Ernst and J. Stanley, eds. *Current Therapy in Vascular Surgery*, 2nd ed. Philadelphia: BC Decker; 1994:227–230.

68

The Clinical Presentation and Diagnostic Evaluation of Chronic Venous Insufficiency

Seshadri Raju, M.D., F.A.C.S.

It is estimated that up to 2% of the general population suffer from severe forms of chronic venous insufficiency. Milder forms are more ubiquitous. The disease has a varied clinical presentation, and the broad spectrum of clinical features has been stratified by a worldwide consensus panel into a classification system based on clinical severity[1] (Table 68–1). A useful functional classification, based on work ability, is presented in Table 68–2.

CLINICAL PRESENTATION

Chronic venous insufficiency affects individuals with a wide range of ages from preadolescents to the elderly. Symptoms are more common and severe among individuals engaged in occupations that require prolonged standing. Patients appear to be particularly uncomfortable when they have to stand on concrete or other hard floors. Occupations that require prolonged sitting with the legs in a dependent, motionless position, such as computer operator and bookkeeper, may also aggravate chronic venous insufficiency. Because chronic venous insufficiency is a posture-related disease in its clinical manifestations, symptoms may ameliorate when work conditions or lifestyles are changed to reduce leg dependency. Retirement or reduction in work hours may partially or completely relieve symptoms. Symptoms and clinical features are often bilateral, although one leg is frequently more symptomatic than the other. The main symptoms are leg pain; fatigue; swelling; stasis skin changes such as discoloration, dermatitis, and lipodermatosclerosis; and ulceration. Varices may be present and may be the chief complaint, especially among cosmetically conscious individuals. Some of the varices may be associated with an itching sensation. Episodes of cellulitis or lymphangitis are the main presenting feature in a small fraction of patients. Recurrent

Table 68–1. Clinical Classification of Chronic Venous Insufficiency

Class 0:	No visible or palpable signs of venous disease
Class 1:	Telangiectases or reticular veins
Class 2:	Varicose veins
Class 3:	Edema
Class 4:	Skin changes ascribed to venous disease (eg, pigmentation, venous eczema, lipodermatosclerosis)
Class 5:	Skin changes as defined above with healed ulceration
Class 6:	Skin changes as defined above with active ulceration

Table 68–2. Functional Classification of Chronic Venous Insufficiency According to Work Disability

Grade 0	No work limitation
Grade 1	Mild discomfort; can walk without support
Grade 2	Discomfort; can work for a full work day with leg support
Grade 3	Unable to work for a full day; restricted to household activities
Grade 4	Unable to do regular household chores; restriction or limitation on such activity
Grade 5	Complications requiring full bed rest or hospitalization

episodes of superficial or deep venous thrombosis also occur in a minority of cases. The combination of pain, swelling, and stasis skin changes is the most common symptom complex, and each of these features is present to a varying degree in most patients with symptomatic chronic venous insufficiency.

Pain is characteristically dependent in nature, becoming worse in the standing position and, less commonly, in the sitting posture with prolonged dependency of the leg. Some patients may characterize the pain as fatigue or discomfort rather than as overt pain. In young women, the menstrual period may exacerbate the pain. The overwhelming majority of patients report that walking or moving the leg is better than standing or sitting still in one position; some have learned to "walk off" the discomfort. Leg elevation typically relieves the pain, and most patients have learned to elevate their legs intermittently during the day, even at work. Many patients sleep with their legs elevated at night as well. In some patients severe pain is triggered by leg dependency and, once started, may continue unabated despite leg elevation and recumbency at night. Most patients use some sort of support device, usually a stocking of some type; such devices vary in their compressive efficiency. Some patients become intolerant of stockings, however, owing to binding, discomfort from heat, or aesthetic or other considerations. Poorly fitting stockings that roll up into a band behind the knee, and the resultant sensation of "cutting off of circulation," are frequent complaints among patients who have abandoned stockings. Even though leg pain is a common symptom, its location varies. Pain is commonly localized to the calf, often expressed as a mixture of fatigue and pain in the calf muscle region. Less commonly, it is expressed as deep pain "in the bone" or along the shin in the distal tibia. Pain may be poorly localized, and some patients may be unable to pinpoint its exact location in the leg. Radiation to proximal regions of the thigh and groin occurs in some patients, and gluteal pain or discomfort should arouse the suspicion of iliac vein obstruction. The pain may be present only when the leg swells and along areas where swelling is present, with a sense of stretching or "bursting" pain in the area.

Open stasis ulcers may be exquisitely painful, especially when the leg is in the dependent position. An inflammatory reaction, or cellulitis, around the ulcer increase the degree of pain. Most patients are surprisingly consistent in quantifying the pain sensation on an analog scale. The frequency of pain varies from 1 or 2 days in a work week to a near-constant pain. Temporizing measures such as leg elevation or use of stockings have ceased to work in the more severely afflicted group, and the pain persists day and night without relief. Use of pain relievers, including nonsteroidals, on a regular basis is quite common, and some patients come to depend on narcotics for pain relief. Painful leg cramps and restless leg syndrome are often associated with chronic venous insufficiency.

Swelling is a common presenting sign. It is initially dependent, coming on after several hours of limb dependence in the standing position. The degree of swelling varies from very mild to extremely severe. In the more severe forms, the swelling is no longer dependent but is continuously present. There may be some reduction in swelling during recumbency at night, but even this disappears with time. Despite descriptions in the literature distinguishing the clinical features of lymphedema from those of venous edema (Stemmer sign), this author has found no feature that is restricted to one condition or the other. It is basically impossible to define the etiology from the clinical appearance of leg edema. Approximately 25% of patients with chronic venous insufficiency have coexisting lymphatic deficiency.[2] In some this is due to recurrent chronic infection in the affected extremity, but in others the basis for lymphatic dysfunction is not clear. An occasional feature in an edematous limb is exudation of large amounts of fluid from excoriating dermatitis or from a small ulcer that constantly drips fluid, much like a lymph fistula. Limb swelling may decrease dramatically with the appearance of the fistula. Typically, these fistulas are episodic, appearing spontaneously and healing after a period of days or weeks.

Stasis skin changes vary from discoloration or cyanosis to hyperpigmentation and dermatitis. The hyperpigmentation is usually along the anterior tibial border but may be more circumferential. It is usually confined to the lower third or two-thirds of the leg but occasionally may be more proximal. Hyperpigmentation, which may be uniform or spotted, is due to hemosiderin deposits and increased melanin production. Stasis dermatitis may also be localized or more diffuse. Scaling may be present. It is usually confined to the lower third or lower two-thirds of the leg (gaiter area), but occasionally it may occur more proximally. In more severe forms the dermatitis is excoriating, with denudation of skin epithelium over a wide area. Loss of hair is common. Some patients present with lipodermatosclerosis with thickening of the skin and subcutaneous tissue, presenting either as a localized patch or a more diffuse, circumferential change in the lower third or two-thirds of the leg.

Frank venous stasis ulceration is typically recurrent but may be continuous, spanning a number of years. Recurrent ulcers that heal and break down repeatedly produce thick scar tissue that appears hypopigmented, surrounded by normally colored skin. Such hypopigmented scars represent ischemic epithelium. Occasionally, such scars are exquisitely tender to the touch and may give the appearance of imminent breakdown. The term *pre-ulcer* is appropriate for skin manifestations with impending breakdown. Stasis ulcers are typically found on the medial side of the leg and are usually single but may be multiple. In extreme cases, they may circumferentially involve the leg. The presence of lateral ulceration should raise the suspicion of short saphenous venous insufficiency. Frank venous statis ulcers should be differentiated from pinpoint skin necrosis over distended varicosities. The presence of an inflammatory reaction, or cellulitis, around the ulcer should be noted. In some patients, a remarkably extensive erythema is present in the affected extremity. A classic lymphangitis may be present, with streaks ascending the leg toward the inguinal region.

Varicosities, when present, may be distributed along the long saphenous, short saphenous, posterior arch, or atypical areas. In extreme cases, a combination of subcutaneous varicosities and spiders may give the appearance of extensive matting in the paramalleolar region and adjoining areas of the foot. Venous ulcers differ from arterial ulcers in that the former are more superficial. Venous ulcers usually do not penetrate the deep fascia. Ulcers may occasionally extend to the foot but seldom encroach on the plantar surface. Skin cracking along the digital margins may be present, especially when there is significant edema. In some patients the ulcer is punctate or vasculitic, but in others it cannot be distinguished from pyoderma gangrenosum. Such ulcers are thought to be an exacerbation of other causative processes due to underlying chronic venous insufficiency.

Recurrent calf venous thrombosis may be a feature of proximal "primary" valvular reflux.[3] Recurrent thrombosis is also a feature of postthrombotic chronic venous insufficiency. In patients exhibiting postthrombotic syndrome, the initiating episode of deep venous thrombosis might have occurred years or even decades before symptom presentation. The thrombotic event might have been related to prior surgery, trauma, fracture, or pregnancy. In a minority of patients, the thrombotic event was silent and the patient has no recollection of related symptoms having occurred in the past.

Pseudothrombosis

Occasionally, patients with chronic venous insufficiency present with pain and discomfort highly suggestive of deep venous thrombosis. The symptoms of pain are rapid in onset, may follow minor trauma, and are commonly associated with development of leg edema. A thorough investigation of the deep venous system, however, including duplex scanning and venography, shows the deep venous system to be free of thrombosis. Such nonthrombotic events resulting in pain and swelling are thought to be due to sudden disequilibrium in the Starling balance. The cause is unknown but may be related to a sudden increase in capillary permeability from low-grade infection or another cause, resulting in sudden decompensation of the Starling balance.

A number of comorbid conditions, particularly rheumatism, arthritis, and morbid obesity, appear to exacerbate the manifestations of chronic venous insufficiency. Among the three major symptoms of chronic venous insufficiency, ie, pain, swelling, and stasis skin changes, pain is by far the most common rea-

son that patients seek medical help. Curiously, pain is sometimes absent in this disease syndrome, with patients presenting with stasis skin changes or an ulcer without pain. Other patients present with painless swelling. A sudden onset of local infection or spreading cellulitis often results in onset of pain in a previously painless ulcer or an edematous extremity. Patients who have had a stasis ulcer for decades without seeking medical help sometimes decide to do so as they become older, because of progressing arthritis or infirmity diminishing their ability to care for the festering ulcer.

DIAGNOSTIC EVALUATION

A full hypercoagulability workup, including assays for antithrombin III, protein C, protein S, anticardiolipin antibody, lupus anticoagulant and activated protein C (APC) resistance, should be completed in patients with chronic venous insufficiency. This information may have etiologic relevance in some patients[4] and may modify perioperative anticoagulation in prospective surgical candidates. When APC resistance is low, the Leiden gene should be sought.

Color duplex instrumentation is now widely available and this modality has superseded all others, both as a screening tool and as a definitive diagnostic technique, in chronic venous insufficiency.[5,6] The presence and location of reflux are easily confirmed. Particular attention should be given to the presence of reflux in the superficial system, ie, long and short saphenous veins and perforators. The deep venous system is also systematically examined. Assessment of the profunda femoral vein by the duplex technique is difficult and prone to errors. Examination for reflux in these venous segments is aided by the use of rapid inflation-deflation cuffs.[7] Use of the cuffs allows calculation of valve closure times (Fig. 68–1). While the utility of this measurement is somewhat controversial, the cuffs provide automation and standardization of the examination technique. Ideally, the patient should be examined in the erect position. In addition to monitoring for reflux, criteria for obstruction, including spontaneity, phasicity, and the response to augmentation maneuvers, should be assessed.

Combined obstruction/reflux is the most common outcome of previous deep venous thrombosis.[8] If any obstruction is found, quantification requires measurement of the arm-foot venous pressure differential and reactive hyperemia.[9] The two techniques, when performed together, confirm the presence of obstruction and provide a method to grade its severity (Table 68–3). Outflow fraction measurement is unreliable in the diagnosis of obstruction because a low outflow fraction may be obtained in the presence of compliance wall changes alone without overt obstruction.[10]

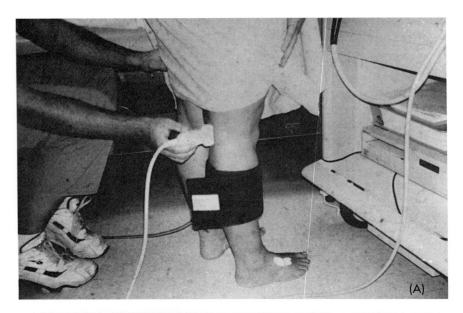

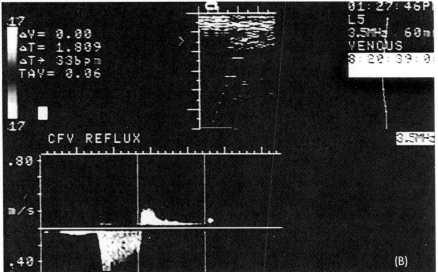

Figure 68–1. (A) Color duplex examination with rapid inflation/deflation cuffs. Note the erect posture for the examination. (B) Reflux in the femoral vein. Valve closure times and average velocity of reflux can be calculated from the tracing. Reflux volume per time unit can be derived from velocity calculations and vessel diameter.

While duplex has been demonstrated to accurately detect the presence of reflux qualitatively, quantification remains more elusive. Measurement of valve closure times, and of several indices based on this measurement, have been disappointing. The grading system based on the number of refluxive venous segments provides a reasonable but imperfect correlation with clinical severity.[5,6] Although it is invasive, ambulatory venous pressure measurement continues to remain the gold standard for measurement of global reflux. In employing this technique, two parameters, ie, postexercise pressure and venous filling time (VFT), are measured. Of the two, VFT appears to be more important because it correlates better with the incidence of venous stasis ulceration than does the measurement of postexercise pressure.[11] Approximately 20% of patients with venous stasis ulceration have normal postexercise

pressure.[12] Photoplethysmography (PPG) has declined in usage because it is not quantitative. Air plethysmography (APG) provides a great deal of physiologic information regarding the calf venous pump that is not available with other techniques or instruments.[13] Arterial inflow into the calf venous pump can be calculated, as well as calf venous pump ejection fraction and residual volume fraction. The venous filling index (VFI-90) gives a measure of passive reflux present when the patient assumes an erect posture after recumbency. Simultaneous ambulatory venous pressure measurement with air plethysmography provides information regarding compliance of the calf venous pump.[10] Ambulatory venous hypertension is multifactorial: reflux is commonly found in patients with ambulatory venous hypertension but other factors, including poor compliance, increased arterial inflow, reduced ejection

Table 68–3. Grading of Obstruction in Chronic Venous Insufficiency

		Arm/Foot Venous Pressure Differential (Normal <4 mm Hg)	Reactive Hyperemia Foot Venous Pressure Elevation (Normal <6 mm Hg)
Grade I*	Fully compensated	<4 mm Hg	<6 mm Hg
Grade II	Partially compensated	<4 mm Hg	>6 mm Hg
Grade III	Partially compensated	>4 mm Hg	>6 mm Hg
Grade IV	Fully decompensated	>4 mm Hg	<6 mm Hg†

*Since pressure parameters for both tests are normal, accurate diagnosis depends on Doppler scanning and/or venography (see text).
†Paradoxical response (see text).
Source: Raju S, Fredericks R. Venous obstruction: an analysis of one hundred thirty-seven cases with hemodynamic, venographic, and clinical correlations. *J Vasc Surg* 1991;14:305–313.

fraction, and decreased venous capacitance, may also be present.[11] Although many of the foregoing abnormalities cannot be corrected when present, the indication of their presence in a patient with ambulatory hypertension does provide a cautionary prognosis for reflux corrective surgery.

If surgery is contemplated, ascending and descending venography are completed in the prospective patient. These contrast studies provide anatomic details of any obstruction that may coexist with reflux, perforator incompetence, and the degree and extent of axial deep venous reflux. From the appearance of ascending and descending venography it may be possible to discern the underlying cause of chronic venous insufficiency, ie, primary versus postthrombotic, but contrast radiography provides only about 60% accuracy in this regard. Final determination of the etiology must await surgical exploration. The degree of reflux present on descending venography can be assessed in one of two ways: the distal extent of reflux (Kistner classification)[14] or the total number of refluxive venous segments present.[5,6] In the latter scoring system, one point each is assigned to the saphenous, superficial femoral, deep femoral, and popliteal venous segments, and a total score of refluxive venous segments present in the individual limb is obtained. Neither method is perfect with regard to hemodynamic correlation, but the latter method does appear to have a better correlation with other measures of reflux.[15] Multisystemic, multilevel reflux is usually present[16] in a severely symptomatic limb with chronic venous stasis, yielding a high score by this classification method. However, some patients with severe reflux remain relatively asymptomatic. A decision to perform surgery, therefore, should not be based on the severity of reflux present in the above investigations, but rather on clinical grounds, ie, clinical severity, the presence of complications, and the failure of conservative management. The selection process may be modified to a certain extent by relevant socioeconomic factors that may render conservative therapy unlikely to succeed (age and occupational factors or comorbid conditions leading to inability to perform or intolerance of regular compressive therapy).

SELECTION OF CANDIDATES FOR SURGICAL INTERVENTION

Once a decision to perform surgery has been made, the above diagnostic workup helps to clarify and localize the pathology. An appropriate surgical approach can then be based on relevant investigations. Among patients presenting with leg swelling, radionucleotide lymphangiography[17] is routinely performed. Although we have not withheld reflux corrective surgery when lymphatic abnormalities are present in patients with chronic venous insufficiency, information on reduced or absent lymphatic function in the operated extremity provides a relevant prognosis for the complete resolution of swelling in the operated extremity.

Symptomatic patients with chronic venous insufficiency may present with pure superficial venous insufficiency, isolated deep venous insufficiency, or a combination of the two. The relative prevalence of these pathologic entities may differ from primary care facilities[18,19] to tertiary centers.[3] Typically, patients with deep venous or combined pathologies are more often seen in tertiary referral practices. In combined superficial and deep venous insufficiency, one or the other component may dominate the clinical presentation. It is important to recognize that the distinction between superficial and deep insufficiency is somewhat artificial in hemodynamic terms. Severe reflux in either system has a global impact on venous function, yet the separation between superficial and deep venous insufficiency has prevailed because symptom presentation in individual patients can be attributed to one or the other system despite some overlap. For example, stasis ulceration is generally related to deep venous reflux but can occasionally result from severe, isolated superficial reflux.[20] The superficial component, ie, varicosities, may be symptomatic, with localized pain, itching, and discomfort or more serious complications, such as thrombosis, localized thrombophlebitis, subcutaneous rupture, or external rupture and hemorrhage through a small eroding ulcer, may be present. While extirpative surgery may provide immediate and specific relief for symptoms related to superficial varicosities, the presence of coincident deep venous reflux in these patients requires careful postoperative follow-up. Deep calf pain, significant leg edema, or stasis skin changes are features generally related to deep venous insufficiency and may not resolve or may recur after a period of remission following superficial extirpative surgery. When combined superficial, perforator, and deep venous pathology is present, it is appropriate to address the superficial and perforator abnormalities first,[18] as the surgical procedures involved are relatively simple and straightforward. Deep venous reconstruction may be reserved for those patients who have persistent or recurrent symptoms after superficial and perforator reflux has been corrected.

REFERENCES

1. Porter JM, Moneta GL, Beebe HG, et al. Reporting standards in venous disease: an update *J Vasc Surg* 1995;21:635–645.
2. Raju S, Fredericks R. Valve reconstruction procedures for non-obstructive venous insufficiency: rationale, techniques, and results in 107 procedures with 2-8 year follow-up. *J Vasc Surg* 1988;7:301–310.
3. Raju S. Venous insufficiency of the lower limb and stasis ulceration: changing concepts and management. *Ann Surg* 1983;197:688–697.
4. Vittore CP, Demos TC. Hereditary deficiency of protein C, protein S and antithrombin III. *Can Assoc Radiol J* 1996;47:251–256.
5. Neglen P, Raju S. A comparison between descending phlebography and duplex Doppler investigation in the evaluation of reflux in chronic venous insufficiency: a challenge to phlebography as the "gold standard." *J Vasc Surg* 1992;16:687–693.
6. Neglen P, Raju S. A rational approach to detection of significant reflux with duplex Doppler scanning and air plethysmography. *J Vasc Surg* 1993;17:590–595.
7. Van Bemmelen PS, Bedford G, Beach K, Strandness DE Jr. Status of the valves in the superficial and deep system in chronic venous disease. *Surgery* 1990;109:730–734.
8. Johnson BF, Manzo RA, Bergelin RO, Strandness DE Jr. Relationship between changes in the deep venous system and the development of the postthrombotic syndrome after an acute episode of lower limb deep vein thrombosis: a one-to-six-year follow-up. *J Vasc Surg* 1995;21:307–313.
9. Raju S, Fredericks R. Venous obstruction: an analysis of one hundred thirty-seven cases with hemodynamic, venographic, and clinical correlations. *J Vasc Surg* 1991;14:305–313.
10. Neglen P, Raju S. Compliance of the normal and postthrombotic calf. *J Cardiovasc Surg* 1995;36:225–231.
11. Raju S, Carr-White PA, Fredericks RK, Neglen PN, Devidas M. Ambulatory venous hypertension: component analysis in 373 limbs. Submitted to *Vasc Surg*.
12. Raju S, Fredericks R. Hemodynamic basis of stasis ulceration—a hypothesis. *J Vasc Surg* 1991;13:491–495.
13. Christopoulos D, Nicolaides AN, Szendro G, et al. Air plethysmography and the effect of elastic compression on venous hemodynamics of the leg. *J Vasc Surg* 1987;5:148–159.
14. Kistner RL, Ferris EB, Randhawa G, et al. A method of performing descending venography. *J Vasc Surg* 1986;4:464–466.
15. Raju S, Fredericks R. Evaluation of methods for detecting venous reflux. *Arch Surg* 1990;125:1463–1467.
16. Raju S. Valve reconstruction procedures for chronic venous insufficiency. *Semin Vasc Surg* 1988;1:101–106.
17. Koren A, Zelikovski A, Melloul M, Reiss R. Isotopic lymphangiography to evaluate lymphedema before and after operative treatment. *Lymphology* 1987;20:96–97.
18. Sethia KK, Darke SG. Long saphenous incompetence as a cause of venous ulceration. *Br J Surg* 1984;71:754–755.
19. Shami SK, Sarin S, Cheatle TR, Scurr JH, Coleridge-Smith PD. Venous ulcers and the superficial venous system. *J Vasc Surg* 1993;17:487–490.
20. Labropoulos N, Leon J, Nicolaides AN, Giannoukas AD, Volteas N, Chan P. Superficial venous insufficiency: correlation of anatomic extent of reflux with clinical symptoms and signs. *J Vasc Surg* 1994;20:953–958.

69

The Surgical Treatment of Chronic Venous Insufficiency: Patient and Procedure Selection and Results

Harold J. Welch, M.D.
Thomas F. O'Donnell, Jr., M.D.

Patients afflicted with venous disease often suffer for years with tired, heavy legs, unsightly varicose veins, hyperpigmentation, and chronic, painful ulcerations. While conservative (ie, nonsurgical) therapy is highly effective in most patients with chronic venous insufficiency (CVI), there remain a number of patients who will request or require surgery to alleviate their symptoms. When evaluating a patient with possible CVI, the physician must answer four questions: (1) Is CVI present? (2) How severe is it? (3) What is the etiology? and (4) What systems are involved? The surgeon must understand the patient's underlying pathology to select the best surgical procedure to correct it. A variety of noninvasive and invasive tests are available to diagnose the cause of the patient's problems and, based on the test results, appropriate intervention can be undertaken.

The classification of CVI was formerly somewhat simple and straightforward. The original system of clinical stratification[1] from Class 0 (normal) through Class 3 (ulceration) allowed one to assess the severity of the patient's symptoms, but it did not address the etiology or pathology of the CVI. The new CEAP (clinical, etiology, anatomic, pathophysiology) system,[2] while more cumbersome, should correct the deficiencies of the original reporting system and allow better comparisons between studies.

PATIENT EVALUATION

Physical Examination

The patient is placed in the upright position, preferably standing on a stool. The limbs are inspected for size discrepancies, edema, pigmentation, lipodermatosclerosis, eczema, ankle flare, varicose veins, and ulcerations. The saphenofemoral junction is palpated for incompetence as the patient is instructed to cough or perform a Valsalva maneuver. Occasionally in limbs with obesity, some veins may not be visible and palpation is the best method to identify abnormal veins in the thigh and calf. Palpation of defects in the subcutaneous tissue of the calf reveals the site of incompetent perforating veins.

The use of tourniquets can aid in determining the level of superficial incompetence and the contribution of the deep venous system to varicose veins. We use the multilevel tourniquet test, with 0.5-inch Penrose drains placed while the patient is supine at four locations: the upper thigh below the saphenofemoral junction, the lower thigh below Hunter's canal, the upper calf, and above the ankle. The patient stands; if calf varicose veins appear, perforator incompetence is present. The tourniquets are then sequentially removed from the bottom to the top, with the clinician looking for filling of the varicose veins. If removal of the ankle tourniquet fills the superficial system, incompetent perforators are suspected. Filling of the lesser saphenous system with removal of the calf tourniquet indicates saphenopopliteal incompetence. Next, the lower thigh tourniquet is released to assess the competence of the Hunterian perforator. If the superficial system remains empty, the high-thigh tourniquet is released to detect incompetence of the saphenofemoral junction.

Tourniquets can also aid the diagnosis of deep venous obstruction and venous claudication, ie, Per-the's test. Iliofemoral venous thrombosis can result in increased flow to superficial collaterals, causing secondary varicose veins. Occlusion of the superficial veins with a tourniquet causes increased discomfort in the leg when the patient exercises.

DIAGNOSTIC TESTS

A number of noninvasive and invasive tests are available to elucidate the underlying pathophysiology. At times, the etiology (ie, reflux or obstruction) can be determined by the history and physical examination, and diagnostic testing can be more focused. Usually, the exact etiology is in question, or both etiologies may coexist so that several tests must be performed for a complete evaluation.

Duplex

Duplex ultrasound is the test of choice in the evaluation of venous disease since it provides both anatomic and hemodynamic information concerning potential venous abnormalities. While it is extensively used to diagnose acute deep venous thrombosis (DVT), the same duplex criteria can apply to chronic obstruction as well. The criteria include spontaneity of flow, phasicity of flow with respiration, augmentation of flow with distal compression, compressibility of the vein with the application of minimal probe pressure, and visualization of the thrombus. The B-mode ultrasound characteristics of the clot are also helpful in determining the age of the clot; older clots are more adherent to the vein wall, have more echogenicity, and have a denser, contracted texture. The vascular technician must be astute, as the development of enlarged collaterals around the thrombosed vein may erroneously be interpreted as the normal vein; thrombus in a duplicated system can also be missed.

Duplex ultrasound is also used to assess venous reflux. While some workers test for reflux by the Valsalva maneuver with the patient supine, we believe it is illogical to test for a pathologic condition caused by gravity in this fashion. Thus, we examine the patient in the upright position, and use the cuff deflation technique, which is more standardized than manual compression techniques. The valve closure time (VCT) is normally less than 0.5 second.[3] A combined superficial femoral and popliteal vein VCT of more than 4.0 seconds is indicative of significant reflux.[4] Duplex ultrasound allows evaluation of specific venous segments, which continuous-wave Doppler and other noninvasive tests do not. We test the greater and lesser saphenous, superficial femoral, profunda femoris, and popliteal veins for reflux. We do not test the tibial veins because of the nonsurgical nature of tibial reflux.

The significance of incompetent perforating veins in the etiology of CVI has been questioned, but for those who believe in their contribution to venous ulcer formation, duplex scanning is an excellent method of localization.

Photoplethysmography/Light Reflection Rheography

Photoplethysmography (PPG) and light reflection rheography (LRR) are similar tests that assess venous reflux by using infrared light reflected off subdermal red blood cells. After the leg is emptied of blood by calf muscle contractions, the length of time for the subdermal venous plexus to refill with blood is calculated. A normal venous refilling time (VRT) is 25 to 30 seconds; shorter times indicate reflux. Tourniquets may be applied and the test repeated to assess the contribution of the superficial system to total leg reflux. These techniques are good screening tools, although they do not provide any anatomic information.

Air Plethysmography

Air plethysmography (APG) utilizes an air-filled vinyl cuff applied to the lower leg to measure volume changes in the calf that result from standardized maneuvers. APG is a valuable tool in the evaluation of CVI, as it can assess several parameters. Reflux is measured by the venous filling index (VFI), and calf muscle pump function is measured by the ejection fraction (EF). Ambulatory venous pressure is indirectly measured by the residual volume fraction (RVF), and obstruction can be assessed using a rapidly deflated thigh cuff to measure the maximum venous outflow fraction (MVO). APG does not give anatomic information but does provide a global assessment of lower limb venous function. We usually combine APG with duplex in our patient evaluation.

Impedance Plethysmography

Impedance plethysmography (IPG) assesses the degree of venous obstruction by measuring the ability of the venous reservoir to expand (venous capacitance) and empty (venous outflow). A thigh cuff is placed and inflated to 50 mm Hg to occlude venous flow. Normal calf expansion is approximately 2 to 3%. Limbs with DVT have less expansion since the capacitance veins are already somewhat filled as a result of the higher venous pressure from the DVT. Venous outflow (MVO) is measured as the thigh cuff is rapidly deflated, limbs with acute DVT have lower venous outflow. Unfortunately, this test is not particularly accurate for thrombosis below the knee, and isolated iliac vein thrombosis may give a flasely negative high MVO.

Arm-Foot Pressure Differential

The minimally invasive arm-foot venous pressure measurement is an excellent hemodynamic test of obstruction and reflux. A vein in the hand and the dorsum of the foot of a supine patient at rest is canulated and connected to a pressure transducer. A normal venous system will have a pressure differential of <4 mm Hg, while patients with phlebographically documented venous thrombosis will have a differential of >4 mm Hg. Recanalization of the thrombus will decrease the differential to <4 mm Hg at rest. The hemodynamics of the recanalization or occlusion can be assessed by inducing reactive hyperemia with a 2-minute thigh cuff occlusion to 300 mm Hg. A normal limb will see a hand-foot venous pressure increase of ≤6 mm Hg within 5 minutes of cuff deflation, while a hemodynamically significant obstruction will increase the hand-foot pressure difference by >6 mm Hg. In limbs with marked, uncompensated venous obstruction, the venous pressure paradoxically rises <6 mm Hg.[5]

Foot venous pressure can also be used to assess venous reflux. While supine, the patient performs a standardized Valsalva maneuver (40 mm Hg for 5 seconds). Significant reflux is present if the foot pressure increases over 4 mm Hg from resting levels.

This test is extremely helpful in determining which patients are candidates for venous bypass surgery based on their hemodynamics and not simply their symptomatology. Additionally, postoperative testing is useful in assessing the efficacy of the surgical procedure.

Ascending Phlebography

While invasive and not without risk, ascending phlebography is the anatomic gold standard, analogous to the arteriogram, and is essential in planning venous surgery. A butterfly needle or angiocatheter is inserted into a vein on the dorsum of the foot. To better fill the deep veins, the needle should be directed toward the toes and not placed too near the ankle. The use of tourniquets above the ankle and below the knee will also preferentially fill the deep system. The patient is on a tilt table, with the weight supported by standing on a wooden block with the contralateral leg. Contrast material is hand injected while spot and/or overhead films are taken in the anteroposterior and lateral projections.

The films are examined for evidence of thrombus, obstruction, and/or recanalization. Possible duplication of the deep venous system is important to know if one is planning an antireflux procedure. The presence of valve structures is sought for possible valvuloplasty. Incompetent perforating veins may be identified on ascending phlebography. Large collaterals bypassing an obstruction are important to visualize, as they may be mistaken for normal anatomy on duplex or continuous-wave Doppler.

Descending Phlebography

Descending phlebography is performed when noninvasive tests are positive for deep venous reflux and reconstructive surgery is contemplated. The patient is placed on a tilt table and either the ipsilateral or contralateral common femoral vein is canulated. The patient is positioned at 70 to 90 degrees, and contrast material is injected while a Valsalva maneuver is performed by the patient. The level of descent of the contrast material is graded according to the Kistner classification. Antireflux surgery is usually reserved for patients with contrast reflux to the below-knee popliteal or tibial vein segments. The presence or absence of reflux in the profunda femoris vein is important to note, as this may affect the results of deep venous reconstruction.

SURGICAL PROCEDURES AND RESULTS

In the vast majority of cases, conservative therapy will be successful in alleviating symptoms and should be the first treatment option. However, there are circumstances, such as varicose veins causing ulcers in a low-risk patient, in which surgery should be recommended as the treatment of choice. While a number of procedures are aimed at correcting reflux in the different venous systems, only venous bypass or transposition provides for relief of obstruction.

Ligation and Stripping of Varicose Veins

While perhaps the most frequent indication for varicose vein surgery is cosmetic, other indications include achy, uncomfortable legs with prolonged standing, recurrent superficial thrombophlebitis, hemorrhage, and skin changes including ulceration.

Among patients with primary varicose veins, ligation and stripping is very effective in alleviating symptoms and preventing recurrence. Preoperative marking of the patient's varicose veins by the operating surgeon is crucial in obtaining good and lasting results. In the past, complete stripping of the greater saphenous vein was routine. This practice has changed to one of selective stripping for several reasons. If the saphenofemoral junction is incompetent and the greater saphenous vein (GSV) is dilated and tortuous, stripping should be performed, but only to just below the level of the knee because stripping of the GSV to the ankle increases the incidence of injury to the saphenous nerve. When the GSV is stripped, it should be done from above downward to decrease the chance of saphenous nerve injury. If the saphenofemoral junction is incompetent but the GSV is not tortuous and only minimally dilated, then simple ligation of the GSV and its tributaries at the saphenofemoral junction will decrease the recurrence rate and minimize the morbidity of the procedure. Despite claims to the contrary, passage of the stripper in the GSV, either antegrade or retrograde, is not always easy. Inability to pass the stripper adequately should lead the surgeon to consider stab avulsion or ligation of the GSV lest the stripper be inadvertently passed into the deep venous system. Obvious perforators that feed varicosities should be ligated to decrease bleeding and recurrences.

Stab avulsion of branch varicosities should always be a cosmetic procedure, as there is no need for long incisions. Depending on the size of the varix, an incision 2 to 4 mm in length is made with a No. 11 blade. The incisions should be vertical except near the knee and ankle, where oblique or transverse incisions are required. The small incisions can easily be closed with Steri-strips or a 5-0 buried absorbable suture. The operated leg should be wrapped with gauze and elastic bandages for 5 days to provide hemostasis and to decrease swelling.

Varicose veins recur in approximately 10 to 20% of patients at 5 years, and in up to 30% at 20 years. The reasons have been extensively researched and include reflux in the distal greater saphenous vein not initially stripped, lesser saphenous reflux, failure to ligate saphenofemoral tributaries, an incompetent accessory saphenous vein, pelvic vein reflux, and incompetent perforating veins. Whatever the hemodynamic reason, the underlying defect in the recurrent varicosities is the same as in the primary varicosities, ie, an abnormality in the vein wall matrix. In recurrent varicose veins, this abnormality becomes clinically evident in veins that were not removed at the initial operation (Table 69–1).

Subfascial Ligation of Incompetent Perforators

Perforating or communicating veins generally direct blood flow from the superficial to the deep system. When the valves of the perforating veins become incompetent, the higher venous pressure generated in the deep system with calf muscle contraction is transmitted to the superficial veins, resulting in varicosities and skin changes. The Hunterian and/or Dodd perforator, located on the medial thigh, if incompetent, will cause the greater saphenous vein to dilate even with an intact saphenofemoral junction. An incompetent Boyd's perforator, located medially just below the knee, can result in a large cluster of varicosities and lipodermatosclerosis. The Cockett perforators communicate between the superficial posterior arch vein and the

deep posterior tibial vein and frequently contribute to venous ulceration. A posterior lateral perforator in the midcalf may lead to ulcerations in the lateral segment of the leg drained by the lesser saphenous vein.

These perforators can be identified by physical examination, ascending phlebography, and duplex ultrasonography. The standard operative approach is the Linton procedure. Using a medial leg incision from below the knee to above the ankle, the dissection is carried down through the fascia and the entire posterior compartment from the medial aspect of the tibia posterolaterally to the fibula is explored. All identifiable perforators are ligated and divided. Alternatively, a posterior "stocking seam" incision can be used, with the distal portion of the incision curved laterally away from the Achilles' tendon. Although these incisions provide excellent exposure, the hospital stay is several days and recovery is prolonged for several weeks. The wound complication rate, with the incisions usually involving the lipodermatosclerotic tissue, may exceed 20%.

Due to the problems associated with the Linton procedure, less invasive procedures have been developed. DePalma utilized stepwise oblique incisions, and Edwards used a shearing phlebotome to divide the medial Cockett perforators. With the improvement in fiberoptics and the development of minimally invasive surgical technology, O'Donnell[6] first utilized laparoscopic instruments for subfascial ligation of incompetent perforators. This technique uses small incisions for the ports in the upper medial aspect of the lower leg away from the underprivileged, diseased gaiter area. The subfascial tissue plane is developed with blunt or balloon dissection and maintained by external traction or CO_2 insufflation. The perforators are clipped with hemaclips and divided. This procedure is performed on an outpatient basis, and the recovery period is minimal. A multicenter registry has shown this to be a safe and effective procedure for subfascial ligation of incompetent perforators[7] (Table 69–2).

Venous Bypass

Most thrombi in the deep venous system resolve or recanalize, but persistent occlusion of the deep system results in venous hypertension and frequently in symptoms of venous claudication. Patients with occlusion of the femoral or iliac veins may complain of a "bursting" sensation in their leg when they walk, in addition to chronic swelling and pain. Evaluation with duplex, plethysmographic venous outflow studies, phlebography, and measurent of hand-foot pressure differentials will identify appropriate candidates for venous bypass.

Several options exist for bypassing an occluded iliac system. The crossover saphenofemoral bypass, originally described by Palma and Esperson in 1960, uses the contralateral GSV. The saphenous vein in the non-affected leg is dissected to the distal thigh and then

Table 69–1. Surgical Results with Varicose Veins

Study	No. of Patients	Length of Follow-up Care (Yr)	Recurrence (%)
Lofgren[13]	1000	10	15
Haeger[14]	578	5	8
Rivlin[15]	2000	>6	7
Hobbs[16]	170	10	29
Chant[17]	100	3	14

Source: From O'Donnell TF Jr, Welch HJ. Chronic venous insufficiency and varicose veins. In: Young JR, Olin JW, Bartholomew JR, eds. *Peripheral Vascular Diseases*, 2nd ed. St Louis; Mosby-Year Book, 1966:514.

Table 69–2. Preliminary North American Registry Results: Subfascial Endoscopic Perforator Surgery (SEPS)

N	Active/Healed Ulcers	Concommitant Varicose Vein Procedure	DVT/PE	Superficial Thrombphlebitis	Wound Infection	Cellulitis	Saphenous Neuralgia	F/U (mean)	Ulcer Healing	Ulcer Recurrence
116	65%/16%	66%	0	3%	7%	2.5%	7.7%*	9.3 mo	78%	6%

*Eight of nine limbs had concomitant procedures
Source: Gloriczki P, Bergan JJ, Menawat SS, et al. *J Vasc Surg* 1997;25:94. Safety, feasibility, and early efficacy of subfascial endoscopic perforator surgery (SEPS): a preliminary report from the North American Registry.

brought through a suprapubic tunnel to be anastomosed to the patent femoral system of the affected limb.(Table 69–3). Alternatively, the contralateral saphenous vein may be removed from the nonaffected leg and used as a femoral-femoral bypass, as the saphenofemoral junction in the nonaffected leg using the Palma procedure may have a poor configuration. Another option is the use of a prosthetic conduit, and we prefer polytetrafluoroethylene (PTFE). This may be used in a femoral-femoral, femoral-iliac, or femoral-caval configuration. Increased blood flow through a venous bypass seems essential for improved patency. An arteriovenous fistula, created in the bypass distal to the proximal anastomosis, is performed by many, including the authors. Postoperatively, the use of intermittent pneumatic compression devices and early ambulation are essential. Postoperative heparin is converted to Coumadin for at least 6 months.

Bypass of an occluded superficial femoral vein with the ipsilateral GSV has been described by Husni. However, Linton showed little sequelae to superficial femoral vein ligation, and today this vein is sometimes harvested as an arterial conduit without detrimental effects. Thus, because the saphenous vein is also frequently unsuitable due to disease or prior stripping, this saphenous vein bypass procedure is rarely performed.

Venous Segment Transfer or Transposition

When the valves of the common and superficial femoral veins are incompetent but the profunda femoris vein or GSV permits no reflux, the proximal end of the superficial femoral vein can be anastomosed to a competent system. This anastomosis can be performed in an end-to-end or end-to-side fashion. However, the saphenous vein is usually involved with the same process and is infrequently available. To date, only Kistner has had good intermediate results, with 78% of patients experiencing a satisfactory outcome at 3 years. The Northwestern group had a high ulcer recurrence rate as a result of failing to treat incompetent perforators concomitantly (Table 69–4).

Vein Valve Transplant

Patients who have severe reflux resulting from post-thrombotic destruction of valves, or rarely from valvu-

Table 69–3. Crossover Saphenofemoral Bypass for Postthrombotic Syndrome

Study	No. of Patients	Results		
		Excellent	Good	Unimproved
Palma[18]	7	57	29	14
Dale[19]	23	43	43	14
May[20]	66	73	0	27
Husni[21]	82	61	15	24
Halliday[22]	50*	76	0	24
O'Donnell[23]	6†	83	17	0

*Patent by Phlebography.
†Patent by B-mode ultrasound.
Source: O'Donnell TF Jr, Welch HJ. Chronic venous insufficiency and varicose veins. In Young JR, Olin JW, Bartholomew JR, eds. *Peripheral Vascular Diseases*, 2nd ed. St Louis: Mosby-Year Book; 1996:515.

lar agenesis, are candidates for vein valve transplantation (VVT). Taheri et al first described the procedure, splicing a segment of brachial vein into the superficial femoral vein.[8] Others have used the axillary vein at this location. Our approach is to transplant a segment of valve bearing axillary vein to the above-knee popliteal vein. We find the axillary vein to be a good size match for the popliteal vein, and others have shown that a competent popliteal vein is important in preventing ulcer formation.[9] A potential cause of VVT failure is subsequent incompetence of the transplanted vein valve segment. Some authors wrap the transplanted segment with PTFE to prevent late dilatation, but we believe this wrap may incite an inflammatory reaction leading to thrombosis. We now usually perform a limited external valvuloplasty of the transplanted segment by placing two 7-0 Prolene sutures at the valve commissures if this segment dilates and is not fully competent prior to transplantation. A recent review of VVT at the New England Medical Center showed a 62% ulcer-free survival at 5 years, with a mean follow-up of 5.3 years.[10] When performed on patients with chronic venous ulcers, VVT has been a relatively durable procedure, providing significant long-term relief of symptoms and ulcers (Table 69–5).

Vein Valvuloplasty

Primary valvular incompetence (PVI) is a condition in which the valve cusp edges are elongated and floppy and do not coapt with retrograde pressure. The diag-

Table 69–4.   Venous Segment Transfer

Study	No. of Limbs	Preoperative Ulcer (%)	Ulcer Healing (%)	Pain Relief (%)
Masuda and Kistner[24]	14	—	80	64
Queral[25]	12	33	100	75
Johnson[26]	12	33	0	25

Source: Adapted from O'Donnell TF Jr, Welch HJ. Chronic venous insufficiency and varicose veins. In: Young JR, Olin JW, Bartholomew JR, eds. *Peripheral Vascular Diseases*, 2nd ed. St Louis: Mosby-Year Book; 1996:517.

Table 69–5.   VVT: Surgical Results

Author	Number	Ulcers (%)	Procedure	Mean F/U (yrs)	Symptom relief	Ulcer Recurrence (%)	VVT Thrombosis (%)
Taheri[8]	66	27	B to F	—	78	6	3
Nash[27]	23	74	B to P	1.5	—	18	0
Raju[28]	18	42	A to F	>2	50	54	—
Eriksson[29]	35	—	A–F(26%)	2.3	—	—	—
			A–P(74%)				
Sottiurai[30]	8	100	B to F	2.8	—	25	0
Cheatle[31]	26	74	A to F	4	48	31	48
Bry[10]	15	93	A to P	5.3	92	21	0

Abbreviations: B, brachial; F, femoral; P, popliteal; A, axillary.
Source: from O'Donnell TF Jr, Welch HJ. Chronic venous insufficiency and varicose veins. In: Young JR, Olin JW, Bartholomew JR, eds. *Peripheral Vascular Diseases*, 2nd ed. St Louis: Mosby-Year Book; 1996:519.

nosis is suggested by reflux documented on duplex ultrasound and descending phlebography and by the presence of valves, without postthrombotic changes on ascending phlebography. Most commonly, in this condition there is an incompetent valve in the proximal superficial femoral vein just below the junction of the profunda femoris vein. There may also be PVI in the popliteal and profunda femoris veins.

Several techniques of valvuloplasty have been described and can be categorized as internal, or open, and external, or closed. Internal valvuloplasty requires a venotomy, either longitudinally through the valve commissure or transversely above the valve cusps. The valve cusps are tightened by running sutures along the cusp edge or by using interrupted sutures in the commissures. After completion of the valvuloplasty, the venotomy is closed and the competency of the repair tested. This is generally done by the "strip test," in which the blood is milked out of the vein from distal to proximal and then observed for reflux at the valve site. We prefer a transverse venotomy, finding it easier to observe suture placement and evaluate competency.

The external valvuloplasty requires two to four sutures placed externally through the valve commissures to "reef" up the abnormally widened commissure angle, and to slightly narrow the vein at the valve sinus. This eliminates the need for a venotomy, which at least theoretically decreases the postoperative thrombotic risk. We believe the use of the angioscope is ideally

suited for external valvuloplasty. The angioscope provides visualization of the vein lumen to make the diagnosis of PVI, guides the proper placement of the sutures, and, most importantly, accurately assesses the adequacy of the repair. External valvuloplasty is faster, and more than one valve can be repaired if desired. However, the vein must be adequately mobilized, often by dividing small side branches, to allow for visualization and repair of the posteriorly oriented valve commissure.

Vein valvuloplasty is the preferred procedure to correct deep venous reflux, as it is simpler and more effective in the long term in the prevention of recurrent ulcers. The long-term ulcer recurrence rate is approximately 30% (Table 69–6).

CONCLUSIONS

Venous ulcers rarely occur in patients with deep venous reflux in the absence of superficial and/or perforator incompetence. The approach to deep venous reflux is open to debate. Several recent studies have shown correction of deep reflux by treating the superficial or perforator systems alone.[11,12] Surgery on the superficial and perforator systems is now performed on an outpatient basis, with little morbidity, and no bridges are burned with this approach. Thus, we prefer to perform deep venous reconstruction with ulcer recurrence after less extensive treatment. However, when operating on

Table 69–6. Valvuloplasty: Surgical Results

Author	No. Limbs	Ulcers (%)	F/U (mo)	Patent (%)	Hemodynamic Improvement (%)
Masuda[24]	51	57	48–252	67	60
Cheatle[31]	52	40	NA	69	NA
Eriksson[29]	22	NA	6–84	100	62
Raju[28]	107	71	24–96	NA	63
Simkin[32]	7	100	NA	NA	50
Sottiurai[30]	20	100	10–73	NA	80
O'Donnell[33]	9	100	2–51	100	100

Abbreviation: NA, not applicable.
Source: O'Donnell TF Jr, Welch HJ, Chronic venous insufficiency and varicose veins. In: Young JR, Olin JW, Bartholomew JR, eds. *Peripheral Vascular Diseases.* 2nd ed. St Louis: Mosby-Year Book; 1996:516.

the deep system, for best long-term results, reflux in the superficial and perforator veins must be eliminated as well.

REFERENCES

1. Porter JM, Rutherford RB, Clagett GP, et al. Reporting standards in venous disease. *J Vasc Surg* 1988;8:172.
2. Porter JM, Moneta GL, et al. The 3rd author is An International Consensus Committee on Chronic Venous Disease. Reporting standards in venous disease: an update. *J Vasc Surg* 1995;21:635.
3. van Bemmelen PS, Bedford G, Beach K, et al. Quantitative segmental evaluation of venous valvular reflux with duplex ultrasound scanning. *J Vasc Surg* 1989;10:425.
4. Welch HJ, Faliakou E, McLaughlin RL, et al. Comparison of descending phlebography with guantitative photoplethysmography, air plethysmography, and duplex quantitative valve closure time in assessing deep venous reflux. *J Vasc Surg* 1992;16:913.
5. Raju S. New approaches to the diagnosis and treatment of venous obstruction. *J Vasc Surg* 1986;4:42.
6. O'Donnell TF. Surgical treatment of incompetent perforating veins. In Bergan JJ, Kistner RL, eds. *Atlas of Venous Surgery*. Philadelphia: WB Saunders; 1992:111.
7. Gloviczki P, Bergan JJ, Menawat SS, et al. Safety, feasibility and early efficacy of subfascial endoscopic perforator surgery (SEPS): A preliminary report from the North American registry. Presented at the 50th annual meeting of the Society for Vascular Surgery, Chicago, June 12, 1996.
8. Taheri SA, Pendergast DR, Lazar E. Vein valve transplantation. *Am J Surg* 1985;150:201.
9. Shull KS, Nicoloides AN, Fernandes e Fernandes J., et al. Significance of popliteal reflux in relationship to ambulatory venous pressure and ulceration. *Arch Surg* 1979;114:1304.
10. Bry JD, Muto PM, Isacsson L, O'Donnell TF. The clinical and hemodynamic results after axillary-to-popliteal vein valve transplantation. *J Vasc Surg* 1995;21:110.
11. Sales CM, Bilof ML, Petrillo KA, Luka NL. Correction of lower extremity deep venous incompetence by ablation of superficial venous reflux. *Ann Vasc Surg* 1996;10:186.
12. Walsh JC, Bergan JJ, Beeman S, Comer TP. Femoral venous reflux abolished by greater saphenous vein stripping. *Ann Vasc Surg* 1994;8:566.
13. Lofgren KA. Postphlebetic syndrome (chronic deep venous insufficiency). In Haimovici H, ed. *Vascular Surgery: Principles and Techniques.* 2nd ed. Appleton-Century-Crofts, Norwalk, CT 1984:979.
14. Haeger K. Five year results of radical surgery for superficial varicies with or without coexisting perforator insufficiency. *Acta Chir Scand* 1966;131:38.
15. Rivlin S. The surgical care of primary varicose veins. *Br J Surg* 1975;62:613.
16. Hobbs JT. Surgery and sclerotherapy in the treatment of varicose veins: a randomized trial. *Arch Surg* 1974;109:793.
17. Chant ADB, Jones HO, Weddel JM. Varicose veins: a comparison of surgery and injection/compression sclerotherapy. *Lancet* 1972;2:1188.
18. Palma ED, Esperson R. Vein transplants and grafts in the surgical treatment of the post-phlebitic syndrome. *J Cardiovasc Surg* 1960;1:94.
19. Dale WA. Crossover vein grafts for relief of iliofemoral block. *Surgery* 1965;57:608.
20. May R. Spakergebnissr nach venosom femoralis bypass. *Vasa* 1974;8:67.
21. Husni EA. Issues in venous reconstruction. *Vasc Diagn Ther* 1981;2:37.
22. Halliday P, Harris J, May J. Femoral-femoral cross-over grafts (Palma operation): a long term follow-up study. In Bergan JJ, Yao JST, eds. *Surgery of the Veins.* New York: Grune & Stratton; 1985:241.
23. O'Donnell TF, Mackey WC, Shepard AD, Callow AD. Clinical, hemodynamic, and anatomic follow-up of direct venous reconstruction. *Arch Surg* 1987;122:474.
24. Masuda EM, Kistner RL. Long-term results of venous valve reconstruction: a four to twenty-one year follow-up. *J Vasc Surg* 1994;19:391.
25. Queral LA, Whitehouse WM, Flinn WR, et al. Surgical correction of chronic deep venous insufficiency by valvular transposition. *Surgery* 1980;87:688.
26. Johnson ND, Queral LA, Flinn WR, et al. Late objective assessment of venous valve surgery. *Arch Surg* 1981;116:1461.
27. Nash T. Long term results of vein valve transplants placed in the popliteal vein for intractable postphlebitic ulcers in pre-ulcer skin changes. *J Cardiovasc Surg* 1988;29:712.
28. Raju S, Fredericks R. Valve reconstruction procedures for nonobstructive venous insufficiency: rationale, techniques, and results in 107 procedures. *J Vasc Surg* 1988;7:301.
29. Eriksson JI, Almgren B. Surgical reconstruction of incompetent deep vein valves. *Uppsala J Med Sci* 1988;93:139.
30. Sottiurai VS. Surgical correction of recurrent venous ulcer. *J Cardiovasc Surg* 1991;32:104.

31. Cheatle TR, Perrin M. Surgical options in the post-thrombotic syndrome. *Phlebology* 1993;8:50.

32. Simkin R, Estembam JC, Bulloj R. Bypass veno-venosos y valvuloplastias en el tratamiento quirugico del sindrome post-trombotico. *Angiologia* 1988;30:4.

33. Welch HJ, McLaughlin RL, O'Donnell TF. Femoral vein valvuloplasty: intraoperative angioscopic evaluation and hemodynamic improvement. *J Vasc Surg* 1992;16:694.

70

Vena Cava Filters

Michael S. Webb, M.D.
Gary S. Dorfman, M.D.

In spite of improvements in the diagnosis and treatment of thromboembolic disease, pulmonary embolism (PE) continues to be a major cause of morbidity and mortality. Estimates suggest that as many as 5 million cases of deep venous thrombosis (DVT) and 750,000 cases of PE occur in the United States annually. These events are the sole cause of 50,000 deaths and are a significant contributing factor in an additional 20,000 deaths each year.[1–5]

Anticoagulation remains the preferred therapy for thromboembolic disease; however, this form of treatment is either ineffective or contraindicated for some patients. Other patients have risk factors predisposing to embolic phenomena in spite of adequate anticoagulation. For these patients, partial interruption of the inferior vena cava (IVC) via percutaneous filter placement has become the procedure of choice to protect against potentially fatal pulmonary emboli.

INDICATIONS

For patients with documented DVT, there are several absolute indications for IVC filter placement. These include (1) contraindications to anticoagulation (Table 70–1), (2) complications of therapeutic anticoagulation requiring discontinuation of such therapy (ie, hemorrhage or heparin-induced thrombocytopenia), (3) progression or recurrence of thromboembolic disease in spite continuous, adequate anticoagulation, and (4) noncompliance with a prescribed anticoagulation regimen.

Patients at increased risk of hemorrhage from long-term anticoagulation because of unsteady gait, syncope, or seizure disorder may benefit from filter placement; however, they should be evaluated on a case-by-case basis. Additional selective indications for filter placement have been adopted for patients with thromboem-

Table 70–1. Contraindications to Anticoagulation

Hemorrhagic stroke or vascular brain neoplasm
Ongoing bleeding from any organ system
Complication of anticoagulation (eg, thrombocytopenia)
Known bleeding tendency
Recent major trauma or surgery
Unsteady gait/tendency to fall
Noncompliance with drug regimen/follow-up
Pregnancy

bolic disease who are deemed to be at high risk of complications of PE despite adequate anticoagulation. These indications include (1) pulmonary embolectomy and/or thrombolysis, (2) DVT in the setting of severe cardiopulmonary disease (chronic obstructive pulmonary disease, massive/chronic PE, cor pulmonale, etc.),[6–10] and (3) free-floating thrombus above the inguinal ligament measuring 5 cm or more.[11–14]

Although long-term outcome data concerning IVC filters are lacking, these devices are generally considered to be safe and effective for patients with traditional indications. These attributes, combined with the relative ease of placement of current systems, have led to increased use IVC filters and proposed expansion of the traditional placement indications. Proponents have suggested the replacement of anticoagulation therapy with caval filtration as primary therapy for DVT in cancer patients.[15–20] Others advocate the use of these devices in patients without documented thromboembolic disease. Settings in which such "prophylactic" use has been proposed include spinal cord injury,[21,22] multitrauma,[23–26] hip fracture,[27] and knee or hip replacement surgery.[28,29] All of these expanded indications remain controversial, and additional studies are required before meaningful conclusions can be drawn regarding their appropriateness.

As filter use has increased, these devices have more frequently been placed in severely ill and elderly patients.[30,31] Some investigators have observed that these patients tend to have relatively high mortality rates in spite of filter placement, and have suggested establishing uniform practice guidelines to ensure the cost-effective use of filters in these populations.[30,32–34]

While caval filters effectively prevent pulmonary embolism, they do nothing to treat the underlying thrombotic process (and may in fact promote thrombus formation). Patients with IVC filters should therefore have conventional anticoagulation therapy initiated/reinitiated as soon as their clinical condition allows.[35]

CONTRAINDICATIONS

There are few absolute contraindications to caval filter placement. Venous thrombosis between the access and deployment sites precludes safe filter deployment. In extreme cases where all routes of access are thrombosed or where there is extensive caval thrombus, thrombolysis may be useful in establishing a suitable route of access or a deployment site. Septic emboli are considered by some to be a contraindication to IVC filtration. Hypercoagulable states are a relative contraindication, as the presence of a foreign body in the vena cava may exacerbate thrombus formation. Patients with severe coagulopathy unresponsive to therapy are relatively poor candidates for percutaneous placement because of the risk of hemorrhage. In such cases, placement of a Simon nitinol filter from an antecubital vein or surgical venotomy and closure should be considered.

THE PERFECT FILTER VERSUS THE AVAILABLE FILTERS

An effective caval filter must be efficient at trapping emboli while maintaining caval patency. The risks of morbidity and mortality of a filter should be less than those posed by thromboembolic disease and no greater than those posed by other treatment options. Although the characteristics of an ideal filter are not universally agreed upon, some are listed in Table 70–2. Ease of placement and other features such as magnetic resonance imaging (MRI) compatibility and the potential for temporary placement are attractive but should not be emphasized over more fundamental performance considerations. That there are six different Food and Drug Administration (FDA)-approved filters marketed for use in the United States, and many more systems on the market in Europe, indicates that the ideal filter has yet to be developed.

Table 70–2. Ideal Filter Characteristics

Biocompatible	Flexible, small-caliber system
Stable	Easily placed
Low impedance	Low cost
Nonthrombogenic	Option for temporary placement
Effective embolus trapping	MRI compatible

STAINLESS STEEL GREENFIELD FILTER

The standard Stainless Steel Greenfield filter (SSGF) (Medi-Tech, Boston Scientific Corp., Watertown, MA) consists of six stainless steel legs that radiate from a central hub, forming a conical shape. The filter is 4.6 cm long and has a maximal diameter of 30 mm at its base. The end of each leg is curved upward 180 degrees to form a hook that serves to anchor the device into the wall of the cava. The leg elements have a zigzag configuration and are spaced 2 mm apart at the apex and 6 mm at the base when expanded in a cava of 28 mm or less (maximum allowable caval diameter is 28 mm). A central hole in the filter apex allows for placement over a guidewire. The conical shape allows for progressive vertical filling in the central portion of the cone so that 70% of the filter can be filled with thrombus, with a reduction in cross-sectional area of only 49%.[36–38] The SSGF causes significant artifact on MRI images; however, it has been shown to be resistant to migration at field strengths of up to 1.5T.[39]

Much has been written about the reduced filtration of this device when deployed more than 15 degrees off the long axis of the vessel; however, this reduction in filtration efficiency is of questionable clinical significance,[40,41] and with proper implantation technique, the problem of tilting can be minimized.

Tadavarthy et al described the first percutaneous placement of the SSGF in 1984.[42] Prior to this time, placement required surgical cutdown. Although the SSGF is still in use, the disadvantages of its large sheath (No. 24 Fr) and its cumbersome deployment system have led most clinicians to abandon this filter for contemporary low-profile systems.

MODIFIED TITANIUM GREENFIELD FILTER

In an effort to minimize both the technical difficulties of placement and access site complications of its predecessor, the 12-F titanium version of the Greenfield filter (TGF) (Medi-Tech, Boston Scientific Corp., Watertown, MA) was developed in 1987. Made from Beta III titanium alloy, it retains the design advantage of the SSGF's conical shape and has similar clot-trapping efficiency and thrombogenicity. The TGF differs from its predecessor in many ways. Its elastic properties allow it to be placed via a No. 14 Fr [outer diameter (OD)] system that is considerably smaller and more flexible than the No. 26 Fr system of the SSGF. Lacking a central apical hole, the titanium version is not deployed over a guidewire. It is broader at its base (38 mm) and exerts a force on the wall of the vena cava greater than that of the SSGF at vessel diameters over 22 mm. It is as inert as stainless steel in tissues, and is resistant to flexion fatigue and corrosion.[36,43] This filter is nonferromagnetic and creates virtually no artifacts on MRI images.[44] The initial TGF had an unacceptable rate of caval perforation and migration.[35,45,46] Modification of the anchoring hooks of the current version have greatly reduced the incidence of these problems.[6,36,47,48] Leg asymmetry and element crossing continue to be noted in 7.4% of deployments using the modified system.[6] This effect has been shown to reduce filtration efficiency in the horizontal but not the vertical position.[49] Severe leg asymmetry and crossing can be corrected with gentle catheter manipulation; however, this maneuver can result in filter migration and is not recommended by the manufacturer. Flushing of each of the Greenfield systems prior to filter deployment may minimize leg crossing and asymmetry.

STAINLESS STEEL GREENFIELD FILTER (NO. 12 FR INTRODUCER)

The latest introduction to the U.S. filter market is a low-profile, over-the-wire stainless steel Greenfield filter (OTWG) (Fig. 70–1). This version is deployed over a stiff 0.035-inch guidewire using a No. 12 Fr introducer. The outer diameter of the introducer sheath is 15 Fr. The filter contains six elements arranged in the characteristic Greenfield conical configuration. It measures 49 mm in height and has a base diameter of 32 mm. Four of the legs end in hooks that point upward, and two legs on opposite sides of the filter terminate in hooks oriented downward. Use of a stiff guidewire is meant to facilitate passage of the OTWG through tortuous venous anatomy. The guidewire may also add some control during filter release. An early redesign incorporates a more flexible introducer tip on the femoral kits that is meant to further minimize technical failures related to inability to navigate tortuous anatomy. A stainless steel device, it creates some local artifact on MRI images.

LGM/VENA TECH

The Lehmann-Girofflier Medical (LGM) or Vena Tech filter (B Braun/Vena Tech, Evanston, IL) was first introduced in 1985. Like the Greenfield filters, the LGM is conical in design. Unlike the Greenfield devices, the filter elements are attached to flat mural-stabilizing side rails designed to optimize centering within the cava, regardless of the angle of deployment. These side rails have numerous small hooks that pro-

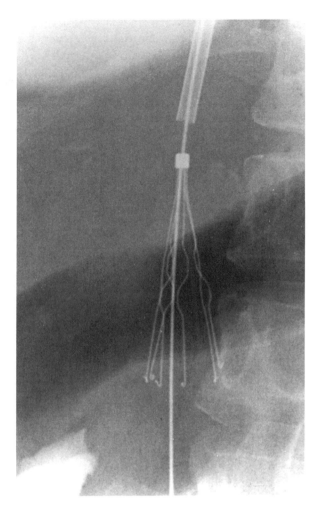

Figure 70–1. No. 12 Fr stainless steel Greenfield filter with No. 12 Fr introducer shown prior to removal of the guidewire. Although the manufacturer suggests using right-sided access, this filter can be successfully deployed from either the left common femoral or internal jugular vein approach. Because of iliocaval and right internal jugluar vein thrombosis, this filter was placed in a suprarenal location using the left internal juglular vein for access.

vide fixation to the caval wall. The LGM is made of Phynox, an alloy of eight metals with properties similar to those of Elgiloy, the material used to make temporary pacing wires. Its ferromagnetic force has been measured to be zero. It creates only minimal MRI artifact, though it does not interfere with the acquisition of diagnostic MRI images of the abdomen.[50]

With the original Vena Tech design, caudal migration and incomplete opening proved to be problematic, and when the LGM was incompletely opened, it filter's clot-trapping ability decreased and the caval thrombosis rate increased.[49,51–54] In 1991, a redesigned Vena Tech Filter was approved by the FDA. This modification alleviated much of the problem of incomplete opening. The newer filter also exerts more force on the wall of the vena cava, reducing the amount of migration compared with the original design. With the redesign came a new No. 12.9 Fr (OD) sheath that is slightly larger than the No. 12 Fr sheath of the original Vena Tech System.[49] This newer sheath is more radiopaque and less prone to kinking—features that help to decrease the technical failure rate. Unlike the other fixed-form filter systems, the LGM is available in a kit that allows the filter to be loaded into its sheath in either orientation. For this reason, the kit is not access site specific.

GIANTURCO-ROEHM BIRD'S NEST FILTER

The Gianturco Roehm Bird's Nest filter (BNF) (Cook, Inc., Bloomington, IN) was first used clinically in 1982. The filter, as originally constructed, suffered from problems of frequent proximal migration and prolapse. The current version of the filter is the result of a 1986 redesign that virtually eliminated the problem. The modified system requires insertion via a No. 14 Fr (OD) sheath.[55] It consists of four fine stainless steel wires that are 25 cm long and 0.018 mm in diameter. These wires are preshaped into a crisscrossing array of nonmatching bends. Each wire is fixed to a strut terminating in a small hook that provides fixation to the caval wall. One of the struts is Z-shaped so that a pusher wire can be attached. Loop stops at the end of each strut prevent IVC perforation. When deployed, the cephalad struts have a V-shaped configuration and the caudal struts are oriented in an inverted V-configuration. Once deployed, the wires of the BNF take on the free-form configuration in the IVC that gives the filter its name. A single kit may be used for either femoral or jugular access. The struts of the filter are easily identified on a plain film; however, the smaller wires that make up the "nest" are often not seen. The filtering efficiency of the device is unrelated to its orientation within the cava. Theoretically, the filter can trap smaller emboli because of the tight meshwork formed by its wires. One potential disadvantage of the filter is its length. At 7 cm, use of the BNF filter in patients with a short segment of usable cava requires the skill developed with experience, to tailor the length of the filter to match that of the IVC. Occasionally, the filter's wires may prolapse beyond the level of the anchoring struts. Mohan et al recently reported a 60% symptomatic IVC occlusion rate in patients with suprarenal wire prolapse.[56] While prolapse may increase the rate of caval thrombosis, it has been shown that the filter remains effective at trapping emboli in the prolapsed configuration.[40] Applying two or three 360 degree twists to the catheter-sheath unit during BNF insertion has been shown to reduce prolapse significantly.[57] The BNF causes significant local artifact and distortion on MRI images; however, there is no significant filter displacement at 1.5T field strength.[58]

SIMON NITINOL FILTER

The Simon nitinol filter (SNF) (Nitinol Medical Technologies, Woburn, MA) is made of a nickel-titanium alloy that has unique thermal shape-memory properties. A soft, straight set of wires when cooled, it instantly resumes a stable, previously imprinted filter shape when warmed to body temperature. The device measures 3.8 cm in length and has a 28-mm dome composed of overlapping loops. Extending below this dome are six legs that diverge radially from the center of the filter. Each of these legs terminates in a small hook that engages the IVC wall. The legs serve as a coarse prefilter and the dome as a fine second filter. With an OD of No. 9 Fr, the SNF has the smallest introducer system of any available filter. It can be deployed in cavae with widths of up to 28 mm;[59] however, the manufacturer suggests a maximum caval diameter of 24 mm if surgery with general anesthesia is planned within 2 weeks of insertion. The device is nonferromagnetic and creates only mild local artifacts on MRI images.[44]

Because of the thermal shape-memory properties of nitinol, which can result in premature activation of the filter shape within the catheter at body temperature, a saline infusion through the sheath is maintained during the deployment process. The small sheath diameter and flexibility of the filter enable the device to pass through acute bends, allowing for placement from access sites as peripheral as the antecubital veins.[60] Once the filter is in the desired location in the vena cava, it is unsheathed and warms to body temperature, rapidly assuming its characteristic shape.

TEMPORARY VENA CAVAL FILTERS

In addition to the permanent filters, there are two other classes of filters that are in use outside the United States: retrievable and temporary filters. The temporary filters must be removed after a limited period of time. Retrievable systems offer the potential for permanent placement if the necessary implantation time exceeds the window for safe explanation. None of the filters commercially available in the United States are designed to be temporary or retrievable. Cope et al reported successful use of a partially deployed BNF to filter the cava temporarily during iliocaval thrombolysis; however, the filter is not specifically designed for such use.[61]

Given the potential for long-term complications related to a permanent indwelling device, the concept of a temporary filter for patients with short-term thromboembolic risks is appealing. If temporary or retrievable filters are to gain widespread acceptance, however, they will have to demonstrate efficacy and complication rates similar to those of their permanent counterparts. In an in vitro study, Stoneham et al showed that two temporary designs have better clot-trapping ability than two widely used permanent filters on the market today.[62] Whether these temporary designs are associated with increased thrombotic complications remains to be seen.

Groups of patients who might benefit from temporary caval filtration include (1) perioperative patients, (2) trauma patients, (3) patients undergoing iliocaval thrombolysis, (4) patients with restricted mobility for limited periods of time, (5) pregnant patients, and (6) patients with complications related to over-anticoagulation.[62]

The devices designed for temporary use are generally tethered to a catheter that is then used to remove the filter[64–67] (Fig. 70–2). Some of the tethered systems allow for infusion of thrombolytic agents at the level of the filter. These filters have a limited useful life, as they must be removed before they are firmly incorporated into the caval wall. Their use should be restricted to patients with very-short-term thromboembolic risks.

Retrievable filters generally have hooks that facilitate capture with a snare catheter.[68–71] The filters are withdrawn into a sheath and then removed from the body. Depending on their design, retrieval can be accomplished from one access site, or may require access from both above and below the filter. In general, these devices cannot be reliably retrieved after 2 to 4 weeks. In patients with a tortuous cava or tilting filter, the retrieval hook may be buried in the IVC wall, which can make capture difficult or impossible.

PATIENT PREPARATION

Once the indication for filter placement has been verified, the patient's laboratory values including coagulation values, platelet count, and hematocrit should be reviewed. Consideration should be given to correcting coagulation in patients with a prothrombin time above 16 and/or platelet counts below 50,000. Patients referred for filter placement may be on heparin. In such cases, we generally continue the heparin until the patient is called to the angiography suite for the procedure. As with any medical procedure, informed consent including the risks, benefits, and alternatives to filter placement must be obtained. Some filter kits now include medical alert devices that identify patients as having an indwelling filter. Patients should be educated regarding their use.

TECHNICAL CONSIDERATIONS

The first step in filter placement is access site selection. This decision should be made after careful consideration of all the available information. The importance of this decision should not be trivialized, as the site chosen may minimize procedural difficulties and influence the type of filter selected.

Access should not be attempted through infected tissue or at sites already known to be thrombosed. Most patients are referred for filter placement after diagnostic imaging has confirmed a site of DVT. Whenever possible, the location and extent of thrombus should be ascertained. This knowledge, in combination with the

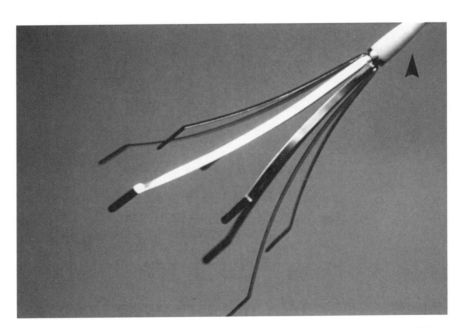

Figure 70–2. The Tempofilter (B Braun/Vena Tech, Evanston, IL) is a tethered filter that has been successfully left in place for periods of up to 6 weeks. The tethering catheter (arrowhead) is buried subcutaneously for the period of implantation and then used to remove the filter at explantation.

information gained from preprocedure venography, prevents inadvertent passage of the introducer system through thrombus, which could result in iatrogenic PE.

Right-sided access is preferred, as the common femoral and internal jugular veins on this side generally provide a straighter path to the IVC. Most interventionalists prefer femoral over jugular access. The reasons include familiarity with the femoral route and the elimination of several complications associated with the jugular approach.

PREDEPLOYMENT VENOGRAPHY

A high-quality inferior vena cavogram prior to filter placement is imperative. This step adds little time to the procedure and is critical to (1) confirm the intracaval position of the catheter, (2) determine IVC patency and diameter, (3) identify and locate the IVC thrombus, (4) map the anatomy of the IVC and its tributaries such as the renal veins, and (5) exclude venous anomalies that might influence filter placement in 10 to 15% of patients.[72,73]

Once access is achieved, a manual injection of contrast material under fluoroscopy through a No. 5 Fr dilator or catheter placed just into the accessed vein is useful to exclude thrombus along the access route. If thrombus is found between the puncture and deployment sites, an alternative puncture site should be selected. The cavogram should be performed with a flush catheter (No. 5 Fr or larger). Unless IVC thrombus dictates otherwise, the catheter should be positioned at the confluence of the iliac veins or in the contralateral common iliac vein just below the IVC bifurcation. Hicks et al have demonstrated the value of performing routine selective renal venography to maximize sensitivity to significant venous anomalies; however, this technique is not universally practiced.[74] The cavogram is acquired in the anteroposterior view using adequate rates and volumes of contrast material (20 cc/sec for 2 seconds) and a filming rate of two or three frames per second. Use of too little contrast material reduces sensitivity to venous anomalies. When possible, patients should perform the Valsalva maneuver during the cavogram to maximize IVC distention.

An accurate measurement of the IVC diameter must be obtained, as only the BNF is suitable for placement in vessels with a corrected diamater greater than 28 mm. (The BNF can be safely deployed in vessels up to 40 mm in diameter.[75]) All other filters on the U.S. market may be safely deployed only if the caval diameter is 28 mm or less. Caval measurement is facilitated by the use of a marker catheter or a radiopaque ruler positioned along the left side of the spine.

The renal and iliac veins are identified by the inflow of unopacified blood from these vessels or by the reflux of contrast into them (Fig. 70–3). Whenever possible, IVC filters should be placed below the level of the low-

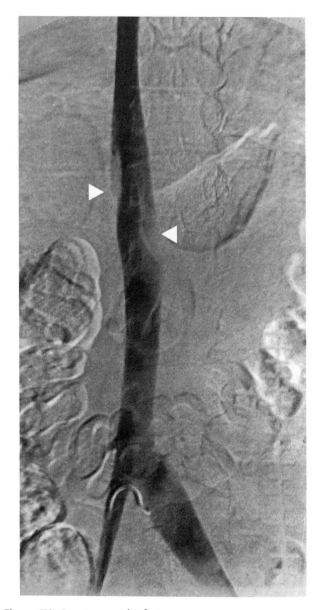

Figure 70–3. A normal inferior vena cavogram demonstrating inflow of unopacified blood from the renal vein (arrowheads) and reflux of contrast material into the normal common iliac veins bilaterally.

est renal vein to reduce the risk of renal vein obstruction related to IVC thrombosis or massive clot capture. Careful renal vein identification minimizes filter misplacements (Fig. 70–4). Placement into a tributary vein can result in thrombosis of the tributary or malalignment of the filter, which can result in loss of filtration efficiency.

Suprarenal placement may be required in cases of renal vein thrombosis, in extensive caval thrombus extending to or above the renal veins, and in the setting of recurrent PE after caval ligation or infrarenal filtration when no upper-extremity DVT is present. Although not universally accepted, suprarenal place-

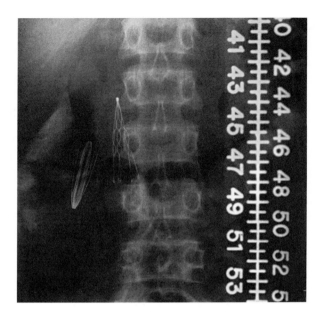

Figure 70–4. Radiograph demonstrating a misplaced Vena Tech filter in the right renal vein with an adjacent titanium Greenfield filter in the caval lumen. Most misplacements can be avoided with careful attention to technique.

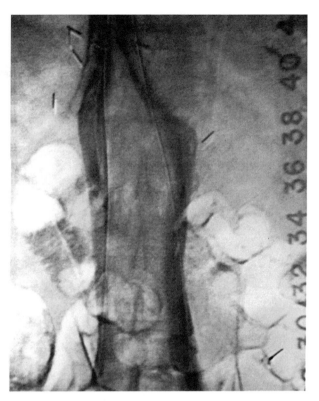

Figure 70–5. Cavogram demonstrating duplication of the IVC. The left IVC terminates at the level of the left renal vein. Infrarenal filters were placed bilaterally.

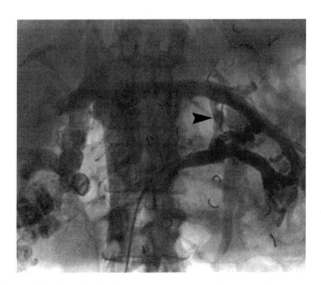

Figure 70–6. Predeployment venogram demonstrating a circumaortic left renal vein. The catheter is positioned in the inferior left renal vein, which passes posterior to the aorta. The superior vein passes anterior to the aorta. Emboli can bypass a caval filter positioned between these two veins via communications at the renal hilum (arrowhead).

ment has also been advocated for pregnant women and women anticipating future pregnancies to avoid compression of the filter by the gravid uterus, which could result in damage to the filter, cava, and surrounding structures. Suprarenal placement in this population also prevents recurrent embolization via an enlarged ovarian vein.

Common venous anomalies that affect filter placement include duplication of the IVC (prevalence 0.2 to 0.3%) (Fig. 70–5), transposition of the IVC (0.2 to 0.5%), circumaortic left renal veins (1.5 to 8.7%) (Fig. 70–6), and multiple renal veins (up to 25% of patients).[76–78] Patients with multiple renal veins may have large hilar communications. Placement of a caval filter between the orifices of these veins results in a persistent conduit for recurrent PE. This is particularly true for circumaortic renal veins in which large hilar communications are common. IVC duplications are identified on femoral venography by a triad of findings: an IVC that appears too narrow, lack of contralateral iliac vein inflow, and termination of the left IVC into the left renal vein. The last may be manifested by increased left renal vein inflow on cavograms performed from the right common femoral vein. Duplications of the IVC necessitate the placement of a filter into each of the cavae unless it can be clearly documented that only one lower extremity is a potential source of emboli.[49]

Finally, venography allows for localization of existing thrombus, which can significantly alter plans for filter placement. Occlusive thrombus above the level of the renal veins may obviate the need for filter placement.

The location and extent of nonocclusive caval thrombus influence the choice of access and deployment sites, which in turn may favor the use of a certain type of filter. For some patients (particularly those with central venous catheters), hemodynamically significant PE can arise from DVT limited to the upper extremities.[79,80] In these settings, superior vena cava filter placement may be called for.[81,82]

FILTER DEPLOYMENT

After the cavogram, the tract is dilated to accommodate the filter delivery system. Dilation can be performed using serial dilators or an appropriately sized angioplasty balloon. Data pertaining to the placement of the SSGF demonstrated that balloon tract dilatation resulted in fewer access site complications compared to dilatation with serial dilators.[83] The advantage of balloon tract dilatation for placement of lower-profile systems has yet to be demonstrated.

During the exchanges related to tract dilatation and introduction of the filter system, care must be taken not to withdraw the guidewire because it could migrate into a caval tributary on readvancement. Similarly, the introducer sheath should not be advanced in the cava unless it is over a wire that is confirmed to be in a caval position. Adhering to these principles helps minimize filter misplacement.

A vertebral landmark identified on the cavogram or a radiopaque scale placed under the patient prior to cavography should be used as a reference for the renal vein level. Prior to deployment, the operator should confirm that the selected filter kit is appropriate for the access and deployment sites chosen. The filter is then deployed. Technical complications are best avoided by proper preparation. Users should have a thorough knowledge of the manufacturer's instructions and be proficient in insertion and deployment of the selected filter. Proficiency is best gained by observing and assisting in filter deployments. Review of available videotapes and practice with models can also be useful. Familiarity with several devices is encouraged, as no single device is appropriate for all clinical situations.

Following filter deployment, hemostasis is achieved using direct pressure, and an abdominal radiograph is taken to document final filter positioning.

POSTPROCEDURE CARE

Vital signs and the puncture site are observed closely for 4 hours. Bed rest is suggested for at least 6 to 8 hours. The patient is instructed to avoid the Valsalva maneuver and heavy lifting for 24 hours. (If needed, stool softeners are given to help avoid straining with bowel movements.) All filter kits come with a filter registration card that should be completed and sent back to the manufacturer.

COMPLICATIONS

Complications associated with all of the available filter devices can be separated into those related to placement technique and those inherent in the filter systems and the underlying disease process.

Inadvertent carotid/vertebral artery puncture, pneumothorax, air embolism, vagus nerve injury, and arrhythmia are procedural complications generally associated with jugular access. Arteriovenous fistula, venous hematoma, filter misplacement, access site thrombosis, and caval perforation are problems that are not necessarily access site specific.

Recurrent PE, IVC thrombosis, IVC perforation, filter fracture, and migration are filter system–related complications encountered with all of the currently available devices. Symptomatic complication rates are quite low. Intuition suggests that the incidence of these complications might vary according to the specific filter; however, differences in patient populations, surveillance methods, and reporting practices make it difficult to quantitate accurately and compare complication rates for the various systems.

One complication that can be minimized with patient and physician education is filter dislodgment related to guidewire entrapment during subsequent central line placement.[84] Patients should be educated to suggest and physicians should learn to use straight guidewires when "blindly" placing central lines in patients with caval filters. This step may not eliminate wire entrapment; however, an in vitro study by Kaufman et al showed no problems with wire entrapment when straight (as opposed to J-tipped) wires were used.[85] The chart should clearly state that the patient has a filter so that appropriate measures can be taken.

FILTER PERFORMANCE

The evaluation of a filter's performance should include determinations of filtration efficacy, caval occlusion rate, and frequency of associated complications such as migration, caval perforation, and access site thrombosis. Criteria such as ease of insertion and MRI compatibility also figure in the overall performance of a device. To date, the majority of published data on the performance of vena cava filters has been based on clinical follow-up using criteria such as death, symptomatic recurrent PE, and lower extremity swelling. Few prospective evaluations have been published in which objective imaging data have been used to verify suppositions made on the basis of clinical information. Clinical follow-up would be acceptable if the outward manifestations of the events of interest were reliable indicators of occurrence or if the performance of the available devices varied greatly. Such is not the case. To illustrate the difference between objective imaging follow-up and clinical follow-up, one need only examine two of the major criteria used to assess filter performance: recurrent PE and caval patency.

The frequent occurrence of asymptomatic PE has been well documented and has been demonstrated in 35 to 51% of DVT patients.[86,87] Likewise, there is ample evidence to show that thrombosis and occlusion of the IVC are often asymptomatic events.[88,89] Additionally, patients with lower extremity DVT are predisposed to develop postphlebitic syndrome, and as many as 79% of patients experience lower extremity swelling due to valve damage related to thrombosis.[89–91] Given these facts, clinical assessment is clearly an unreliable indicator of recurrent PE and caval patency. The same can be said of clinical assessment of other criteria of interest including filter migration, access site thrombosis, and caval perforation. As the incidence of PE is not reflected by the manifestation of clinical symptoms, objective evaluation is needed if meaningful differences in filter performance are to be detected. The logistical problems associated with this type of data collection have prevented this type of analysis of the currently available filters.

RECURRENT PE/TRAPPING EFFICACY

Attempts to categorize caval filters by their trapping efficiency are understandable. The assumption that recurrent PE results from a filter's inability to trap emboli, however, is not necessarily valid. At least five other mechanisms exist for PE after filter placement: (1) occlusion of the IVC due to trapped emboli, with extension of thrombus cephalad; (2) nonocclusive propagation of thrombus along the wall of the cava through the filter; (3) nonocclusive embolus trapped within the filter, with subsequent cephalad propagation through the filter; (4) formation of thrombus at a site above the level of the filter (including renal and upper extremity veins); and (5) placement of a filter above collateral channels not recognized or developed at the time of predeployment venography.

Many in vitro and in vivo models have been devised to assess the clot-trapping efficiency of each of the available filters.[40,41,54,92–96] While all of these models suffer from design deficiencies of some form, they seem to indicate that the filtration effectiveness of all of the FDA-approved devices is comparable for all but the smallest experimental emboli.

As with much of the data in the filter literature, reported rates of recurrent PE are difficult to interpret because of varying survey techniques and inadequate follow-up. Nevertheless, the data suggest a similar rate of recurrent PE for all of the available devices—generally ranging from 2.7 to 4%.[6,51,54,55,59,97–100]

CAVAL THROMBOSIS

IVC occlusion after filter placement may occur as a result of thrombus formation within the filter, trapping of sufficient thrombus to occlude the filter, extrinsic compression on the cava, or by intimal hyperplasia that may be induced by the presence of the filter. Using IVC thrombosis/occlusion as a measure of filter performance is somewhat controversial. As the filtration efficiency of a filter increases, so does its impedance and its tendency to cause caval occlusion. Because no one has yet determined what constitutes a significant PE, we do not know what the ideal threshold for clot capture should be. This ideal threshold likely varies, depending on the clinical situation. Patients with little respiratory reserve might benefit from a filter with high trapping efficacy; however, patients with no comorbid cardiopulmonary disease might be better served by a filter that sacrifices filtration efficiency for better long-term caval patency.

With follow-up to 12 years, the caval patency rate for the SSGF has been reported to be 96%;[97] however, only 27% of the patients in the study had objective follow-up to determine caval patency. One study evaluated patients with SSGFs who underwent scanning for reasons unrelated to the previously placed filters. Twenty-nine percent of these patients had clinically unsuspected total occlusion of the IVC, and all of these patients had normal cavae prior to filter placement.[101]

In a series of 146 patients prospectively studied after LGM filter placement, patency was 92% at 2 years, 80% at 4 years, and 70% at 6 years. The recurrent PE rate was 3.5%.[98] It was postulated that the delayed occlusions may be secondary to retraction of clot trapped within the filter or intimal hyperplasia caused by the presence of the filter. It an in vivo sheep model, the clot-trapping efficiency of the LGM filter was shown to be higher than that of the TGF; however, the LGM filter was the more likely of the two filters to occlude.[15] The clinical significance of these findings is debatable; however, they do illustrate that criteria for optimal filter design may be incompatible and that trade-offs must be made for any given system.

A symptomatic caval occlusion rate of 9% was reported in the original series of 103 patients receiving SNFs.[59] A relatively small series of patients ($n = 24$) with malignancies experienced a symptomatic occlusion rate of 21%.[102] In the latter series, hypercoagulable states related to malignancy may account for the relatively high number of occlusions. These symptomatic occlusion rates are higher than those generally reported for the other FDA-approved devices.

IVC patency rates greater than 97% and recurrent PE rates less than 3% were reported in an early series of patients after BNF placement. These data were gathered from telephone and questionnaire contact made with 440 of 481 patients who had their filters in place for 6 months or more. Imaging follow-up was performed on only 40 patients. Seven of the 37 (19%) patients who underwent ultrasound or angiographic follow-up had documented occlusion of the vena cava, and two of the three patients who underwent pulmonary angiography had evidence of recurrent PE.[55] Another study reported an IVC occlusion rate of 21% after BNF placement.[103] Yet another study reported that with follow-up of 2 to 40 months, no IVC occlusions occurred in 37 of 61 patients imaged with ultrasound.[104]

These data underscore the need for better information concerning the long-term efficacy and complications of all caval filters. Data should be prospectively gathered and based on objective imaging information. Given the differences in patient populations and experimental techniques, it is difficult to know the significance of patency rates reported by the various studies. In general, rates of symptomatic IVC occlusion range from 2.9 to 9%.[6,53,55,59,97,98] Non-filter-related factors that might alter the incidence of caval thrombosis include the amount of residual clot below the filter, adjunctive anticoagulant therapy, and the presence of hypercoagulable states.

SELECTION OF A FILTER

As no significant differences in efficacy or associated complications have been conclusively established among the available filters, operator familiarity and facility with a device are often what dictate filter selection. Situations do exist, however, in which clinical circumstances suggest or even dictate the use of one filter design over the others.

The SNF has a clear advantage over the other devices in situations in which tortuous venous anatomy needs to be negotiated. This is the only available filter that can be placed via access sites as peripheral as the antecubital veins.

In the settings of a low-lying renal vein, incomplete caval thrombosis, and suprarenal or superior vena cava placement, there may only be a short segment of usable cava in which to deploy a filter. Situations such as this call for a filter with a small caval footprint, and one of the Greenfield devices should be considered.

Placement of a single BNF in the oversized IVC is favored over bilateral iliac devices because of the potentially increased risk of iliac thrombosis associated with the latter approach.[94] Measuring 70 mm long, the BNF is not suitable for patients in whom the length of usable cava is limited. In the unusual setting of a IVC more than 28 mm in diameter where there is not a sufficient length of usable IVC for the deployment of a BNF, dual common iliac vein filters can be placed.

MRI of all the available filters is considered to be safe; however, the ability to obtain diagnostic information about the filter and the surrounding tissues varies greatly among the devices. For patients with known abdominal pathology that may require future MRI evaluation, the TGF, SNF, or LGM filter should be selected.

The LGM and BNF are the only low-profile sysems that require a single kit for either femoral or jugular access routes. This flexibility may be appealing to institutions where few filters are placed and inventory costs need to be minimized.

CONCLUSIONS

IVC filter placement is a valuable method of PE prophylaxis in patients with DVT who cannot be anticoagulated, who have failed anticoagulation therapy, or who remain at significant risk for complications of PE in spite of adequate anticoagulation. Because caval filters do nothing to treat (and may exacerbate) the underlying thrombotic process, patients with IVC filters should have conventional anticoagulation therapy initiated as soon as their clinical condition allows.

The relative safety and ease of placement of contemporary filters have resulted in their expanded use—often outside of traditional guidelines. Liberalization of filter indications may be warranted; however, such determinations should be supported by prospective investigation.

Although the published data show no clear differences in clinical outcome to suggest the superiority of one filter design over another, the relative strengths and weaknesses of the available filters often lead to the selection of a particular device. Studies of currently available filters continue, and new devices are constantly being introduced into the clinical arena. Soon temporary devices are likely to be commercially available in the United States. As large-scale, prospective trials are conducted, perhaps clear difference in efficacy and complication rates among the various permanent and temporary filters will emerge. Until then, selection should be based on personal experience, a working understanding of the available filters, and detailed knowledge of the patient's anatomy and clinical circumstances.

REFERENCES

1. Harmon B. Deep venous thrombosis: a prospective on anatomy and venographic analysis. *J Thorac Imaging* 1989;4:15–19.
2. Schuman LM. The epidemiology of thromboembolic disorders: a review. *J Chronic Dis* 1965;18:815–845.
3. Dalen JE, Albert JS. Natural history of pulmonary emboli. *Prog Cardiovasc Dis* 1975;17:257–270.
4. Evans AJ, Sostmann HD, Knilson MH, et al. Detection of deep venous thrombosis: prospective comparison of MR imaging with contrast venography. *AJR* 1993;161:131–139.

5. Freiman DG, Suyemoto J, Wessler S. Frequency of pulmonary thomboembolism in man. *N Engl J Med* 1965; 290:1278–1286.

6. Greenfield LJ, Cho KJ, Proctor M, et al. Results of a multicenter study of the modified hook titanium Greenfield filter. *J Vasc Surg* 1991;14:253–257.

7. Stewart JS, Greenfield LJ. Transvenous caval filtration and pulmonary embolectomy. *Surg Clin North Am* 1982; 62:411–430.

8. Golueke PJ, Garrett WV, Thompson JE, et al. Interruption of the vena cava by means of the Greenfield filter: expanding the indications. *Surgery* 1988;103:111–117.

9. Rohrer MJ, Scheidler MG, Wheeler HB, et al. Extended indications for placement of an inferior vena cava filter. *J Vasc Surg* 1989;10:44–50.

10. Pomper SR, Lutchman G. The role of intracaval filters in patients with COPD and DVT. *Angiology* 1991;42:85–89.

11. Dorfman GS. Percutaneous inferior vena cava filters. *Radiology* 1990;174:987–992.

12. Simon M, Palestrant AM. Transvenous devices for management of pulmonary embolism. *Cardiovasc Intervent Radiol* 1980;3:308–318.

13. Norris SC, Greenfield LJ, Herrmann JB. Free-floating iliofemoral thrombus: a risk of pulmonary embolism. *Arch Surg* 1985;120:806–808.

14. McCollum C. Vena caval filters: keeping big clots down. *Br Med J* 1987;294:1566.

15. Hubbard KP, Roehm JO Jr, Abbruzzese JL. The bird's nest filter, an alternative to long-term oral anticoagulation in patients with advanced malignancies. *Am J Clin Oncol* 1994;17(2):115–117.

16. Cohen JR, Tenenbaum N, Citron M. Greenfield filter as primary therapy for deep venous thrombosis and/or pulmonary embolism in patients with cancer. *Surgery* 1991;109:12–15.

17. Cohen JR, Grella L, Citron M. Greenfield filter instead of heparin as primary treatment for deep venous thrombosis of pulmonary embolism in patients with cancer. *Cancer* 1992;70:1993–1996.

18. Whitney BA, Kerstein MD. Thrombocytopenia and cancer: use of the Kimray-Greenfield filter to prevent thromboembolism. *South Med J* 1987;80:1246–1248.

19. Calligaro KD, Bergen WS, Haut MJ, et al. Thromboembolic complications in patients with advanced cancer: anticoagulation versus Greenfield filter placement. *Ann Vasc Surg* 1991;5:186–189.

20. Olin JW, Young JR, Graor RA, et al. Treatment of deep vein thrombosis and pulmonary emboli in patients with primary and metastatic brain tumors. *Arch Intern Med* 1987;147:2177–2179.

21. Wilson JT, Rogers FB, Wald SL. Prophylactic vena cava filter insertion in patients with traumatic spinal cord injury: preliminary results. *Neurosurgery* 1994;35(2):234–239.

22. Jarrell BE, Posuniak E, Roberts J, et al. A new method of management using the Kimray-Greenfield filter for deep venous thrombosis and pulmonary embolism in spinal cord injury. *Surg Gynecol Obstet* 1983;157:316–320.

23. Rogers FB, Shackford SR, Ricci MA, et al. Routine prophylactic vena cava filter insertion in severely injured trauma patients decreases the incidence of pulmonary embolism. *J Am Coll Surg* 1995;180(6):641–647.

24. Khansarinia S, Dennis JW, Veldenz HC, et al. Prophylactic Greenfield filter placement in selected high-risk trauma patients. *J Vasc Surg* 1995;22(3):231–235.

25. Rodriguez JL, Lopez JM, Proctor MC, et al. Early placement of prophylactic vena cava filters in injured patients at high risk for pulmonary embolism. *J Trauma* 1996;40(5):797–802.

26. Rosenthal D, McKinsey JF, Levy AM, et al. Use of the Greenfield filter in patients with major trauma. *Cardiovasc Surg* 1994;2:52–55.

27. Fullen WD, Miller EG, Steele WF, et al. Prophylactic vena cava interruption in hip fractures. *J Trauma* 1973;13:403–410.

28. Vaughn BK, Knezevich S, Lombardi AV, et al. Use of the Greenfield filter to prevent fatal pulmonary embolism associated with total hip and knee arthroplasty. *J Bone Joint Surg* 1989;71:1542–1548.

29. Emerson RH, Cross R, Head WC. Prophylactic and early therapeutic use of the Greenfield filter in hip and knee joint arthroplasty. *J Arthroplasty* 1991;6:129–135.

30. Crystal KS, Kase DJ, Scher LA, et al. Utilization patterns with inferior vena cava filters: surgical versus percutaneous placement. *J Vasc Intervent Radiol* 1995;6(3):443–448.

31. Walsh DB, Birkmeyer JD, Barrett, JA, et al. Use of vena cava filters in the Medicare population. *Ann Vasc Surg* 1995;9(5):483–487.

32. McLoughlin RF, Sirkis H, So CB, et al. Severity of disease score as a predictor of mortality after caval filter insertion. *J Vasc Intervent Radiol* 1995;6(5):715–719.

33. Starok MS, Common AA. Follow-up after insertion of bird's nest inferior vena cava filters. *Can Assoc Radiol J* 1996;47(3):189–194.

34. Lossef SV, Barth KH. Outcome of patients with advanced malignancies receiving vena caval filters. *J Vasc Intervent Radiol* 1995;6(2):273–277.

35. Harris EJ Jr, Kinny EV, Harris EJ Sr, et al. Phlegmasia complicating prophylactic percutaneous inferior vena caval interruption: a word of caution. *J Vasc Surg* 1995;22(5):606–611.

36. Greenfield LJ, DeLucia A. Endovascular therapy of venous thromboembolic disease. *Surg Clin North Am* 1992;72(4):969–989.

37. Greenfield LJ, McCurdy JR, Brown PP, et al. A new intracaval filter permitting continued flow and resolution of emboli. *Surgery* 1973;73:599.

38. Brown PP, Peyton MD, Elkins RC, et al. Experimental comparison of a new intracaval filter with the Mobin-Udin umbrella device. *Circulation* 1974;50(2 Suppl):272–276.

39. Teitelbaum GP, Bradley WG, Klein BD. MR imaging artifacts, ferromagnitism, and magnetic torque of intravascular filters, stents, and coils. *Radiology* 1988;166:657–664.

40. Katsamouris AA, Waltman AC, Delichatsios MA, et al. Inferior vena cava filters: in vitro comparison of clot trapping and flow dynamics. *Radiology* 1988;166:361–366.

41. Thompson BH, Cragg AH, Smith TP, et al. Thrombus trapping efficiency of the Greenfield filter in vivo. *Radiology* 1989;172:979–981.

42. Tadavarthy SM, Castaneda-Zuniga W, Salamonowitz E, et al. Kimray-Greenfield filter: percutaneous introduction. *Radiology* 1984;151:525–526.

43. Greenfield LJ, Savin MA. Comparison of titanium and stainless steel Greenfield vena cava filters. *Surgery* 1989;106:820–828.

44. Teitelbaum GP, Ortega HV, Vinitski S, et al. Low artifact intravascular devices: MR imaging evaluation. *Radiology* 1988;168:713–719.

45. Ramchandani P, Koople HA, Zeit RM. Splaying of titanium Greenfield inferior vena cava filter. *AJR* 1990; 155:1103–1104.

46. Teitelbaum GP, Jones DL, van Breda A, et al. Vena caval filter splaying: potential complication of use of the titanium Greenfield filter. *Radiology* 1989;173:809–814.

47. Greenfield LJ, Cho KJ, Tauscher JR. Evolution of hook design for fixation of the titanium Greenfield filter. *J. Vacs Surg* 1990;12(3):345–353.

48. Greenfield LJ, Cho KJ, Pais So, et al. Preliminary clinical experience with the titanium Greenfield vena cava filter. *Arch Surg* 1989;124:657–659.

49. Hicks ME, Dorfman GS. Vena caval filters. In Strandness DE, Van Breda A, eds. *Vascular Diseases: Surgical and Interventional Therapy*. New York: Churchill Livingstone; 1994:1017–1043.

50. Kiproff PM, Deeb ZL, Contractor FM, et al. Magnetic resonance characteristics of the LGM vena cava filter: technical note. *Cardiovasc Intervent Radiol* 1991;14:254–255.

51. Ricco JB, Crochet D, Sebilotte P, et al. Percutaneous transvenous caval interruption with the "LGM" filter: early results of a multicenter trial. *Ann Vasc Surg* 1988;3:242–247.

52. Reed RA, Teitelbaum GP, Taylor FC, et al. Incomplete opening of LGM (Vena Tech) filters inserted via the transjugular approach. *JVIR* 1991;2:441–445.

53. Murphy TP, Dorfman GS, Yedlicka JW, et al. LGM vena cava filter: objective evaluation of early results. *JVIR* 1991;2:107–115.

54. Korbin CD, Reed RA, Taylor FC, et al. In vitro flow phantom analysis and clot-capturing ability of incompletely opened Vena Tech-LGM vena caval filters. *Cardiovasc Intervent Radiol* 1993;16(1):3–6.

55. Roehm JOF, Johnsrude IS, Barth MH, et al. The bird's nest inferior vena cava filter: a progress report. *Radiology* 1988;168:745–749.

56. Mohan CR, Hoballah J, Sharp WJ, et al. Comparative efficacy and complications of vena cava filters. *J Vasc Surg* 1995;21:235–246.

57. Roehm JO Jr, Thomas JW. The twist technique: a method to minimize wire prolapse during bird's nest filter deployment. *J Vasc Intervent Radiol* 1995;6(3):455–459.

58. Watanabe AT, Teitelbaum GP, Gomes AS, et al. MR imaging of the bird's nest filter. *Radiology* 1990;177:578–579.

59. Simon M, Athathanasoulis CA, Kim D, et al. Simon nitinol inferior vena cava filter: initial clinical experience: *Radiology* 1989;172:99–103.

60. Kim D, Schlam BW, Porter DH, et al. Insertion of the Simon nitinol caval filter: value of the antecubital vein approach. *AJR* 1991;57:521–522.

61. Cope C, Baum RA, Duszak RA Jr. Temporary use of a bird's nest filter during iliocaval thrombolysis. *Radiology* 1996;198(3):765–767

62. Stoneham GW, Burbridge BE, Millward SF. Temporary inferior vena cava filters: in vitro comparison with permanent IVC filters. *JVIR* 1995;6:731–736.

63. Venbrux AC. Temporary inferior vena cava filters. In Trerotola SO, Savader SJ, Durham JD, eds. *Venous Interventions*. Society of Cardiovascular and Intervention Radiology, Fairfax, VA; 1995:293–299.

64. Quilliet LE. Removable inferior vena cava filter: Filcard RF02. Results of multicenter pilot study. Presented at the International Symposium on Vena Cava Filters, Potiers, France, 1992.

65. Thery C, Asseman P, Amrouni N, et al. Use of a new removable vena cava filter in order to prevent pulmonary embolism in patients submitted to thrombolysis. *Eur Heart J* 1990;11:334–341.

66. Nagawa N, Cragg AH, Smith TP, et al. A retrievable nitinol vena cava filter: experimental and initial clinical results. *JVIR* 1994;5:507–512.

67. Vorwerk D, Schmitz-Rode T, Schurmann K, et al. Use of a temporary caval filter to assist percutaneous iliocaval thrombectomy: experimental results. *JVIR* 1995;6:737–740.

68. Irie T, Yamauchi T, Makita K, et al. Retrievable IVC filter: preliminary in vitro and in vivo evaluation. *JVIR* 1995;6:449–454.

69. Neuerburg J, Gunther RW, Rassmussen E, et al. New retrievable percutaneous vena cava filter: experimental in vitro and in vivo evaluation, *CVIR* 1993;16:224–229.

70. Millward SF, Bormanis J, Burbridge BE, et al. Preliminary clinical experience the Gunther temporary inferior vena cava filter. *JVIR* 1994;5:863–868.

71. Epstein DH, Darcy MD, Henter DW, et al. Experience with the Amplatz retrievable vena cava filter. *Radiology* 1989;172:105–110.

72. Martin KD, Kempczinski RF, Fowl RJ. Are routine cavograms necessary before Greenfield filter placement? *Surgery* 1989;106:647–650.

73. Mejia EA, Saroyan RM, Balkin PW, et al. Analysis of inferior venacavography before Greenfield filter placement. *Ann Vasc Surg* 1989;3:232–235.

74. Hicks ME, Malden ES, Vesely TM, et al. Prospective anatomic study of the inferior vena cava and renal veins: comparison of selective renal venography with cavography and relevance in filter placement. *J Vasc Intervent Radiol* 1995;6(5):721–729.

75. Reed RA, Teitelbaum GP, Taylor FC, et al. Use of the Bird's nest filter in oversized inferior vena cavae. *JVIR* 1991;2:447–450.

76. Chuang VP, Mena E, Hoskins PA. Congenital anomalies of the inferior vena cava. Review of embryogenesis and presentation of a simplified classification. *Br J Radiol* 1974;47:206–213.

77. Layton BT, Shaff MI, Mazer M, et al. Major venous anomalies of the inferior vena cava and renal veins: a radiographic and pictorial essay. *Semin Intervent Radiol* 1990;7(2):86–92.

78. Jones WP, D'Souza VJ, Herrera M, et al. An atlas of commonly encountered vascular variants. *Semin Intervent Radiol* 1990;7(4):236–262.

79. Diebold J, Lohrs V. Venous thrombosis and pulmonary embolism: a study of 58039 autopsies. *Pathol Res Pract* 1991;187:260–266.

80. Monreal M, Lafoz E, Ruiz J, et al. Upper extremity deep venous thrombosis and pulmonary embolism: a prospective study. *Chest* 1991;99(2):280–283.

81. Black MD, French GJ, Rasuli P, et al. Upper extremity deep venous thrombosis, Underdiagnosed and potentially lethal. *Chest* 1993;103(6):1887–1890.

82. Ascer E, Gennaro M, Lorensen E, et al. Superior vena caval Greenfield filters: indications, techniques, and results. *J Vasc Surg* 1996;23(3):498–503.

83. Dorfman GS, Esparza AR, Cronan JJ. Percutaneous large bore venotomy and tract creation: comparison of sequential dilator and angioplasty balloon methods in a porcine model—preliminary report. *Invest Radiol* 1988;23:441–446.

84. Loesberg A, Taylor FC, Awh MH. Dislodgement of inferior vena cava filters during "blind" insertion of central venous catheters. *AJR* 1993;161(3):637–638.

85. Kaufman JA, Thomas JW, Geller SC, et al. Guide-wire entrapment by inferior vena cava filters: in vitro evaluation. *Radiology* 1996;198(1):71–76.

86. Dorfman GS, Cronan JJ, Tupper TB, et al. Occult pulmonary embolism: a common occurrence in deep venous thrombosis. *AJR* 1987;148:263–266.

87. Huisman MV, Buller HR, ten Cate JW, et al. Unexpected high prevalence of silent pulmonary embolism in patients with deep venous thrombosis. *Chest* 1989;95:498–502.

88. Moran JM, Kahn PC, Callow AD. Partial versus complete caval interruption for venous thromboembolism. *Am J Surg* 1969;117:471–479.

89. Strandness DE, Langlois Y, Cramer M, et al. Long-term sequelae of acute venous thrombosis. *JAMA* 1983;250:1289–1292.

90. Lindner DJ, Edwards JM, Phinney ES, et al. Long-term hemodynamic and clinical sequelae of lower extremity deep vein thrombosis. *J Vasc Surg* 1986;4:436–442.

91. Mudge M, Hughes LE. The long-term sequelae of deep vein thrombosis. *Br J Surg* 1978;65:692–694.

92. Robinson JD, Madison MT, Hunter DW, et al. In vitro evaluation of caval filters. *Cardiovasc Intervent Radiol* 1988;11:346–351.

93. Burke PE, Michna BA, Harvey CF, et al. Experimental comparison of percutaneous vena caval devices: titanium Greenfield filter versus bird's nest filter. *J Vasc Surg* 1987;6:66–70.

94. Korbin CD, Reed RA, Taylor FC, et al. Comparison of filters in an oversized vena caval phantom: intracaval placement of a bird's nest filter versus biiliac placement of Greenfield, Vena Tech-LGM, and Simon nitinol filters. *JVIR* 1992;3:559–564.

95. Millward SF, Marsh JL, Pon C, et al. Thrombus trapping efficiency of the LGM (Vena Tech) and titanium Greenfield filters in vivo. *JVIR* 1992;3:102–106.

96. Palestrant AM, Prince MR, Simon M. Comparative in vitro evaluation of the nitinol inferior vena cava filter. *Radiology* 1982;145:351–355.

97. Greenfield LJ, Michna BA. Twelve year clinical experience with the Greenfield vena cava filter. *Surgery* 1988;104:706–712.

98. Crochet DP, Stora O, Ferry D, et al. Vena Tech-LGM filter: long-term results of a prospective study. *Radiology* 1993;188:857–860.

99. Taylor FC, Awh MH, Kahn CE, et al. Vena Tech vena cava filter: experience and early follow-up. *JVIR* 1991;2:435–440.

100. Millward SF, Marsh J, Peterson RA, et al. LGM (Vena Tech) vena cava filter: clinical experience in 64 patients. *JVIR* 1991;2:429–433.

101. Johnson CM, McKusick MA. Computed tomography of Greenfield filters abstract B-069. SCVIR 1991 annual meeting program. Reston, VA: Society of Cardiovascular and interventional Radiology; 1991:167.

102. Grassi CJ, Matsumoto AH, Teitelbaum GP. Vena caval occlusion after Simon nitinol filter placement: identification with MR imaging in patients with malignancy. *JVIR* 1992;3:535–539.

103. Ferris EJ, McCowan TC, Carver DK, et al. Percutaneous inferior vena cava filters: Follow up of seven designs in 320 patients. *Radiology* 1993;188:851–856.

104. Lord RSA, Ben I. Early and late results after Bird's Nest filter placement in the inferior vena cava. Clinical and duplex ultrasound follow-up. *Aust NZ J Surg* 1994;64:106–114.

71

Catheter-Directed Thrombolysis for Lower Extremity Deep Vein Thrombosis

Mark W. Mewissen, M.D.
Signe H. Haughton, B.A., C.C.R.C.

Deep vein thrombosis (DVT) of the lower limb is a serious, even life-threatening condition requiring treatment primarily to avoid the morbidity and mortality associated with its most serious acute complication, pulmonary embolism (PE). Most primary care physicians and specialists have long recognized that anticoagulation alone is the treatment of choice to guard against acute PE, but unfortunately, few are fully aware of the delayed complication of acute DVT, postthrombotic syndrome (PTS), which can occur months to years following acute DVT.[1] Furthermore, while heparin is of value in reducing thrombus propagation and the incidence of PE,[2] it does not prevent the manifestation of PTS, reported in up to two-thirds of patients following an episode of acute DVT.[3,4] Many reports have shown that systemic thrombolytic therapy can reestablish patency in acutely thrombosed veins, thereby preventing valvular damage, which can lead to PTS. More recently, catheter-directed regional thrombolysis has been reported to predictably lyse acute deep vein thrombus in selected patients, alleviating acute limb pain and swelling.[5] However, the long-term benefits of such aggressive therapy are not yet known.

NATURAL HISTORY OF LOWER EXTREMITY DVT

PTS affects up to 4% of the population and most patients who suffer from acute DVT.[1-3,6] Its manifestations, including chronic leg pain, edema, hyperpigmentation, and, in advanced cases, venous stasis ulcers, occur in up to two-thirds of patients following an episode of acute DVT.[4] An increasing prevalence of severe PTS is seen over years. Ambulatory venous hypertension, the underlying pathophysiology of PTS, is gener-

ally accepted as the hemodynamic mechanism that accounts for the development of these sequelae. Theoretically, this could result from venous valvular incompetence and/or chronic venous outflow obstruction.[7]

Current noninvasive diagnostic technology has been of increasing interest and importance during the past decade and has clearly enhanced our knowledge of the natural history of acute DVT. For instance, duplex ultrasonography offers an opportunity to acquire both anatomic and physiologic information using gray scale imaging combined with pulsed Doppler waveform analysis. Because the technique has the advantage of visualizing the entire venous system of the lower extremity, serial examinations have provided important objective information on venous patency, recanalization, and valvular reflux following acute DVT. Natural history studies employing duplex ultrasound technology have shown that postthrombotic limbs are more likely to have a combination of reflux and residual obstruction than either abnormality alone[7] and that the risk of developing reflux in veins involved by thrombus is more than twice that in uninvolved veins. Caps[8] recently showed that as many as one-third of venous segments that develop reflux were uninvolved by the initial acute thrombosis and that incompetent venous segments tend to develop when upstream veins have not fully recanalized (ie, remain at least partially obstructed). Other studies have shown that recanalization of venous thrombi commonly occurs and that early recanalization preserves valve function. In a long-term ultrasound follow-up study of 113 patients treated with conventional anticoagulation for acute DVT, Meissner et al showed that the time required to complete recanalization was related to the ultimate development of reflux.[9] In that study, complete recanalization took 2.3

to 7.3 times longer in venous segments developing reflux than in segments in which valves remained competent. It is now generally accepted that venous thrombi commonly recanalize or undergo spontaneous lysis and that the difference in outcome between individuals is probably related to differences between intrinsic coagulation and fibrinolytic systems.

From these studies, it can be theorized that initial therapy targeted at complete elimination of the acute thrombus should aid in protecting the hemodynamic integrity of venous valves and protect limbs against PTS.

GOALS OF TREATMENT

Elimination of the embolic potential of existing thrombus, restoration of unobstructed flow, prevention of further thrombosis, and preservation of venous valve function are the ideal goals of therapy for acute DVT. Meeting these goals will not only prevent PE but will also minimize the long-term sequelae of venous hypertension and the development of PTS. Multiple treatment options including anticoagulation, surgical venous thrombectomy, and thrombolytic therapy achieve these goals to a variable degree. For instance, while anticoagulation with heparin followed by Coumadin therapy is effective in minimizing PE, recurrent thrombotic episodes continue to occur and PTS is not prevented.[10] In fact, with anticoagulation alone, restoration of venous patency relies solely on individual endogenous fibrinolysis. furthermore, even with therapeutic heparin anticoagulation, 30 to 40% of patients develop extension of their DVT and only 20 to 25% have a venographic evidence of partial thrombolysis.[11,12] Treatment strategies aimed at eliminating or reducing the risk of PTS should focus on preserving valvular function and eliminating the risk of continued venous obstruction following acute DVT. Surgical removal by means of thrombectomy techniques combined with creation of arteriovenous fistulas have been employed successfully in Europe and the United States,[13,14] but overall, such procedures have not been commonly performed. Thrombolytic agents are an attractive form of early therapy because they eliminate obstructive thrombus in the deep veins and should therefore help provide protection against PTS. The perceived benefits of early, rapid recanalization in preserving valve function serve as the rationale for the use of lytic therapy to treat acute DVT.[15,16]

THROMBOLYTIC THERAPY: RATIONALE

In a pooled analysis of 13 randomized studies, Comerota and Aldridge found that only 4% of patients treated with heparin had significant or complete lysis compared to 45% of patients randomized to systemic streptokinase therapy.[17] Furthermore, in the heparin group, as many as 82% had either no venographic evidence of lysis or clearly demonstrated thrombus extension compared to 37% in the streptokinase group. Similarly, in an analysis of pooled data from six trials judged to have proper randomization, systemic thrombolysis was 3.7 times more effective in producing some degree of lysis than was heparin.[18] From these data, we see there is excellent objective evidence that systemic thrombolysis is more effective than anticoagulation in promoting early lysis.

Two studies reported a late clinical outcome following randomization to either anticoagulation or systemic streptokinase for acute lower limb DVT.[19,20] Although the follow-up periods in both studies were different, 1.6 years[19] versus 6.5 years,[20] the majority of patients with severe symptoms of PTS received anticoagulation alone. In both reports, the majority of patients who received streptokinase were free of PTS. Although both studies suffer from small sample sizes and lack of objective measures to grade PTS, it is nonetheless suggested that systemic thrombolysis achieves better anatomic and clinical outcomes than anticoagulation alone.

Long-term improved venous hemodynamics and preservation of valvular function have not been well documented following systemic lytic therapy. In a long-term, randomized follow-up study,[21] popliteal venous valve incompetence, measured by direct Doppler examination, was more common in patients randomized to anticoagulation versus systemic streptokinase. Nine percent of patients successfully lysed had an incompetent valve compared with 77% of those who were not lysed. This study, however, has not yet been published in a peer-reviewed journal.

CATHETER-DIRECTED THROMBOLYSIS

Background

Over the past 10 years, catheter-directed thrombolysis techniques have established effectiveness in the endovascular treatment of acute limb ischemia secondary to acute native arterial and bypass graft thrombotic occlusions.[22] Delivering thrombolytic agents by means of low-profile infusing catheters and guidewires placed directly into the occlusion under fluoroscopic guidance offers several advantages over systemic lytic therapy. Because highly concentrated plasminogen activators can be delivered directly into the thrombus, treatment duration can be reduced, complete lysis rates improved, and fewer bleeding episodes and other complications associated with systemic therapy can be expected. In addition, the technique allows for supplemental endovascular treatment of uncovered hemodynamic lesions by means of balloon angioplasty or stent techniques.[23]

Similar regional catheter-based lytic treatments have been recently applied in the treatment of iliofemoral

DVT.[5,14] In a series of 25 patients treated with catheter-directed thrombolysis for iliofemoral DVT by Semba and Dake,[5] complete lysis was achieved in 18 (72%) patients, and swelling was successfully reduced in all but 1. Only one patient suffered a bleeding complication of heme-positive stools. After the drug was discontinued, there were no significant adverse sequelae. This initial report suggests that catheter-directed lytic therapy in patients with lower extremity DVT can achieve significant lysis of clot and may be associated with low complication rates.

Choice of Lytic Agent

Although most published DVT thrombolysis trials have used systemic streptokinase, urokinase and recombinant tissue plasminogen activator (rt-PA) are two other lytic agents in common use today. The differences between these agents are based on clinical study results, with reports on thrombolytic activity and fibrinolytic specificity pertaining to each agent. For instance, Graor et al showed that streptokinase was associated with the slowest rate of clot dissolution and that rt-PA induced the most rapid rate of thrombolysis.[24] In a recent laboratory study, Ouriel et al objectively confirmed an advantage of rt-PA over streptokinase and urokinase with respect to early reperfusion, but this benefit did not persist because lysis rates between rt-PA and urokinase equalized during the latter reperfusion period.[25] These findings corroborate the observations of Meyerowitz et al in a randomized clinical study comparing rt-PA and urokinase.[26] Also, in the STILE trial,[27] a prospective, randomized trial designed to evaluate surgery versus thrombolysis for ischemia of the lower extremity, there was no significant difference between rt-PA and urokinase in terms of lytic efficacy or outcome.

These observations, taken in conjunction with economic considerations, suggest that urokinase may be the most appropriate agent in catheter-directed venous thrombolysis.

Contraindications to Lytic Therapy

Absolute Contraindication

Active internal bleeding
Recent (<2 months) cerebrovascular accident or other active intracranial process
Recent eye operation
Recent central nervous system surgery
Severe allergic reaction to thrombolytic agent

Relative Major Contraindications

Recent (<10 days) major surgery, obstetric delivery, organ biopsy, previous puncture of noncompressible vessels
Recent serious gastrointestinal bleeding
Recent serious trauma

Severe arterial hypertension (≥200 mm Hg systolic blood pressure or ≥110 mm Hg diastolic blood pressure)

Relative Minor Contraindications

Recent minor trauma, including cardiopulmonary resuscitation
High likelihood of a left heart thrombus, for example, mitral disease with atrial fibrillation
Bacterial endocarditis
Hemostatic defects including those associated with severe hepatic or renal disease
Pregnancy
Age over 75 years
Diabetic hemmorrhagic retinopathy

Technique

With the patient prone on the angiographic table, we prefer the ipsilateral popliteal venous approach because it is invariably difficult to penetrate an occluded superficial femoral vein from above due to venous valves that prevent safe catheter and guidewire manipulations. The popliteal vein is easily accessed under ultrasound guidance, even when thrombosed. A coaxial infusing system consisting of a No. 5 Fr multi-sidehole catheter and an infusing wire is placed directly into the occlusion, and its position is confirmed by venography. From this approach, the valves are easily traversed without risk of damaging the valve leaflets. Urokinase therapy is initiated at 150,000 to 200,000 (total) units/hr, evenly split between the infusing ports. As a general practice, we rarely employ a total urokinase dose of more than 200,000 units/hr, regardless of the thrombus burden or the number of involved extremities. During the thrombolytic infusion, we concurrently administer an intravenous heparin infusion at a rate of 500 to 1000 units/hr following a 5000-unit bolus of heparin.

In our experience as well as that of others,[5] completes lysis can be achieved in over 75% of limbs infused, with a mean urokinase administration of about 5 million units (Mu). It is now recognized that on the venous side, substantially more lytic agent is necessary to attain complete lysis compared to the dose required for the arterial system. Patients are monitored in the intensive care unit or in a stepdown unit, like those receiving thrombolytic treatment for acute PE or an arterial occlusion.

VENOUS REGISTRY

Objectives

A national multicenter Venous Registry involving over 70 medical centers began accumulating data on patients with symptomatic lower limb DVT in an attempt to define the potential role of lytic therapy more precisely, not only in alleviating early symptoms, but also in determining its short- and long-term impact on clinical outcome and valvular competence. The Registry was recently closed after enrollment of nearly 500 patients. Although late follow-up data have not yet been gathered for final analysis, several early observations are available on the technique and the early venographic outcome based on interim data collected from the first 68 evaluable patients.

Patients, Technique, and Early Results

Of the 68 evaluable cases, a complete set of venographic evaluations, as well as follow-up duplex scans of at least 10 to 14 days, were available and served as the basis for this interim evaluation.

Thirty-five percent of the patients had a prior history of DVT. Sixty-five percent presented with acute symptoms ($\leq$10 days), 24% had chronic symptoms ($\geq$10 days), and 12% presented with both acute and chronic symptoms. Right and left limbs were equally affected, and five patients had bilateral involvement. Access sites used for direct thrombolysis included the right internal jugular vein in 26 patients (38%), the common femoral vein in 33 (49%), and the popliteal vein in 19 (28%). A pedal (systemic) approach was used in 17 patients (25%). According to more recent data, the popliteal vein has become the access site of choice in the majority of cases. In 47% of the 68 cases, thrombi involved both supra- and infrainguinal venous segments. Isolated infrainguinal thrombus was found in 29%. Other sites accounted for the remaining 24%. Of these, five patients (7%) presented with massive thrombosis of both inferior vena cava and iliofemoral venous systems.

Direct intrathrombic thrombolysis thrombolysis was performed in 69 limbs (75%), and pedal/systemic infusion was performed in 17 (25%). Of the patients in the pedal/systemic infusion group, 13 had a combination of the two techniques, and 4 patients received a pedal infusion alone without catheter-directed delivery.

Duration of urokinase infusion for the systemic infusion group was longer than for the direct infusion group, 75.7 hours versus 48.6 hours, respectively. The amount of urokinase used also varied between the two groups, 12.8 Mu in the pedal/systemic group and 7.4 Mu in the direct infusion group. At this interim point, there was statistical significance between the techniques in both the amount of urokinase infused and the duration of lytic therapy ($p < 0.05$).

Following lysis, adjunctive stents were used to maintain venous patency in 34 limbs (49%). This suggests that an acute venous thrombotic event may be precipitated by an underlying venous compression or an underlying chronic venous lesion such as those associated with May-Thurner syndrome. This was true for the

majority of patients with iliofemoral DVT (53%). In such cases, balloon angioplasty alone has not provided adequate hemodynamic relief of chronic iliac vein lesions. Although the long-term benefit of metallic stents in the iliac veins is not known, based on this initial experience, stents have become an adjunctive form of treatment for the relief of uncovered chronic lesions following lytic therapy.

Major bleeding complications occurred in seven patients (10%), with six requiring transfusion. One subdural hematoma occurred during therapy for a thrombus that developed after a fall and initial treatment with t-PA. There were no reports of symptomatic pulmonary embolism occurring during infusion therapy.

Of the 73 limbs treated, complete lysis (no residual thrombosis on venogram), partial lysis (residual thrombus), and failure (unchanged from the pre-lysis venogram) occurred in 48%, 38%, and 14%, respectively. Placement of the infusion devices into the thrombus and completion (rather than premature termination) of the infusion were significantly associated with successful lytic outcomes. While technique, pedal/systemic versus catheter-directed, was not shown to be statistically significant at the 95% confidence level, there was a trend toward significance in its association with lytic success. Finally, there was a trend in favor of complete lysis achieved in limbs with acute DVT (<10 days) and no prior history of DVT on the symptomatic limb.

Case Study

A 62-year-old retired woman presented to the emergency room with a painful left leg and increased swelling over the previous 6 days. The patient was born with a congenital hip dislocation and occassionally used a cane for ambulation. Her prior medical history was otherwise noncontributory. She denied having any chest pain but admitted to experiencing a brief episode of shortness of breath the night prior to admission. She denied having fever, chills, nausea/vomiting, or any periods of inactivity or sitting for prolonged periods of time.

Duplex ultrasound indicated acute DVT involving the left common femoral vein extending to the popliteal vein. Initial laboratory studies were normal. The patient received a 5000-unit bolus of heparin in the emergency room in addition to an IV heparin drip at a rate of 1000 units/hr. The electrocardiogram showed mild sinus tachycardia, and the chest x-ray showed no acute changes.

The patient was admitted to the hospital and catheter-directed thrombolytic therapy was considered, given the patient's good health and absence of contraindications.

Under ultrasound guidance, a No. 6 Fr sheath was placed in the left popliteal vein. Contrast medium was injected manually, and limited venography identified

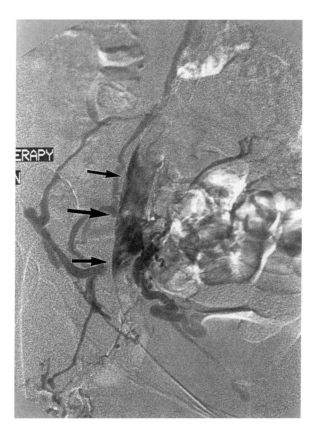

Figure 71–1. Digital subtraction venography of the left lower extremity demonstrating acute iliofemoral thrombosis (black arrows).

thrombosis of the entire iliofemoral-to-popliteal segment (Fig. 71–1). Urokinase was infused at a rate of 150,000 units/hr, evenly split between the sheath and two ports of a coaxial system embedded in the occlusion. Intravenous heparin was concomitantly administered at a rate of 1000 units/hr to maintain the partial thromboplastin time between 50 and 80.

Twenty-four hours after initiation of lysis and administration of 3 Mu of urokinase, the patient's symptoms improved significantly. Venography showed marked lysis in the previously thrombosed iliofemoral segment; however, residual thrombosis persisted. This thrombus was gently macerated using a 6-mm and an 8-mm balloon angioplasty catheter. Urokinase was restarted and continued overnight.

After a total of 5.3 Mu of urokinase, follow-up venography demonstrated complete absence of clot in the popliteal, superficial femoral, common femoral, and iliac veins (Fig. 71–2A–C). Significant stenosis was uncovered at the level of the common iliac vein, with a mean pressure gradient in excess of 6 mm Hg (Fig. 71–2D). A 12mm x 40mm Wallstent was deployed and further expanded with a 12-mm baloon (Fig. 71–3). Urokinase was discontinued, and the left popliteal vein sheath was left in place for continued heparin infusion. The patient experienced no complications. The following morning, the sheath was removed and hemostasis was achieved without difficulty.

At 3 months of follow-up the patient remains symptom free, and the deep veins remain patent and competent by duplex sonography.

PATIENT SELECTION FOR LOWER EXTREMITY DVT

Patients with acute iliofemoral DVT and a life expectancy not reduced by a fatal illness are likely to suffer from severe postthrombotic sequelae and should benefit most from lytic therapy.

Any patient who presents with phlegmasia cerulea dolens, irrespective of age or underlying disease state, should be considered for treatment unless an obvious contraindication exists.

Young, active patients with acute (<10 days), isolated infrainguinal DVT, documented by ultrasound or venography, may benefit from lytic therapy, except for those with a contraindication or those with isolated thrombosis of the tibial veins.

Hopefully, final analysis of the Venous Registry data will identify variables that will influence the late outcome and help to identify more precisely patients most likely to benefit from lytic therapy.

CONCLUSION

From recent reports as well as interim Venous Registry data, it appears that thrombolytic therapy administered

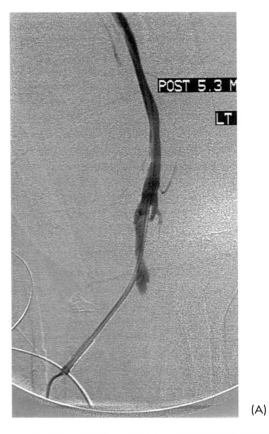

(A)

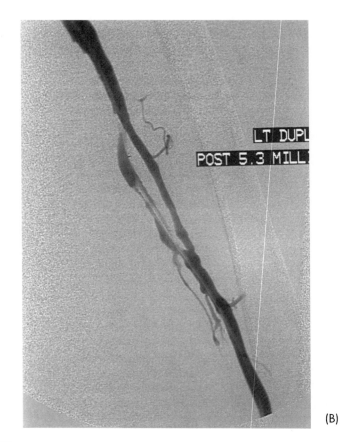

(B)

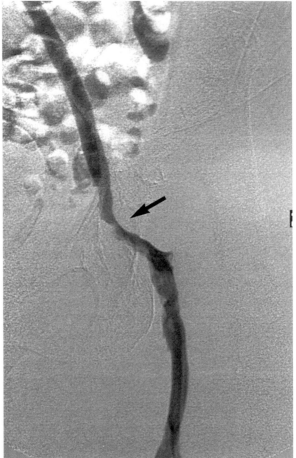

(C)

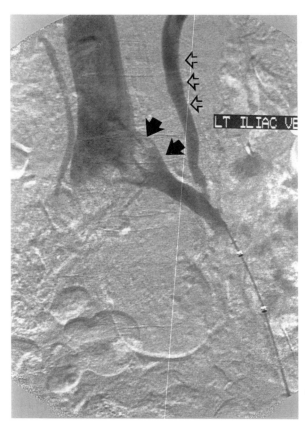

(D)

← **Figure 71-2.** Following administration of 5.3 Mu of urokinase, venography performed via a popliteal vein sheath demonstrates (A) a patent popliteal vein; (B) a patent superficial femoral vein; and (C) patent common femoral and external iliac veins; note the irregularities at the level of the common femoral vein (black arrow), not hemodynamically significant by intravenous pressure measurements; (D) focal stenosis at the left iliocaval junction (black arrows), probably as a result of iliac arterial compression (May-Thurner). Also note the hypertrophied venous collateral (open black arrows), indicative of the hemodynamic significance of the lesion.

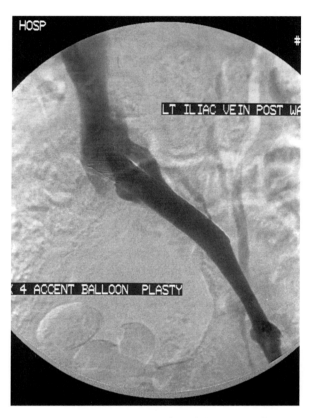

Figure 71-3. Iliac venous outflow following Wallstent placement (12 mm x 4 cm), relieving the obstruction, as demonstrated by lack of collateral filling.

by means of catheter-based techniques is superior to systemic infusion methods in achieving complete lysis, with resulting early clinical improvement. Whether this form of treatment will prove to preserve long-term valvular integrity in selected patients remains speculative. A randomized trial comparing anticoagulation alone versus catheter-directed thrombolysis followed by anticoagulation will be necessary to assess objectively the impact of lytic therapy on deep vein valve function and the incidence of PTS.

REFERENCES

1. O'Donnell TF, Browse NL, Burnand KG, et al. The socioeconomic effects of an iliofemoral thrombus. *J Surg Res* 1977;22:483–488.
2. Heparin and PE.
3. Markel A, Manzo RA, Bergelin RO, et al. Valvular reflux after deep vein thrombosis: incidence and time of occurrence. *J Vasc Surg* 1992;15:377–384.
4. Strandness DE, Langlois Y, Cramer M, et al. Long-term sequelae of acute venous thrombosis. *JAMA* 1983; 250:1289–1292.
5. Semba CP, Dake MD. Iliofemoral deep venous thrombosis: aggressive therapy with catheter-directed thrombolysis. *Radiology* 1994;191:487–494.
6. Coons WW, Willis PW, Keller JB. Venous thromboembolism and other venous disease in the Tecumseh Community Health Study. *Circulation* 1973;48:839–846.
7. Johnson BF, Manzo RA, Bergelin RO, et al. Relationship between changes in the deep venous system and the development of the postthrombotic syndrome after an acute episode of lower limb deep vein thrombosis: a one-to six-year follow-up. *J Vasc Surg* 1995;21:307–312.
8. Caps MC, Manzo RA, Bergelin RO, et al. Venous valvular reflux in veins not involved at the time of acute deep vein thrombosis. *J Vasc Surg* 1995;22:524–531.
9. Meissner MH, Manzo RA, Bergelin RO, et al. Deep venous insufficiency: the relationship between lysis and subsequent reflux. *J Vasc Surg* 1993;18:596–608.
10. Meissner MH, Caps MC, Bergelin RO, et al. Propagation, rethrombosis, and new thrombus formation after acute deep venous thrombosis. *J Vasc Surg* 1995;22:558–567.
11. Strandness DE. Thrombus propagation and level of anticoagulation. *J Vasc Surg* 1990;12:497–498.
12. Krupski WC, Bass A, Dilley RB, et al. Propagation of deep venous thrombosis by duplex ultrasonography. *J Vasc Surg* 1990;12:467–475.
13. Plate G, Einarsson E, Ohlin P, et al. Thrombectomy and temporary arterio-venous fistula in acute iliofemoral venous thrombosis. *J Vasc Surg* 1984;1:867–876.
14. Comerota A, Aldridge SC, Cohen G, et al. A strategy of aggressive regional therapy for acute iliofemoral venous thrombosis with contemporary venous thrombectomy or catheter-directed thrombolysis. *J Vasc Surg* 1990;20:244–254.
15. Truebstein G. Can thrombolysis prevent postphlebitic syndrome and thromboembolic disease? *Haemostasis* 1986;3:38–50.
16. Kakkar VV, Howe CT, Laws JW, et al. Late results of treatment of deep vein thrombosis. *Br Med J* 1969;1:810–811.
17. Comerota A, Aldridge SC. Thrombolytic therapy for deep venous thrombosis: a clinical review. *CJS* 1993;36:359–364.
18. Goldhaber SZ, Buring JE, Lipnick RJ, et al. Pooled analysis of randomized trials of streptokinase and heparin in phlebographically documented acute deep venous thrombosis. *Am J Med* 1984;76:393–397.
19. Elliot MS, Immelman EJ, Jeffrey P, et al. A comparative randomized trial of heparin versus streptokinase in the treatment of acute proximal venous thrombosis: an interim report of a prospective trial. *Br J Surg* 1979;66:838–843.
20. Arnesen H, Heilo A, Jakobsen E, et al. A prospective study of streptokinase and heparin in the treatment of deep vein thrombosis. *Acta Med Scand* 1978;203:457–463.

21. Jeffrey P, Immelman E, Amoore J. Treatment of deep vein thrombosis with heparin or streptokinases long-term venous function assessment (abstract No. S20.3). In: *Proceedings of the Second International Vascular Symposium*, 1989.

22. Kandarpa K. Technical determinant of success in catheter-directed thrombolysis for peripheral arterial occlusions. *J Vasc Interv Radiol* 1995;18:367–372.

23. Ouriel K, Shortell CK, De Weese JA, et al. A comparison of thrombolytic therapy with operative revascularization in the initial treatment of acute peripheral arterial ischemia. *J Vasc Surg* 1994;19:1021–1030.

24. Graor RA, Olin J, Bartholomew JR, et al. Efficacy and safety of intraarterial local infusion of streptokinase, urokinase, or tissue plasminogen activator for peripheral arterial occlusion: a retrospective review. *J Vasc Med Biol* 1990;2:310–315.

25. Ouriel K, Welch EL, Shortell CK, et al. Comparison of streptokinase, urokinase, and recombinant tissue plasminogen activator in an in vitro model of venous thrombolysis. *J Vasc Surg* 1995;22:593–597.

26. Meyerovitz MF, Goldhaber SZ, Regan K, et al. Recombinant tissue type plasminogen activator versus urokinase in peripheral and graft occlusions: a randomized trial. *Radiology* 1990;175:75–78.

27. The STILE Investigators. Results of a prospective randomized trial evaluating surgery versus thrombolysis for ischemia of the lower extremity: the STILE trial. *Ann Surg* 1994;220:251–268.

72

Transvenous Catheter Pulmonary Embolectomy: Indications, Technique, and Results

Mary C. Proctor, M.S.,
Lazar J. Greenfield, M.D.

Pulmonary embolism (PE) is a preventable cause of morbidity and mortality affecting more than 100,000 patients in this country each year. Implementation of clinical practice guidelines for treating PE could significantly reduce this complication and the related direct and indirect costs. Although prophylaxis, diagnosis, and treatment of PE have been widely explored in the literature, the evidence favoring any particular intervention is still evolving. This situation is probably related to the multifactorial causation of thromboembolism and the variable risk-benefit profile of the available interventions.

PE is easier to prevent than to diagnose or treat. In some cases, the first symptom is death, with diagnosis made at autopsy.[1] The differential diagnoses include myocardial infarction, pneumonia, and atelectasis.[2] The process of evaluating a hospitalized patient with recent onset of chest pain and dyspnea can require

time that the patient with acute, massive PE does not have.[3] The early use of pulmonary angiography and rapid intervention may be the patient's only hope.

Levels of PE acuity are differentiated on the basis of hemodynamic data, degree of pulmonary occlusion, and arterial blood gases (Table 72–1). The choice of treatment should be based on the patient's classification, which also suggests the prognosis. PE is classified as minor if the extent of pulmonary artery (PA) occlusion is less than 30% and there is little hemodynamic disturbance. These patients tend to do well with an intravenous course of heparin and 3 to 6 months of Coumadin. As occlusion increases to 50%, patients present with dyspnea. Both PA and central venous pressures increase. These patients often require pharmacologic circulatory support but usually respond to resuscitation. When more than 50% of the PA bed is occluded, patients may present in shock with an arte-

Table 72–1. Stratification of PE

Category	Signs and Symptons	Gases	PA Occlusion (%)	Hemodynamics
Minor	Anxiety Hyperventilation	PaO_2 <80 mm Hg $PaCO_2$ < 35 mm Hg	20–30	Tachycardia
Major	Dyspnea Collapse	PaO_2 < 65 mm Hg $PaCO_2$ < 30 mm Hg	30–50	CVP elevated, PA > 20 mm Hg Responds to resuscitation
Massive	Dyspnea Shock	PaO_2 < 50 mm Hg $PaCO_2$ < 30 mm Hg	> 50	CVP elevated, PA > 25 mm Hg Requires pressors, inotropes
Chronic	Dyspnea Syncope	PaO_2 < 70 mm Hg $PaCO_2$ 30–40 mm Hg	> 50	CVP elevated, PA > 40 mm Hg Fixed low cardiac output

Abbreviations: PaO_2, partial pressure of oxygen in arterial blood; $PaCO_2$, partial pressure of carbon dioxide in arterial blood; CVP, central venous pressure.
Source: Veith FJ, ed. *Current Critical Problems in Vascular Surgery*, Vol 6. Quality Medical; 1994:94. Used by permission of Quality Medical Publishing, Inc., St. Louis.

rial oxygen pressure (PaO_2) below 50%, requiring vassopressors or inotropes to maintain cardiac output. It is this group with massive PE that has the highest risk of mortality. Unless the condition is rapidly diagnosed and aggressively treated, the patient is unlikely to survive. The final class of PE consists of those patients who have acute PE superimposed on chronic, recurrent embolic events. The PA pressure is elevated markedly, and symptoms of cor pulmonale may be present.

TREATMENT

There are four possible methods of therapy: anticoagulation, thrombolytic therapy with urokinase or tissue plasminogen activator, open surgical embolectomy, and transvenous catheter embolectomy.[3] Heparin is the standard therapy because its antithrombotic and anticoagulant properties help to stabilize the embolus and prevent extension. It is normally administered for 5 days, and relief of symptom is usually seen within 12 to 24 hours. However, while this is adequate for patients with asymptomatic or minor PE, it is not likely to be effective in patients with massive occlusion.

Thrombolytic agents have been used to treat PE since the 1970s.[4] They have been shown to reduce the size of PE more rapidly than heparin during the first several hours of treatment, although controlled studies have demonstrated no improvement in overall mortality. Lytic therapy requires several hours to clear the embolus and may not work rapidly enough to correct hemodynamic instability and to prevent death. In addition, many hospitalized patients have a contraindication to thrombolysis due to recent surgery, trauma, or hypocoagulability, which precludes its use.[5] Even patients without these contraindications are subject to the risk of hemorrhagic complications including stroke. Finally, the cost of lytic therapy is extremely high. For all of these reasons, it is not an ideal therapy for patients with major or massive PE.

Pulmonary Embolectomy

Historically, open surgical pulmonary embolectomy was the standard of care for patients with massive PE.[6] The first approach was described by Trendelenburg in 1908 but was never completed successfully. Kirschner finally performed the first successful embolectomy by thoracotomy in 1924. This procedure has a very high mortality rate, with survival rates of 10%. By placing the patient on cardiopulmonary bypass prior to embolectomy, Sharp was able to lower mortality by 30%.[7] DelCampo reported a series of 650 pulmonary embolectomies with a survival rate of 60% when bypass was used compared to 49% when done without bypass.[8] Despite these improvements, the procedure remains risky in patients who are in shock, as it requires general anesthesia, a sternotomy, and the use of total cardiopulmonary bypass. It also requires a specially trained surgical team and sophisticated surgical equipment, none of which are found at the majority of community hospitals.

Others have reported more promising results. Kieng et al[9] described results in 134 patients that compare favorably with the outcome of thrombolytic therapy Jamieson reported results in 150 cases, with a low surgical mortality of 8.7%.[10] Clearly, patient selection is the most important determinant of the outcome because patients who are hemodynamically stable, as opposed to unstable, are most likely to survive with or without the procedure.

As the use of catheters for intravenous procedures became commonly accepted, the door was opened for the development of a transvenous approach to pulmonary embolectomy (Fig. 72–1). The initial work by Greenfield and colleagues[11,12] in an animal model demonstrated that embolectomy was effective in restoring pulmonary surfactant and PA flow. Recovery of gas exchange occurred within 30 minutes. Evaluation of this technique in dogs demonstrated that removal of even one experimental embolus resulted in large

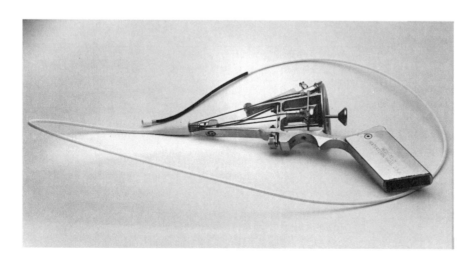

Figure 72–1. The Greenfield pulmonary embolectomy catheter and control handle.

decreases in PA pressure and resistance. These studies confirmed the concept of a critical degree of pulmonary vascular obstruction from a combination of mechanical obstruction and vasoactive substances released from the platelets.

The initial clinical experience with catheter embolectomy demonstrated a lower mortality than with open embolectomy.[13] Two of the deaths that occurred in the first 10 patients were due to recurrent embolism prior to caval clipping.[7] This led Greenfield and colleagues to develop a transvenous vena caval filter that could be placed at the time of embolectomy.[12] Its conical design traps potentially fatal PE while maintaining flow through the vena cava, thus allowing lysis of the trapped emboli. From 70 to 80% of the filter volume could be filled without significant reduction in caval flow.[14]

The original embolectomy device consisted of a rigid suction cup attached to a No. 8.5 Fr balloon catheter. This was inserted into the femoral or jugular vein through an operative venotomy and advanced through the PA to the thrombus under fluoroscopy. The location of the embolus was confirmed by low-volume injections of contrast medium. This early device was modified following the first 10 cases. The balloon was found to be unnecessary, and maneuverability was improved by the use of a steerable catheter guided by a "joy stick." The rigid metal cup was replaced with a radiopaque plastic cup.

Once the catheter cup is aligned with the thrombus, suction is applied using a large syringe. Attachment by aspiration of the embolus is confirmed when a vacuum is created. If blood returns, the catheter must be repositioned. The blood from the syringe can be returned to the patient. Once the embolus is attached, the entire unit is withdrawn through the venotomy. The procedure is repeated until no further thrombi are located or until hemodynamic stability is established.

While many transvenous procedures are done percutaneously using a sheath, catheter embolectomy should never be done in this manner. The suction cup usually attaches to the embolus in a folded position, as shown in Figure 72–2. If an attempt is made to withdraw the catheter through the sheath, the embolus may be knocked off or the rigid sheath may slice through it, allowing reembolization. The open venotomy can be controlled with umbilical tape, and the vein can distend to allow removal of the catheter and folded embolus intact.

Continuous electrocardiographic monitoring should be maintained throughout the procedure to detect any cardiac arrhythmia, which can develop from irritation of the conduction system as the catheter is advanced through the right side of the heart. Adjusting the posi-

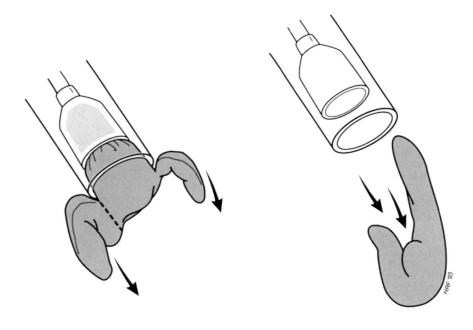

©1993 University of Michigan

Figure 72–2. Use of a percutaneous sheath may dislodge or fragment an embolus, resulting in recurrent embolization. (Reprinted with permission of the University of Michigan.)

tion of the catheter will usually eliminate this problem. In addition, blood pressure should be monitored regularly to determine the hemodynamic response to reduction of the thrombus. As the occlusion is relieved, vasopressor agents must be titrated. The progress of the procedure can be monitored by repeated measurement of PA pressure and cardiac output. In addition, the patient's level of consciousness should be monitored; it will increase as the patient becomes hemodynamically stable. Standby anesthesia should be available if the patient is not intubated.

As suggested above, the hemodynamic response usually occurs prior to any improvement in respiratory function, and it may not be possible to remove the patient from the ventilator for several hours. If no emboli are removed after 30 minutes and the patient continues to require hemodynamic support, open embolectomy ought to be considered.[15] Additionally, operative intervention is necessary when the patient requires chest compression and the catheter procedure cannot be performed. In all other situations, transvenous catheter embolectomy should be the initial procedure of choice once the diagnosis is confirmed angiographically.

The major advantage of the procedure is that the obstruction of the PA is rapidly removed, leading to reversal of right ventricular dilation, right heart failure, and ischemia (Fig. 72–3). When the effects of right ventricular dysfunction are reversed, the patient's immediate and long-term prognosis are improved. Additional advantages include the efficiency of a minor surgical procedure performed under local anesthesia in the angiography suite at the time of pulmonary angiography. Embolectomy does not require extensive training or sophisticated equipment. It is significantly less expensive than operative embolectomy, and the recovery period is far shorter. Overall, the cost effectiveness is well balanced compared to either operative embolectomy or thrombolytic therapy.

RESULTS

We have managed 50 embolectomy patients over a period of 26 years. These 24 females and 26 males had a mean age of 52 years. Thrombus was successfully removed in 76% of all cases, and 90% of the procedures were performed during the past 10 years. The majority of procedures were performed from the femoral vein, although the last 18 involved a jugular approach, which we now prefer. The traditional indication was for hemodynamically unstable patients with massive PE. As we gained experience with this procedure and established its safety and efficacy, we successfully extended the indications to include four patients with major PE requiring weaning from ventilatory support.[16]

Timsit et al have reported a similar experience with this technique at the Laennec Hospital in France. Between 1982 and 1989 they treated 18 patients, with successful embolus extraction in 11. They demonstrated a statistically significant association between the success of the procedure and the time from the first episode of PE, as well as the duration of hemodynamic impairment, with p values of 0.0004 and 0.003, respectively.[17]

While catheter embolectomy is effective in patients with major and massive PE, it has not been successful in patients with chronic PE and chronic pulmonary hypertension. Once the embolus has become adherent to the vessel, it cannot be successfully removed by this method. If fresh thrombus has embolized in addition to the chronic one, a small measure of relief may be achieved with embolectomy, but the results have not been impressive.

During the past several years, new devices and methods of transvenous embolectomy have been suggested. Brady et al performed embolectomy using a No. 8 Fr diagnostic catheter to fragment and disperse the fragments distally,[18] but their outcomes could not be achieved by other investigators.[19] Cope described modifications of the Greenfield device that involved using a sheath to introduce the catheter, but risks with this approach have been described elsewhere.[16,20] Animal studies have been done to evaluate a rapidly spinning blade that macerated the thrombus, but it was unsuccessful for two reasons. The blade did significant damage to the endothelial and muscular layers of the PA wall, and as the thrombus was destroyed, hemolysis developed. A complex device was evaluated that confined the thrombus within a chamber, where it was macerated and evacuated through a catheter. A third device confined a rotating blade within a wire basket that protected the vessel walls during clot destruction. None of these devices combine the safety and efficacy of the Greenfield embolectomy catheter, and they have not become commercially available. Modifications of the Greenfield device are ongoing and include the use of intravascular ultrasound for locating the thrombus and incorporation of new catheter technologies to enhance maneuverability.

While improving the device increases the safety and efficacy of the procedure, diagnosing the condition rapidly and identifying those patients who will die without emergent intervention improves survival. Pulmonary angiography is the diagnostic gold standard. However, echocardiography is being used increasingly to identify those patients with PE who are experiencing cardiac failure from a massive PA occlusion. If these patients can be differentiated from those with less severe effects and undergo embolectomy, the effects of the PE on the right side of the heart can be minimized. Patients who demonstrate right ventricular dilation are

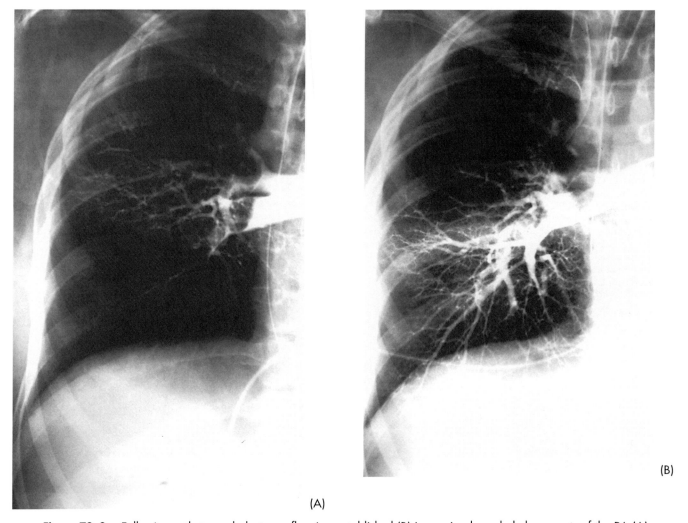

(A)

(B)

Figure 72–3. Following catheter embolectomy, flow is reestablished (B) in previously occluded segments of the PA (A).

at risk for decreased coronary perfusion, ischemia, and worsening right-sided heart failure.[21] Nazeyrollas et al demonstrated that echocardiography had a 6% false-positive rate and a 13% false-negative rate.[22] Given these findings, echocardiography may be useful in facilitating decision making in treating these critical patients.

The efficacy of the Greenfield transvenous embolectomy device has been demonstrated for appropriately selected patients. As new technologies are developed, they need to be fully evaluated in both animal and human clinical trials. These evaluations should include safety, efficacy, long-term outcomes, and cost-benefit assessments, as many of these new technologies involve highly complex materials.

REFERENCES

1. Morgenthaler TI, Ryu JH. Clinical characteristics of fatal pulmonary embolism in a referral hospital. *Mayo Clin Proc* 1995;70:417–424.

2. Hampson NB. Pulmonary embolism: difficulties in the clinical diagnosis. *Semin Respir Infect* 1995;10(3):123–130.

3. Tapson VF. Massive pulmonary embolism. Diagnostic and therapeutic strategies. *Clin Chest Med* 1995;16(2):329–340.

4. Goldhaber SZ. Thrombolytic therapy in venous thromboembolism. Clinical trials and current indications. *Clin Chest Med* 1995;16(2):307–320.

5. Levine MN. Thrombolytic therapy for venous thromboembolism. Complications and contraindications. *Clin Chest Med* 1995;16(2):321–328.

6. Scannell J. The surgical management of acute massive pulmonary embolism. *Prog Cardiovasc Disc* 1967;9:488–494.

7. Langham M, Greenfield LJ. Transvenous catheter embolectomy for life-threatening pulmonary thromboembolism. *Infect Surg* 1986;5(12):694–701.

8. Del Campo C. Pulmonary embolectomy: a review. *Can J Surg* 1985;28(2):111–113.

9. Kieny R, Charpentier A, Kieny T. What is the place of pulmonary embolectomy today? *J Cardiovasc Surg* 1991;32:549–554.

10. Bradley MJ, Spencer PA, Alexander L, Milner GR. Colour flow mapping in the diagnosis of the calf deep vein thrombosis. *Clin Radiol* 1993;47:399–402.
11. Greenfield LJ, Pearce H, Nichols R. Recovery of respiratory function and lung mechanics following experimental pulmonary embolectomy. *J Thorac Cardiovasc Surg* 1968;55(2):160–168.
12. Greenfield LJ, Reif M, Guenter C. Hemodynamic and respiratory responses to transvenous pulmonary embolectomy. *J Thorac Cardiovasc Surg* 1971;62(6):890–897.
13. Greenfield LJ, Bruce T, Nichols N. Transvenous pulmonary embolectomy by catheter device. *Ann Surg* 1971;174:881–886.
14. Stewart J, Greenfield LJ. Transvenous vena caval filtration and pulmonary embolectomy. *Surg Clin North Am* 1982;62(3):411–429.
15. Greenfield LJ. Intraluminal techniques for vena caval interruption and pulmonary embolectomy. *World J Surg* 1978;2:45–59.
16. Greenfield LJ, Proctor MC, Williams D, Wakefield T. Long-term experience with transvenous catheter pulmonary embolectomy. *J Vasc Surg* 1993;18:450–458.
17. Timsit J, Reynaud P, Meyer G, Sors H. Pulmonary embolectomy by catheter device in massive pulmonary embolism. *Chest* 1991;100(3):655–658.
18. Brady AJB, Crake T, Oakley C. Percutaneous fragmentation and dispersion versus pulmonary embolectomy by catheter device in massive pulmonary embolism. *Chest* 1991;102:1305–1306.
19. Meyer G, Diehl JL, Reynaud P, Sors H. Percutaneous fragmentation and dispersion versus pulmonary embolectomy by catheter device in massive pulmonary embolism. Reply. *Chest* 1992;102:1306.
20. Cope C. Venous cannula for emergency catheter pulmonary embolectomy. *Radiology* 1986;161(20):553–560.
21. Lualdi JC, Goldhaber SZ. Right ventricular dysfunction after acute pulmonary embolism: pathophysiologic factors, detection, and therapeutic implications. *Am Heart J* 1991;130(6):1276–1282.
22. Nazeyrollas P, Metz D, Chapoutot L, et al. Diagnostic accuracy of echocardiography—Doppler in acute pulmonary embolism. *Int J Cardiol* 1995;47(3):273–280.

73

Venous Stents: Indications, Technique, Results

Josef Rösch, M.D.
Bryan D. Petersen, M.D.
Paul C. Lakin, M.D.

Venous stents are very effective devices for the treatment of obstructions of large veins, particularly of the superior vena cava (SVC), inferior vena cava (IVC), and their major branches. A wide variety of pathologic conditions can result in large vein obstructions. Neoplastic masses compress and sometimes directly invade the veins; inflammatory or traumatic lesions and irradiation result in perivascular fibrosis. These are the most common external causes of large vein obstructions. As for internal causes, iatrogenic consequences of diagnostic or therapeutic indwelling catheters and dialysis shunts are the most common. Progressive obstructions, whether of external or internal origin, result in compromised blood flow and often lead to a secondary thrombosis that converts a partial into a complete obstruction—an occlusion.

Obstructions of large veins have severe circulatory consequences: venous hypertension with congestion and edema in the draining area of the involved veins and subsequent development of characteristic clinical congestive syndromes, such as the SVC and IVC syndromes, thoracic "inlet" syndrome, May-Thurner syndrome, and Budd-Chiari syndrome.

Percutaneous transluminal angioplasty (PTA) is much less effective in the treatment of venous obstructions than it is in the arterial system. It may temporarily relieve uncomplicated stenoses of the SVC caused by indwelling catheters, membranous obstructions of the IVC, or stenoses of subclavian or iliac veins secondary to dialysis shunts. However, the majority of large vein obstructions, whether neoplastic, inflammatory, or postirradiation in origin, do not respond well to PTA. The stenosis may distend during balloon inflation, but

it recoils immediately. Placement of an expandable stent keeps the lumen open and prevents elastic recoil and thus is a much better therapeutic option. For uncomplicated obstructions of large veins, stenting is the primary treatment of choice.[1-14] In venous obstructions complicated by thrombosis or in venous occlusions, stenting should be preceded by local fibrinolytic therapy.[8,9,11,12]

LOCAL FIBRINOLYSIS

Local fibrinolytic therapy is an effective and relatively safe technique for dissolving thrombus complicating anatomic venous obstructions. Urokinase, the fibrinolytic agent of choice, is injected in high doses directly into the clot via a small-lumen, multiple-side-hole catheter(s). With thrombosis of the axillary, subclavian, innominate, or iliac veins, a loading dose of 250,000 IU urokinase is used first to lace the clot; this is followed by continued infusion at a rate of 60,000 to 100,000 IU/hr. With SVC or IVC thromboses extending into its branches, two catheters are introduced bilaterally into the thrombosed veins. The loading dose is doubled in such cases (250,000 IU through each catheter) and followed by a dose of 40,000 to 60,000 IU/hr into each catheter, depending on the patient's weight and general condition. During local fibrinolysis, systemic heparin is administered to maintain the partial thromboplastin time at 1.5 times normal. Follow-up studies are done at 8- to 12-hour intervals and the position of the infusion catheter is adjusted, depending on the progress of lysis.

The duration of the local fibrinolytic infusion required for a complete lysis varies, but lysis is usually

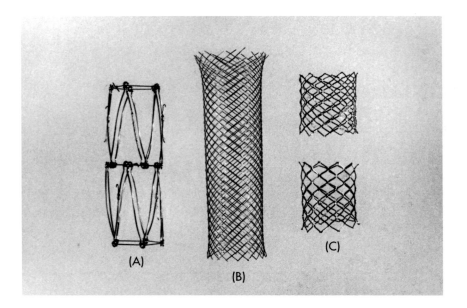

Figure 73–1. Three types of expandable stents used for venous stenting: (A) self-expandable Gianturco-Rösch Z stent, (B) self-expandable Wallstent, and (C) balloon-expandable Palmaz stents.

completed in 12 to 48 hours; occasional patients require up to 72 hours of infusion.

EXPANDABLE STENTS

Expandable stents currently available for venous stenting include the Gianturco-Rösch Z stent (Z-stent) (Cook, Inc., Bloomington, IN), the Wallstent (Schneider, USA, Inc., Minneapolis, MN), and the Palmaz stent (Johnson and Johnson Interventional, Inc., Warren, NJ). (Fig. 73–1). Although the self-expanding Z-stents and Wallstents, as well as the balloon-expandable Palmaz stents, are well suited for venous stenting, each stent has advantages and disadvantages in the venous system.

The *Z-stent* is commercially available as both a biliary and a tracheo-bronchial stent in diameters ranging from 8 to 35 mm. With the Z-stent, the maximal expansile force is in the central portion of the body, with less expansile force at the ends of the stent. Single-body Z-stents tend to "migrate" to a position either above or below a lesion. Therefore, double-body Z-stents should be used in short stenoses. They tend to center with the junction of the stents at the level of the tightest stenosis. For long stenoses, multibody Z-stents are optimal. The Z-stents have minimum surface area and can be placed across inflowing veins with no risk of occlusion. The bare Z-stents are sufficient in the majority of cases. With an obstruction caused by an intraluminal tumor or direct tumor ingrowth, the Z-stent covered with Dacron offers the best results.[15]

The *Wallstent* is available in diameters ranging from 5 to 24 mm. The main advantages of the Wallstent are their ready availability in longer lengths and the relatively small size of their delivery system. They are also relatively flexible and easily introduced. Their current disadvantage is their relatively low expensile force in

larger sizes, especially when they are not fully expanded. If they are not appropriately centered in the stenosis, they tend to "migrate" from the stenotic portion to a more dilated portion of the vein.

The *Palmaz stent* is balloon expandable and available in diameters of up to 12 mm, although they can be overdilated to a larger diameter. Their principal advantage is the predictability of their location on release and therefore the ability for precise placement. Their disadvantage is their susceptibility to plastic deformation due to compression. Strong extrinsic compression may result in narrowing or occlusion of the stented lumen. Therefore, Palmaz stents are not suitable for any location that is subject to compression, particularly in the subclavian and femoral regions.

In choosing a stent, it is essential to select a stent of the proper size to prevent its migration. The stent's diameter should be 15 to 20% larger than the normal diameter of the stented vessel. The stent should also be long enough to extend at least 2 cm both proximal and distal to the stented stenosis. Stent flexibility and compressibility are additional factors to consider in making a selection. The flexible Wallstent should be used in areas of motion such as the distal external iliac vein or the femoral vein. The self-expandable stents should also be placed in areas of potential extrinsic compression such as the subclavian vein.

For stent placement, femoral, subclavian, and jugular approaches are suitable. First, the stenosis should be dilated with a balloon. This is useful for introduction of the introductory sheath and evaluation of the character of the lesion and its extent for proper stent placement. With multiple stent placement, we usually place the more cranial stent first. When stenting the SVC bifurcation, we stent first the left brachiocephalic vein and then the SVC. In this way, we achieve direct contact of both stents. With stenting of the IVC bifurcation, we start by placing a stent in the IVC and follow with stents in the common iliac veins.

The patients undergo heparin anticoagulation during the stent placement procedure. The majority of patients, except those with hemodialysis shunts, receive continuous anticoagulation therapy after stent placement for 2 months until full stent endothelialization occurs. Patients with obstructions caused by malignancies and those requiring fibrinolytic therapy before stent placement receive long-term anticoagulation.

RESULTS

Venous stent placement has immediate clinical effects. In our 88 patients with large vessel obstructions in whom we generally used Z-stents, stent placement resulted in expansion of the obstructive lesions, regardless of their severity, and establishment of normal blood flow, with rapid relief of congestive symptoms. In patients with SVC syndrome, cyanosis of the face disappeared and a normal complexion returned shortly after stent placement. Facial edema and headache regressed within 24 hours, and truncal and upper extremity edema resolved in 2 to 3 days. Lower extremity swelling and ascites in IVC obstructions usually took slightly longer to resolve: 3 to 7 days after stenting.

Long-term results depend on the character of the obstruction, ie, whether it is caused by a malignant tumor or a benign process or is related to a dialysis fistula. Of our 88 patients, 53 had large vein obstructions related to malignant tumors, 19 to benign processes, and 16 to dialysis shunts.

Malignant Tumor Obstructions

Of 53 patients with obstructions caused by malignancies, tumors of the lung and mediastinum accounted for obstruction of the SVC and its branches, resulting in severe SVC syndrome in 26 patients. Stents in these patients were placed primarily in the SVC, but in many patients they also extended into the innominate and subclavian veins. In 23 patients with hepatomegaly secondary to metastases causing IVC stenosis, ascites, and severe edema of the lower extremities, stents were placed in the narrowed intrahepatic portion of the IVC and in one patient in hepatic veins as well. Four patients with pelvic tumors and unilateral lower extremity edema had stents placed in the iliac veins.

Stent placement provided excellent palliation. The majority (46 patients, 87%) did not have recurrence until their death or to the present time (from 8 days to 26 months; mean, 4 months) Fig. 73–2. Recurrence was observed in only seven (13%) patients due to tumor ingrowth and secondary thrombosis. Local fibrinolysis, PTA, and new stent placement established assisted patency, resulting in symptom relief in the five treated patients, with follow-up of 6 months.

Benign Venous Obstructions

In 19 patients with benign lesions, large vein obstruction was caused by postirradiation or idiopathic fibrosis, indwelling catheters, trauma, cirrhosis and Budd-Chiari syndrome. Stents were placed into the SVC, IVC and innominate, subclavian, hepatic, portal, and iliac veins. Stent placement, the definitive treatment for these patients with benign venous obstructions, resulted in long-term palliation, with complete regression of their symptoms. Seventeen patients had no recurrence of their congestive symptoms to the present time or to their death. Seven patients are still living 24 to 82 months (mean, 54 months) after stent placement Fig. 73—3. Ten died from 1 to 37 months (mean, 11 months) after stent placement secondary to their underlying disease or of unrelated causes. Two patients who had symptom recurrence due to intimal hyperplasia responded well to PTA and/or placement of a second stent, with assisted patency of up to 37 months.

Obstructions Related to Dialysis Shunts

Sixteen of our patients had obstructions related to arteriovenous dialysis shunts, with severe stenoses involving the brachiocephalic or subclavian vein. Stent placement extended the life of the fistula, but primary patency was less than that in patients with other types of benign venous stenosis. Only two patients had a normal diameter lumen up to 13 months after placement. In the other 14 patients, the stent lumen narrowed due to intimal hyperplasia. Repeated PTA, atherectomy, and/or new stent placement kept stented veins open and shunts functioning up to 79 months.

COMPLICATIONS

With proper stent sizing and placement we avoided stent migration, a complication that has been reported in the literature.[1] Early in our series, when we did not use heparin anticoagulation during the procedure, stents in two patients clotted during prolonged placement procedures. This thrombosis was successfully treated by short (2 to 3 hours) local urokinase infusion, and the stents remained open afterward. Four patients with local fibrinolytic therapy prior to stent placement had a large neck or groin hematoma at the catheter insertion site.

SUMMARY

Stent placement has great potential in the treatment of large vein obstructions. It is a simple, percutaneous, low-risk procedure that immediately relieves obstruction and results in rapid resolution of patients' congestive syndromes. In patients with malignancies, stent placement is an excellent palliative treatment and provides long-term relief in the majority of patients. In

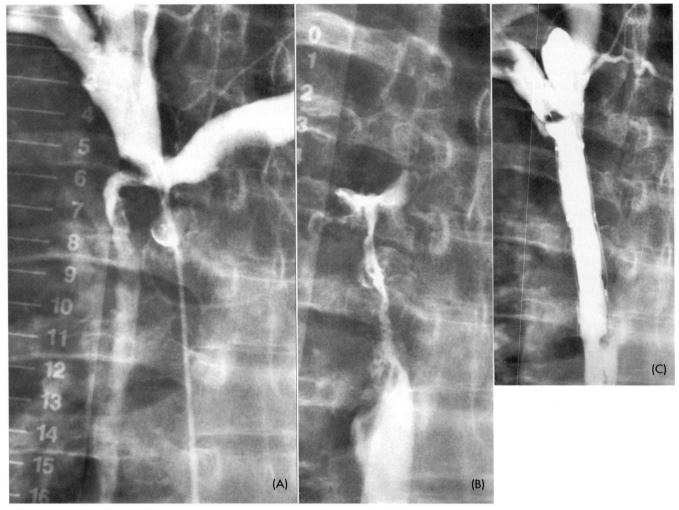

Figure 73–2. Obstruction of the SVC in a 64-year-old man with squamous cell carcinoma extending into the mediastinum and severe SVC syndrome. The patient had already been treated with maximum-dose radiation. After stent placement, he was asymptomatic for 11 months until his death due to tumor metastases. (A,B) Initial venograms show severe obstruction of the SVC secondary to direct tumor ingrowth. (C) Superior vena cavogram after placement of a Z-stent shows good stent expansion and excellent SVC patency.

patients with benign lesions, stent placement is a definitive treatment of large vein obstructions. Patients with obstructions related to an arteriovenous dialysis shunt benefit from stent placement because it significantly prolongs the life of the shunt. Local fibrinolytic therapy is an essential adjunct prior to stent placement in patients with venous obstructions complicated by superimposed thrombosis.

REFERENCES

1. Carrasco CH, Charnsangavej C, Wright K, Wallace S, Gianturco C. Use of Gianturco self-expanding stent in stenoses of the superior and inferior vena cava. *JVIR* 1992;3:409–419.
2. Dondelinger RF, Goffette P, Kurdziel JC, Roche A. Expandable metal stents for stenoses of the vena cava and large veins. *Semin Interven Radiol* 1991;8:252–263.
3. Antonucci F, Salomonowitz E, Stuckmann G, et al. Placement of venous stents: clinical experience with self-expanding prosthesis. *Radiology* 1991;183:493–497.
4. Elson JD, Becker GJ, Wholey MH, Ehrman KO. Vena caval and central venous stenoses: management with Palmaz balloon-expandable intraluminal stents. *JVIR* 1991;2:215–223.
5. Furui S, Sawada S, Irie T, et al. Hepatic inferior vena cava obstruction: treatment of two types with Gianturco expandable metallic stents. *Radiology* 1990;176:665–670.
6. Kishi K, Sonomura T, Mitsuzane K, et al. Self-expandable metallic stent therapy for superior vena cava syndrome: clinical observations. *Radiology* 1993;189:531–535.
7. Oudkerk M, Heystraten FM, Stoter G. Stenting in malignant vena caval obstruction. *Cancer* 1993;71:142–146.
8. Putnam JS, Uchida BT, Antonovic R, Rösch J. Superior vena cava syndrome associated with massive thrombosis: treatment with expandable wire stents. *Radiology* 1988;167:727–728.

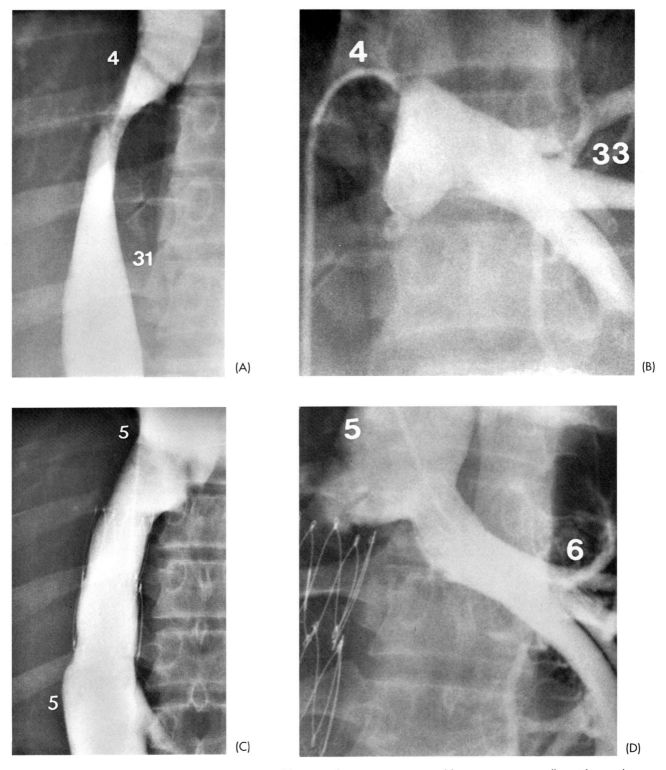

(A)

(B)

(C)

(D)

Figure 73–3. Budd-Chiari syndrome in a 26-year-old man with massive ascites and lower extremity swelling. The syndrome was caused by thrombosis of the right hepatic vein, severe stenosis of the left hepatic vein, and compression of the intrahepatic IVC. After the patient received Z-stents in the IVC and left hepatic vein, his ascites and lower extremity edema resolved. He has since been doing well, with no recurrence of symptoms, 6 years after stent placement. (A) Inferior vena cavogram reveals tight stenosis of the intrahepatic IVC portion, with a pressure gradient of 27 mm Hg. (B) Selective left hepatic venogram reveals severe ostial stenosis of the left hepatic vein, with a pressure gradient of 29 mm Hg. (C) Follow-up inferior vena cavogram 2 months after stent placement shows excellent expansion of the upper IVC, with no pressure gradient. (D) Follow-up left hepatic venogram after stent placement shows excellent expansion of the vein ostium and only a 1-mm pressure gradient.

9. Rösch J, Bedell JE, Putnam J, Antonovic R, Uchida B. Gianturco expandable wire stents in the treatment of superior vena cava syndrome recurring after maximum-tolerance radiation. *Cancer* 1987;60:1243–1246.

10. Trerotola SD, Lund GB, Samphilipo MA, et al. Palmaz stent in the treatment of central venous stenosis: safety and efficacy of redilation. *Radiology* 1994;190:379–385.

11. Rösch J, Uchida BT, Hall LD, et al. Gianturco expandable stents in the treatment of superior vena cava syndrome. *Cardiovasc Intervent Radiol* 1992;15:319–327.

12. Rösch J, Keller PS, Uchida BT, Barton RE. Interventional management of large venous obstruction. In: Strandness DE, Van Breda A, eds. *Vascular Diseases, Surgical and Interventional Therapy*. New York: Churchill Livingstone; 1994:999–1015.

13. Trerotola SO. Axillosubclavian veins and superior vena cava. In: Savader SJ, Trerotola SO, eds. *Venous Interventional Radiology with Clinical Perspectives*. New York: Thieme; 1996;269–284.

14. Mitchel SE. Inferior vena cava. In: Savader SJ, Trerotola SO, eds. *Venous Interventional Radiology with Clinical Perspectives*. New York: Thieme; 1996:285–297.

15. Chin DH, Petersen BD, Timmermans H, Rösch J. Stent-graft in management of superior vena cava syndrome. *Cardiovasc Intervent Radiol* 1996;19:302–304.

74

Long-Term Central Venous Catheters: Placement and Management

Donald F. Denny, Jr., M.D.

In the past 20 years, the use of long-term vascular access devices has increased dramatically. The introduction and development of tunneled silicon catheters by Broviac et al[1] and Hickman et al[2] was followed by the development of implantable ports.[3] An industry centered on venous access and outpatient therapy has burgeoned. Parenteral nutrition, antibiotics, and analgesia are provided in the home by visiting nurses, hospice programs, and commercial enterprises. Ambulatory chemotherapy programs have become the norm. In 1994, the global market for venous access devices was $410,420,000. Of this, $231,400,000 was in the United States alone (personal communication, Bard Incorporated). The market continues to expand rapidly, with an expected annual growth rate of (peripherally inserted control catheters (PICCs)) (personal communication, Sims Deltec).

The choices for access have expanded. Advances in sonography including color Doppler imaging assist placement in patients with unusual anatomy. With improved imaging and access technology, alternative access to the central veins using the inferior vena cava (IVC) or collateral veins in cases of occlusion of the subclavian vein, jugular vein, or superior vena cava (SVC) is possible when the primary access veins are occluded. Smaller catheters and ports intended for peripheral access to the central veins have been developed; the placement of these devices is simplified with fluoroscopic or ultrasound guidance. We have improved our understanding of the causes and treatment of catheter-related thrombosis and infection. This chapter reviews recent developments in access devices, access techniques, and the management of these devices and their associated complications.

ACCESS DEVICES

Access devices are characterized by the number and size of the catheter lumens and by whether an external connector or an implantable port terminates the catheter. Several factors must be considered before deciding which access method and device to use for a specific patient. First is the purpose for which the catheter is intended. The most common primary applications are chemotherapy, parenteral alimentation, antibiotic therapy, and hemodialysis. Other uses include transfusion, plasmapheresis, and patient-controlled analgesia. A single-lumen catheter can be used for any of these purposes on an intermittent or continuous basis. Multiple, simultaneous applications favor the use of a multilumen catheter, most often a two-lumen system. The risk of infection increases with the number of lumens, perhaps due to increased handling by personnel.[4] An implantable port is preferred when the need for access is intermittent because the intact skin protects the device from damage and infection when the device is not in use and because the implantable device interferes less with the patient's lifestyle. An external catheter is commonly used for continuous access or when high catheter flows are needed. Access to the central veins can be either central, usually via the subclavian or jugular veins, or peripheral via an extremity vein. High-flow, large-lumen catheters must be placed from a central rather than a peripheral approach due to their size. Peripheral access is generally limited to catheters 7 French or smaller.

The patient's preferences should play an important part in the choice of a device. The repeated needle punctures required to access a port may be intolerable to some. A small peripheral port in the arm may be preferred when the location or larger size of a chest port is undesirable. Normal lifestyle activities may be a determinant. For example, a peripheral or central port is less restrictive for recreational activities such as swimming than an external catheter.

External Catheters

Long-term external catheters are constructed of silicon rubber or polyurethane. They are usually tunneled subcutaneously between the vein access site and the skin exit site. Within the tunnel, a Dacron cuff is attached to the catheter. Over a 6-week period after placement, connective tissue grows into the interstices of the cuff, providing mechanical stability and a barrier to infection. For shorter-term protection, an antimicrobial cuff (VitaCuff, Bard Inc., Salt Lake City, UT) composed of collagen impregnated with silver ions has been developed. The silver ions provide an immediate chemical barrier to infection, while swelling of the collagen cuff to two or three times the dry volume assists in immediate mechanical stability. Dissolution of the collagen over approximately 6 weeks leaves the Dacron cuff for long-term protection. In a randomized, multicenter trial of 234 catheters using the collagen cuff, Maki et al[5] reported a drop in catheter-related sepsis from 3.7% to 1.0% of patients, and in a study of ICU patients, Flowers et al[6] reported a decrease from 13.8% to 0%.

More recent publications have questioned the need for routine tunneling. As originally envisioned, the tunnel protects against bacterial seeding of the vascular system from the skin. However, recent reports comparing nontunneled CVCs to tunneled ones suggest that there may be no benefit to tunneling.[7] As a result, there has been a rise in the use of nontunneled catheters for long-term access.[8,9] Eliminating the tunnel simplifies the procedure and reduces patient discomfort and procedure cost. Tunneling will continue to be used to allow a choice of exit site that is comfortable and convenient for the patient.

The user must choose between a valved catheter (eg, Groshong, Bard Inc.) and a nonvalved configuration. Valved catheters have a two-way valve at the tip of the catheter, which allows blood drawing and infusion but prevents blood from entering when the catheter is not in use. This feature may decrease the chance of catheter thrombosis and eliminates the need for heparin in the flush solution. Delmore et al[10] reported no cases of catheter occlusion in 72 Groshong catheters used for a median of 191 days. However, in a comparison of Hickman and Groshong catheters in cancer patients, Pasquale et al[11] found a significantly higher frequency of catheter malfunction with the Groshong. Single-lumen Groshong catheters are available in 3.5 to 8.0 French sizes and double-lumen catheters in 5.0 to 9.5 French sizes.

The nonvalved catheters differ primarily in the number, size, and configuration of the lumens. The single-lumen catheters for pediatric patients (eg, Broviac, Bard) have an intravascular portion of 2.7 to 6.6 French; the extravascular, subcutaneous portion is larger to resist kinking and breakage. Multilumen catheters usually have asymmetric lumens; the largest is used for infusion of viscous products and for drawing blood. Typical sizes are 8 to 13 French.

Long-term cuffed dialysis catheters have two lumens with staggered end holes. Examples include the Hickman (Bard) 13.5 French double-lumen catheter in lengths of 28 to 40 cm and the 11.5 French Soft-Cell catheter (Vas-Cath, Ontario, Canada). Depending on the flow requirements, access catheters as large as 21 French are used.

It is important to consider the length of the catheter is high-flow applications. Catheter flow is a function of lumen size and catheter length. Dialysis and plasmapheresis catheters are available in lengths of 20 to 40 cm. This is suitable for routine jugular and subclavian access but may restrict alternative access routes such as the translumbar approach to the IVC (see below).

PICCs are 2 to 6 French in size and are constructed of silicone elastomer or polyurethane. They have one or two lumens and are designed for placement via the arm. PICCs may be valved or not. The main advantages of a PICC are the lower risk of peripheral versus central access, the potential preference of the patient for arm rather than chest placement, and the possibility for bedside placement by trained nurses. Disadvantages include the smaller lumen size and hence restricted flow rate, the need for intact venous anatomy for successful placement, and the potential for catheter-related venous thrombosis of the extremity. These catheters are usually not tunneled. The longevity of these catheters is uncertain. PICC lines are suitable for short- and intermediate-term therapy lasting for weeks to months and may be suitable for long-term access in many patients. Infusion can be either continuous or intermittent. These catheters are commonly used for chemotherapy and antibiotic therapy for osteomyelitis or endocarditis.

Although designed for bedside placement, a PICC is placed more reliably when fluoroscopic guidance is available. Andrews et al[12] placed a 5 French silicon catheter into the basilic or brachial vein 73 times in 70 patients using fluoroscopic guidance, with 99% success, and recommended fluoroscopic guidance for patients with inadequate peripheral veins or when the patient wishes to avoid a catheter placed across the elbow. Cardella et al reported PICC placement in 305 patients; access was successful in 74% of 150 patients treated at the bedside versus 98.7% in 155 patients treated fluoroscopically.[13]

Implantable Ports

Implantable ports are available in single- or dual-lumen configurations, with a preattached or attachable silicon rubber or polyurethane catheter, with or without a valve. The ports are made of plastic or titanium; access is through a compressed silicon disk designed for 1000 to 2000 accesses with a noncoring needle (Fig. 74–1). Plastic ports produce minimal radiographic and computed tomography (CT) artifacts and do not interfere with radiation therapy portals. Plastic and titanium are both compatible with magnetic resonance imaging (MRI), although there is less imaging artifact in the volume around plastic ports. Implantable ports may be more convenient and comfortable for patients than external catheters, need to be flushed less frequently, and are protected by the skin when not in use. Single-lumen ports come in 6 to 10 French catheter sizes. Double-lumen ports are available with 10 to 13 French catheters. Central ports are placed in a subcutaneous pocket over the upper chest wall. The catheter is placed either percutaneously or by cutdown into the jugular, subclavian, or cephalic vein.

It is difficult to determine if ports become infected less often than external catheters. Most reports have not been randomized and have not directly compared devices in the same groups of patients. Studies supporting port use include the prospective comparison study reported by Ross et al.[14] When the external catheters were used, there were 0.13 exit site infections and 0.03 cases of bacteremia per 100 patient days. Using the implanted devices, there were 0.06 pocket infections and no cases of bacteremia per 100 patient days. Other studies support the advantages of implantable systems in other groups of patients.[3,15] On the other hand, ports are more complicated to implant and are more costly.

The most common use for implantable ports is in the care of patients requiring chemotherapy. While intensive parenteral support may be needed in these patients, it is usually on an intermittent basis. The benefit of a port in patients who require continuous therapy is questionable. A report by Pomp et al[16] supports the use of ports for home parenteral nutrition based on the low rate of major complications, such as sepsis, and on a preference for a port by their patients who had had a previous external catheter.

Small ports have been developed for arm placement and for children (Fig. 74–2). Andrews et al.[17] used a plastic cone-shaped port attached to a 5 French polyurethane catheter in 35 patients, with excellent short- and long-term results. In this series, ports were used for chemotherapy, blood transfusion, and blood sampling.

Another port designed for peripheral access to the central veins is the PAS Port (Sims Deltec, St. Paul, MN). This is a small, lightweight, low-profile titanium port attached to a 5.7 French polyurethane catheter (Fig. 74–2). The catheter is advanced to the SVC, and the port is placed medial or lateral to the biceps muscle or in the forearm. The small size decreases the incision length and dissection required for placement.

Several manufacturers have subsequently developed ports specifically intended for arm placement, includ-

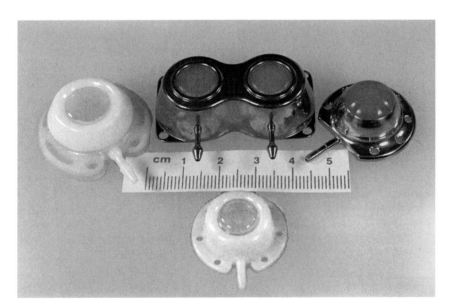

Figure 74–1.   Central ports. Back, left to right: Bard plastic MRI, Deltec dual lumen, and Bard dome ports. Front: Bard small plastic MRI port. (Reprinted from Denny DF Jr: Central venous access, in Taveras JM, Ferucci JT, eds. *Radiology: Diagnosis, Imaging, Intervention.* Philadelphia: JB Lippincott; 1995; chap 150, Fig 5, p 7, with permission.)

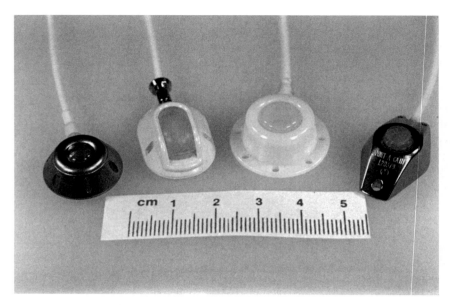

Figure 74–2.   Peripheral ports. Left to right: Cook Vital port, MediTech R-port, Bard small plastic MRI, Deltec PASPort. The Bad small MRI port is a central port shown for comparison to the ports designed for peripheral placement. (Reprinted from Denny DF Jr: Central venous access, in Taveras JM, Ferucci JT, eds. *Radiology: Diagnosis, Imaging, Intervention.* Philadelphia: JB Lippincott; 1995: chap 150, Fig 2, p 4, with permission.)

ing Bard, MediTech, Cook, and Strato. The preliminary success, longevity, and complication rates for peripheral ports are comparable to those for the larger central ports.[18–20]

ACCESS TECHNIQUES

The standard surgical technique for placement of external catheters and ports requires an operating room with local or general anesthesia. Fluoroscopic guidance is encouraged. Bedside placement of tunneled catheters has been described. Teaching videotapes available from the catheter and port manufacturers demonstrate routine placement. Routine placement techniques for central venous access devices using the subclavian and jugular veins has been reviewed by Mauro and Jaques.[21]

Imaging techniques are particularly useful for peripherally inserted central catheters and ports; alternative access when the subclavian veins, jugular veins, or SVC are occluded; and sonographic guidance for central and peripheral vein access.

Sonographic Guidance

Sonographic guidance is helpful both before and during routine subclavian and jugular vein access. Lameris et al[22] reported a drop in subclavian puncture complications from 10% to 0% when sonographic guidance was used. Mallory et al[23] used sonographic guidance for internal jugular vein puncture in the intensive care unit and found a drop in access failure from 35% to 0%.

Scanning prior to puncture detects venous thrombosis and variant anatomy. Procedure guidance is performed by aligning a 5- to 7.5-MHz linear array transducer along the course of the vein. The vein is usually larger than the adjacent artery, is thinner-walled, and varies with respiration (Fig. 74–3). The vein is compressible if not impeded by bone. Doppler analysis, if available, further distinguishes vein from artery. The access needle is introduced in the plane of the transducer. The transducer is positioned to visualize the needle and vein simultaneously. The tip of the needle will deflect and then puncture the vein wall. Using sonography, the operator can avoid unnecessarily deep needle passes that may puncture the pleura or artery. Sonography is particularly helpful in cases of obesity, postsurgical scarring, previous thrombophlebitis, or coagulopathy. Sonography may also be helpful in making the subclavian vein puncture more laterally, avoiding the compression and fracture of the catheter between the clavicle and first rib, the "pinch-off" syndrome.[24] While reports have described specially treated needle tips for improved sonographic visualization during organ biopsy or drainage, routine 18- to 21-gauge needles are easily seen during subclavian or jugular venipuncture.

The high incidence of central vein catheterization may justify using an ultrasound device designed specifically for central and peripheral venous access. An example is the SiteRite (Dymax, Pittsburgh, PA), a compact, portable, battery-powered ultrasound machine with a 3-inch screen. The unit has a guidance

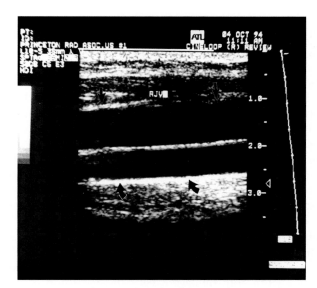

Figure 74–3. Ultrasound study of the jugular vein. The vein (arrows) is larger and thinner-walled than the adjacent artery (curved arrows). The vein is easily compressible, and its size varies with respiration.

tool attached to the transducer that simplifies venipuncture. In a randomized study, inexperienced first- and second-year residents successfully performed 23 catheterization procedures (92%) using this device for guidance versus only 12 procedures (44%) using standard anatomic landmarks.[25]

Peripherally Inserted Central Catheters and Ports

Bedside placement of a PICC uses the veins of the antecubital fossa or forearm, but these veins are often thrombosed due to repeated blood tests and placement of peripheral IV catheters. The basilic, cephalic, or brachial veins are almost always preserved above the antecubital fossa and can be visualized fluoroscopically by peripheral injection of contrast material or by using sonography. Imaging guidance plus the use of a variety of guidewires and catheters may allow successful completion of an otherwise impossible procedure in cases of obstructed or variant anatomy. The placement of a PICC or peripheral port requires only local anesthesia and minimal surgery. IV sedation can often be avoided, which permits immediate discharge of the patient after the procedure, without the need to monitor the patient in a recovery room.

Recent publications recommend the use of carbon dioxide (CO_2) for venography. Advantages include lack of toxicity and avoidance of allergic reactions.[26] While CO_2 is more cumbersome to use and harder to see, these limitations are minimal in arm venography.

Venospasm has been a common problem limiting peripheral vein catheterization. This can be avoided by preprocedure use of 100 μg nitroglycerin intravenously or sublingually. In addition, the use of a small-gauge access needle and a very-soft-tipped 0.018-inch (0.46-

mm) guidewire is recommended (eg, Micropuncture Peel-Away Introducer, Cook Inc., Bloomington, IN).

Venous access is performed at the level of the mid-upper arm, far enough above the elbow and below the axilla to avoid interfering with arm motion or clothing.[27] The basilic vein is preferred due to its larger size. With the use of the upper arm instead of the forearm, the device is less obtrusive. The port is placed medial or lateral to the biceps muscle. This can be at the site of vein access or tunneled for convenience a short distance away.

Alternative Access Routes

Central vein access in cases of occlusion of the jugular vein, subclavian vein, or SVC has been a frequent subject of reports in surgery and radiology publications. Thoracotomy with direct catheter placement in the right atrium, SVC, or azygos vein was an early alternative. Arteriovenous fistulas were created but were subject to early closure. Direct placement of a catheter in the IVC by open surgical technique has been reported.[28,29]

Percutaneous catheterization of the IVC using a translumbar approach is easily performed using C-arm fluoroscopy. Direct IVC catheterization is analogous to translumbar aortography. The IVC is generally more lateral and superficial than the aorta and more oval in shape.[30] A preoperative CT scan is helpful in planning the best position and angle for placement of a needle in the IVC. Placement of an IVC catheter from a femoral vein approach is used in the occasional patient with difficult access but is not routinely necessary. The technique described by Kenney et al[31] is used. The approach is from a point over the right iliac crest at a cephalad oblique angle, entering the IVC below the renal veins at the L2 to L3 level. A 21-gauge needle is used with a very-soft-tipped, 0.018-inch (0.46-mm) guidewire (eg, Neff access kit, Cook, Inc.) for initial dilator placement. After exchange for a heavy duty guidewire, the track is dilated and a peel-away sheath is placed, with its tip in the right atrium. The sheath chosen should be 1 or 2 French larger than the desired catheter. A tunnel is created between the sheath entry point and the proposed skin exit site. This is usually in the flank or the anterolateral right chest below the right breast. The catheter is pulled through the tunnel and trimmed to the desired length. It is introduced through the sheath to the right atrium or high IVC, and the sheath is peeled away. Special considerations apply for high-flow catheters used for dialysis and plasmapheresis. Because these catheters are shorter than those used for other purposes, a more lateral or posterolateral exit site and a shorter intravascular length may be used.

The catheter should be flushed immediately with heparin. The back incision is closed using subcuticular technique, and an anchoring silk suture is tied around the catheter at the exit site. The anchor suture is left in place for 3 weeks while the Dacron cuff is fixed by ingrowth of connective tissue.

Depending on the type of catheter used, the order and technique for tunneling and catheter length trimming may need to be adjusted. For example, the Groshong catheter is placed in the vein prior to tunneling its back end to the exit site. If an implantable port is used from this approach, it should be anchored over the lower ribs with nonabsorbable sutures to stabilize the port.

One difficulty associated with the procedure is the tendency of the sheath to kink at the point of entry into the IVC. The chance of this happening can be decreased by making an oblique track to minimize the angle at the junction between the sheath and the IVC. If a kink prevents passage of the catheter, the operator can pass a guidewire tht has a low coefficient of friction (eg, Terumo glidewire, MediTech Inc., Boston MA) through the catheter to stiffen it. The catheter and the wire can be advanced as a unit into and through the sheath. If this procedure is still not successful, the guidewire may be advanced in front of the catheter through the kink. The sheath is then retracted so that it is just entering the IVC and is no longer bent; then the catheter and guidewire can be advanced together.

We[32] reported successful use of the translumbar IVC route in seven procedures in six patients with 6 to 12 French catheters, with no case of subsequent catheter malposition or IVC thrombus. Lund et al[33] placed 46 catheters in 40 patients, with sizes ranging from 9.6 to 14.4 French. IVC thrombus occurred in eight patients, and two thrombi were occlusive. All thrombi were successfully lysed with urokinase. Catheter malposition was found at follow-up in five patients: four catheters were repositioned angiographically, and one resumed its position spontaneously. The patient's position, respiratory motion, coughing, sneezing, and vomiting all may cause the catheter to move. Successful placement in infants and children has been reported.[32,34,35]

The transhepatic route directly to the IVC or via a hepatic vein has been used. Although reports are limited,[34-37] this route appears to have few complications and good long-term results. The approach is analogous to that of transhepatic cholangiography and biliary drainage from a right lateral direction. Alternatively, a subcostal approach can be used. Ultrasound and CT are used in procedure planning. Ultrasound is useful for intraprocedural guidance and helps to avoid major intrahepatic vascular structures such as the portal vein. A peel-away sheath is used. The access catheter is tunneled a short distance to a convenient exit site over the chest or abdomen. Any standard external catheter or port can be placed via this approach. Care

should be taken to leave a sufficient length of catheter within the IVC to avoid inadvertent malposition during respiratory excursion of the liver. Some degree of slack at the entry point into the liver may be advisable. In the pediatric age group, patient growth may greatly shorten the intravascular portion. Hepatic vein rather than direct IVC access may be preferred in these patients.[35]

Even in cases of extensive central vein occlusion, including the IVC, alternative routes of percutaneous catheterization often can be found. Small-vessel catheteriztion systems including 21-gauge needles, 0.016-inch (0.41-mm) platinum or gold tipped guidewires, and small sheaths are used for cannulation and passage of catheters through collateral networks to the central veins. A combined surgical and radiologic approach may be considered in complex cases. Meranze et al[38] described a patient with SVC occlusion between the right atrium and the azygos vein and occlusion of the left subclavian vein, venous return was via the azygos vein to the IVC. The right subclavian vein had been previously thrombosed and was now recanalized but narrow. A hypertrophied intercostal vein was catheterized from the right subclavian vein through the SVC and the azygos vein. A stone basket was exchanged for the catheter. After surgical cutdown of the intercostal vein over the stone basket, a silicon rubber catheter was grasped and pulled from the intercostal vein to the high-flow azygos system.

COMPLICATIONS AND MANAGEMENT

Procedure Complications

The most common procedure complication of peripheral access is puncture of the brachial artery. This occurs due to the proximity of the artery to the basilic vein. The basilic vein, being the largest vein, is the one most often chosen for access. This complication can be avoided by careful palpation of the artery at the site chosen for access. In the lower third of the upper arm, the vein is superficial to the artery and is separated by a fascial plane. This is the safest zone for access of the basilic vein. Using the cephalic vein, if it is large enough, avoids the risk of arterial puncture entirely. Recognition of arterial puncture may be delayed; the distal arm pulses may be intact even with placement of a catheter through both walls of the brachial artery. Development of a large arm hematoma or pulsatile bleeding from the catheter entry site should prompt the diagnosis.

Minor bruising at a peripheral entry site is common. Peripheral access is often used in patients with coagulopathy or thrombocytopenia because this route does not risk injuring vital structures such as the lung, pleura, or subclavian or carotid artery.

There are a variety of procedure complications specific to centrally placed catheters. Arterial puncture and pneumothorax are the two most frequent; less common problems are arteriovenous fistula, mediastinal hemorrhage, cardiac tamponade, hemothorax, hydrothorax, and air embolism.

The principal procedure complication of port placement is hematoma. A small amount of local bruising at the pocket site can be expected in most patients. However, the pocket should not be closed until all active bleeding is controlled. Hematoma causes local pain and disfigurement. It also provides an excellent medium for bacterial growth and port infection. Presence of a hematoma will prevent successful use of the port if the access disk cannot be palpated. Adequate coagulation indices and platelet count should be ensured prior to placing a port.

Mechanical Complications

Mechanical problems requiring specific consideration in long-term access are usually related to breakage of the access device either within or external to the patient. Catheter migration or fragmentation is an occasional problem that can be treated by catheter redirection and retrieval using snares, guidewires, and catheters. In the past, catheter fragmentation most often occurred at the time of placement, during the insertion of the plastic catheter directly through a metal needle. The incidence of this problem dropped following the change from needle to sheath introduction. Delayed fragmentation is most often seen in pinch-off syndrome, a problem specific to the subclavian vein route. It results from repeated catheter compression or fixation by the subclavius muscle or costoclavicular ligament and occurs in catheters whose entry point into the vein is too medial. In a review by Lafreniere, the mean time to fracture was 6.5 months.[24] Pinch-off syndrome is usually discovered after the catheter has fractured, either due to a nonfunctioning catheter or as an unexpected finding on a chest radiograph. Radiographs prior to fracture may show abrupt angulation or compression of the catheter at the point of fixation.[39] Examination of the catheter fragments show a characteristic "fish mouth" appearance at the fracture site.

The tip of the catheter may erode into or through the wall of the SVC. This usually occurs with catheters placed via the left internal jugular or subclavian veins.[40] The catheter tip erodes at the junction between the left brachiocephalic vein and the SVC, where the abrupt angulation of the vein may cause the tip to lie against the right lateral wall of the SVC. Initially, this may cause positional inability to aspirate blood through the catheter. Subsequently, the patient may feel pain in the chest or neck during infusion due to extravasation into the mediastinum. Diagnosis is performed by a venogram.

Unlike external catheters, the connection of the infusion needle to the port cannot be directly inspected. If the needle is not in the port, or only partially in, the infusate may leak subcutaneously. The clinical effect will depend on the material being infused. To avoid this complication, the port should be aspirated prior to infusion. If there is no blood return, extra caution must be taken to ensure correct needle position and port function. Any complaint of local, chest, or neck pain should be carefully investigated. This problem is less common with peripheral ports because they are usually more superficial and easily palpable. The hubs and external tubing of external catheters are subject to wear and tear from repeated use. They are occasionally damaged by needles used for access. Repair kits are available, avoiding a lengthy and expensive replacement session.

Thrombotic Complications

Thrombotic complications occur in 3.7 to 10% of patients.[41] Asymptomatic thrombosis of the subclavian and jugular veins following catheter placement may occur in 30 to 50% of patients. Thrombosis may develop despite rigorous adherence to flushing and heparin protocols. Many patients are hypercoagulable, particularly those with malignant tumors. Other factors promoting thrombosis are venous irritation caused by some chemotherapeutic agents and hyperalimentation fluids and by the catheters themselves, as well as venous stasis caused by tumor compression. Catheter thrombosis and venous thrombosis may occur independently of each other (Fig. 74–4). Kim et al have described the various radiographic appearances of catheter-related thrombosis.[42]

Thrombotic complications are best treated by avoidance. Flush protocols for the specific catheter in use should be closely followed. For external catheters, 3 to 5 mL of heparin 100 U/mL is generally used. Concentrations of 10 U/mL are effective and are commonly used in children. A larger flush volume than normal may be needed for longer or larger catheters. External catheters should be flushed after each use and weekly when not in use. Prepared packs containing saline and heparin solution are available for home use by patients. Valved catheters are flushed with 10 to 20 mL of saline instead of heparin. Ports are flushed with 3 mL of heparin solution after each use and monthly when not in use. Ports with valved catheters are flushed with 20 mL of saline instead of heparin.

Prophylactic use of 1 mg warfarin daily may prevent catheter-related thrombosis. In a prospective, randomized trial, Bern and colleagues[43] reported that thrombosis developed in 15 of 40 patients not receiving warfarin versus 4 of 42 patients in whom warfarin treatment was begun 3 days before catheter placement and continued for 90 days afterward. No bleeding compli-

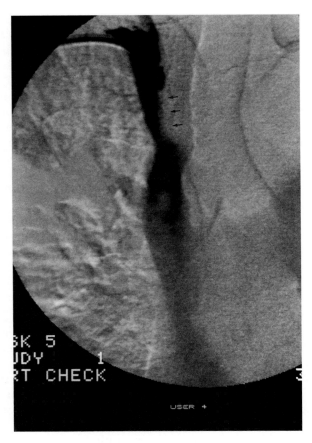

Figure 74–4. Mural thrombus. Central catheter injection shows an area of narrowing along the left border of the brachiocephalic vein (arrows) caused by a mural thrombus. There is retrograde filling of the brachiocephalic vein proximal to the thrombus and antegrade filling of the SVC. Catheter function is unaffected.

cations or detectable changes in coagulation tests occurred in the patients receiving warfarin. We have adopted this protocol for our oncology patients and for any other patients known to be hypercoagulable.

Early recognition of catheter occlusion improves the chance for successful treatment. The initial sign is usually the inability to aspirate blood from the catheter. This is usually due to the fibrin sheath that forms around all intravascular catheters or it may be due to a thrombus at the catheter tip (Fig. 74–5). Inability to aspirate blood from the catheter may also result when the tip of the catheter is against the vein wall. In this circumstance, having the patient change the position of the arm or head to perform a Valsalva maneuver will often correct the problem. If blood cannot be aspirated from a catheter that has been functioning well previously, tip occlusion should be suspected. If untreated, progressive thrombosis may cause increasing resistance to injection and finally catheter occlusion.

Occluded catheters should be promptly treated with a fibrinolytic agent. Outpatient treatment with urokinase, 5000 U in 1.8 mL (Abbokinase Open-Cath,

Abbott Laboratories, North Chicago, IL), via the catheter will usually reopen the clogged device in 30 to 60 minutes. The dose may be repeated if necessary. Leaving the urokinase in overnight has been successful. Continued catheter dysfunction should prompt a radiographic contrast study by catheter injection to verify proper position and mechanical integrity. In a report by Haire and colleagues,[44] 29 of 30 catheters that failed to reopen after bolus injections of 5000 U urokinase were successfully reopened with a 12-hour urokinase infusion of 40,000 U/hr, without bleeding complications; all 17 totally occluded catheters were reopened. For external catheters with refractory occlusion, a combination of guidewire manipulation and urokinase infusion will often salvage the catheter. Recent reports have described the use of a wire snare for stripping the fibrin sheath from an occluded catheter.[45] The snare is introduced via a catheter from a remote site, usually the femoral vein. Short-term patency rates are good, but long-term benefits are undetermined.

Venous thrombosis may occur around the catheter either secondary to tip thrombus or independent of catheter function. In some patients, chronic vein irritation at the tip of the catheter causes a venous stricture (Fig. 74–6). This may subsequently thrombose, causing acute obstructive signs and symptoms. Clinical onset of central venous obstruction is manifest by arm or facial

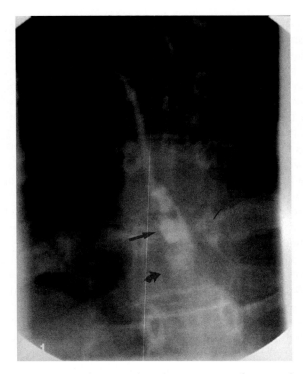

Figure 74–5. Catheter tip thrombus. Injection of a central catheter shows an area of contrast stain (arrow) extending from the tip. Faint opacification of the SVC (curved arrow) shows that the catheter obstruction is partial. Blood could not be aspirated from the catheter.

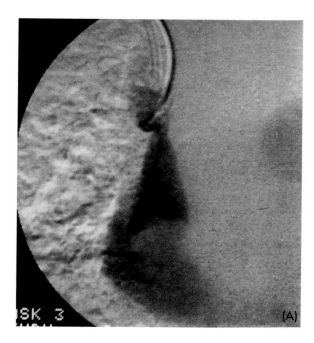

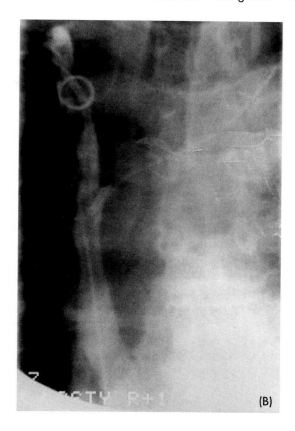

Figure 74–6.   SVC stricture. (A) SVC catheter injection shows a severe stricture at the tip of a port catheter. (B) After a snare was used to retract the port catheter, the stricture was dilated and a stent was placed.

swelling, cyanosis, venous distention, and superficial venous collaterals. For peripheral access, there is a small risk of thrombophlebitis of the arm vein through which the catheter passes. This manifests as a red, indurated cord along the course of the vein. The lower arm may swell if venous return is compromised. The arm is treated with elevation and warm soaks. If thrombophlebitis extends to the axillary or central veins, heparin should be given. Depending on the severity of symptoms, heparin may be used even if thrombosis does not extend centrally.

In the evaluation of catheter malfunction, it should be kept in mind that a contrast catheter study will usually give information only on the catheter tip and downstream vein; it does not allow evaluation of the vein through which the catheter passes. In cases of suspected thrombophlebitis, both a contrast study through the catheter and a peripheral venogram or sonogram may be required to fully evaluate the extent of thrombosis and to guide further therapy. Patients with venous occlusion at the catheter tip may often be treated successfully with urokinase infusion through the catheter rather than a peripheral vein, with both relief of symptoms and restoration of catheter function. Traditional teaching mandates removal of a catheter from a thrombosed vein. However, in many patients, alternative venous access may be severely restricted. If the vein can be reopened using fibrinolytic therapy, both venous function and the catheter can be saved. If the vein can-

not be reopened, a functioning catheter may still be left in place if the signs and symptoms of thrombophlebitis improve with therapy and in the absence of signs of septic thrombophlebitis. In the series of Haire et al,[44] in the six patients with catheter occlusion and subclavian vein thrombosis, the venous obstruction became asymptomatic when treated with anticoagulants alone, while the catheter was treated only with urokinase.

Septic thrombophlebitis is a more serious complication. This should be suspected in the setting of thrombophlebitis with fever, leukocytosis, purulent drainage, or positive blood cultures. Removal of the device is mandatory.[46] Local treatment, heparin, and antibiotics are used.

Infectious Complications

Catheter-related infection is a common problem.[47,48] The frequency of catheter-related infections is between 10 and 30%, with a rate of 1 to 3 per 1000 catheter days. Infection may occur early or late and is potentially catastrophic despite the availability of specific antibiotics. Not all infections in patients with long-term venous catheters are due to the device. Documenting that the catheter is itself involved or at fault may be difficult. Semiquantitative culture of the catheter using the technique of Maki et al[49] is considered positive when culture shows more than 15 colony-forming units. Cooper and Hopkins[50] have described a technique using Gram stain of the catheter tip. However, both of these techniques require removal of the access device. Quantitative blood cultures from the catheter and a peripheral site may allow diagnosis with the catheter in place. Weightman et al[51] showed that patients with catheter-related sepsis had at least a 10-fold increase in colony counts from specimens drawn from the catheter compared with peripheral blood. Non-tunneled external catheters may be replaced over a guidewire. Culture of the tip of the replaced catheter may assist in diagnosis; at the same time, access is preserved.

There is a strong correlation between catheter-related thrombosis and infection. Raad et al discovered that in 31 patients with mural thrombi of a catheterized vein found postmortem, 7 had antemortem catheter-related septicemia versus none of the 41 patients without mural thrombus.[52] It is likely that the fibrin sheath that forms over the intravascular portion of the catheter plays an important role not just in thrombosis but also in infecton. Electron microscopy of catheters removed postmortem has shown bacteria embedded within the fibrin matrix of patients without evidence of antemorten infection.[52] Thrombolytic therapy has been proposed as an adjunct to treatment; while there are favorable case reports, a beneficial effect has yet to be shown in larger randomized trials.[53]

Strict adherence to sterile technique during placement must be followed by a systematic approach to clean catheter care and use. Many patients are immunocompromised because of their underlying disease, immunosuppressive therapy, or chemotherapy and are at higher risk for infection. In general, placement of a port or tunneled catheter should be deferred in septic patients: because there is a higher risk of bacterial seeding of the catheter, the additional surgery needed to place and remove these devices is not justified. Catheter thrombosis itself increases the risk of infection. Multilumen catheters may be more prone to infection than single-lumen devices, perhaps because of the increased handling of the device by personnel.[4] However, other factors such as disease and illness severity may be more important determinants than the number of lumens.

Infection in the first 3 to 5 postoperative days is often due to infection of the subcutaneous track or pocket caused by intraoperative contamination. The use of prophylactic antibiotics at the time of catheter placement is debated, with conflicting opinions and differing practice patterns. A single dose of a broad-spectrum antibiotic with coverage of normal skin flora, such as 1 g cephazolin, is in common use, but this cannot take the place of rigorous sterile technique. Delayed infection often starts at the catheter exit site or in the pocket where it is entered by the access needle, but it may also come via hematogenous seeding from a distant site. Catheter infections are caused by skin flora in 50 to 70% of cases and are thought to develop by contiguous spread from the exit site, to the tunnel, to the endovascular space. Hub contamination and luminal colonization are other recognized routes. The most common organism isolated is *Staphylococcus epidermidis*, found in 25 to 50% of cases. *S. aureus* is isolated in 25% of cases. *Candida* species are found in 5 to 10% of cases. Early recognition of superficial infection at the skin exit site of the catheter or access needle may help save the access device. Signs of erythema, pain, or exudate should receive immediate treatment. These signs may be minimal or absent in patients with neutropenia. In a review of Hickman catheter infections in patients with malignant tumors, Press et al[46] reported that only 15.4% of patients with exit site infections required catheter removal, as opposed to 69% with tunnel infections and 100% with septic thrombophlebitis or septicemia.

Depending on the causal agent, the severity of infection, and the difficulty of reestablishing venous access, catheter-related sepsis may be treated without device removal. If signs fail to improve in 48 to 72 hours or if infection recurs after cessation of a course of appropriate antibiotics, the device should be removed. Catheter infections caused by fungal species and tunnel or pocket infections caused by *Pseudomonas* are difficult to eradicate without catheter removal.

Clear, semipermeable plastic dressings have been associated with increased exit site colonization and catheter-related infections.[54] Based on this finding and on the increased cost of the plastic dressing, our routine is a dry gauze dressing changed three times weekly. The use of antibiotic and iodophor ointments at the exit site has been studied. The common triple-antibiotic ointment, polymixin-neosporin-bacitracin, has been associated with an increased prevalence of fungal colonization at the exit site and perhaps an increase in *Candida*-related catheter infections. The iodophor preparation is active against both bacteria and fungi and is preferred. More recently, favorable reports using chlorhexidine have been published.[55]

REFERENCES

1. Broviac JW, Cole JJ, Scribner BH. A silicone rubber atrial catheter for prolonged parenteral hyperalimentation. *Surg Gynecol Obstet* 1973;136:602–606.
2. Hickman RO, Buckner CD, Clift RA, Sanders JE, Stewart P, Thomas ED. A modified right atrial catheter for access to the venous system in marrow transplant recipients. *Surg Gynecol Obstet* 1979;148:871–875.
3. Brothers TE, von Moll LK, Niederhuber JE, Roberts JA, Walker-Andrews S, Ensminger WD. Experience with subcutaneous infusion ports in three hundred patients. *Surg Gynecol Obstet* 1988;166:295–301.
4. Early TF, Gregory RT, Wheeler JR, et al. Increased infection rate in double lumen versus single lumen Hickman catheters in cancer patients. *South Med J* 1990;83:34–36.
5. Maki DG, Cobb L, Garman JK, Shapiro JM, Ringer M, Helgerson RB. An attachable silver-impregnated cuff for

the prevention of infection with central venous catheters: a prospective, randomized multicenter trial. *Am J Med* 1988;85:307–314.

6. Flowers RH III, Schwenzer KJ, Kopel RF, et al. Efficacy of an attachable subcutaneous cuff for the prevention of intravascular catheter-related infection. *JAMA* 1989;261:878–883.

7. Andrivet P, Bacquer A, Vu Ngoc C, et al. Lack of clinical benefit from subcutaneous tunnel insertion of central venous catheters in immunocompromised patients. *Clin Infect Dis* 1994;18:199–206.

8. Raad I, Davis S, Becker M, et al. Low infection rate and long term durability of nontunneled silastic catheters. *Arch Intern Med* 1993;153:1791–1796.

9. Openshaw KL, Picus D, Hicks ME, Darcy MD, Vesely TM, Picus J. Interventional radiologic placement of Hohn central venous catheters: results and complications in 100 consecutive patients. *JVIR* 1994;5:111–115.

10. Delmore JE, Horbelt DV, Jack BL, Roberts DK. Experience with the Groshong long-term central venous catheter. *Gynecol Oncol* 1989;34:216–218.

11. Pasquale MD, Campbell JM, Magnant CM. Groshong versus Hickman catheters. *Surg Gynecol Obstet* 1992;174:408–410.

12. Andrews JC, Marx MV, Williams DM, Sproat I, Walker-Andrews SC. The upper arm approach for placement of peripherally inserted central catheters for protracted venous access. *AJR* 1992;158:427–429.

13. Cardella JF, Fox PS, Lawler JB. Interventional radiologic placement of peripherally inserted central catheters. *J Vasc Intervent Radiol* 1993;4:653–660.

14. Ross MN, Haase GM, Poole MA, et al. Comparison of totally implanted reservoirs with external catheters as venous access devices in pediatric oncologic patients. *Surg Gynecol Obstet* 1988;167:141–144.

15. Greene FL, Moore W, Strickland B, et al. Comparison of a totally implantable access device for chemotherapy (Port-a-cath) and long term percutaneous catheterization (Broviac). *South Med J* 1988;81:580–583.

16. Pomp A, Caldwell MD, Albina JA. Subcutaneous infusion ports for administration of parenteral nutrition at home. *Surg Gynecol Obstet* 1989;169:329–333.

17. Andrews JC, Walker-Andrews SC, Ensminger WD. Long-term central venous access with a peripherally placed subcutaneous infusion port: initial results. *Radiology* 1990;176:45–47.

18. Pearl JM, Goldstein L, Ciresi KF. Improved methods in long term venous access using the P. A. S. Port™. *Surg Gynecol Obstet* 1991;173:313–315.

19. Morris P, Buller R, Kendall S, Anderson B. A peripherally implanted permanent central venous access device. *Obstet Gynecol* 1991;78:1138–1142.

20. Kahn ML, Barboza RB, Kling GA, Heisel JE. Initial experience with percutaneous placement of the PAS Port implantable venous access device. *J Vasc Intervent Radiol* 1991;3:459–461.

21. Mauro MA, Jaques PF. Radiologic placement of long-term central venous catheters: a review. *J Vasc Intervent Radiol* 1993;4:127–137.

22. Lameris JS, Post PJM, Zonderland HM, Gerritsen PG, Kappers-Klunne MC, Schutte HE. Percutaneous placement of Hickman catheters: comparison of sonographically guided and blind techniques. *AJR* 1990;155:1097–1099.

23. Mallory DL, McGee WT, Shawker TH, et al. Ultrasound improves the success rate of internal jugular vein cannulation: a prospective, randomized trial. *Chest* 1990;98:157–160.

24. Lafreniere R. Indwelling subclavian catheters and a visit with the "pinched-off" sign. *J Surg Oncol* 1991;47:261–264.

25. Gualtieri E, Deppe SA, Sipperly ME, Thompson DR. Subclavian venous catheterization: greater success rate for less experienced operators using ultrasound guidance. *Crit Care Med* 1995;23:692–697.

26. Hahn ST, Pfammatter T, Cho KJ. Carbon dioxide gas as a venous contrast agent to guide upper-arm insertion of central venous catheters. *Cardiovasc Intervent Radiol* 1995;18:146–149.

27. Hovsepian DM, Bonn J, Eschelman DJ. Techniques for peripheral insertion of central venous catheters. *JVIR* 1993;4:795–803.

28. Boddie AW. Translumbar catheterization of the inferior vena cava for long term angioaccess. *Surg Gynecol Obstet* 1989;168:55–57.

29. Voeller GR, Frederick RC, Luther RW. Direct transcaval placement of both a Greenfield filter and a Hickman catheter. *Surgery* 1990;107:110–112.

30. Cazenave FL, Glass-Royal MC, Teitelbaum GP, Zuurbier R, Zeman RK, Silverman PM, CT analysis of a safe approach for translumbar access to the aorta and inferior vena cava. *AJR* 1991;156:395–396.

31. Kenney PR, Dorfman GS, Denny DF Jr. Percutaneous inferior vena cava cannulation for long term parenteral access. *Surgery* 1985;97:602–605.

32. Denny DF Jr, Greenwood LH, Morse SS, Lee GK, Baquero J. Inferior vena cava: translumbar catheterization for central venous access. *Radiology* 1989;170:1013–1014.

33. Lund GB, Lieberman RP, Haire WD, Martin VA, Kessinger A, Armitage JO. Translumbar inferior vena cava catheters for long term venous access. *Radiology* 1990;174:31–35.

34. Robertson L, Jaques P, Mauro M, Azizkhan RG, Robards J. Percutaneous inferior vena cava placement of tunneled silastic catheters for prolonged vascular access in infants. *J Pediatr Surg* 1990;25:596–598.

35. Azizkham RG, Taylor LA, Jacques PF, Mauro MA, Lacey SR. Percutaneous translumbar and transhepatic inferior vena caval catheters for prolonged venous access in children. *J Pediatr Surg* 1992;27:165–169.

36. Crummy AB, Carlson P, McDermott JC, Andrews D. Percutaneous transhepatic placement of a Hickman catheter. *AJR* 1989;153:1317–1318.

37. Kaufman JA, Greenfield AJ, Fitzpatrick GF. Transhepatic cannulation of the inferior vena cava. *J Vasc Intervent Radiol* 1991;2:331–334.

38. Meranze SG, McLean GK, Stein EJ, Jordan HA. Catheter placement in the azygos system: an unusual approach to venous access. *AJR* 1985;144:1075–1076.

39. Hinke DH, Zandt-Stastny DA, Goodman LR, Quebbeman EJ, Krzywda EA, Anddris DA, Pinch-off syndrome: a complication of implantable subclavian venous access devices. *Radiology* 1990;177:353–356.

40. Duntley P, Siever J, Korwes ML, Harpel K, Heffner JE. Vascular erosion by central venous catheters. Clinical features and outcome. *Chest* 1992;101:1633–1638.

41. Moss JF, Wagman LD, Riihimaki DU, et al. Central venous thrombosis related to the silastic Hickman-Broviac catheters in an oncologic population. *J Parenter Enteral Nutr* 1989;13:397–400.

42. Kim FM, Burrows PE, Hoffer FA, Chung T. Interpreting the results of pediatric central venous catheter studies. *Radiographics* 1996;16:747–754.
43. Bern MM, Lokich JJ, Wallach SR, et al. Very low doses of warfarin can prevent thrombosis in central venous catheters: a randomized prospective trial. *Ann Intern Med* 1990;112:423–428.
44. Haire WD, Lieberman RP, Lund GB, Edney J, Wieczorek BM. Obstructed central venous catheters: restoring function with a 12 hour infusion of low dose urokinase. *Cancer* 1990;66:2279–2285.
45. Nazarian GK, Myers TV, Bjarnason H, et al. Applications of the Amplatz snare device during interventional radiologic procedures. *AJR* 1995;165:673–678.
46. Press OW, Ramsey PG, Larson EB, Fefer A, Hickman RO. Hickman catheter infections in patients with malignancies. *Medicine* 1984;63:189–200.
47. Toltzis P, Goldman DA. Current issues in central venous catheter infection. *Annu Rev Med* 1990;41:169–176.
48. Clarke DE, Raffin TA. Infectious complications of indwelling long-term central venous catheters. *Chest* 1990;97:966–972.
49. Maki DG, Weise CE, Sarafin HW. A semiquantitative culture method for identifying intravenous catheter-related infection. *N Engl J Med* 1977;296:1305–1309.
50. Cooper GL, Hopkins CC. Rapid diagnosis of intravascular-associated infection by direct Gram staining of catheter segments. *N Engl J Med* 1985;312:1142–1147.
51. Weightman NC, Simpson EM, Speller DCE, Mott MG, Oakhill A. Bacteremia related to indwelling central venous catheters: prevention, diagnosis and treatment. *Eur J Clin Microbiol Infect Dis* 1988;7:125–129.
52. Raad II, Luna M, Khalil SAM, Costerton JW, Lam C, Bodey GP. The relationship between the thrombotic and infectious complications of central venous catheters. *JAMA* 1994;271:1014–1016.
53. Jones GR, Konsler GK, Dunaway RP, Lacey SR, Azizkhan RG. Prospective analysis of urokinase in the treatment of catheter sepsis in pediatric hematology-oncology patients. *J Pediatr Surg* 1993;28:350–357.
54. Conly JM, Grieves K, Peters B. A prospective, randomized study comparing transparent and dry gauze dressings for central venous catheters. *J Infect Dis* 1989;159:310–319.
55. Maki DG, Ringer M, Alvarado CJ. Prospective randomized trial of povidone-iodine, alcohol, and chlorhexidine for prevention of infection associated with central venous and arterial catheters. *Lancet* 1991;338:339–343.

Index